Skeletal Muscle Pathology

For Churchill Livingstone

Publisher: Timothy Horne
Editorial Co-ordination: Editorial Resources Unit
 Copy Editor: Paul Singleton
 Indexer: Jill Halliday
Production Controller: Lesley W. Small
Design: Design Resources Unit
Sales Promotion Executive: Hilary Brown

Skeletal Muscle Pathology

Edited by

Frank L. Mastaglia MD (WA) FRACP FRCP

Professor of Neurology, University of Western Australia;
Consultant Neurologist, Queen Elizabeth II Medical Centre,
Perth, Western Australia

and

Lord Walton of Detchant Kt TD MA MD DSc FRCP
Honorary Fellow, Green College,
Oxford; former Professor of Neurology,
University of Newcastle upon Tyne

SECOND EDITION

CHURCHILL LIVINGSTONE
EDINBURGH LONDON MADRID MELBOURNE NEW YORK AND TOKYO 1992

CHURCHILL LIVINGSTONE
Medical Division of Longman Group UK Limited

Distributed in the United States of America by Churchill
Livingstone Inc., 650 Avenue of the Americas, New York,
N.Y. 10011, and by associated companies, branches and
representatives throughout the world.

First edition 1982
Second edition 1992

ISBN 0-443-04241-1

British Library Cataloguing in Publication Data
A catalogue record for this book is available from the British
Library.

Library of Congress Cataloging in Publication Data
A catalog record for this book is available from the Library of
Congress.

The
publisher's
policy is to use
**paper manufactured
from sustainable forests**

Printed and bound in Great Britain by
Butler & Tanner Ltd, Frome and London

Preface to the Second Edition

Since the first edition of this book was published in 1982, much new information has emerged about the pathological changes which may occur in human skeletal muscle in health and disease and many new techniques have been introduced, especially in the fields of immunopathology and immunocytochemistry. We therefore considered that it would be timely to bring the book up to date ten years after the appearance of the first edition in order to draw together all of this new information and to bring it to the attention of general pathologists, neuropathologists, neurologists and indeed all of those interested in human neuromuscular disease and in its diagnosis and management.

A completely new chapter on muscle biopsy by Dr Roger Pamphlett has been introduced in this edition, and we have rearranged the remaining chapters in what we believe to be a more logical sequence. We are delighted that many of those who wrote for the first edition have willingly agreed to bring their chapters completely up to date. We thank Drs Adams, Aström, Dawkins, Garlepp, Hall, McDonald, Pleasure and van Unnik for their contributions to the first edition, and we welcome as new authors Drs Borg, DiMauro, Hays, Hughes, Johnson, Kendall-Taylor, Lisak, Pamphlett and Ricci. We believe that this work is now thoroughly up to date and trust that it will prove to be a valuable reference source to all of those working in the field.

As in the first edition, much material, including many illustrations, previously published elsewhere is included in this volume and we are very grateful to the many authors, editors and publishers who have given us permission to reproduce this material. Full acknowledgement of original sources is given in individual figure captions or at the end of each chapter. We also thank the staff of Churchill Livingstone for their continual encouragement and support during the various stages in preparation of the book and, as always, we are deeply indebted to our respective secretaries, Mrs Sheila Moncrieff and Miss Rosemary Allan for their efficient and capable help, which has enabled us to complete the work after a surprisingly short interval following the commissioning of the individual revised chapters.

Perth, Western Australia   F.L.M.
Oxford, England   J.N.W.
1992

Preface to the First Edition

It is now some 30 years since the classical monograph by Adams, Denny-Brown and Pearson entitled *Diseases of muscle: a study in pathology* was first published, heralding the modern era of myology and myopathology. This masterly treatise has since gone through a number of further editions, the latest being written by Professor R. D. Adams himself. That work, and the more recent *Disorders of voluntary muscle* edited by one of us (JNW), which first appeared in 1964, have been, and still are, major sources of reference for clinicians and pathologists confronted with problems in muscle disease. A third monograph by Dubowitz, Brooke and Neville entitled *Muscle biopsy: a modern approach*, which dealt with muscle biopsy interpretation, emphasizing the application of histochemical and ultrastructural techniques, subsequently appeared in 1973 and has also fulfilled an important role, as have several other publications, too numerous to list, which have dealt with various aspects of neuromuscular disease, but have not been primarily concerned with pathology.

When we were approached by Churchill Livingstone in 1978 about the possibility of editing a multi-author text on muscle pathology, we were therefore in some doubt as to the need for such a publication. But after much thought and after earnest consultations with interested colleagues we eventually decided to go ahead with the venture with the aim of producing a comprehensive volume on muscle pathology dealing with the histological, histochemical and ultrastructural changes and with the fundamental biochemistry and immunology of neuromuscular diseases insofar as they affect skeletal muscle, in order to complement the information included in the three works mentioned above. Our objective has been to produce a book which will be useful not only to clinicians, neuropathologists and research workers who are actively involved in the field of muscle disease but also to the general pathologist who, from time to time, may need to refer to such a volume to help him in interpreting the changes in samples of muscle which may come to him. We were satisfied that we should combine the expertise of many leading workers in the neuromuscular field by constructing a multi-author volume in order to give greater depth to the work. Suitable contributors from 11 different countries were eventually chosen, thus providing truly international coverage.

Inevitably there have been some unforeseen and unavoidable delays, partly due to our wish to find authoritative authors for all of the chapters and partly to the variable time taken for completion of different contributions. We are especially indebted to the authors who accepted our invitation and who have gone to so much effort to produce well-illustrated and up-to-date reviews of their subject material; without them it would never have been possible to produce such a broadly based work. We also appreciate the willingness of many authors, editors and publishers to allow us to reproduce in this volume much material, including many illustrations, which has previously been published elsewhere. Acknowledgements to the sources from which such original material has been derived are given in the individual figure captions or Acknowledgements sections, but as editors we wish to express to all of them our thanks. We are very grateful, too, to Mr Andrew Stevenson of Churchill Livingstone and to other members of his staff for their help at various stages in the preparation of the book. We owe a deep debt of gratitude to Mrs Heather Russell for her help in editing the chapters and in particular for her painstaking checking of the individual reference lists. Finally we are deeply indebted to our secretaries, Mrs Pamela McBryde and Miss Rosemary Allan, for their unfailing help and support in bringing the book to completion.

Perth, Western Australia   F. L. M.
Newcastle upon Tyne, England   J. N. W.
1982

Contributors

Eduardo Bonilla MD
Associate Professor of Neurology, Department of Neurology, Columbia University College of Physicians and Surgeons, New York, USA

Kristian Borg MD PhD
Associate Professor, Department of Neurology, Karolinska Hospital, Stockholm, Sweden

C Coërs MD
Honorary Professor, Department of Neurology, Hospital Brugmann, Brussels, Belgium

S M Chou MD PhD
Head, Neuropathology Section, Cleveland Clinic Foundation; Former Professor and Director of Neuropathology Laboratory, West Virginia University Medical Center, West Virginia, USA

Michael J Cullen MA DPhil
Principal Research Associate, Muscular Dystrophy Research Laboratories, Regional Neurological Centre, Newcastle General Hospital, Newcastle upon Tyne, UK

Salvatore DiMauro MD
Professor of Neurology, MDA H Houston Mewitt Clinical Research Center for Muscular Dystrophy and Related Diseases, Columbia University College of Physicians and Surgeons, New York, USA

Michel Fardeau MD
Director of Research, CNRS; Director, Research Group for Neuromuscular Biology and Pathology (INSERM), Paris, France

D G F Harriman MD FRCP FRCPath
Former Reader in Neuropathology, University of Leeds, Leeds, UK

Arthur P Hays MD
Associate Professor of Clinical Neuropathology, Department of Pathology, Division of Neuropathology, Columbia University College of Physicians and Surgeons, New York, USA

Peter Hudgson FRCP FRACP
Consultant Neurologist, Regional Neurosciences Centre, Newcastle General Hospital; Senior Lecturer in Neurology, University of Newcastle upon Tyne, Newcastle upon Tyne, UK

J T Hughes MD DPhil FRCP FRCPath
Emeritus Fellow, Green College, Oxford; Honorary Consultant Neuropathologist to the Oxfordshire Health Authority, UK

F G I Jennekens MD
Division of Neuromuscular Diseases, University Hospital Utrecht, Utrecht, The Netherlands

Felix Jerusalem MD
Professor and Head of Department of Neurology, University of Bonn, Bonn, Germany

M A Johnson PhD
Research Lecturer in Neuromuscular Disease, Muscular Dystrophy Research Laboratories, Regional Neurological Centre, Newcastle General Hospital Newcastle upon Tyne, UK

Byron A Kakulas MD(Hon) (Athens) MD(WA) FRACP FRCPath FRCPA
Professor of Neuropathology, Royal Perth Hospital, Perth, Western Australia

Pat Kendall-Taylor MD FRCP
Professor of Endocrinology and Consultant Physician, Department of Medicine, Royal Victoria Infirmary and University of Newcastle upon Tyne, Newcastle upon Tyne, UK

D N Landon MB BS BSc
Reader in Neurocytology, Institute of Neurology,
London, UK

Robert P Lisak MD
Professor and Chairman, Department of
Neurology, Wayne State University School of
Medicine; Chief of Neurology, Harper Hospital;
Neurologist-in-Chief, Detroit Medical Center,
Detroit, USA

Frank L Mastaglia MD(WA) FRACP FRCP
Professor of Neurology, University of Western
Australia; Consultant Neurologist, Queen
Elizabeth II Medical Centre, Perth, Western
Australia

John A Morgan-Hughes MD FRCP
Consultant Physician, National Hospital for
Neurology and Neurosurgery, London, UK

Ikuya Nonaka MD
Head, Division of Ultrastructural Research,
National Institute of Neuroscience, National
Center of Neurology and Psychiatry, Tokyo,
Japan

Roger Pamphlett MB ChB BSc(Med) FRACP MRCPath
Senior Lecturer, University of Sydney, Sydney,
New South Wales, Australia

Enzo Ricci MD
Visiting Postdoctoral Fellow, Department of
Neurology, Columbia University College of
Physicians and Surgeons, New York, USA;
Department of Neurology, Universita' Cattolica
del Sacro Cuore, Rome, Italy

Harvey B Sarnat MS MD FRCP(C)
Professor of Paediatrics, Pathology and Clinical
Neurosciences, University of Calgary Faculty of
Medicine and Alberta Children's Hospital,
Calgary, Alberta, Canada

Eijiro Satoyoshi MD
President, National Center of Neurology and
Psychiatry, Tokyo, Japan

Henning Schmalbruch MD
Senior Lecturer, Institute of Neurophysiology,
University of Copenhagen, Copenhagen, Denmark

Michael Swash MD FRCP MRCPath
Consultant Neurologist, The Royal London
Hospital and St Mark's Hospital, London; Senior
Lecturer in Neuropathology, The London
Hospital Medical College, London, UK

Fernando M S Tomé MD PhD
Directeur de Récherche, INSERM U 153, Paris,
France

Lord Walton Kt TD MA MD DSc FRCP
Dr de l'Univ (Hon Aix-Marseille) DSc
(Hon Leeds) DSc (Hon Leicester) DSc
(Hon Hull) DCL (Hon Newcastle) MD (Hon
Sheffield) Hon FACP Hon FRCP (Edin) Hon
FRCP (Canada) Honorary Fellow and former
Warden, Green College, Oxford; former Professor
of Neurology, University of Newcastle upon
Tyne; Honorary Consulting Neurologist, Oxford
District and Regional Hospitals, UK

Contents

1. Skeletal muscle — normal morphology, development and innervation

D. N. Landon

INTRODUCTION

Striated skeletal muscle is the major tissue component of the mammalian body, and contributes between 40 and 50% to its total weight. The constituent cells of all types of muscle possess structural modifications that fit them for their specialized function of converting chemical energy into mechanical work. These structural features achieve their most elaborate and complex expression in striated skeletal muscle. Such muscle is, with few exceptions, under voluntary nervous control, in contrast to cardiac and visceral muscle, and is concerned with providing the mechanical effort that enables the organism to move within, and interact with, its physical environment. The account of the morphology of skeletal muscle that follows will concentrate upon the relationship of its structure at various levels of organization to this primary function, but the large contribution made by striated muscle to the body's content of water (80%) and of intracellular ions such as potassium, and its functions as a store of energy rich compounds, as a reservoir of protein and as a source of body heat, give it a major role in the general metabolism of the organism which should not be overlooked. Fuller accounts of many of the topics covered may be found in recent reviews by Squire (1981), Schmalbruch (1985) and Cullen & Landon (1988).

HISTOLOGY

An individual skeletal muscle consists of a bundle of muscle 'fibres' within a connective tissue framework. These fibres are elongated multinucleate syncytia, up to 10 cm or more in length, with diameters in the range of 10–100 μm. Some authors prefer to call such structures 'muscle cells' as they consist of a single protoplasmic mass within one cell membrane, but the terms 'muscle fibre' and 'myofibre' have long-standing currency in this connotation and will be used here to avoid confusion. Muscle fibres in general run from one end of a muscle, or muscle fasciculus, to the other, without interruption or overlap with others, but the pennate arrangement of most muscles in the body ensures that few fibres exceed 10 cm in length, and that they are considerably shorter than the overall length of the muscle of which they form a part. The reported dissection of individual muscle fibres up to 34 cm long from a human sartorius muscle (Lockhart & Brandt 1937–38) lacks histological confirmation that the strands dissected consisted of single uninterrupted fibres.

The striated muscle fibres that constitute an individual muscle are bound together by collagenous connective tissue, and this is usually divided into three components for purposes of description. The epimysium provides a tough elastic envelope of orientated collagen fibrils; it delimits the muscle from adjacent structures, and at its end merges with tendon, aponeurosis or periosteum. Deep extensions of this layer of organized collagen subdivide the enclosed muscle fibres into smaller fascicles; these septa are referred to collectively as the perimysium. Finally, the individual muscle fibres are separated one from another by an interlacing network of fine collagen fibrils, the endomysium (Fig. 1.1). The combination of endomysial reticulin and the basal lamina of the muscle fibre, a continuous amorphous collagenous envelope closely adherent to the cell membrane (see Fig. 1.4), is visible by light microscopy as a

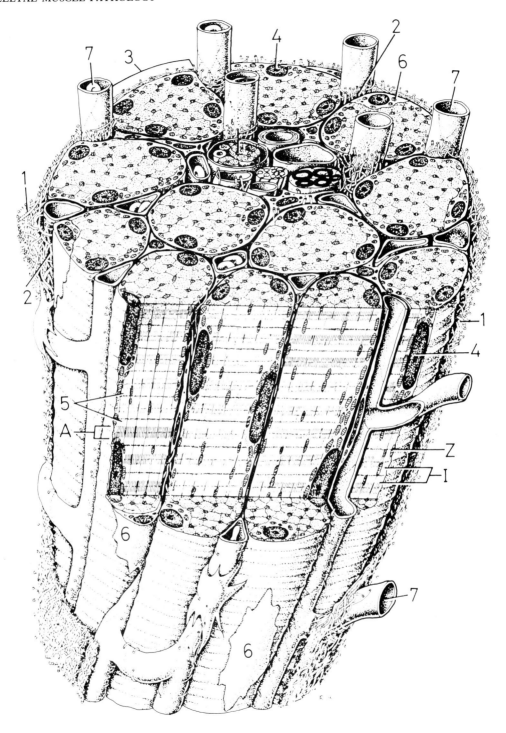

Fig. 1.1 A diagrammatic representation of a small fascicle of myofibres. It is bounded externally by the perimysium (1), a feltwork of collagen fibrils, which is continuous with a mesh of finer collagen fibrils, the endomysium (2), between the individual myofibres (3). The myofibres themselves contain elongated nuclei (4) and contractile myofibrils (5); small myosatellite cells (6) are closely applied to their external surfaces. Also shown are the numerous longitudinally running capillaries (7) with short transverse interconnections. (Figure 126 from Krstić 1978, by kind permission of the author and publishers)

diaphanous tube following removal of the muscle fibre, as a consequence of acute trauma or cellular degeneration, and was named the 'sarcolemma' by Bowman (1840). The term has subsequently been adopted by many writers as a synonym for the muscle cell plasmalemma; this is an unfortunate development in some respects, as it is frequently necessary to distinguish between these two components, particularly when discussing the cellular events that occur during muscle degeneration and regeneration. In this account the term sarcolemma will be given its original meaning, and the cell membrane of the muscle fibre will be referred to as the plasmalemma.

The collective importance of the sarcolemmal tubes as a connective tissue scaffold for striated muscle has been demonstrated by the experiments of Hall-Craggs (1974), and others, who have shown that massive myonecrosis, induced by chemical or physical means that do not disrupt the connective tissue of muscle, can be followed by regeneration of a complete muscle virtually indistinguishable from its original state; and by those of Vracko & Benditt (1972), in which excised muscle segments were re-implanted at right angles to their natural orientation: the regenerating myofibres followed the original connective tissue planes of the implant, and were uninfluenced by the natural axis of the muscle within which they lay. The normally very attenuated endomysial sheaths of muscle fibres, virtually invisible by light microscopy, become much thickened and more obvious in a number of pathological conditions, in particular in those involving chronic inflammatory change and repeated episodes of myonecrosis.

Individual myofibres are often portrayed as cylinders, but this view reflects the inadequacy of structural preservation afforded by conventional histological techniques using paraffin-embedded material, and the study of well-prepared frozen sectioned, or aldehyde-fixed, resin-embedded muscle has provided unequivocal evidence that the natural profiles of myofibres within a transversely sectioned muscle fascicle form an assembly of interlocking irregular polygons (Figs. 1.1 and 1.2). Measurements of the mean and range of muscle fibre diameters have shown that these vary with species and the particular muscle sampled, as well as with age (Brooke & Engel 1969b, Moore et al 1971), sex (Brooke & Engel 1969a) and the degree

of muscular development of the individual examined (Gollnick et al 1972, Costill et al 1976). Autopsy studies by Aherne et al (1971) and Polgar et al (1973) have provided values for fibre size in a number of the major muscle groups in man, and similar data obtained from biopsy specimens have been described by Brooke & Engel (1969a,b), Reniers et al (1970) and Reske-Nielsen et al (1970). Large proximal muscles tend to contain fibres with a larger mean diameter; conversely, small distal muscles, concerned with more delicate movements, contain small fibres. Children have smaller fibres than adults, and women have smaller fibres than men of comparable age; systematic physical training induces an increased mean fibre diameter in both sexes. In true transverse sections of myofibres, the ratio of the longest to the shortest diameter is in general less than two to one in normal muscle; flattened, acutely angulated fibres in which this ratio is exceeded usually indicate pathological change.

In longitudinal sections the most striking features of the microscopical appearance of skeletal muscle fibres are their transverse striations, from which they derive their alternative name. These alternating light and dark bands have a mean periodicity in the range of 1.5–3.0 µm in human biopsy specimens, depending upon the degree of muscle shortening; the structural basis for this banding and the nomenclature of its components are described in detail below. Also visible by light microscopy are the nuclei of the myofibre which lie at its surface, immediately beneath the plasmalemma (Fig. 1.1). They contain evenly dispersed chromatin and one or two conspicuous nucleoli, and are elongated ellipsoids in form, with their (12–15 µm) long axes parallel to the axis of the myofibre. These intrinsic myonuclei number 50–100/mm of myofibre length, and at least one or two are usually visible therefore in any transverse section of normal thickness. Very few occupy a more central position within the fibre, the upper value for normal generally being taken to be 3% (Greenfield et al 1957, Schmitt 1978); increases above this level are a consistent feature of a number of myopathies, or may alternatively be indicative of past episodes of fibre degeneration and regeneration. It has relatively recently been established through the use of electron microscopy, that a proportion of the apparent population of myofibre nuclei visible by light microscopy are extrinsic to the fibres and belong to small flattened myosatellite cells lying between the inner aspect of the myofibre basal lamina and its plasmalemma (see Fig. 1.4), indenting the surface of the latter in such a manner that the external contour of the fibre is undisturbed (Mauro 1961, Muir et al 1965). Similar cells have been found in many vertebrate species. They are numerous in young animals, their incidence relative to that of intrinsic nuclei diminishing with age; the values for normal human material are over 10% in children and 2–5% in adults. The fine structure of myosatellite cells and their possible roles in muscle development and repair are described and illustrated below (see Fig. 1.17).

Red and white muscle

It has long been recognized that the skeletal muscles of the vertebrate body do not form a single homogeneous population, and are divisible on the basis of several morphological and physiological characteristics into at least two major subgroups. The most obvious visible difference between these is their varying degree of red colouration, which Kuhne (1865) showed to be due to an intrinsic pigment, later termed myoglobin, and not to the greater density of blood capillaries also found within 'red' muscles. Ranvier (1873) subsequently showed that 'red' and 'white' muscles differed in their physiological properties: red muscle both contracted and relaxed more slowly than white, and required lower frequencies of electrical stimuli to generate a smooth tetanic response. Histological differences between the two types of muscle were also recognized early, the fibres constituting typical red muscles generally being found to be of small diameter and rich in granular sarcoplasm (Knoll 1891). It was later discovered that the increased myoglobin content of red muscles, and thus their capacity to attract and hold oxygen, was associated with increased activity of the cytochrome oxidase system responsible for the aerobic synthesis of energy-rich compounds (Lawrie 1952); white muscles were found to lack these properties and to be more efficient in the anaerobic synthesis of energy-rich materials, of which they usually contained stores

in the form of glycogen (Lawrie 1953). Such studies, and the known anatomical distribution of identifiable red and white muscles in a wide range of vertebrate species (red fibres lying in a deeper plane, nearer to the trunk or limb axis than white fibres and spanning single joints), led to a consensus view that 'red' muscles, though more slowly contracting, are responsible for the sustained powerful activity required by postural functions, such activity being continuously fuelled by aerobic glycolysis; white muscles, capable of rapid powerful actions, but lacking staying-power because of the rundown with activity of their relatively limited stores of energy-rich compounds and the accumulation of lactic acid, are used preferentially for more vigorous intermittent activity (Dawson & Romanul 1964, Romanul 1964, Needham 1971, Close 1972).

Muscle fibre histochemistry

The identification of functional and metabolic differences between individual muscles was followed by the recognition that most are composed of fibres which can, in turn, be shown to possess a range of metabolic activities, and that the 'redness' or 'whiteness' of a muscle thus reflects the sum of the properties of its constituent fibres. Detection of the metabolic characteristics of individual myofibres depended upon the development of histochemical techniques and their application to frozen-sectioned, fresh or fixed muscle (Padykula 1952, Padykula & Herman 1955, Wachstein & Meisel 1955). Using such methods, Ogata (1958a, b) and Nachmias & Padykula (1958) were able to distinguish three fibre types in the muscles of a range of vertebrates, according to their staining reactions for succinic dehydrogenase and cytochrome oxidase activity, and their fat content: 'red' fibres stained strongly for all three components, while 'intermediate' and 'white' fibres stained progressively more weakly. Dubowitz & Pearse (1960) later showed that there is a reciprocal relationship between the staining reaction for oxidative enzymes and phosphorylase in human myofibres, the smaller red fibres staining strongly for the former, while the larger white fibres gave a more positive phosphorylase reaction. Engel (1962) subsequently showed that in unfixed muscle the large white fibres, poor in oxidative enzymes and rich in phosphorylase, stained more strongly for myosin ATPase activity after preincubation at pH 9.4, than did the small red fibres, and he used this difference as the basis of a scheme of classification for human striated muscle fibres: type 1 fibres were defined as small, red, rich in oxidative enzymes and poor in phosphorylase and ATPase activity at pH 9.4, while the larger type 2, white, fibres showed the direct inverse of these properties.

Stein & Padykula (1962) proposed a three-fibre classification based on their studies of rat muscle, in which the distribution of the reaction product, as well as the overall intensity of the staining, were utilized as criteria for distinguishing fibre types. Their type A fibres corresponded to the large white type 2 fibres of Engel, and type C to the typical small red type 1 fibres; type B constituted a class with characteristics intermediate between those of A and C. The application of a wider range of histochemical reactions to animal muscle by others resulted in a further subdivision of these classes, in one instance into at least eight fibre types (Romanul 1964), but such classifications have proved difficult to apply to human muscle. The most widely adopted system of fibre-typing for this purpose is the Brooke & Kaiser (1970) modification of the system proposed by Engel (1962) in which type 2 fibres are differentiated into two major subgroups, 2A and 2B, according to their staining behaviour when subjected to acid preincubation before the ATPase staining reaction. Preincubation at pH 4.3 or below reverses the ATPase staining pattern seen after alkali preincubation, type 1 (oxidative) fibres staining intensely and type 2 (phosphorylase-positive) fibres remaining unstained. Preincubation between pH 4.6 and 4.3 produces a third ATPase staining pattern (Fig. 1.2a) in which type 1 and some of the type 2 (2B) fibres stain, while others (2A) remain unstained. Parallel staining for oxidative enzymes and glycogen reveals that the fibres unstained at pH 4.6 (2A) represent an intermediate class of fibre (Fig. 1.2b), having both oxidative and glycolytic properties (Close 1972, Dubowitz & Brooke 1973).

More recently immunocytochemical studies have shown that at least five myosin isoenzyme heavy chains can be consistently detected in developing and mature mammalian skeletal muscle. The embryonic isoenzyme is successively replaced by neonatal, and either slow- or fast-twitch forms as these fibres differentiate, the fifth slow tonic isoenzyme being expressed in the primary myotubes during development and in the nuclear bag intrafusal fibres of muscle spindles (q.v.); others have been reported. These myosin heavy-chain isoenzymes may occur in association with a larger number of light-chain isoenzymes, to yield a continuum of potential fibre types (Staron & Pette 1987, Pette & Staron 1988) which, when combined with polymorphisms of tropomyosin (Bronson & Schachat 1982) and troponin (Dhoot & Perry 1980), provides some explanation for the metabolic heterogeneity of muscle fibres (Pette 1985), and their capacity to respond to variations in functional demand by changes in their phenotypic expression. Fibre types delineated by myosin ATPase and metabolic enzyme histochemistry therefore represent peaks in a continuous distribution of properties which may be expected to vary with species, stage of development and use.

Fibre type and function

Physiological experiments on animal muscle have reinforced the usefulness of fibre-type classifications based on histochemical profiles. Close (1967) demonstrated motor units in rat muscle having fast, slow and intermediate contraction times, and Barnard et al (1971) showed that contraction speed correlates directly with ATPase staining intensity, following preincubation at pH 9.4. Burke et al (1971) were also able to classify cat motor units into three classes, using as criteria both contraction speed and resistance to fatigue: individual units were slow, fatigue-resistant (S); fast, fatigue-resistant (FR); or fast, rapidly fatiguable (FF). The fibre types corresponding to these units were found to have the histochemical characteristics of type 1, type 2A and type 2B respectively. The major properties of fibres so classified in human muscle are listed in Table 1.1.

The finding that the muscle fibres innervated by a single motor neurone possess identical histochemical characteristics and uniform physiological properties (Kugelberg & Edström 1968, Burke et al 1971) serves to emphasize the importance of the functional interrelationship existing between these two components of the 'motor unit'. Cross-innervation experiments in which the nerve supply to a predominantly 'fast' muscle (EDL) was transposed with that of a 'slow' muscle such as soleus (Buller et al 1960b, Dubowitz 1967, Romanul & van der Meulen 1967) have demonstrated the lability of the histochemical and functional characteristics of mature myofibres, and their capacity to adopt the properties of a different fibre type under the influence of innervation by a foreign nerve. This influence was initially considered to be mediated by a trophic substance liberated from the nerve terminals, but experiments (Lömo 1976, Buller & Pope 1977) have shown that the imposition of abnormal patterns of activity on muscles by artificial stimulation, applied either directly or via their natural nerve supply, will mimic the earlier results obtained by cross-innervation, and it now appears that the pattern of use to which a myofibre is naturally subject has the predominant influence in determining its structure and physiological properties, and thus its histochemical 'type'.

Edström & Kugelberg (1968a) subjected single ventral root fibres in the rat to prolonged stimulation, and were subsequently able to identify the individual component myofibres of the motor units supplied by detecting the depletion of their glycogen stores in PAS-stained transverse sections of the muscle. They found that the fibres that constitute a motor unit are not grouped together in close proximity within the muscle, but are dispersed throughout a much larger volume of muscle among the fibres of other units. Given the uniform characteristics of fibres comprising each motor unit, this observation explains the chequer-board variation in histochemical staining intensity (Jennekens et al 1971b) seen in transverse sections of most muscles (Fig. 1.2). The origin of this dispersion of the individual fibres of each motor unit during muscle development is still a subject for debate and will be considered in greater detail later, but it has become evident from a computer simulation study (Willison 1980) that the arrangement seen in mature muscle is not a random one, and that the adjacencies of the constituent fibres of each unit have been minimized during their ontogeny. The functional advantages to the animal of this arrangement may include dispersion of

muscle action currents to avoid self-excitation, and spread of the contractile force generated by a unit across a significant proportion of the cross-section of the muscle. This may be expected to smooth the effects of recruitment of additional motor units with increasing muscular effort, and to improve the sensitivity of feedback to the central nervous system from muscle and tendon sensory receptors (q.v.). The observations of Gregory & Proske (1979), that individual tendon-organs in the cat medial gastrocnemius muscle can be activated by the contraction of many different motor units, support such a suggestion. It has been inferred that similar dispersion of the individual myofibres of a motor unit also occurs in man, on the basis of observations on biopsies from patients suffering from myokymia, a condition in which a small proportion of motor units undergo repetitive spontaneous discharge. Glycogen-depleted myofibres were found scattered throughout the muscle sample, and these were arranged in a number of groups, each of a single fibre type (Williamson & Brooke 1972). The anatomical and physiological properties of motor units in mammalian muscle have been reviewed by Buchthal & Schmalbruch (1980).

As has been pointed out earlier, the balance of the proportion of myofibres within any individual muscle having fast or slow contraction characteristics, and corresponding metabolic properties, varies from one muscle to another; the extremes of this spectrum are represented by white and red muscles respectively, but even these consist of a mixture of myofibre types. Furthermore, the numerical proportions of the different types are not constant throughout the cross-sectional area of any given muscle, white fast-twitch anaerobic fibres tending to predominate in the superficial aspects of limb muscles and red oxidative fibres in their deeper portions (Denny-Brown 1929, Jennekens et al 1971a, Johnson et al 1973, Pullen 1977). The large variations in the proportions of the different fibre types in samples of similar muscles from different subjects, found by Brooke & Engel (1969a) and Johnson et al (1973), probably reflect the inherent histochemical mutability of striated muscle fibres referred to above, and their capacity to adapt their biochemical and physiological properties to the range of functional loads

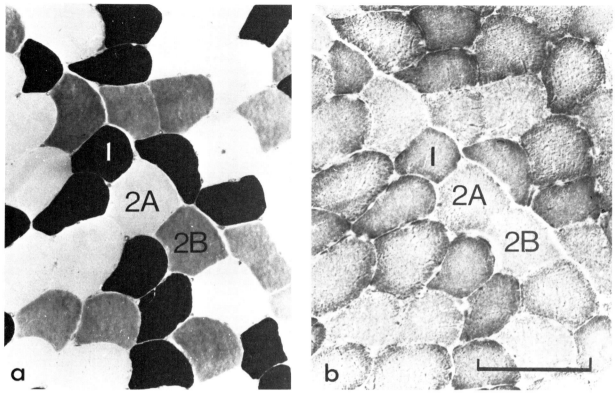

Fig. 1.2 Serial transverse frozen sections of normal human muscle stained for (a) ATPase activity at pH 4.6, and (b) DPNH activity. Three muscle fibre types are evident, scattered in a chequerboard distribution. In (a) the small intensely staining fibres are type 1 (slow, oxidative), the pale fibres type 2A (fast, oxidative), and those showing intermediate staining intensity type 2B (fast, glycolytic). Comparison with (b) shows that, in general, the type 1 fibres have a high uniform DPNH activity; the type 2A fibres have an intermediate level of activity and a coarse granular distribution; and type 2B fibres have the lowest activity. Scale bar = 100 μm. (Micrographs kindly provided by Dr J. A. Morgan-Hughes, Institute of Neurology, London)

Table 1.1 A classification of fibre types applicable to human muscle

Fibre type	1(S)	2A(FR)	2B(FF)
Size	Small	Intermediate	Large
Myoglobin content	High	High	Low
Energy metabolism	Oxidative	Oxidative/glycolytic	Glycolytic
Glycogen content (PAS)	Low	High	Intermediate
Lipid content	High	Intermediate	Low
Mitochondria	Many	Many	Few
Local capillary density	High	High	Low
Enzyme activites:			
(1) ATPase, pH 9.4	Low	Moderate to high	High
ATPase, pH 4.6–4.4	High	Low	Intermediate
ATPase, below pH 4.3	High	Low	Low
(2) Oxidative (SDH, NADH-TR)	High	Intermediate	Low
(3) Phosphorylase	Low	High	High
"Physiological characteristics:			
(1) Speed of contraction	Slow	Intermediate to fast	Fast
(2) Resistance to fatigue	High	Intermediate	Low

"Based on animal experiments

placed upon them by different individuals. Confirmation that shifts in the percentages of the different fibre types present within the same muscle occur with training or inactivity in human volunteers has been reported by Costill et al (1976), Andersen & Henricksson (1977) and Jansson et al (1978). Such sources of variability must be taken into account when assessing the significance of the proportions of the individual fibre types found in human muscle biopsy specimens. The potential for variations between species in the proportions of fibre types within the same muscle, and the relationship of such variation to function, is well illustrated by the work of Gauthier & Padykula (1966) on the diaphragms of 30 different mammals. In small animals such as the mouse, which has a rapid respiration rate, small-diameter, mitochondria-rich myofibres predominated, whereas the diaphragm of a large animal such as a cow, with a slow respiration rate, consisted almost entirely of large-diameter 'white' fibres. Correlation of the histochemical properties of myofibres with their fine structure is discussed in a subsequent section.

Vasculature

Muscles receive a rich blood supply from branches of regional arteries. While these may vary somewhat between individuals in number and anatomical arrangement, the supply to each muscle is usually a closed system without connections to adjacent structures. Within the muscle the afferent vessels break up to supply an extensive capillary network between the myofibres. The capillaries have a predominantly longitudinal orientation (Fig. 1.1), linked by short transverse branches, and are most numerous in those regions of the muscle rich in 'oxidative' myofibres. Their endothelial cells generally possess numerous pinocytic vesicles (Fig. 1.3), but lack 'tight junctions' at their contiguous margins and are freely permeable to tracers such as horseradish peroxidase. Capillary pericytes, stellate cells with slender branches which closely encircle the external surface of the endothelial cells, and have a filament-rich cytoplasm resembling that of smooth muscle myocytes, are relatively common and can on occasion be seen to be innervated by slender non-myelinated nerve

fibres. The capillary basal lamina covers the external contour of the endothelial cells, or endothelial cells plus periocytes, and is a 20–30 nm thick layer of amorphous collagen in both small animals and young human subjects. Thickening and reduplication of the basal lamina is common in the elderly, however, and similar changes are seen in a wide range of muscle disorders in younger patients (Siperstein et al 1968, Vracko 1970, Jerusalem et al 1974).

THE FINE STRUCTURE OF THE MYOFIBRE

Muscle cell plasmalemma

Over the greater part of the myofibre surface the plasmalemma provides a smooth, electrically excitable envelope for the multinucleate syncytium of sarcoplasm and its contained myofibrils. It is indented here and there by myosatellite cells (q.v.) lying between it and its adjacent basal lamina, and is connected by small pores (20–40 nm diameter) in a semi-regular fashion to the contiguous membranes of the subsurface caveolae and tubules of the transverse tubular system (see below). The plasmalemma is related on its external surface to the basal lamina of the myofibre, an extracellular layer composed largely of amorphous type IV collagen, 20–30 nm thick, that adheres closely to its external contour (Fig. 1.4). Other components include fibronectin and laminin (Sanes 1982). The basal lamina is separated from the apparent cell surface by an electron-lucent interval, 10–15 nm wide, representing an unstained portion of the glycocalyx of the muscle plasma membrane to which it is closely bound. Reduplication of the basal lamina is occasionally seen, and is indicative of past episodes of muscle cell degeneration and repair, either partial or complete. Separation of the basal lamina from the muscle cell surface may occur after recovery from transient episodes of cell swelling induced, for example, by ischaemia and at the sites of exocytosis of cellular debris from damaged fibres. The basal lamina constitutes the boundary between the muscle fibre and the connective and vascular tissue compartment of the muscle, and it may function as a diffusion barrier for large molecules (Oldfors & Fardeau 1983).

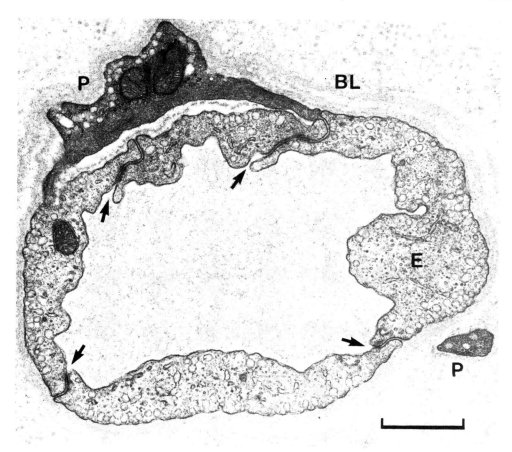

Fig. 1.3 A human muscle capillary. The endothelial cells (E) contain numerous pinocytotic vesicles, and their margins (arrows) lack tight junctional complexes. External to the endothelial cells are processes of a pericyte (P) and a somewhat thickened and reduplicated basal lamina (BL). Scale bar = 1 μm

The chemical composition of the muscle plasma-lemma (sarcolemma) has been determined in a number of species, such as the rabbit (Madeira & Antunes-Madeira 1973) in which the isolated membrane has been shown to be 63% protein and 17.3% lipid. The latter consisted of neutral lipid, cholesterol and cholesterol esters, the proportion of cholesterol being highest in slow-twitch fibres (Fischbeck et al 1982), and phospholipids of which the major components were lecithin 43%, phosphatidylethanolamine 24%, sphingomyelin 23% and lysolecithin 10%. Similar values have been found in other species.

Two consistent regional variations are observable in the morphology of the muscle cell surface. One is at the insertion of the muscle into tendon or bone, where the individual myofibres taper and develop irregular surface ridges and grooves, to end as a mass of finger-like projections and intervening invaginations which provide a greatly increased surface area for the attachment of the connective tissues. The plasmalemma bounding this myotendinous junctional region is marked by a layer of conspicuous electron density in the immediately adjacent sarcoplasm; this material merges with the terminal Z discs of the myofibrils and appears to provide the point of insertion for the I filaments of the last sarcomere into the cell membrane at the end of the myofibre (Ishikawa 1979). The subplasmalemmal density at the

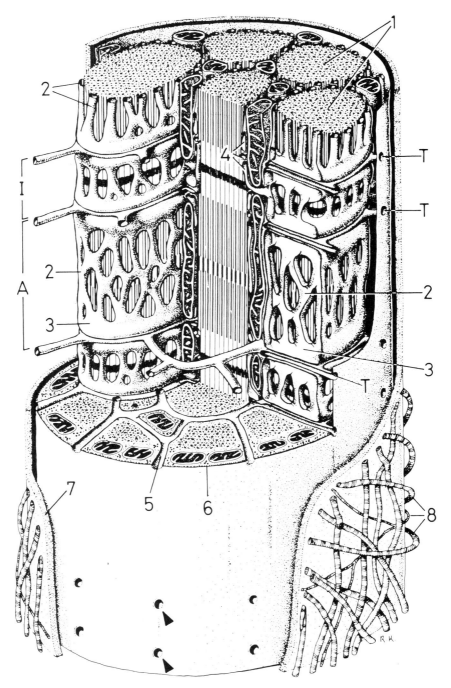

Fig. 1.4 A diagrammatic dissection of a single mammalian myofibre. The myofibrils (1), with their arrays of thick and thin filaments and A and I bands, are ensheathed by complex sacs of sarcoplasmic reticulum; these are divided into central fenestrated zones (2) and terminal cisternae (3). The transverse tubular system (T) makes contact with the terminal cisternae of the sarcoplasmic reticulum at the triads (4) around each myofibril, and at the myofibre surface is continuous (5), via subsurface caveolae (not shown) with the plasmalemma (6). The fibre is surrounded externally by an amorphous extracellular component, the basal lamina (7), which, with the endomysial collagen/reticulin fibrils (8), together constitute the sarcolemma. (Figure 129 from Krstić 1978, by kind permission of the author and publishers)

myotendinous junction resembles that seen at the crests of the postjunctional folds of the motor end-plate (q.v.); it is of interest that this region has been found to possess raised levels of acetylcholin-esterase and acetylcholine receptor activity when compared with the remainder of the extra-junctional plasma membrane. These properties may be considered to be an atavism and evidence of incomplete differentiation associated with the role of the ends of the fibres in growth in length. The second major regional specialization of the plasmalemma, the neuromuscular junction, is con-sidered in detail below.

Some more subtle variations in the structure of muscle cell plasma membranes at the macromole-cular level have been described by Ellisman et al (1976). They have reported that freeze–fracture preparations of fibres from rat extensor digitorum longus muscles showed aggregates of 6 nm particles in square arrays within the P face of the extra-junctional plasmalemma in most muscle fibres examined. The density of occurrence of these aggregates appeared to be a function of distance from the neuromuscular junction; it was low in a 15 μm band immediately adjacent to its margin, increasing to a maximum of 15–30 μm^2 at 0.5–1 mm from the end-plate, and declining to 3–15 μm^2 at a distance of 2–4 mm. Examination of comparable regions of soleus muscle fibres showed a virtual absence of such arrays, only 10% of fibres possessing them, and then at very low densities. Schmalbruch (1979a) has described similar square arrays of 6–7 nm particles in the P faces of membranes from adult human muscle fibres, but not in those from a 22-week fetus, and it is clear that they appear late in the development of fast-twitch fibres (Hudson et al 1982), and in the rat require innervation up to 30 days postnatal for their full expression (Sirken & Fischbeck 1985). In the adult fibres the numbers of arrays present showed a bimodal distribution, with the largest arrays being found in the fibres in which they were most numerous. The high and low peaks of this distribution were considered to cor-respond to fast- and slow-twitch fibres respectively. Both fetal and adult fibres possessed scattered single 6–7 nm particles, in equal frequency.

Experimental reinnervation of a slow muscle by a fast muscle nerve, for example of soleus by the nerve to extensor digitorum longus in the rat (Ellisman et al 1978), results in the development of 6 nm particle arrays in the plasma membranes of the slow myofibres, in a similar density and with a similar gradient of frequency with distance from the neuromuscular junction, to that normally seen in fast-twitch fibres. While this finding suggests that the formation of the square arrays of particles is, like so many other aspects of myofibre morphology, neurally induced, their sizes and numbers are not affected by denervation of normally innervated fibres, at least in the short term (Tachikawa & Clementi 1979). Ellisman et al (1976) suggest that the presence or absence of square arrays in membranes from fast- and slow-twitch muscle fibres may reflect a characteristic of difference other than the well-recognized spectrum of metabolic properties usually employed to define muscle fibre types (see above), and relate to dif-ferences in the basic membrane properties of fast- and slow-twitch muscle fibres. They point out that the concentration and distribution of the particle arrays cannot be correlated directly with differ-ences in excitability, because similar structures have been reported in cells that do not conduct propagated action potentials; they propose, as an alternative, that the observed variation may be related to known differences between the membranes of the extensor digitorum longus and soleus muscles in the efficiency of their sodium/potassium electrogenic pumping mechanisms, and their adenyl cyclase activities (Festoff et al 1977). Other, larger (10 nm) particles occur within both the P and E faces of the muscle plasmalemma. They are not preferentially associated with a parti-cular fibre-type, but changes in their numbers and distribution have been claimed to occur in dener-vated and dystrophic muscle (Schotland et al 1981), and after prolonged hypoxia (Schmalbruch 1980). It has been claimed that up to 50% of these 10 nm particles may represent sodium/potassium-ATPase molecules (Pumplin & Fambrough 1983).

The proteolipid membrane and intrinsic protein particles which constitute the plasmalemma are related on their deep surface to a superficial layer of sarcoplasm which, in regions between the sub-surface caveolae of the T system (q.v.), shows enhanced staining in conventional electron-microscopic preparations. It contains a number of species of fibrous proteins thought to play a structural role in strengthening the plasmalemma and subjacent layer of sarcoplasm, and linking both to the underlying myofibrils. These proteins include desmin, a 50 000 mol. wt subunit of the 10 nm intermediate filaments which also form a network around individual myofibrils and link the edges of contiguous Z-discs to maintain their lateral registration; vinculin, a protein with similar functions which is transiently expressed during development and fibre regeneration; and the recently discovered protein dystrophin (Hoffman et al 1987). The last is a dumbbell-shaped rod 100–120 nm long with a molecular weight of 400 000, which forms a network of homodimers linked to the integral membrane proteins of the plasmalemma, and also probably interacts with other cytoskeletal proteins including spectrin and ankyrin. The particular interest of dystrophin is that it has been shown to be the protein product of the gene on the X-chromosome deleted or disrupted in Duchenne and Becker muscular dystrophy, and its absence or reduction respectively in these diseases may increase the fragility of the plasmalemma, and thus the susceptibility of the fibre to damage by minor trauma or metabolic stress (Menke & Jockusch 1991).

The myofibrils

The major subcellular components of the muscle fibre are the myofibrils, which occupy 85–90% of its total volume. They are irregular polygons in cross-section, with a mean diameter of approximately 1 μm in most muscles, and they are of indefinite length, matching that of the myofibre of which they form a part. Each myofibril is composed of serially repeating segments of identical structure — the sarcomeres — the precise lateral alignment of which, from one myofibril to the next, gives to the fibre as a whole its characteristic cross-striations. An individual sarcomere consists of a dark central band 1.5–1.6 μm long, flanked by two paler bands, the lengths of which vary with the state of shortening of the myofibre. The more dense central 'A' (anisotropic) band is crossed at its mid-point by a dark, narrow transverse line, the 'M' line or band, bordered by a paler band of variable width, the 'H' zone (Fig. 1.5). The A

band is composed of a regular hexagonal array of filaments 15–18 nm in diameter at their mid-point tapering at either end, the principal constituent of which is the protein myosin. The pale 'I' (isotropic) bands on either side of the A band are divided at their mid-points by a narrow dense line, the 'Z' line or disc. The I band is also constructed of parallel filaments, varying in length from 1.0 to 1.35 μm in different vertebrate species, but these are more slender (7 nm diameter) and less regular in their arrangement than those of the A band. They each consist of paired α-helices of chains of a 'globular' protein, actin, in combination with a second globular protein, troponin, and a long-chain protein, tropomyosin. At the Z line the I filaments of the two halves of one I band form regularly arranged square lattices and find a common attachment in the dense matrix material of the Z line. The Z lines thus mark the longitudinal boundaries of the individual sarcomeres, which each consist of one A band and two half I bands (Fig. 1.6a). The free ends of the I filaments interdigitate between the elements of the hexagonal A-band lattice, in such a manner that each I filament occupies the centre of a triangular space between three adjacent A filaments. Contraction of a myofibre is brought about by the shortening of the sarcomeres that make up its constituent myofibrils, and this is accomplished, in turn, by a sliding movement of the I filaments towards the centre of the A band, which, if carried to its physiological limit, will result in extinction of the I bands and apposition of the Z lines to the ends of the A filaments. During relaxation following a contraction this sliding movement is reversed, and will continue until the normal resting length of the sarcomere, generally 2.5–3.0 μm, has been restored. The H zone, like the I band, varies in width with sarcomere length, as it represents that portion of the A-filament lattice unoccupied by I filaments, the central ends of the latter forming its margins. The generation of the forces that give rise to the inward movement of the I filaments within the A band, and thus to sarcomere shortening during muscular contraction, is attributed to cyclic interactions between cross-bridges arising from the myosin molecules of the A filaments, and the actin molecules of the I filaments (Huxley H E 1971). Contraction is triggered by a

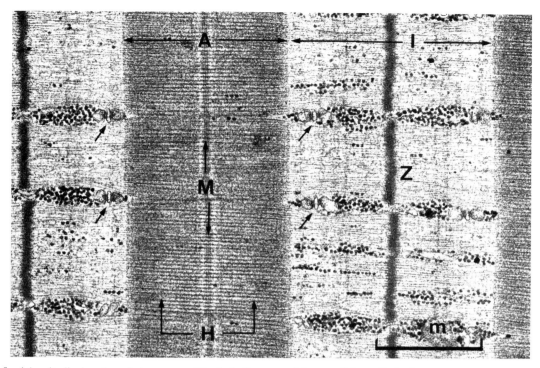

Fig. 1.5 A longitudinal section of a human myofibre including parts of four parallel myofibrils. Dark A bands (A) alternate with pale I bands (I), the latter being bisected at their mid-points by narrow dense Z lines (Z). The thick filaments of the A band possess a set of fine transverse cross-striations at their centres, the M line (M). The thin filaments of the I bands interdigitate with those of the A band, and their central ends delimit the H zone (H). Triads, junctions between the sarcoplasmic reticulum and the transverse tubules running circumferentially around each myofibril, two to each sarcomere, are marked with arrows. The dense granules between myofibrils and within the I bands are glycogen: one mitochondrion is shown (m). Scale bar = 1 μm

local increase in calcium ions released from the sarcoplasmic reticulum (q.v.), and its energy requirements are met by the local hydrolysis of ATP. The roles of the various elements of the sarcomere in the contraction process, and details of their chemical composition and structure, are described below.

The components of the sarcomere

The A band

The anisotropic band of the sarcomere consists of a regular parallel array of 'thick' myofilaments, 15–18 nm in diameter, the principal constituent of which is the protein myosin. These A filaments are 1.5–1.6 μm long, the exact value depending upon the method of tissue preparation but showing very little variation between mammalian species

(1.57 μm in cryosectioned human muscle: Sjöström & Squire 1977), and each is linked to its immediate neighbours at its mid-point by stable cross-bands, the M line, to form a regular hexagonal lattice. Along most of its length, each filament carries a series of regularly arranged side projections or 'cross-bridges'. These cross-bridge regions extend from the ends of the filaments to a point approximately 80 nm from their midpoints, leaving a smooth central zone, 160 nm long (Sjöström & Squire 1977) which includes the M line; this is the 'pseudo-H' zone or 'bare zone'.

The myosin molecules, of which the A filament is largely composed, are rod-shaped, 170 nm, two-stranded, α-helices bearing two pear-shaped heads at one end (Elliott & Offer 1978). Each is a hexamer comprised of two heavy chains of approximately 200 000 daltons and four light chains of 20 000 daltons each: the two heavy chains

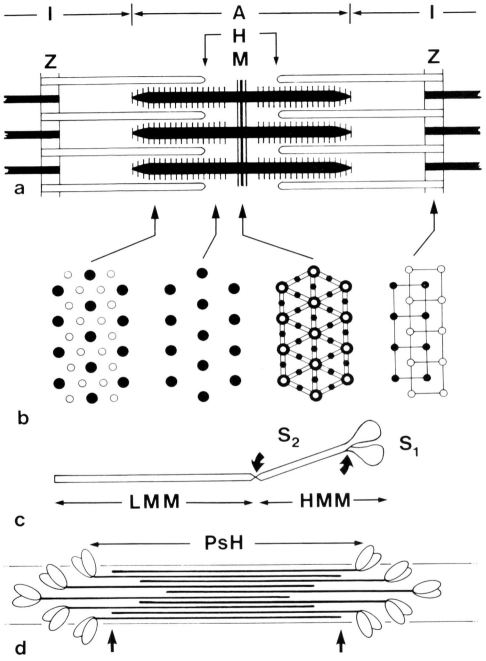

Fig. 1.6 (a) A diagram of the structure of the sarcomere. The A band (A) is composed of an hexagonal lattice of thick filaments bearing projections, linked together at their mid-points by the M-line bridges (M). The I filaments of each half I band (I) arise from the Z discs (Z) as a regular square array, and interdigitate with the A filaments to form a second hexagonal lattice. The interval between the central ends of the two sets of I filaments constitutes the H zone (H). The appearances of representative cross-sections through the sarcomere at the points indicated are illustrated in (b). (c) shows the components of the myosin molecule. A rod-shaped shaft of light meromyosin (LMM) is joined by a flexible link to heavy meromyosin (HMM), which consists of two pear-shaped heads (the S_1 subunits) and a straight shaft (the S_2 subunit). The sites on the molecule susceptible to enzymic attack are indicated by curved arrows. (d) A schematic view of the central region of a thick filament to illustrate the antiparallel packing of the myosin molecules, with their heads projecting from the surface of the filament. The region between the most central sets of heads is the 'bare' or 'pseudo-H zone' (PsH); arrows mark the somewhat shorter region of overlap of the shafts of the myosin molecules from the two halves of the thick filament

wind around each other in a coiled coil of helices to form the tail of the molecule, and then fold separately to produce the two heads. The four light chains are of two chemically distinct classes, one of each being associated with each head (Craig & Knight 1983). The light chains of the fast-twitch fibres appear to differ from those of slow muscle, and this difference is reflected in their actomyosin ATPase activities. The shaft of this molecule can be broken by tryptic digestion into two components: light meromyosin (LMM), a straight length of two-chain α-helix approximately 90 nm long and having a molecular weight of 150 000; and heavy meromyosin (HMM), which consists of the remaining 40 nm of the shaft of the molecule and its two attached globular heads, and has a molecular weight of about 350 000. The heads, in which reside the actin-binding and ATPase activities of the molecule, may in turn be separated from the helical component by further enzyme digestion to produce the S_1 and S_2 subunits of HMM respectively (Fig. 1.6c). Huxley (1963) has shown that the shafts of the myosin molecules stack together to form the shaft of the A filament in such a manner that the paired heads lie on its surface, and that the myosin molecules in each half of one A filament are arrayed with opposite polarities, the heads pointing towards the two ends of the filament; the region of overlap of the two arrays of LMM tails gives rise to the central bare zone (Fig. 1.6d). The A filaments taper towards their distal ends, and X-ray diffraction studies have demonstrated that the myosin heads are arranged around them in a semi-regular helix (Craig & Offer 1976a) with pairs of heads on opposite sides of the shaft at intervals of 14.3 nm, each successive pair being rotated by 120° about the axis of the shaft relative to its nearest neighbours, to give an overall axial repeat of 43.0 nm (Huxley & Brown 1967). Solubility studies have shown that HMM subfraction 2, the short component of the shaft adjacent to the globular heads, does not share the propensity of both whole myosin and LMM to form ordered aggregates under physiological conditions. It has therefore been suggested that HMM may interact only weakly with adjacent myosin molecules in vivo and that its junction with LMM may act as a flexible joint, permitting the HMM component of each myosin molecule to lie at a variable angle to the shaft of the whole A filament (Huxley 1969, Lowey et al 1969, Trinick & Elliott 1979). Biochemical aspects of the substructure of the myosin molecule have been reviewed by Gergely (1988).

A bands prepared by a variety of different techniques show consistent patterns of cross-banding. A semi-regular series of fine striations, 14–15 nm apart, are visible throughout the A band including the pseudo-H zone, and these are considered to represent either the structure of the LMM backbone of the thick filament (Hanson et al 1971), or, in the cross-bridge zone, a combined pattern generated by the cross-bridges and the periodicity of the LMM tails (Craig 1977, Sjöström & Squire 1977). Superimposed upon these fine cross-striations over the central two-thirds of the thick filaments are a series of broader stripes, having a periodicity of around 43.0 nm, matching that of the major repeat of the myosin heads along the length of the individual filaments in the cross-bridge zone. It has been established that these bands represent the location of non-myosin protein components of the A filaments (Fig. 1.7b). Artificial A filaments of a variety of lengths, both longer and shorter than native A bands, can be generated by the precipitation of purified myosin from salt solutions (Huxley 1963), and an early report that the non-myosin components of the A filaments repeated at intervals of 44.2 nm (Huxley 1967) led to a suggestion that the lack of direct correspondence between this repeat and the 43 nm repeat of myosin could result in a 'vernier' type of interaction between the two components, and that this could, in turn, be responsible for establishing the remarkably constant length of A filaments in vertebrate muscle (Huxley & Brown 1967). A similar role has been assigned to the more recently identified non-myosin A-band component titin (see below). It is now clear that it is the structure of the myosin backbone of the A filament that determines the location of the non-myosin protein bands (Craig 1977, Sjöström & Squire 1977), and that the 44.2 nm periodicity can be ascribed to the effects of interference arising within the thickness of the A filament array on the basic 43.0 nm repeat (Rome et al 1973, Craig & Megerman 1979).

A total of nine transverse striations have been

a

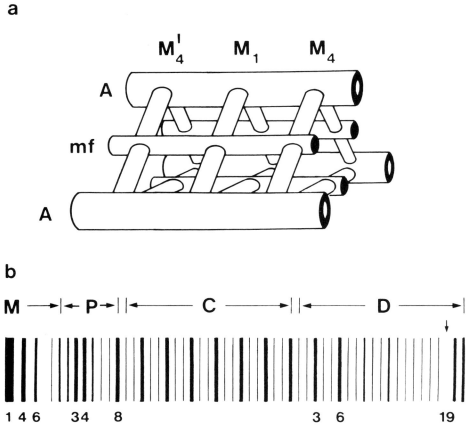

b

Fig. 1.7   (a) A schematic view of the unit cell of a three-line M band. Adjacent thick (A) filaments are linked by cross-bridges at M_1 and M'_4, M_4; at their mid-points these cross-bridges incorporate a second set of slender longitudinal M filaments (mf). In five-line M bands a further set of cross-bridges is present at M'_6 and M_6. (Redrawn after Luther & Squire 1978). (b) A diagrammatic representation of the cross-striation pattern of one half of an A band. The seven prominent stripes in the C region represent the location of the non-myosin C protein; additional non-myosin proteins are believed to be located in both the proximal (P 3–4 and 8) and distal (D 3 and 6) zones (see text). The intervening regular pattern of fine striations represents the repeating structure of the myosin backbone of the thick filament and its cross-bridges. It has been suggested that the loss of a stripe at D 19 (arrow) indicates the absence of a pair of cross-bridges at this location. (Based on data in Sjöström & Squire 1977, Craig & Megerman 1979)

recognized in each half of the pseudo-H zone, and these have been numbered M1 to M9 from the filament centre outwards (Sjöström & Squire 1977, Luther & Squire 1978). The central band (M_1), and a pair flanking it at an interval of 22 nm (M4), are particularly prominent in most preparations, and collectively constitute the histological M line. Slow-twitch muscular activity is associated with the appearance of a second pair of dense bands (M6) at 43.7 nm from the filament centre, to give a five-banded M line (Sjöström & Squire 1977). Studies of the three-dimensional structure of the M line have shown that its constituent bands represent the positions of substantial cross-bridges that link each A filament to its six nearest neighbours in a hexagonal array. When the A band is viewed in transverse section, each of these bridges shows a thickening at its mid-point, and these have been interpreted to indicate the existence of a set of short, small-diameter (4–5 nm), longitudinally orientated M filaments mid-way between each A filament. A model structure of a three-banded M line incorporating these components was described by Knappeis & Carlsen (1968). The major features of this model were confirmed by Luther & Squire (1978) (Fig. 1.7a) who suggested that there may be an additional cross-linking component between adjacent M filaments at the position of line M3, that would account for the consistent appearance of interfilament staining at this region in their frog muscle preparations. They also proposed that a weaker, inter-A filament cross-linkage may exist at line M9, immediately adjacent to the central margin of the myosin cross-bridge zone. These observations and models are not compatible with that proposed by Pepe (1975), in which each A filament is linked to only two of its neighbours at any one level by diametrically opposed pairs of M bridges. A number of non-myosin M proteins have been isolated, but their exact locations and functions within the intact M line are at present uncertain. Examples are M-protein, a 150 000 mol.wt component of M line extracts that has been ascribed a structural role in the M cross-bridges (Chowrashi & Pepe 1979); myomesin, a 185 000 mol.wt protein also associated with the M-line cross-bridges (Grove et al 1984, 1989); and the MM isoenzyme of creatine kinase which co-migrates with a 42 000 mol.wt M-line component (Walliman et al 1979). No functional significance can be attached at present to the differing M-line structures observed in fast- and slow-twitch mammalian myofibres, but the presence of an M line appears to be conditional upon the arrangement of the A filaments into a superlattice with dimensions $\sqrt{3}$ times larger than that of the smallest possible hexagonal lattice, in which next-nearest, rather than nearest, neighbours have an identical axial orientation. Some invertebrate muscles that lack M lines have been shown by X-ray diffraction to have randomly orientated thick filaments (Wray et al 1975), and it has been proposed that organization into a superlattice is necessary if the M-bridge bonding sites are to be correctly positioned relative to one another (Craig 1977).

Variation in the intensity of the transverse banding of the cross-bridge region in both sectioned and negatively stained A bands permits its division into 17, approximately equal, 43 nm segments grouped into three zones (Fig. 1.7b). These are a 'P' or proximal zone consisting of the three 43 nm sections immediately adjacent to the pseudo-H or bare zone; a more distal, seven-banded 'C' zone; and a 'D' or distal zone that lacks the broad stripes of its more central neighbours, and possesses a semiregular pattern of fine lines 14–15 nm apart in negatively stained preparations (Sjöström & Squire 1977). The C zone is so-called from the presence in this region of the most abundant of the non-myosin A-band proteins, C protein. This material has been isolated and purified (Offer et al 1973), and has been shown to be an elongated 25 nm monomer lacking any helical component, with a molecular weight of 140 000. It has no ATPase or calcium-binding activity, and while it does not affect the ATPase activity of myosin, it inhibits actomyosin ATPase. It has also been reported recently that C protein, alone of the A-band non-myosin proteins, can compete with HMM-S$_1$ for binding sites on F actin (Moos et al 1978). Antibody-staining studies have shown that C protein is bound strongly and solely to the seven major bands in the C zone, and that these have the same 43 nm repeat as the underlying myosin backbone of the thick filament (Pepe & Drucker 1975, Craig & Offer 1976a). As C protein does not bind to HMM-subfraction 1 (Starr & Offer 1978) it is thought to be attached to the tails of the myosin molecules constituting the shaft of the thick filament. The known properties of C protein, and the tenacity and specificity with which it binds to a restricted zone on the A band, have prompted a number of suggestions that it has a structural role in the A filaments; however, the original proposal, referred to above, that C and other non-myosin proteins serve to control the length of the thick filaments, is not supported by recent evidence (Pepe 1975, 1979, Craig & Megerman 1979). Its restricted attachment to the mid-zone of the cross-bridge region may, however, be linked to a re-arrangement of the shafts of the myosin molecules within the thick filament that is thought to occur within the same region (Pepe 1979). The possible functional consequences of the capacity of C protein to bind to both myosin and actin are discussed by Moos et al (1978).

The bands of the P zone of the cross-bridge region also represent sites of attachment of non-myosin proteins to the thick filaments (Pepe 1975). One of these, H protein, has been isolated from crude extracts of C protein and has been shown by antibody staining to be located exclusively on band 8 at the distal edge of the P zone (Craig &

Megerman 1979). A second, unnamed, contaminant of C-protein extracts appears to bind solely to more proximal bands (3 and 4), at the junction of the first and second sections of the P zone. It is likely that the D zone also contains non-myosin protein components, although in smaller quantities, but these have yet to be identified (Fig. 1.7b). A consistent feature of the outermost part of the D zone is a pale transverse striation visible immediately inside the distal margin of stained, sectioned A bands. The pallor of this region relative to adjacent portions of the A band is enhanced in sarcomeres treated with labelled anti-HMM-S_1 and antimyosin serum, indicating that the gap probably represents a loss of one set of myosin cross-bridges at this site (Craig & Offer 1976b, Pepe 1979). Absence of a pair of cross-bridges at the third 14.3 nm repeat from the filament tip is compatible with the model by Pepe & Dowben (1977) of the packing of the myosin molecules within the tapering end of the A filament. The detailed structure of the thick filament and its relationship to the process of muscular contraction has been reviewed by Squire (1981).

The I band

The principal component of the thin myofilaments that characterize the I band of the sarcomeres is the protein actin. In its monomeric form (G actin) this is an asymmetrical ellipsoid, consisting of two distinct and roughly globular domains separated by a cleft, with overall dimensions of $6.7 \times 4.0 \times 3.7$ nm, with a molecular weight of about 45 000. These monomers are assembled into a filamentous polymer (F actin), a right-handed, two-stranded helix 6–7 nm in diameter, twisted so that there are 13–15 actin molecules for every full rotation of the helix with their long axes nearly aligned with the helix of the filament (Milligan et al 1990). The centre-to-centre spacing of the monomers along each chain is 5.46 nm, and the units of the two strands are staggered relative to one another by one half period, 2.73 nm (Fig. 1.8a). The exact pitch of the helix varies with the source of the filaments, one half-rotation being 36.0 nm in vertebrate striated muscle (Huxley & Brown 1967), and up to 38.5 nm in insect flight muscle (Miller & Tregear 1972). The grooves on either side of the two chains of actin molecules are occupied by a second I-filament protein, tropomyosin. This is a rod-shaped molecule, consisting of two, approximately equal, left-handed α-helices, 38.5 nm long with a total molecular weight of 66 000, units of which assemble head-to-tail to form a pair of continuous spiral strands along the length of each I filament (Cohen et al 1971, Ebashi 1980). Each tropomyosin molecule is attached to exactly seven actin monomers via their inner domains, and it is this relationship, rather than the more variable pitch of the actin helix, that defines the functional unit of the I filament, and thus of the contractile regulatory system (see below). The outer domain of the actin molecule provides the main attachment site for the S_1 myosin head. The biochemistry of the I filaments and striated muscle actin has been reviewed by Gergely (1988).

F-actin strands prepared in vitro are of indefinite length (Hanson 1973), but within the intact sarcomere the I filaments have a constant and well-defined length that varies from 1.0 to 1.35 μm, according to the method of preparation and animal species studied (Huxley 1963, Sjöström & Squire 1977). The I filaments are attached at one end to the Z line, which bisects the I band at its mid-point, in a regular square 22 nm array; at the other end they penetrate the hexagonal lattice of the A band, where each occupies a trigonal point between three adjacent thick filaments to form a second, interlocking, hexagonal lattice (Fig. 1.6b). The free central margin of the whole I-filament assembly delimits the lateral border of the H band, the exact location of which will vary with the state of shortening of the sarcomere. The affinity of the actin helix for myosin has been demonstrated by treating I bands isolated from homogenized muscle with HMM-S_1 subfragments (Huxley 1963). The individual I filaments become 'decorated' with regularly arranged arrowheads of S_1 subunits every 35–37 nm. The arrowheads are always directed towards the free ends of the filaments, and therefore point in opposite directions on the two sides of the Z line, indicating that the filaments are structurally polarized. This method has been used to demonstrate the widespread occurrence of actin in the form of 5–6 nm microfilaments in a wide range of cell types (Ishikawa et al 1969); it has been found that

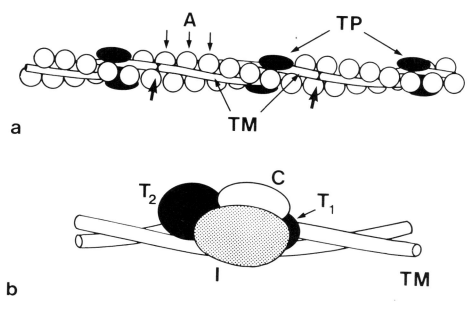

Fig. 1.8 (a) A diagrammatic view of a section of an I filament. A double chain of globular actin monomers (A) is wound in a right-handed helix, the grooves between the two chains containing a second double helix of the filamentous protein tropomyosin (TM), to which they are attached. A third protein component, troponin (TP) is situated as a series of globular complexes at regular intervals along the filament, attached to a single specific binding site on each tropomyosin molecule. Arrows indicate the junctions between adjacent tropomyosin molecules. (b) The components of a troponin complex attached to the tropomyosin double helix (TM). The calcium-binding properties of the complex are contained in the C subunit. (Redrawn after Ebashi 1980)

individual actin filaments always possess a uniform polarity, and that its direction is identical in all filaments where these are grouped into strands. Actin or microfilaments attached to submembrane densities, such as those that occur at the muscle plasmalemma at the myotendinous junction or at intercellular contacts of the zona adhaerens type, also show a consistent polarity, with the HMM-S_1 arrowheads directed away from their point of attachment, as in the Z disc (Ishikawa 1979).

I bands in sectioned and stained muscle (Huxley 1967), and F actin strands polymerized from unpurified actin by precipitation with divalent cations (Hanson 1973), both show regular transverse striations with a period of approximately 40 nm, and a similar periodicity has been reported in X-ray diffraction images of unfixed muscle (Huxley & Brown 1967). It is now known from antibody-staining studies (Pepe 1966, Ohtsuki et al 1967) that these cross-striations represent the location of the third I-filament protein — troponin (Ebashi et al 1968). This is a globular structure with a molecular weight of approximately 80 000

and is composed of three major subunits I, C and T having molecular weights of approximately 24 000, 20 000 and 37 000 respectively. Troponin C has a strong affinity for calcium ions, each molecule having two pairs of binding sites: the high-affinity sites competitively binding Mg^{2+}, the other two being specific for Ca^{2+}. Calcium ion affinity is enhanced by interactions between the components of the troponin complex; these may involve conformational changes, which may in turn play an essential role in the interactions between the thick and thin myofilaments during muscle activity. One troponin complex is attached to a specific point on each tropomyosin molecule in the grooves of the actin helix (Fig. 1.8b) to give the observed periodicity of 38.5 nm along the I filaments (Ohtsuki 1975, 1979). The properties of troponin and its roles in the regulation of muscular contraction are reviewed by Ebashi (1980) and Gergely (1988). In addition to its filaments, the I band contains unstructured interstitial material of moderate electron density and largely unknown composition. In many species concentrations of this substance can occur adjacent to the Z disc, giving rise to a broad transverse band, the 'N$_1$' line (Page 1968, Franzini-Armstrong 1970a). The line is better defined and closer to the Z disc in shortened sarcomeres (Page 1968); its position may reflect the point of maximum incursion of the I filaments into the A-band lattice during normal contractile activity. A second, N$_2$ line, is often visible further from the Z disc, approximately midway between it and the A/I junction in relaxed fibres. Both bands have recently been identified as sites of concentration of the high-molecular-weight polypeptide nebulin (600–800 kd) which accounts for 3% of myofibrillar mass and binds strongly to alpha-actinin (Nave et al 1990), but monoclonal antibody binding studies indicate that nebulin is also located at other intermediate positions along the I filaments up to 1.0 μm from the Z disc (Wang & Wright 1988). It has been proposed that nebulin constitutes a set of inextensible filaments attached at one end to the Z disc, running in parallel with both the I filaments and the titin filaments (q.v.) below.

It has been suspected for a number of years that the well-characterized thick and thin filaments of the sarcomere are augmented by accessory filamentous proteins, and that these may contribute to the longitudinal elasticity of the myofibril (Maruyama & Yamamoto 1979). Convincing morphological evidence for the existence of such parallel elastic filaments has been difficult to obtain (Hoyle 1983), but recent experiments involving chemical removal of the I filaments have demonstrated the presence of 4 nm fine filaments connecting the ends of the A filaments to the Z discs (Wang and Ramirez-Mitchell 1983, Funatsu et al 1990, Salviati et al 1990). These filaments appear to be built up of very high molecular weight polypeptides, a major component of which, titin (connectin), has been isolated and characterized (Maruyama et al 1977, Maruyama 1986, Wang et al 1979, Wang 1982). The molecular weight of titin has been variously estimated to be between 1 and 2.8 million daltons, and it appears to consist of a long (900 nm), very thin rod with a single globular head, which associate as dimers or higher oligomers via their head regions (Nave et al 1989). Mild protein digestion of myofibrils, which releases only titin, results in a loss of resting tension and

disruption of the 4 nm filaments (Funatsu et al 1990), and immunocytochemical studies indicate that the titin molecules extend throughout each half sarcomere, with the globular head ends anchored close to the M-line, and their tails attached to the Z disc (Furst et al 1988, Nave et al 1989, Salviati et al 1990). Dynamic studies appear to indicate that the central portion of the titin filaments are firmly attached to the A filaments, and that within the normal range of sarcomere extension their elasticity resides in the I band, in the portion between the N$_1$ line and the ends of the A filaments (Horowits et al 1989, Pierobon-Bormioli et al 1989). The elastic titin filaments appear to be independent of the I filaments, and it has been suggested that they may be responsible for maintaining the mechanical continuity of the sarcomere (Maruyama et al 1989).

The Z disc

The Z line or disc is an optically and electron-dense transverse structure (the membrane of Krause) which divides each I band at its mid-point and constitutes the boundary between adjacent sarcomeres. Electron microscopy of sections cut at a shallow angle to the plane of the Z disc shows that immediately adjacent to the disc the filaments of each half I band lose their apparently haphazard arrangement and become organized into a regular 22 nm square array, the square lattices so formed on the two surfaces of the disc being offset, one from another, by 50% along both axes. Each I filament is therefore positioned opposite the centre of a square formed by the ends of four filaments from the I band on the opposite side of the disc (Fig. 1.6). In longitudinal sections the terminal 20–30 nm portions of the I filaments appear to thicken as they approach the disc, showing increased electron-density and merging with the amorphous dense material of the Z disc itself. While there is general agreement concerning these appearances among those who have studied the fine structure of the Z discs in striated muscle of higher vertebrate species, many diverse explanations have been proposed for its internal structure, and for the mode of attachment of the I filaments.

Knappeis & Carlsen (1962), who studied frog muscle fixed in osmium tetroxide, considered that the I filaments terminate at the surface of the disc, and that each gives rise to four finer Z filaments which pass diagonally through the thickness of the Z disc and connect it to the four nearest I filaments of the next sarcomere. When viewed along the axes of the I filaments, these Z filaments form the boundaries of a second set of squares, measuring 15.5 nm on each side, rotated at 45° with respect to the I-filament square lattice adjacent to the disc (Fig. 1.9a). The appearances of longitudinal sections were compatible with this arrangement of connecting fibrils, showing either a zig-zag pattern in which each I filament was connected by a pair of short oblique links to the tips of the two nearest I filaments in the next sarcomere, or I filaments aligned end-to-end with an intervening dense zone of complex structure. Franzini-Armstrong & Porter (1964) later reported essentially similar structural patterns in the muscles of several different species, but placed greater emphasis on the amorphous dense material within the disc. They proposed that this constituted a membrane, pulled in opposite directions by the attached tips of the I filaments from the two sarcomeres, the consequent deformation producing thickened ridges corre-

sponding to the electron-dense lines seen by Knappeis & Carlsen (1962) and interpreted by them as Z filaments. Reedy (1964) subsequently demonstrated a basket-weave appearance in transverse sections of osmium tetroxide-fixed rat muscle (Fig. 1.10a); he explained this by a modification of the Knappeis & Carlsen (1962) model in which the 'weave' was achieved by tangential engagement of the Z filaments with the tips of the I filaments (Fig. 1.9a), the I filaments themselves being four stranded helices having the same-handedness on the two faces of the disc. The final model based solely on osmium-fixed muscle (larval newt tail) was that proposed by Kelly (1967). He made use of stereo-electron micrographs and reported the presence of a system of loops of I filaments or I-filament components within the thickness of the Z disc, in which an element of one I filament looped around the tip of a nearby I filament of the next sarcomere and then returned to its own side, to form one component of an I filament immediately adjacent to that from which it had first arisen. Translated into a wire model, this arrangement results in an interlocking square mesh of filaments within the Z disc, each one of which represents half of either the double-stranded actin helix, or its companion double helix of tropomyosin. If the looping filaments are given an appropriate curvature and inclination to the I-filament axis, this model will also mimic both the zig-zag Z line seen in longitudinal sections, and the Reedy 'basket-weave' when viewed en face.

Routine use of glutaraldehyde in place of osmium tetroxide as a primary fixative for muscle subsequently led to the recognition of a second pattern of filament linkage within the Z disc (Fardeau 1969a,b, Landon 1969, 1970b, Macdonald & Engel 1971). The large 'woven' lattice of Z filaments disposed at 45° to the planes of the I-filament array, seen in osmium-fixed material and described above, was replaced in aldehyde-treated tissue by a regular small square lattice of 5 nm-wide elements with a period of 11 nm and axes coinciding with those of the files of I filaments (Fig. 1.9b). The appearance of longitudinal sections also differed, the classical zig-zag pattern being replaced by either interdigitation of the ends of the I filaments through the thickness of the

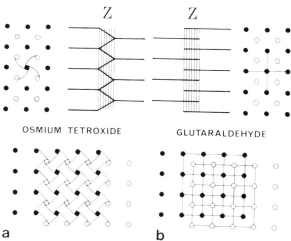

Fig. 1.9 A diagrammatic view of the internal structure of Z discs in longitudinal and transverse section following primary fixation (a) in osmium tetroxide, and (b) in glutaraldehyde. Transected I filaments arising from one side of a disc are shown as open circles, and those from the adjacent sarcomere by closed circles; the matrix material is represented by fine vertical hatching. For details see text

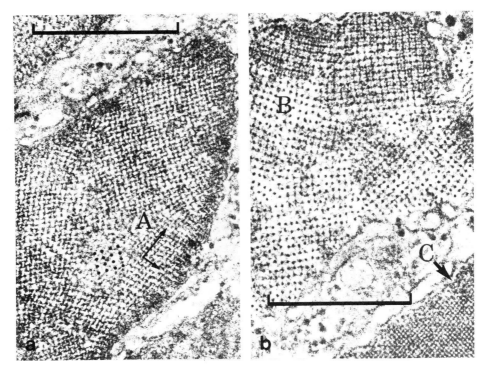

Fig. 1.10 The fine structural appearances of Z discs in transversely sectioned myofibres. (a) Muscle fixed in osmium tetroxide showing the large 'woven' pattern of I-filament interconnections (A), the axes of the weave (small arrows) being offset by 45° from the axes of alignment of the I filaments adjacent to the disc (dots). (b) A slightly oblique section through a Z disc fixed in glutaraldehyde in which the I filament square lattice on one side of the disc merges with a small square lattice having the same axes but half the period (B). A uniform area of the small lattice pattern can be seen at (C), and represents a section through the mid-plane of an adjacent disc. Scale bar = 0.5 μm

disc, or their apparent continuity from one sarcomere to the next. Examination of stereo-pairs of electron micrographs of sections passing through the plane of the disc at a shallow angle (Landon 1970b) were interpreted as showing that the small regular 11 nm-square lattice was the product of the superimposition of two larger lattices of twice that period (i.e. 22–24 nm), the one out of register with the other by half its repeat along each axis. These basic 22–24 nm lattices appeared to be formed by a dense cross-linkage of the terminal portions of the I filaments throughout the thickness of the Z disc, each with its immediate neighbours from the same sarcomere, the interdigitation of the I filaments from the two sarcomeres determining the registration of the two lattices (Fig. 1.10b). No looping configurations were observed.

It was proposed that the glutaraldehyde-fixed structure could be transformed into that seen following osmium tetroxide fixation by realignment of the cross-linking elements, in such a manner that they were no longer connected to the I filaments of the same sarcomere but rotated through 45° in a transverse plane and linked with the tips of the I filaments of the adjacent sarcomere (Landon 1970b). This process would have the effect of 'unlocking' the two lattices, allowing the interdigitating I filaments to slide apart until tethered by the linking filaments. In their new position these would correspond to the Z filaments of Knappeis & Carlsen (1962), and give rise to the narrow zig-zag Z line and large single woven lattice characteristic of osmium-fixed muscle. Other workers have considered a structural transformation of this extent to be improbable, and have proposed alternative models to account for the small (11 nm) lattice configuration (Macdonald & Engel 1971, Rowe 1971, Kelly & Cahill 1972, Ullrick et al 1977). The small lattice has been reported to be absent from fast fish muscle, whatever method of fixation is employed (Franzini-Armstrong 1973b).

Both Rowe (1971) and Macdonald & Engel (1971) have proposed looping filament models comparable to that suggested by Kelly (1967), but neither provides completely satisfactory images of both the large woven and small square lattices, or the basis for a convincing explanation of their interconvertibility. Rowe's model does, however, provide a parallel with the multiple linkages between I filaments seen in longitudinal sections of the Z discs of slow-twitch rat myofibres, an arrangement that is not explained by other models (Rowe 1973). Macdonald & Engel (1971) also proposed and favoured an alternative model without loops, based on the Z-filament structure reported by Knappeis & Carlsen (1962), in which paired connecting filaments arising from the tips of each I filament were acutely angled at their mid-points to yield a configuration in plan view resembling a diametrically opposed pair of limbs from a swastika, and suggested that sets of such units could collectively mimic the small square lattice image. This pattern can, in their model, be converted into the large woven lattice without altering the basic connections of the linking elements, by moving the ends of the I filaments belonging to the two sarcomeres apart along their long axes, or by increasing their lateral separation. The model of Kelly & Cahill (1972) also employed curved Z filaments, with the connections and relationships proposed by Knappeis & Carlsen (1962), to reproduce the large woven lattice but they suggested that the small square lattice was the product of superimposed condensations of Z-disc matrix material linking adjacent I filaments of the same sarcomere, and did not represent filamentous connections (Fig. 1.11). They proposed that the two patterns normally coexist, the small square lattice being the more prominent in glutaraldehyde tissue in which the Z-disc matrix material is better preserved and the I filaments interdigitate, and

that the large woven lattice and zig-zag Z line of osmium tetroxide-fixed tissue result from extraction of some of the matrix material and movement apart of the ends of the I filaments. An optical diffraction analysis of electron micrographs of canine cardiac Z bands and Z rods by Goldstein et al (1977, 1979) has confirmed the existence of both the small square and large woven lattice structures in the Z bands. The average edge dimension of the large I-filament square lattice in transverse sections was 23.9 nm, and an axial periodicity of 38.0 nm was detected along the overlapped ends of the I filaments in longitudinal sections. Lastly, Ullrick et al (1977) published a looping-filament model in which three connecting filaments originate from the end of each I filament and are bent so as to form three of the four legs of a swastika. The loops arising from adjacent sarcomeres are apposed, but not interwoven, and each returns to its own sarcomere to join two other similar filaments at the tip of an immediately adjacent I filament. They also presented an alternative model in which each I filament gives rise to two rather than three branches, but in each case they considered that the large woven lattice represents the 'natural' condition of the Z disc, and that the small square lattice is a consequence of fixation-induced shrinkage.

The number and variety of models proposed for the Z disc are an index of the difficulties that have been experienced in attempting to obtain unequivocal morphological evidence of its structure, and if the various patterns described reflected merely differential extraction of materials, or the artefactual realignment of connecting filaments as a consequence of differing fixation procedures, they would be of relatively little general interest. Evidence is available, however, from structural studies of fixed tissue (Reedy 1967, Franzini-Armstrong 1973b) and from X-ray diffraction experiments on living muscle (Elliott et al 1967, Huxley & Brown 1967), that I-filament spacing in the ordered zone adjacent to the Z disc is related to sarcomere length, and increases with sarcomere shortening. Added interest is given to these dimensional changes by a theory of muscular contraction put forward by Ullrick (1967) in which he proposed that the contractile force in muscle is

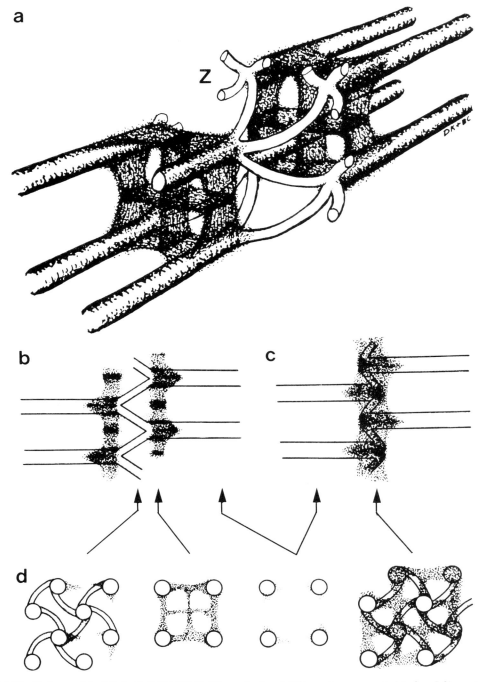

Fig. 1.11   (a) The Z-disc model of Kelly & Cahill (1972). The ends of each I filament are connected to four I filaments of the next sarcomere by obliquely disposed Z filaments (Z), in the manner proposed by Knappeis & Carlsen (1962). The small square lattice is considered to be composed of condensations of matrix material between the ends of the I filaments. Differences in the degree of overlap of the ends of the I filaments (b and c), consequent upon different fixation procedures, were held to be responsible for controlling whether the image of the large 'woven' (b) or small square (c) lattice pattern predominated in section including the central regions of the disc (d). (Modified from Kelly & Cahill 1972, and reproduced by kind permission of the authors and the editor of the Anatomical Record)

generated by active radial expansion of the Z discs, shortening of the fixed-volume sarcomeres (Elliott et al 1963) being an inevitable consequence of increase in their diameter.

Experiments designed to test the relationship between I-filament spacing and Z-disc lattice pattern, on the one hand, and the length and contractile state of the sarcomeres to which they belong, on the other (Landon 1970c), have shown that the Z discs of rat muscle fixed in situ while contracting in response to a tetanizing electrical stimulus possess a high proportion of the large woven lattice pattern—a pattern seldom seen in the same muscles similarly fixed at rest, and wholly absent from muscles fixed in a relaxed state immediately following a short tetanizing stimulus (Fig. 1.12). The change from the small square to the large woven lattice, observed in the muscles fixed

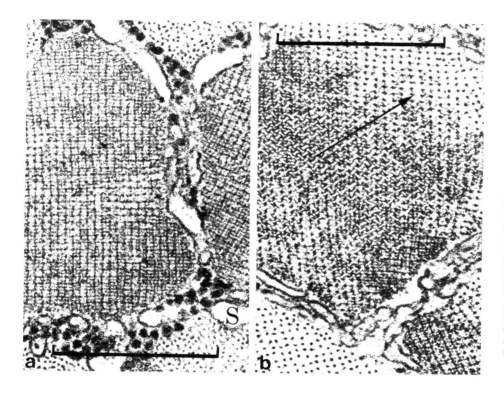

Fig. 1.12 Muscle fixed in glutaraldehyde (a) in a relaxed state immediately following a 10-second tetanic contraction, and (b) while actively contracting. The Z discs of the relaxed muscle possess a uniform fine square lattice pattern of ~ 11 nm period: in the contracting muscle this is largely replaced by a larger 'woven' pattern, similar to that seen following osmium tetroxide fixation, with axes offset at 45° from those of the I-filament lattice (arrow). (S) indicates the dilated sarcoplasmic reticulum of the post-tetanic muscle. The changes in Z-lattice pattern and I-filament spacing consequent upon contraction are shown diagrammatically below (c). Scale bar = 0.5 μm

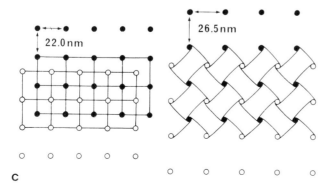

while contracting, was accompanied by an increase in the I-filament spacing at the disc from 22.0 nm to 26.5 nm, a dimensional change not far removed from that reported by Elliott et al (1967) on the basis of X-ray diffraction studies of living, contracting toad muscle (19.7–30.0 nm) or by Yu et al (1977) who studied frog sartorius muscle (21.8 to 26.7 nm with change in sarcomere length from 3.0 to 2.0 μm), when allowance is made for the tissue shrinkage inevitably associated with preparation for electron microscopy (Reedy & Barkes 1974). Electron-microscopic confirmation of comparable change in Z-disc lattice dimensions with change in sarcomere length was provided by Davey (1976), who showed that the sarcomere length dependency of the Z lattice is similar to that of the A filament lattice. These observations thus provide prima facie evidence that the Z disc can undergo transitory and reversible changes in both its radial dimensions and internal structure during muscular contraction in vivo, and that the fine square and coarse woven lattices represent alternative and interconvertible forms of Z-disc structure that correspond to the relaxed and contracted states of the sarcomere respectively (Landon 1970c). It is not currently known, however, whether the increase in I-filament spacing and lattice transformation are actively associated with the contractile process per se, or are passive corollaries of sarcomere shortening, comparable to the well-recognized increase in the spacing of the A- and I-filament arrays in the A band with muscle shortening (Elliott et al 1963, 1967, Brandt et al 1967) as suggested by Davey (1976).

If it is accepted that both Z-disc lattice patterns exist in vivo, and represent alternative functional states, the construction of a convincing model of Z-disc structure becomes a matter of considerable interest. It is difficult to do full justice to the various models listed above within the space available, and the reader is referred to the original papers cited for fuller information, but it is the writer's view that none provides a wholly convincing description of Z-disc structure. Any successful model must, inter alia: (1) make adequate allowance for the matrix material which constitutes, by weight, the major component of the disc; (2) be capable of rapid reversible transformation between the two basic lattice patterns;

and (3) be compatible with a range of different Z-line thicknesses. The last point, hitherto largely ignored in this discussion, is of some importance as mammalian Z lines vary in thickness with muscle fibre type, slow-twitch fibres having Z lines approximately twice the thickness (90–100 nm) of fast-twitch fibres (40–50 nm). Details of the measurements obtained from different species, and the relationship of these values to histochemical fibre-type are discussed at greater length in a later section (p. 38). Several of the models outlined above are based on observations of very thin Z lines from very fast fish or amphibian muscle (Knappeis & Carlsen 1962, Kelly 1967, Franzini-Armstrong 1973b), and do not seem compatible with thicker structures. The multiple looping systems postulated by Rowe (1971, 1973) and Hoyle (1983), on the other hand, can mimic the appearances seen in longitudinal sections of thick mammalian Z discs, but the regular systematic interweaving of single cytoplasmic filaments required by these models is inherently implausible; no comparable arrangement has been described in any other cell type. A model fulfilling the conditions listed above could be constructed, however, by linking two interdigitating square arrays of I filaments by sets of paired angulated filaments having the configuration suggested in the second model proposed by Macdonald & Engel (1971), the linkage between I filaments of the same sarcomere being reinforced by matrix at the surface of the disc. This model seems capable of predicting all of the morphological features of the mammalian Z disc so far described, including the small square and large woven lattice patterns seen at small and large I-filament spacings respectively, and the pennate appearance of the interdigitating ends of the I filaments often visible in longitudinal sections. If the connecting filaments are attached at intervals of 20–25 nm along the overlapping ends of the I filaments, the model also permits a stepwise increase in Z-disc thickness by 20–25 nm increments, which closely resembles that described in human muscle in the different fibre types (Schmalbruch & Kamieniecka 1974, Payne et al 1975). See also the review by Schmalbruch (1985).

The chemical composition of the Z disc has also been a source of controversy. The striking similarity of the 40 nm orthorhombic lattice of negatively stained tropomyosin crystals (Huxley 1963) to the I-filament square lattice at the surface of the disc, initially led to the suggestion that a tropomyosin net, or nets, constituted the 'back-bone' of the Z disc, and that the I filaments were attached to the corners of each square of the tropomyosin mesh via their individual tropomyosin double helices. It was later shown that none of the polymorphic forms of tropomyosin crystal that can be prepared artificially has a symmetry truly· comparable to that of the Z-disc lattices, and that the tropomyosin mesh cannot be distorted to fit the Z disc without altering the basic pattern of its connections (Caspar et al 1969). This conclusion was reinforced by immune staining (Endo et al 1966) and chemical extraction experiments (Stromer et al 1967, 1969), which showed that Z lines contain only minor concentrations of either tropomyosin or actin. Another major protein constituent of skeletal muscle, isolated by Ebashi et al (1964) and named α-actinin, was subsequently proposed as a Z-line constituent on the grounds of its pronounced cross-linking affinity for actin (Briskey et al 1967). Alpha-actinin has since been demonstrated by immunological staining to be confined strictly to the lattice regions of Z lines in striated muscle (Masaki et al 1967, Schollmeyer et al 1974), and to contribute approximately 50% of their total mass (Suzuki et al 1976). It has been isolated from skeletal, cardiac and smooth muscle, and consists of asymmetrical rod-shaped particles, 4×40 nm, which are probably homodimers of a 100 000 mol. wt polypeptide chain (Suzuki et al 1976, Singh et al 1977). Antibodies raised against skeletal muscle α-actinin cross-react with very similar α-actinin-like molecules in other cells (Jockusch 1979); it has therefore been possible to show that such molecules are present in many cell types, and are restricted to sites of increased cytoplasmic electron-density associated with actin or micro-filament bundles. Their occurrence at the focal points of fibroblast stress fibres (Lazarides 1976), at cleavage furrows in dividing cells (Fujiwara et al 1978), and at the submembrane densities of organized intercellular junctional complexes (Craig & Pardo 1979), provide evidence that α-actinin has a widespread structural function within cells, of which its location in the Z disc is but one example. The actin or microfilament bundles

arising from sites of α-actinin concentration always possess a uniform polarity when 'decorated' with HMM-S_1 subunits, with arrowheads pointing away from the dense zone (Ishikawa 1979). This feature, and the finding that α-actinin binds selectively to the ends of actin filaments at physiological temperatures in vitro (Goll et al 1972), suggests that it is responsible for the polarization of the native I filaments of the sarcomere (Huxley 1963). It is not known whether α-actinin resides in the filamentous or matrix components of the Z disc, but the latter is favoured by Schollmeyer et al (1974).

Some additional insight into Z-disc structure has been obtained from studies of dense rod-like abnormalities at the Z line, 'nemaline' rods or 'rod bodies', that are relatively common in diseased and denervated muscle (Shy et al 1963, Price et al 1965, Engel & Gomez 1967). These have a regular lattice structure and appear to be formed by longitudinal outgrowths of Z-disc material into the I bands, which distort the normal arrangements of myofilaments in the contiguous sarcomeres. In longitudinal sections orthogonal to the plane of the rod lattice, the internal structure can be seen to be directly comparable to that of a normal Z disc, consisting of a regular series of dense parallel filaments, 6–7 nm in diameter and stacked at 11–12 nm intervals. These are continuous with the thin filaments of the adjacent I band, alternate members of the series being connected to the same I band, and the whole assembly shows a transverse periodicity of 20–30 nm (Fig. 1.13a). The internal structure of the rods seen in transverse sections closely resembles the small square lattice pattern of the Z disc, having the same (11–12 nm) periodicity, and differs only in having a more pronounced accentuation of the corners of the squares (Fig. 1.13b), a feature that may be attributed to the presence of dense longitudinal filaments at those sites which, in a transversely cut rod, will extend throughout the full thickness of the section. The essential structural identity of Z discs and rod bodies was confirmed by Goldstein et al (1977) in optical diffraction analyses of the two structures in canine cardiac muscle. Attempts to detect actin and tropomyosin within the rods by antibody-staining methods have proved unsuccessful, but the longitudinal filaments bind HMM-S_1 subunits

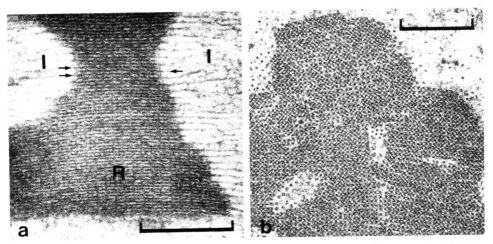

Fig. 1.13 The appearances of axial (a) and transverse (b) sections through a nemaline rod in human muscle. Thin filaments leave the I band (I) and interdigitate (arrows) with those from the adjacent sarcomere within the thickness of the rod (R). In transverse section they appear to be arranged in a regular small square lattice closely resembling the small lattice of the Z discs of relaxed muscle (see text). Scale bars = 0.25 μm

and are therefore assumed to contain an actin helix, the antigenic properties of which are masked by other components (Yamaguchi et al 1978, Jockusch et al 1980). Rods react strongly, however, to anti-α-actinin (Jockusch et al 1980) and, as in the Z disc, the α-actinin present seems to be associated with the matrix component rather than the filaments; treatment of rods with calcium-activated protease removes the matrix and releases α-actinin, leaving the filament lattice largely intact (Stromer et al 1976, Yamaguchi et al 1978).

Other protein species restricted to the vicinity of the Z discs may be responsible for the exact lateral registration of the sarcomeres across the width of the myofibre, and thus for the regularity of its transverse striation. Filamentous connections having the characteristics of 10 nm 'intermediate' filaments have been reported between the margins of adjacent Z discs in sectioned muscle (see for example Thornell et al 1980), being particularly conspicuous in atrophic fibres in which the inter-myofibrillar sarcoplasm is increased, and it has been shown that complete Z lines can be released from muscle fibres dissociated in a blender after extraction of actin and myosin. These lines consist of transverse assemblies of Z discs, held together into a net by a fine filamentous mesh at their margins (Lazarides & Granger 1978). Immune staining of both intact muscle and Z nets for the

presence of desmin (Lazarides & Balzer 1978), otherwise known as skeletin (Small & Sobieszek 1977), a 50 000 mol. wt protein thought to be the major constituent of intermediate filaments, has shown that it is confined to the edges of the Z discs and to the filamentous sarcoplasm between their contiguous edges (Lazarides et al 1979, Thornell et al 1980). It seems reasonable, therefore, to ascribe the maintenance of transverse order across the width of the myofibre to this cytoskeletal network of intermediate filaments linking adjoining edges of individual Z discs, and the perimeter of the whole Z-line assembly to the plasmalemma. Intermediate filaments have a much more widespread distribution in developing muscle cells (Bennett et al 1979) and can be a prominent feature of diseased and regenerating muscle fibres (Edström et al 1980).

Leptomeres

Leptomeres, also known as 'leptomeric fibrils', 'striated bodies' and 'microladders', have been reported as inclusions within myofibres from a wide range of vertebrate species (Ruska & Edwards 1957, Mair & Tomé 1972). They are striped structures of variable overall dimensions with a regular internal periodicity of 120–200 nm, and appear to be composed of alternating bands of microfilaments and dense matrix (Fig. 1.14). They seem to have no preferred orientation and may occur anywhere within the myofibres, but are most commonly found in the superficial sarcoplasm abutting upon the plasmalemma. Leptomeres are particularly abundant in skeletal or cardiac muscle fibres that have been in some way modified for special functions, examples being the intrafusal myofibres of the muscle spindles (Gruner 1961, Katz 1961, Landon 1966, Scalzi & Price 1971) and the fibres of cardiac conducting tissue (Page et al 1969, Viragh & Challice 1969, Bogusch 1975). They are occasionally, but by no means invariably, associated with the lateral margins of Z discs, and while they have been ascribed mechanical functions in certain situations (Thornell et al 1976), it is doubtful if they possess this property generally.

Their appearance suggests that they are composed of laterally aligned bundles of actin microfilaments, interspersed with α-actinin-rich dense patches analogous to those seen at the junctions of fibroblast stress fibres, but such speculations require confirmation by immunocytochemical staining. Leptomeres have been reported to occur in large numbers in the rare Zebra Body myopathy (Lake & Wilson 1975).

Muscular contraction

The sliding-filament theory of muscular contraction (Huxley & Niedergerke 1954, Huxley & Hanson 1954), in which the actin and myosin components of muscle are postulated to be organized into separate filaments and to move past

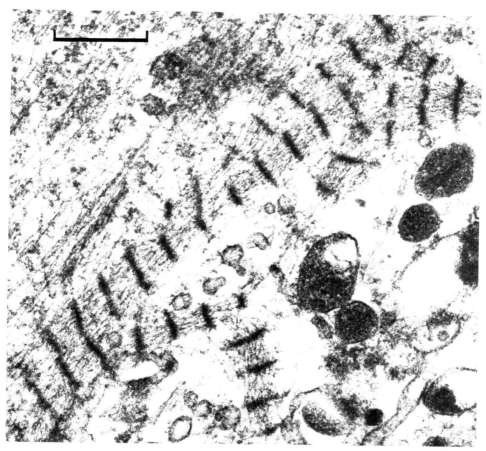

Fig. 1.14 A leptomere in a cultured human myotube. It appears to be composed of a bundle of fine filaments linked by periodic dense transverse striations at approximately 190 nm intervals. Scale bar = 0.5 μm

one another during contraction, is now the generally accepted explanation for the mechanics of sarcomere shortening (see Needham 1971 for a review of earlier theories). It must be emphasized, however, that hypotheses concerning the mechanisms by which the forces responsible for this movement are generated form no part of the sliding-filament theory per se, and are still, in some important respects, speculative. Currently, the most widely favoured hypothesis is that of Huxley (1957), in which the I filaments are drawn into the A-band lattice by cyclical force-generating interactions between the myosin cross-bridges and specific binding sites on the actin molecules of the thin filaments. However, a number of other mechanisms have been proposed, of which those of Ullrick (1967) and of Elliott et al (1970), which exploit the constant-volume characteristics of the sarcomere and the effects of short-range electro-static interactions between the myofilaments, are but two examples.

Much experimental evidence has been obtained to support the widely accepted view that activation of the contraction mechanism is brought about by a local increase in the calcium ion concentration (Ebashi 1980), released from the terminal cisternae of the sarcoplasmic reticulum in response to change in the electrical state of the transverse tubular system connecting the internal regions of the myofibre with the plasmalemma. The calcium ion so released is bound by calcium affinity sites on the troponin-C molecule, and this reaction is believed to cause a conformational change in the troponin complexes that is transmitted to the tropomyosin double helix of the thin filament. The shift induced in the position of the tropomyosin relative to the adjoining actin helix unblocks binding sites on the actin monomers that are masked in the resting state by steric hindrance, permitting their interaction with the myosin heads on the cross-bridges (Hazelgrove 1972, Huxley 1972). In the Huxley (1957) hypothesis, revised and extended by Huxley & Simmons (1971), attachment of the myosin heads to the actin sites is seen as a transient event, resulting in cooperative hydrolysis of ATP, followed by detachment of the cross-bridges, the energy released powering a force-generating movement of the myosin head units. Serial repetition of this process, each myosin

head engaging a succession of actin monomers along an adjacent thin filament in a ratchet-like fashion, will, collectively, have the effect of driving the thin filament array deeper into the A-band lattice, thus causing the sarcomere to shorten. Gordon et al (1966) showed that the isometric tension developed in a muscle fibre when activated correlates well with the degree of overlap of the thin filaments with the cross-bridge zones on the A filaments, supporting the concept that actin/cross-bridge interactions are responsible for generating contractile force. In relaxation, calcium ion is withdrawn from the myofilament lattice into the sarcoplasmic reticular cisterns by a calcium/magnesium activated ATPase pump; this results in a shift in the arrangement of the troponin and tropomyosin components of the thin filaments that inactivates the actin-binding sites. Several aspects of these mechanisms have yet to be verified experimentally.

In rigor, a state of sustained shortening brought about by a deficiency of ATP, most of the myosin heads are attached to actin-binding sites, and the condition is usually equated with the end of the 'power stroke' of the normal contraction mechanism; however, it has yet to be shown unequivocally that generation of force during normal contractile activity is indeed accomplished while the myosin and actin molecules are attached to one another (Huxley 1979). The evidence indicates that, on the contrary, cross-bridge order diminishes during activation (Huxley HE 1971, 1972), only 20% of the cross-bridges being attached to thin filaments at any instant in frog muscle contracting isometrically (Huxley & Brown 1967); that fewer cross-bridges are attached during active shortening than under isometric conditions (Huxley & Simmons 1973); and that loss of cross-bridge order with activation extends into the central regions of the A filaments where there is no overlap with I filaments (Huxley HE 1971). Furthermore, not all actin monomers appear to be involved in cross-bridge interactions, the points of attachment in invertebrate muscle forming a regular pattern that seems to bear a constant relationship to the locations of the troponin complexes along the I filament (Wray et al 1978).

Huxley & Simmons (1971) proposed a model to account for cross-bridge movement, in which the myosin heads move the actin filaments by oscillating elastically in a hinge-like manner about their junction with the HMM shaft. The mechanism probably involves several steps, and is complicated by the need to accommodate its geometry to the increase in the transverse spacing of the A-band lattice that occurs with sarcomere shortening, a consequence of the fixed-volume characteristics of the myofibril (Elliott et al 1963, 1967, Brandt et al 1967). The force-generating cross-bridges are thus required to work over increasing interfilament distances with sarcomere shortening, e.g. from 19 mm to 26 nm in frog muscle in which sarcomere length was reduced from 3.6 μm to 2.0 μm (Elliott et al 1963). Huxley (1969) proposed that the myosin heads could maintain an appropriate working distance from the actin filaments if the HMM-S$_2$ subunits of the myosin molecules were to swing out from the shaft of the thick filament by a hinge at the junction with their LMM components. Appropriate movements of the cross-bridges away from the thick filament backbone have been shown by X-ray diffraction to accompany activation (Hazelgrove 1975), a change, like the perturbation of the central cross-bridges, that seems to be independent of cross-bridge interaction with actin. It is not known what part, if any, the non-myosin proteins of the A filament play in the contractile mechanism. The increases in I-filament spacing and Z-disc dimensions that accompany sarcomere shortening and expansion of the A-band lattice, and their possible role in the contraction process, were described above. These reversible changes also tend to maintain the parallel alignment of the thick and thin myofilaments throughout the normal range of sarcomere lengths, the optimal geometry for transmitting tension along the axis of the myofibre. Other reviews of the possible mechanisms and kinetics of muscle contraction, not mentioned above, are those of A. F. Huxley (1971), White & Thorson (1975), Squire (1981) and Craig (1986).

The sarcoplasm

The cytoplasm of the myofibre, the sarcoplasm, intervenes as a thin layer between the plasmalemma and the external surfaces of the outermost myofibrils, and fills the interstices between the myofibrils in the core of the fibre. Apart from mitochondria, and the membrane systems of the T tubules and sarcoplasmic reticulum (described separately below), the interstitial sarcoplasm contains occasional free ribosomes, small cisternae of the rough endoplasmic reticulum and droplets of neutral lipid, along with microtubules and intermediate filaments. Lipid droplets lie between the myofibrils adjacent to the mitochondria and occur more often in slow-twitch oxidative muscle fibres, but they are never a conspicuous component of normal human muscle. The microtubules have a generally longitudinal orientation, but a regular spiral arrangement around the myofibrils has been described in mammalian heart muscle (Goldstein & Entman 1978). The 10 nm intermediate filaments, identified with the protein termed skeletin (Small & Sobieszek 1977) or desmin (Lazarides & Balzer 1978), are inconspicuous in adult muscle studied by conventional electron-microscopic techniques, but appear to be preferentially located at the Z-line region and to surround and interconnect adjacent Z discs, a location confirmed by immunohistochemical studies (Lazarides et al 1979, Thornell et al 1980). The subplasmalemmal layer of sarcoplasm also contains a scattering of free ribosomes, intermediate filaments and microtubules, together with occasional pinocytotic and coated uptake vesicles associated with the plasmalemma, and the membranes of the subsurface caveolae and outer ends of the T tubules. This external component of the sarcoplasm is expanded in the perinuclear regions, where it often contains increased numbers of ribosomes and Golgi membrane systems, and at the neuromuscular junction where it provides a sole-plate for the motor nerve terminal; the morphology of the neuromuscular junction is described in detail later. Other structures found in the sarcoplasm of normal adult human muscle include lipofuscin granules, compact heterogeneous masses of neutral lipid and autolysed cellular debris, and myelin figures, variable-sized secondary lysosomes packed with concentric phospholipid membranes.

Internal membrane systems of muscle fibres

The transverse tubules and sarcoplasmic reticulum

are two closely interrelated sets of internal membrane systems that play important parts in the excitability and functional activation of skeletal muscle fibres; the structures and distribution of the two systems have been extensively explored in the skeletal muscles of many vertebrate and invertebrate species. Descriptions by Revel (1962), Peachey (1965), Fawcett & McNutt (1969) and Franzini-Armstrong (1973a) give more detailed accounts of the anatomy of these systems than space permits in this chapter.

The transverse tubular system

The transverse tubules are fine tubular extensions of the muscle-cell plasma membrane, which penetrate into and traverse the sarcoplasm between the myofibrils, branching and interconnecting one with another as they do so, to form a series of networks across the transverse plane of the fibre (Fig. 1.4). They are flattened in transverse section with external dimensions of their short and long axes in the ranges of 25–35 nm and 90–130 nm respectively (Cullen et al 1984), but they are subject to swelling or shrinkage in response to change in tonicity of the extracellular fluid (Davey & O'Brien 1978). They arise during development as invaginations of the surface membrane (Ezerman & Ishikawa 1967), but in mature mammalian skeletal muscle their connections to the fibre surface are only rarely visible, as they are effected via irregularly sacculated subsurface caveolae (Fig. 1.15b). Nevertheless, continuity of the extracellular space with the tubular lumen can be readily demonstrated with electron-opaque tracer materials such as horseradish peroxidase (Fig. 1.15a); the method has also been used in conjunction with high-voltage electron microscopy to show the three-dimensional structure of the transverse tubules in frog muscle (Peachey & Eisenberg 1978). The number and arrangement of the tubule nets within a fibre reflect the sarcomeric segmentation of its myofibrils, and differ between mammals and lower vertebrates: the latter possess only one tubular system per sarcomere, which lies in the plane of the Z disc, whereas the former have two, one on the A-band side of each A- and I-band junction. Longitudinal tubules connecting adjacent T-tubule nets can sometimes be found,

though relatively infrequently, but it has become clear from the studies of Peachey & Eisenberg (1978) that, in frog muscle at least, their paucity does not imply that each tubule system constitutes an independent planar net across the thickness of the myofibre, as adjacent networks are interconnected in a helical fashion along its length, in parallel with the helical arrangement demonstrable in the myofibril cross-striations. The transverse tubular nets have been calculated to contribute betwen 0.1 and 0.5% to the total fibre volume (Eisenberg 1983), but such a figure, and their relatively inconspicuous appearance in conventional sectioned preparations, belie their importance to the muscle cell, as their contribution to the total surface area is very considerable, amounting in frog muscle to as much as seven times that of the plasmalemma with which they are in continuity (Peachey 1965, Mobley & Eisenberg 1975). Somewhat lower values for the ratio of the areas of T-tubule membrane to plasmalemma were found in human muscle (Hoppeler et al 1973) and guinea-pig muscle (Eisenberg & Kuda 1976), and in the latter the fast-twitch fibres have more than twice the T-tubule membrane surface-to-volume ratio of slow-twitch fibres. The role of the transverse tubular system as an extension of the surface membrane was emphasized by Thesleff et al (1979), who demonstrated its involvement in uptake endocytosis and lysosomal activation in denervated and dystrophic avian and mammalian muscle. Abnormal 'honeycomb' structures apparently derived from the transverse tubular system are not uncommon in denervated and atrophic muscle fibres, and can be shown by the use of electron-opaque tracers to retain their continuity with the extracellular space.

The lumina of the T tubules of skeletal muscle generally have no obvious content in conventional electron-microscopic preparations and, as noted above, are easily penetrated by fine particulate tracers placed within the extracellular space. The rather larger-diameter T tubules of cardiac muscle do, however, contain extensions of the basal lamina (Fawcett & McNutt 1969), and the striking stainability of the T-tubule lumina of skeletal muscle with osmium ferrocyanide fixatives in the presence of phosphate ions (Forbes et al 1977) suggests that they may also contain a less readily

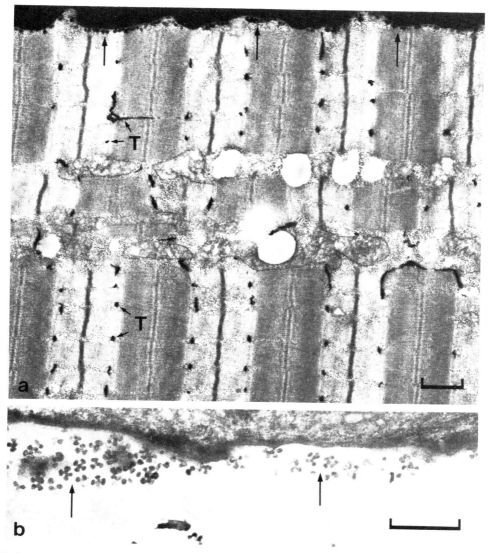

Fig. 1.15 (a) A longitudinal section through a human myofibre stained by the method of Forbes et al (1977) to demonstrate the distribution of the T system. The electron-dense osmium-ferricyanide reaction product fills the extracellular space, the subsurface caveolae (arrows) and the T-tubular component of the triads (T). (b) A tangential section through the surface of a myofibre in a similar preparation illustrating the lobulated form of the subsurface caveolae. Scale bars = 1 μm

visible, yet significant, content of glycoprotein. This is supported by the occasional finding of an amorphous central lamina within the lumen of tubules in conventional electron-microscopic preparations. The presence of such macromolecules within the tubule lumen could reduce its conductivity below the value calculated from its apparent electron-optical dimensions, and provide an explanation for experimental evidence that both

sodium and potassium diffusion coefficients are reduced within the transverse tubular system (Barry & Adrian 1973).

Sarcoplasmic reticulum

The major internal membrane system of the muscle cell is the sarcoplasmic reticulum. This is thought to be derived from the rough endoplasmic reticulum during development (Ezerman & Ishikawa 1967) but its membranes do not carry ribosomes in mature muscle fibres. It consists of a series of flattened fenestrated sacs around and between the external aspects of each myofibril (Figs 1.4, 1.16). The degree of development and structural complexity of the reticulum within individual fibres correlates with their mechanical properties, being most extensive and elaborate in fast-twitch fibres (Pellegrino & Franzini 1963, Page 1965, 1969, Schiaffino et al 1970). The aggregate surface area of the sarcoplasmic reticular membranes is very large, and has been calculated to approach 135 times that of the cell plasmalemma in frog fast-twitch fibres (Peachey 1965). Somewhat lower figures have been obtained in quantitative studies of mammalian muscle fibres (Eisenberg & Kuda 1976).

The longitudinal arrangement of the sarcoplasmic reticulum reflects that of the T tubules and myofibril sarcomeres. In amphibia and fish, a single cylindrical sarcoplasmic reticular sac encompasses each sarcomere and extends from one Z disc to the next; in mammals, reptiles and birds, the number of sarcoplasmic reticular units is doubled, successive sacs being related to A and I bands alternately along the length of each myofibril; those opposite the I bands span the Z discs and are thus shared by neighbouring sarcomeres. Each cylindrical sac has a central more-or-less fenestrated zone, depending upon species and fibre type, and continuous unfenestrated components at each end, which are known as the terminal cisternae or lateral sacs (Fig. 1.16). Quantitative studies of the sarcoplasmic reticulum in mammalian muscle (Eisenberg & Kuda 1976) have shown that the proportion of the total volume of the myofibre occupied by the terminal cisternae is greatest in fast-twitch glycolytic, type 2B fibres, and least in slow-twitch oxidative type 1 fibres, with an intermediate value in type 2A fast-twitch oxidative/glycolytic fibres. The volume of the longitudinal component of the sarcoplasmic reticulum is also larger in the type 2B fibres, but no differences are apparent between type 1 and type 2A. The strongest correlation with muscle fibre type is shown by the surface density of the terminal cisterns (Eisenberg 1983).

In conventional electron-microscopic prepara-

tions the terminal cisternae usually contain an amorphous to finely granular matrix material, which is not seen within the fenestrated central zones of the sarcoplasmic reticular sacs; histochemical studies have shown that this material has a strong affinity for calcium ions (Costantin et al 1965). Biochemical analysis of isolated sarcoplasmic reticular membranes (Meissner et al 1973) has permitted the separation and identification of their constituent proteins. One major component, contributing two-thirds of the protein present, has been identified with the membrane-associated Ca^{2+},Mg^{2+} ATPase responsible for scavenging Ca^{2+} ion from the sarcoplasm and pumping it across the sarcoplasmic reticular membranes into the lumina of the sarcoplasmic reticular cisternae during muscle relaxation (Martenosi 1982). The other major protein constituent of the sarcoplasmic reticulum is water-soluble, with a high proportion of acid amino acid residues, and has a strong affinity for Ca^{2+} ions. It has been identified with the calcium binding material, calsequestrin, found within the terminal cisternae (Maclennan & Wong 1971, Maclennan & Holland 1975). The in situ localization of these two components has been achieved using immunofluorescence techniques (Jorgensen et al 1979), the Ca^{2+} ATPase being found throughout the I bands and at the centre of each A band, and the calsequestrin at the A/I interface, the position of the sarcoplasmic reticular terminal cisternae. The regions of the sarcoplasmic reticular membranes rich in Ca^{2+} ATPase have been shown to possess a layer of increased electron density in the immediately adjacent cytoplasm in tannic acid-treated preparations (Somlyo 1979), and to be rich in 8.5 nm P face intramembranous particles when studied by freeze-fracture replication. The latter are more numerous in fast-contracting myofibres (Franzini-Armstrong 1980, 1983), and particle frequency has been directly related to Ca^{2+} ATPase activity (Martonosi et al 1980).

Sarcoplasmic reticular—transverse tubular junctions

The faces of adjacent sarcoplasmic reticular terminal cisternae do not abut directly upon one another, but enter jointly into a close and consistent structural relationship with the T tubule

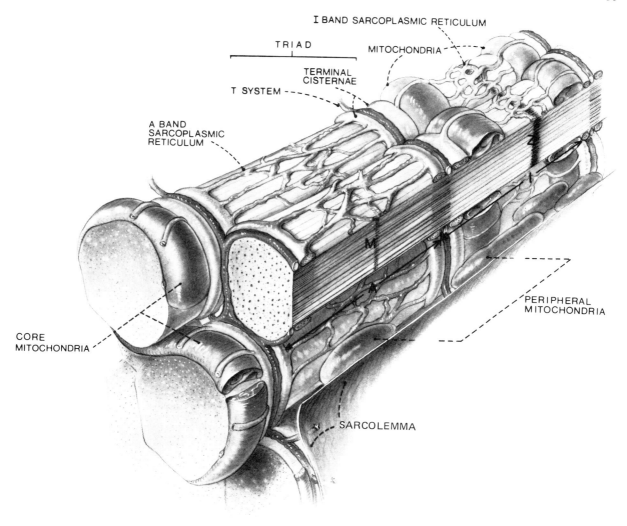

Fig. 1.16 A diagrammatic representation of the relationship of the sarcoplasmic reticulum, T system and mitochondria to the myofibrils of mammalian muscle. (From Eisenberg et al 1974, reproduced by kind permission of the authors and the editor of the Journal of Cell Biology)

that lies between them, either at the level of the Z line in amphibia and fish, or at the A/I junctions in mammalia, reptiles and birds. This combination of a single T tubule and two laterally aligned terminal sarcoplasmic reticular cisternae is referred to as a 'triad' (Fig. 1.16), and it has been calculated that in frog-fast-twitch fibres some 80 per cent of the T-system membrane is related to the sarcoplasmic reticulum in this fashion (Peachey 1965). A more simple arrangement of 'dyads', in which a single sarcoplasmic reticular terminal

cisterna is associated with each T tubule, can be found in slow-twitch mammalian fibres (Cullen et al 1984), and is the rule in lower animal orders such as the arthropods; more complex 'pentads' and 'heptads' are present as a normal component of some fast-contracting mammalian muscles (Revel 1962). Similar pentads and heptads are seen in atrophic and denervated fibres in diseased human and animal muscle. In primitive chordates such as *Amphioxus* the terminal sarcoplasmic reticular cisternae are directly related to the plasmalemma at the surface of the cell, without the intervention of a T tubule, and a similar arrangement can be found in developing mammalian myotubes.

The sarcoplasmic reticular membrane forming the wall of the terminal cisterna adjacent to the T tubule is termed the junctional SR and has a regularly scalloped structure with a 30 nm periodicity when sectioned in its long axis. Transverse sections of the triad show that this appearance is due to the existence of paired outward projections of the sarcoplasmic reticular membrane, sometimes referred to as sarcoplasmic reticular feet, which span the 10–20 nm gap between the two membranes and appear to make intimate contact with the wall of the T tubule to which they are opposed, as if to form a series of 'spot welds' (Kelly 1969). The tightness of the apposition of the two membrane systems at these points of contact is still a matter for debate: amorphous material has been reported to intervene between the two membranes in frog muscle (Franzini-Armstrong 1970b) and can often be seen in mammalian muscle, but a later study by Franzini-Armstrong (1971), in which fine particulate materials were applied to 'skinned' frog-muscle fibres, indicated that the majority of the interface at the triad is accessible to such tracers. Neither freeze–fracture (Franzini-Armstrong 1974, 1980) nor conventional microscopical techniques provide any support for past suggestions that the sarcoplasmic reticular and the T-tubule lumina are continuous at their points of contact, but Somlyo (1979) has reported the presence of bridges between the two membranes in tannic acid-fixed triads, with a periodicity matching that of the sarcoplasmic reticular feet, which she has interpreted as representing phospholipid connections between their outer leaflets, while Rayns et al (1975) have described bridging particles in freeze–fracture preparations. More recently, Franzini-Armstrong (1980, 1984) has demonstrated the presence of regularly arranged groups of four intramembranous particles within the 'P face' of the T tubules of toadfish swim-bladder muscle and frog slow-tonic muscle. These particles are disposed in two parallel rows in a distribution matching that of the sarcoplasmic reticular feet, but with twice the spacing along the rows. She argues that the corre-

spondence between the particle aggregates and the feet is indicative of a large complex spanning the T-tubule membrane, junctional gap, and sarcoplasmic reticular membrane. The general arrangement and relationships of the membrane systems in a mammalian muscle fibre are illustrated diagrammatically in Figure 1.16.

The functional significance of this intimate relationship between the T system and sarcoplasmic reticulum, and between the latter and the contractile elements of the sarcomere, have been the subject of extensive study and are reviewed by Costantin (1975). Depolarization of the muscle cell surface membrane, initiated either at the neuromuscular junction, or artificially elsewhere along the fibre (Huxley A F 1971), is followed by an inward spread of depolarization along the transverse tubular system. The arrival of this signal at the triads stimulates the rapid release of calcium ion from its sites of sequestration within the sarcoplasmic-reticular terminal cisternae into the adjacent sarcoplasm, and this in turn results in activation of the contractile mechanism of the sarcomere (see above). Relaxation from the contracted state follows a longer time-course and is achieved by the active, enzyme-mediated return of calcium ion into the sarcoplasmic reticulum, the more rapid relaxation of fast-twitch fibres correlating with their more extensive and elaborate sarcoplasmic-reticular membranes (Rosenbluth 1969, Schiaffino et al 1970, Eisenberg & Kuda 1976), their higher content of associated Ca^{2+}, Mg^{2+}-activated ATPase (Jorgensen et al 1979) and their much greater content of parvalbumin, a soluble Ca^{2+}-binding protein, which scavenges calcium ion directly from the cytosol. The recent studies of the structural relationship between the sarcoplasmic reticular and transverse tubular systems, referred to above, appear to rule out the existence of any direct connection between the sarcoplasmic reticular cisternae and the T-tubule lumen capable of transmitting ionic current (Kelly 1969), despite suggestions that the sarcoplasmic reticulum is to some extent accessible to small ions and molecules in the extracellular space (Birks & Davey 1969, 1972), and evidence of transient changes in sarcoplasmic reticulum volume following brief episodes of tetanus (Landon 1982a). The models of the excitation–contraction coupling process currently in favour therefore invoke a capacitance effect, whereby charge movement occurring within the T-tubule membrane induces an approximately tenfold increase in the sarcoplasmic reticular membrane permeability to Ca^{2+} above the resting value (Schneider & Chandler 1973, Adrian & Almers 1976). The further suggestion that these charge movements involve shifts of macromolecular dipoles within the adjacent membranes of the two systems (Adrian 1978), and the relationship of such dipoles to the observed intramembranous particles (Franzini-Armstrong 1980), remain matters for speculation. The molecular mechanisms responsible for the active transport of calcium by the sarcoplasmic reticulum have been reviewed by Tada et al (1978). More extensive reviews of the structure and interrelationships of the sarcoplasmic reticular and transverse tubular systems may be found in Schmalbruch (1985) and Cullen & Landon (1988).

Mitochondria

The mitochondria of the myofibre are, in general, sausage-shaped structures with a mean diameter of about 0.1 nm, but their overall size and shape is subject to considerable variation and some are extensively branched. Most possess simple transverse cristae, but zig-zag forms can also be seen; irregularly branched or concentric cristae occur in a number of myopathic conditions. Mitochondria are found between the myofibrils and within the subplasmalemmal sarcoplasm, and in the latter situation occur in clusters in association with the myonuclei and with the sole-plates of the neuromuscular junctions, particularly those of small animals. The intermyofibrillar mitochondria are situated predominantly within the I-band regions, partly or completely encircling the myofibrils adjacent to the Z line (Fig. 1.16), but a small proportion are longitudinally aligned between the sarcomeres of adjacent myofibrils. The muscle fibres of children contain, on average, a higher mitochondrial volume fraction (4.5%) than those of adults (3.4%) (Jerusalem et al 1975), and those of men (5.2%) contain more than those of women (4.1%) (Hoppeler et al 1973) as do those of long-distances runners when compared with matched untrained controls (Fridén et al 1984).

Shafiq et al (1966) and Ogata & Murata (1969) found greater numbers of larger mitochondria in type 1 slow-twitch muscle fibres, in their qualitative fine structural studies of human muscle, confirming the established histochemical evidence of high levels of mitochondrial enzyme activity in the same fibre type, and differences in numbers of mitochondrial profiles and their size have been used to distinguish myofibre types at an ultrastructural level (Payne et al 1975). Quantitative studies of human muscle, however, have failed to provide objective evidence of consistent differences in the mitochondrial volume fractions of the various myofibre types (Cullen & Weightman 1975, Jerusalem et al 1975), but this failure may merely reflect inadequacies in the relatively simple stereological methods employed. The association of increased mitochondrial numbers with small-diameter slow-twitch fibres is more readily apparent in animal muscle (Gauthier & Padykula 1966, Gauthier 1969, Schiaffino et al 1970), and its reality has been confirmed by a number of quantitative studies. The mitochondrial volume fractions of guinea-pig red (soleus) and white (vastus) fibres are 5% and 1.9% respectively (Eisenberg et al 1974, Eisenberg & Kuda 1975) and comparable figures were obtained from the rat soleus (6.6%) and medial gastrocnemius (2.1%) muscles (Stonnington & Engel 1973; means of the values from transverse and longitudinal sections), and from the red (4.9%) and white (1.6%) fibres of the cat gastrocnemius (Kamieniecka & Schmalbruch 1980). In the guinea-pig some 80–85% of the mitochondrial volume fraction of both red and white fibres is contained within a superficial zone, 1 μm thick, immediately beneath the plasmalemma (Eisenberg & Kuda 1976). Fast red (type 2A) fibres in general possess larger individual mitochondrial profiles than either the slow (type 1) or fast glycolytic (type 2B) fibres, but their orientation is predominantly longitudinal and contrasts with transverse orientation of the mitochondria of the slow, type 1 fibres (Eisenberg & Kuda 1976). Estimates of mitochondrial numbers within muscle fibres, as distinct from volume fractions, are of little practical value and can rarely be obtained with any accuracy, because of the wide variations in mitochondrial size and shape, particularly in type 1 fibres.

The mitochondria of skeletal muscle can contain a range of inclusions: small dense calcium-containing granules are a normal component of the matrix, and larger spherical, osmiophilic inclusions are not uncommon in diseased muscle. Far more striking are the so-called paracrystalline inclusions of apparently protein nature which occupy the potential space between the inner and outer mito-chondrial membranes, or its extension within the folds of the inner membrane which form the cristae. These have been much described and illustrated, and appear to be of two distinct varieties (Morgan-Hughes et al 1977, Hammersen et al 1980, Stadhouders 1981, Cullen & Landon 1988). The more common of the two is the 'parking lot' or type I inclusion, which has a distinctive and complex structure which yields highly variable appearances in electron-micrographs depending upon its orientation relative to the plane of section (Schmalbruch 1983). The type 2 crystals are dense rectangular or elongated rhomboidal bodies with an internal structure which is a regular fine lattice (Morgan-Hughes et al 1977). The type I crystals in general tend to occupy and distend that part of the intramembrane space which forms the core of the mitochondrial cristae, whereas the type 2 crystals usually lie between the inner and outer membranes of the mitochondrial wall, often in chains which displace the matrix and cristae to the ends of the mito-chondrion and to short segments between adjacent crystals. Type I crystals can however on occasion be found in an intramural position, and small type 2 crystals may occur within the cristae. Despite their early recognition and well-characterized morphology the composition and functional signi-ficance of the paracrystalline mitochondrial inclusions have yet to be determined. Attention has been drawn (Landon 1982b) to the structural similarity between type I crystals and isolated cytochrome oxidase crystals (Maniloff et al 1973), but Bonilla et al (1975), and more recently Sato et al (1990) have been unable to obtain electron-histochemical or immunocytochemical evidence that the crystals possess cytochrome oxidase activity. Immunoreactivity for mitochondrial creatine kinase has however been demonstrated in the crystals by Stadhouders et al (1990).

Paracrystalline inclusions may be found occa-sionally in normal human muscle of all ages, but more commonly in the elderly, and they are a regular feature of the pathology of a number of disease states (DiMauro 1979, Carafoli & Roman 1980, Stadhouders 1981) (see also Morgan-Hughes —Chapter 10 this volume), not all of which may involve a primary disturbance of mitochondrial function (Engel & Dale 1968, Chou 1969, Fardeau 1970). Their appearance may also be induced experimentally by ischaemia (Hanzlikova & Schiaffino 1977, Heine & Schaeg 1979), by the administration of mitochondrial poisons including the uncoupling agent 2, 4–dinitrophenol (Melmed et al 1975, Sahgal et al 1979) or the respiratory chain inhibitor diphenyleneiodonium (Byrne et al 1982), and the drug Zidovudine (AZT).

Fine structure and histochemical fibre type

Several attempts have been made to correlate dif-ferences in the fine structure of muscle fibres with their subdivision into fibre types by histochemical means. Fibre-type identifications employing features visible by both light and electron micro-scopy, such as numbers and distribution of mito-chondria, presence or absence of lipid or glycogen, in animals (see for example Shafiq et al 1969, Pellegrino & Franzini 1963, Landon 1970b, Schiaffino et al 1970), and in man (Shafiq et al 1966, Ogata & Murata 1969, Schmalbruch & Kamieniecka 1974, Payne et al 1975, Prince et al 1981) have allowed a degree of correlation with such fine structural features as the extent of the sarcoplasmic reticulum and the dimensions of the M and Z lines, but where quantitative approaches have been applied to the study of human muscle the results have often proved inconclusive (Cullen & Weightman 1975, Jerusalem et al 1975). More recent fine structural studies, in animals, of muscles or portions of muscles composed of a single muscle fibre type (Gauthier 1969, Eisenberg & Kuda 1976, Salmons et al 1978), or of fibres previously typed by histochemical means (Eisenberg & Kuda 1977) have, however, served to confirm and amplify the results obtained by earlier, less direct methods and, in conjunction with the use of stereological techniques (Eisenberg 1983), have placed such findings on a more secure quantitative basis. A number of the fine structural differences between the major fibre types have been referred to above in describing individual subcellular organelles; some others are summarized below.

The width of the Z line has been noted by a number of observers to vary with putative muscle fibre type (Gauthier 1969, Landon 1970b, Schiaffino et al 1970, Duchen 1971, Shafiq et al 1971, Garamvölgyi 1972, Schmalbruch & Kamieniecka 1974), but the values obtained have varied with the species or muscle studied and the criteria employed by different observers to define the limits of the measured structure (Cullen & Weightman 1975, Salmons et al 1978, Schmalbruch 1985). It is clear, however, that in any particular muscle the widest Z lines are found in slow-twitch oxidative (type 1) fibres and the narrowest in the fast-twitch glycolytic (type 2B) fibres, with the type 2A, fast-twitch oxidative/glycolytic fibres having intermediate values. The mean values for Z-line width, obtained from a number of different human muscles include those by Payne et al (1975) and typed in accordance with their mito-chondrial content, were 95 nm (type 1), 74 nm (type 2A) and 54 nm (type 2B); Schmalbruch & Kamieniecka (1974) obtained mean values of 104 nm (type 1), 84 nm (type 2A) and 74 nm (type 2B), from five specimens of human brachial biceps muscle, and values of 128 nm (type 1), 104 nm (type 2A) and 88 nm (type 2B) were obtained by Sjöström et al (1982a) from histoche-mically defined fibres. Corresponding figures obtained from rat muscle fibres (typed by mito-chondrial content, quantity and distribution of sarcoplasmic reticulum, and the presence or absence of glycogen) were in the ranges 63–110 nm (type 1), 43–70 nm (type 2A) and 30–55 nm (type 2B) (Gauthier 1970, Landon 1970b, Schiaffino et al 1970), and slow- and fast-contracting rabbit muscle fibres have Z-line widths of 80 and 40 nm respectively (Salmons et al 1978). Mean values for Z-line width of 89 nm (Cullen & Weightman 1975) and 85 nm (Jerusalem et al 1975) have been obtained from random samples of human muscle fibres of undefined histochemical or functional type; in the former case a positive association was found between Z-line width and volume of sarco-plasm, and in the latter there was some suggestion of a positive correlation with mitochondrial

volume; Schmalbruch & Kamieniecka (1974) found a significant negative correlation between Z-line width and numbers of triads. Z-line widths are difficult to measure with accuracy in conventional thin sections, and may be subject to preparative artefact, but the finding of consistent differences in Z-line width in cryosectioned human muscle (Sjöström & Squire 1977) supports the conclusion that a range of Z-line dimensions exist in vivo, the absolute values of which will depend upon the method of preparation of the tissue and the muscle and species studied. In any one preparation the upper and lower limits of the measured range of values may, therefore, be expected to correspond to slow type 1 and fast type 2B fibres respectively, but other independent criteria will be required to identify fibres containing Z lines of intermediate widths (Eisenberg 1983).

The dimensions of the M band at the centre of the A band have also been reported to show con-sistent differences between fibre types. Payne et al (1975) found broad M lines, 89 nm wide, in fibres rich in mitochondria and possessing wide Z lines, and narrow (59 nm) M lines in fibres with few mitochondria and narrow Z lines; these were equated with type 1 and type 2B fibres respec-tively. A third group of fibres with a mean M-line width of 79 nm were identified as type 2A. The M band consists of three or five parallel lines or 'bridges' (Knappeis & Carlsen 1968), the outer-most pair of which show considerable variation in their staining intensity in different fibres (Cullen & Weightman 1975), and it is not clear from their report how Payne et al (1975) defined the limits of the structures they measured. Sjöström & Squire (1977) and Sjöström et al (1982a) have since shown that myofibres in cryosectioned human muscle are divisible into two classes according to whether they show three or five M-band bridging lines. In the former study, fibres with three lines were identified as type 2 fast-twitch from their narrow Z lines, few mitochondria and content of glycogen, and those with five lines as type 1 slow-twitch fibres; no attempt was made to subdivide the type 2 fibre group. Densitometric studies of negatively stained cryosectioned A bands gave values of 22 and 43.7 nm for the separation of the inner and outer pairs of M bridges from the mid-point of the central line; as the individual M lines are 8 nm wide, the maximum width for a three-line M band is 52 nm, and 95.4 nm for a five-line band. It is not clear what structures could have given rise to the intermediate M-line widths recorded by Payne et al (1975). Sjöström et al (1982b) used M-line structure as the criterion of fibre type in classifying the fibres of human anterior tibialis and vastus lateralis muscles, and found that 83% of fibres were identified correctly using Z-line width, but that mitochondrial content was an unreliable indicator correlating with M-line width in only 37% of fibres.

It will be apparent from the foregoing that sufficient information is now available, concerning the ranges of variation in the fine structure of the different myofibre types, to permit the assignment of functional characteristics to most of the individual fibres in the muscles of the more commonly studied mammalian and avian species, with a fair degree of confidence, but it must be emphasized that such differences are only relative, and that absolute quantitative values for any measured feature cannot be extrapolated with safety between species, or even from one muscle to another within an individual species. Given these limitations, *type 1* slow-twitch oxidative fibres may be defined as those in any given muscle having a smaller than average diameter, a high content of mitochondria with a predominantly transverse orientation, relatively inconspicuous sarcoplasmic reticulum and triads, five-line M bands and broad Z lines, negligible glycogen and occasional intermyofibrillar lipid droplets. *Type 2B* fast-twitch glycolytic fibres will have diameters in the upper range of those of the muscle as a whole, contain few small mito-

chondria, have a well-developed sarcoplasmic reticulum with numerous and conspicuous terminal cisternae and T tubules, three-line M bands and narrow Z line, and some intermyofibrillar glycogen, but little lipid. *Type 2A* fast-twitch, oxidative/glycolytic fibres may be expected to contain abundant mitochondria with predominantly longitudinal orientation, some in subplasmalemmal aggregations, and show a development of the sarcoplasmic reticulum and triads comparable with, or somewhat exceeding, that of the type 1 fibres, three- or five-line M bands, Z lines of intermediate width, and both glycogen and lipid within the sarcoplasm. A summary comparison of the characteristics of the three principal fibre types is provided in Table 1.2. Most, if not all, of these characteristics are liable to alteration as a consequence of artificially induced changes in contractile activity (Salmons et al 1978, Eisenberg & Salmons 1979), exercise (Prince et al 1981), disuse or disease.

MONONUCLEATED CELLS ASSOCIATED WITH STRIATED MUSCLE FIBRES

Myosatellite cells

Myosatellite cells are small, flattened mononucleate cells of fusiform outline closely applied to the surface of striated muscle fibres (Mauro 1961, Muir et al 1965, Campion 1984, Schmalbruch 1985). They are considered by many to represent a persisting population of myoblastic stem cells, the source both of the additional myofibre nuclei required during the hypertrophic phase of muscle

Table 1.2 Summary of the distinguishing features of muscle fibre types visible in conventional electron microscopic preparations

Fibre type	1	2A	2B
Z Disc	Thick, 85–105 nm	Intermediate, 45–85 nm	Thin, 35–55 nm
M Line	Wide, 5-line 95 nm	Intermediate, 3- or 5-line, 50–95 nm	Narrow, 3-line, 50 nm
Mitochondria	Numerous, transverse	Numerous, longitudinal	Few, transverse
SR and triads	Inconspicuous	Intermediate	Well developed
Glycogen	Little	Moderate	Conspicuous
Lipid	Consistent intermyofibrillar droplets	Sparse, subplasmalemmal droplets	Absent

growth (Ishikawa 1966, Church 1969, Moss & Leblond 1971), and of the myoblasts responsible for regenerative repair of damaged muscle fibres in situ (Reznik 1969), in re-implanted minced muscle (Snow 1979), and in vitro (Bischoff 1979). Myosatellite cells appear to be evenly distributed along the length of the myofibres (Muir 1970, Schultz 1979), but not necessarily at random as they are seen more frequently in close association with intrinsic myonuclei than might be expected to occur by chance (Teravainen 1970, Ontell 1974), and their common occurrence adjacent to the soleplates of neuromuscular junctions has led to the description by Kelly (1978) of a specific class of 'perisynaptic satellite cells'. An increased incidence of myosatellites is also found in association with the polar intracapsular regions of the intrafusal myofibres of muscle spindles (Landon 1966). They lie beneath the myofibre basal lamina in a matching depression in the fibre surface (Fig. 1.17), and this close relationship to the myofibre plasmalemma and inclusion within the contour of the fibre ensures that myosatellite cells can usually be identified with confidence only by electron microscopy, the technique to which they owe their initial discovery (Mauro 1961). Ontell (1974) has, however, reported successful identification of satellite cells in stained plastic sections, and Lawrence & Mauro (1979) have described their appearance in isolated frog muscle fibres in vitro using Nomarski optics. Myosatellite cell numbers decline with age both in animals (Allbrook et al 1971) and in man, contributing more than 10% of the apparent total of myofibre nuclei in young human subjects, falling to 2–3% in normal muscle from mature individuals. Myosatellite cell numbers in normal muscle in a range of species, and their change with age, have been reviewed by Schmalbruch (1985). Increased numbers of myosatellites are found in denervated (De Recondo et al 1966, Hess & Rosner 1970, Aloisi et al 1973, Ontell 1974, Schultz 1978) and mildly traumatized muscle (Teravainen 1970), and also in regenerating diseased muscle (Shafiq et al 1967, Mair & Tomé 1972, Chou & Nonaka 1977, Lipton 1979, Wakayama & Schotland 1979). It is not at present certain that all of the increased numbers of mononucleate cells in a satellite position seen in these conditions result from the multiplication of pre-existing myosatellite cells. It has been suggested that some, and possibly even a major proportion, are derived from intrinsic myonuclei that separate with a small surrounding portion of sarcoplasm from the reactive or degenerating myofibres, and resume an independent existence as myosatellites (Hess & Rosner 1970, Reznik 1970, Mastaglia et al 1975a). Myosatellite cells can be liberated from adult animal muscle fibres for study in vitro by enzymatic destruction of their basal laminae (Bischoff 1974), and a quantitative technique for obtaining myogenic cells from adult human muscle has been described by Yasin et al (1977).

The fine structure of the myosatellite cells reflects their lack of obvious differentiated function (Fig. 1.17). Their nuclei are usually, but not invariably, asymmetrically disposed with respect to the cytoplasm, one tail of which is often considerably longer and more attenuated than the other (Franzini-Armstrong 1979), and are smaller than the true myonuclei. They contain conspicuous masses of clumped peripheral heterochromatin (Ishikawa 1966, Conen & Bell 1970) and lack nucleoli. The ratio of cytoplasmic to nuclear volume is low and the polar regions of the cytoplasm contain few organelles; free ribosomes, small vesicles, longitudinally arranged microtubules, and fine and intermediate filaments predominate. The perinuclear region of the cytoplasm contains small numbers of small-diameter short mitochondria and occasional rough endoplasmic reticular sacs and Golgi membrane systems, together with glycogen, myelin figures and lipofuscin granules in older human subjects. Paired centrioles (Muir 1970, Conen & Bell 1970, Mair & Tomé 1972), one of which is often associated with a cilium, are frequently seen in the perinuclear cytoplasm. The apposed plasma membranes of the myosatellite and myofibre usually show an abundance of attached pinocytotic vesicles. Intercellular attachments of the 'adhaerens' type also occur, although infrequently, the two membranes having a uniform separation of ~15 nm, increased on occasion by the presence of lamellated extracellular masses of phospholipid material between the two membranes. True myosatellite cells as defined above seldom, if ever, contain organized arrays of myofilaments; cells in a satellite position in which such nascent myofibrils occur can almost

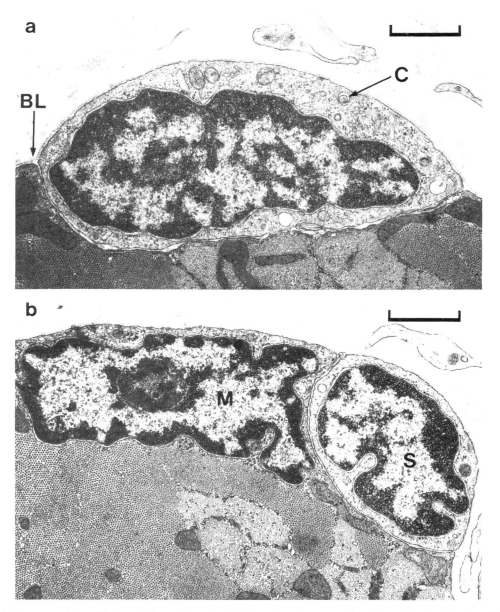

Fig. 1.17   (a) A myosatellite cell lying within an indentation in the surface of a rat myofibre, beneath its basal lamina (BL). The dense nucleus containing clumped chromatin, and undifferentiated cytoplasm are characteristic of such cells. The section includes a vestigial cilium at (C). (b) An example of the not uncommon association of a myosatellite cell (S) with an intrinsic myonucleus (M). Scale bars = 1 μm

invariably be shown by serial sectioning to be part of a small multinucleate satellite myotube or myofibre (Aloisi 1970, Landon 1970a, Ontell 1977).

Other mononuclear cells

Not all cells situated beneath the basal lamina of a myofibre are necessarily myosatellites, and other cell types to be considered are macrophages, leucocytes and fibroblasts. Macrophages of characteristic morphology are a common feature of diseased or traumatized muscle containing degenerating myofibres; they may be found in the perimysial or endomysial connective tissue, or amid the myoplasmic debris within the basal lamina of a degenerating fibre. They are easily distinguished from myosatellite cells by their dense heterochromatic nuclei, dense cytoplasmic matrix rich in primary and secondary lysosomes, and ruffled cell border. Neutrophil polymorphonuclear leucocytes may also be found within the sarcolemmal tube in the early stages of myofibre degeneration (Fig. 1.18a), but have never been reported beneath the basal lamina of an intact fibre in normal tissue. A third class of cell, much less easily distinguished from myosatellites on grounds of morphology, are the 'invasive' (Franzini-Armstrong 1979) or 'free' cells (Schiaffino et al 1979) originally described by Mastaglia et al (1975b) and tentatively identified by them as lymphocytes or monocytes. These cells have less obviously heterochromatic nucleoplasm than typical haematogenous macrophages; they have pale, relatively undifferentiated cytoplasm, large cytoplasmic pseudopodia and a smooth unruffled cell surface. They may be found in the process of traversing the myofibre basal lamina, in various stages of penetration into the interior of the fibre, or wholly enclosed by myoplasm (Mastaglia et al 1975b). The defect in the basal lamina through which they enter is small and there is no evidence of damage to the myofibre plasma membrane, which appears to adapt itself to the shape of the invading cell (Fig. 1.18b). It has been suggested that penetration is achieved by expansion of pre-existing T tubules (Franzini-Armstrong 1979). Transient invasion of one cell by another has been recorded in other systems (Humble et al 1956), and has been termed emperipolesis; the case of the 'invasive' cell and the myofibre may represent an aspect of the body's mechanism for the immune surveillance of its tissues. If such wandering lymphocytes or monocytes can remain quiescent beneath the myofibre basal lamina without expressing their invasive potential, they will be effectively indistinguishable on cytological grounds from genuine

myosatellites, and their true incidence will be difficult to assess. Fibroblasts, or fibroblast-like cells, have been reported to occur in direct contact with the myofibre surface, beneath its basal lamina, in regenerating muscle (Shafiq et al 1967, Trupin et al 1979). The characteristics by which fibroblasts are usually recognized in tissue sections include their interstitial location within the connective tissue compartment, their large angular nuclei containing dispersed chromatin and an obvious nucleolus, extensive flattened cytoplasmic processes containing well-developed rough endoplasmic reticular cisternae distended by a finely granular content, extensive Golgi systems and lack of basal lamina (Fig. 1.19a). The identification of fibroblasts within the basal laminae of intact myofibres, referred to above, rest upon the presence of a well-developed rough endoplasmic reticulum within the cells observed. It is possible, however, that such examples represent activated myosatellite cells, in which the rough endoplasmic reticular cisternae are a prominent feature (Fig. 1.19b).

MUSCLE DEVELOPMENT

Histogenesis

Striated muscle of mammals develops in the embryo from somatic mesoderm, the trunk and body-wall muscles from the metamerically segmented paraxial myotomes and the limb muscles from unsegmented splanchnopleure, differentiation following a proximodistal and cephalocaudal progression. Condensations of mesenchyme appear at the sites of future muscle masses in the limb buds of the human embryo at the sixth week of gestation and by the eighth week the primordia of most individual muscles are clearly defined. These are composed of groups of small 'myotubes', multinucleate syncytia containing a central chain of rounded nuclei within a peripheral shell of basophilic cytoplasm bearing the first traces of cross-striation, lying within a loose connective-tissue stroma. Few cytological or fine structural data are available concerning the exact sequence of events that leads to the appearance of the first myotubes, but it is clear from studies of later stages of myogenesis in vivo, and by analogy

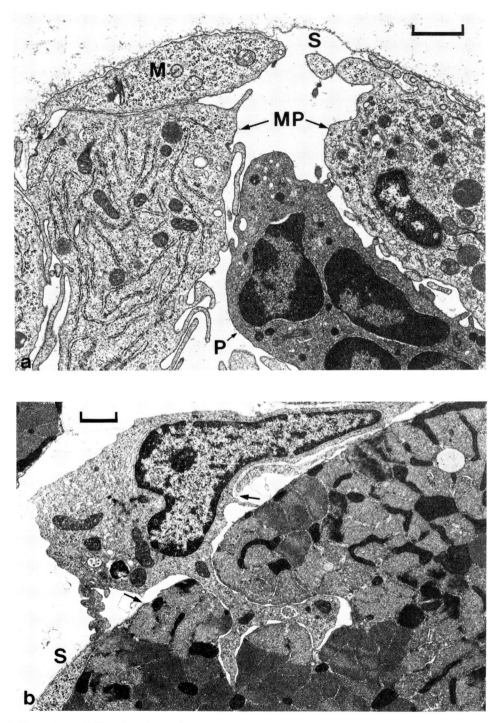

Fig. 1.18 (a) Macrophages (MP) and a polymorphonuclear leucocyte (P) within the persisting sarcolemma (S) of a degenerating myofibre. A myoblastic cell rich in polysomes is also visible (M). (b) an extrinsic cell invading the substance of an apparently intact myofibre. The edges of the ruptured basal lamina are indicated by arrows; part of a true myosatellite cell is visible at (S). Scale bars = 1 μm

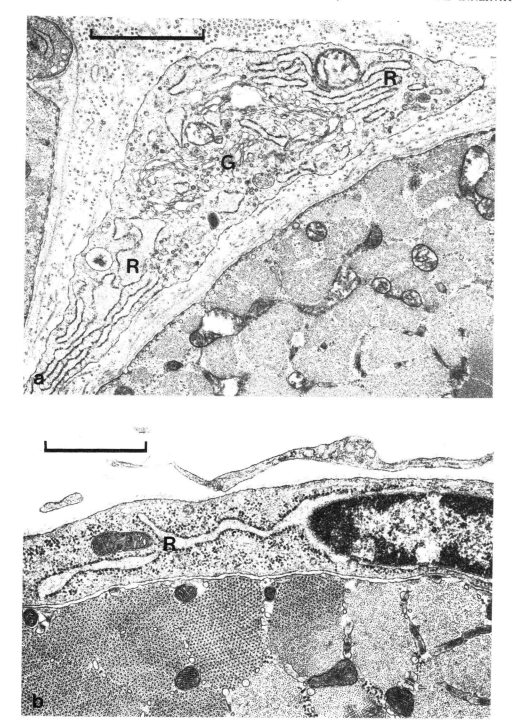

Fig. 1.19   (a) An endomysial fibroblast in human muscle; it lacks a basal lamina, and contains abundant Golgi complexes (G) and extensive rough endoplasmic reticular cisterns (R) with a finely granular content. Scale = 2 μm. (b) An activated myosatellite cell beneath the basal lamina of a rat myofibre. Such cells commonly contain a few large rough endoplasmic reticular cisternae (R) connected to the nuclear envelope, and may be mistaken for fibroblasts. Scale bar = 1 μm

from similar processes observed in vitro, that myotubes are formed by the coalescence or fusion of a number of myogenic stem cells, 'myoblasts', into one multinucleate unit. Earlier suggestions that muscle cell nuclei increase in number by mitotic or 'amitotic' division without cytokinesis can now be discounted.

Once formed, the population of myotubes increases rapidly, and its individual members increase in length, girth and content of nuclei. A rapid increase in the number of myotubes/myofibres within limb muscles of the human fetus continues until the fourth postnatal month (Montgomery 1962). The myofibre population has been reported to undergo a steady decline thereafter throughout childhood and adult life (Morpurgo 1898, Tello 1917, Montgomery 1962), but Adams & de Reuck (1973), who examined fibre numbers in three muscles from 46 different individuals, reported a gradual rise between birth and the end of the fifth decade, the total increase amounting to 80–100% of the neonatal total. At older ages, muscle fibre numbers showed a progressive fall. By contrast, small mammals show no evidence of a significant increase in myofibre numbers after the immediate neonatal period (Goldspink & Rowe 1968). The mechanism responsible for increase in myotube/myofibre numbers has also been a source of controversy; some have held that proliferation is achieved by splitting of existing myotubes (MacCallum 1898, Tello 1922, Cuajunco 1942), others, that the new myotubes arise by fusion of members of a local, continually dividing population of stem cells (Morpurgo 1898, Meves 1909, Couteaux 1941). The latter view is now clearly correct, and the processes involved are described below. Individual myotubes/myofibres increase in length in the developing human embryo pari passu with the changing dimensions of the limb and trunk segments within which they lie; it seems from animal experiments (see below) that this is accomplished by incorporating additional sarcoplasm, sarcomeres and membrane constituents into the tips of the fibres and not by interstitial insertion along their length.

Studies of muscle development in chickens and small mammals, both in vivo and in tissue culture, have greatly extended our knowledge of the details of these processes. In the rat the first myotubes appear at the 14th to 15th day of gestation: they are identified by their central columns of nuclei containing prominent nucleoli, and syncytial cytoplasm rich in ribosomes, sarcotubular membranes, glycogen granules, lipid droplets and small clumps of myofilaments. These myotubes occur in small groups separated by loose connective tissue, consisting of a reticulum of angular mesenchymal fibroblasts in a structureless matrix; each member of a group is closely related to a number of less-differentiated muscle cells (Kelly & Zacks 1969a). These cells are divisible into two classes (Fig. 1.20): (i) true mononucleate myoblasts, which are rounded cells characterized by small dense nuclei without nucleoli and with cytoplasm containing rough endoplasmic reticular cisternae within a matrix filled with free ribosomes; (ii) multinucleate myofilament-containing muscle cells that represent the initial stage in formation of the next generation of myotubes. Both varieties lie within the basal lamina of the established myotube against which they abut (Kelly & Zacks 1969a). Only the mononucleate myoblasts show mitosis, and it has been shown experimentally that some such cell divisions are 'critical' or 'quantal' (Holtzer 1970), in the sense that one or both of the daughter cells are thereafter irrevocably committed to differentiation and fusion, either with other postmitotic myoblasts to form a new myotube, or with an existing myotube to add to its complement of nuclei and cytoplasm. In tissue cultures of muscle cells, the switch from myoblast proliferation to fusion requires a certain minimal density of cells and seems to be promoted by accumulation within the culture medium of a diffusable polypeptide with a high molecular weight (Konigsberg 1971). The shift into the postmitotic phase is signalled by a prolongation of the G_1 portion of the mitotic cycle, retention of diploid DNA, and the start of synthesis of muscle-specific proteins (Stockdale & Holtzer 1961, Pearson 1981) including specific membrane antigens (Walsh & Ritter 1981). Some authors, in discussing these events, have adopted a nomenclature that distinguishes between 'presumptive' or 'premyoblasts', members of the continuously replicating population of stem cells, and true myoblasts that have left the mitotic cycle and are committed to

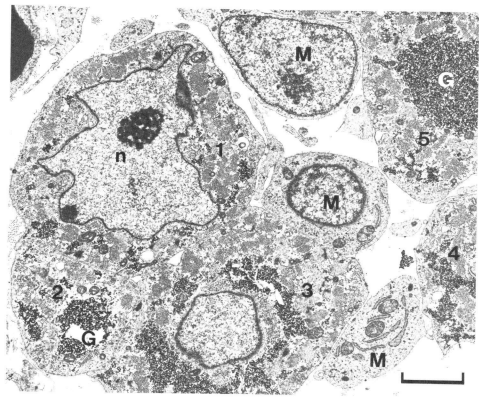

Fig. 1.20 A transverse section through a cluster of myotubes in m. gastrocnemius of an 8-week-old human fetus. The closely opposed myotubes (1–5) possess large nuclei containing dispersed chromatin and prominent nucleoli (n), developing myofibrils, and large stores of granular glycogen (G). The adjacent mononuclear myoblasts (M) have cytoplasm rich in polysomes and denser, more granular nuclei. Scale bar = 2 μm

fusion (Bischoff & Holtzer 1969). This functional distinction is not matched by any clear-cut pattern of structural change, and all mononuclear myogenic cells will therefore be referred to as myoblasts in this account of the morphology of developing muscle. It is probable, however, that the appearance within some of these myoblasts of proliferating rough endoplasmic reticulum from the nuclear envelope, and a rudimentary nucleolus attached to the peripheral heterochromatin, represent structural modifications associated with the onset of pre-fusion differentiation in 'post-quantal' cells.

Myoblast fusion

Direct evidence of myoblast fusion has been obtained by light-microscopic time-lapse cinema-tography (Cooper & Konigsberg 1961), but convincing fine structural images of this process are rare. Shimada (1971) has illustrated focal breakdown of the adjacent membranes of laterally aligned chick myoblasts in tissue culture that leads to the formation of cytoplasmic bridges between the cells, with subsequent breakdown of the residual membrane into vesicles resulting in their complete coalescence. An analogous process has been described by Lipton & Konigsberg (1972) in cultured quail muscle, with the difference that a single initial pore, created by a small focal area of membrane fusion, was considered to expand by lateral extension without further membrane breakdown, until the two cells were confluent. Discontinuous lengths of paired membranes, between areas of cytoplasm containing differing patterns of myofibril content, can be seen in rat myofibres regenerating in vivo (Landon, unpublished observations); such appearances are assumed to represent an incomplete stage of fusion between two regenerating myotubes, and identification of the individual contributions of fused myogenic cells to their joint cytoplasm, on the basis of their differing content of ribosomes, has been reported by Ross et al (1970). Myoblasts will, under normal circumstances, fuse only with other myogenic cells; the specific membrane properties responsible for such recognition can be destroyed, and cell fusion inhibited, by substances that alter the structure of the cell surface.

Myotube proliferation

Subsequent differentiation, which in the rat extends from the 17th day of gestation to the end of the second postnatal week, results in the appearance of a series of generations of additional myotubes. At their earliest stage of development these take the form of small flattened multinucleate bands closely adherent to one of the more developed myotubes. Their nuclei possess nucleoli and their cytoplasm contains plentiful polysomes, Golgi membrane stacks and slender bundles of thick and thin myofilaments organized into myofibrils. A striking feature of the interface between the new myotube and its more mature neighbour is the presence of finger- or keel-like projections from the surface of the former, that lie within reciprocal invaginations of the cell membrane and cytoplasm of the older myotube (Kelly & Zacks 1969a, Landon 1970a, 1971). These projections extend deep into the substance of the established myotube and are frequently found in close proximity to its nuclei (Fig. 1.21); both the invading and invaginated cell surfaces bear coated uptake vesicles. Quantitative studies of this phenomenon (Landon 1971) have shown that these contacts are most complex morphologically during the early stages of the differentiation of the new myotube as judged by its content of myofilaments, being most elaborate when these occupy approximately 9% of the cross-sectional area of the myotube cytoplasm. Increase in myofilament content above this level is associated with a diminution in the numbers and size of the projections, none being found on myotubes having

a myofilament content exceeding 35%. An almost identical structural arrangement is found in human fetal muscle, with the minor difference that the maximum complexity of the contact zones is associated with a somewhat higher (15%) filament content (Landon, unpublished observations). True mononucleate myoblasts very seldom engage in such complex surface contacts with myotubes (Ontell 1977); suggestions that the phenomenon may represent a stage in the fusion of adjacent cells receive no support from the results of serial sectioning large numbers of contacts and their examination using a tilting specimen stage (Landon 1970a, Ontell 1979). The increased area of membrane contact, the close relationship of the projections on the new myotubes to the nuclei of its more differentiated neighbour, and the frequent presence of coated vesicles on the apposed membranes (Fig. 1.22), suggest a role for the more mature 'primary' myotube in the promotion or control of the early stages of differentiation of the 'secondary' myotube, possibly by the transfer of messenger materials between them.

Continued differentiation of the secondary myotubes involves increases in diameter, nuclear number and myofilament content, and their separation from the primary myotubes. The last process is frequently accompanied by the appearance of columns of myoblasts interposed between the adjacent primary and secondary myotubes and within their common basal lamina; these are the progenitors of the tertiary and later generations of myotubes, and there is evidence (Kelly & Zacks 1969a) that such cells preferentially associate with the smallest, and thus by inference the least mature, of the existing myotubes. The new myotube resulting from their fusion will thus lie alongside, and differentiate in association with, a secondary myotube, in the manner described above for the primary and secondary generations (Fig. 1.23). Maturation of the primary myotubes to myofibres occurs concurrently with the proliferation of secondary myotubes, and is accompanied by peripheral migration of the nuclei to a subplasmalemmal position, synthesis of contractile proteins and their assembly into larger and more numerous myofibrils, maturation of the sarcotubular system, and the establishment of motor innervation. The development of primary

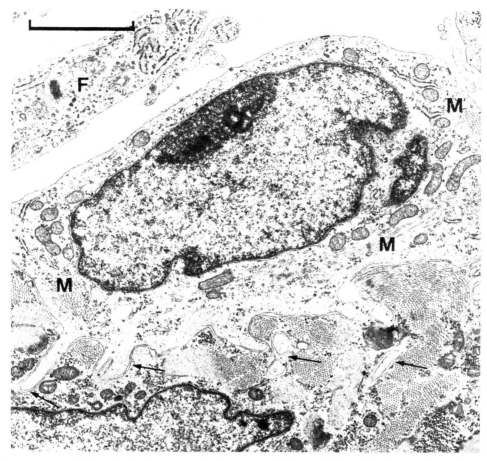

Fig. 1.21 A young myotube from developing rat muscle. Nascent myofibrils are visible within the cytoplasm (M), and numerous processes on its deep surface (arrows) penetrate into clefts in the surface of the more mature myotube upon which it lies. (F) = fibroblast. Scale bar = 2 μm

myotubes is not, however, dependent upon innervation, unlike the secondary and subsequent generations which appear to have an absolute requirement for both innervation ánd contractile activity for their maturation and maintenance (Harris 1981), denervation at birth causing a permanent deficit in fibre numbers even in muscles which later become re-innervated (McArdle & Sansone 1977, Betz et al 1980).

In the rat, the shift from the intrauterine environment at birth is marked by loss of most of the lipid droplets and stores of glycogen granules that are a prominent feature of the fetal myotubes (Schiaffino & Hanzlikova 1972). The lipid droplets are extruded by the muscle cells into the inter-

stitium, where they may be found in some numbers during the first two postnatal days, before their removal by macrophage activity.

Development of the contractile apparatus

Primitive myofibrils appear early in the postfusion development of mammalian myotubes and may be found in avian muscle in mononucleate myoblasts before fusion (Stockdale & Holtzer 1961). Actin production appears to start at an early stage in both avian and mammalian myogenesis, and the first actin filaments form an irregular feltwork beneath the plasmalemma of prefusion myoblasts. Thereafter muscle-specific proteins are expressed

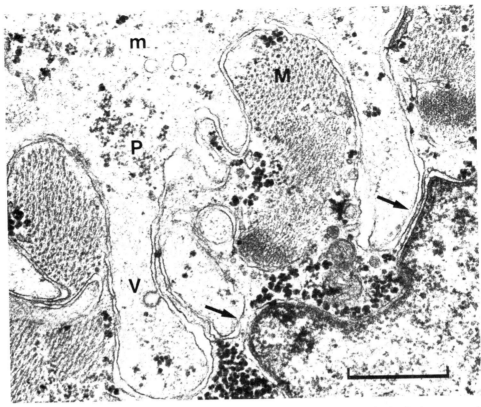

Fig. 1.22 The apposed surfaces of a young myotube (m) and its more mature neighbour (M) in developing rat muscle. The processes of the former possess coated uptake vesicles (V), and contain polysomes (P) and a meshwork of microfilaments. At their tips they come into intimate contact with the nuclear envelope of the more mature myotube (arrows). Scale bar = 1 μm

in a consistent order, first desmin, to be followed by titin, muscle-specific actin, myosin heavy chains and lastly nebulin (Furst et al 1989). The desmin becomes incorporated into the 10 nm intermediate filaments which are widespread in early post-fusion myotubes (Ishikawa et al 1968); their numbers diminish as the myofibrils become established (Bennett et al 1979), but some persist in the vicinity of the Z-discs and play a part in the transverse alignment of the sarcomeres in the mature myofibre (Thornell et al 1980). The newly synthesized high-molecular-weight titin molecules appear to be stable and to be rapidly integrated into the myotube cytoskeleton (Isaacs et al 1989), and it has been suggested that the elastic filaments with their high titin content may function as important initial organizers of the main myofibrillar protein arrays and may also have a role in

determining the length of the A filaments (Furst et al 1989, Handel et al 1989, Colley et al 1990). Organized bundles of I filaments attached to small dense primordia of Z-band material are later found in the more superficial parts of the myotube cytoplasm (Heuson-Stiennon 1965), coinciding in time of appearance, but not necessarily in direct association, with the first small regular arrays of A filaments (Fischman 1967). Subsequent radial growth of these early myofibrils appears to be accomplished by the addition of further filamentous and Z-band components to their periphery (Morkin 1970), and also possibly by the coalescence of adjacent strands. Myofibril growth is accompanied by a fall in the numbers of free ribosomes (Dessouky & Hibbs 1965), and the appearance of long spiral polysomes in close association with the peripheral filaments of the nascent A bands (Allen

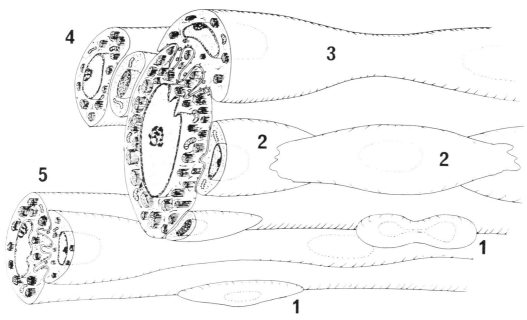

Fig. 1.23 A schema illustrating the production of new myotubes during the hyperplastic phase of myogenesis. Mononucleate myoblasts (1), adherent to the surface of pre-existing myotubes, proliferate and differentiate to form chains of overlapping spindle-shaped cells (2). These cells fuse, and the resulting myotube (3) begins to synthesize contractile proteins, and develops a close morphological relationship with the surface of its more mature neighbour. This contact is lost with further differentiation (4), and the two myotubes become separated by proliferation of myoblasts between their opposed surfaces. Repetition of these processes (5) gives rise to successive generations of new myotubes

& Pepe 1965, Larson et al 1973), suggesting that the myosin subunits of the A filaments are synthesized in situ.

The two components of the sarcotubular system, the transverse tubules and the sarcoplasmic reticulum, are identifiable from the earliest stages of myotube differentiation and appear to develop simultaneously (Ezerman & Ishikawa 1967, Schiaffino & Margreth 1969). The smooth flattened sacs of sarcoplasmic reticulum arise as outgrowths of the rough endoplasmic reticulum of the early myotube, and the T tubules from invaginations of the plasmalemma. The latter generate an extensive system of branched tubules within the subplasmalemmal cytoplasm, from which further branches penetrate between the myofibrils where they make triadic contacts with units of the sarcoplasmic reticulum (Walker & Schrodt 1968, Kelly 1971, 1980). In the rat the sarcoplasmic reticulum has, by the second postnatal week, become organized into segments, in register with the A and I bands of the sarcomeres alternately, and

extensive triadic junctions are visible between the T tubules and the terminal cisternae of the sarcoplasmic reticulum opposite the interfaces between each A and I band. The adult differences in the extent and arrangement of the sarcoplasmic reticulum in fast- and slow-twich fibres develop somewhat later in postnatal life (Luff & Atwood 1971, Schmalbruch 1985).

Histochemical differentiation

Little evidence of a systematic variation in the histochemical staining properties of developing myofibres is visible in the human fetus until the fifth month of gestation. Minor differences in the intensity of myofibrillar ATPase and phosphorylase staining occur earlier (Fenichel 1966, Kamieniecka 1968), but these appear to reflect quantitative differences in the myofibril content of myotubes at differing stages of development. The first suggestion of the adult checkerboard pattern of fibres with different histochemical properties appears at 15–20 weeks' gestation and is complete between 26 (Martin & Joris 1970) and 30 weeks (Fenichel 1966, Dubowitz 1968). All developing myotubes and myofibres initially possess high oxidative enzyme, phosphorylase and myofibrillar ATPase activity, but at 18 weeks' gestation, or shortly thereafter, some of the largest fibres show a reduction in the activity of the latter two enzymes while retaining their oxidative properties. These large fibres are scattered more or less evenly through the more numerous population of smaller ATPase-positive fibres, and are considered to be the histochemical equivalent of the basophilic B fibres described by Wohlfart (1937). At 18 weeks' gestation they constitute 4–5% of the fibre population, but continued growth of the smaller acidophilic A fibres during subsequent development, and an increase in the total numbers of fibres with type 1 characteristics, result in the disappearance of the B fibres as a distinct class by 30 weeks' gestation. The B fibres have been proposed as a source of type 1 fibres, but their numbers are always small and they probably represent merely the largest and most conspicuous members of the emerging type 1 fibre population. Studies on animal muscle have provided convincing evidence that most type 1 fibres originate from the conversion of the histochemical characteristics of members of the primitive type 2 fibre population that predominates at earlier stages of development; major increases in the proportion of type 1 fibres in the muscles of pigs, rats and guinea-pigs are accompanied by only minor increases in total fibre numbers within individual muscles, or identifiable muscle fascicles (Karpati & Engel 1968, Cooper et al 1970, Kelly & Schotland 1972). This shift in the histochemical properties of individual fibres is associated with changes in their myosin and troponin isoenzyme patterns (Trayer & Perry 1966, Gauthier et al 1978, Dhoot & Perry 1980, Rubinstein & Kelly 1981, Bronson & Schachat 1982, Pette & Staron 1988), and the differentiation of distinct fast and slow contractile characteristics (Buller et al 1960a, Close 1964). It is probable that the type 1 fibres of human muscle likewise originate from fibres that initially possessed high ATPase activity, the change accompanying maturation of their innervation and the development of distinct phasic and tonic

modes of contractile activity, but direct evidence that this is the case is currently lacking. Hormonal influences on skeletal muscle development have been reviewed by Rubinstein et al (1988).

Muscle fibre growth

In small mammals, such as the rat and mouse, the pattern of muscle fibre growth is markedly biphasic, hyperplasia predominating in the first period of development, from the start of myogenesis until the end of the second postnatal week, at which time the production of new myotubes ceases abruptly, to be succeeded by a lengthy phase of fibre hypertrophy. The point of transition coincides with achievement by the myofibres of mononeuronal innervation, and acquisition by the young animal of sufficient coordinated motor activity for it to assume an independent mobile existence. A similar, but less clear-cut, biphasic development occurs during the fetal period in larger animals (Ashmore et al 1972). In the human fetus the initial rapid increase in myotube numbers begins to decline at approximately the 21st week of gestation, i.e. at a crown–rump length of around 22 cm (Stickland 1981), the change again coinciding with the onset of the transformation of myotubes into myofibres and the beginning of their phase of hypertrophy; however, in man, as in other large mammals, new myotubes continue to be formed until well into the postnatal period (Montgomery 1962, Burleigh 1974), and probably throughout most of adult life (Adams & de Reuck 1973). Muscle fibres in full use from early in development grow most rapidly, those of the diaphragm having a mean diameter twice that of limb muscle fibres in the neonatal child (Bowden & Goyer 1960). Growth of the limb muscles subsequently catches up with that of the diaphragm as the child becomes more active, their fibres being of approximately equal diameter by one year of age.

Not all myotubes that are formed continue to grow and differentiate to maturity; large degenerating myotubes are a common feature of human fetal muscle of between 10 and 16 weeks' gestation (Webb 1972, Landon, unpublished observations). Similar degeneration of a part of the cell population is a normal concomitant of organogenesis in other systems, but the precipitating factors in any individual myotube, and the relationship of the phenomenon to the progress of innervation, are unknown. Detailed reviews of the growth and development of human muscle have been given by Mastaglia (1974) and Malina (1978).

The observed increases in muscle fibre numbers occurring during fetal and postnatal development are achieved through the generation of new myotubes, by a continuation of the processes of fusion and differentiation of mononucleate myoblasts associated with existing myofibres, described above. The persistence into adult life within muscles of such a stem population of myoblast/satellite cells also provides the basis for the capability of normal striated muscle to regenerate damaged or necrotic fibres. Budding or splitting of existing muscle fibres (Cuajunco 1942), or the lengthening of short fibres that do not initially extend the full length of the developing muscle (Montgomery 1962), have also been proposed as mechanisms for increase in fibre number. The contribution of the latter process is likely, however, to be slight, as developing myofibres generally extend the full length of the muscle belly (Bridge & Allbrook 1970). Groups of two or more closely adherent myofibres, having a joint cross-sectional profile appropriate to a single fibre, and fibres partly divided by narrow longitudinal clefts, can be found in both normal and pathological muscle, although they are most common in the latter. Such appearances have been cited as evidence that fibres may multiply by splitting during growth, or to compensate for increased load or the loss of other fibres (van Linge 1962, Schwartz et al 1976, Bradley 1979). It can sometimes be shown by serial sectioning that such cleft fibres, or groups of fibre profiles, unite at another level into a single homogeneous fibre; this provides evidence that individual fibres can indeed be 'split', in the sense of being divided into two or more smaller parallel branches at any point along their length. However, these observations reveal nothing about the mechanism responsible for such divisions; it is the writer's view that fibres do not split in the dynamic sense of the word, and that the phenomenon of fibre splitting probably represents incomplete fusion of clusters of small myofibres, regenerating within the persisting

sarcolemmal tube of a single fibre that has previously undergone partial or total degeneration (Hall-Craggs & Lawrence 1970, Schmalbruch 1976, 1979b).

Increase in nuclear number and fibre diameter

The hypertrophic phase of muscle growth, in which the predominant changes are increase in fibre diameter and length, is associated with an increase in the numbers of nuclei within each myofibre. Early suggestions that this increase could be attributed to mitotic, or amitotic, division of the original population of nuclei contributed by the myoblasts whose fusion gave rise to the fibre, can now be discounted. No convincing demonstration of mitosis of true muscle nuclei (all of which are diploid, Strehler et al 1963) has ever been reported, and there is an equal lack of evidence that mammalian somatic cell nuclei ever divide in an amitotic manner. The satellite cells of muscle divide continuously, however, throughout the period of active myogenesis (Hellmuth & Allbrook 1973). This dividing cell population can be labelled with ^{3}H thymidine, and it has been shown by Moss & Leblond (1970, 1971) that a substantial proportion of the labelled daughter nuclei derived from satellite cell divisions are subsequently incorporated into myofibres as true muscle nuclei. Similar results have been obtained by implanting clonal cultures of labelled myoblasts into normal muscle of the original donor (Lipton & Schultz 1979). There is now, therefore, little doubt that the observed increase in numbers of myofibre nuclei during fibre growth is brought about by the fusion of mononucleate cells with the growing fibres, and that this population of stem cells can be identified with the satellite cells. During the most active phase of myogenesis, about 50% of the products of satellite cell division fail to fuse with myofibres (Hellmuth & Allbrook 1973), maintaining a constant satellite cell population equivalent to approximately one-third of the numbers of true myonuclei (Schultz 1974, Landon, unpublished observations). Satellite cell numbers decline thereafter to the adult level of about 5% of the total myofibre nuclear number in small animals, and to 1–2% in man.

Increase in myofibre nuclear numbers is associated with increase in fibre diameter. The relationship between fibre cross-sectional area and total nuclear number is linear during much of the postnatal development of chicken muscle (Moss 1968); this finding may imply the existence of a critical upper limit to the mass of sarcoplasm that can be supplied by the genetic apparatus of each myonucleus. Much of the increase in myofibre cross-sectional area is attributable to increase in the numbers of their contained myofibrils. These have a bimodal diameter distribution in growing muscle, and it has been suggested that myofibrils may have an optimal maximal diameter of 1–1.2 μm, and that they may proliferate by subdivision when this value is exceeded (Goldspink 1970). Fine structural appearances compatible with the occurrence of longitudinal division of individual myofibrils are common during postnatal growth (Goldspink 1970) and in muscles responding to release from immobilization (Shear 1975), or undergoing work hypertrophy. These take the form of longitudinal clefts partly dividing large myofibrils in the A- and I-band regions, and areas of disorganization in Z discs. The process involved has been termed 'myofibril splitting' (Goldspink 1970) but the use of this phrase raises similar problems of semantics to those discussed above in connection with the splitting of myofibres. Longitudinal division of myofibrils during growth of a fibre may indeed be a dynamic event in which the myofilament lattice is ripped apart by an imbalance of the tensile forces set up during contraction, as suggested by Goldspink (1970, 1971), but the evidence available would equally well support involvement of more subtle remodelling processes, the effects of which may be directed towards maintaining a ratio of myofibril mass to sarcoplasmic reticulum surface area that optimizes calcium ion kinetics during excitation and relaxation. The precise value of this ratio would be influenced by the specific contractile characteristics of each individual fibre, and its state of development. Observed differences in myofibril size and shape, and degrees of separation at the A band, in adult fast- and slow-twitch fibres, lend some support to this view and are less easily explained on a purely mechanical basis. The role of contractile function as a determinant of muscle growth has been reviewed by Zak (1981).

Growth in myofibre length

The increases in myofibre numbers and diameter during development, described above, are accompanied by growth in length of the individual fibres of each muscle, to match the changing dimensions of the whole organism. A small part of this increase in length has been attributed to a reduction in the extent of overlap of the thick and thin myofilaments under resting conditions with growth (Goldspink & Rowe 1968), resulting in an increase in mean sarcomere length. No differences have been reported in the lengths of the A and I filaments themselves, when neonatal and adult limb muscle fibres are compared, and most of the increase in myofibre length with growth must therefore be achieved by adding additional sarcomeres (Close 1964, 1972). Histological studies in which markers were inserted into growing muscles (Kitiyakara & Angevine 1963), and autoradiographic experiments using isotope-labelled precursors of myofilament protein (Griffin et al 1971, Williams & Goldspink 1971), have shown that these additional sarcomeres are incorporated into the ends of the growing myofibre at the myotendinous junction. An alternative view has been advanced by Schmalbruch (1968, 1985), who has proposed that additional intercalated sarcomeres may develop at sites of Z-line disruption or streaming, and extend progressively across the width of the myofibre. There is no evidence, however, that Z-line abnormalities are more common in children and adolescents than in adults, indeed the reverse, and increase in Z-line abnormalities has been convincingly shown usually to be associated with excessive or unusual functional loads (Fridén 1984). Nevertheless, a somewhat comparable division of the A band at the M-line has been described in crab striated muscle by Jahromi & Charlton (1979), a new Z-line appearing in the gaps so formed to create two sarcomeres where one had existed before. Immobilization of growing mouse muscle at a shortened length results in a decrease in the rate of addition of sarcomeres, normal numbers being recovered when the restriction is removed (Williams & Goldspink 1971, 1973). Experiments in the cat have shown that a similar adjustment of sarcomere numbers to functional length occurs in adult muscle (Tabary et al

1972). A number of aspects of muscle fibre growth have been reviewed by Goldspink (1980).

INNERVATION OF MUSCLE AND THE NEUROMUSCULAR ENDORGANS

The nerves to individual limb muscles of mammals generally enter their deep surfaces, in company with a major component of the arterial supply to that muscle, and there divide into a number of subsidiary branches which ramify and further subdivide within the central region of the muscle belly. The bundles of nerve fibres comprising each branch are enclosed by perineurial sheaths continuous with that of the parent nerve, the number of layers of perineurial cells diminishing progressively in such a way that the finest branches may consist of a single myelinated nerve fibre within a unilamellar sheath (Fig. 1.24). Myelinated and unmyelinated axons are present within this system

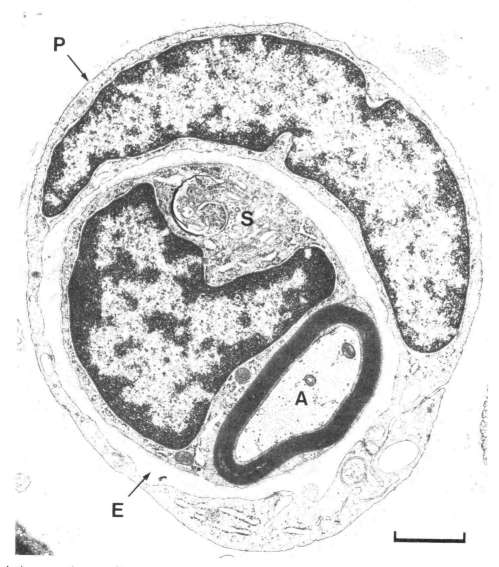

Fig. 1.24 An intramuscular nerve fibre near its termination within the end-plate region of a rat soleus muscle. The myelinated axon (A) and its Schwann cell (S) are surrounded by a narrow collagen-containing endoneurial space (E) and are ensheathed by a single perineurial cell layer (P). Scale bar = 1 μm

in approximately equal proportions and are divisible into three basic categories: (1) myelinated somatic efferent (motor) fibres innervating the myofibres; (2) myelinated and unmyelinated somatic afferent (sensory) fibres from muscle spindles, Golgi tendon organs, Pacinian and paciniform corpuscles, and free unencapsulated nociceptive terminals; and (3) unmyelinated autonomic efferent fibres. At least two-thirds of the total of somatic fibres are afferent, and a large proportion of these are unmyelinated (Boyd & Davey 1968). For a schematic summary of the innervation of muscle, see Figure 1.29.

The motor innervation of muscle

The motor, somatic efferent fibres of a muscle nerve arise either from clusters of neurones in lamina IX of the ventral grey columns of the spinal cord, or from the motor cranial nerve nuclei in the brain stem. The structure and functional relationships of these anterior horn motor neurones have been reviewed by Conradi (1976). They show a bimodal size distribution with peaks at 20 and 40–50 μm mean diameter (van Buren & Frank 1965), and the existence of this dual population of cells is reflected in a similarly bimodal distribution of the diameters of the nerve fibres to which they give rise, whether measured in the ventral roots or in distal nerve branches adjacent to the muscle supplied (Boyd & Davey 1962). The large-diameter group is composed of α-fibres, which innervate fast motor units exclusively, and β-fibres, which are distributed to both slow motor units and certain of the intrafusal myofibres of the muscle spindle (q.v.). The small-diameter group contains the γ-fibres; these supply the remainder of the muscle spindle intrafusal myofibres. Nerve fibres taper in the course of their passage to their distal terminals, and this leads to different values being obtained for efferent fibre diameter spectra in the ventral roots and in the nerves to individual muscles. The large-fibre group have diameters ranging from 12–20 μm in the lumbar ventral roots of the cat, but these diminish to 10–15 μm in the nerve to the medial gastrocnemius (Boyd & Davey 1962). The small-diameter group also show a reduction in size, from 3–8 μm in the roots to 2–7 μm in the

muscle nerve. This tapering process is presumably accelerated in the group of large fibres by the considerable degree of branching of individual fibres that occurs proximal to their entry into the muscle (Gilliatt 1966); little branching of the small-diameter fibres is seen until close to their points of termination at the muscle spindles (Barker 1974). In many muscle nerves the γ-efferents can be divided into two subgroups, consisting of those with slender, 3–4 μm diameter, thinly myelinated fibres and a second group of stouter, 6–7 μm diameter, thickly myelinated fibres (Boyd 1962), but clear evidence that these represent two functionally distinct classes of γ-fibre has yet to be obtained (Matthews 1972).

The neuromuscular synapse

The essential histological and fine structural features of the neuromuscular synapse are illustrated in Figures 1.25 and 1.26. The myelinated motor nerve fibre ends as an unmyelinated terminal segment, its length and degree of branching varying with species, age and muscle fibre type. The two extremes of this variation are represented by the junctions on the slowly contracting muscle fibres of amphibia, reptiles and birds, in which the unmyelinated terminal region of the axon may ramify over a considerable length of muscle fibre, making multiple points of synaptic contact, and the neuromuscular junctions on fast-twitch mammalian muscle fibres where the terminal is typically restricted to a number of short branches within a single discrete motor end-plate (Fig. 1.25). The unmyelinated portion of the axon leading from the end of the last segment of the myelin sheath, and its terminal arborization, are ensheathed and covered on their external surfaces by a prolongation of the Schwann cell covering of the nerve fibre, the terminal cells on the superficial surface of the motor end-plate sometimes being referred to as the 'teloglia'. Despite the presence of this continuous cover, the interface between nerve and muscle fibre at the neuromuscular junction provides a potential portal of entry for extraneous materials of large molecular weight into the endoneurial space of the parent

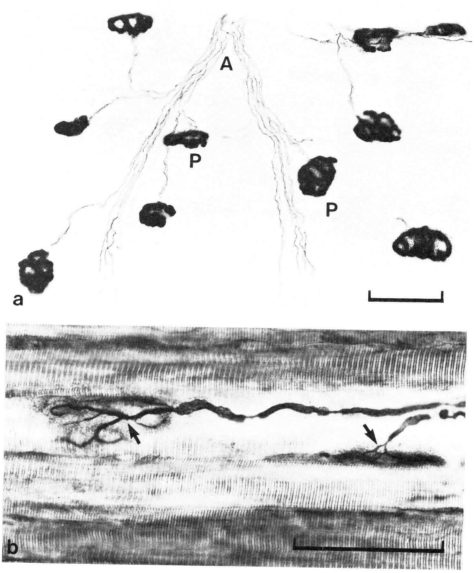

Fig. 1.25   (a) The appearance and distribution of neuromuscular synapses in the end-plate zone of a rat soleus muscle. Slender silver-impregnated axons (A) provide an individual supply to compact sole-plates (P) stained for acetylcholinesterase by the method of Koelle and Friedenwald. (b) Neuromuscular junctions in a rat soleus muscle in which the acetylcholinesterase has been demonstrated by the bromindoxylacetate technique. The silver-stained axons break up into a number of fine branches (arrows) within the end-plate regions which are delimited by the finely granular acetylcholinesterase stain. The end-plate on the right is viewed in profile, and can be seen to be raised above the general contour of the muscle fibre (the Doyère eminence). Scale bars = 100 μm. (From preparations kindly supplied by Professor L. W. Duchen and Dr S. Gomez of the Institute of Neurology, London)

nerve, and is freely permeable to tracers, such as horseradish peroxidase, that are excluded by the perineurial sheath.

Accumulation of peripheral sarcoplasm at the site of the neuromuscular junction results in its elevation above the general contour of the muscle

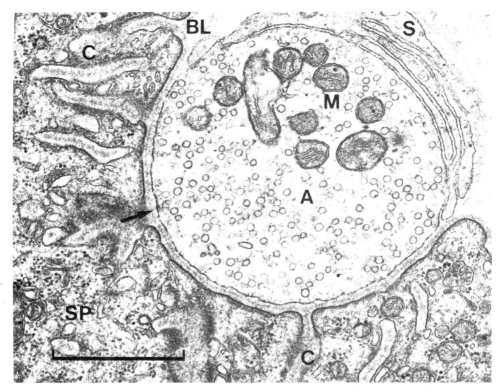

Fig. 1.26   A portion of a motor end-plate from a rat soleus muscle. The axon terminal (A) is covered on its external aspect by Schwann cell processes (S) and contains numerous clear synaptic vesicles and mitochondria (M). It is separated from the myofibre sole-plate (SP) by a layer of basal lamina, extensions of which fill the postsynaptic clefts (C). An arrow indicates a site of increased density on the presynaptic membrane associated with vesicle release. Scale bar = 1 μm

fibre, to produce the 'Doyère eminence' or sole-plate. When sectioned, the end-plate sarcoplasm generally contains one or more nuclei, rough and smooth endoplasmic reticular and Golgi membrane systems, and mitochondria; the latter are particularly numerous in the motor end-plates of small mammals, but are less conspicuous at the human neuromuscular junction. In higher vertebrates the ramifications of the nerve terminals are sunk into 'gutters' in the surface of the sole-plate, and their respective plasma membranes are separated from one another by an extension of the basal lamina covering the remainder of the muscle fibre. The floors and walls of these gutters are marked by numerous postjunctional folds separated by secondary postsynaptic clefts of varying depth and structural complexity, the lumina of which are filled by extensions of the basal lamina material that separates the adjacent nerve and muscle

membrane (Fig. 1.26). The presence of the post-synaptic clefts in the sole-plate considerably increases the postsynaptic membrane area, the ratio of pre- to postsynaptic areas being approximately 1:10 in both human intercostal and rat limb muscle (Engel & Santa 1971, Engel et al 1976). The morphology of this postsynaptic apparatus shows consistent differences in slow- and fast-twitch mammalian fibres; the former in general possess simple, shallow postsynaptic clefts; the latter larger numbers of deeper and more elaborately branched clefts (Padykula & Gauthier 1970, Gauthier 1976).

The motor nerve terminal

The axoplasm of the nerve terminals lying within the postsynaptic gutters is bounded by a plasma membrane, the axolemma, and has a high content of organelles. The most conspicuous of these are mitochondria and clear synaptic vesicles, 45–50 nm in diameter, but elements of the smooth endoplasmic reticulum, secondary lysosomes, coated vesicles and large dense-cored vesicles are also usually visible, together with neurofilaments and microtubules at and near the junction of the terminal proper with the terminal non-myelinated segment of its parent motor axon. The synaptic vesicles, which on average occupy some 15% of the axon terminal volume, are not uniformly distributed throughout the terminal axoplasm, and in sectioned material they often seem to aggregate around spots or ribbons of increased electron density, distributed along those parts of the axolemma facing the postsynaptic muscle membrane (Fig. 1.26). Freeze–fracture preparations have demonstrated that such densities are flanked by parallel pairs of double rows of 10 nm intramembranous particles set in a 20 nm square array, 40 nm apart, which are believed to be voltage-sensitive calcium channels (Pumplin et al 1981). These so-called 'active zones' (Couteaux & Pécot-Dechauvassine 1970) are considered to play a part in the release of acetylcholine quanta from the synaptic vesicles into the extracellular space between the adjacent nerve and muscle membranes, in a manner analogous to that postulated for the presynaptic dense web at interneural synapses (Akert et al 1972). In amphibia, they lie opposite, and parallel with, the mouths of the secondary postsynaptic clefts in the sole-plate; their ribbon-like nature and the tendency for synaptic vesicles to attach to the axolemma alongside them have been well demonstrated in freeze–fracture preparations of frog neuromuscular junctions (Sandri et al 1977). Heuser (1977) and Heuser et al (1979) have illustrated the sequential attachment and opening of synaptic vesicles in similar preparations that have been rapidly frozen within milliseconds of stimulation of the motor nerve. In mammals the 'active zones' are shorter than those seen in amphibia, and differ in both orientation and location, lying opposite the convexities of the postsynaptic folds, rather than at the mouths of the clefts, and at right angles to their long axes. A further difference is that vesicle release appears to occur between the paired double rows of particles in mammalia, i.e. in the zone of electron density,

rather than on the lateral side of each member of a pair, as occurs in the frog (Ellisman et al 1976).

Neurotransmitter release

In the past there has been some dispute concerning the mechanism of transmitter release at synapses, including argument as to whether the so-called synaptic vesicles do in fact contain acetylcholine quanta, and a suggestion that they may not exist as vesicles in unfixed tissue but may represent the products of artefactual disruption of pre-existing tubular membrane systems (Gray 1976). There is now, however, a current consensus favouring both their in vivo reality and their functional role in the storage and rapid, massive release of acetylcholine (Ceccarelli & Hurlbut 1980). It must be emphasized, however, that quantal release of neurotransmitter constitutes a minor proportion of the total liberated at the end-plate, the majority (possibly as much as 90%) being released in a non-quantal fashion (Katz & Miledi 1977). The synaptic vesicles are considered to originate either from recycled elements of the plasmalemma, or by continuous budding from the terminal network of the axonal smooth endoplasmic reticulum (Droz et al 1979). However formed, they subsequently accumulate acetylcholine by unknown mechanisms and pass to the presynaptic membrane under the influence either of Brownian motion (Katz 1969) or of positive directional forces associated with microtubules (Gray 1978). Nerve action potentials arising at the terminal induce changes in the calcium ion permeability of the presynaptic membrane, which activates the protein calmodulin (DeLorenzo et al 1979, Hooper and Kelly 1984) causing fusion of the synaptic vesicles with the axolemma in the regions of the active zones and release of their acetylcholine content into the extracellular space between the nerve and muscle membranes. Convincing evidence of stages in this process is seldom seen in fixed, sectioned preparations, possibly because efficient ejection of multiple quanta within a short time-span requires rapid integration of the synaptic vesicles into the presynaptic axolemma. Physiological evidence supporting the vesicular hypothesis of acetylcholine release at the neuromuscular synapse has been reviewed by Katz (1978) and Jones (1987).

Clark et al (1972) used the venom of the black widow spider to induce massive releases of acetylcholine quanta from the neuromuscular nerve terminal, and showed that this results in depletion of the vesicle content of the axon terminals and an increase in the area of the presynaptic cell membrane, consequent upon fusion of synaptic vesicles with the axolemma. The subsequent fate of this additional membrane material has been explored by Heuser & Reese (1973), among others, using the exogenous tracer, horseradish peroxidase, and they have shown that the excess membrane introduced into the axolemma by vesicle discharge is taken back into the terminals via coated vesicles. These form at any point around the terminal perimeter and then pass into the axoplasm, where they seem to fuse with elements of the smooth endoplasmic reticulum; it is possible, but not proved, that their components are thereafter re-utilized to form new synaptic vesicles. One effect of the presynaptically acting elapid snake venom toxins, e.g. β-bungarotoxin (Lassignal & Heuser 1977, Landon et al 1980) is to block some aspect of this uptake sequence; its application to either amphibian or mammalian neuromuscular junctions results in coated vesicles accumulating along the axolemma, free within the axoplasm, and adherent to the axonal smooth endoplasm reticulum.

Postsynaptic structures

The structure of the postsynaptic side of the neuromuscular junction has been briefly referred to above, and is illustrated in Figure 1.26. Acetylcholine released from the synaptic vesicles diffuses across the synaptic cleft and activates chemosensitive receptors situated on the infolded membranes of the postsynaptic muscle plasmalemma (Fertuk & Salpeter 1974, Barnard et al 1975). These receptors are molecular entities possessing both binding sites for acetylcholine and all of the other components necessary to generate the ion channels mediating the acetylcholine response, but are themselves electrically insensitive (Fambrough 1979). The evidence currently available suggests that the receptor is a pentameric integral membrane glycoprotein with an aggregate molecular weight of 275 kd. The four distinct constituent subunits have molecular weights calculated from amino acid sequences (Numa et al 1984), of 50116 (α), 53681, (β), 56279 (γ) and 57565 (δ), two of the α units combining with one each of the others to form a ring around a central pit or channel 1.5–2 nm in diameter (Ross et al 1977). The two α units appear not to be contiguous, and to be separated by the γ unit. Only the α subunits carry acetylcholine binding sites, but all four subunit types are required to make a functional ligand-gated ion channel; it is thought that the β unit may be selectively involved in receptor localization. The whole receptor complex is roughly cylindrical, having overall dimensions of 8×11 nm, with the long axes of the subunits (the central regions of which appear to be hydrophobic helices) spanning the postsynaptic membrane, to give extensive hydrophilic extracellular and cytoplasmic domains. Such a structural arrangement is well adapted to provide the protein-bounded aqueous channel for selective conduction of small cations necessary for its combined functions of receptor and ion-conductor. The biochemistry and molecular biology of the acetylcholine receptor have been reviewed by Karlin (1980), Conti-Tronconi & Raftery (1982) and Anderson (1987).

While it was at one time proposed that the acetylcholine receptors are dispersed uniformly across the entire extent of the postsynaptic muscle membrane covering the primary and secondary postsynaptic clefts of the sole-plate, there is now good evidence that they are restricted to the juxtaneural crests of the postsynaptic folds. The postsynaptically acting snake venom, α-bungarotoxin, has a potent and specific blocking effect on acetylcholine receptors and, when labelled with [125]I (Fambrough et al 1973) or conjugated to horseradish peroxidase (Lentz et al 1977), has been used to determine the ultrastructural localization of the receptors within the end-plate. Such experiments result in staining of the juxtaneural crests and adjacent outer 25% of the postsynaptic folds, the deeper parts of the fold being devoid of stainable receptors. Morphological studies of sectioned neuromuscular junctions prepared by conventional methods have shown that the muscle cell membrane covering the corresponding regions of the folds stains more densely, and appears thicker than that deep within the postsynaptic clefts; in very thin sections or lipid-extracted material, the juxtaneural membrane contains irregularly spaced densities of 11–14 nm diameter. Freeze–fracture preparations of mouse neuromuscular junctions have demonstrated rows of particles of similar size within the juxtaneural thickenings of the postsynaptic membrane. As these constitute the only major class of intramembrane particle within the juxtaneural muscle membrane, and are confined to areas that bind α-bungarotoxin, they are taken to represent the morphological equivalent of the functional acetylcholine receptor (Rash & Ellisman 1974). No differences have been detected in either the distribution or packing density of these particles (about 10 000/μm^2) in fast- and slow-twitch muscle neuromuscular junctions (Heuser & Salpeter 1979, Hirokawa & Heuser 1982), despite the obvious differences in their gross morphology, referred to earlier; their constant numbers and semi-regular arrangement have been ascribed to the stabilizing effect of a network of filaments and other electron-dense materials within the sub-plasmalemmal cytoplasm on the crests of the postjunctional folds which include 43-, 58- and 270-kDa proteins peculiar to this region (Rosenbluth 1974, Ellisman et al 1976, Couteaux 1981, Burden 1987).

A further component of the postjunctional system is the enzyme acetylcholinesterase, which is required to hydrolyse acetylcholine released from the nerve terminal and thus allow the rapid repolarization of the postsynaptic membrane. With a molecular weight of approximately 300 000, it is also a candidate for identification with some of the 11–14 nm intramembranous particles on the crests of the postjunctional folds, and close proximity of chemoreceptor and transmitter inactivator within the excitable membrane have obvious theoretical attractions. However, motor end-plates stained histochemically for acetylcholinesterase activity, or selectively labelled with radioisotopes and examined using quantitative electron-microscopic autoradiography (Salpeter 1967), consistently show that the reaction product is predominantly extracellular and extends throughout the postjunctional clefts; it is not restricted merely to the electron-dense portions of the postjunctional membrane at the juxtaneural crests of the folds. The reaction product is coarse and thus does not

allow precise localization (Fig. 1.25), but confirmatory evidence of the largely extracellular location of acetylcholinesterase has been obtained from enzyme digestion studies of motor end-plates, in which the basal lamina has been removed with collagenase, taking with it 50% of the end-plate acetylcholinesterase activity, of which 85% could be recovered enzymatically intact (Hall & Kelly 1971). Muscle fibres so treated show no significant alteration in either their basic electrical properties or the electron-microscopic appearance of the postsynaptic plasmalemma, and it is thus unlikely that the acetylcholinesterase removed had formed an integral component of the membrane. It is probable, therefore, that the active acetylcholinesterase molecules are bound to constituents of the basal lamina throughout the extent of the postjunctional cleft (McMahan et al 1978). The synthesis, processing, transport and location of the various molecular forms of acetylcholinesterase have been reviewed by Rotundo (1987).

The motor end-plate proper is surrounded by an electrically inexcitable perijunctional band, about 200–500 μm wide, that shows evidence of appreciable acetylcholine sensitivity. The concentration of receptors is, however, very much lower than that found at the postjunctional membrane of the end-plate itself, by at least three orders of magnitude, and the region contains no evident submembrane densities. At the edge of the perijunctional zone the fall-off in chemosensitivity is abrupt, but in most muscles so far examined a sparse scattering of extrajunctional receptors is detectable throughout the electrically excitable membrane which covers the remainder of the muscle cell surface. Extrajunctional receptors have been found to differ from end-plate receptors in a number of physical and pharmacological properties, and are considered to represent a distinct molecular species (Fambrough 1979). Denervation, experimental inactivation or disuse of skeletal muscle results in a rapid increase in acetylcholine sensitivity throughout the whole extent of the extrajunctional muscle cell plasmalemma. This increase in chemosensitivity is accompanied by a parallel increase in numbers of α-neurotoxin binding sites, indicating the appearance of additional receptor molecules. It is now clear that this increase is not caused by the release and spread of existing receptors from the postjunctional membrane, as the level of activity at the end-plate persists relatively unchanged for many days following denervation (Levitt-Gilmour and Salpeter 1986); it must therefore be ascribed to de novo synthesis of additional receptors, but it is not known whether these are in all respects identical to the extrajunctional receptors of normal muscle. Muscle activity induced artificially, either through the motor nerve or by direct stimulation of the muscle (Lömo & Westgaard 1975), inhibits or reverses increases in extrajunctional acetylcholine sensitivity, and thus appears to have a direct inhibitory effect on receptor biosynthesis. Factors concerned in the synthesis and turnover of acetylcholine receptors have been reviewed by Salpeter (1987).

Motor end-plate development

The first histological evidence of innervation of the proximal limb muscles in the human fetus can be found at, or slightly before, the 10th week of gestation (Tello 1917, Cuajunco 1942), although patches of acetylcholinesterase activity have been reported to occur on human myotubes from as early as the eighth week. The entering nerve fibres ramify among the myotubes of the primordial muscle and end as simple knob-like terminals on their central regions. Electron microscopy has shown that these endings consist of simple rounded axon terminals that abut against apparently unmodified areas of the muscle plasmalemma and its overlying basal lamina. The nerves supplying these endings consist of bundles of fine unmyelinated axons, ensheathed as a group by accompanying Schwann cells; they subsequently acquire individual Schwann-cell sheaths but remain unmyelinated until after the 16th week (Fidzianska 1971). The nerve terminals become thicker and more branched with further development, assuming a compact, plate-like structure within a raised sole-plate, but do not attain their fully mature form until a few months after birth.

Fine structural studies of rat muscle have provided a more detailed picture of the process of end-plate formation. Unequivocal evidence of developing neuromuscular junctions can be found at the 18th day of gestation in both intercostal

muscles (Teravainen 1968, Kelly & Zacks 1969b) and the medial gastrocnemius (Landon, unpublished observations); the occurrence of these contacts coincides with the first appearance of localized acetylcholinesterase activity (Kelly & Zacks 1969b). Small areas of close membrane contact between developing neurites and myotubes, without intervention of a basal lamina or apparent postjunctional specialization, have been reported to occur 2 days earlier (Kelly & Zacks 1969b) but it is not clear what relationship these bear to the 18-day junctions, as similar close contacts can also be found between neurites and other cell types at this stage of development. Slender bundles of fine unmyelinated axons, enclosed within a common Schwann-cell sheath, end as small bulbous terminals containing 45–50 nm clear vesicles and small mitochondria, in close proximity to the surfaces of the larger myotubes. Patchy increases in the density of contiguous portions of the myotube plasmalemma, thickening of the interposed basal lamina with remodelling of its constituents (Anderson 1986), and the presence of aggregations of mitochondria and other cell organelles in the subjacent sarcoplasm, signal the first appearance of the sole-plate (Fig. 1.27). These changes are accompanied by the first appearance of clusters of acetylcholine receptors. Peripheral sole-plate nuclei and the first shallow postjunctional folds have appeared by birth (Fig. 1.28); by the 10th–14th postnatal days the terminal branches of the axon have become segregated into individual grooves in the sole-plate, and the postjunctional folds approximate to their adult condition in number, extent and degree of branching. The development of the motor end-plate has been reviewed by Bennett (1983).

The constant and restricted anatomical situation of the motor end-plate zone of a mature muscle is explicable in terms of its ontogeny. Initial nerve–muscle contacts occur at a developmental stage at which the myotubes are only some 300–400 μm long, and possess a surface membrane evenly supplied with acetylcholine receptors and uniformly receptive to innervation. The establishment of a neuromuscular synapse at any point on such a myotube results in the remainder of the cell membrane becoming refractory to further attempts at innervation, and restriction of the incorporation

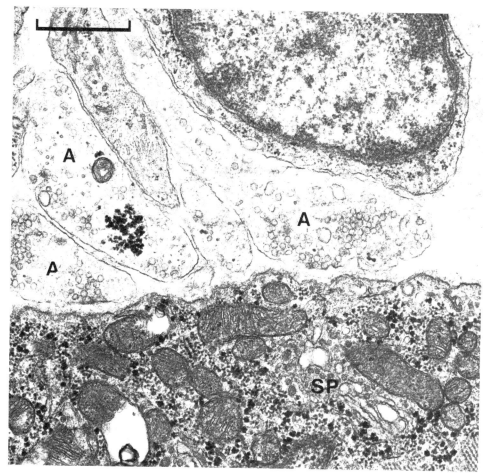

Fig. 1.27   An early stage in the development of a neuromuscular junction in m. gastrocnemius of a fetal rat. A cluster of axon terminals (A), containing collections of clear vesicles, make contact with a primitive sole-plate (SP) lacking postsynaptic folds. Scale bar = 1 μm

of further acetylcholine receptor molecules to the synaptic region (Bennett & Pettigrew 1975). Subsequent growth in length of the two ends of the myotube/myofibre will take place within this context of established central innervation, only the tips of the fibre retaining traces of the early generalized distribution of acetylcholine receptors and acetylcholinesterase activity. The end-plate zone of the mature muscle thus defines the site and extent of the original myotubes at the period at which they became innervated. Subsequent generations of myotubes develop in association with the central, most differentiated portions of their more mature neighbours, and show a similar

gradation of maturation from their centres to their poles (see earlier section; Kelly & Zacks 1969a, Landon 1970a, 1971). They also first become sufficiently differentiated to be receptive to innervation in their central regions, and these lie within the already established end-plate zone of the muscle.

Polyneuronal innervation

While it is clear that, in mammalian muscle, only one end-plate develops on each myotube during normal ontogeny in vivo (Lubinska & Zelená 1966, Bennett & Pettigrew 1974), it has recently

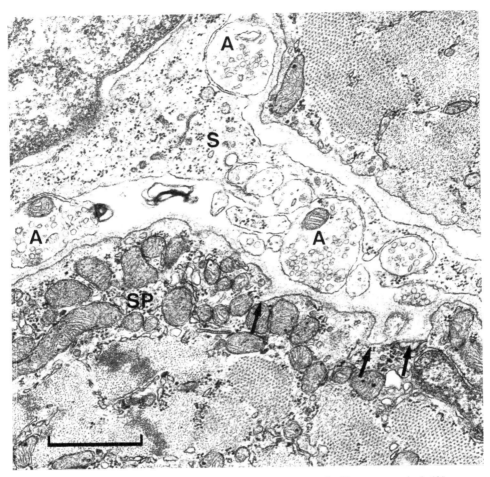

Fig. 1.28   A later stage of motor end-plate development in early postnatal rat muscle. The axon terminals (A) are more numerous and are scattered over a wider area on the surface of the developing sole-plate (SP), which possesses a few rudimentary postsynaptic clefts (arrows). The axon terminals are covered on their external surfaces by Schwann cell processes (S). Scale bar = 1 μm

become apparent from both physiological (Redfern 1970) and anatomical studies (Bennett & Pettigrew 1974) that, for a period during development, each of these single end-plates normally receives transient simultaneous innervation by terminals from several different neurones. Up to five or six independent neurites may be found converging upon any individual end-plate in both cat and rat muscle at birth, but an abrupt decline in this polyneuronal innervation occurs after the 10th postnatal day, and only a single input remains by day 16 (Brown et al 1976). This loss of innervation seems to be the result of a controlled withdrawal of axon sprouts by all of the participating neurones without occasioning denervation of any myotube,

one of the original simple bulbous endings developing a complex terminal aborization while the others regress (Riley 1977, O'Brien et al 1978, Bixby 1981). No fine structural evidence of axon terminal degeneration has been found to account for this loss of synaptic input (Korneliussen & Jansen 1976, Riley 1981), and it is assumed that the redundant primitive terminals, and the neurites from which they originate, retract and are absorbed into their parent axons. Reduction in muscle activity by nerve blockade or tenotomy has been shown to prolong the phase of polyneuronal innervation (Benoit & Changeux 1975, Thompson et al 1979, Brown et al 1982); conversely, the achievement of mononeuronal innervation is accelerated by enhanced activity, either natural or artificially induced (O'Brien et al 1978, Zelena et al 1979). This phenomenon has attracted much attention in recent years and has been reviewed by van Essen (1982), Hopkins and Brown (1984) and Betz (1987).

Dispersion of the motor unit

The apparently non-random dispersion of the component myofibres of one motor unit (Willison 1980) among a population innervated by other neurones has been referred to above, but the mechanism by which this arrangement is achieved during ontogeny remains a matter for speculation. One possible explanation lies in the observation that functional innervation of mammalian muscle begins at an early stage of its development, and precedes the appearance of the full complement of myofibres. Successive generations of myotubes (Kelly & Zacks 1969a, Landon 1970a, 1971) become available for innervation as muscle fibre numbers increase. Because each develops in close physical association with a myotube belonging to one of the preceding generations, these are dispersed between neighbouring myotubes and myofibres at different stages of development. Ingrowing motor axons, whose entry into the muscle is spread over a considerable period of embryogenesis (Weiss 1941), therefore encounter myotubes in a spectrum of developmental stages and degrees of prior innervation, and only some may be in a suitable state to accept innervation. Such asynchronous innervation of fibres that will be adjacent in the mature muscle may ensure the dispersal of the myofibres of any individual motor unit throughout a relatively large volume of other muscle fibres (Lubinska, quoted by Engel 1970, Kelly & Schotland 1972).

Transient polyneuronal innervation may provide a mechanism by which this simple, hierarchic dispersal of motor nerve terminals can be modified, possibly profoundly, but the factors that determine which endings are retained and which rejected at any one end-plate are obscure. Each motor neurone seems to have a normal upper limit to the numbers of myofibres it can innervate in fully differentiated muscle (Jansen et al 1975), a ratio that is temporarily increased five-fold during the

phase of polyneuronal innervation; it is possible that selection of which terminals should survive may depend upon gradients of maturity of central connections and functional activity within the motor neurone pool. Alternatively, selection may be peripheral and governed by local competition between axon terminals for some essential trophic connection with the myofibres, or by differential susceptibility to the metabolic consequences of contractile activity (Vrbova et al 1988). These phenomena offer a fertile field for future experiment.

Sensory innervation of muscle

The afferent elements of the muscle nerves have their cell bodies in the dorsal spinal root or cranial root ganglia. The sensory ganglion cells are divisible into two classes — small darkly staining cells and larger pale cells — and these are believed to give rise to unmyelinated and myelinated peripheral processes respectively (Lieberman 1976). The afferent nerve fibres have been divided into four groups (Lloyd 1943) denoted by the Roman numerals I–IV, of which I–III represent the three peaks of the trimodal myelinated afferent fibre-diameter spectrum, and group IV the non-myelinated afferents. Group I contains the largest fibres (12–20 μm diameter) and comprises the Ia afferents from the muscle spindles and Ib tendon-organ afferents (Fig. 1.29). Group II (6–12 μm diameter) contains the secondary terminal afferents from muscle spindles and some fibres from Pacinian corpuscles, and group III (1–6 μm diameter) the afferents from the smaller paciniform and unencapsulated 'free' endings. The non-myelinated group IV axons terminate as free endings in the interstitial connective tissues and are the most numerous component, contributing two-thirds of the total sensory innervation (Stacey 1969). The experimental evidence and methods of study that substantiate this classification are reviewed by Barker (1974).

Muscle spindles

Muscle spindles are collections of a few small-diameter muscle fibres enclosed within a cellular and connective tissue capsule, the swollen centre and tapering ends of which give the spindle its name (Fig. 1.29). Essentially similar structures can be found throughout the skeletal musculature of terrestrial and amphibious vertebrates; the few exceptions to this generalization are either cranial muscles or those which do not move joints. Spindles were originally considered to be sites of pathological change, or embryonic 'rests' of immature myotubes, but their consistent association with intramuscular nerve fascicles led Kerschner (1888) to propose that they might be complicated end-organs serving muscular sense. This supposition was confirmed by the observations of Ruffini (1898) upon the complex nerve-terminal ramifications around the central (equatorial) regions of the spindle muscle fibres, and the demonstration by Sherrington (1894) that these endings were of sensory origin. Numerous subsequent studies of the anatomy of muscle spindles (Barker 1948, Boyd 1962, Cooper & Daniel 1963, Barker et al 1970) reviewed by Barker (1974), and studies of their function (Matthews 1933, Leksell 1945, Cooper 1961, Matthews 1964, Granit 1970, Boyd 1976), have established that these organs act as length–tension receptors in parallel with the extrafusal myofibres comprising the bulk of the muscle, and that the properties of the central sensory region can be modulated by the contractile activity of the poles of the small intrafusal muscle fibres. The latter are under efferent nervous control largely independent of the supply to the extrafusal fibres, providing a dimension of freedom that enables the spindle to play an important part in the servo-assistance mechanisms believed to govern integrated muscular activity (see reviews by Matthews 1972, 1977).

The density of supply of muscle spindles differs in different muscle groups within the body, the ratio of spindles to extrafusal muscles being greater in the axial musculature of the trunk and in distal limb muscles than in those of the limb girdles. The very rich supply of spindles in the intrinsic muscles of the hand, the rotator muscles of the limbs and the short suboccipital muscles, suggests an association between spindle density and refinement of movement, a suggestion in agreement with the proposal by Cooper (1966) that the numbers of spindles within a muscle are directly proportional to those of its constituent motor units.

Muscle spindles are not uniformly distributed throughout the mass of extrafusal fibres in most muscles, and tend to lie predominantly within the deeper or more axial zones, richest in type 1 and type 2A oxidative extrafusal fibres (Yellin 1969); this association with the parts of the muscles most involved in sustained postural activity may well be of functional importance.

The capsule and connective tissue

The capsule of the muscle spindle represents an extension of the perineurium enclosing the nerve fibres that innervate the equatorial regions of the intrafusal muscle fibres. It is about 200 μm in diameter at its mid-point and 3–4 mm long overall. It consists of 9–15 or more layers of flattened pavement epithelia-like cells, tightly adherent at their contiguous edges, and separated one from another by thin interposed layers of fine collagen fibrils. The numbers of layers of cells diminish progressively towards the poles of the spindle until reduced to a tube one cell thick, from the ends of which some intrafusal fibres project into the general endomysial connective tissue space. The capsule has been shown to be an active and selective diffusion barrier (Alexeev 1976, Hunt et al 1978), and to be more permeable to intravascular high-molecular-weight tracers at the poles than at the equator (Dow et al 1980). As the intrafusal fibres traverse the dilated central zone of the capsule they are further enclosed by an attenuated inner 'axial sheath' (Fig. 1.30), first described by Sherrington (1894). The space between this inner investment and the main capsule is filled by a fluid with a high content of hyaluronic acid (von Brzezinski 1962). The claim (Sherrington 1894), that this 'lymph space' is in direct communication with the regional lymphatic system, has never been confirmed; from the standpoint of fluid mechanics, it is more probably a closed system, the osmotic activity of its high-molecular-weight content serving to maintain a positive turgor within the capsule. The distended equatorial region of the capsule and its enclosed fluid contents may insulate the sensitive central regions of the intrafusal fibres from mechanical stresses other than those delivered by tension along their long axes. Distension of the subcapsular

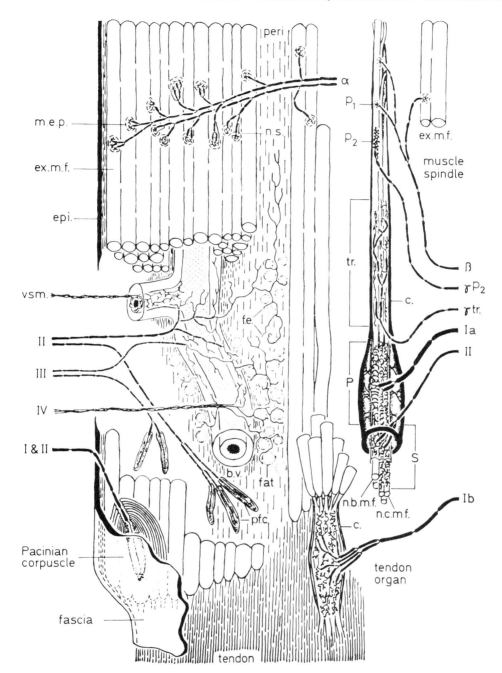

Fig. 1.29   A diagram summarizing the motor and sensory innervation of mammalian striated muscle and its associated connective tissue. Nerve fibres on the right-hand side are exclusively concerned with muscle innervation: those on the left innervate other tissues also. Roman numerals refer to groups of myelinated (I, II, III) and non-myelinated (IV) sensory fibres; Greek letters refer to motor fibres. The spindle pole is cut short to about half its length, the extracapsular portion being omitted, (b.v.) blood vessel; (c) capsule; (epi.) epimysium; (ex.m.f.) extrafusal muscle fibres; (f.e.) free endings; (n.b.m.f.) nuclear-bag muscle fibre; (n.c.m.f.) nuclear-chain muscle fibre; (n.s.) nodal sprout; (m.e.p.) motor end-plate; (P) primary ending; (p₁,p₂) two types of intrafusal end-plates; (peri.) perimysium; (pf.c.) paciniform corpuscle, (S) secondary ending; (t.r.) trail ending; (vsm.) vasomotor fibres. (From Barker 1974, by kind permission of the author and publishers)

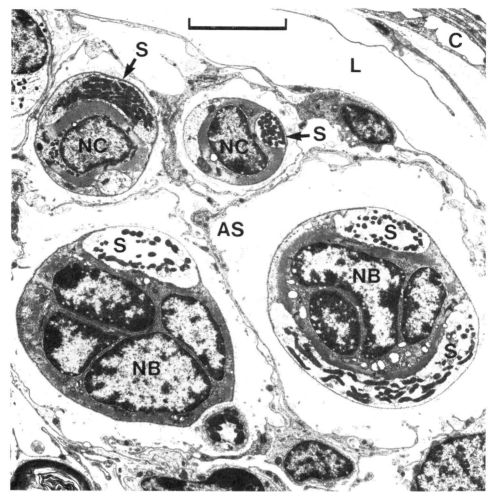

Fig. 1.30   A transverse section through the equatorial regions of a neuromuscular spindle from a mouse hind-limb muscle. Two nuclear bag (NB) and two nuclear chain (NC) intrafusal fibres are visible, each enwrapped by sensory nerve terminals (S). They lie within individual compartments of the axial sheath (AS), itself lying within the 'lymph' space (L) bounded by the multilamellar capsule (C). (Preparation kindly supplied by Dr L. Quieroz, Institute of Neurology, London) Scale bar = 5 μm

space and thickening of the capsule wall may occur in several muscle and neuromuscular diseases (Cazzato & Walton 1968, Swash Ch. 19, this volume).

The collagenous connective tissue of the capsule, and the fine reticulin coverings of the intrafusal fibres, are augmented by elastin, an otherwise inconspicuous component of skeletal muscle (Cooper & Daniel 1963, Landon 1966, Cooper & Gladden 1974). Longitudinal networks of elastin fibres surround the nuclear bag fibres; these are thickest and most elaborate within the poles of the

capsule and over the extracapsular portions of the intrafusal fibres, and are more sparsely distributed over the bags at the equator. It has been reported that nuclear bag fibres innervated by 'static' γ-efferent fibres (see below) possess a more substantial network of elastin filaments than those innervated by 'dynamic' fibres, and that these filaments continue into the extrafusal connective tissue as a substantial elastic tendon (Gladden 1976). Relatively few elastic fibres are found around nuclear chain fibres, and are concentrated in their equatorial regions. Granit (1970) has suggested that the elastin component of the spindle may have a significant role in assisting its elastic recoil on release from tension, and may provide an important parallel elastic component to the intrafusal fibres during stretch.

Blood supply

Capillaries can be found coursing between the layers of the capsule wall in most spindles. In some species, including man, the cat and the rabbit, these may penetrate into the subcapsular space and travel for some distance close to the axial bundle of intrafusal fibres (Cooper & Daniel 1963, Corvaja et al 1969, Barker 1974). It has been shown that, in the rabbit, these vessels constitute a separate and exclusive micro-circulation to the spindles (Miyoshi & Kennedy 1979). Furthermore, the endothelial cells of the intracapsular capillaries differ from those in the rest of the muscle in having a few pinocytotic vesicles, and tight junctions impermeable to horseradish peroxidase (Kennedy & Yoon 1979). Thus in most respects they more closely resemble the endoneurial capillaries of peripheral nerves (Miyoshi et al 1979) than the capillaries of extrafusal muscle, emphasizing the essentially endoneurial character of the intracapsular space.

Intrafusal myofibres

In most spindles, 3–14 or more intrafusal fibres are contained within a single capsule, but tandem spindles can occur in which two longitudinally aligned capsules share some intrafusal fibres in common, each capsule being associated with a zone of sensory innervation. Spindles in small muscles generally contain fewer intrafusal fibres than those in larger limb muscles, and small animals have fewer intrafusal fibres in their spindles than large animals. The intrafusal fibres themselves are usually 10–20 μm in diameter and, in most mammals, are readily distinguishable into two morphological classes — nuclear bag fibres and nuclear chain fibres (Boyd 1962, Cooper & Daniel 1963). The former are the larger, being at least twice the diameter of the nuclear chain fibres, and are consistently longer, usually extending for several millimetres into the body of the

muscle beyond the polar ends of the capsule. Their principal distinguishing feature is replacement of the myofibrils in the equatorial regions by massed myonuclei — hence the term 'nuclear bag' (Fig. 1.30). The two ends of this zone are continuous with a myotube region, in which longitudinal chains of central nuclei are surrounded by a continuous shell of myofilaments; more polar still, the nuclei decrease in frequency and adopt a coventional subplasmalemmal site. Not all of the myofibrils are lost over the nuclear bag region, longitudinal continuity between the two contractile poles being maintained by a few slender myofibrils that span the bag (Cooper & Daniel 1963, Landon 1966, 1974). Nuclear chain fibres are always of smaller diameter than nuclear bag fibres (approximately 10 μm), are usually coextensive with the capsule, and contain a central chain of elongated nuclei surrounded by an unbroken shell of myofibrils. As in the nuclear bag fibres, the central nuclei of the chain fibre give way to more sparsely distributed subplasmalemmal nuclei in the polar regions. Chain fibres normally outnumber bag fibres by a ratio of about two to one. Myosatellite cells are often found in association with the polar intracapsular regions of both bag and chain fibres (Landon 1966).

Histochemistry

Histochemical studies in man and in many other animal species have demonstrated the existence of either two (Henneman & Olson 1964, Nyström 1967, Spiro & Beilin 1969) or three (Ogata & Mori 1964, Wirsén & Larsson 1964, Yellin 1969) distinct classes of intrafusal fibre. Subsequent use of the Guth & Samaha (1970) technique to demonstrate actomyosin ATPase after acid or alkaline preincubation (James 1971, Ovalle & Smith 1972, Harriman et al 1975) has confirmed the validity of a division of intrafusal fibres into three types, namely nuclear chain fibres and two varieties of nuclear bag fibre. Ovalle & Smith (1972) termed the two types of nuclear bag fibre 'bag 1' and 'bag 2' and showed that, while the first contained moderate quantities of only the acid-stable, alkaline-labile form of ATPase, 'bag 2' fibres contained ATPase that was stable under both acid and alkaline conditions; with acid preincubation, 'bag

2' fibres always stained more heavily than 'bag 1' fibres. Bag 2 intrafusal fibres are usually grouped with the chain fibres in cat spindles, leaving the bag 1 fibres relatively isolated (Butler 1980, Milburn 1984). Nuclear chain fibres contained substantial quantities of only the acid-labile, alkaline-stable form of ATPase (see Table 1.3). Harriman et al (1975) reported variable quantities of acid-stable ATPase in the polar regions of chain fibres, but otherwise agreed with the findings of Ovalle & Smith (1972). The activities of both phosphorylase and succinic dehydrogenase have been found to be lowest in the larger bag fibres (bag 1) and highest in the chain fibres, with the smaller bag fibres (bag 2) having variable intermediate properties (Yellin 1969). Other oxidative

enzymes (e.g. NADH) are present in high concentrations throughout all three classes of intrafusal fibre (Harriman et al 1975). Immunocytochemical studies of muscle spindles, using antibodies against myosin heavy-chain isoenzymes and M-band proteins, have introduced additional complexities into the classification of intrafusal fibres (Eriksson and Thornell 1990). In human spindles dynamic bag 1 and static bag 2 fibres in general react with all myosin isoenzymes (embryonic, neonatal, slow-twitch, fast-twitch and slow tonic), and with all M-band antibodies apart from anti-M-protein which only stains local sites along bag 1 fibres. Nuclear chain fibres react strongly for all antibodies except for slow-twitch and slow-tonic isoenzymes. The slow-tonic isoenzyme is expressed

Table 1.3 Summary of mammalian intrafusal myofibre characteristics

Characteristics	Intrafusal myofibre type		
	Bag 1 (slow, dynamic)	Bag 2 (fast, static)	Chain (fast, static)
Structure			
Central nucleation	Bag	Bag	Chain
Length	Extend well beyond limits of capsule		Approx, coextensive with capsule
Diameter:			
Intracapsular	12–23 mm	10–16 mm	4–13 mm
Polar	14–20 mm	10–16 mm	7–12 mm
Associated elastin	Moderate; poles > equator	Substantial; poles + extracapsular tendon	scanty; equator > poles
Mitochondria	Few, small	Few, intermediate	Numerous, large
Sarcoplasmic reticulum	Inconspicuous	Moderate	Abundant
M line:			
Equator	Absent	Faint, double	Present
Poles	Present (except rat)	Present	Present
Innervation			
Sensory	Primaries, Group Ia, predominate		Secondaries, Group II predominate
Motor″	β and γ dynamic (γ static?)	γ static	γ static (β static?)
Histochemistry			
Oxidative enzymes	Moderate/high	Moderate/high	High
ATPase, pH 9.4	Low	Intermediate	High
pH 4.35	Intermediate	High	Low
Phosphorylase	Low	Intermediate	High
PAS	Low/moderate	Moderate	Moderate/high
Functional properties			
Afferent response to stretch	Dynamic	Static	Static
Contraction speed	Slow	Fast	Fast
Development			
Order of appearance of intrafusal myofibres	Second (first?)″	First (second?)″	Last

″See text.

early in development and is claimed to be a reliable marker for developing bag fibres (Thornell and Pedrosa 1990).

Fine structure

The histological and histochemical differences between the various classes of intrafusal fibres are reflected in their fine structure (Landon 1966, Corvaja et al 1969, Banker & Girvin 1971, Ovalle 1971, 1972). Nuclear chain fibres most closely resemble slow-twitch type 1 extrafusal fibres. Their myofibrils have the appearance of discrete units in transverse section and are surrounded by substantial amounts of sarcoplasm rich in sarcoplasmic reticulum, glycogen and large mitochondria. Sarcotubular triads and pentads are numerous and the centre of each A band is marked by a distinct M line. In 'typical' nuclear bag fibres (Barker & Stacey 1970), i.e. bag 1 fibres, the proportions of sarcoplasm and its contained organelles are much reduced, with the consequence that the mass of myofilaments lacks clear-cut separation into myofibrils, merging together into a more or less continuous 'felden struktur'. The mitochondria are fewer in number and smaller, the sarcotubular contacts take the form of dyads or triads and are sparsely distributed, and the M line is either absent (Landon 1966), or replaced by a pair of faint parallel densities (Ovalle 1971, 1972, Banks et al 1977). In the nuclear bag region the myofilaments are greatly reduced in number, but a few persist in the form of slender myofibrils and provide tenuous longitudinal continuity between the more substantial mass of myofilaments of the myotube regions flanking the central bag. The 'intermediate' or bag 2 fibres vary in their fine structure in different species, but in general more closely resemble nuclear chain fibres than the 'typical' bag 1 fibre. The myofibrils are better defined than in the latter, the sarcoplasmic reticulum and sarcotubular junctions are more abundant, the mitochondria larger and more frequent, and the sarcomeres possess a well-defined M line throughout the longitudinal extent of the fibre. Leptomeres (q.v.) occur relatively frequently in all types of intrafusal fibre in most of the animal species examined (Gruner 1961, Landon 1966, Corvaja et al 1969, Ovalle 1972). The major

structural, histochemical and functional characteristics of mammalian intrafusal fibres are summarized in Table 1.3. Minor deviations from the pattern described occur in several species, and some of these have been reviewed by Barker (1974) and Barker et al (1976a). Areas of close contact have been observed by electron microscopy between adjacent nuclear chain fibres in cat spindles (Corvaja et al 1967, Adal 1969, Butler 1980) and similar contacts are also to be found in rat and man; the phenomenon is of unknown functional significance, but may be responsible for reports, based on light microscopy, that intrafusal fibres split or branch. At their ends, within the polar regions of the spindle capsule, the nuclear chain fibres break up into short tails within local aggregations of connective tissue at the surface of an adjacent nuclear bag fibre or the inner wall of the capsule. Such insertions provide the mechanism by which tension within the muscle may be transmitted to the nuclear chain fibres, enclosed as they are within the capsule, and may also furnish the means by which contraction of the nuclear chain fibres unloads the central regions of the nuclear bag fibres with which they lie in parallel (Cooper 1961, Boyd 1976).

Sensory innervation

The nuclear bag and chain regions of the intrafusal fibres are closely related to the terminals of sensory nerves, arising from neurones in the spinal or cranial root ganglia. These are of two varieties and are distinguishable by their morphology and the calibre of their parent axons. Large-diameter group Ia afferents enter the equator of the spindle and divide beyond the last node of Ranvier, by way of two or more dichotomous divisions, into a number of stout, non-myelinated branches. These end by enwrapping the central bag or chain zones of the intrafusal fibres in a semi-regular annulospiral fashion, to constitute the so-called 'primary' sensory endings (Fig. 1.30). Other smaller-diameter afferent group II fibres accompany the large Ia fibres into the subcapsular space, and then pass to the para-equatorial regions to either side of the zone innervated by the primary annulospiral terminal, where they lose their myelin sheaths and end as short irregular annulospiral terminals or fine arborescences—the latter being the 'flower sprays' of Ruffini (1898). The majority of these 'secondary' endings are located on the nuclear chain fibres, with only occasional branches passing to the nuclear bag fibres.

The primary nerve terminals lack a Schwann cell covering and are closely applied to the surface of the bag and myotube regions of the intrafusal myofibres, lying beneath the basal lamina in a trough or gutter on their surface. On the nuclear bag fibres the edges of this trough are frequently prolonged into sarcoplasmic 'lips' partly enclosing the external aspect of the nerve terminal (Landon 1966, Adal 1969, Corvaja et al 1969). The fine structure of the axoplasm within the sensory ending differs from that of its parent axon in a manner similar to that seen in other mechanoreceptors, consisting of fluffy amorphous electron-dense material containing a few centrally placed bundles of neurofilaments and neurotubules, and large numbers of small mitochondria and small clear vesicles, 20–100 nm diameter. Such sensory nerve contacts also differ from motor nerve terminals in their lack of an intervening layer of basal lamina between the contiguous nerve and muscle cell membranes, and the absence of any recognizable subneural apparatus, the only organized inter-cellular contacts being limited to occasional maculae adhaerentes. The secondary sensory terminals have a similarly close relationship to the surfaces of the nuclear chain fibres, but have no deep troughs for their reception on the intrafusal fibres; the axoplasm of the major coils and bulbs of these endings has a similar fine structure to that described in the primary terminals (Corvaja et al 1969). The connecting stalks of the 'flower sprays' resemble slender non-myelinated nerve fibres, containing neurotubules, neurofilaments and occasional small mitochondria and vesicles, both empty and dense-cored (Landon 1974). The morphological features described above suggest that the sensory nerve terminal is a distinct entity, with biophysical properties that differ from those of its parent axon, and that it is securely tethered to the surface of the intrafusal fibres and must therefore comply with changes in the longitudinal and radial dimensions of the regions in which it lies during applied stretch or intrafusal fibre contraction.

Motor innervation

The details of the connections and functional properties of the motor innervation of mammalian muscle spindles have long been a source of controversy (Boyd 1962, Barker et al 1970, Matthews 1972, Barker 1974). It is now established, however, that intrafusal efferent nerves are derived from two distinct sources; small-diameter branches of β-efferent axons, most of whose terminals supply slow-twitch extrafusal fibres, and small-diameter γ-efferent axons with an exclusively intrafusal distribution (Fig. 1.29). The β-terminals seem to be situated solely on nuclear bag fibres, ending as compact neuromuscular synapses with nucleated sole-plates, the 'p₁' plates of Barker (1967), that differ little from extrafusal motor end-plates (Barker et al 1980). The γ-fibres, on the other hand, are distributed to all classes of intrafusal fibre and end in two types of terminal, clearly distinguishable in metal-impregnated light-microscopic preparations. These take the form either of large patches of knob-like nerve endings without any obvious underlying sole-plate, or of fine, diffuse thread-like endings—the 'p₂' plates and 'trail' endings respectively of Barker (1967); p₂ plates can supply either bag or chain fibres but the bag fibre supply generally predominates. Branched fibres leading to p₂ plates on both bag and chain fibres have also been reported (Barker et al 1970). Trail endings often supply both bag and chain fibres within any individual spindle or, less frequently, either type separately. They are characterized by a mainly juxta-equatorial position, extensive ramifying terminals, and the common occurrence of long unmyelinated preterminal axons. Each of these classes of efferent ending was once claimed to have a distinctive and characteristic fine structure; p₁ terminals possessed sole-plates well provided with deep branched post-synaptic folds; p₂ plates had shallow sole-plates with short wide unbranched folds; while trail endings showed no evidence of postsynaptic specialization (Adal & Barker 1967, Barker et al 1970). Later studies have demonstrated that such features do not provide a reliable basis upon which to identify intrafusal motor terminals; smooth and folded postsynaptic membranes can occur in all classes of terminal and on each kind of intrafusal fibre

(Barker et al 1978). The motor innervation of adult rat spindles has been described by Walro and Kucera (1985).

Afferent response, efferent innervation and intrafusal fibre type

The muscle spindle is a stretch receptor of great sensitivity, capable of responding both to change in length and to rate of change in length, the velocity sensitivity of the sensory ending being signalled by an increasing rate of afferent discharge with increasing velocity of stretch (Matthews 1933). Much of this velocity sensitivity, the 'dynamic' component, is contributed by the primary sensory ending; the secondaries are largely insensitive to velocity and produce only a 'static' response to change in muscle length (Cooper 1961, Matthews 1964). As the secondary endings are largely confined to the nuclear chain fibres, the dynamic component of the afferent response has been attributed to the nuclear bag fibre and ascribed, by analogy with the properties of slowly contracting extrafusal fibres, to its supposedly greater 'viscosity' when stretched (Matthews 1964, 1972). The constituent nerve fibres of the efferent innervation to the muscle spindle have also been shown to have either dynamic or static characteristics, according to the effect of their stimulation on the afferent discharge generated in response to a simple 'ramp' stretch. Both kinds of γ-efferent excite the primary ending under isometric conditions, but whereas dynamic efferent fibres increase the velocity response at the beginning and end of the applied stretch, the static efferents reduce the velocity response and enhance the primary discharge at the new sustained length (Crowe & Matthews 1964). Where one fusimotor nerve fibre branches to supply two or more spindles it induces the same dynamic or static effect on the primary afferent discharge of each, indicating that the effect is either a specific property of that nerve fibre, or that each efferent is exclusively distributed to a functionally distinct class of intrafusal myofibre. The latter view has provided the basis for the model of spindle innervation and function proposed by Boyd (1962), and elaborated by Matthews (1964, 1972), in which two types of intrafusal myofibre, nuclear bag and nuclear chain, are

separately innervated by dynamic and static γ-efferents respectively, the β-efferents to the nuclear bag fibres providing a second, purely dynamic, component.

While this scheme has provided a useful working hypothesis, it could not be reconciled initially with the complex spindle 'wiring systems' described by Barker and his colleagues in a number of species (Barker 1974), or with the unequivocal physiological evidence of static γ-efferent innervation of nuclear bag fibres (Brown & Butler 1973, Barker et al 1976b). These difficulties have now been resolved by the discovery that there are two distinct varieties of nuclear bag fibre, with different mechanical characteristics and independent innervation. Dynamic fusimotor axons always innervate bag 1 fibres while static axons innervate bag 2 or chain fibres, or both together (Boyd 1976, Boyd et al 1977, Emonet-Dénand et al 1977, Laporte 1978). The primary sensory terminals on the bag 1 fibres therefore mediate the dynamic component of the primary afferent response, while those on the bag 2 and chain fibres are responsible for static sensitivity. Some degree of overlap of primary afferent innervation between dynamic and static intrafusal fibres has been observed in the rat (Diwan and Milburn 1986, Walro and Kucera 1985, 1988), and in fusimotor innervation in monkeys and man (Kucera 1985, 1986), but not to an extent that would invalidate the basic pattern described above.

Development

Histological studies in man (Cuajunco 1927, 1940) and other species (Tello 1917, Zelená 1957, 1959, Marchand & Eldred 1969) have shown that recognizable neuromuscular spindles are present in striated muscles from an early stage of development. The primary afferent axons are among the first nerve fibres to enter the growing muscle; in the rat (Zelená 1957, 1959) these have made contact with myotubes adjacent to the neurovascular axis of the muscle by the 17th and 18th days of gestation. Initially, only one or two intrafusal myotubes are visible within the developing capsule, but their numbers increase with subsequent development, four or five being present a week after birth. The primary sensory terminals at first consist of only incomplete turns and short spiral sections, but when the subcapsular space appears, 2–3 weeks after birth, the ending has achieved its mature annulospiral form. Development of the fusimotor innervation lags behind that of the primary afferent system and is not detectable until the first or second postnatal day.

Fine structural studies of developing rat muscle (Landon 1972, Milburn 1973) have shown that initial simple contacts between large unmyelinated intramuscular nerve terminals and apparently undifferentiated single myotubes, at 18–19 days' gestation, lead to encirclement of the myotube by the nerve terminal and the concurrent extension of the nerve sheath to form a unilamellar capsule around the innervated region. Subsequent proliferation and fusion of satellite myoblasts associated with the innervated myotube give rise to a succession of further, intracapsular myotubes, in a manner similar to that which occurs in extrafusal myogenesis (Kelly & Zacks 1969a, Landon 1970a, 1971). At birth, the original myotube and its next-formed companion have developed nuclear bags, and a subsequent generation of smaller-diameter nuclear chain myotubes has appeared by the third postnatal day. The young intrafusal fibres remain in a tightly packed bundle, locked together by filipodial extensions of their superficial cytoplasm, until 3–6 days after birth, the sensory nerve terminal enwrapping the external surface of the entire bundle (Fig. 1.31). Lateral separation of the individual intrafusal fibres during the second postnatal week is accompanied by their acquisition of individual sensory innervation, the development of an axial sheath distinct from the multilamellar capsule, and the first appearance of a distinct subcapsular space. A similar developmental sequence has been described in the spindles of the cat by Butler (1980) and Milburn (1984). Earlier suggestions that the intrafusal fibres proliferate by splitting (Cuajunco 1927, Marchand & Eldred 1969), or by the incorporation of additional extrafusal myotubes within the capsule (Cuajunco 1940) are explained by this late separation of the full complement of bag and chain fibres. Little information is available concerning the development of the fusimotor innervation to the spindle, but small intracapsular neuromuscular junctions of simple morphology have been reported at 1 hour

(Milburn 1973) and 12 hours (Landon 1972) after birth, in the rat, and between the 41st and 43rd days of fetal life in the cat (Barker and Milburn 1981).

While it has been shown that nuclear bag fibres differentiate before nuclear chain fibres during the development of the spindle (Cuajunco 1927, Landon 1972, Milburn 1973), the order of appearance of the bag 1 and bag 2 fibres has yet to be established with certainty. Milburn (1973), whose description preceded the general adoption of the bag 1, bag 2 nomenclature, identified the first nuclear bag fibre to appear as a 'typical' bag fibre, with predominantly glycolytic metabolism and without M lines, and the second as an 'intermediate' fibre with high oxidative activity and typical M lines. Typical and intermediate bag fibres (Barker & Stacey 1970) have been equated by Ovalle & Smith (1972) with bag 1 and bag 2 fibres respectively — an identification with which Barker (1974) concurs. However, Barker et al (1976a) and Banks et al (1977) have subsequently quoted Milburn (1973 and personal communication) to the effect that the first intrafusal fibre to appear is a bag 2 fibre. Unequivocal identification of individual nuclear bag fibres during their early development is difficult, because of the absence of unambiguous cytological markers until the 12th postnatal day in the rat (Milburn 1973), and distinctions based on diameter differences in single transverse sections are hampered by the lack of lateral registration between corresponding portions of the adjacent nuclear bag fibres. A possibly more plausible developmental sequence, and one that agrees with the original description by Milburn (1973), is bag 1, bag 2, chain. The first intrafusal fibre to develop, bag 1, would then retain the more primitive histochemical and functional characteristics, predominant primary sensory innervation and an extracapsular motor supply, the arrival within the muscle of the parent axons of which will precede that of the smaller-diameter γ-efferents. The fast-twitch, bag 2 and chain fibres would develop later, their appearance coinciding with the arrival of the smaller-diameter group II afferent and γ-efferent axons. Such a sequence, modified by a minor degree of cross-innervation, could provide the basis for an ontogenetic explanation of the adult pattern of

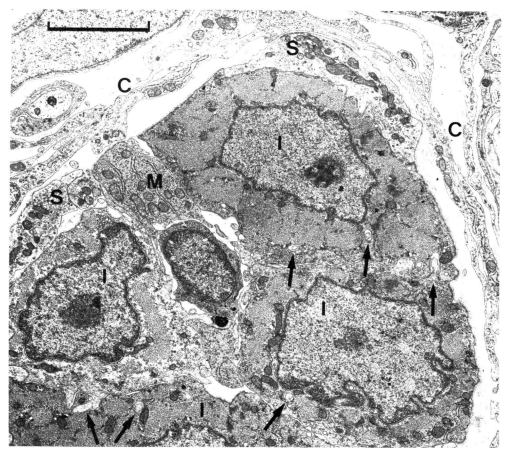

Fig. 1·31 A developing neuromuscular spindle in m. gastrocnemius from a 2.5-day-old rat. The intrafusal fibres (I) and residual myoblasts (M) form a tight cluster within a common basal lamina, locked together in places by filipodia (arrows); the whole is enwrapped by the developing sensory nerve terminal (S). There is no lymph space at this stage of development, the cells of the capsule (C) being closely applied to the surface of the infrafusal fibre bundle. Scale bar = 3 μm

intrafusal innervation. The observed gradation in complexity of the fusimotor terminals — simple, widely ramifying trail endings in the para-equatorial regions and more complex and circum-scribed 'plate' endings at the poles — may reflect the declining influence of the sensory terminals on the metabolic and functional activities of the intra-fusal fibres with increasing distance from the equator (Landon 1974), a view supported by Butler's (1988) observations on the differing morphology of end-plates on bag and chain fibres re-innervated by α-motor neurons.

The indispensability of the sensory innervation to both spindle development and the maintenance of the normal equatorial anatomy of the intrafusal

fibres, has been demonstrated repeatedly (Sherrington 1894, Tower 1932, Zelená 1964). Rat hind-limb muscles denervated by nerve crush at birth, fail to develop muscle spindles if re-innervation is delayed beyond the first week (Zelená & Hnik 1960); conversely, maintenance of afferent innervation in a muscle subjected to pro-longed de-efferentation preserves the equatorial regions of the intrafusal fibres, despite complete atrophy of the extrafusal muscle (Zelená 1962), and in neonatal spindles results in the production of supernumerary intrafusal fibres (Soukup and Zelená 1990). More recent studies of the effects of neonatal excision of the lumbosacral spinal cord on the development of rat muscle spindles (Zelená

& Soukup 1973, 1974) have shown that the intra-fusal myofibres are capable of both histochemical and ultrastructural differentiation in the absence of efferent innervation. The three intrafusal fibre types defined by the ATPase reaction were clearly distinguishable 40 days after operation, as were the normal M-line differences between bag and chain fibres, and this differentiation extended into their polar regions. The extrafusal fibres in the same muscles were atrophic and lacked evidence of fibre-type differentiation. Fusimotor innervation thus appears to play a very restricted part in the histogenesis of the mammalian muscle spindle. Transient denervation of rat muscles at slightly later stages of development can result in spindles with abnormally few intrafusal fibres, lacking obvious equatorial nucleation (Schiaffino & Pierobon-Bormioli 1976), or the partial escape of an intrafusal fibre from the 'juvenescent' influence of the sensory innervation, one polar extension adopting the dimensions and characteristics of an extrafusal fibre (Werner 1973a, b). Bag fibres have been shown to be more resistant to efferent dener-vation than chain fibres (Adams & de Reuck 1973, Schröder 1974, Kucera 1977). In the rat, the ontogenetic influence of the sensory nerve appears to be greatest during the period of normal myoge-nesis and to decline later in life: intrafusal fibres that have been made to undergo a cycle of degeneration and regeneration within an intact capsule, as a consequence of bupivacaine intoxi-cation, fail to develop their original degree of equatorial nucleation despite early sensory re-innervation (Milburn 1976). Transient denerva-tion of mature muscle spindles results in an increase in the numbers of intrafusal myofibres (Schröder et al 1979).

The Golgi tendon organ

A second category of encapsulated sensory nerve terminal is found at musculotendinous and musculo–aponeurotic junctions in birds and mammals; it was definitively described by Golgi (1880). These fusiform structures consist of a number of the component collagen fascicles of the tendon adjacent to its attachment to the muscle, enclosed by a cellular, multilamellar capsule, and innervated at their widest point by a myelinated Ib afferent axon, 7–15 μm in diameter, arising from the intramuscular nerve trunk (Fig. 1.32). As in the muscle spindle, the perineurial sheath of the entering nerve is continuous (and homologous) with the capsule, but there is no equivalent of the subcapsular space of the spindle, longitudinal septa derived from the inner wall of the capsule dividing the enclosed space into a number of subcompart-ments (Bridgman 1968, 1970). The afferent nerve fibre loses its myelin sheath on entry into the capsule and divides into a widely branching arborescence of non-myelinated terminals between the tendon fascicles. Each tendon organ usually receives independent and exclusive innervation by a single Ib afferent fibre, but branched fibres supplying several receptor organs, and dual inner-vation of one, are also seen occasionally (Barker 1974). The sizes of tendon organs, and the number of myofibres to which their tendinous components are attached, vary with species and body size. In the rat the capsules are about 0.5 mm long and 50 μm in diameter, with five or six attached muscle fibres, whereas in man they average 1.5 mm in length and 120 μm in diameter, and are in longitudinal continuity with 10–20 myofibres (Bridgman 1970). The physiolo-gical observations of Gregory & Proske (1979) suggest that these attached myofibres belong to a number of different motor units. The 'in series' situation of the tendon organ, and the inextensibi-lity of its connective tissue components, ensure that it predominantly senses changes in muscle tension, and its response to stimulation is typical of a slowly adapting mechanoreceptor. Quantita-tive data concerning the numbers and distribution of tendon organs in the cat are given by Swett & Eldred (1960) and Barker (1974).

Fine structural studies of tendon organs (Merrillees 1962, Schoultz & Swett 1972, 1974) confirmed the existence of a close and complex relationship between the terminals of the afferent nerve fibre and the tendon fascicles enclosed by the capsule. The terminals, in part ensheathed by Schwann cells, elsewhere separated from the connective tissue space merely by a basal lamina, weave their way between the collagen fibre bundles, which themselves spiral, branch and reunite (Fig. 1.32). The nerve terminal cytoplasm has the amorphous, moderately electron-dense

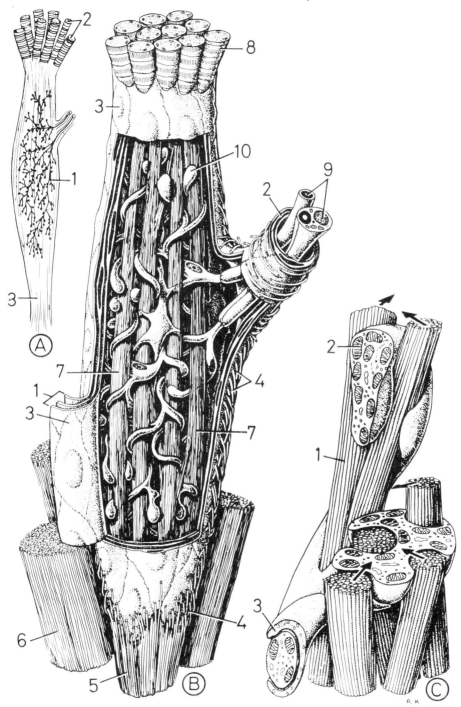

Fig. 1.32 Diagrams illustrating the structure of the Golgi tendon organ. (A) The terminal arborization of the Ib afferent nerve fibre (1) ramifies between the collagen fibres of the tendon, interposed between the ends of the myofibres (2) and its insertion (3). (B) The capsule of the organ (1) is continuous with the perineurial sheath of the incoming nerve (2) and is composed of layers of flattened cells (3) and an external collagen sheath (4). Some fine branches of the collagen bundles of the tendon (5 and 6) traverse the intracapsular space (7) and are attached proximally to the tips of the myofibres (8). The incoming nerve fibres (9) end as a complex arborization (10) between and around these fine collagen bundles. (C) Arrows indicate the forces generated when the spirally running collagen bundles (1) of the interior of the tendon organ straighten under tension, and compress the sensory terminals (2) that are largely bare of Schwann cell (3) cover. (Figure 184 from Krstić 1978, by kind permission of the author and publishers)

cytoplasm and rich content of mitochondria and small vesicles typical of a mechanoreceptor; Schoultz & Swett (1972) suggested that tensile forces applied to the collagen strands will cause them to straighten and thus to twist and pinch the large surface areas of the axonal branches trapped between them.

Development

The development of the tendon organ in the chick, cat and man has been described by Tello (1917) and by Zelená & Soukup (1977) in the rat. Fibres from the muscle nerve grow out beyond the motor end-plate zone to the region of the developing myotendinous junction, and there branch around the ends of the myotubes. Tello described the occurrence of transient bulb- or ring-like contacts between these neurites and the myotubes in silver preparations, and Zelená (1976) has reported fine structural evidence of neuromuscular connections between undoubted afferent axon terminals and the ends of the extrafusal myofibres in developing myotendinous junctions of the rat, up to the fifth postnatal day. These contacts are later lost, but persistence into adult life of somewhat similar contacts between afferent nerve terminals and the ends of myofibres at the myotendinous junction is seen in the palisade endings on extraocular muscles (Dogiel 1906). These endings are also encapsulated and have been described as 'myotendinous cylinders'; their structure in the rhesus monkey has been described by Ruskell (1978). In the developing Golgi tendon organ the afferent terminals continue to branch amid an increasing mass of connective tissue within the developing capsule, until the adult form of the organ has been achieved (Tello 1917).

The fine structural study by Zelená & Soukup (1977) of developing rat tendon organs showed that their first appearance at 20–21 days' gestation lags behind that of the muscle spindles (18 days), and that the receptor body is formed during the first postnatal week by proliferation of Schwann cells and fibroblasts around the extensively branched afferent nerve terminal. Additional spiral bundles of collagen fibrils are assembled between the Schwann cells and the developing terminals; these become linked to the tips of the myofibres and the collagen bundles of the tendon or aponeurosis. The capsule is first apparent at the second postnatal day, and the muscle fibre tips have withdrawn from this by the end of the first postnatal week. Subsequent constriction of the neck of the capsule at either pole, and growth in length, results in a structurally mature tendon organ by 2–3 weeks after birth. Tendon organs do not depend upon normal muscle function for their development, and differentiate in normal numbers and size after neonatal tenotomy (Zelená 1963), but they are, like the muscle spindles and other receptor organs, wholly dependent upon intact sensory innervation for their induction and morphogenesis; they do not develop in muscles de-afferented at birth (Zelená 1975).

Pacinian corpuscles, paciniform and free endings

Pacinian corpuscles are cylindrical or ovoid structures composed of a central rod-like axon terminal, surrounded by a capsule constructed from many regular, concentric layers of cells, interspersed with fine collagen fibrils and layers of basal lamina. They are innervated by large, fast-conducting group I or group II afferent axons, and function as rapidly adapting mechanoreceptors with a particular role in vibration sensitivity. The details of their microscopic and fine structure have been described by Pease & Quilliam (1957), Munger (1971), Spencer & Schaumburg (1973) and Bannister (1976), and their physiological properties have been reviewed by Loewenstein (1971). Pacinian corpuscles are widely distributed throughout the subcutaneous and deep connective tissues of the body; those innervated through muscle nerves are situated in the intermuscular fascial planes and on the surfaces of tendons, aponeuroses and interosseus septa, but seldom within muscle tissue itself. Paciniform endings are smaller versions of the Pacinian corpuscle with thinner capsules, 4–10 layers of cells in all, and a more elongated, cylindrical form. They are distributed in a similar manner to the Pacinian corpuscles through the connective tissues of the musculoskeletal system, including the myotendinous junction where they may be closely associated with Golgi tendon organs. The development of interosseus Pacinian corpuscles is described by Zelená (1978). Paciniform endings function as rapidly adapting mechanoreceptors, and are supplied by group II or group III afferent axons. Free nerve endings are largely derived from group IV non-myelinated afferent axons, less frequently from groups II and III, and very occasionally group I, myelinated afferents. They can be found throughout the connective tissue of muscles and their associated fasciae, aponeuroses and tendons (Stacey 1969). They end as fine beaded terminals on blood vessels and among the fat cells and collagen bundles of the interstitial tissues; they are assumed to have a nociceptive function and to respond to stimuli such as sustained deep pressure.

A comprehensive bibliography of reports up to 1977 on the morphology, pathology, physiology and pharmacology of muscle receptors may be found in Eldred et al (1967, 1977).

ACKNOWLEDGEMENTS

I wish to acknowledge my gratitude to Mr H. W. J. Long and Mr B. S. Young for their expert technical assistance in preparing material used to illustrate this chapter; and to Mrs R. Maynard and Mrs J. Humphreys for preparing the typescript.

I am grateful to the authors, editors and publishers referred to in the captions to various figures which have been reproduced from previous publications for their permission to include such material in this chapter.

REFERENCES

Adal M N 1969 The fine structure of the sensory region of cat muscle spindles. Journal of Ultrastructure Research 26: 332

Adal M N, Barker D 1967 The fine structure of cat fusimotor endings. Journal of Physiology 192: 50

Adams R D, De Reuck J 1973 Metrics of muscle. In: Kakulas B A (ed) Basic research in myology. Excerpta Medica, Amsterdam, vol 1, p 3

Adrian R H 1978 Charge movement in the membrane of striated muscle. Annual Review of Biophysics and Bioengineering 7: 85

Adrian R H, Almers W 1976 Charge movement in the membrane of striated muscle. Journal of Physiology 254: 339

Aherne W, Ayyar D R, Clarke P A, Walton J N 1971 Muscle fibre size in normal infants, children and adolescents. An autopsy study. Journal of the Neurological Sciences 14: 171

Akert K, Pfenninger K, Sandri C, Moor H 1972 Freeze etching and cytochemistry of vesicles and membrane complexes in synapses of the central nervous system. In: Pappas G D, Purpura D P (eds) Structure and function of synapses. Raven Press, New York, p 67

Alexeev N P, 1976 A study of the permeability of the outer capsule of the frog muscle spindle to potassium ions using ion-selective micro-electrodes. Tsitilogiya 18: 629

Allbrook D B, Han M F, Hellmuth A E 1971 Population of muscle satellite cells in relation to age and mitotic activity. Pathology 3: 233

Allen E R, Pepe F A 1965 Ultrastructure of developing muscle cells in the chick embryo. American Journal of Anatomy 116: 115

Aloisi M 1970 Patterns of muscle regeneration. In: Mauro A, Shafiq S A, Milhorat A T (eds) Regeneration of striated muscle and myogenesis. Excerpta Medica, Amsterdam, p 180

Aloisi M, Mussini I, Schiaffino S 1973 Activation of muscle nuclei in denervation and hypertrophy. In: Kakulas B A (ed) Basic research in myology. Excerpta Medica, Amsterdam, vol 1, p 338

Andersen P, Henriksson J 1977 Training-induced changes in the subgroups of human type II skeletal muscle fibres. Acta Physiologica Scandinavica 99: 123

Anderson M J 1986 Nerve-induced remodelling of muscle basal lamina during synaptogenesis. Journal of Cell Biology 102: 863

Anderson D J 1987 Molecular biology of the acetylcholine receptor: structure and regulation of biogenesis. In: Salpeter M M (ed) The vertebrate neuromuscular junction. Alan R Liss, New York, p 285

Ashmore C R, Robinson D W, Rattray P, Doerr L 1972 Biphasic development of muscle fibres in the foetal lamb. Experimental Neurology 37: 241

Banker B Q, Girvin J P 1971 The ultrastructural features of the mammalian muscle spindle. Journal of Neuropathology and Experimental Neurology 30: 155

Banks R W, Harker D W, Stacey M J 1977 A study of mammalian intrafusal muscle fibres using a combined histochemical and ultrastructural technique. Journal of Anatomy 123: 783

Bannister L H 1976 Sensory terminals of peripheral nerves. In: Landon D N (ed) The peripheral nerve. Chapman and Hall, London, p 396

Barker D 1948 The innervation of the muscle spindle. Quarterly Journal of Microscopical Science 89: 143

Barker D 1967 The innervation of mammalian skeletal muscle. In: de Reuck A V S, Knight J (eds) Ciba Foundation symposium on myotactic, kinesthetic and vestibular mechanisms. Churchill, London, p 3

Barker D 1974 The morphology of muscle receptors. In: Hunt C C (ed) Muscle receptors: handbook of sensory physiology, Springer, Berlin, vol III/2, p 2

Barker D, Milburn A 1981 Development of cat spindles. Journal of Physiology 325: 85

Barker D, Stacey M J 1970 Rabbit intrafusal muscle fibres. Journal of Physiology 210: 70

Barker D, Stacey M J, Adal M N 1970 Fusimotor innervation

in the cat. Philosophical Transactions of the Royal Society of London; B 258: 315

Barker D, Banks R W, Harker D W, Milburn A, Stacey M J 1976a Studies of the histochemistry, ultrastructure, motor innervation and regeneration of mammalian intrafusal muscle fibres. In: Homma S (ed) Understanding the stretch reflex. Progress in Brain Research 44: 67

Barker D, Emonet-Dénand F, Harker D W, Jami L, Laporte Y 1976b Distribution of fusimotor axons to intrafusal muscle fibres in cat tenuissimus spindles as determined by the glycogen depletion method. Journal of Physiology 261: 49

Barker D, Bessou P, Jankowska E, Pagés B, Stacey M J 1978 Identification of intrafusal muscle fibres activated by single fusimotor axons and injected with fluorescent dye in cat tenuissimus spindles. Journal of Physiology 275: 149

Barker D, Emonet-Dénand F, Laporte Y, Stacey M J 1980 Identification of the intrafusal endings of skeletofusimotor axons in the cat. Brain Research 185: 227

Barnard D A, Dolly J O, Porter C W 1975 The acetylcholine receptor and the ionic conductance modulation system of skeletal muscle. Experimental Neurology 48: 1

Barnard R J, Edgerton V R, Furukawa T, Peter J B 1971 Histochemical, biochemical and contractile properties of red, white and intermediate fibers. American Journal of Physiology 220: 410

Barry P H, Adrian R H 1973 Action potential in transverse tubules and its role in the activation of skeletal muscle. Journal of Membrane Biology 14: 243

Bennett G S, Fellini S A, Toyama Y, Holtzer H 1979 Redistribution of intermediate filament subunits during skeletal myogenensis and maturation in vitro. Journal of Cell Biology 82: 577

Bennett M R 1983 Development of neuromuscular synapses. Physiological Reviews 63: 915

Bennett M R, Pettigrew A G 1974 The formation of synapses in striated muscle during development. Journal of Physiology 241: 515

Bennett M R, Pettigrew A G 1975 The formation of neuromuscular synapses. Cold Spring Harbor Symposium on Quantitative Biology 40: 409

Benoit P, Changeux J P 1975 Consequences of tenotomy on the evolution of multi-innervation in developing rat soleus muscle. Brain Research 99: 354

Betz W J 1987 Motoneuron death and synapse elimination in vertebrates. In: Salpeter M M (ed) The vertebrate neuromuscular junction. Alan R Liss, New York, p 117

Betz W J, Caldwell J H, Ribchester R R 1980 The effects of partial denervation at birth on the development of muscle fibres and motor units in rat lumbrical muscle. Journal of Physiology 303: 265

Birks R I, Davey D F 1969 Osmotic responses demonstrating the extracellular character of the sarcoplasmic reticulum. Journal of Physiology 202: 171

Birks R I, Davey D F 1972 An analysis of volume changes in the T tubules of frog skeletal muscle exposed to sucrose. Journal of Physiology 222: 95

Bischoff R 1974 Enzymatic liberation of myogenic cells from adult rat muscle. Anatomical Record 180: 645

Bischoff R 1979 Tissue culture studies on the origin of myogenic cells during muscle regeneration in the rat. In: Mauro A (ed) Muscle regeneration. Raven Press, New York, p 13

Bischoff R, Holtzer H 1969 Evidence for obligatory mitosis during myogenesis. Journal of Cell Biology 43: 13a

Bixby J L 1981 Ultrastructural observations on synaptic elimination in neonatal rabbit skeletal muscle. Journal of Neurocytology 10: 81

Bogusch G 1975 Electron microscopic observations on leptomeric fibrils and leptomeric complexes in the hen and pigeon heart. Journal of Molecular and Cellular Cardiology 7: 733

Bonilla E, Schotland D L, DiMauro S, Aldover B 1975 Electron cytochemistry of crystalline inclusions in human skeletal muscle mitochondria. Journal of Ultrastructure Research 51: 404

Bowden D H, Goyer R A 1960 The size of muscle fibres in infants and children. Archives of Pathology 69: 188

Bowman W 1840 On the minute structure and movements of voluntary muscle. Philosophical Transactions of the Royal Society of London p 457

Boyd I A 1962 The structure and innervation of the nuclear bag muscle fibre system and the nuclear chain muscle fibre system in mammalian muscle spindles. Philosophical Transactions of the Royal Society of London; B 245: 81

Boyd I A 1976 The response of fast and slow nuclear bag fibres and nuclear chain fibres in isolated cat muscle spindles to fusimotor stimulation and the effect of intrafusal contraction on the sensory endings. Quarterly Journal of Experimental Physiology 61: 203

Boyd I A, Davey M R 1962 The groups of origin in the nerves to skeletal muscle of the γ_1 and γ_2 fusimotor fibres present close to, and within, mammalian muscle spindles. In: Barker D (ed) Symposium on muscle receptors. Hong Kong University Press, Hong Kong, p 191

Boyd I A, Davey M R 1968 Composition of peripheral nerves. Livingstone, Edinburgh

Boyd I A, Gladden M H, McWilliam P N, Ward J 1977 Control of dynamic and static nuclear bag fibres by γ and β axons in isolated cat muscle spindles. Journal of Physiology 256: 133

Bradley W G 1979 Muscle fiber splitting. In: Mauro A (ed) Muscle regeneration. Raven Press, New York, p 215

Brandt P W, Lopez E, Reuben J P, Grundfest H 1967 The relationship between myofilament packing density and sarcomere length in frog striated muscle. Journal of Cell Biology 33: 255

Bridge D T, Allbrook D 1970 Growth of striated muscle in an Australian marsupial (Setonyx brachyurus). Journal of Anatomy 106: 285

Bridgman C F 1968 The structure of tendon organs in the cat: a proposed mechanism for responding to muscle tension. Anatomical Record 162: 209

Bridgman C F 1970 Comparisons in structure of tendon organs in the rat, cat and man. Journal of Comparative Neurology 138: 369

Briskey E J, Seraydarian K, Mommaerts W F H M 1967 The modification of actomyosin by α-actinin. II. The interaction between α-actinin and actin. Biochimica et biophysica acta 133: 424

Bronson D D, Schachat F H 1982 Heterogeneity of contractile proteins. Differences in tropomyosin in fast, mixed, and slow skeletal muscles of the rabbit. Journal of Biological Chemistry 257: 3937

Brooke, M H, Engel W K 1969a The histographic analysis of human muscle biopsies with regard to fiber types. I. Adult male and female. Neurology (Minneapolis) 19: 221

Brooke M H, Engel W K 1969b The histographic analysis of human muscle biopsies with regard to fiber types. IV. Children's biopsies. Neurology (Minneapolis) 19: 591

Brooke M H, Kaiser K K 1970 Muscle fiber types: how many and what kind? Archives of Neurology (Chicago) 23: 369

Brown M C, Butler R G 1973 Depletion of intrafusal muscle fibre glycogen by stimulation of fusimotor fibres. Journal of Physiology 229: 25

Brown, M C, Jansen J K S, van Essen D 1976 Polyneuronal innervation of skeletal muscle in new-born rats and its elimination during maturation. Journal of Physiology 261: 387

Brown, M C, Hopkins W G, Keynes R J 1982 Short-and long-term effects of paralysis on the motor innervation of two different neonatal mouse muscles. Journal of Physiology 329: 439

Buchthal F, Schmalbruch H 1980 Motor unit of mammalian muscle. Physiological Reviews 60: 90

Buller A J, Pope R 1977 Plasticity in mammalian skeletal muscle. Philosophical Transactions of the Royal Society of London, B 278: 295

Buller A J, Eccles J C, Eccles R M 1960a Differentiation of fast and slow muscles in the cat hind limb. Journal of Physiology 150: 399

Buller A J, Eccles J C, Eccles R M 1960b Interactions between motoneurones and muscles in respect of the characteristic speeds of their responses. Journal of Physiology 150: 417

Burden S J 1987 The extracellular matrix and subsynaptic sarcoplasm at nerve-muscle synapses. In: Salpeter M M (ed) The vertebrate neuromuscular junction. Alan R Liss, New York, p 163

Burke R E, Levine D N, Zajac F E, Tsairis P, Engel W K 1971 Mammalian motor units: physiological–histochemical correlation in three types in cat gastrocnemius. Science 174: 709

Burleigh I G 1974 On the cellular regulation of growth and development in skeletal muscle. Biological Reviews 49: 267

Butler R 1980 The organization of muscle spindles in the tenuissimus muscle of the cat during late development. Developmental Biology 77: 191

Butler R 1988 Evidence for transdifferentiation of alpha motoneuron terminals during reinnervation of muscle spindles. In: Hnik P, Soukup T, Vesjada R, Zelena J (eds) Mechanoreceptors, development, structure and function. Plenum Press, New York, p 105

Byrne E, Hayes D J, Morgan-Hughes J A, Clark J B 1982 Some effects of experimentally induced mitochondrial lesions on the function and metabolic content of rat muscle. Proceedings of the Vth International Congress on Neuromuscular Diseases, Marseille 1982 (Abst) 35: 3

Campion D R 1984 The muscle satellite cell: a review. International Review of Cytology 87: 225

Carafoli E, Roman I 1980 Mitochondria and disease. Molecular Aspects of Medicine 3: 295

Caspar D L D, Cohen C, Longley W 1969 Tropomyosin: crystal structure, polymorphism and molecular interactions. Journal of Molecular Biology 41: 87

Cazzato, G, Walton J N 1968 The pathology of the muscle spindle. A study of biopsy material in various muscular and neuromuscular diseases. Journal of the Neurological Sciences 7: 15

Ceccarelli B, Hurlbut W P 1980 Vesicle hypothesis of the release of quanta of acetylcholine. Physiological Reviews 60: 396

Chou S M 1969 'Megaconial' mitochondria observed in a case of chronic polymyositis. Acta Neuropathologica (Berlin) 12: 68

Chou S M, Nonaka I 1977 Satellite cells and muscle regeneration in diseased human skeletal muscles. Journal of the Neurological Sciences 34: 131

Chowrashi P K, Pepe F A 1979 M-band proteins: evidence for more than one component. In: Pepe F A, Sanger J W, Nachmias V T (eds) Motility in cell function. Academic Press, New York, p 419

Church J C T 1969 Satellite cells and myogenesis; a study in the fruit bat web. Journal of Anatomy 105: 419

Clark A W, Hurlbut W P, Mauro A 1972 Changes in the fine structure of the neuromuscular junction of the frog caused by black widow spider venom. Journal of Cell Biology 52: 1

Close R 1964 Dynamic properties of fast and slow skeletal muscles of the rat during development. Journal of Physiology 173: 74

Close R 1967 Properties of motor units in fast and slow skeletal muscles of the rat. Journal of Physiology 193: 45

Close R I 1972 Dynamic properties of mammalian skeletal muscles. Physiological Reviews 52: 129

Cohen C, Caspar D L D, Parry D A D, Lucas R M 1971 Tropomyosin crystal dynamics. Cold Spring Harbor Symposium on Quantitative Biology 36: 205

Colley N J, Tokuyasu K T, Singer S J 1990 The early expression of myofibrillar proteins in round postmitotic myoblasts of embryonic skeletal muscle. Journal of Cell Science 95: 11

Conen P E, Bell C D 1970 Study of satellite cells in mature and fetal human muscle and rhabdomyosarcoma. In: Mauro A, Shafiq S A, Milhorat A T (eds) Regeneration of striated muscle and myogenesis. Excerpta Medica, Amsterdam, p 194

Conradi S 1976 Functional anatomy of the anterior horn motor neuron. In: Landon D N (ed) The peripheral nerve. Chapman & Hall, London, p 279

Conti-Tronconi B M, Raftery M A 1982 The nicotinic cholinergic receptor: correlation of molecular structure with functional properties. Annual Review of Biochemistry 51: 491

Cooper S 1961 The response of the primary and secondary endings of muscle spindles with intact motor innervation during applied stretch. Quarterly Journal of Experimental Physiology 46: 389

Cooper S 1966 Muscle spindles and motor units. In: Andrews B L (ed) Control and innervation of skeletal muscle. Thomson and Co, Dundee, p 9

Cooper S, Daniel P M 1963 Muscle spindles in man: their morphology in the lumbricals and the deep muscles of the neck. Brain 86: 563

Cooper S, Gladden M H 1974 Elastic fibres and reticulin of mammalian muscle spindles and their functional significance: Quarterly Journal of Experimental Physiology 59: 367

Cooper W G, Konigsberg I R 1961 Dynamics of myogenesis in vitro. Anatomical Record 140: 195

Cooper C C, Cassens R G, Kastenschmidt L L, Briskey E J 1970 Histochemical characterization of muscle differentiation. Developmental Biology 23: 169

Corvaja N, Marinozzi V, Pompeiano O 1967 Close appositions and junctions of plasma membranes of intrafusal muscle fibres in mammalian muscle spindles. Pflügers Archiv für die gesamte Physiologie des Menschen und der Tiere 296: 337

Corvaja N, Marinozzi V, Pompeiano O 1969 Muscle spindles in the lumbrical muscle of the adult cat. Archives italiennes de biologie 107: 365

Costantin L L 1975 Contractile activation in skeletal muscle.

Progress in Biophysics and Molecular Biology 29: 199
Costantin L L, Franzini-Armstrong C, Podolsky R J 1965 Localization of calcium-accumulating structures in striated muscle fibers. Science 147: 158
Costill D L, Daniels J, Evans W, Fink E W, Krakenbuhl G, Saltin B 1976 Skeletal muscle enzymes and fiber composition in male and female track athletes. Journal of Applied Physiology 40: 149
Couteaux R 1941 Recherches sur l'histogenèse du muscle strié des mammifères et la formation des plaques motrices. Bulletin Biologique de la France et de la Belgique (Paris) 2: 8
Couteaux R 1981 Structure of the subsynaptic sarcoplasm in the interfolds of the frog neuromuscular junction. Journal of Neurocytology 10: 947
Couteaux R, Pécot-Dechauvassine M 1970 Vesicules synaptiques et poches au niveau des 'zones actives' de la jonction neuromusculaire. Comptes rendus hebdomadaires des séances de l'Académie des sciences 271D: 2346
Craig R 1977 Structure of A-segments from frog and rabbit skeletal muscle. Journal of Molecular Biology 109: 69
Craig R 1986 The structure of the contractile filaments. In: Engel A G, Banker B Q (eds) Myology. McGraw-Hill, New York, p 73
Craig R, Knight P 1983 Myosin molecules, thick filaments and the actin-myosin complex. In: Harris J R (ed) Electron Microscopy of proteins. Macromolecular structure and function, vol 4, p 97
Craig R, Megerman K 1979 Electron microscope studies on muscle thick filaments. In: Pepe F A, Sanger J W, Nachmias V T (eds) Motility in cell function. Academic Press, New York, p 91
Craig R, Offer G 1976a The location of C-protein in rabbit skeletal muscle. Proceedings of the Royal Society of London; B 192: 451
Craig R, Offer G 1976b Axial arrangement of crossbridges in thick filaments of vertebrate skeletal muscle. Journal of Molecular Biology 102: 325
Craig S W, Pardo J V 1979 Alpha-actinin localization in the junctional complex of intestinal epithelial cells. Journal of Cell Biology 80: 203
Crowe A, Matthews P B C 1964 The effects of stimulation of static and dynamic fusimotor fibres on the response to stretching of the primary endings of muscle spindles. Journal of Physiology 174: 109
Cuajunco F 1927 Embryology of the neuromuscular spindle. Carnegie Institute Washington Publications, Contributions to Embryology 19: 45
Cuajunco F 1940 Development of the neuromuscular spindle in human fetuses. Carnegie Institute Washington Publications, Contributions to Embryology 28: 95
Cuajunco F 1942 Development of the human motor end plate. Carnegie Institute Washington Publications, Contributions to Embryology 30: 127
Cullen M J, Landon D N 1988 The ultrastructure of the motor unit. In: Walton J N (ed) Disorders of voluntary muscle. Churchill Livingstone, Edinburgh, p 27
Cullen M J, Weightman D 1975 The ultrastructure of normal human muscle in relation to fibre type. Journal of the Neurological Sciences 25: 43
Cullen M J, Hollingworth S, Marshall M W, 1984 A comparative study of the transverse tubular system of the rat extensor digitorum longus and soleus muscles. Journal of Anatomy 138: 297
Davey D F 1976 The relation between Z-disk lattice spacing and sarcomere length in sartorius muscle fibres from Hyla cerula. Australian Journal of Experimental Biological and Medical Sciences 54: 441
Davey D F, O'Brien G M 1978 The sarcoplasmic reticulum and T-system of rat extensor digitorum longus muscles exposed to hypertonic solutions. Australian Journal of Experimental Biology and Medical Science 56: 409
Dawson D M, Romanul F C A 1964 Enzymes in muscle. II. Histochemical and quantitative studies. Archives of Neurology (Chicago) 11: 369
DeLorenzo R J, Freedman S D, Yoke W R, Maurer S C 1979 Stimulation of Ca^{2+}-dependent neurotransmitter release and presynaptic nerve terminal protein phosphorylation by calmodulin and a calmodulin-like protein isolated from synaptic vesicles. Proceedings of the National Academy of Sciences of the USA 76: 1838
Denny-Brown D E 1929 The histological features of striped muscle in relation to its functional activity. Proceedings of the Royal Society of London; B 104: 371
De Recondo J, Fardeau M, Lapresle J 1966 Étude au microscope électronique des lesions musculaires d'atrophie neurogène par atteinte de la corne antérieure. Revue Neurologique 114: 169
de Reuck J, van der Eecken H, Roels H 1973 Biometrical and histochemical comparison between extra- and intrafusal muscle fibers in dennervated and re-innervated rat muscle. Acta Neuropathologica (Berlin) 25: 249
Dessouky D A, Hibbs R G 1965 An electron microscope study of the development of the somatic muscle of the chick embryo. American Journal of Anatomy 116: 523
Dhoot G K, Perry S V 1980 The components of the troponin complex and development in skeletal muscle. Experimental Cell Research 127: 75
DiMauro S 1979 Metabolic myopathies. In: Vinken, P J, Bruyn G W (eds) Handbook of clinical neurology, vol 41. North Holland, Amsterdam, p 175
Diwan F H, Milburn A 1986 The effects of temporary ischaemia on rat muscle spindles. Journal of Embryology and experimental Morphology 92: 223
Dogiel A S 1906 Die Endigungen der sensiblen Nerven in der Augenmuskeln und deren Sehen beim Menschen und der Saugetieren. Archiv für Mikroskopische Anatomie und Entwicklungsmechanik 68: 501
Dow P R, Shinn S L, Ovalle W K 1980 Ultrastructural study of a blood-muscle spindle barrier after systemic administration of horseradish peroxidase. American Journal of Anatomy 157: 375
Droz B, Koening H L, Di Gamberardino L, Courand J Y, Chretien M, Souyri F 1979 The importance of axonal transport and endoplasmic reticulum in the function of the cholinergic synapse in normal and pathological conditions. Progress in Brain Research 49: 23
Dubowitz V 1967 Cross-innervated mammalian skeletal muscle: histochemical, physiological and biochemical observations. Journal of Physiology 193: 481
Dubowitz V 1968 Developing and diseased muscle. SIMP Research Monograph No. 2, Heinemann, London
Dubowitz V, Brooke M H 1973 Muscle biopsy: a modern approach. W B Saunders, London
Dubowitz V, Pearse A G 1960 A comparative histochemical study of oxidative enzyme and phosphorylase activity in skeletal muscle. Histochemie 2: 105
Duchen L W 1971 An electron microscopic comparison of motor end-plates of slow and fast skeletal muscle fibres of the mouse. Journal of the Neurological Sciences 14: 37
Ebashi S 1980 Regulation of muscle contraction. Proceedings of the Royal Society of London B 207: 259

Ebashi S, Ebashi F, Maruyama K 1964 A new protein factor promoting contraction of actomyosin. Nature 203: 645

Ebashi S, Kodama A, Ebashi F 1968 Troponin. I. Preparation and physiological function. Journal of Biochemistry 64: 465

Edström L, Kugelberg E 1968a Histochemical composition, distribution of fibers and fatiguability of single motor units. Journal of Neurology, Neurosurgery and Psychiatry 31: 424

Edström L, Kugelberg E 1968b Properties of motor units in the rat anterior tibial muscle. Acta Physiologica Scandinavica 73: 543

Edström L, Thornell L-E, Eriksson A 1980 A new type of hereditary distal myopathy with characteristic sarcoplasmic bodies and intermediate (skeletin) filaments. Journal of the Neurological Sciences 47: 171

Eisenberg B R 1983 Quantitative ultrastructure of mammalian skeletal muscle. In: Peachey L D, Adrian R H (eds) Handbook of physiology, section 10: skeletal muscle. American Physiological Society, Bethesda, p 73

Eisenberg B R, Kuda A M 1975 Stereological analysis of mammalian skeletal muscle. II. White vastus muscle of the adult guinea pig. Journal of Ultrastructure Research 51: 176

Eisenberg B R, Kuda A M 1976 Discrimination between fiber populations in mammalian skeletal muscle by using ultra-structural parameters. Journal of Ultrastructure Research 54: 76

Eisenberg B R, Kuda A M 1977 Retrieval of cryostat sections for comparison of histochemistry and quantitative electron microscopy in a muscle fiber. Journal of Histochemistry and Cytochemistry 25: 1169

Eisenberg B R, Salmons S 1976 Ultrastructural correlates of fibre type transformation in rabbit skeletal muscle. Journal of Physiology 301: 16P

Eisenberg B R, Kuda A M, Peter J B 1974 Stereological analysis of mammalian skeletal muscle. I. Soleus muscle of the adult guinea-pig. Journal of Cell Biology 60: 732

Eldred E, Yellin H, Gadbois L, Sweeney S 1967 Bibliography on muscle receptors: their morphology, pathology and physiology. Experimental Neurology, Supplement 3: 1

Eldred E, Yellin H, DeSantis M, Smith C M 1977 Supplement to bibliography on muscle receptors: their morphology, pathology, physiology and pharmacology. Experimental Neurology 55: 1

Elliott A, Offer G 1978 Shape and flexibility of the myosin molecule. Journal of Molecular Biology 123: 505

Elliott G F, Lowy J, Worthington C R 1963 An X-ray and light diffraction study of the filament lattice of striated muscle in the living state and rigor. Journal of Molecular Biology 6: 295

Elliott G F, Lowy J, Millman B M 1967 Low angle X-ray diffraction studies of living striated muscle during contraction. Journal of Molecular Biology 25: 31

Elliott G F, Rome E M, Spencer M 1970 A type of contraction hypothesis applicable to all muscles. Nature 226: 417

Ellisman M H, Rash J E, Staehelin L A, Porter K R 1976 Studies of excitable membranes. II. A comparison of specializations at neuromuscular junctions and nonjunctional sarcolemmas of mammalian fast and slow twitch muscle fibers. Journal of Cell Biology 68: 752

Ellisman M H, Brooke M H, Kaiser K K, Rash J E 1978 Appearance in slow muscle sarcolemma of specializations characteristic of fast muscle after reinnervation by a fast muscle nerve. Experimental Neurology 58: 59

Emonet-Dénand F, Laporte Y, Matthews P B C, Petit J 1977 On the subdivision of the static and dynamic fusimotor actions on the primary endings of the cat muscle spindle.

Journal of Physiology 268: 827

Endo M, Nonomura Y, Mosaki T, Ohtsuki I, Ebashi S 1966 Localization of native tropomyosin in relation to striation patterns. Journal of Biochemistry 60: 605

Engel A G, Gomez M R 1967 Nemaline (Z-disk) myopathy: observations on the origin, structure and solubility properties of the nemaline structures. Journal of Neuropathology and Experimental Neurology 26: 601

Engel A G, Dale A J D 1968 Autophagic glycogenosis of late onset with mitochondrial abnormalities: light and electronmicroscopic observations. Proceedings of the Mayo Clinic 43: 233

Engel A G, Santa T 1971 Histometric analysis of the ultrastructure of the neuromuscular junction in myasthenia gravis and in the myasthenic syndrome. Annals of the New York Academy of Sciences 183: 46

Engel A G, Tsujihata M, Lindstrom J M, Lennon V A 1976 The motor end-plate in myasthenia gravis and in experimental autoimmune myasthenia gravis. A quantitative ultrastructural study. Annals of the New York Academy of Sciences 274: 60

Engel W K 1962 The essentiality of histo- and cytochemical studies of skeletal muscle in the investigation of neuromuscular disease. Neurology (Minneapolis) 12: 778

Engel W K 1970 Selective and non-selective susceptibility of muscle fiber types. Archives of Neurology (Chicago) 22: 97

Eriksson P O, Thornell L E 1990 Human muscle spindle fibre types as revealed with antibodies against isomyosins and M-band proteins. Journal of the Neurological Sciences 98 (suppl): 48

Ezerman E B, Ishikawa H 1967 Differentiation of the sarcoplasmic reticulum and the T-system in developing chick skeletal muscle. Journal of Cell Biology 35: 405

Fambrough D M 1979 Control of acetylcholine receptors in skeletal muscle. Physiological Reviews 59: 165

Fambrough D M, Drachman D B, Satyamurti S 1973 Neuromuscular junction in myasthenia gravis: decreased acetylcholine receptors. Science 182: 293

Fardeau M 1969a Ulstrastructure des fibres musculaires squelettiques. Presse Médicale 77: 1341

Fardeau M 1969b Étude d'une nouvelle observation des 'nemaline myopathy'. II. Données ultrastructurales. Acta neuropathologica (Berlin) 13: 250

Fardeau M 1970 Ultrastructural lesions in progressive muscular dystrophies: a critical study of their specificity. In: Canal N, Scarlato G, Walton J N (eds) Muscle diseases. Excerpta Medica, Amsterdam, p 98

Fawcett D W, MacNutt N S 1969 The ultrastructure of the cat myocardium. I. Ventricular papillary muscle. Journal of Cell Biology 42: 1

Fenichel G M 1966 A histochemical study of developing human skeletal muscle. Neurology (Minneapolis) 16: 741

Fertuk H C, Salpeter M M 1974 Localization of acetylcholine receptor by ^{125}I-labelled, bungarotoxin binding at mouse motor endplates. Proceedings of the National Academy of Sciences of the USA 71: 1376

Festoff B W, Oliver K L, Reddy N B 1977 In vitro studies of skeletal muscle membranes: adenyl cyclase of fast and slow-twitch muscle and the effects of denervation. Journal of Membrane Biology 32: 331

Fidzianska A 1971 Electron microscope study of the development of human foetal muscle, motor endplate and nerve. Acta neuropathologica (Berlin) 17: 234

Fischbeck K H, Bonilla E, Schotland D L 1982 Freeze-fracture analysis of plasma membrane cholesterol in fast- and slow-twitch muscles. Journal of Ultrastructure Research 81: 117

Fischman D A 1967 An electron microscope study of myofibril formation in embryonic chick skeletal muscle. Journal of Cell Biology 32: 557

Forbes M S, Plantholt B A, Sperelakis N 1977 Cytochemical staining procedures selective for sarcotubular systems of muscle: modifications and applications. Journal of Ultrastructure Research 60: 306

Franzini-Armstrong C 1970a Details of the I band structure as revealed by the localization of ferritin. Tissue and Cell 2: 327

Franzini-Armstrong C 1970b Studies of the triad. I. Structure of the junction in frog twitch fibers. Journal of Cell Biology 47: 488

Franzini-Armstrong C 1971 Studies of the triad. II. Penetration of tracers into the junctional gap. Journal of Cell Biology 49: 196

Franzini-Armstrong C 1973a Membranous systems in muscle fibers. In: Bourne G H (ed) The structure and function of muscle. Academic Press, New York, p 532

Franzini-Armstrong C 1973b The structure of a simple Z line. Journal of Cell Biology 58: 630

Franzini-Armstrong C 1974 Freeze fracture of skeletal muscle from the tarantula spider. Journal of Cell Biology 61: 501

Franzini-Armstrong C 1979 A description of satellite and invasive cells in frog sartorius. In: Mauro A (ed) Muscle regeneration. Raven Press, New York, p 233

Franzini-Armstrong C 1980 Structure of sarcoplasmic reticulum. Federation Proceedings 39: 2403

Franzini-Armstrong C 1983 Disposition of Ca ATPase in SR membrane from skeletal muscle. Journal of Cell Biology 97: 260a

Franzini-Armstrong C 1984 Freeze–fracture of frog slow tonic fibers. Structure of surface and internal membranes. Tissue and Cell 16: 647

Franzini-Armstrong C, Porter K R 1964 The Z-disc of skeletal muscle fibrils. Zeitschrift für Zellforschung und Mikroskopische Anatomie 61: 661

Fridén J 1984 Changes in human skeletal muscle induced by long-term eccentric exercise. Cell and Tissue Research 236: 365

Fridén J, Sjöström M, Ekblom B 1984 Muscle fiber type characteristics in endurance trained and untrained individuals. European Journal of Applied Physiology and Occupational Physiology 52: 266

Fujiwara K, Porter M E, Pollard T D 1978 Alpha-actinin localization in the cleavage furrow during cytokinesis. Journal of Cell Biology 79: 268

Funatsu T, Higuchi H, Ishiwata S 1990 Elastic filaments in skeletal muscle revealed by selective removal of thin filaments with plasma gelsolin. Journal of Cell Biology 110: 53

Furst D O, Osborn M, Nave R, Weber K 1988 The organization of titin filaments in the half-sarcomere revealed by monoclonal antibodies in immunoelectron microscopy: a map of ten non-repetitive epitopes starting at the Z line extends close to the M line. Journal of Cell Biology 106: 1563

Furst D O, Osborn M, Weber K 1989 Myogenesis in the mouse embryo: differential onset of expression of myogenic proteins and the involvement of titin in myofibril assembly. Journal of Cell Biology 109: 517

Garamvölgyi N 1972 Slow and fast muscle cells in human striated muscle. Acta biochimica et biophysica academiae scientiarum hungaricae 7: 165

Gauthier G F 1969 On the relationship of ultrastructural and cytochemical features to colour in mammalian skeletal muscle. Zeitschrift für Zellforschung und Mikroskopische Anatomie 95: 462

Gauthier G F 1970 The ultrastructure of three fiber types in mammalian skeletal muscle. In: Briskey E J, Cassens R G, Marsh B B (eds) The physiology and biochemistry of muscle as a food. University of Wisconsin Press, Madison, vol. 2, p 103

Gauthier G F 1976 The motor end-plate: structure. In: Landon D N (ed) The peripheral nerve. Chapman and Hall, London, p 464

Gauthier G F, Padykula H A 1966 Cytological studies of fiber types in skeletal muscle. A comparative study of the mammalian diaphragm. Journal of Cell Biology 28: 333

Gauthier G F, Lowey S, Hobbs A W 1978 Fast and slow myosin in developing muscle fibres. Nature 274: 25

Gergely J 1988 Biochemical aspects of muscular structure and function. In: Walton J (ed) Disorders of Voluntary Muscle. Churchill Livingstone, Edinburgh, p 109

Gilliatt R G 1966 Axon branching in motor nerves. In: Andrew B L (ed) Control and innervation of skeletal muscle. Thomson and Co, Dundee, p 53

Gladden M H 1976 Structural features relative to the function of intrafusal muscle fibres in the cat. In: Homma S (ed) Understanding the stretch reflex, Progress in Brain Research 44: 51

Goldspink G 1970 The proliferation of myofibrils during muscle fibre growth. Journal of Cell Science 6: 593

Goldspink G 1971 Changes in striated muscle fibres during contraction and growth with particular reference to myofibril splitting. Journal of Cell Science 9: 123

Goldspink G 1980 Growth of muscle. In: Goldspink D F (ed) Development and specialization of skeletal muscle. Cambridge University Press, Cambridge, p 19

Goldspink G, Rowe R W D 1968 The growth and development of muscle fibres in normal and dystrophic mice. In: Research in muscular dystrophy. Pitman Medical Publishing, London, p 116

Goldstein M A, Schroeter J P, Sass R L 1977 Optical diffraction of the Z lattice in canine cardiac muscle. Journal of Cell Biology 75: 818

Goldstein M A, Entman M L 1978 Microtubules in mammalian heart muscle. Journal of Cell Biology 79: 183

Goldstein M A, Schroeter J P, Sass R L 1979 The Z lattice in canine cardiac muscle. Journal of Cell Biology 83: 187

Golgi C 1880 Sui nervi dei tendini dell'uomo e di altri vertebrait e di un nuovo organo nervoso terminale musculotendineo. Memorie della Academia delle scienze di Torino 32: 359

Goll D E, Suzuki A, Temple J, Homes G R 1972 Studies on purified alpha-actinin. I. Effects of temperature and tropomyosin on the alpha-actinin/F-actin interaction. Journal of molecular Biology 67: 469

Gollnick P D, Armstrong R B, Saubert G W, Piehl K, Saltin B 1972 Enzyme activity and fiber composition in skeletal muscles of untrained and trained men. Journal of Applied Physiology 33: 312

Gordon A M, Huxley A F, Julian F J 1966 The variation in isometric tension with sarcomere length in vertebrate muscle fibres. Journal of Physiology 184: 170

Granit R 1970 The basis of motor control. Academic Press, London

Gray E G 1976 Problems of understanding the substructure of synapses. Progress in Brain Research 45: 207

Gray E G 1978 Synaptic vesicles and microtubules in frog

motor endplates. Proceedings of the Royal Society of London B 203: 219

Greenfield J G, Shy G M, Alvord E C Jr, Berg L 1957 An atlas of muscle pathology in neuromuscular diseases. Livingstone, Edinburgh

Gregory J E, Proske U 1979 The responses of Golgi tendon organs to stimulation of different combinations of motor units. Journal of Physiology 295: 251

Griffin G E, Williams P E, Goldspink G 1971 Region of longitudinal growth in striated muscle fibres. Nature 232: 28

Grove B K, Kurer V, Lehner C L, Doetchman T C, Perriard J-C, Eppenberger H M 1984 A new 185 000 dalton skeletal muscle protein detected by monoclonal antibodies. Journal of Cell Biology 98: 518

Grove B K, Cerny L, Perriard J-C, Eppenberger H M, Thornell L E 1989 Fiber type-specific distribution of M-band proteins in chicken muscle. Journal of Histochemistry and Cytochemistry 37: 447

Gruner J E 1961 La structure fine du fuseau neuromusculaire humain. Revue Neurologique 104: 490

Guth L, Samaha F J 1970 Procedure for the histochemical demonstration of actomyosin ATPase. Experimental Neurology 28: 365

Hall Z W , Kelly R B 1971 Enzymatic detachment of endplate acetylcholinesterase from muscle. Nature (New Biology) 239: 62

Hall-Craggs E C B 1974 Rapid degeneration and regeneration of a whole skeletal muscle following treatment with bupivacaine (Marcain). Experimental Neurology 43: 349

Hall-Craggs E C B, Lawrence C A 1970 Longitudinal fibre division in skeletal muscle: a light and electron microscope study. Zeitschrift für Zellforschung und mikroskopische Anatomie 109: 481

Hammersen F, Gidlof A, Larsson J, Lewis D H 1980 The occurrence of paracrystalline mitochondrial inclusions in normal human skeletal muscle. Acta Neuropathologica (Berlin) 49: 35

Handel S E, Wang S M, Greaser M L, Schultz E, Bulinski J C, Lessard J L 1989 Skeletal muscle myofibrillogenesis as revealed with a monoclonal antibody to titin in combination with detection of alpha- and gamma-isoforms of actin. Developmental Biology 132: 35

Hanson J 1973 Evidence from electron microscopic studies on actin paracrystals concerning the origin of the cross-striation in the thin filaments of vertebrate skeletal muscle. Proceedings of the Royal Society of London B 183: 39

Hanson J, O'Brien E J, Bennett P M 1971 Structure of the myosin-containing filament assembly (A-segment) separated from frog skeletal muscle. Journal of Molecular Biology 58: 865

Hanzlikova V, Schiaffino S 1977 Mitochondrial changes in ischaemic skeletal muscle. Journal of Ultrastructure Research 60: 121

Harriman D G F, Parker P L, Elliott B J 1975 The histochemistry of human intrafusal muscle fibres. Journal of Anatomy 119: 206

Harris A J 1981 Embryonic growth and innervation of rat skeletal muscles. 1. Neural regulation of muscle fibre numbers. Philosophical Transactions of the Royal Society of London B 293: 257

Hazelgrove J C 1972 X-ray evidence for a conformational change in the actin-containing filaments of vertebrate striated muscle. Cold Spring Harbor Symposium on Quantitative Biology 37: 341

Hazelgrove J C 1975 X-ray evidence for conformational changes in the myosin filament of vertebrate striated muscle. Journal of Molecular Biology 92: 113

Heine H, Schaeg G 1979 Origin and function of 'rod-like' structures in mitochondria. Acta Anatomica (Basel) 103: 1

Hellmuth A E, Allbrook D 1973 Satellite cells as the stem cells of skeletal muscle. In: Kakulas B A (ed) Basic research in myology. Excerpta Medica, Amsterdam, p 343

Henneman E, Olson C B 1964 Relations between structure and function in the design of skeletal muscles. Journal of Neurophysiology 28: 581

Hess A, Rosner S 1970 The satellite cell bud and myoblast in denervated mammalian muscle fibers. American Journal of Anatomy 129: 21

Heuser J E 1977 Synaptic vesicle exocytosis revealed in quick-frozen frog neuromuscular junctions treated with 4-aminopyridine and given a single electrical shock. In: Cowan W M, Ferrendelli J A (eds) Society for Neuroscience Symposia. Society for Neuroscience, Bethesda, vol 2, p 215

Heuser J E, Reese T S 1973 Evidence of recycling of synaptic vesicle membrane during transmitter release at the frog neuromuscular junction. Journal of Cell Biology 57: 315

Heuser J E, Salpeter M M 1979 Organization of acetylcholine receptors in quick-frozen, deep etched, and rotary-replicated *Torpedo* postsynaptic membranes. Journal of Cell Biology 82: 150

Heuser J E, Reese T S, Dennis M J, Jan Y, Jan L, Evans I 1979 Synaptic vesicle exocytosis captured by quick freezing and correlated with quantal transmitter release. Journal of Cell Biology 81: 275

Heuson-Stiennon J A 1965 Morphogenèse de la cellule musculaire striée, étudiée au microscope électronique. I. Formation des structures fibrillaires. Journal de Microscopie 4: 657

Hirokawa N, Heuser J E 1982 Internal and external differentiations of the postsynaptic membrane at the neuromuscular junction. Journal of Neurocytology 11: 487

Hoffman E P, Brown R H, Kunkel L M 1987 Dystrophin: the protein product of the Duchenne muscular dystrophy locus. Cell 51: 919

Holtzer H 1970 Proliferation and quantal cell cycles in the differentiation of muscle, cartilage and red blood cells. In: Padykula H A (ed) Gene expression in somatic cells. Academic Press, New York, p 69

Hooper J E, Kelly R B 1984 Calcium-dependent calmodulin binding to cholinergic synaptic vesicles. Journal of Biological Chemistry 259: 141

Hopkins W G, Brown M C 1984 Development of nerve cells and their connections. Cambridge University Press, Cambridge UK

Hoppeler H, Luthi P, Claassen H, Weibel E R, Howald H 1973 The ultrastructure of the normal human skeletal muscle: a morphometric analysis on untrained men, women and well-trained orienteers. Pfluegers Archiv für die Gesamte Physiologie des Menschen und der Tiere 344: 217

Horowits R, Podolsky R J 1987 The positional stability of thick filaments in activated skeletal muscle depends on sarcomere length: evidence for the role of titin filaments. Journal of Cell Biology 105: 2217

Horowits R, Maruyama K, Podolsky R J 1989 Elastic behaviour of connection filaments during thick filament movement in activated skeletal muscle. Journal of Cell Biology 109: 2169

Hoyle G 1983 Muscles and their neural control. John Wiley, New York

Hudson C S, Dyas B K, Rash J E 1982 Changes in number and distribution of orthogonal arrays during postnatal muscle development. Developmental Brain Research 4: 91

Humble J G, Jayne W H, Pulvertaft R J V 1956 Biological interaction between lymphocytes and other cells. British Journal of Haematology 2: 283

Hunt C C, Wilkinson R A, Fukami Y 1978 Ionic basis of the receptor potential in primary endings of mammalian muscle spindles. Journal of General Physiology 71: 683

Huxley A F 1957 Muscle structure and theories of contraction. Progress in Biophysics 7: 255

Huxley H E 1963 Electron microscopic studies on the structure of natural and synthetic protein filaments from striated muscle. Journal of Molecular Biology 7: 281

Huxley H E 1967 Recent X-ray diffraction and electron microscope studies of striated muscle. Journal of General Physiology 50: 71

Huxley H E 1969 The mechanism of muscle contraction. Science 164: 1356

Huxley A F 1971 The activation of striated muscle and its mechanical response. Proceedings of the Royal Society of London B 178: 1

Huxley H E 1971 The structural basis of muscular contraction. Proceedings of the Royal Society of London B 178: 131

Huxley H E 1972 Factors controlling the movement and attachment of the crossbridges in muscle. Cold Spring Harbor Symposium on Quantitative Biology 37: 341

Huxley A F 1974 Muscular Contraction. Journal of Physiology 243: 1

Huxley H E 1979 concluding remarks. In: Sugi H, Pollack G H (eds) Cross-bridge mechanism in muscle contraction. University of Tokyo Press, Tokyo, p 651

Huxley H E, Brown W 1967 The low angle X-ray diagram of vertebrate striated muscle and its behaviour during contraction and rigor. Journal of Molecular Biology 30: 383

Huxley H E, Hanson J 1954 Changes in the cross-striations of muscle during contraction, stretch and their structural interpretation. Nature 173: 973

Huxley A F, Niedergerke R 1954 Structural changes in muscle during contraction. Nature 173: 971

Huxley A F, Simmons R M 1971 Proposed mechanism of force generation in striated muscle. Nature 233: 533

Huxley A F, Simmons R M 1973 Mechanical transients and the origin of muscular force. Cold Spring Harbor Symposium on Quantitative Biology 37: 669

Isaacs W B, Kim I S, Struve A, Fulton A B 1989 Biosynthesis of titin in cultured skeletal muscle cells. Journal of Cell Biology 109: 2189

Ishikawa H 1966 Electron microscopic observations of satellite cells with special reference to the development of mammalian skeletal muscle. Zeitschrift für Anatomie und Entwicklungsgeschichte 125: 43

Ishikawa H 1979 Identification and distribution of intracellular filaments. In: Hatano S, Ishikawa H, Sato H (eds) Cell motility: molecules and organization. University Park Press, Baltimore, p 417

Ishikawa H, Bischoff R, Holtzer H 1968 Mitosis and intermediate sized filaments in developing skeletal muscle. Journal of Cell Biology 38: 538

Ishikawa H, Bischoff R, Holtzer H 1969 Formation of arrowhead complexes with heavy meromyosin in a variety of cell types. Journal of Cell Biology 43: 312

Jahromi S S, Charlton M P 1979 Transverse sarcomere splitting. Journal of Cell Biology 80: 736

James N T 1971 The histochemical demonstration of three types of intrafusal fibre in rat muscle spindles. Histochemical Journal 3: 457

Jansson E, Sjödin B, Tesch P 1978 Changes in muscle fibre type distribution in man after physical training. Acta Physiologica Scandinavica 104: 235

Jennekens F G I, Tomlinson B E, Walton J N 1971a The sizes of the two main histochemical fibre types in five limb muscles in man. An autopsy study. Journal of the Neurological Sciences 13: 281

Jennekens F G I, Tomlinson B E, Walton J N 1971b Data on the distribution of fibre types in five human limb muscles. An autopsy study. Journal of the Neurological Sciences 14: 245

Jerusalem F, Rakusa M, Engel A G, Macdonald R D 1974 Morphometric analysis of skeletal muscle capillary ultrastructure in inflammatory myopathies. Journal of the Neurological Sciences 23: 391

Jerusalem F, Engel A G, Peterson H A 1975 Human muscle fiber fine structure: morphometric data on controls. Neurology (Minneapolis) 25: 127

Jockusch B M 1979 Alpha actinin-like proteins. In: Hatano S, Ishikawa H, Sato H (eds) Cell motility: molecules and organization. University Park Press, Baltimore, p 121

Jockusch B M, Veldman H, Griffiths G W, van Oost B A, Jennekens F G I 1980 Immunofluorescence microscopy of a myopathy. Experimental Cell Research 127: 409

Johnson M A, Polgar J, Weightman D, Appleton D 1973 Data on the distribution of fibre types in 36 human muscles. An autopsy study. Journal of the Neurological Sciences 18: 111

Jones S W 1987 Presynaptic mechanisms at vertebrate neuromuscular junctions. In: Salpeter M M (ed) The vertebrate neuromuscular junction Alan R Liss, New York, p 187

Jorgensen A O, Kalnins V, Maclennan D H 1979 Localization of sarcoplasmic reticulum proteins in rat skeletal muscle by immunofluorescence. Journal of Cell Biology 80: 372

Kamieniecka Z 1968 Stages of development of human foetal muscles with reference to some muscular diseases. Journal of the Neurological Sciences 7: 319

Kamieniecka Z, Schmalbruch H 1980 Neuromuscular disorders with abnormal muscle mitochondria. In: Bourne G H, Danielli J F (eds) International Review of Cytology Vol 65. Academic Press, New York, p 321

Karlin A 1980 Molecular properties of nicotinic acetylcholine receptors. Cell Surface Reviews 6: 191

Karpati G, Engel W K 1968 Histochemical investigation of fiber type ratios with myofibrillar ATPase reaction in normal and denervated skeletal muscle. American Journal of Anatomy 122: 145

Katz B 1961 The terminations of the afferent nerve fibre in the muscle spindle of the frog. Philosophical Transactions of the Royal Society of London B 243: 221

Katz B 1969 The release of neurotransmitter substances, Liverpool University Press, Liverpool.

Katz B 1978 The release of the neuromuscular transmitter and the present state of the vesicular hypothesis. In: Porter R (ed) Studies in neurophysiology. Cambridge University Press, Cambridge, p 1

Katz B, Miledi R 1977 Transmitter leakage from motor nerve endings. Proceedings of the Royal Society of London B 196: 59

Kelly D E 1967 Models of muscle Z-band fine structure based on a looping filament configuration. Journal of Cell Biology 34: 827

Kelly D E 1969 The fine structure of skeletal muscle triad junctions. Journal of Ultrastructure Research 29: 37

Kelly A M 1971 Sarcoplasmic reticulum and T tubules in differentiating rat skeletal muscle. Journal of Cell Biology 49: 335

Kelly A M 1978 Perisynaptic satellite cells in the developing and mature rat soleus muscle. Anatomical Record 190: 891

Kelly A M 1980 T tubules in neonatal rat soleus and extensor digitorum longus muscles. Developmental Biology 80: 501

Kelly D E, Cahill M A 1972 Filamentous and matrix components of skeletal muscle Z-disks. Anatomical Record 172: 623

Kelly A M, Schotland D L 1972 The evolution of the 'checkerboard' in a rat muscle. In: Banker B Q, Przybylski R J, Van der Meulen J P, Victor M (eds) Research in muscle development and the muscle spindle. Excerpta Medica International Congress Series No. 240, p 32

Kelly A M, Zacks S I 1969a The histogenesis of rat intercostal muscle. Journal of Cell Biology 42: 135

Kelly A M, Zacks S I 1969b The fine structure of motor endplate morphogenesis. Journal of Cell Biology 42: 154

Kennedy W R, Yoon K S 1979 Permeability of muscle spindle capillaries and capsule: a horseradish peroxidase study. Muscle and Nerve 2: 101

Kerschner L 1888 Beiträge zur Kenntnis der sensiblen Endorgane. Anatomische Anzeiger 3: 288

Kitiyakara A, Angevine D M 1963 A study of the pattern of post embryonic growth of m. gracilis in mice. Developmental Biology 8: 322

Knappeis G G, Carlsen F 1962 The ultrastructure of the Z disc in skeletal muscle. Journal of Cell Biology 13: 323

Knappeis G G, Carlsen F 1968 The ultrastructure of the M-line in skeletal muscle. Journal of Cell Biology 38: 202

Knoll P 1891 Über protoplasmaarne und protoplasmareiche Muskulatur. Deukschriften der Osterreichischen Akademie der Wissenschaften 58: 633

Konigsberg I R 1971 Diffusion-mediated control of myoblast fusion. Developmental Biology 26: 133

Korneliussen H, Jansen J K S 1976 Morphological aspects of the elimination of polyneuronal innervation of skeletal muscle fibres in newborn rats. Journal of Neurocytology 5: 591

Kristić R V 1978 Die Gewebe des Menschen und der Säugetiere. Springer Verlag, Berlin

Kucera J 1977 Splitting of the nuclear bag fiber in the course of muscle spindle denervation and reinnervation. Journal of Histochemistry and Cytochemistry 25: 1102

Kucera J 1985 Characteristics of the motor innervation of muscle spindles in the monkey. American Journal of Anatomy 173: 113

Kucera J 1986 Reconstruction of the nerve supply to a human muscle spindle. Neuroscience Letters 63: 180

Kucera J, Dorovini-Zis K, Engel W K 1978 Histochemistry of rat intrafusal muscle fibres and their motor innervation. Journal of Histochemistry and Cytochemistry 26: 973

Kugelberg E, Edström L 1968 Differential histochemical effects of muscle contractions on phosphorylase and glycogen in various types of fibres: relation to fatigue. Journal of Neurology, Neurosurgery and Psychiatry 31: 415

Kuhne W 1865 Farbstoff der Muskeln. Archiv für Pathologische Anatomie und Physiologie 33: 79

Lake B D, Wilson J 1975 Zebra body myopathy. Clinical, histochemical and ultrastructural studies. Journal of the Neurological Sciences 24: 437

Landon D N 1966 Electron microscopy of muscle spindles. In: Andrew B L (ed) Control and innervation of skeletal muscle. Thomson and Co, Dundee, p 96

Landon D N 1969 The fine structure of the Z disc of rat striated muscle. Journal of Anatomy 106: 172P

Landon D N 1970a Observations on the morphogenesis of rat skeletal muscle. Journal of Anatomy 107: 385

Landon D N 1970b The influence of fixation upon the fine structure of the Z-disk of rat striated muscle. Journal of Cell Science 6: 257

Landon D N 1970c Change in Z-disk structure with muscular contraction. Journal of Physiology 211: 44P

Landon D N 1971 A quantitative study of some of the fine structural features of developing myotubes in the rat. Journal of Anatomy 110: 170

Landon D N 1972 The fine structure of the equatorial regions of developing muscle spindles in the rat. Journal of Neurocytology 1: 189

Landon D N 1974 The muscle spindle. In: Beck F, Lloyd J B (eds) The cell in medical science. Academic Press, London, vol 2, p 511

Landon D N 1982a The excitable apparatus of skeletal muscle. In: Culp W J, Ochoa J (eds) Abnormal nerves and muscles as impulse generators. Oxford University Press, Oxford, p 607

Landon D N 1982b Skeletal muscle — normal morphology, development and innervation. In: Mastaglia F L, Walton J N (eds) Skeletal muscle pathology, 1st edn. Churchill Livingstone, Edinburgh, p 1

Landon D N, Westgaard R H, MacDermot J, Thompson E J 1980 The morphology of rat soleus neuromuscular junctions treated in vitro with purified β-bungarotoxin. Brain Research 202: 1

Laporte Y 1978 The motor innervation of the muscle spindle. In: Porter R (ed) Studies in neurophysiology. Cambridge University Press, Cambridge, p 45

Larson P F, Fulthorpe J J, Hudgson P 1973 The alignment of polysomes along myosin filaments in developing myofibrils. Journal of Anatomy 116: 327

Lassignal N L, Heuser J E 1977 Evidence that β-bungarotoxin arrests synaptic vesicle recycling by blocking coated vesicle formation. Neuroscience Abstracts 3: No. 1192

Lawrence T, Mauro A 1979 Identification of satellite cells in vitro in frog muscle fibers by Nomarski optics. In: Mauro A (ed) Muscle regeneration. Raven Press, New York, p 275

Lawrie R A 1952 The activity of the cytochrome system in muscle and its relation to myoglobin. Biochemical Journal 55: 298

Lawrie R A 1953 The relation of energy-rich phosphate in muscle to myoglobin and to cytochrome-oxidase activity. Biochemical Journal 55: 305

Lazarides F 1976 Actin, alpha actinin and tropomyosin interaction in the structural organisation of actin filaments in non-muscle cells. Journal of Cell Biology 68: 202

Lazarides E, Balzer D R 1978 Specificity of desmin to avian and mammalian muscle cells. Cell 14: 429

Lazarides E, Granger B L 1978 Fluorescent localization of membrane sites in glycerinated chicken skeletal muscle fibers and the relationship of these sites to the protein composition of the Z disc. Proceedings of the National Academy of Sciences of the United States of America 75: 3683

Lazarides E, Hubbard B D, Granger B L 1979 Studies on the structure, interaction with actin, and function of desmin and intermediate filaments in chicken muscle cells. In: Hatano S, Ishikawa H, Sato H (eds) Cell motility: molecules and organization. University Park Press, Baltimore, p 521

Leksell L 1945 The action potential and excitatory effects of the small ventral root fibres to skeletal muscle. Acta physiologica scandinavica 10 (Suppl 31): 1

Lentz T L, Mazurkiewicz J R, Rosenthal J 1977 Cytochemical localization of acetylcholine receptors at the neuromuscular junction by means of horseradish peroxidase-labelled α-bungarotoxin. Brain Research 132: 423

Levitt-Gilmour T A, Salpeter M M 1986 Gradient of extrajunctional acetylcholine receptors early after denervation of mammalian muscle. Journal of Neuroscience 6: 1606

Lieberman A R 1976 Sensory ganglia. In: Landon D N (ed) The peripheral nerve. Chapman and Hall, London, p 188

Lipton B H 1979 Skeletal muscle regeneration in muscular dystrophy. In: Mauro A (ed) Muscle regeneration. Raven Press, New York, p 31

Lipton B H, Konigsberg I R 1972 A fine structural analysis of the fusion of myogenic cells. Journal of Cell Biology 53: 348

Lipton B H, Schultz E 1979 Developmental fate of skeletal muscle satellite cells. Science 205: 1292

Lloyd D P C 1943 Neuronal patterns controlling transmission of ipsilateral hind limb reflexes in the cat. Journal of Neurophysiology 6: 293

Lockhart R D, Brandt W 1937–8 Length of striated muscle fibres. Journal of Anatomy 72: 470

Loewenstein W R 1971 Mechano-electric transduction in the pacinian corpuscle. Initiation of sensory impulses in mechanoreceptors. In: Loewenstein W R (ed) Handbook of sensory physiology. Springer Verlag, Berlin, vol 1, p 269

Lömo T 1976 The role of activity in the control of membrane and contractile properties of skeletal muscle. In: Thesleff S (ed) Motor innervation of muscle. Academic Press, New York, p 289

Lömo T, Westgaard R H 1975 Control of ACh sensitivity in rat muscle fibers. Cold Spring Harbor Symposium on Quantitative Biology 40: 263

Lowey S, Slayter H S, Weeds A G, Baker H 1969 Substructure of the myosin molecule. I. Subfragments of myosin by enzymic degradation. Journal of Molecular Biology 42: 1

Lubinska L, Zelená J 1966 Formation of new sites of acetylcholine esterase activity in denervated muscles of young rats. Nature 210: 39

Luff A R, Atwood H L 1971 Changes in the sarcoplasmic reticulum and transverse tubular system of fast and slow skeletal muscles of the mouse during postnatal development. Journal of Cell Biology 51: 369

Luther P, Squire S 1978 Three-dimensional structure of the vertebrate muscle M-region. Journal of Molecular Biology 125: 313

McArdle J J, Sansone F M 1977 Re-innervation of rat fast and slow twitch muscle following nerve crush at birth. Journal of Physiology 271: 567

MacCallum J B 1898 On the histogenesis of the striated muscle fibre and the growth of the human sartorius muscle. Johns Hopkins Hospital Bulletin 9: 208

Macdonald R D, Engel A G 1971 Observations on organization of Z-disk components and on rod-bodies of Z-disk origin. Journal of Cell Biology 48: 431

Maclennan D H, Holland P C 1975 Calcium transport in sarcoplasmic reticulum. Annual Review of Biophysics and Bioengineering 4: 377

Maclennan D H, Wong P T S 1971 Isolation of a calcium-sequestering protein from sarcoplasmic reticulum. Proceedings of the National Academy of Sciences of the United States of America 68: 1231

McMahan U J, Sanes J S, Marshall L M 1978 Cholinesterase is associated with the basal lamina at the neuromuscular junction. Nature 271: 172

Madeira V M C, Antunes-Madeira M C 1973 Chemical composition of sarcolemma isolated from rabbit skeletal muscle. Biochimica et biophysica acta 298: 230

Mair W G P, Tomé F M S 1972 Atlas of the ultrastructure of diseased human muscle. Churchill Livingstone, Edinburgh

Malina R M 1978 Growth of muscle tissue and muscle mass. In: Falkner F, Tanner J M (eds) Human growth. 2. Postnatal growth. Baillière Tindall, London, p 273

Maniloff J, Vanderkooi G, Hayashi H, Capaldi R A 1973 Optical analysis of electron micrographs of cytochrome oxidase membranes. Biochimica et biophysica acta 298: 180

Marchand E R, Eldred E 1969 Postnatal increase of intrafusal fibers in the rat muscle spindle. Experimental Neurology 25: 655

Martin L, Joris C 1970 Histoenzymological and semiquantitative study of the maturation of the human muscle fibre. In: Walton J N, Canal N, Scarlato G (eds) Disease of muscle. International Congress Series No. 199. Excerpta Medica, Amsterdam, p 657

Martonosi A N 1982 Regulation of cytoplasmic calcium concentration by the sarcoplasmic reticulum. In: Schotland D L (ed) Disorders of the motor unit. John Wiley, New York, p 565

Martonosi A, Roufa D, Ha D-B, Boland R 1980 The biosynthesis of sarcoplasmic reticulum. Federation Proceedings 39: 2415

Maruyama K 1986 Connectin: an elastic filamentous protein of striated muscle. International Review of Cytology 104: 81

Maruyama K, Yamamoto K 1979 Contribution of connectin to the parallel elastic component of muscle. In: Sugi H, Pollack G H (eds) Cross-bridge mechanism in muscle contraction. University of Tokyo Press, Tokyo, p 319

Maruyama K, Matsubara S, Natori R, Nonomura Y, Kimura S, Ohashi K, Murakami F, Handa S, Eguchi G 1977 Connectin, an elastic protein from muscle. Characterization and function. Journal of Biochemistry 82: 317

Maruyama K, Matsuno A, Higuchi H, Shimaoka S, Kimura S, Shimizu T 1989 Behaviour of connectin (titin) and nebulin in skinned muscle fibres released after extreme stretch as revealed by immunoelectron microscopy. Journal of Muscle Research and Cell Motility 10: 350

Masaki T, Endo M, Ebashi S 1967 Localization of 6S component of alpha actinin at the Z-band. Journal of Biochemistry 62: 630

Mastaglia F L 1974 The development and growth of the skeletal muscles and connective tissues. In: Davis J A, Dobbing J (eds) Scientific foundations of paediatrics. Heinemann, London, p 348

Mastaglia F L, Dawkins R L, Papadimitriou J M 1975a Morphological changes in skeletal muscle after transplantation. Journal of the Neurological Sciences 25: 227

Mastaglia F L, Papadimitriou J M, Dawkins R L 1975b Mechanisms of cell mediated myotoxicity. Journal of the Neurological Sciences 25: 269

Matthews B H C 1933 Nerve endings in mammalian muscle. Journal of Physiology 78: 1

Matthews P B C 1964 Muscle spindles and their motor control. Physiological Reviews 44: 219

Matthews P B C 1972 Mammalian muscle receptors and their central actions. Edward Arnold, London

Matthews P B C 1977 Muscle afferents and kinaesthesia. British Medical Bulletin 33: 137

Mauro A 1961 Satellite cell of skeletal muscle fibres. Journal of Biophysical and Biochemical Cytology 9: 493

Meissner G, Conner G E, Fleisher S 1973 Isolation of sarcoplasmic reticulum by zonal centrifugation and purification of Ca^{2+}-pump and Ca^{2+}-binding proteins. Biochimica et biophysica acta 298: 246

Melmed C, Karpati G, Carpenter S 1975 Experimental mitochondrial myopathy produced by in vivo uncoupling of oxidative phosphorylation. Journal of the Neurological Sciences 26: 305

Menke A, Jockusch H 1991 Decreased osmotic stability of dystrophin-less muscle cells from the mdx mouse. Nature, London 349: 69

Merrillees N C R 1962 Some observations on the fine structure of a Golgi tendon-organ of a rat. In: Barker D (ed) Symposium on muscle receptors. Hong Kong University Press, Hong Kong, p 199

Meves F 1909 Uber Neubildung quergestreifter Muskelfasern nach Beobachtungen am Huhnerembryo. Anatomische Anzeiger 34: 161

Milburn A 1973 The early development of muscle spindles in the rat. Journal of Cell Science 12: 175

Milburn A 1976 The effect of the local anaesthetic bupivacaine on the muscle spindle of the rat. Journal of Neurocytology 5: 425

Milburn A 1984 Stages in the development of cat muscle spindles. Journal of Embryology and Experimental Morphology 82: 177

Miller A, Tregear R T 1972 Structure of insect fibrillar flight muscle in the presence and absence of ATP. Journal of Molecular Biology 70: 85

Milligan R A, Whittaker M, Safer D 1990 Molecular structure of F-actin and location of surface binding sites. Nature 348: 217

Miyoshi T, Kennedy W R 1979 Microvasculature of rabbit muscle spindles. Archives of Neurology (Chicago) 36: 471

Miyoshi T, Kennedy W R, Yoon K S 1979 Morphometric comparison of capillaries in muscle spindles, nerve, and muscle. Archives of Neurology (Chicago) 36: 547

Mobley B A, Eisenberg B R 1975 Sizes of components in frog skeletal muscle measured by methods of stereology. Journal of General Physiology 66: 31

Montgomery R D 1962 Growth of human striated muscle. Nature 195: 194

Moore M J, Rebeiz J J, Holden M 1971 Biometric analyses of normal skeletal muscle. Acta neuropathologica (Berlin) 19: 51

Moos C, Mason C M, Besterman J M, Feng I-N M, Dubin J H 1978 The binding of skeletal muscle C-protein to F-actin, and its relation to the interaction of actin with myosin subfragment 1. Journal of Molecular Biology 124: 571

Morgan-Hughes J A, Darveniza P, Kahn S N, Landon D N, Sherratt R M, Land J M, Clark J B 1977 A mitochondrial myopathy characterized by a deficiency in reducible cytochrome b. Brain 100: 617

Morkin E 1970 Postnatal muscle fiber assembly; localization of newly synthesized myofibrillar proteins. Science 167: 1499

Morpurgo B 1898 Uber die postembryonale Entwicklung der quergestreiften Muskeln von weissen Ratten. Anatomische Anzeiger 15: 200

Moss F P 1968 The relationship between the dimensions of the fibres and the number of nuclei during normal growth of skeletal muscle in the domestic fowl. American Journal of Anatomy 122: 555

Moss F P, Leblond C P 1970 Nature of dividing nuclei in skeletal muscle of growing rats. Journal of Cell Biology 44: 459

Moss F P, Leblond C P 1971 Satellite cells as the source of nuclei in muscles of growing rats. Anatomical Record 170: 421

Muir A R 1970 The structure and distribution of satellite cells. In: Mauro A, Shafiq S A, Milhorat A T (eds) Regeneration of striated muscle, and myogenesis. Excerpta Medica, Amsterdam, p 91

Muir A R, Kanji A H M, Allbrook D B 1965 The structure of satellite cells in skeletal muscle. Journal of Anatomy 99: 435

Munger B L 1971 Patterns of organization of peripheral sensory receptors. In: Loewenstein W R (ed) Handbook of sensory physiology. Springer Verlag, Berlin, vol 1, p 523

Nachmias V T, Padykula H A 1958 A histochemical study of normal and denervated red and white muscles of the rat. Journal of Biophysical and Biochemical Cytology 4: 47

Nave R, Furst D O, Weber K 1989 Visualization of the polarity of isolated titin molecules: a single globular head on a long thin rod as the M band anchoring domain? Journal of Cell Biology 109: 2177

Nave R, Furst D O, Weber K 1990 Interaction of alpha-actinin and nebulin in vitro. Support for the existence of a fourth filament system in skeletal muscle. FEBS Letters 269: 163

Needham D M 1971 Machina carnis. Cambridge University Press, Cambridge

Numa S, Noda M, Takahashi H, Tanabe T, Toyosato M, Furutani S 1984 Molecular structure of the nicotinic acetylcholine receptor. Cold Spring Harbor Symposium on Quantitative Biology 48: 57

Nyström B 1967 Muscle spindle histochemistry. Science 155: 1424

O'Brien R A D, Östberg J C, Vrbová G 1978 Observations on the elimination of polyneuronal innervation in developing mammalian skeletal muscle. Journal of Physiology 282: 571

Offer G, Moos C, Starr R 1973 A new protein of the thick filaments of vertebrate skeletal myofibrils. Extraction, purification and characterization. Journal of Molecular Biology 74: 653

Ogata T 1958a A histochemical study of the red and white muscle fibers. Part I. Activity of the succinoxidase system in muscle fibers. Acta medicinae Okayama 12: 216

Ogata T 1958b A histochemical study of the red and white muscle fibers. Part II. Activity of the cytochrome oxidase in muscle fibers. Acta medicinae Okayama 12: 228

Ogata T, Mori M 1964 Histochemical study of oxidative enzymes in vertebrate muscles. Journal of Histochemistry and Cytochemistry 12: 171

Ogata T, Murata F 1969 Cytological features of three fiber types in human striated muscle. Tohoku Journal of Experimental Medicine 99: 225

Ohtsuki I 1975 Distribution of troponin components in the thin filament studied by immunoelectron microscopy. Journal of Biochemistry 77: 633

Ohtsuki I 1979 Molecular arrangement of troponin-T in the thin filament. Journal of Biochemistry 86: 491

Ohtsuki I, Masaki T, Nonomura Y, Ebashi S 1967 Periodic distribution of troponin along the thin filament. Journal of Biochemistry 61: 817

Oldfors A, Fardeau M 1983 The permeability of the basal lamina at the neuromuscular junction. An ultrastructural study of rat skeletal muscle using particulate tracers. Neuropathology and Applied Neurobiology 9: 419

Ontell M 1974 Muscle satellite cells. Anatomical Record 178: 211

Ontell M 1977 Neonatal muscle: an electron microscopic study. Anatomical Record 189: 669

Ontell M 1979 The source of 'new' muscle fibers in neonatal muscle. In: Mauro A (ed) Muscle regeneration. Raven Press, New York, p 137

Ovalle W K 1971 Fine structure of rat intrafusal muscle fibres. The polar region. Journal of Cell Biology 51: 83

Ovalle W K 1972 Fine structure of rat intrafusal fibres. The equatorial region. Journal of Cell Biology 52: 382

Ovalle W K, Smith R S 1972 Histochemical identification of three types of intrafusal muscle fibers in the cat and monkey based on the myosin ATPase reaction. Canadian Journal of Physiology and Pharmacology 50: 195

Padykula H A 1952 The localization of succinic dehydrogenase in tissue sections of the rat. American Journal of Anatomy 91: 107

Padykula H A, Gauthier G F 1970 The ultrastructure of the neuromuscular junctions of mammalian red, white, and intermediate skeletal muscle fibers. Journal of Cell Biology 46: 27

Padykula H A, Herman E 1955 The specificity of the histochemical method for adenosine triphosphate. Journal of Histochemistry and Cystochemistry 3: 170

Page S G 1965 A comparison of the fine structures of frog slow and twitch muscle fibres. Journal of Cell Biology 26: 477

Page S G 1968 Fine structure of tortoise skeletal muscle. Journal of Physiology 197: 709

Page S G 1969 Structure and some contractile properties of fast and slow muscle of the chicken. Journal of Physiology 205: 131

Page E, Power B, Fozzard H A, Meddoff D A 1969 Sarcolemmal evaginations with knob-like or stalked projections in Purkinje fibres of the sheep's heart. Journal of Ultrastructure Research 28: 288

Payne C M, Stern L Z, Curless R G, Hannapel L K 1975 Ultrastructural fibre typing in normal and diseased human muscle. Journal of the Neurological Sciences 25: 99

Peachey L D 1965 The sarcoplasmic reticulum and transverse tubules of the frog's sartorius. Journal of Cell Biology 25: 209

Peachey L D, Eisenberg B R 1978 Helicoids in the T system and striations of frog skeletal muscle fibres seen by high voltage electron microscopy. Biophysics Journal 22: 145

Pearson M L 1981 Muscle differentiation in cell culture: a problem in somatic cell and molecular genetics. In: Leighton T, Loomis W F (eds) An introduction to recent research on experimental systems. Academic Press, New York

Pease D C, Quilliam T A 1957 Electron microscopy of the pacinian corpuscle. Journal of Biophysical and Biochemical Cytology 3: 331

Pellegrino C, Franzini C 1963 An electron microscopic study of denervation atrophy in red and white skeletal muscle fibers. Journal of Cell Biology 17: 327

Pepe F A 1966 Some aspects of the structural organization of the myofibril as revealed by antibody-staining methods. Journal of Cell Biology 28: 505

Pepe F A 1975 Structure of muscle filaments from immunohistochemical and ultrastructural studies. Journal of Histochemistry and Cytochemistry 23: 543

Pepe F A 1979 The myosin filament: molecular structure. In: Pepe F A, Sanger J W, Nachmias V T (eds) Motility in cell function. Academic Press, New York, p 103

Pepe F A, Dowben P 1977 The myosin filament. V. Intermediate voltage electron microscopy and optical diffraction studies of the substructure. Journal of Molecular Biology 113: 199

Pepe F A, Drucker B 1975 The myosin filament. III. C-protein. Journal of Molecular Biology 99: 609

Pette D 1985 Metabolic heterogeneity of muscle fibres. Journal of Experimental Biology 115: 179

Pette D, Staron R S 1988 Molecular basis of the phenotypic characteristics of mammalian muscle fibres. In: Plasticity of the neuromuscular system. Wiley, Chichester (Ciba Foundation Symposium 138), p 22

Pierobon-Bormioli S, Betto R, Salviati G 1989 The organization of titin (connectin) and nebulin in the sarcomeres: an immunocytolocalization study. Journal of Muscle Research and Cell Motility 10: 446

Polgar J, Johnson M A, Weightman D, Appleton D 1973 Data on fibre size in 36 human muscles. An autopsy study. Journal of the Neurological Sciences 19: 307

Price H M, Gordon G B, Pearson C M, Munsat T L, Blumberg J M 1965 New evidence of excessive accumulation of Z-band material in nemaline myopathy. Proceedings of the National Academy of Sciences of the United States of America 45: 1398

Prince F P, Hikida R S, Hagerman F C, Staron R S, Allen W H 1981 A morphometric analysis of human muscle fibres with relation to fibre types and adaptations to exercise. Journal of the Neurological Sciences 49: 165

Pullen A H 1977 The distribution and relative sizes of three histochemical fibre types in the rat tibialis anterior muscle. Journal of Anatomy 123: 1

Pumplin D W, Fambrough D M 1983 ($Na^+ + K^+$)—ATPase correlated with a major group of intramembrane particles in freeze-fracture replicas of cultured chick myotubes. Journal of Cell Biology 97: 1214

Pumplin D W, Reese T S, Llinas R 1981 Are the presynaptic active zone particles the calcium channels? Proceedings of the National Academy of Sciences USA 78: 7210

Ranvier L A 1873 Des muscles rouges et des muscles blancs chez les rongeurs. Comptes rendus hebdomadaires des séances de l'Académie des sciences 77: 1030

Rash J E, Ellisman M H 1974 Studies of excitable membranes. I. Macromolecular specializations of the neuromuscular junction and the nonjunctional sarcolemma. Journal of Cell Biology 63: 567

Rayns D G, Devine C E, Sutherland C 1975 Freeze fracture studies of membrane systems in vertebrate muscle. I. Striated muscle. Journal of Ultrastructure Research 50: 306

Redfern P A 1970 Neuromuscular transmission in newborn rats. Journal of Physiology 209: 701

Reedy M K 1964 The structure of actin filaments and the origin of the axial periodicity in the I substance of vertebrate striated muscle. Proceedings of the Royal Society of London B 160: 458

Reedy M K 1967 Personal communication, quoted by Elliott, Lowy & Millman (1967)

Reedy M K, Barkes A E 1974 Disordering of myofibril structure due to fixation, dehydration and embedding. Journal of Cell Biology 63: 282a

Reniers J, Martin L, Joris C 1970 Histochemical and quantitative analysis of muscle biopsies. Journal of the Neurological Sciences 10: 349

Reske-Nielsen E, Coërs C, Harmsen A 1970 Qualitative and quantitative histological study of neuromuscular biopsies from healthy young men. Journal of the Neurological Sciences 10: 369

Revel J P 1962 The sarcoplasmic reticulum of the bat cricothyroid muscle. Journal of Cell Biology 12: 571

Reznik M 1969 Thymidine ^{3}H uptake by satellite cells of regenerating skeletal muscle. Journal of Cell Biology 40: 568

Reznik M 1970 Satellite cells, myoblasts and skeletal muscle regeneration. In: Mauro A, Shafiq S A, Milhorat A T (eds) Regeneration of skeletal muscle, and myogenesis. Excerpta Medica, Amsterdam, p 133

Riley D A 1977 Spontaneous elimination of nerve terminals from the end-plates of developing skeletal myofibers. Brain Research 134: 279

Riley D A 1981 Ultrastructural evidence for axon retraction during spontaneous elimination of polyneuronal innervation of the rat soleus muscle. Journal of Neurocytology 10: 425

Romanul F C A 1964 Enzymes in muscle. I. Histochemical studies of enzymes in individual muscle fibres. Archives of Neurology (Chicago) 11: 355

Romanul F C A, van der Meulen J 1967 Slow and fast muscles after cross-innervation. Enzymatic and physiological changes. Archives of Neurology (Chicago) 17: 387

Rome E, Offer G, Pepe F A 1973 X-ray diffraction of muscle labelled with antibody to C-protein. Nature (New Biology) 244: 152

Rosenbluth J 1969 Sarcoplasmic reticulum of an unusually fast-acting crustacean muscle. Journal of Cell Biology 42: 534

Rosenbluth J 1974 Substructure of the amphibian motor endplate. Evidence for a granular component projecting from the outer surface of the receptive membrane. Journal of Cell Biology 62: 755

Ross K F A, Jans D E, Larson P F, Mastaglia F L, Parsons R, Fulthorpe J J, Jenkison M, Walton J N 1970 Distribution of ribosomal RNA in fusing myoblasts. Nature 226: 545

Ross M J, Klymkowsky M W, Agard D A, Stroud R M 1977 Structural studies of membrane-bound acetylcholine receptor from Torpedo californica. Journal of Molecular Biology 116: 635

Rotundo R L 1987 Biogenesis and regulation of acetylcholinesterase. In: Salpeter M M (ed) The vertebrate neuromuscular junction. Alan R Liss, New York, p 247

Rowe R W 1971 Ultrastructure of the Z-line of skeletal muscle fibers. Journal of Cell Biology 51: 674

Rowe R W 1973 The ultrastructure of Z-disks from white, intermediate, and red fibres of mammalian striated muscle. Journal of Cell Biology 57: 261

Rubinstein N A, Kelly A M 1981 Development of muscle fiber specialization in the rat hind limb. Journal of Cell Biology 90: 128

Rubinstein N A, Lyons G E, Kelly A M 1988 Hormonal control of myosin heavy chain genes during development of skeletal muscles. In: Plasticity of the neuromuscular system. Wiley, Chichester (Ciba Foundation Symposium 138), p 35

Ruffini A 1898 On the minute anatomy of the neuromuscular spindles of the cat, and on their physiological significance. Journal of Physiology 23: 190

Ruska H, Edwards G A 1957 A new cytoplasmic pattern in striated muscle fibres and its possible relation to growth. Growth 21: 73

Ruskell G L 1978 The fine structure of innervated myotendinous cylinders in extraocular muscles of rhesus monkeys. Journal of Neurocytology 7: 693

Sahgal V, Subramani V, Hughes R, Shah H, Singh H 1979 On the pathogenesis of the mitochondrial myopathies: an experimental study. Acta Neuropathologica (Berlin) 46: 177

Salmons S, Gale D, Sreter F 1978 Ultrastructural aspects of the transformation of muscle fibre type by long-term stimulation: changes in Z discs and mitochondria. Journal of Anatomy 127: 17

Salpeter M M 1967 Electron microscope autoradiography as a quantitative tool in enzyme cytochemistry. I. The distribution of acetylcholinesterase at motor endplates of a vertebrate twitch muscle. Journal of Cell Biology 32: 379

Salpeter M M 1987 Development and neural control of the neuromuscular junction and of the junctional acetylcholine receptor. In: Salpeter M M (ed) The vertebrate neuromuscular junction. Alan Liss, New York, p 55

Salviati G, Betto R, Ceoldo S, Pierobon-Bormioli S 1990 Morphological and functional characterization of the endosarcomeric elastic filament. American Journal of Physiology 259: C 144

Sanes J R 1982 Laminin, fibronectin and collagen in synaptic and extrasynaptic portions of muscle fiber basement membrane. Journal of Cell Biology 9: 442

Sato T, Seki K, Hirawake H, Nakamura S, Horai S, Ozawa T 1990 Immunocytochemistry of mitochondria. Journal of the Neurological Sciences 98: 58

Sandri C, van Buren J M, Akert K 1977 Membrane morphology of the vertebrate nervous system. Progress in Brain Research 46. Elsevier, Amsterdam

Scalzi H A, Price H M 1971 The arrangement and sensory innervation of the intrafusal fibers in the feline muscle spindle. Journal of Ultrastructure Research 36: 375

Schiaffino S, Hanzlikova V 1972 Autophagic degradation of glycogen in skeletal muscles of the newborn rat. Journal of Cell Biology 52: 41

Schiaffino S, Margreth A 1969 Coordinated development of the sarcoplasmic reticulum and T-system during postnatal differentiation of rat skeletal muscle. Journal of Cell Biology 41: 855

Schiaffino S, Hanzlikova V, Pierobon S 1970 Relations between structure and function in rat skeletal muscle fibers. Journal of Cell Biology 47: 107

Schiaffino S, Pierobon Bormioli S 1976 Morphogenesis of rat muscle spindles after nerve lesion during early postnatal development. Journal of Neurocytology 5: 319

Schiaffino S, Pierobon Bormioli S, Aloisi M 1979 Fiber branching and formation of new fibers during compensatory muscle hypertrophy. In: Mauro A (ed) Muscle regeneration. Raven Press, New York, p 177

Schmalbruch H 1968 Noniusperioden und Langen Wachstum der quergestriefen Muskelfaser. Zeitschrift für Mikroskopische Anatomie Forschung 79: 493

Schmalbruch H 1976 Muscle fibre splitting and regeneration in diseased human muscle. Neuropathology and Applied Neurobiology 2: 3

Schmalbruch H 1979a 'Square arrays' in the sarcolemma of human skeletal muscle fibres. Nature 281: 145

Schmalbruch H 1979b Manifestations of regeneration in myopathic muscles. In: Mauro A (ed) Muscle regeneration. Raven Press, New York, p 201

Schmalbruch H 1980 Delayed fixation alters the pattern of intramembrane particles in mammalian muscle fibers. Journal of Ultrastructure Research 70: 15

Schmalbruch H 1983 The fine structure of mitochondrial abnormalities in muscle diseases. In: Scarlato G, Cerri C (eds) Mitochondrial pathology in muscle diseases. Piccin, Padua, p 41

Schmalbruch H 1985 Skeletal muscle. Springer-Verlag, Berlin

Schmalbruch H, Kamieniecka Z 1974 Fiber types in human brachial biceps muscle. Experimental Neurology 44: 313

Schmitt H P 1978 Quantitative analysis of voluntary muscles from routine autopsy material, with special reference to the problem of remote carcinomatous changes ('neuromyopathy'). Acta neuropathologica (Berlin) 43: 143

Schneider M F, Chandler W K 1973 Voltage-dependent charge movement in skeletal muscle: a possible step in excitation–contraction coupling. Nature 242: 244

Schollmeyer J V, Goll D E, Stromer M H, Dayton W, Singh I, Robson R M 1974 Studies on the composition of the Z-disk. Journal of Cell Biology 63: 303a

Schotland D L, Bonilla E, Wakayama Y 1981 Freeze–fracture studies of muscle plasma membrane in human muscular dystrophy. Acta Neuropathologica (Berlin) 54: 189

Schoultz T W, Swett J E 1972 The fine structure of the Golgi tendon organ. Journal of Neurocytology 1: 1

Schoultz T W, Swett J E 1974 Ultrastructural organization of the sensory fibers innervating the Golgi tendon organ. Anatomical Record 179: 147

Schröder J M 1974 The fine structure and de- and reinnervated muscle spindles. I The increase, atrophy and 'hypertrophy' of intrafusal muscle fibres. Acta Neuropathologica (Berlin) 30: 109

Schröder J M, Kemme P T, Scholz L 1979 The fine structure of denervated and reinnervated muscle spindles: morphometric study of intrafusal fibres. Acta Neuropathologica (Berlin) 46: 95

Schultz E 1974 A quantitative study of the satellite cell population in postnatal mouse lumbrical muscle. Anatomical Record 180: 589

Schultz E 1978 Changes in satellite cells in growing muscle following denervation. Anatomical Record 190: 229

Schultz E 1979 Quantification of satellite cells in growing muscle using electron microscopy and fiber whole mounts. In: Mauro A (ed) Muscle regeneration. Raven Press, New York, p 131

Schwartz M S, Sargeant M, Swash M 1976 Longitudinal fibre splitting in neurogenic muscular disorders. Its relation to the pathogenesis of 'myopathic' change. Brain 99: 617

Shafiq S A, Gorycki M A, Goldstone L, Milhorat A T 1966 Fine structure of fiber types in normal human muscle. Anatomical Record 156: 283

Shafiq S A, Gorycki M, Mauro A 1967 An electron microscopic study of regeneration and satellite cells in human muscle. Neurology (Minneapolis) 17: 567

Shafiq S A, Gorycki M A, Milhorat A T 1969 An electron microscope study of fibre types in normal and dystrophic muscles of the mouse. Journal of Anatomy 104: 281

Shafiq S A, Askanas V, Milhorat A T 1971 Fiber types and preclinical changes in chicken muscular dystrophy. Archives of Neurology (Chicago) 25: 283

Shear C R 1975 Myofibril proliferation in developing skeletal muscle. In: Bradley W G, Gardner-Medwin D, Walton J N (eds) Recent advances in myology. Excerpta Medica, Amsterdam, p 364

Sherrington C S 1894 On the anatomical constitution of nerves of skeletal muscles; with remarks on recurrent fibres in the ventral spinal nerve root. Journal of Physiology 17: 211

Shimada Y 1971 Electron microscope observations on the fusion of chick myoblasts in vitro. Journal of Cell Biology 48: 128

Shy G M, Engel W K, Somers J E, Wanko T 1963 Nemaline myopathy — a new congenital myopathy. Brain 86: 793

Singh I, Goll D E, Robson R M, Stromer M H 1977 N- and C-terminal amino acids of purified alpha actinin. Biochimica et biophysica acta 491: 29

Siperstein M D, Unger R H, Madison L L 1968 Studies of muscle capillary basement membranes of normal subjects, diabetic and prediabetic patients. Journal of Clinical Investigation 47: 1973

Sirken S M, Fischbeck K H 1985 Freeze–fracture studies of denervated and tenotomized rat muscle. Journal of Neuropathology and Experimental Neurology 44: 147

Sjöström M, Squire J M 1977 The fine structure of the A- band in cryo-sections. Journal of Molecular Biology 109: 49

Sjöström M, Kidman S, Henriksson-Larsen K, Angquist K-A 1982a Z- and M-band appearance in different histochemically defined types of human skeletal muscle fibres. Journal of Histochemistry and Cytochemistry 30: 1

Sjöström M, Angqvist K-A, Bylund A-C, Friden J, Gustavsson L, Schersten T 1982b Morphometric analysis of human muscle fibre types. Muscle and Nerve 5: 538

Small J V, Sobieszek A 1977 Studies on the function and composition of the 10-nm (100 A) filaments of vertebrate smooth muscle. Journal of Cell Science 23: 243

Snow M H 1979 Origin of regenerating myoblasts in mammalian skeletal muscle. In: Mauro A (ed) Muscle regeneration. Raven Press, New York, p 91

Somlyo A V 1979 Bridging structures spanning the junctional gap at the triad of skeletal muscle. Journal of Cell Biology 80: 743

Soukup T, Zelená J 1990 Myogenesis in rat muscle spindles after neonatal deafferentation. Journal of the Neurological Sciences 98 (suppl.): 48

Spencer P S, Schaumburg H H 1973 An ultrastructural study of the inner core of the pacinian corpuscle. Journal of Neurocytology 2: 217

Spiro A J, Beilin R L 1969 Human muscle spindle histochemistry. Archives of Neurology (Chicago) 20: 271

Squire J 1981 The structural basis of muscular contraction. Plenum Press, New York

Stacey M J 1969 Free endings in the skeletal muscle of the cat. Journal of Anatomy 105: 231

Stadhouders A M 1981 Mitochondrial ultrastructural changes in muscular diseases. In: Busch H F M, Jennekens F G I, Scholte H R (eds) Mitochondria and muscular diseases. Mefar, Netherlands, p 113

Stadhouders A, Jap P, Walliman T 1990 Biochemical nature of mitochondrial crystals. Journal of the Neurological Sciences 98: 304

Staron R S, Pette D 1987 The multiplicity of myosin light and heavy chain combinations in histochemically typed single fibres of rabbit soleus muscle. Biochemical Journal 243: 687

Starr R, Offer G 1978 The interaction of C-protein with heavy meromyosin and subfragment-2. Biochemical Journal 171: 813

Stein J M, Padykula H A 1962 Histochemical classification of individual skeletal muscle fibers of the rat. American Journal of Anatomy 110: 103

Stickland N C 1981 Muscle development in the human foetus as exemplified by m. sartorius: a quantitative study. Journal of Anatomy 132: 557

Stockdale F E, Holtzer H 1961 DNA synthesis and myogenesis. Experimental Cell Research 24: 508

Stonnington H H, Engel A G 1973 Normal and denervated muscle. Neurology (Minneapolis) 23: 714

Strehler B L, Konigsberg I R, Kelly F E, 1963 Ploidy of myotube nuclei developing in vitro as determined with a recording double-beam micro-spectrophotometer. Experimental Cell Research 32: 232

Stromer M H, Hartshorne D J, Rice R V 1967 Removal and reconstruction of Z-line material in striated muscle. Journal of Cell Biology 35: 623

Stromer M H, Hartshorne D J, Mueller H, Rice R V 1969 The effects of various protein fractions on Z- and M-line reconstruction. Journal of Cell Biology 40: 167

Stromer M H, Tabatabai L B, Robson R M, Goll D E, Zeece M G 1976 Nemaline myopathy—an integrated study: selective extraction. Experimental Neurology 50: 402

Suzuki A, Goll D E, Singh I, Allen R E, Robson R M, Stromer M H 1976 Some properties of purified skeletal muscle alpha actinin. Journal of Biological Chemistry 251: 6860

Swett J E, Eldred E 1960 Distribution and numbers of stretch receptors in medial gastrocnemius and soleus muscles of the cat. Anatomical Record 137: 453

Tabary J C, Tabary C, Tardieu C, Tardieu G, Goldspink G 1972 Physiological and structural changes in the cat's soleus muscle due to immobilization at different lengths by plaster casts. Journal of Physiology 224: 231

Tachikawa T, Clementi F 1979 Early effects of denervation on the morphology of junctional and extrajunctional sarcolemma. Neuroscience 4: 437

Tada M, Yamamoto T, Tonomura Y 1978 Molecular mechanism of active calcium transport by sarcoplasmic reticulum. Physiological Reviews 58: 1

Tello J F 1917 Genesis de las terminaciones nerviosas motrices y sensitivas. Trabajos del Labortorio de investigaciones biológicas de la Universidad de Madrid 15: 101

Tello J F 1922 Die Entstehung der motorischen und sensiblen Nervendigungen. Zeitschrift für die Gesamte Anatomie 64: 348

Teravainen H 1968 Development of the myoneural junction in the rat. Zeitschrift für Zellforschung und Mikroskopische Anatomie 87: 249

Teravainen H 1970 Satellite cells of striated muscle after compression injury so slight as not to cause degeneration of the muscle fibres. Zeitschrift für Zellforschung und Mikroskopische Anatomie 103: 320

Thesleff S, Libelius R, Lundquist I 1979 Endocytosis as inducer of degenerative changes in skeletal muscle. In: Kidman A D, Tomkins J M (eds) Muscle, nerve and brain degeneration. Excerpta Medica, Amsterdam, p 119

Thompson W, Kuffler D P, Jansen J K S 1979 The effect of prolonged, reversible block of nerve impulses on the elimination of polyneuronal innervation of new-born rat skeletal muscle fibers. Neuroscience 4: 271

Thornell L-E, Pedrosa F 1990 Development of muscle spindles involves special myogenic cell lineages and neurogenic influence. Journal of the Neurological Sciences 98 (suppl): 46

Thornell L-E, Sjöström M, Andersson K-E 1976 The relationship between mechanical stress and myofibrillar organization in heart Purkinje fibres. Journal of Molecular and Cellular Cardiology 8: 689

Thornell L-E, Edström L, Eriksson A, Henrikson K-G, Angquist K-A 1980 The distribution of intermediate

filament protein (skeletin) in normal and diseased human skeletal muscle. Journal of the Neurological Sciences 47: 153

Tower S S 1932 Atrophy and degeneration in the muscle spindle. Physiological Reviews 33: 90

Trayer I P, Perry S V 1966 The myosin of developing skeletal muscle. Biochemische Zeitschrift 345: 87

Trinick J, Elliott A 1979 Electron microscopic studies of thick filaments from vertebrate skeletal muscle. Journal of Molecular Biology 131: 133

Trupin G L, Hsu L, Hsieh Y-H 1979 Satellite cell mimics in regenerating skeletal muscle. In: Mauro A (ed) Muscle regeneration. Raven Press, New York, p 101

Ullrick W C 1967 A theory of contraction for striated muscle. Journal of Theoretical Biology 15: 53

Ullrick W C, Toselli P A, Saide J D, Phear W P C 1977 Fine structure of the vertebrate Z-disc. Journal of Molecular Biology 115: 61

van Buren J M, Frank K 1965 Correlation between the morphology and potential field of a spinal motor nucleus in the cat. Electroencephalography and Clinical Neurophysiology 19: 112

van Essen D C 1982 Neuromuscular synapse elimination: structural, functional and mechanical aspects. In: Spitzer N C (ed) Neuronal development. Plenum Press, New York, p 333

van Linge B 1962 The response of muscle to strenuous exercise. Journal of Bone and Joint Surgery 44B: 711

Viragh S Z, Challice C E 1969 Variations in filamentous and fibrillar organization and associated sarcolemmal structures in cells of the normal mammalian heart. Journal of Ultrastructure Research 28: 321

von Brzezinski D K 1962 Untersuchungen zur Histochemie der Muskelspindeln. I Mitteilung: Topochemie der Polysaccharide. Acta histochemica; Zeitschrift für Histologische Topochemie 12: 75

Vracko R 1970 Skeletal muscle capillaries in diabetics: a quantitative analysis. Circulation 41: 271

Vracko R, Benditt E P 1972 Basal lamina: the scaffold for orderly cell replacement. Observations on regeneration of injured skeletal muscle fibres and capillaries. Journal of Cell Biology 55: 406

Vrbova G, Lowie M B, Evers J 1988 Reorganization of synaptic inputs to developing skeletal muscle fibres. In: Plasticity of the neuromuscular system. Wiley, Chichester (Ciba Foundation Symposium 138), p 131

Wachstein M, Meisel E 1955 The distribution of demonstrable succinic dehydrogenase and of mitochondria in tongue and skeletal muscle. Journal of Biophysical and Biochemical Cytology 1: 483

Wakayama Y, Schotland D L 1979 Muscle satellite cell populations in Duchenne dystrophy. In: Mauro A (ed) Muscle regeneration. Raven Press, New York, p 121

Walker S M, Schrodt G R 1968 Triads in skeletal muscle fibers of 19-day fetal rats. Journal of Cell Biology 37: 564

Walliman T, Pelloni G, Turner D C, Eppenberger H M 1979 Removal of the M-line by treatment with Fab' fragments of antibodies against MM-creatine kinase. In: Pepe F A, Sanger J W, Nachmias V T (eds) Motility in cell function. Academic Press, New York, p 415

Walro J M, Kucera J 1985 Motor innervation of intrafusal fibers in rat muscle spindles: incomplete separation of dynamic and static systems. American Journal of Anatomy 173: 55

Walro J M, Kucera J 1988 Sensory 'cross-terminals' between dynamic and static intrafusal fibres in rat muscle spindles. In: Hnik P, Soukup T, Vesjada R, Zelena J (eds) Mechanoreceptors, development, structure and function. Plenum Press, New York, p 105

Walsh F S, Ritter M A 1981 Surface antigen differentiation during myogenesis in culture. Nature 289: 60

Wang K 1982 Myofilaments and myofibrillar connections: role of titin, nebulin, and intermediate filaments. In: Pearson M L, Epstein H F (eds) Muscle Development: molecular and cellular control. Cold Spring Harbor Laboratories, Cold Spring Harbor, New York, p 439

Wang K, Ramirez-Mitchell R 1983 A network of transverse and longitudinal intermediate filaments is associated with sarcomeres of adult vertebrate skeletal muscle. Journal of Cell Biology 96: 562

Wang K, Wright J 1988 Architecture of the sarcomere matrix of skeletal muscle: immuno-electron microscope evidence that suggests a set of parallel inextensible nebulin filaments anchored at the Z line. Journal of Cell Biology 107: 2199

Wang K, McClure J, Tu A 1979 Titin; major myofibrillar components of striated muscle. Proceedings of the National Academy of Sciences of the United States of America 76: 3698

Wang S M, Greaser M L, Schultz E, Bulinski J C, Lin J J, Lessard J L 1988 Studies on cardiac myofibrillogenesis with antibodies to titin, actin, tropomyosin and myosin. Journal of Cell Biology 107: 1075

Webb J N 1972 The development of human skeletal muscle with particular reference to muscle cell death. Journal of Pathology 106: 221

Weiss P 1941 Nerve patterns: the mechanics of nerve growth. Growth 5: 163

Werner J K 1973a Duration of normal innervation required for complete differentiation of muscle spindles in newborn rats. Experimental Neurology 41: 214

Werner J K 1973b Mixed intra- and extrafusal muscle fibres produced by temporary denervation in newborn rats. Journal of Comparative Neurology 150: 279

White D C S, Thorson J 1975 The kinetics of muscle contraction. Pergamon Press, Oxford

Whiting A, Wardale J, Trinick J 1989 Does titin regulate the length of muscle thick filaments? Journal of Molecular Biology 205: 263

Williams P E, Goldspink G 1971 Longitudinal growth of striated muscle fibres. Journal of Cell Science 9: 751

Williams P E, Goldspink G 1973 The effect of immobilization on the longitudinal growth of striated muscle fibres. Journal of Anatomy 116: 45

Williamson E, Brooke M H 1972 Myokymia and the motor unit. Archives of Neurology (Chicago) 26: 11

Willison R G 1980 Arrangement of muscle fibers of a single motor unit in mammalian muscles. Muscle and Nerve 3: 360

Wirsén C, Larsson K S 1964 Histochemical differentiation of skeletal muscle in foetal and newborn mice. Journal of Embryology and Experimental Morphology 12: 759

Wohlfart G 1937 Uber das Vorkommen verschiedner Arten von Muskelfasern in der Skelettmuskulatur des Menschen und einiger Säugetiere. Acta psychiatrica et neurologica, Supplement 12: 1

Wray J S, Vibert P J, Cohen C 1975 Diversity of cross-bridge configurations in invertebrate muscles. Nature 257: 561

Wray J, Vibert P, Cohen C 1978 Actin filaments in muscle: pattern of myosin and tropomyosin/troponin attachments. Journal of Molecular Biology 124: 501

Yamaguchi M, Robson R M, Stromer M H, Dahl D S, Oda T 1978 Actin filaments form the backbone of nemaline myopathy rods. Nature 271: 265

Yasin R, Van Beers G, Nurse K C E, Al-Ani S, Landon D N, Thompson E J 1977 A quantitative technique for growing human adult skeletal muscle in culture starting from mononucleated cells. Journal of the Neurological Sciences 32: 347

Yellin H 1969 A histochemical study of muscle spindles and their relationship to extrafusal fibre types in the rat. American Journal of Anatomy 125: 31

Yu L C, Lymn R W, Podolsky R J 1977 Characterization of a non-indexible equatorial X-ray reflection from frog sartorius muscle. Journal of Molecular Biology 115: 455

Zak R 1981 Contractile function as a determinant of muscle growth. In: Dowben R M and Shay J W (eds) Cell and muscle motility, vol I. Plenum Press, New York, p 1

Zelená J 1957 The morphogenetic influence of innervation on the ontogenetic development of muscle spindles. Journal of Embryology and Experimental Morphology 5: 283

Zelená J 1959 Effect of innervation on the development of skeletal muscle. Bavakova Sbirka 12: 1

Zelená J 1962 The effect of denervation on muscle development. In: Gutmann E (ed) The denervated muscle. Publishing House of the Czechoslovak Academy of Sciences, Prague, p 103

Zelená J 1963 Development of muscle receptors after tenotomy. Physiologia bohemoslovenica 12: 30

Zelená J 1964 Development, degeneration and regeneration or receptor organs. Progress in Brain Research 12: 175

Zelená J 1975 The role of sensory innervation in the development of mechanoreceptors. In: Iggo A, Ilyinsky O B (eds) Somatosensory and visceral receptor mechanisms. Elsevier, Amsterdam, p 59

Zelená J 1976 Sensory terminals on extrafusal muscle fibres in myotendinous regions of developing rat muscles. Journal of Neurocytology 5: 447

Zelená J 1978 The development of Pacinian corpuscles. Journal of Neurocytology 7: 71

Zelená J, Hnik P 1960 Absence of spindles in muscles of rats reinnervated during development. Physiologia bohemoslovenica 9: 373

Zelená J, Soukup T 1973 Development of muscle spindles deprived of fusimotor innervation. Zeitschrift für Zellforschung und Mikroskopische Anatomie 144: 435

Zelená J, Soukup T 1974 The differentiation of intrafusal fibre types in rat muscle spindles after motor denervation. Cell and Tissue Research 153: 115

Zelená J, Soukup T 1977 The development of Golgi tendon organs. Journal of Neurocytology 6: 171

Zelená J, Vyskocil F, Jirmanova I 1979 The elimination of polyneuronal innervation of end-plates in developing rat muscles with altered function. Progress in Brain Research 49: 365

2. Muscle biopsy

R. Pamphlett

INTRODUCTION

The biopsy of skeletal muscle poses two problems not encountered in handling other tissues: first, since muscle is contractile in nature it needs to be handled in a way that prevents damage and artefactual change. Secondly, routine paraffin sections of muscle are seldom of great use, and frozen sections with a battery of histological and histochemical stains are needed for accurate diagnosis. Because of these special requirements, every centre that handles muscle has developed its own techniques for biopsy and tissue processing. Many laboratories have strongly-held views, based on long experience, that their technique is the 'correct' one, so it is unwise to prescribe any particular method as being the only one worth trying. In this chapter some basic principles of muscle biopsy and tissue processing will be described, and the methods that we have found to give reliable results will be outlined.

INDICATIONS FOR MUSCLE BIOPSY

Most muscle biopsies are performed for one of two reasons. The first is as part of the investigation of a clinically suspected neuromuscular disorder after other tests have proved non-diagnostic. The second is to attempt to make a histological diagnosis of a systemic disease, such as sarcoidosis or polyarteritis nodosa, in which muscle may be affected microscopically without any muscular symptoms being present. Muscle biopsy may also be performed for research into normal physiology or to gain an understanding of the pathophysiology of various neuromuscular diseases.

Close cooperation between the clinician and the pathologist is essential at all stages of muscle biopsy, since muscle reacts in a rather restricted way to a number of insults, and an aetiological diagnosis based on histology alone is not common. Some clinicians who regard the pathologist as the final diagnostic arbiter may hold unrealistically high expectations of the muscle biopsy and may become disillusioned after receiving ten successive reports of 'non-specific' changes. Therefore physicians not familiar with muscle pathology may need to be reminded what information can reasonably be expected to be gleaned from a histological examination of muscle. Overall, the diagnostic yield of muscle biopsy is high in neurogenic disorders, inflammatory myopathies, and congenital myopathies, moderate in metabolic myopathies, and low in endocrine myopathies and disorders of the neuromuscular junction.

Nothing reduces the enthusiasm and curiosity of a pathologist more than inadequate clinical details, so the whole procedure may be a waste of time and money if the only information available is '? muscle weakness'. The minimum the person looking at the biopsy needs to know are the patient's age, sex, relevant family history, symptoms and signs, current medications, and results of muscle enzyme activity, electromyography, and nerve conduction studies. A request form can be designed with these points included and distributed to clinicians who order muscle biopsies.

CHOICE OF MUSCLE TO BIOPSY

Since a severe chronic muscle disorder leads eventually to a non-specific 'end-stage' histological appearance, the ideal muscle to biopsy is one only moderately affected by the disease. This may be difficult to gauge clinically, but in chronic myopathies an apparently normal muscle is often involved microscopically, while in acute diseases a severely affected muscle may still yield diagnostic pathological changes if the process has not gone on long enough to give an 'end-stage' appearance.

In most centres only a few muscles, for example the lateral quadriceps and biceps brachii, are routinely biopsied so that familiarity is obtained with the normal fibre size and type distributions in these muscles. Other muscles can be sampled if a particular muscle is focally affected by the disease or for cosmetic reasons (a triceps scar is less noticeable than a biceps brachii one). When a muscle that is infrequently biopsied is being looked at histologically the normal fibre size and type distribution must be known, since these can vary markedly from muscle to muscle (Polgar et al 1973, Johnson et al 1973). If specimens of both muscle and peripheral nerve are required the gastrocnemius muscle and sural nerve can be sampled through the same incision. For examination of motor end-plates special techniques are required (see later and Ch. 17).

In patients who have a patchy disease such as polymyositis, non-invasive procedures such as technetium pyrophosphate muscle scans (Yonker et al 1987) or magnetic resonance imaging (Kaufman et al 1987) may locate active regions of pathology suitable for biopsy. Another situation in which pre-biopsy muscle imaging is useful is in patients who have either selective involvement of certain muscles in a limb, or severely atrophic muscles with extensive replacement by fatty tissue. In these patients either computed tomography or real-time ultrasound can locate viable muscle suitable for biopsy (Heckmatt & Dubowitz 1987, Fremion 1988). Ultrasound has the advantage of being quick and suitable for outpatient biopsies.

BIOPSY TECHNIQUE

Muscle can be biopsied in three ways: using an open (surgical) technique, with a needle, or with a conchotome (alligator forceps). A major controversy at present in muscle pathology concerns the choice of biopsy technique. Some workers adhere to the open method (Heffner 1984), some have switched to performing needle biopsies only (Dubowitz 1985), while others use combinations of techniques such as needle and conchotome biopsies (Dietrichson et al 1987). Many centres, ourselves included, use both open and needle or conchotome methods, according to the clinical diagnosis and to the muscle chosen for biopsy.

1. Open biopsy

This is probably still the most frequently performed method, and is the gold standard for all other techniques. As with all 'minor' repetitive surgical procedures the tendency is for the most junior member of the surgical team to be assigned to the muscle biopsy list, the result often being the removal of inadequate, traumatized tissue. This can be avoided if an experienced surgical colleague can be persuaded to perform all your open muscle biopsies. A regular theatre list for muscle biopsies should be arranged, preferably early in the week. The laboratory can then prepare itself well in advance and a technician can plan to be in theatre to assist the surgeon and receive the specimen.

Although the operation is usually performed under local anaesthesia, for young children and highly anxious adults a general anaesthetic may be required. It must be remembered that not only patients with malignant hyperthermia but also those with Duchenne dystrophy may react adversely to halothane and succinylcholine administration (Karpati & Watters 1980), and that general anaesthesia is potentially hazardous in any patient with weak respiratory muscles.

In the operating theatre the skin over the muscle to be sampled is cleaned and local anaesthetic is infiltrated into the skin and subcutaneous tissue, but not into the muscle itself. A 4 to 8 cm incision is made through the skin in the direction of the muscle fibres, and the subcutaneous tissue and muscle fascia is opened to expose the muscle. In some conditions, such as eosinophilic fasciitis, the surgeon should be asked specifically to include fascia together with the muscle. All muscle samples should be taken from the muscle belly, and not near a tendon where structural differences in the myofibres may cause diagnostic confusion (see later).

Three muscle samples are usually taken, for

resin (plastic), cryostat, and paraffin sections respectively. If the muscle is kept at resting length it makes the semithin, electron-microscopic, and paraffin sections easier to assess, so two types of clamps have been devised:

(a) One type of clamp is closed over the partially separated muscle bundle when still in continuity with the rest of the muscle, and the ends just outside the clamp are severed. A simple clamp of this type can be made from a children's tongue holder (Guys' pattern) by removing part of the distal loop, or a clamp can be specially constructed (Fig. 2.1). A more versatile instrument consists of two artery forceps united by a steel band; small or large forceps with different tip separations can hold muscle bundles of different sizes (Harriman 1984). An advantage of these clamps is that an adequate amount of muscle has to be removed by the surgeon to fit the clamp. For small samples, suitable especially for electron microscopy, a separate clamp can be fastened on to the muscle in situ using special forceps (Fig. 2.2) (Bardosi & Zobel 1985). In theory there should be a difference in the degree of stretch between muscles such as the quadriceps (which is relaxed with the knee extended during biopsy) and the biceps brachii (which is stretched with the arm extended during biopsy) but in practice this is insignificant.

(b) With the second type of clamp the muscle bundle is first removed by the surgeon, then placed in the jaws of the clamp and stretched slightly by turning a screw to separate the jaws (Fig. 2.1). Many surgeons prefer this method since in situ muscle clamps can be awkward to handle. If these forceps are not available a ligature can be tied to each end of a muscle bundle which is then stretched gently over a glass slide or a spatula broken down to size.

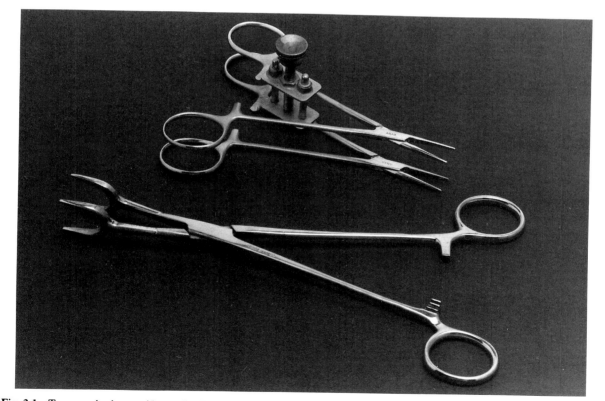

Fig. 2.1 Two muscle clamps. Above: the distance between these two forceps can be changed with the screw mechanism. Below: a simple custom-made clamp (×0.6)

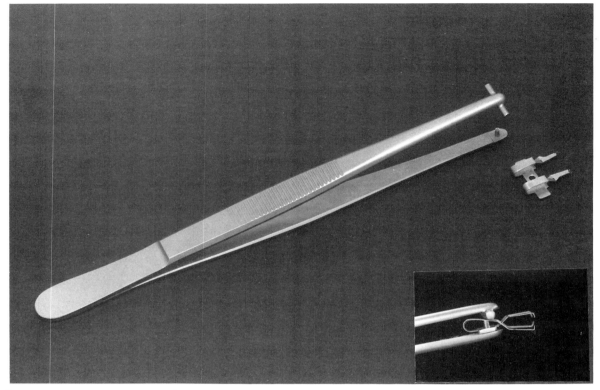

Fig. 2.2   Separate clamps can be manipulated in these specially-designed forceps. At rest the jaws of the clamps are closed (×0.9). Inset: pressure on the forceps opens the jaws of the clamp

Some experience is required with these stretching techniques to avoid overstretching the muscle and causing muscle fibre rupture. Stapling the free muscle bundle to a piece of balsa wood has been suggested as another method to prevent contraction (Siegel & Weiss 1988).

The specimen for resin embedding and electron microscopy is taken first because for ultrastructural assessment the fibres should be minimally disturbed. The direction of the muscle fibres is noted and a thin bundle (about 1.0 cm in the longitudinal plane × 0.2 × 0.2 cm) is gently separated in the longitudinal plane and placed in one of the clamps. The end of the clamp containing the muscle bundle is submerged in glutaraldehyde. A larger bundle (about 2 × 0.5 × 0.5 cm) is similarly removed for formalin fixation. The largest segment for cryostat sections (about 2 cm long by 1 cm

thick) is removed and placed on a saline-moistened gauze swab in a container. There is no need to stretch the muscle for the transverse cryostat sections if between 10 to 15 minutes passes to allow the muscle to relax before freezing. This delay does not affect routine histochemical stains adversely. Further small segments are removed as required for microbiological, biochemical, immunological or cell culture techniques.

After local bleeding is controlled, the fascia and subcutaneous tissue are closed with interrupted absorbable sutures. The skin can be closed with an absorbable subcutaneous running stitch to avoid having to remove sutures at a later date. A plaster is put over the cleaned wound and a pad and bandage is firmly applied to help prevent intramuscular bleeding. The procedure is usually painless, though some patients feel minor discomfort while the muscle is being handled. The patient can move the limb gently immediately after the operation. Complications such as intramuscular haematoma, muscle herniation through the fascia, and wound infection are rare.

2. Needle biopsy

Since the invention of the first needle biopsy instrument by Duchenne in 1868 the basic design has been modified in various ways. One of the most popular needles is that designed by Bergstrom (1962) based on a synovial biopsy needle. It consists of a sharp-tipped hollow outer needle with a small window near the tip. A cylinder with a sharp edge fits tightly into the needle. Either because of the intrinsic tension in the muscle, or by squeezing the muscle externally, a small portion protrudes into the window. This is guillotined by the inner cylinder and removed with a probe. The Bergstrom needle is still used with good results in many centres (Heckmatt et al 1984).

It is somewhat difficult to manipulate the two

parts of this needle and to squeeze the muscle at the same time. This problem was solved by the Baylor needle (Nichols et al 1968) in which two finger rings are attached to the outer shaft and a ring for the thumb is attached to the cutting cylinder. This type of needle can be operated with one hand, leaving the other hand free to manipulate the muscle. A later modification was the addition of a vacuum attachment, the suction drawing a larger piece of muscle into the needle lumen (Edwards et al 1983). The muscle sample is prevented from being drawn into the vacuum tubing by an aspirator trap, and with this needle three or four pieces of muscle can be guillotined in quick succession from the same site. Another needle is the Kellogg biopsy instrument (Pamphlett et al 1985) in which only the distal 1.5 cm of the inner cylinder is hollow, so that once suction is applied the portion of muscle guillotined stays within the distal hollow section (Fig. 2.3). This reduces trauma to the specimen and obviates the

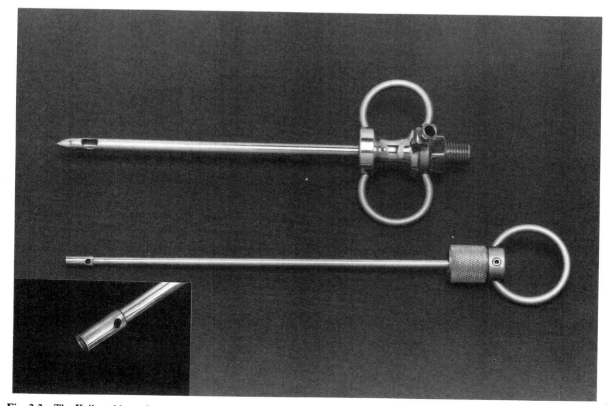

Fig. 2.3 The Kellogg biopsy instrument. The inner cylinder (below) fits into the hollow outer needle (above) (×0.72). Inset: the distal 0.5 cm of the inner cylinder is hollow and has a cutting edge and an aperture to transmit the negative pressure

need for an aspirator trap. Disposable needles such as the Tru-Cut (Travenol) can be tried (Fukuyama et al 1981) but most workers find the samples obtained too small.

Needles are made with varying outside diameters (usually from 3 to 5 mm), and for children and small muscles the distance between the window and the needle tip can be reduced to lessen the amount of muscle which has to be penetrated. In all the non-disposable instruments it is important to keep the cutting edge sharp since an incompletely guillotined muscle causes tearing of fibres on withdrawal of the needle and considerable discomfort.

Because the biopsy is blind it is imperative to have a good anatomical knowledge of the region to avoid damage to larger nerves and blood vessels. The preferred muscle for needle biopsy is the lateral quadriceps since the main muscle bulk at this site is at some distance from the large arteries and nerves. It is difficult to be certain that it is the

vastus lateralis that is being biopsied since the vastus intermedius lies immediately below it. This is of some importance because the proportion of fibre types differs in these two muscles, the deeper vastus intermedius having a greater proportion of type I fibres (Edgerton et al 1975, Mahon et al 1984).

Some workers perform a coagulation profile on all patients before needle biopsy. We do so only on those patients in whom there is a clinical suspicion that a bleeding disorder may be present. Most adults do not need sedation before the biopsy, but the anxious patient may benefit from 10 mg of diazepam half an hour beforehand. In children, especially those between the ages of 1 and 12 years, sedative premedication is usually needed.

The method described here is for biopsy of the lateral quadriceps using the Kellogg biopsy instrument. Either a completely sterile or a 'no-touch' technique can be used, the latter being convenient

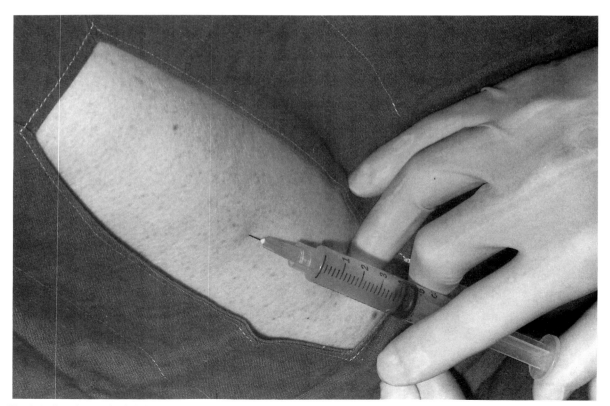

Fig. 2.4 Local anaesthetic is injected superficially into the lateral thigh

for outpatient work. The skin over the lateral quadriceps is cleaned and local anaesthetic (1% lignocaine without adrenaline) is injected into the skin and subcutaneous tissue 10 to 15 cm above the knee (Fig. 2.4). A 0.5 cm incision is made in the skin using a number 11 scalpel blade (Figs 2.5, 2.6). The small amount of bleeding stops after a short period of local pressure. The needle is inserted (with the window closed) perpendicularly through the skin incision to a depth of between 3 to 5 cm into the muscle (Fig. 2.7). The outer needle can be marked at one-centimetre intervals to measure the depth of penetration. Negative pressure from a portable vacuum pump can be applied when the window of the needle is opened, or more conveniently a 20 ml syringe can be attached to the needle and the syringe plunger withdrawn (Fig. 2.8). The window is then closed, guillotining the contained piece of muscle. The needle is withdrawn and the muscle sample re-moved from the hollow cylinder with a sterile

needle. The procedure can be repeated two or three times at different angles and depths, using the same skin incision for entry.

The technician who is to process the muscle samples should be present while the biopsies are performed so that the adequacy of each sample can be assessed under magnification. If the sample is inadequate another can be taken straight away, thus avoiding the need to recall the patient later for a further biopsy. The wound is closed with a plaster strip, since stitches are not required. Pressure is maintained on the wound site for five minutes to help prevent haematoma formation.

Each biopsy takes about 10 seconds to perform, and the whole procedure lasts 15 to 20 minutes, after which the patient can walk about the room. Patients describe varying degrees of discomfort. Most feel a sense of pressure as the needle is being pushed through the muscle and a momentary sharp pain as the muscle is being cut. This is often followed by local muscle stiffness for up to 24

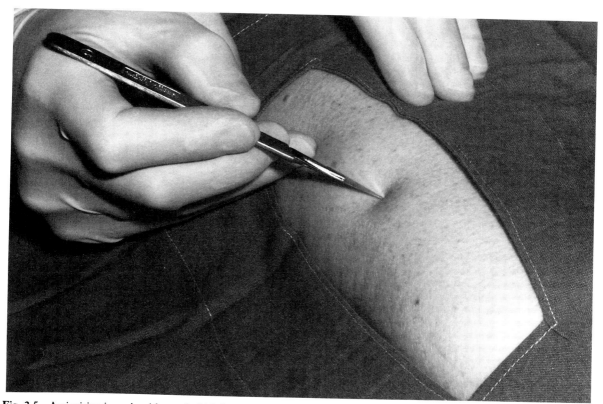

Fig. 2.5 An incision is made with a scalpel blade

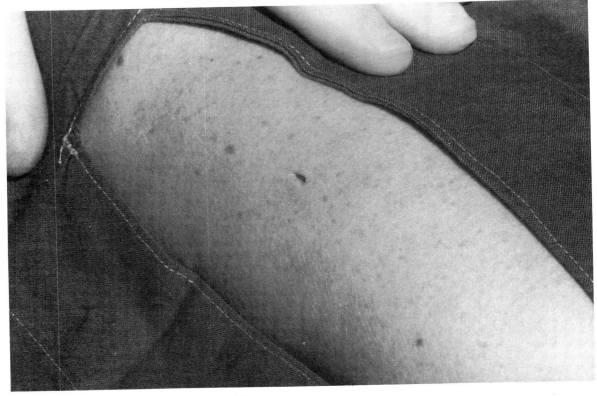

Fig. 2.6   The 0.5 cm incision will leave no appreciable scar

hours, usually not enough to limit mobility. Hardy Swedes go cross-country skiing immediately after needle muscle biopsies (Hultman 1967).

Potential complications are bleeding, wound infection, and damage to peripheral nerves. In fact complication rates are very low. In 800 needle biopsies Edwards et al (1983) had three cases of intramuscular haematoma and one minor wound infection, and no complications were reported in 674 children who had needle biopsies performed by Heckmatt et al (1984).

3. Conchotome biopsy

The conchotome biopsy is a procedure claimed to be intermediate between needle and open biopsy, and therefore called the 'semi-open' technique, though in fact it is much closer to a needle than to an open biopsy. The conchotome was originally designed as a nasal forceps to remove nasal conchae. It is a type of alligator forceps, the Weil-Blakesley size 3 being the most suitable for adult muscle biopsy (Fig. 2.9). Local anaesthetic is injected into the skin and a 0.5 cm incision is made through the skin, subcutaneous tissue, and fascia. The fascial incision is needed for the blunt tip of the closed jaws to pass easily into the muscle. Once inserted, the conchotome is advanced for 2 to 3 mm into the muscle with the jaws open. The jaws are closed, twisted through 180° to ensure that all the muscle fibres are severed, and withdrawn. This instrument enables biopsies to be taken from small muscles since unlike the needles there is no dead space between the tip and the sampling aperture.

The method has been popular in Scandinavia for some time (Radner 1965, Lindholm 1968), and has recently been used with good results in the United Kingdom (Dietrichson et al 1987). In a series of 959 patients Henriksson (1979) found

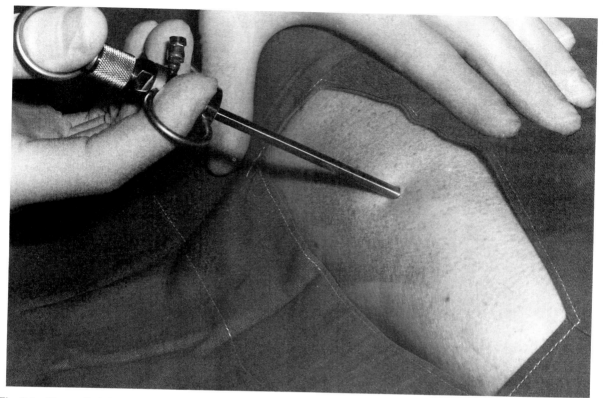

Fig. 2.7 The needle is inserted through the incision into the muscle with the window closed (inner cylinder pushed in)

only 19 biopsies impossible to evaluate because of artefact or too little tissue, and specimens were usually double the size of those from the needle method. In the 222 conchotome biopsies performed by Dietrichson et al (1987) adequate material was obtained for diagnostic purposes in all cases. These workers often sampled the tibialis anterior muscle and found that this muscle frequently yielded diagnostic information when proximal muscles were severely wasted.

CHOICE OF BIOPSY TECHNIQUE

After it is decided that a muscle biopsy is indicated, which method should be tried, open, needle or conchotome? Many workers, especially those performing only occasional biopsies, still opt for open biopsy, its main advantage being that a large amount of muscle is obtained so that the possibility of missing changes due to a patchy disease is reduced. An open biopsy is necessary if a disease affecting medium-sized blood vessels (such as polyarteritis nodosa) is being sought, or if special techniques such as motor point biopsy or in-vitro pharmacological testing are required. There are, however, disadvantages to open biopsy. An operating theatre and surgeon have to be arranged in good time. In obese patients a large skin incision has to be made in order to get adequate muscle exposure, and in small children with abundant subcutaneous tissue a relatively large incision is similarly required.

Needle muscle biopsy has many advantages. There is no appreciable scar. The apparatus is transportable so that the biopsy can be performed in the outpatient department, the ward, or the intensive-care unit. The procedure can usually be performed the same day it is requested, and the clinician can, if necessary, have a light microscopic report within 24 hours. Needle biopsies are suit-

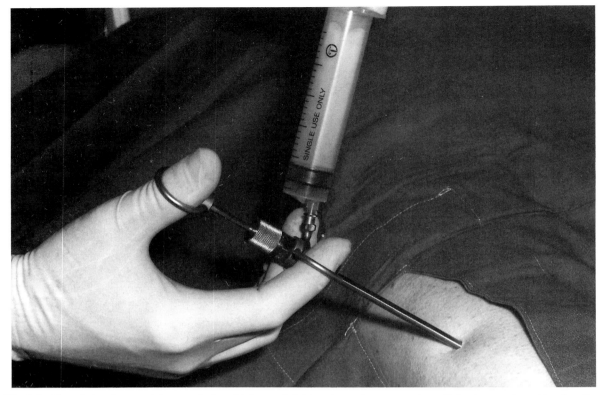

Fig. 2.8 The window is opened (inner cylinder withdrawn slightly) and negative pressure is applied using a syringe. Muscle will be sucked into the window and can be guillotined by pushing the inner cylinder in again

able for children (Curless & Nelson 1975, Fukuyama et al 1981, Heckmatt et al 1984) as well as adults. Since the needle procedure is less invasive than open biopsy clinicians feel more justified in asking for biopsies for less well-defined problems such as muscle pain. Repeated needle examinations can be performed to assess the course of a disease or its response to treatment.

The main concern over needle muscle biopsies is how often a patchy lesion will be missed with the smaller sample. To help overcome this problem the muscle can be biopsied at different angles and depths, or different muscles can be biopsied at the same session. In studies comparing simultaneous open and needle biopsies in 6 and 33 patients respectively the two procedures gave equal diagnostic yields (Porro et al 1969, Fukuyama et al 1981).

There is invariably some sarcomere contraction seen on electron microscopy of needle samples and subtle myofilament changes may be difficult to interpret. As long as this contraction is recognized for what it is (and a change such as basal lamina folding must not be misinterpreted as indicating fibre atrophy) most ultrastructural pathology can be readily diagnosed with needle samples.

The conchotome may be useful if distal muscles or proximal muscles of small bulk need to be sampled. The conchotome usually gives more tissue than a needle. In patients who have had both needle and conchotome biopsies the majority have preferred the conchotome method (Dietrichson et al 1987).

Ideally, all three techniques should be available so that a choice can be made as to which is suitable for the individual patient. Our practice has been to perform a needle biopsy when there is any doubt as to which technique to use. If a

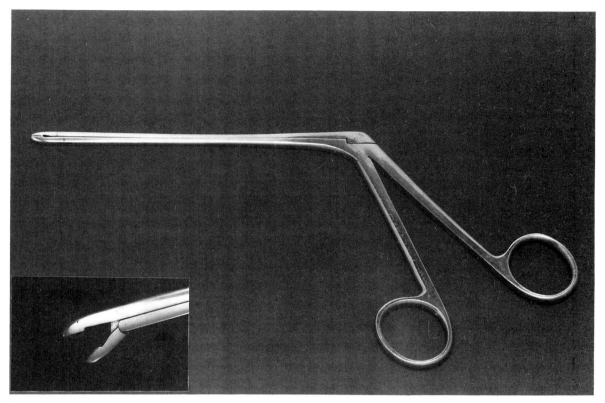

Fig. 2.9   The conchotome. The forceps is inserted into the muscle with the jaws closed (×0.72). Inset: the jaws are opened to bite off a piece of muscle

diagnosis is obtained the patient has been saved an open biopsy; if no diagnosis is made open biopsy can be resorted to.

SPECIMEN PROCESSING AND STAINING

The muscle samples are usually processed for cryostat, paraffin and resin (plastic) sections.

1. Cryostat sections

(a) Processing

The specimen is trimmed to a block not more than 0.8 cm^3 so that freezing will be reasonably uniform throughout the tissue. It is then orientated for transverse sections and attached to a cryostat chuck with an adhesive such as OCT compound (Tissue Tek). Muscle cannot simply be immersed in liquid nitrogen because rapid freezing

is prevented by a layer of gaseous nitrogen that forms around and insulates the tissue, the result being 'ice-crystal artefact'. The usual method of reducing ice crystal formation is to immerse the sample for 5 to 10 seconds in a small beaker of isopentane (a rapid heat conductor) which has been cooled in liquid nitrogen to a temperature of between −160°C and −170°C, a temperature at which the isopentane becomes syrupy. Although easy in theory the technique requires skill since the muscle may suffer either ice-crystal artefact (the isopentane is not cool enough or the muscle is taken out too soon) or the block may crack (the isopentane is too cold or the muscle is left in for too long). Some workers find that an easier technique, in which the timing is less critical, is to drop the sample for a few seconds into hexane cooled to −70°C in acetone and solid carbon dioxide (Filipe & Lake 1983).

When a distant hospital asks advice on transporting a muscle sample, one suggestion is to dust the muscle liberally with talc or starch powder (as provided with surgical gloves) and to drop it into liquid nitrogen. The powder acts as a rapid heat conductor and prevents the gaseous nitrogen layer forming. An alternative is to have the referring hospital send the muscle cooled on ice, since samples can be kept for up to about 24 hours at 0°C without essential loss of histological or histochemical quality (Heene & Haar 1984, Braund & Ambling 1988).

After the muscle has been frozen it is transferred to a cryostat for sectioning. A cryostat is a rotary microtome kept at a low temperature (usually −20°C) in a freezer box. For optimal sections great care has to be taken to ensure that the microtome knife is kept sharp and that the anti-roll bar which keeps the sections flat is correctly aligned. Sections between 5 and 10 μm thick are cut, air-dried, and mounted on coverslips before staining.

The remaining muscle can be stored for a short time at −20°C but for longer storage a lower temperature, either in a freezer at −70°C or in liquid nitrogen, is required. We prefer long-term storage in liquid nitrogen, since, despite alarm systems, freezers can occasionally suffer from power failures that can destroy samples collected over many years.

For the smaller specimens obtained from needle and conchotome biopsies a greater degree of technical skill is required to handle and orientate the tissue. Some form of magnification is needed for fibre orientation, preferably a dissecting microscope with a cold light source. The largest specimen is selected for cryostat sections. Once orientated, the muscle is placed on an orange stick with the muscle fibres parallel to the stick. The stick with attached muscle can then be frozen in the isopentane and liquid nitrogen. The frozen muscle is easily lifted off the stick and attached to a cryostat chuck with a small amount of OCT. For resin embedding, small orientated slivers of muscle can be attached to an orange stick and immersed in glutaraldehyde. Specimens for paraffin embedding are processed similarly to open biopsies. Figure 2.10 shows the size of a typical specimen taken by needle biopsy.

(b) Staining

Cryostat sections can be stained in two ways: with a modified general histological stain (such as haematoxylin and eosin or Gomori trichrome), or with histochemical techniques designed to identify specific cell contents such as glycogen, enzymes and lipids. Details of individual histological or histochemical methods are available elsewhere (Pearse 1985, Dubowitz 1985).

(i) Routine stains. A vast array of histological and histochemical techniques is now available, but for the routine screening of most disorders the following seven stains suffice:

Haematoxylin and eosin (H&E). A good general morphological stain. Stains muscle fibres pink, nuclei blue, fibrous connective tissue light pink and mitochondria blue, so the 'ragged-red' fibres of a mitochondrial myopathy will be 'battered-blue' on a cryostat H&E section. Regenerating fibres, with their high content of RNA, also stain blue.

Modified Gomori trichrome. Stains myofibres dark green, fibrous connective tissue light green, and mitochondria red. Useful for general morphology, variations in mitochondrial number and distribution ('ragged-red' fibres), rod bodies, cytoplasmic bodies, and the inclusions of inclusion body myositis. The myelin of intramuscular nerves stains red. If the sections are damaged by rough handling or lift off the slide, dramatic red staining will ensue which an inexperienced observer could interpret as a florid mitochondrial myopathy.

Myofibrillary ATPase at routine (9.4), reversed (4.2) and intermediate (4.6) pH. The routine (dark fibres type 2) and reversed (dark fibres type 1) ATPase stains reveal the distribution of the main fibre types. For fibre subtypes 2A and 2B an ATPase at pH 4.6 is performed, preferably on serial sections with the other ATPase stains. The ATPase also demonstrates a loss of myofibrillary elements in 'unstructured' cores. The pH for each stain will vary slightly in different laboratories, and in the same laboratory in altered climatic conditions, so the optimal pH has to be worked out by trial and error. The stains fade after a while, but colour is maintained if the slides are kept refrigerated.

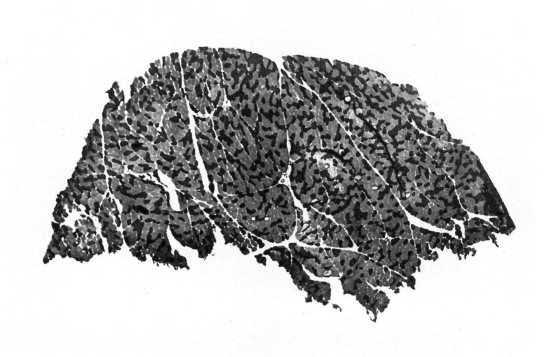

Fig. 2.10   Size of a needle biopsy specimen. ATPase pH 9.4 (×12)

NADH–tetrazolium reductase (NADH–TR) and succinic dehydrogenase (SDH). Most laboratories perform one of these, our own preference being for the SDH. The NADH–TR stains mitochondria and sarcoplasmic reticulum so any architectural changes in the myofibrillary pattern are readily seen. SDH is an intramitochondrial protein and shows clumped mitochondria dramatically. Tubular aggregates stain with NADH–TR but not with SDH.

Periodic acid–Schiff (PAS), with and without diastase. This stains glycogen a magenta colour (that can be removed with diastase) and other polysaccharides. Staining of glycogen is more intense if the sections are protected from water by a thin layer of celloidin. A celloidin coat is advisable in all suspected cases of glycogen storage disease (Fig. 2.11).

Acid phosphatase. Stains lysosomes and is thus a marker for macrophages (Fig. 2.12). In lysosomal storage disorders such as acid maltase deficiency this stain is strongly positive. The stain is negative

in normal muscle and is a sensitive indicator of fibre damage.

Oil red O. Stains neutral lipid red. This stain is more specific than Sudan Black B, which stains neutral lipids, complex lipids, and organelle membranes. An increased intrafibre lipid content may be suspected if numerous small 'holes' are seen within the fibres on H&E stains. The amount of intrafibre lipid varies from case to case, presumably in line with fat metabolism elsewhere in the body. In some young children with no detectable lipid enzyme abnormalities numerous large fat globules may be present, particularly in type 1 fibres, so a diagnosis of lipid storage myopathy needs always to be supported biochemically.

(ii) Other stains. In some centres a selection of the following stains may be performed routinely, but we reserve them for cases in which either the clinical findings or the results of the previous stains have suggested further stains are needed.

Phosphorylase. Can detect an absence of this

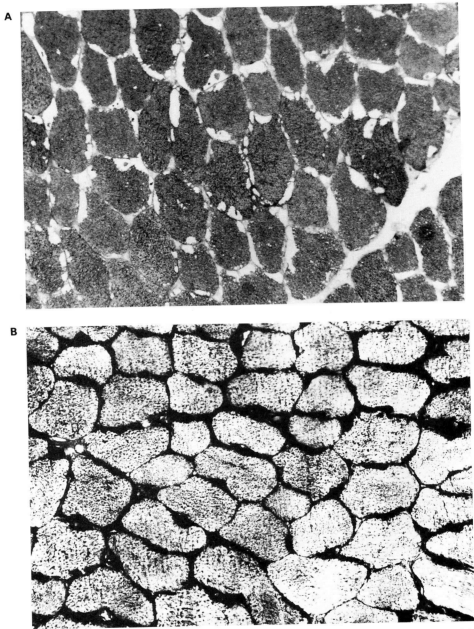

Fig. 2.11   Protection of PAS sections. (a) Cryostat section of muscle from a case of McArdle's disease stained with PAS only. Most of the subsarcolemmal glycogen has been washed out during processing. (b) PAS with celloidin coat (same case). The glycogen stains darkly (×88)

enzyme in McArdle's disease. The colour fades rapidly (it can be restored by treating with iodine) and caution needs to be exercised in diagnosing McArdle's disease if the phosphorylase stain is older than a few days. Some laboratories perform this stain routinely because the histological changes in McArdle's disease may be subtle.

Phosphofructokinase. Absence of this enzyme is

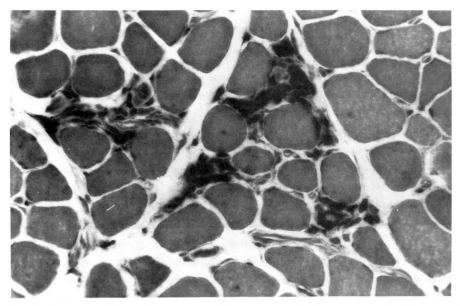

Fig. 2.12 Stain for acid phosphatase. Macrophages phagocytosing necrotic muscle fibres are easily identified by their dark (red) staining. Duchenne muscular dystrophy. (×175)

sought in a glycogen storage disorder when the phosphorylase is normal.

Myoadenylate deaminase (AMP deaminase). We perform this stain in patients with exertional myalgia, mindful of the continuing controversy surrounding the importance of this enzyme in muscle pathology (Shumate et al 1979).

Cytochrome c oxidase. This stain is performed if a mitochondrial myopathy is suspected clinically or found microscopically, or if a low cytochrome oxidase is discovered on muscle biochemistry. Some workers use this stain routinely, since in both the fatal infantile and encephalomyopathic forms of cytochrome c oxidase deficiency ragged red fibres may be absent (Nonaka et al 1988).

Verhoeff–van Gieson. A combination histological stain that demonstrates increased interfibre collagen (pink). Muscle fibres stain yellow. It also stains elastic fibres (black) so that necrosis in a blood vessel wall is easily appreciated. Better results are obtained when this stain is performed on paraffin sections.

(iii) Immunocytochemistry. Immunocyto-chemistry allows visualization of antigens within tissue, but its usefulness in the routine diagnosis of muscle disorders is still in its infancy. The technique involves producing a labelled antibody to the antigen being sought, and the methods, for both light and electron microscopy, and the wide range of antigens that can now be localized in muscle have been reviewed elsewhere (Fitzsimons and Sewry 1985).

The ATPase activities of the subtypes of 'fast' and 'slow' myosin are used routinely to classify fibres into types 1, 2A, 2B and 2C histochemically. Antibodies to fast and slow myosins can now identify antigenic fibre types 1 and 2, though the correspondence to the histochemical typing is only approximate, as shown in Figure 2.13. Type 2 fibres can be further subtyped into types 2A and 2B by myosin antibodies (Pierobon-Bormioli et al 1981). However, the antigenic typing is complex, since individual fibres may contain more than one type of myosin, as is the case in histochemical type 2C fibres that contain antigenic types 1 and 2 myosin (Pierobon-Bormioli et al 1981).

Regenerating fibres may be distinguished from mature fibres by their content of fetal myosins (Sartore et al 1982), though this is not completely straightforward as shown in Figure 2.13. In future, antibodies to myosin may be able to establish how many subtypes of muscle fibre exist; new subtypes

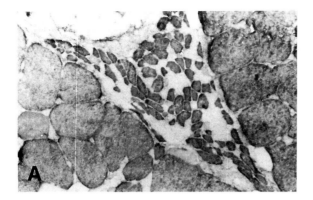

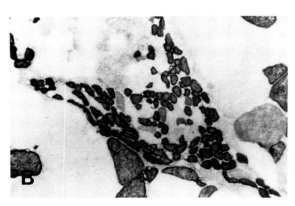

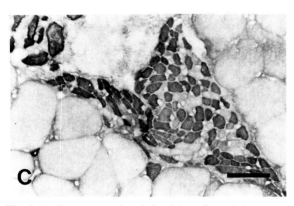

Fig. 2.13 Immunocytochemical staining of myosin in muscle of a 3-year-old boy with spinal muscular atrophy.
(a) Monoclonal antibody to fast myosin (N0Q7.5.2b) gives uniform staining of large fibres and patchy staining of atrophic fibres. (b) With monoclonal antibody to slow myosin (N0Q7.5.4D) a few large fibres stain positively, while small fibre staining is patchy. (c) With polyclonal antibody to fetal myosin a subpopulation of the atrophic fibres contain the fetal myosin while the large fibres are unstained. Sections stained by the indirect method, secondary antibodies labelled with HRP. Bar = 50 μm. Micrographs courtesy of Dr J. Dangain and Dr J. F. Y. Hoh. Monoclonal antibodies supplied by Dr R. Fitzsimons

continue to be identified (Gorza 1990). Other applications may be to decide whether small fibres are immature, atrophic, or regenerating, and to assess whether fibres on a section that stains uniformly with histochemical stains are in fact of only one fibre type.

Another antigen that can now be immunohistochemically localized in muscle is the protein dystrophin. Dystrophin is found in normal individuals at the sarcolemma of the muscle fibres, whereas it is absent in patients with Duchenne muscular dystrophy (Bonilla et al 1988a), and appears to show a mosaic pattern of positive and negative fibres in carriers of Duchenne dystrophy (Bonilla et al 1988b).

2. Paraffin sections

(a) Processing

The specimen to be embedded in paraffin is fixed at resting length in 10% formalin for 24 hours. The blocks are dehydrated in alcohol, cleared in xylene, embedded in paraffin wax, and 5- to 7-μm thick longitudinal and transverse sections are cut.

Many muscle laboratories no longer produce paraffin sections, but longitudinal sections (difficult to cut from frozen muscle) can be made from paraffin blocks so that changes such as segmental fibre necrosis, contraction bands and nuclear chains can be seen. Thin (down to 3 μm) sections can be cut from paraffin blocks with clearer cytological detail than that obtainable with cryostat sections. This is important for example in vasculitis where diagnostic destructive changes in the vessel wall may be obscured in thicker sections. Finally, large sections of muscles can be cut and if a patchy disease process is being sought all the tissue can be embedded and serial or step sections examined.

(b) Staining

Paraffin-embedded tissue has been fixed in formalin and heated to 60°C, processes which deactivate most enzymes. During dehydration in alcohol, lipids and material such as the basophilic granular inclusions of inclusion body myositis are dissolved out. Nevertheless, a number of informative stains can still be performed on paraffin sections:

Haematoxylin and eosin, and Verhoeff-van Gieson. As described for cryostat sections, these give a good overall view of muscle fibres, collagen, and blood vessels, especially with the cytological detail available with the thinner paraffin sections.

Stains for infectious agents. Although some parasites in muscle can be seen on H&E sections, in many infective conditions special stains are needed to demonstrate the invading organism. If the organism is unknown, three screening stains can be performed: a Gram stain for bacteria, a methenamine silver stain for fungi, and a Ziehl–Neelsen stain for acid-fast bacilli. Stains for less common agents are described in detail elsewhere (Bancroft & Cook 1984).

A new method of promise is in situ hybridization, in which hybridization of a nucleic acid probe to nucleic acids within histological preparations permits a high degree of spatial localization of sequences complementary to that probe (Haase et al 1984). This technique can show direct infection of muscle fibres by viruses such as the retrovirus HTLV-1 (Wiley et al 1989). The hybridization can be performed on either cryostat or paraffin sections (Burns et al 1986).

Fibre typing in paraffin sections. A major disadvantage of paraffin sections has been that different fibre types could not be distinguished. Recently however, Bardosi et al (1989) have used specific antisera raised against lectins (endogenous sugar receptors) to show accurate fibre typing of type 1, 2A and 2B fibres on formalin-fixed, paraffin-embedded muscle biopsy specimens.

3. Resin (plastic) sections

The thin bundle of muscle in a clamp or on an orange stick is fixed overnight in cold 3% glutaraldehyde buffered in cacodylate, and small (not more than 1 mm thick) blocks are taken for transverse and longitudinal sections. The blocks are post-fixed in osmium tetroxide, dehydrated in alcohol, and embedded in a resin ('plastic') such as Spurr's. Semithin (as opposed to ultrathin) sections of 1 μm thickness are cut with a glass knife and stained with toluidine blue.

With resin-embedded material shrinkage of fibres is minimal, and with such thin sections the cytological detail is superior to that obtained with paraffin or cryostat sections (Fig. 2.14). Appearances similar to those of low-power electron micrographs can be obtained with 1000× light magnification and oil immersion. A further advantage of semithin sections is that any interesting features can be further studied with electron microscopy, using ultrathin sections from the appropriately trimmed resin block. Toluidine blue stains some substances metachromatically, so mast cell granules and the sulphatides of metachromatic leucodystrophy will stain red.

4. Electron microscopy

Electron microscopy is time-consuming and costly, so in most departments it is performed only on selected muscle biopsies. A reasonable compromise is to embed specimens from all biopsies in resin and to proceed to electron microscopy only if clinically indicated (for example a suspected mitochondrial myopathy) or if a structural abnormality is found on light microscopy that warrants further study.

If an abnormality is seen on a cryostat section, the frozen block can be thawed and then fixed and processed for electron microscopy. Although the ultrastructure will not be as detailed as when the tissue has been immersed immediately in glutaraldehyde, this method is adequate for the characterization of, for example, parasites in muscle (Fig. 2.15) (Pamphlett and O'Donague 1990).

BASIC INTERPRETATION OF MUSCLE BIOPSIES

A systematic approach will ensure that no pathological changes are overlooked when the muscle slides are examined. The following features should be sought with the routine stains:

1. Overall architecture of muscle bundles (roughly triangular, round, or distorted)
2. Muscle fibre size (normal, atrophic, or hypertrophic). An eyepiece micrometer is needed to measure fibre diameters
3. Fibre shape (polygonal, angular, or round)

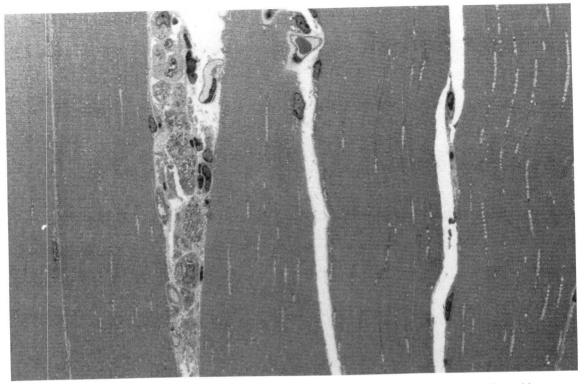

Fig. 2.14 Resin-embedded longitudinal section of muscle, stained with toluidine blue. Portion of a necrotic fibre with macrophages is seen on the left. Delicate capillaries are visible. All muscle fibres contain rows of vacuoles. From a case of AIDS-associated myopathy (×225)

4. Fibre types (size of different types, checkerboard or grouped patterns, predominance of one type)
5. Internal nuclei (normally in fewer than 3% of fibres)
6. Focal abnormalities in fibres:
   (a) Necrosis, phagocytosis, or regeneration
   (b) Vacuoles (simple, or rimmed with basophilic material)
   (c) Inclusions (rods, cytoplasmic bodies, or tubular aggregates)
   (d) Architectural changes (cores, targets, moth-eaten fibres, lobulated fibres, mitochondrial clumping, ring fibres, or split fibres)
7. Enzyme deficiencies (abnormal intrafibre glycogen or fat)
8. Interstitium (fibrous connective tissue, fat, blood vessels, nerves, muscle spindles, inflammation, amyloid)

A simple but often neglected technique is that of examining the sections under crossed polarizers. Abnormal birefringent substances that may be found in muscle are amyloid stained with Congo red, foreign bodies, or crystals such as those of oxalic acid (Fig. 2.16).

After these features have been looked for, the following questions can be asked:

1. Are the appearances normal or a variant of normal? Points to remember are the smaller fibres in children (Aherne et al 1971, Oertel 1988), the effects of physical exercise on fibre size and type (Jansson et al 1978), and the finding of small fibres with internal nuclei near a muscle tendon (Fig. 2.17). Intramuscular nerves have been mistaken for parasites, and muscle spindles for groups of atrophic fibres. The size and proportion of fibre types varies not only between different muscles but also at

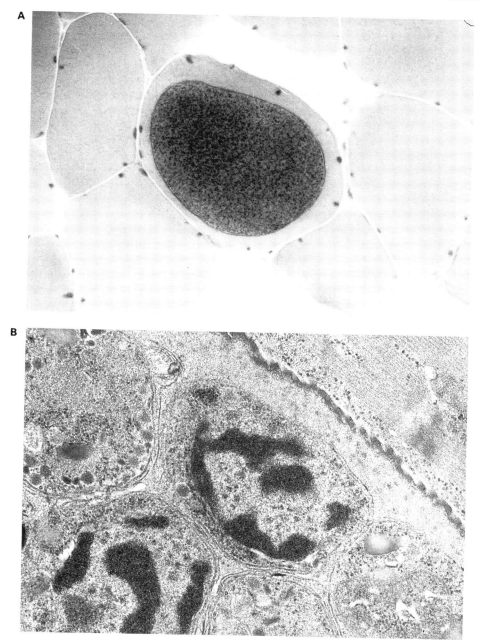

Fig. 2.15   Electron microscopy from frozen tissue. (a) A large parasitic cyst in the muscle of a man with myalgia H&E (×175). (b) On electron microscopy the cyst wall and cystozooites are clearly seen, confirming the diagnosis of *Sarcocystis* infection (×31 500)

different sites within the same muscle (Mahon et al 1984), so that subtle changes in overall fibre size and distribution of fibre types need to be interpreted with caution. Small neurovascular bundles can be mistaken for groups of inflammatory cells, especially if the blood vessel is difficult to identify (Fig. 2.18). However, the cells in these bundles do not

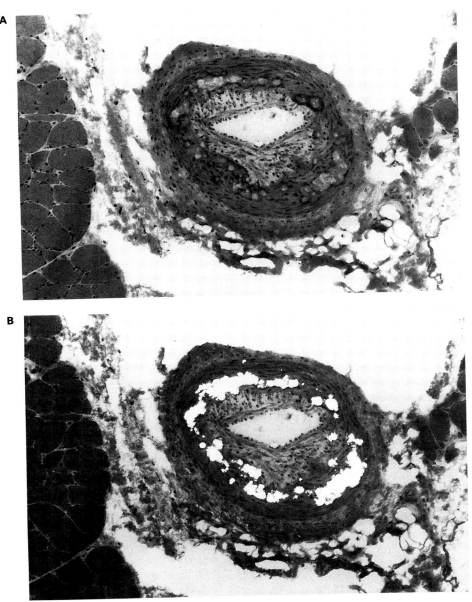

Fig. 2.16 Use of polarized light in a case of oxalosis. (a) Faint irregular bodies occupy the media of an intramuscular artery. (b) Under polarized light the bodies (oxalic acid crystals) exhibit brilliant birefringence. (H&E, ×56)

invade muscle fibres, and the acid phosphatase stain for macrophages is usually negative.

2. Could the appearances be due to artefact? The vacuoles caused by ice-crystal damage may lead to a diagnosis of a vacuolar myopathy, but ice-crystal change is usually patchy (Fig. 2.19), with a gradation from smaller to larger vacuoles across a number of fibres (Fig. 2.20). Large, darkly-staining fibres seen on transverse section may be due to contraction artefact (Fig. 2.21). However, if the fibres have been held at resting length during fixation, any contraction

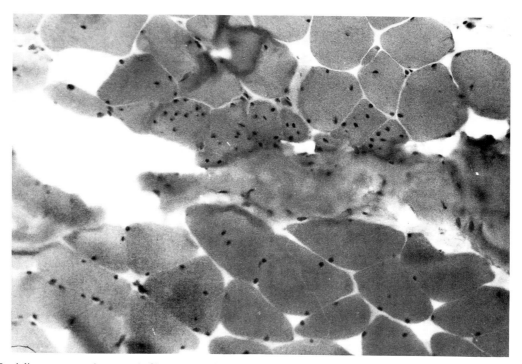

Fig. 2.17 Adjacent to a tendon, muscle fibres are small and contain numerous internal nuclei (H&E ×100)

bands seen can be considered real and not due to tissue handling (Lotz & Engel 1987). If a needle has been previously inserted into the biopsied muscle, an erroneous diagnosis of an inflammatory myopathy may be made. Clues to this injury are an elongated track containing inflammatory cells (unfortunately seen only rarely) (Fig. 2.22) and the monophasic nature of the muscle necrosis and regeneration. Crush artefact is common around the edges of needle biopsies and only fibres internal to the outer rim of tissue should be taken into consideration for diagnostic purposes.

3. Can the changes be fitted into a broad diagnostic category? Diagnostic patterns are: (i) normal muscle, (ii) mild, non-diagnostic changes, (iii) neuropathic changes, and (iv) myopathic changes.

4. Can a specific diagnosis be made? This will be discussed in the following chapters.

5. Are any further tests needed? More specialized stains or electron microscopy may be indicated, depending on the clinical diagnosis or the results of the routine stains.

SPECIALIZED TECHNIQUES

1. Biochemistry

Biochemical analysis can be performed on open or needle muscle biopsies, but the number of tests on needle samples is limited by the amount of tissue obtained. Nevertheless, it is possible to screen for a variety of abnormalities on the smaller specimens and diagnose a number of enzyme deficiencies. Biochemical and chemical methods are especially useful to confirm the results of qualitative histochemical stains.

Mitochondrial enzyme activity can be assessed by spectrophotometry, the reduction of added cytochrome c being used to measure levels of cytochrome c oxidase, succinate cytochrome c reductase, pyruvate plus malate cytochrome c reductase, 2-oxoglutarate cytochrome c reductase, and glutamate cytochrome c reductase (Gohil et al 1981). Quantitative measurement of the various cytochromes requires an open biopsy specimen. Needle samples also give enough tissue to measure fatty acid metabolism (free and esterified carnitine, carnitine acyl transferase), glycogen metabolism

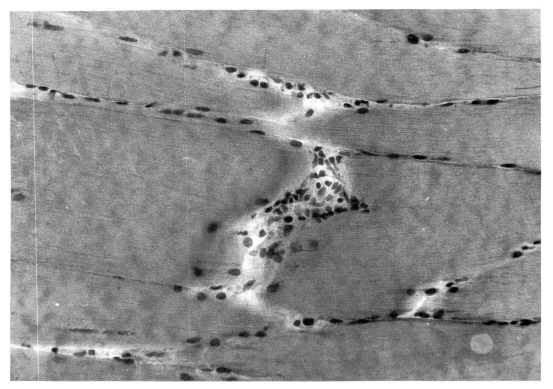

Fig. 2.18   A neurovascular bundle can resemble an infiltrate of inflammatory cells (H&E, ×153)

(quantitative glycogen content, phosphorylase, phosphofructokinase, and acid maltase), and levels of myoadenylate deaminase.

A recent advance has been the measurement of the protein dystrophin in muscle biopsy samples (Hoffman et al 1988). Low or absent levels are found in Duchenne dystrophy, and an abnormal-molecular-weight dystrophin occurs in Becker dystrophy. Muscle tissue is needed for the test since no components of blood have detectable levels of this protein. Only a small amount of frozen muscle (less than 0.1 g) is needed for the Western blot analysis; the length of time the muscle has been kept frozen, the type of muscle biopsied, and the age of the patient do not seem to be important.

2. Quantification

With the advent of time-saving computerized equipment the quantification of muscle fibre size and type distribution has become a routine pro-cedure in many laboratories. The methods and problems of estimating muscle fibre size are summarized by Aherne & Dunhill (1982). The 'least diameter' measurement for estimating fibre size is one frequently used in practice (Dubowitz 1985).

There are three approaches to measuring fibre sizes and type distribution. In the first, a photo-graph is taken and the diameter of a defined number of fibres is measured with a ruler. This method is obviously laborious and requires much technician time. The second method is to use a semi-automatic image analyser such as the Kontron MOP. This consists of an electronic drawing board on which individual fibre circumferences or least diameters are outlined, and according to the programme in the microprocessor, information such as fibre size and type distribution can be analysed and recorded. A third method utilizes an automatic image analyser, such as the Quantimet 970 (Cambridge Instruments), that enables features of interest to be selected by grey-level

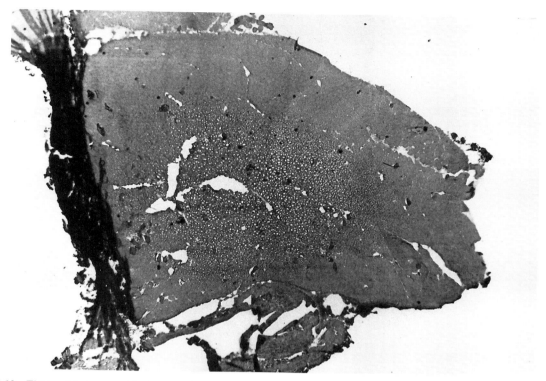

Fig. 2.19 The small holes caused by ice-crystal artefact are characteristically more severe in deeper levels of the sample, while the outer rim is spared. The section has folded on the left, a common problem with cryosections. (Modified Gomori trichrome, ×15)

contrast, and measurements to be made of size, number, shape, position or orientation of these features. Some new image analysis systems are also able to differentiate between features of different colours. These automatic instruments are fast, but they are costly and require considerable expertise to programme and operate.

The quantitative results may reveal abnormalities not apparent on routine observation (Maunder-Sewry & Dubowitz 1981, Stanstedt et al 1982). It can however be difficult to assess the pathological significance of subtle changes that can be picked up only on quantification, given the variation in fibre types and sizes even within single muscles (Elder et al 1982, Lexell et al 1983, Mahon et al 1984).

3. Biopsy for motor end-plates

The anatomical distribution of end-plates varies in different muscles; they may be confined to a thin transverse or parabolic band across the muscle or they may be distributed throughout the muscle (Aquilonius et al 1984). Many workers sample short muscles to increase the chance of finding end-plates, and a popular site is the external intercostal muscle (Stern et al 1975), though this requires considerable surgical expertise to avoid causing a pneumothorax. We have recently been sampling the extensor digitorum brevis muscle (Pamphlett 1991), the disadvantage being that the patient has to rest the foot for a few days post-biopsy. From these small muscles a thin strip of muscle is fixed in glutaraldehyde at resting length in a clamp. Pairs of adjacent strips are dissected from this bundle, and end-plates are localized in one of each pair with cholinesterase staining (Engel 1970). Small blocks can then be taken from the end-plate zone of the adjacent unstained strip and processed for electron microscopy. Muscle sampling using an electrical stimulator to locate the end-plate zone is described in Chapter 18.

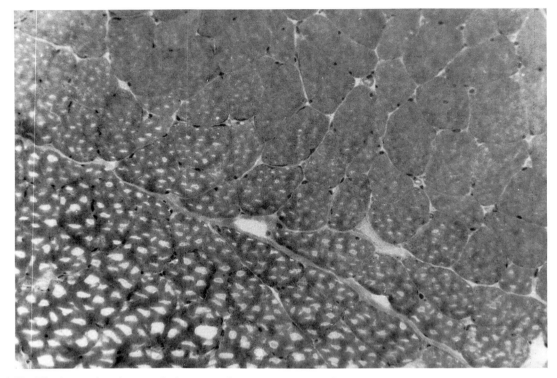

Fig. 2.20 The damage from ice-crystals shows a gradient across the muscle fibres. (Modified Gomori trichrome, ×102)

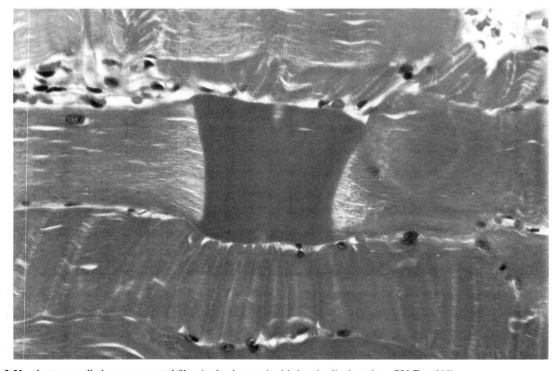

Fig. 2.21 A segmentally hypercontracted fibre is clearly seen in this longitudinal section. (H&E, ×212)

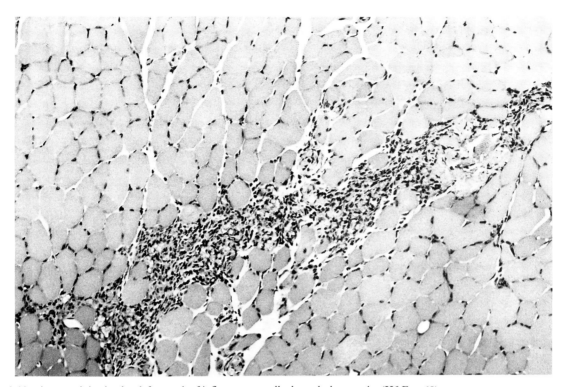

Fig. 2.22 A recent injection has left a track of inflammatory cells through the muscle. (H&E, ×68)

4. Other techniques

Among the plethora of special techniques that can now be applied to muscle are in vitro testing for sensitivity to anaesthetic agents (Ellis et al 1971) and tissue culture (Witkowski 1977). Comments on immunocytochemistry used to locate a number of antigens are given in Fitzsimons & Sewry (1985).

REFERENCES

Aherne W A, Dunhill M S 1982 Methods of estimating fibre size. In: Morphometry. Arnold, London, pp 103–117

Aherne W, Ayyar D R, Clarke P A, Walton J N 1971 Muscle fibre size in normal infants, children and adolescents. An autopsy study. Journal of the Neurological Sciences 14: 171

Aquilonius S M, Asmark H, Gillberg P G, Nandedkar S, Olsson Y, Stalberg E 1984 Topographical localization of motor endplates in cryosections of whole human muscles. Muscle and Nerve 7: 287

Bancroft J D, Cook H C 1984 Infective agents in tissue. In: Manual of histological techniques. Churchill Livingstone, Edinburgh, pp 203–217

Bardosi A, Zobel H J 1985 A new clamp for muscle and nerve biopsy. Muscle and Nerve 8: 725

Bardosi A, Dimitri T, Wosgien B, Gabius H J 1989 Expression of endogenous receptors for neoglycoproteins, especially lectins, that allow fiber typing on formaldehyde-fixed, paraffin-embedded muscle biopsy specimens. Journal of Histochemistry and Cytochemistry 37: 989

Bergstrom J 1962 Muscle electrolytes in man. Scandinavian Journal of Clinical and Laboratory Investigation 14 (suppl 68): 11

Bonilla E, Samitt C E, Miranda A F et al 1988a Duchenne muscular dystrophy: deficiency of dystrophin at the muscle cell surface. Cell 54: 447

Bonilla E, Schmidt B, Samitt C E et al 1988b Normal and dystrophin-deficient muscle fibers in carriers of the gene for Duchenne muscular dystrophy. American Journal of Pathology 133: 440

Braund K G, Ambling K A 1988 Muscle biopsy samples for histochemical processing: alterations induced by storage. Veterinary Pathology 25: 77

Burns J, Redfern D R, Esiri M M, McGee J O 1986 Human and viral gene detection in routine paraffin embedded tissue by in situ hybridisation with biotinylated probes: viral localisation in herpes encephalitis. Journal of Clinical Pathology 39: 1066

Curless R G, Nelson M B 1975 Needle biopsies of muscle in

infants for diagnosis and research. Developmental Medicine and Child Neurology 17: 592

Dietrichson P, Coakley J, Smith P E M, Griffiths R D, Helliwell T R, Edwards R H T 1987 Conchotome and needle percutaneous biopsy of skeletal muscle. Journal of Neurology, Neurosurgery, and Psychiatry 50: 1461

Dubowitz V 1985 Muscle biopsy. A practical approach. Bailliere Tindall, London

Edgerton V R, Smith J L, Simpson D R 1975 Muscle fibre type populations of human leg muscle. Histochemical Journal 7: 259

Edwards R H T, Round J M, Jones D A 1983 Needle biopsies of skeletal muscle: a review of 10 years' experience. Muscle and Nerve 6: 676

Elder B C G, Bradbury K, Roberts R 1982 Variability of fibre type distributions within human muscles. Journal of Applied Physiology 53: 1473

Ellis F R, Keany M P, Harriman D G F et al 1971 Screening for malignant hyperpyrexia. British Medical Journal 3: 559

Engel A G 1970 Locating motor end plates for electron microscopy. Mayo Clinic Proceedings 45: 450

Filipe M I, Lake B D 1983 Histochemistry in pathology. Churchill Livingstone, Edinburgh, p 301

Fitzsimons R, Sewry C A 1985 Immunocytochemistry. In: Dubowitz V (ed) Muscle biopsy. A practical approach. Balliere Tindall, London, pp 184–207

Fremion A S 1988 The value of guided needle muscle biopsy. Journal of Child Neurology 3: 75

Fukuyama Y, Suzuki Y, Hirayama Y et al 1981 Percutaneous needle muscle biopsy in the diagnosis of neuromuscular disorders in children. Histological, histochemical and electron microscopic studies. Brain and Development 3: 277

Gohil K, Jones D A, Edwards R H T 1981 Analysis of muscle mitochondrial function with techniques applicable to needle biopsy samples. Clinical Physiology 1: 195

Gorza L 1990 Identification of a novel type 2 fiber population in mammalian skeletal muscle by combined use of histochemical myosin ATPase and anti-myosin monoclonal antibodies. Journal of Histochemistry and Cytochemistry 38: 257

Haase A, Brahic M, Stowring L, Blum H 1984 Detection of viral nucleic acids by in situ hybridization. Methods in Virology 7: 189

Harriman D G F 1984 Diseases of muscle. In: Adams J H, Corsellis J A N, Duchen L W (eds) Greenfield's neuropathology. Arnold, London, p 1029

Heckmatt J Z, Dubowitz V 1987 Ultrasound imaging and directed needle muscle biopsy in the diagnosis of selective involvement in muscle disease. Journal of Child Neurology 2: 205

Heckmatt J Z, Moosa A, Hutson C, Maunder-Sewry C A, Dubowitz V 1984 Diagnostic needle muscle biopsy: a practical and reliable alternative to open biopsy. Archives of Disease in Childhood 59: 528

Heene R, Haar F 1984 Mailing muscle biopsy samples for histochemical processing. Conditions and morphometric approach to the alterations induced by storage. Journal of Neurology 231: 176

Heffner R R Jr 1984 Muscle biopsy in the diagnosis of neuromuscular disease. Seminars in Diagnostic Pathology 1: 114

Henriksson K G 1979 'Semi-open' muscle biopsy technique: a simple outpatient procedure. Acta Neurologica Scandinavica 59: 317

Hoffman E P, Fischbeck K H, Brown R H et al 1988

Characterization of dystrophin in muscle-biopsy specimens from patients with Duchenne's or Becker's muscular dystrophy. New England Journal of Medicine 318: 1363

Hultman E 1967 Studies on muscle metabolism of glycogen and active phosphate with special reference to exercise and diet. Scandinavian Journal of Clinical and Laboratory Investigation 19 (suppl 94): 18

Jansson E, Sjodin B, Tesch P 1978 Changes in muscle fibre type distribution in man after physical training. Acta Physiologica Scandinavica 104: 235

Johnson M A, Polgar J, Weightman D, Appleton D 1973 Data on the distribution of fibre types in thirty-six human muscles. An autopsy study. Journal of the Neurological Sciences 18: 111

Karpati G, Watters G V 1980 Adverse anesthetic reactions in Duchenne dystrophy. In: Angelini C, Danielli G A, Fontanari D (eds) Muscular dystrophy research: advances and new trends. Excerpta Medica, Amsterdam, pp 206–217

Kaufman L D, Gruber B L, Gerstman D P, Kaell A T 1987 Preliminary observations on the role of magnetic resonance imaging for polymyositis and dermatomyositis. Annals of the Rheumatic Diseases 46: 569

Lexell J, Hendriksson-Larsen K, Sjostrom M 1983 Distribution of different fibre types in human skeletal muscles. Acta Physiologica Scandinavica 117: 115

Lindholm T 1968 The influence of uraemia and electrolyte disturbances on muscle action potentials and motor nerve conduction in man. Acta Medica Scandinavica (suppl 491): 23

Lotz B P, Engel A G 1987 Are hypercontracted muscle fibers artifacts and do they cause rupture of the plasma membrane? Neurology 37: 1466

Mahon M, Toman A, Willan P L T, Bagnall K M 1984 Variability of histochemical and morphometric data from needle biopsy specimens of human quadriceps femoris muscle. Journal of the Neurological Sciences 63: 85

Maunder-Sewry C A, Dubowitz V 1981 Needle muscle biopsy for carrier detection in Duchenne muscular dystrophy. Journal of the Neurological Sciences 49: 305

Nichols B L, Hazlewood C F, Barnes D J 1968 Percutaneous needle biopsy of quadriceps muscle: potassium analysis in normal children. Journal of Pediatrics 72: 840

Nonaka I, Koga Y, Shikura K et al 1988 Muscle pathology in cytochrome c oxidase deficiency. Acta Neuropathologica (Berlin) 77: 152

Oertel G 1988 Morphometric analysis of normal skeletal muscles in infancy, childhood and adolescence: an autopsy study. Journal of the Neurological Sciences 88: 303

Pamphlett R 1991 Looking for lead at endplates in motor neurone disease. Medical Journal of Australia 154: 637

Pamphlett R, O'Donague P 1990 Sarcocystis infection of human muscle. Australian & New Zealand Journal of Medicine 20: 705

Pamphlett R, O'Donague P 1990 Sarcocystis infection of human muscle. Australian & New Zealand Journal of Medicine (in

Pamphlett R, Harper C, Tan N, Kakulas B A 1985 Needle muscle biopsy: will it make open biopsy obsolete? Australian and New Zealand Journal of Medicine 15: 199

Pearse A G E 1985 Histochemistry. Theoretical and applied, 4th edn. Churchill Livingstone, Edinburgh

Pierobon-Bormioli S, Sartore S, Dalla Libera L, Vitadella M, Sciaffino S 1981 'Fast' isomyosins and fiber types in mammalian skeletal muscle. Journal of Histochemistry and Cytochemistry 29: 1179

Polgar J, Johnson M A, Weightman D, Appleton D 1973 Data

on fibre size in thirty-six human muscles: an autopsy study. Journal of the Neurological Sciences 19: 307

Porro R S, Webster H de F, Tobin W 1969 Needle biopsy of skeletal muscle: a phase and electron microscopic evaluation of its usefulness in the study of muscle disease. Journal of Neuropathology and Experimental Neurology 28: 229

Radner S 1965 Instruments for percutaneous muscle biopsy. Journal Stille-Werner 21, Stockholm

Sartore S, Gorza L, Schiaffino S 1982 Fetal myosin heavy chains in regenerating muscle. Nature 298: 294–296

Shumate J B, Katnik R, Ruiz M et al 1979 Myoadenylate deaminase deficiency. Muscle and Nerve 2: 213

Siegel I M, Weiss L A 1988 Stapling muscle biopsy specimens to prevent artifacts. Journal of the American Medical Association 260: 338

Stanstedt P, Nordell L E, Hendriksson K G 1982 Quantitative analysis of muscle biopsies from volunteers and patients with neuromuscular disorders. Acta Neurologica Scandinavica 66: 130

Stern L Z, Gruener R, Anderson R M 1975 External intercostal muscle biopsy. Archives of Neurology 32: 779

Wiley C A, Nerendberg M, Cros D, Soto-Aguilar M C 1989 HTLV-1 polymyositis in a patient also infected with the human immunodeficiency virus. New England Journal of Medicine 320: 992

Witkowski J A 1977 Diseased muscle cells in culture. Biological Reviews 52: 431

Yonker R A, Webster E M, Edwards N L et al 1987 Technetium pyrophosphate muscle scans in inflammatory muscle disease. British Journal of Rheumatology 26: 267

3. Pathological reactions of skeletal muscle

M. J. Cullen   M. A. Johnson   F. L. Mastaglia

INTRODUCTION

Skeletal muscle undergoes pathological reactions that are common to other tissues but it also has two special characteristics which uniquely influence its reaction to injury or disease. First, every muscle fibre is a syncytium formed as a result of the fusion of several hundreds or thousands of component myoblasts, and secondly, by far the greatest part of its volume is occupied by contractile filaments.

The first property means that an injury may, initially at least, affect only a small part of a fibre, and that in disease a genetic lesion may be manifested at different times in different parts of the fibre. As a skeletal muscle fibre is typically several hundred times longer than it is broad, it is not uncommon to find one segment of its length showing pathological changes while the rest appears normal.

The second property is associated with the functional specialization of skeletal muscle as a force-generating tissue so that more than 80% of its volume is occupied by contractile myofibrils. The myofibrils contract and relax in response to calcium fluxes out of and into the sarcoplasmic reticulum (SR) such that the free calcium concentration in the sarcoplasm oscillates between about 10^{-8} to 10^{-5} M. The free concentration in the extracellular fluid, in contrast, is always several orders higher at $\sim 10^{-3}$ M. Maintenance of the low intracellular calcium concentration is dependent on the functional integrity of the plasma membrane, and any injury or disease which alters or damages the plasma membrane may result in an uncontrolled entry of extracellular calcium which, in turn, causes activation of the myofibrils and therefore gross changes in the morphology of the fibre. The changes will be essentially secondary to the initial lesion: one of the major problems in interpreting muscle pathology is in distinguishing these secondary responses from other more basic abnormalities.

Another problem is in distinguishing truly pathological changes from artefacts of processing. Splits in hypertrophied fibres, for example, cannot always be distinguished in histological sections from fractures arising during processing or sectioning. Another common artefact is the formation of contraction bands, usually in fibres at the edge of a biopsy where the muscle has been inexpertly handled. These bands can be indistinguishable from the clumps of overcontracted myofibrils caused by the pathological calcium influx referred to above.

A third problem met in trying to assess the importance of morphological changes in pathological muscle is one of sampling. In terms of trauma to the patient, the smaller the piece of tissue taken for biopsy the better, but the smaller the biopsy the greater is the possibility of obtaining a non-representative sample and perhaps even of missing an area significant for diagnosis. This is a more important consideration in electron microscopy than in histology or histochemistry because the sample size is necessarily far smaller.

A fourth consideration concerns the specificity of the pathological changes which are found. Most, if not all, the changes which are encountered are not specific to any one disease entity. One of the commonest myofibrillar changes, for example, is Z-band streaming, which is seen in many conditions and which is also seen to a limited extent in normal healthy muscle. Accumulation of glycogen is another non-specific change that is very variable in extent and can be seen to some degree in normal muscle. Nevertheless, the pattern of abnormalities in a muscle can be characteristic of a particular disease; in assessing a biopsy for diagnosis, therefore, the whole spectrum of changes which are seen has to be taken into account.

In this chapter we are not so much concerned with describing the changes associated with particular conditions, which will be dealt with in subsequent chapters, but with describing the cellular reactions of muscle to disease. For this purpose, a muscle can be considered to be a collection of individual myofibres which may be affected in different or similar ways, but which do not influence each other in their reactions. The first section deals with the general reactions of the myofibre as a whole, where every component may be expected to be involved. The second section deals with reactions of individual components of the fibres.

BASIC PATHOLOGICAL REACTIONS

Atrophy and hypotrophy

Atrophy is one of the most common responses of a muscle fibre to loss of neural influences, to processes which prevent normal contractile activity, and to various pathological stimuli. It involves a phase of negative growth and regression in volume. Hypotrophy, on the other hand, is less common and involves an arrest or slowing of normal growth of the muscle fibre.

Patterns of atrophy

Muscle fibre atrophy is a common finding in a variety of chronic myopathies, both inherited and acquired, but the most striking degrees of atrophy result from denervation of muscle due to anterior horn cell and peripheral nerve disorders.

A number of different patterns of muscle fibre atrophy are recognizable with the light microscope. Atrophy of randomly distributed single fibres is a very non-specific finding which, on its own, has no diagnostic significance. In chronic myopathies, too, such as the muscular dystrophies or the inflammatory myopathies, atrophic fibres are usually randomly distributed and the atrophic process is usually a non-selective one, involving both major fibre types. In some cases of dermatomyositis, a characteristic atrophy of the most peripheral fibres in muscle fascicles occurs ('perifascicular' atrophy) (see Ch. 12 and Fig. 3.1). In denervation, the atrophic process is generally a non-selective one which may involve both type 1 and type 2 fibres, and a number of different histological patterns are found according to the speed of evolution and completeness of the denervating process (see Ch. 16). If a muscle is totally denervated, for example following division of its motor nerve, all of the constituent fibres undergo a reduction in size. More often, however, in situations of partial denervation, the atrophic fibres are distributed between fibres of normal size, either singly or in groups of variable numbers. For reasons which are not well understood, denervated muscle fibres are often angulated in shape, appearing to be indented by the surrounding normal fibres. This is not so in biopsies from infants, however, in which denervated fibres are usually rounded rather than angulated. Although in animals type 2 fibres show a more marked degree of atrophy than type 1 fibres after nerve section, in man the different fibre types usually atrophy to about the same extent after denervation, although occasionally there may be preferential atrophy of type 1 or more often of type 2A or type 2B fibres (Karpati 1979).

In a number of situations the atrophic process may involve selectively either the type 1 or the type 2 muscle fibres. Selective type 1 fibre atrophy is relatively uncommon and occurs in myotonic dystrophy as well as in 'centronuclear' myopathy

Fig. 3.1 Perifascicular atrophy in juvenile dermatomyositis; myofibrillar ATPase, alkaline pre-incubation. ×132

Fig. 3.2 Type 1 fibre hypotrophy in centronuclear myopathy; myofibrillar ATPase, pH 4.3 pre-incubation. ×338

Fig. 3.3 Type 2B fibre atrophy in steroid myopathy; myofibrillar ATPase, pH 4.6 pre-incubation. ×132

Fig. 3.1

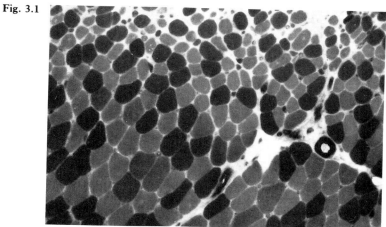

Fig. 3.2

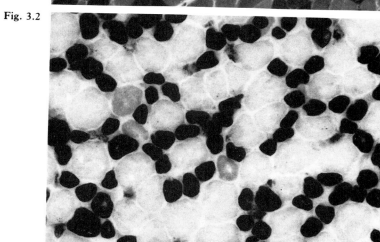

Fig. 3.3

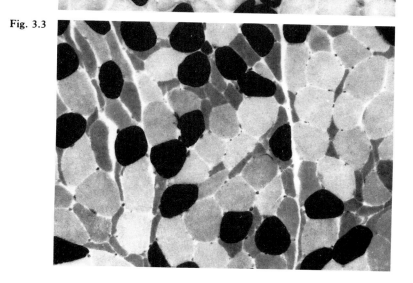

(Fig. 3.2), nemaline myopathy, and some cases of congenital fibre-type disproportion (Dubowitz & Brooke 1973). In the last three disorders, and in the neonatal form of myotonic dystrophy in which type 1 fibre atrophy may also occur (Argov et al 1980a), the term hypotrophy is probably more appropriate than atrophy, as the type 1 fibres may never have reached a normal size. Selective type 2 fibre atrophy (Fig. 3.3) is, by contrast, one of the commonest abnormalities found in muscle biopsies and is quite non-specific, being found in a variety of conditions including myasthenia gravis, polymyositis, polymyalgia rheumatica, connective tissue diseases, corticosteroid myopathy and Cushing's disease, in various metabolic disorders including osteomalacia and primary hyperparathyroidism, and in cachectic states.

Morphological changes in atrophic fibres

In conventional histological preparations, atrophic fibres may be indistinguishable from the normal fibres in everything but their size and shape. More detail of atrophic fibres can frequently be seen in toluidine blue-stained 1 μm plastic sections (Fig. 3.4) but the fine-structural characteristics can be distinguished only under the electron microscope. One of the commonest features is the irregularity of the fibre outline, which is thrown into folds, particularly at the 'angles' of the fibres (Fig. 3.5). Exterior to the peripheral folds, the redundant basal lamina is also cast into complex folds (Figs. 3.5, 3.6). It is generally accepted that this results from a pulling away of the plasma membrane from the basal lamina which maintains its original size. This is a very useful feature in distinguishing atrophic from regenerating or hypotrophic fibres, because growing or non-atrophying fibres are surrounded by a cohesive basal lamina (Fig. 3.5).

In certain situations, histochemical techniques would show changes in atrophic muscle fibres. For example, in denervation, oxidative enzyme preparations often show increased activity and there is also increased activity with the non-specific esterase technique, whereas glycogen and phosphorylase are lost at an early stage (Karpati 1979).

The myofibrils in atrophic fibres are usually thinner than in normal fibres (Fig. 3.7) and may become mis-aligned and disrupted in late-stage atrophy. The sarcoplasmic reticulum (SR) and T system may become extremely prominent (Fig. 3.8) and the transverse tubules and the associated triads commonly change to a longitudinal orientation (Fig. 3.8). There is frequently an accumulation of autophagic vacuoles and the lipofuscin residue of lysosomal action. More details of the changes in ultrastructure are given in the appropriate sections later in the chapter.

Cellular mechanisms

The mechanisms underlying myofibre atrophy are poorly understood. Shrinkage of a cell or tissue may be brought about either by an enhancement of the normal rate of protein degradation or by a reduction in protein synthesis or by both processes occurring simultaneously. Studies on relative

---

Fig. 3.4 Atrophic muscle fibres (arrows) located singly between the normal fibres in a case of congenital myotonic dystrophy. Toluidine blue stained 1 μm section. ×560

Fig. 3.5 Two small fibres in a case of Werdnig-Hoffmann disease. The upper fibre is atrophic and has a wavy outline and many folds of redundant basal lamina (BL). The lower fibre is hypotrophic and has a closely adherent basal lamina. ×5600

Fig. 3.6 An atrophic fibre with an associated satellite cell (Sat) in a case of spinal muscular atrophy. The atrophic fibre has a smooth outline compared with that in Figure 3.4. BL = redundant basal lamina. ×6730. (Reproduced from Mastaglia & Hudgson (1981) with kind permission of Churchill Livingstone)

Fig. 3.7 Part of an atrophic fibre from a case of Werdnig–Hoffmann disease. Note the narrowness of some of the myofibrils (Mf). ×11 995

Fig. 3.8 Part of an atrophic fibre from a case of motor neuron disease. Note the 'sexad' (composed of three elements of the T system and three elements of the sarcoplasmic reticulum) and the longitudinal orientation of the two triads (Tr). T = T system. SR = sarcoplasmic reticulum. ×22 420

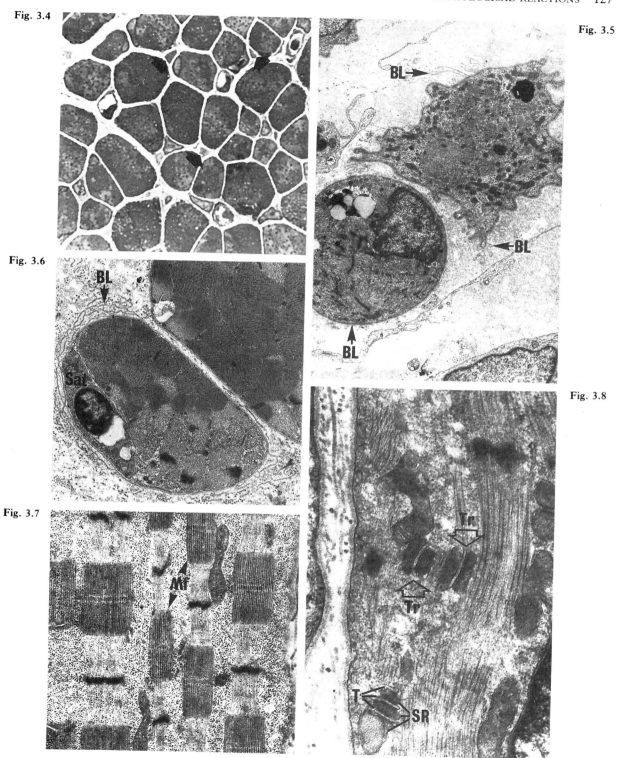

Fig. 3.4

Fig. 3.5

Fig. 3.6

Fig. 3.7

Fig. 3.8

turnover rates of the myofibrillar proteins in experimental animals and in man have shown considerable heterogeneity between individual proteins (Millward 1980). In the I filaments, actin seems to turn over more slowly than troponin and tropomyosin, and in the A filaments the myosin heavy chains turn over more slowly than the light chains. During myofibre atrophy where, at least in the early stages, the relative amounts of the contractile proteins appear unaltered, the relative rates of turnover of each protein must be unchanged. In those pathological conditions where there is a relative accumulation of one type of filament, the rates of turnover must get out of step.

The identification of the enzymes involved in muscle protein degradation is still uncertain. The proteinases which have been shown to be present in muscle and which are able to break down myofibrillar proteins are calcium-activated proteinase (CAP), cathepsin B and cathepsin D (Bird et al 1980). CAP selectively degrades troponins T and I, tropomyosin, C protein and M protein, but not myosin, actin or α-actinin. Zeece & Katoh (1989) compared the speed with which different myofibrillar proteins were degraded by cathepsin D in vivo at 37°C and pH 5.5. Titin and almost all proteins with a molecular weight greater than the myosin heavy chains (including M- and C-protein) were degraded most rapidly. Actin, tropomyosin, troponins T and I, and myosin light chains LC1 and LC2 were degraded more slowly. Neither α-actinin nor desmin were degraded by cathepsin D under these conditions.

Schwartz & Bird (1977) found that the degradation of actin and myosin by cathepsin B was less extensive than that by cathepsin D. They calculated that at pH 5.0, in the amounts found in rat skeletal muscle, cathepsins B and D theoretically could degrade all the native myosin in 6–9 days. However, the mechanisms of protein degradation in skeletal muscle are still not well understood (Guarnieri et al 1989). Different proteolytic systems are probably active in skeletal muscle under different conditions. Basal degradative processes may differ from increased proteolysis during fasting or in disease states such as trauma, sepsis or diabetes (Furuno & Goldberg 1986).

Cathepsins B and D are lysosomal and if, as is generally accepted, there is lysosomal involvement in muscle protein breakdown there must be some way of introducing those proteins into the lysosomes. Myofibrillar material within lysosomes has not been observed under the electron microscope. It has therefore been suggested that CAP, which is sarcoplasmic, serves to break down myofilaments into smaller pieces that could be managed by digestive vacuoles (Dayton et al 1976, Cullen & Pluskal 1977, Goll et al 1978). One problem with this potential mechanism is that CAP appeared to require millimolar levels of calcium for optimum activity (2–3 orders of magnitude greater than free calcium in the sarcoplasm). However Dayton et al (1981) later showed that there were two forms of CAP, one of which has a low calcium requirement. The K_ms for calcium for the low and high requiring forms are 0.45 μM and 0.74 mM respectively. Dayton et al suggested that the low calcium requiring form was active during normal protein turnover. It is also reasonable to suppose that in necrotic fibres, where calcium reaches millimolar levels, the high calcium requiring form becomes active. This is compatible with the loss of the Z-line and I-band often observed in necrotic fibres (Cullen & Fulthorpe 1982).

Clearly, our understanding of the underlying mechanism of myofibre atrophy is still largely speculative. The conditions that produce atrophy are well documented and the morphological end-results can be observed and measured. However, we are still largely ignorant of the intermediate stages involving the activation and role of the cellular proteinases. It is not known, for example, whether there is a common mechanism involved in the different conditions which bring about atrophy, or whether each situation is unique. If the latter is the case, then present research is as yet only touching the surface of this topic.

Hypotrophy

The term hypotrophy is applicable to fibres of small size which have never reached a normal size as a result of an arrest in the normal maturation processes. As already indicated, the small type 1 fibres found in nemaline myopathy, centronuclear myopathy (Fig. 3.2) and in congenital fibre type disproportion, fall into this category and it has been postulated that the impairment of maturation in these situations may be due to a defective neural influence during myogenesis (Engel et al 1968, Argov et al 1980b). Similarly, small fibres with features suggestive of a maturational arrest may also be found in neonatal myotonic dystrophy (Sarnat & Silbert 1976) and in Werdnig-Hoffman disease (Fidzianska 1976). Characteristically, hypotrophic fibres have a closely adherent basal lamina (Fig. 3.5) in contrast to atrophic fibres. Other morphological features include the presence of internally situated and at times central myonuclei producing a myotube-like appearance, and frequent satellite cells (Farkas-Bargeton et al 1978).

Hypertrophy

Muscle hypertrophy may occur physiologically as a response to an increased work-load in individuals with a high level of physical activity, may be hormonally induced (e.g. by anabolic steroids or growth hormone), and may also occur in certain disease states. The term hypertrophia musculorum vera has been used in occasional individuals with pronounced generalized muscular hypertrophy in the absence of myotonia or impairment of muscle function. The physiological hypertrophy which occurs in athletes as a result of physical training may involve both major fibre types (Prince et al 1977) but with endurance training there is a selective hypertrophy of type 1 fibres. With sprint and strength-training, both fibre types increase in size but the type 2 fibres more so than the type 1 fibres (Saltin et al 1976, Staron et al 1989). It is possible that differences in the level of physical activity and in exercise patterns account in part for the relative differences in fibre-type sizes in men and women, type 2 fibres being larger in men than in women, but a hormonal effect is more probably the cause.

In pathological states the most marked degrees of muscular hypertrophy are encountered in myotonia congenita and in the more slowly progressive forms of muscular dystrophy (e.g. the Becker and limb-girdle varieties). Muscle fibre hypertrophy also occurs in long-standing hypothyroidism and in acromegaly. In the latter condition, both fibre types undergo hypertrophy (Mastaglia, 1973). Muscle fibre hypertrophy,

which is presumably of a compensatory nature, is also encountered in states of chronic partial denervation as in some forms of spinal muscular atrophy (Fig. 3.9), and also occurs briefly in the early stages of denervation in certain muscles such as the diaphragm.

Muscle fibre hypertrophy results principally from an increase in the numbers of myofibrils. The basic mechanisms involved in the laying down of new myofibrils are incompletely understood. Longitudinal splitting of myofibrils, once they reach a certain size, may be one of the ways in which the numbers of myofibrils are increased (Goldspink 1972). Satellite cells have been noted to be more prominent in hypertrophic human muscle (Reger & Craig 1968) and incorporation of these cells into the muscle fibre syncytium may be a way of increasing the myonuclear complement.

Internal migration of sarcolemmal nuclei and longitudinal splitting (Fig. 3.10) may occur in muscle fibres which have undergone work or

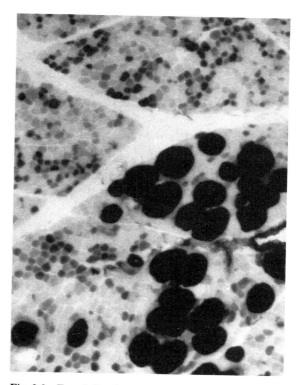

Fig. 3.9 Type 1 fibre hypertrophy in infantile SMA; myofibrillar ATPase, pH 4.3 pre-incubation. ×190

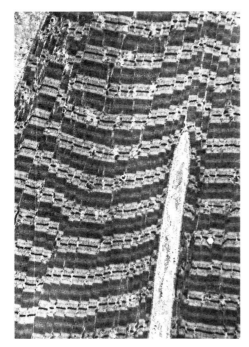

Fig. 3.10 Longitudinal splitting of a muscle fibre in a case of Duchenne muscular dystrophy. ×2670

compensatory hypertrophy and such changes may be prominent in chronic myopathies and in chronic denervating conditions (Mastaglia & Walton 1971b, Schwartz et al 1976). Longitudinal splitting of muscle fibres is the likely basis for the apparent increase in muscle fibre numbers seen with the light microscope in some experimental studies of compensatory work hypertrophy. The factors responsible for splitting of hypertrophic fibres are not known. However, the observation in transverse sections that a myonucleus is commonly present at the apex of the cleft dividing the muscle fibre suggests that nuclear migration plays a part (Swash et al 1978). It seems likely that splitting is an adaptive response which occurs when the fibre reaches a critical size at which supplies of oxygen and exchange of metabolites are no longer efficient.

True hypertrophy of a muscle must be distinguished from pseudohypertrophy in which the volume of muscle may be increased because of fatty infiltration, an inflammatory process such as cysticercosis, or the presence of a tumour (Adams et al 1962). The prominent enlargement of the muscles of the calves, which occurs in the

Duchenne form of muscular dystrophy and which is commonly referred to as pseudohypertrophy, appears to be due to a combination of true hypertrophy of muscle fibres and an increase in the amount of interstitial fibrous connective tissue and adipose tissue (Mastaglia 1970).

Measurement of fibre size

The quantitative assessment of the extent of atrophy and hypertrophy is important in the diagnosis of neuromuscular disease. On simple observation of muscle sections, it is easy to mistake, for example, a population consisting of normal-diameter and hypertrophied fibres for one consisting of, respectively, atrophied and normal-diameter fibres. Where necessary, subjective observation should be followed by objective assessment. The first pre-requisite is access to appropriate data on normal muscle fibre size. In using published normal data, it is important to check that methods of muscle preparation are compatible since it is obviously inappropriate to compare measurements made on frozen sections with those made on fixed material.

Frozen sections are used wherever possible since differentiation of muscle fibre types is often necessary. Well-orientated material is to be preferred but any obliqueness is taken into consideration when measuring techniques based on the calculation of orthogonal diameters are used (Song et al 1963). Computer-aided image analysis systems have enabled routine measurements of samples of 200–300 fibres per biopsy to be made quickly and with a high degree of accuracy.

The normal range of fibre diameters in adult male subjects is approximately 40–80 μm and that for females 30–70 μm (Brooke & Engel 1969a). Size differences between type 1 and type 2 fibres exist, usually being more pronounced in males than in females; however, these differences are relatively small and are usually ignored in routine diagnostic work. The assessment of biopsies from infants and children is made with reference to normal growth curves (Brooke & Engel 1969b). At no time does the normal human muscle fibre population in one individual show a greater than 3-fold variation in fibre size and is less variable in children than in adults.

Conventional statistical analysis, based on calculation of mean diameter and standard deviations is less useful in diagnostic practice than histographic studies of fibre size distributions. Normal muscle fibre populations show a unimodal size distribution, any size difference between type 1 and type 2 fibres being insufficient to be reflected in the overall distribution. The random fibre atrophy and/or hypertrophy seen in many myopathies manifests itself as an increase in range, which may be up to 20-fold in chronic myopathic disorders, but which is not necessarily associated with any change in mean diameter. In contrast neurogenic disorders, involving synchronous atrophy or hypertrophy of the component fibres of whole motor units, frequently show markedly bimodal or trimodal size distributions. The incidence of atrophy and hypertrophy can be assessed objectively by means of the calculation of 'atrophy and hypertrophy factors' (Brooke & Engel 1969c; see Chapter 16). This technique takes into consideration both the relative numbers of affected fibres and the degree of abnormality shown by individual fibres, and is thus a useful indication of the prevalence of atrophy and/or hypertrophy in muscle biopsies.

Fibre type proportions

The proportions of type 1 and type 2 fibres differ widely in normal human muscles in accordance with their differing physiological roles. In general, postural muscles such as m. soleus contain a predominance of type 1 fibres whereas muscles such as m. triceps, which serve a mainly phasic function, contain a predominance of type 2 fibres. The range of fibre type proportions for any one muscle tends to vary considerably between normal individuals, so that ranges based on 95% confidence limits are quite broad. Normal ranges for type 1 percentage in the most commonly biopsied muscles are as follows: biceps 34–51%, deltoid 43–63%, gastrocnemius 37–51%, quadriceps 28–48%, tibialis anterior 62–84% (Johnson et al 1973b). If the fibre type constitution of a biopsy falls outside these normal ranges, a pathological process may be suspected. An abnormal type 1 fibre predominance is often found in hypothyroid subjects, whereas type 2 predominance often

results from hyperthyroidism (see Chapter 13). In dysthyroid states, changes in fibre type constitution arise as a result of physiological conversion of muscle fibres. However, abnormal fibre type constitution can be the result of selective loss of one particular fibre type. For example, selective necrosis of type 2 fibres has been postulated in Duchenne muscular dystrophy (Webster et al 1988) and may account, at least in part, for the type 1 predominance seen in biopsies from patients in later phases of this disorder. However, in many chronic myopathies it is probable that some type 2 motor units undergo conversion to type 1 in response to the altered physiological demands of muscles whose range of activity is severely compromised.

In addition to abnormalities of numerical fibre type constitution, the spatial distribution of fibre types can also become abnormal, especially in neurogenic disorders (see Chapter 16). The spatial distribution in normal human muscles is random (Fig. 3.11) and any departure from a random arrangement can be assessed objectively by using quantitative techniques such as the 'enclosed fibre counting' (EFC) method (Jennekens et al 1971, Johnson et al 1973b) or calculation of the 'co-dispersion index' (CDI) (Lester et al 1983). Instances of uniform fibre type grouping such as are found in chronic anterior horn cell disorders (Fig. 3.12) are often so striking as to render statistical analysis unnecessary, but quantitative methods are useful for assessment of equivocal biopsies.

It must be borne in mind that some non-random distributions may arise as a result of mechanisms other than denervation. For example, clustered regenerating fibres may be subject to non-random reinnervation, resulting in uniform fibre type grouping of limited extent. Fibre splitting may also give rise to sizeable clusters of fibres of uniform type but not to large-scale grouping. In chronic myopathies it is possible that depletion of muscle fibres as a result of necrosis is not a totally random process from the spatial viewpoint, and may contribute to minor abnormalities of fibre type distribution. Profound changes in numerical fibre type constitution do not in themselves imply prior denervation and reinnervation since they may occur as a result of physiological fibre type con-

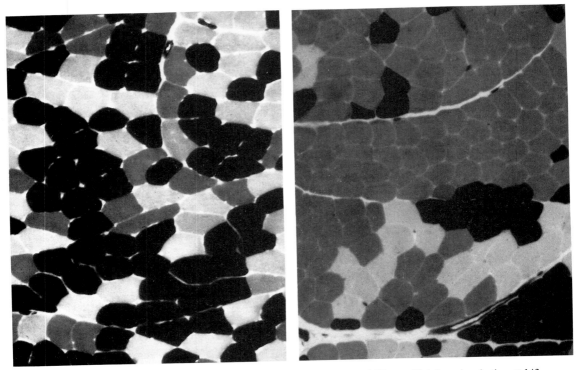

Fig. 3.11   Normal random spatial distribution of muscle fibre types; myofibrillar ATPase, pH 4.6 pre-incubation. ×142

Fig. 3.12   Uniform fibre type grouping due to re-innervation; myofibrillar ATPase, pH 4.6 pre-incubation. ×142

version without any physical remodelling of motor units. Quantitative methods such as the CDI or EFC techniques assess uniform fibre type grouping in the context of the particular fibre type constitution of the individual muscle under analysis. Physiological fibre type interconversion should not result in any departure from the normal random spatial distribution whereas remodelling of motor units will almost always have this effect.

Necrosis and regeneration

Necrosis

As in the case of other cell types, necrosis of muscle fibres may occur as a result of an acute injury of either intrinsic or extrinsic origin, leading to irreversible damage and death of the cell. The concept of cell death is more difficult to apply to the muscle fibre because of its multi-nucleated state and linear form. It is relatively

uncommon for the full length of a muscle fibre to undergo necrosis and, more often, the injury is confined to a segment of variable length in which the nuclei and cytoplasmic organelles are destroyed while the major portion of the fibre remains intact (*segmental necrosis*).

The factors which lead to such a segmental form of injury are poorly understood but, on the basis of observations upon dystrophic muscle (Mokri & Engel 1975), and after experimental micropuncture lesions (Karpati & Carpenter 1982), it seems likely that one cause of segmental necrosis might be a focal injury to the plasma membrane of the muscle fibre. A massive rise in intracellular calcium levels is thought to occur after such an injury and is thought to be the major factor responsible for triggering off the chain of events leading to irreversible metabolic and structural changes in the muscle fibre. It seems that the surviving portions of the muscle fibre must be able to synthesize new membranes to separate them from

Fig. 3.13

Fig. 3.14

Fig. 3.15

Fig. 3.16

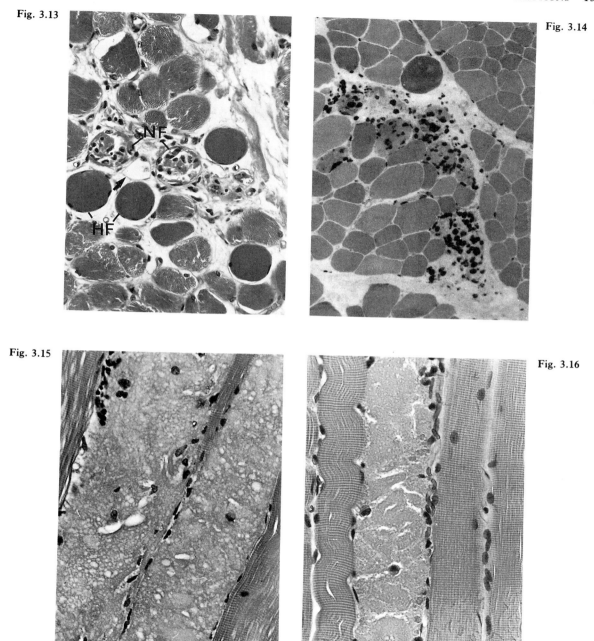

Fig. 3.13 Hyaline fibres (HF) and necrotic fibres (NF) undergoing phagocytosis in a case of Duchenne dystrophy. Note the empty sarcolemmal tube (arrow). Haematoxylin and eosin. ×210. (Reproduced by permission of the Medical Department, The British Council)

Fig. 3.14 Phagocytosis of muscle fibres in Becker muscular dystrophy; non-specific esterase. ×114

Fig. 3.15 Two necrotic fibres in a case of hypothyroid myopathy. H&E, ×270

Fig. 3.16 A necrotic fibre in a case of mitochondrial myopathy. H&E, ×270

the irreversibly damaged segment and to maintain osmotic homeostasis. The nature of the minimal injury which will lead to segmental necrosis is not clear but morphological observations indicate that lesser forms of injury do not necessarily lead to necrosis of the entire cross-sectional area of the muscle fibre. Thus, in certain circumstances, necrosis and phagocytosis may be confined to the central part of the fibre.

Necrosis may result from a variety of extrinsic insults to the muscle fibre, including trauma, ischaemia, extremes of temperature, and toxic agents including factors liberated by sensitized lymphoid cells; on the other hand it may result from genetically determined intrinsic derangements in the muscle fibre, as in the muscular dystrophies or hereditary defects of muscle metabolism. A fundamental distinction must be made between the *selective* muscle fibre necrosis which occurs in the muscular dystrophies and acquired metabolic, nutritional and inflammatory myopathies, in which the basal lamina of the muscle fibre (and the endomysium) remain intact and serve as a scaffolding for regeneration of the necrotic segment, and the *non-selective* type of damage which occurs after trauma, haemorrhage, ischaemia or certain forms of infection, in which the interstitial tissues are also damaged (*pan-necrosis*) and the continuity of the basal lamina and endomysium of individual muscle fibres may be lost. In the latter situation, effective regeneration of damaged muscle fibres is less likely to occur.

Morphological changes in necrotic fibres

The histological appearances in fibres which have been irreversibly injured are, in general, fairly stereotyped but vary to some extent according to the nature of the injury and to the method of tissue preparation and staining. The classical appearances of Zenker's hyaline degeneration and of waxy and granular degeneration were described in fixed paraffin-embedded tissues (Adams et al 1962). The light-microscopic changes form a continuum, the final stage of which is the complete removal of the contents of the muscle fibre by phagocytic cells (*myophagia*) (Figs 3.13, 3.14).

The earliest stage is that seen in so-called hyaline ('opaque', 'dark', 'hypercontracted', 'hyper-reactive') fibres (Fig. 3.13), which in histological sections are excessively rounded, increased in calibre and show loss of detail of individual myofibrils. They stain more darkly than the normal muscle fibres in sections stained with haematoxylin and eosin, trichrome, picro-Mallory, PTAH, PAS and for oxidative enzymes. These fibres are also typically 'calcium-positive' in sections stained for calcium by the GBHA, von Kossa or alizarin red methods. In longitudinal sections and with the electron microscope it is apparent that in hyaline fibres there is marked hypercontraction of the myofibrils leading to the formation of contraction clumps or knots in one portion of the fibre, and to tearing apart of the myofibrils in neighbouring segments of the fibre. The appearances of such fibres in transverse section therefore change at different levels. A section through a contraction clump will produce the appearance of a hyaline or opaque fibre, while a section taken further along the fibre from where the myofibrils have been displaced might show a complete absence of contractile elements (Fig. 3.13).

There has been some debate as to the significance which should be placed on the finding of hyaline fibres in histological specimens, as they may be produced artefactually even in normal muscle when the tissue is not handled with sufficient care at the time of removal, or if it is placed in certain fixatives containing alcohol or ammonia (Adams et al 1962). In spite of this, it is clear that hyaline fibres of this type may be found even in unfixed cryostat sections of carefully handled tissue, particularly in the Duchenne form of muscular dystrophy (Cullen & Fulthorpe 1975), suggesting that in such circumstances they represent a genuine pathological change occurring in vivo. This view is further supported by the finding of phagocytic cells in portions of the fibre adjoining hypercontracted segments in serial transverse sections of some hyaline fibres in Duchenne dystrophy (Nonaka & Sugita 1980).

The intermediate stages of breakdown of the muscle fibre may present various appearances under the light microscope. Characteristically, in unfixed cryostat sections stained with haematoxylin and eosin, the intensity of staining is reduced and histochemical techniques show an early loss of enzyme activity and glycogen. The contents of the fibre undergo progressive disorganization and fragmentation, which usually occurs in parallel with the appearance of mononuclear phagocytic cells within the necrotic segment. A number of different appearances may be recognized in sections of paraffin-embedded material (Figs 3.15–3.18). One which is seen most typically in Duchenne dystrophy consists of a breakdown of the contents of the fibre into hyaline waxy clumps. A second appearance, which is seen particularly with very acute toxic forms of muscle damage, consists of a marked fragmentation and dissolution of muscle fibres even in the apparent absence of significant numbers of mononuclear phagocytic cells. Another type of change, which we have noted particularly in certain metabolic myopathies and which has recently also been described in some patients with the immunodeficiency syndrome and myopathy (Panegyres et al 1990), consists of a finely granular or microvesicular appearance, the latter being due to dilatation of the sarcotubular systems. Whether these varied appearances represent different stages in the breakdown sequence of the muscle fibre, or whether they reflect differences in the nature of the injury to the fibre and the tempo of the necrobiotic process is not clear.

Patterns of muscle fibre necrosis

For practical purposes the following patterns of muscle fibre damage, which take account of both the spatial and temporal distribution of the muscle lesions, can be considered (Kakulas 1975).

Monophasic monofocal injuries. Focal injuries to the muscle as a result of external trauma, needle insertion or ischaemic infarction would come under this category.

Monophasic polyfocal. Multiple lesions throughout the skeletal musculature resulting from a single metabolic or toxic insult fall into this category. Situations in which this pattern of muscle damage occurs include acute forms of intoxication due to drugs or venoms (Figs 3.18–3.20) or metabolic derangements such as severe hypokalaemia.

The term *acute rhabdomyolysis* is sometimes used when there is extensive muscle fibre necrosis with myoglobinuria which may lead to acute renal failure. This may be caused by alcohol or a variety of drugs (Mastaglia & Argov 1981), snake venoms (Rowland et al 1969), viral infections (see Ch. 12), and certain inborn metabolic defects of muscle such as myophosphorylase deficiency, phosphofructokinase deficiency and carnitine palmityltransferase deficiency.

Polyphasic polyfocal. Into this category fall the chronic progressive human myopathies such as muscular dystrophy and polymyositis in which muscle fibre necrosis occurs randomly throughout the skeletal musculature over a prolonged period. As a result, necrotic and regenerating muscle fibre lesions of different ages are seen at different sites in a muscle and in different muscles (Figs 3.13, 3.21).

Regeneration

The ability of skeletal muscle to regenerate after injury is well established. Regeneration occurs as a sequel to necrosis and in a healthy muscle with an intact innervation and blood supply will lead to functional and structural reconstitution of the muscle provided that the injurious agent is no longer active. So active is the regenerative potential of skeletal muscle fibres that in amphibia and small mammals whole muscles may be reformed after excision and mincing into small fragments (Carlson 1970). The crucial factors in determining the effectiveness of regeneration are whether or not the scaffolding formed by the basal lamina of the muscle fibre and surrounding tissues remains intact, and whether or not the basic pathological process subsides. The most effective regeneration occurs when the basal lamina and endomysium remain intact; the new fibres will then be formed within the original *sarcolemmal tubes* and will therefore have an orderly orientation in parallel with the remaining fibres in the muscle (*isomorphic regeneration*). In contrast, after trauma, haemorrhage, or infection, the basal lamina and endomysium may also be disrupted and regeneration will be less orderly and less effective (*anisomorphic regeneration*) (Adams et al 1962). In such situations the continuity of damaged muscle fibres will not necessarily be restored and the newly formed fibres will often be surrounded by proliferating

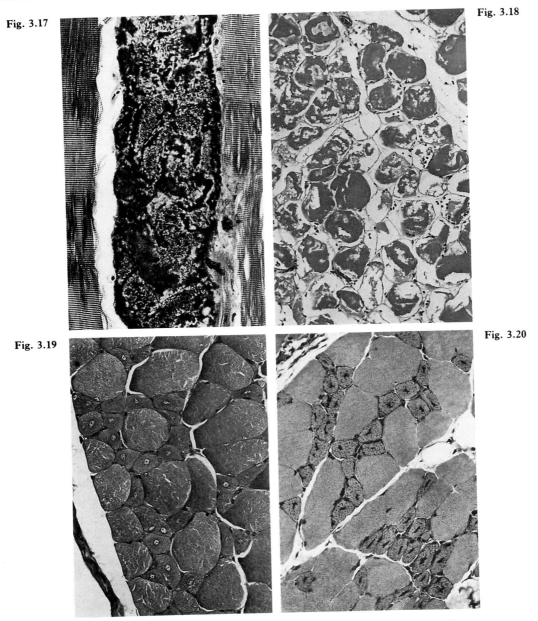

Fig. 3.17

Fig. 3.18

Fig. 3.19

Fig. 3.20

Fig. 3.17   A necrotic fibre in a case of hypothyroid myopathy. Phosphotungstic acid haematoxylin. ×270

Fig. 3.18   Acute rhabdomyolysis due to envenomation by the brown mulga snake, *Pseudechis australis*. H&E, ×140

Fig. 3.19   Regenerating myofibres at the late myotube stage with central vesicular nuclei in mouse muscle 7 days after exposure to *P. australis* venom. H&E, paraffin-embedded, ×270

Fig. 3.20   Regenerating myofibres at the late myotube stage with central vesicular nuclei in mouse muscle 7 days after exposure to *P. australis* venom. H&E. Cryostat section. ×270

fibroblasts and take on the appearance of so-called *muscle giant cells*. Such a proliferation of muscle cells and connective tissues after trauma to a muscle may give rise to a localized swelling or pseudotumour (see Chs 21 and 22).

The integrity of the basal lamina is also important for rapid regeneration because constituents of its synaptic portion are involved in organizing differentiation of the new neuromuscular junction (see Basal lamina, p 144).

Mechanisms of regeneration. Muscle fibres regenerate from mononucleated myogenic stem cells (*myoblasts*), which are themselves not affected by the original injury to the muscle fibre and which subsequently undergo mitotic division and fuse to form *myotubes* (Fig. 3.22). Whole new myofibres may be formed by the fusion of these myotubes or, if the necrosis is segmental, by the fusion of the myotubes with the viable stumps of the fibres. This has been termed *discontinuous regeneration* to distinguish it from so-called continuous regeneration where growth is thought to occur by elongation of the surviving segments by the recruitment of nuclei and cytoplasm from the stumps. Evidence for continuous regeneration has largely come from light-microscopic work on the regeneration of amphibian limbs (Hay 1971) and whether it is important in mammalian muscle is unclear, although some workers still favour it (Astrom & Adams 1988).

Source of myogenic cells. For a long time the site of origin of the new myoblasts was the source of considerable argument, but about 30 years ago, by use of the electron microscope, a population of cells was discovered that lay between the plasma membrane and basal lamina of the muscle fibre (Katz 1961; Mauro 1961). These were termed *satellite cells* (for review, see Campion 1984). A combination of electron-microscopic, tissue-culture (Bischoff 1979, Konigsberg et al 1975) and autoradiographic techniques (Snow 1977, 1978; Hsu et al 1979, Trupin & Hsu 1979) has now shown beyond doubt that the satellite cells (Figs 3.23, 3.24) are the major, and probably the only, source of new myoblasts in regenerating skeletal muscle. Interestingly, cardiac muscle, which does not possess satellite cells, is unable to regenerate.

Morphological characteristics. Regenerating muscle cells have a number of distinctive charac-teristics which enable them to be recognized with the light and the electron microscope (Figs 3.25–3.28). With the light microscope, the most distinctive features in sections stained with haematoxylin and eosin are the basophilia of the cytoplasm, which reflects the high content of ribonucleic acid, and the appearance of the nuclei which are large, with dispersed chromatin (so-called 'vesicular' nuclei), and have a prominent nucleolus. The high content of cytoplasmic RNA may also be demonstrated by other staining techniques, such as the cresyl violet and azure B methods, and is reflected in the finding of numerous ribosomes and polyribosomes in the cytoplasm with the electron microscope.

Myoblasts are thin, spindle-shaped mononu-cleated cells which characteristically lie on the inner aspect of the basal lamina of the degenerating muscle fibre. They are richly endowed with mitochondria and, as a consequence, the cytoplasm reacts intensely in histochemical preparations demonstrating activity of oxidative enzymes. The multinucleated myotubes are also seen peripher-ally in necrotic muscle fibres, closely applied to the basal lamina, and a number of these may line the inside of the sarcolemmal tubes. In the myotubes the myofibrils assume their normal longitudinal and transverse orientation in the peripheral portions of the myotube on either side of the central myonuclei. As a result, parallel cross-striations may be recognized with the light microscope in longitudinal sections. Other features seen with the electron microscope in regenerating muscle cells are the presence of longitudinally orientated microtubules and prominent Golgi apparatus.

While the early stages of regeneration occur within the confines of the original basal lamina, once the myotubes reach a certain stage of development they acquire a new basal lamina which is first seen in areas where the developing fibre is no longer in contact with the old basal lamina (Vracko & Benditt 1972). At later stages of maturation the myonuclei assume a peripheral position in the fibre, but still show chromatin dispersion and a prominent nucleolus, while myofibrils increase in numbers and are more tightly packed within the sarcoplasm, which retains an excessive degree of basophilia. This allows such

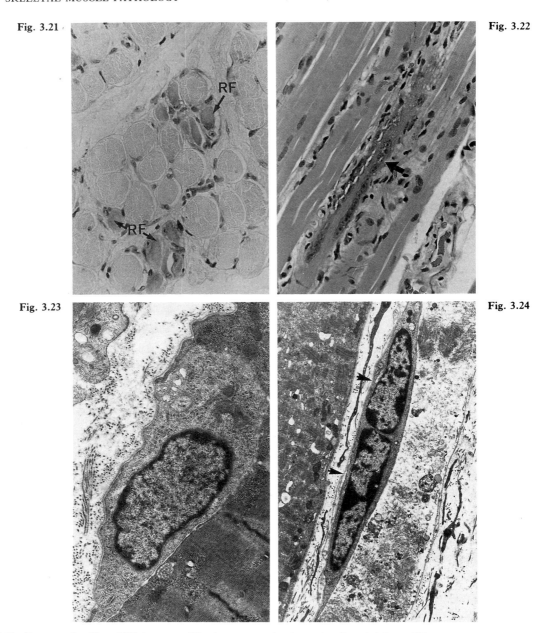

Fig. 3.21

Fig. 3.22

Fig. 3.23

Fig. 3.24

Fig. 3.21 Regenerating fibres (RF) in a case of Duchenne muscular dystrophy. Cresyl violet. ×270

Fig. 3.22 Regeneration in a case of alcoholic myopathy. Late myotube (arrow) with a chain of nuclei with prominent nucleoli. H&E ×270

Fig. 3.23 A satellite cell (Sat) lying outside the plasma membrane and inside the basal lamina (BL) in a case of Duchenne muscular dystrophy. Hc = honeycomb structure. ×10 700

Fig. 3.24 A binucleate cell lying beneath the basal lamina (arrows) of a necrotic fibre in a case of polymyositis. ×6700

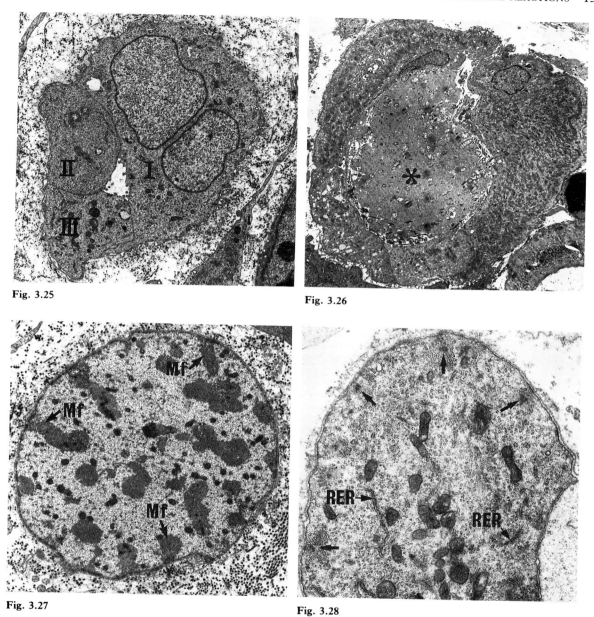

Fig. 3.25

Fig. 3.26

Fig. 3.27

Fig. 3.28

Fig. 3.25 Transverse section through a regenerating fibre in a case of dermatomyositis. The profile (I) containing two nuclei is a myotube. The other two profiles (II and III) are myoblasts or early myotubes. ×6665

Fig. 3.26 A regenerating fibre in a case of dermatoymyositis. Regeneration is at a later stage than in Figure 3.25 with considerable myofibril development, although a large portion of the necrotic parent fibre (asterisk) remains in the centre ×3395

Fig. 3.27 A regenerating fibre in a case of polymyositis with well-defined myofibrils (Mf) which are commonly associated with the plasma membrane. ×12 575

Fig. 3.28 Part of a regenerating fibre in mdx mouse muscle. The cytoplasm contains clusters of ribosomes, rough endoplasmic reticulum (RER) and nascent myofibrils (arrows) at the fibre periphery. ×9960

fibres to be recognized even when they have reached an advanced stage of maturation. With the electron microscope a double basal lamina may be seen and may allow the fibre to be identified as recently regenerated.

Regenerating fibres have a high content of oxidative enzymes such as succinate dehydrogenase and NADH tetrazolium reductase, but do not show phosphorylase activity until late in maturation. Although they have a high level of myofibrillar ATPase activity, there is no differentiation into distinct fibre types until the very late stages of maturation; until then, only fibres with type 2c characteristics (with both acid-stable and acid-labile ATPase activity) are seen (Reznik 1972; Snow 1973).

Autophagy

Autophagy, or self-digestion, is a normal physiological activity of living cells and is a mechanism for the turnover of cytoplasmic constituents, for disposing of redundant components and for using them as emergency sources of energy. The process becomes stimulated and is particularly important when the tissue is exposed to unfavourable conditions such as starvation, dietary deficiency or inhibition of protein synthesis. The presence of large numbers of autophagic vacuoles is a sign that the myofibre is stressed or diseased. When the stress is prolonged, autophagy may be followed by death and necrosis of the fibre.

At the cellular level, autophagy involves the envelopment and isolation of a portion of the cytoplasm by membranes derived probably from the smooth endoplasmic reticulum or Golgi apparatus. The resulting vacuole, with its contents, is then thought to fuse with another autophagic vacuole or with a primary lysosome which acts as a source of acid hydrolases necessary for the digestion of the contents. The contents of the vacuoles can be extremely heterogeneous. Mitochondria can frequently be identified because of their characteristic appearance but other membranous organelles, glycogen and lipid are also commonly seen. The sequestered material is hydrolysed to indigestible debris or to soluble intermediates such as small dipeptides or amino acids which can be re-used or released from the cell.

Autophagy has been widely studied in several types of cell, especially hepatocytes, neurones and epithelial cells (see Holtzman 1976 for review) and in experimental situations can be put on a firm quantitative basis with the estimation of autophagic vacuole half-lives (Mortimore & Schworer 1977, Pfeifer 1978). However, in the field of muscle pathology the study of autophagy, except in certain experimental situations, has not advanced beyond the descriptive stage, despite being a very common phenomenon. Autophagic vacuoles are seen in a wide variety of neuromuscular diseases where there is myofibre breakdown, whether it be myopathic or neurogenic in origin, including muscular dystrophy (Milhorat et al 1966, Santa 1969, Neville 1973), myotonic dystrophy (Schröder & Adams 1968), distal myopathy (Markesbery et al 1977, Nonaka et al 1985, Borg et al 1989), polymyositis (Shafiq et al 1967a, Mastaglia & Walton 1971a), nemaline myopathy (Nonaka et al 1989) and idiopathic inflammatory myopathy (Carpenter et al 1978). They have also been described in patients with intermittent claudication (Teräväinen & Makitie 1977) and in many toxic and metabolic myopathies (Rewcastle & Humphrey 1965; Howes et al 1966, Engel & Dale 1968, Engel 1973, Bardosi et al 1990). The two features which are characteristic and which are common to the autophagic vacuoles in all these conditions is that they are membrane-bound and the contents show evidence of breakdown or condensation. The contents are diverse. In the distal myopathy described by Markesbery et al (1977) the vacuole contents are vesicular and granular. In the autophagic vacuoles shown in Figure 3.29 from a case of polymyositis, and in those described by Teräväinen & Makitie (1977) there is both granular and membranous material.

Evidence of autophagy is perhaps most frequently seen when myofibre atrophy is known to be occurring, for example after experimental denervation (Schiaffino & Hanzlikova 1972, Cullen & Pluskal 1977). Figure 3.30 shows a small autophagic vacuole in a rat EDL muscle which has been denervated for 15 days. The vacuole contains some unidentifiable debris and a mitochondrion identifiable by the double membrane. A similar vacuole is seen in a rat soleus muscle (Fig. 3.31) in which atrophy occurred following administration of dexamethasone. Autophagic vacuoles are usually found towards the periphery of the muscle fibres

(Figs 3.29, 3.30). From here the contents are subsequently expelled to the extracellular space. Figure 3.29 shows the contents of several autophagic vacuoles in various stages of exocytosis. The surface topography of the fibres can become extremely convoluted at these areas of exocytosis (Terävainen & Makitie 1977, Cullen et al 1979). Autophagic debris is sometimes seen in expanded T-tubules and it is likely that in this situation exocytosis has ocurred into the tubule which acts as a gutter to the extracellular space (Kelly et al 1986, Engel & Banker 1986).

The source of the isolating membranes which delimit the autophagic vacuoles is not firmly established. In muscle there are three potential membrane contributors: the T system, the SR and the Golgi apparatus. A contribution by the Golgi apparatus towards the membranes of autophagic vacuoles has not generally been observed, although Engel (1970a) showed continuity between the Golgi membranes and the membranes of the autophagic vacuoles in type 2 glycogenosis. This is somewhat surprising because, although the Golgi apparatus has been observed to provide membranes

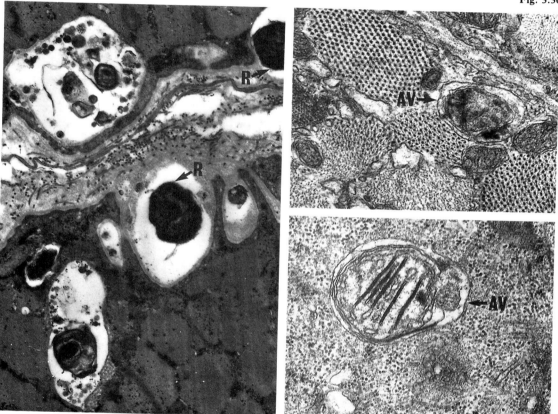

Fig. 3.29

Fig. 3.30

Fig. 3.31

Fig. 3.29 Residual bodies (R) being extruded at the periphery of two myofibres in a case of polymyositis. The outer 'vacuoles' are lined with a basal lamina indicating that they are continuous with the plasma membrane. ×16 725

Fig. 3.30 An autophagic vacuole (AV) in a rat extensor digitorum longus muscle. The vacuole contains a mitochondrion and other, unidentifiable, debris. ×37 725

Fig. 3.31 An autophagic vacuole (AV) in the soleus muscle of a dexamethasone-fed rat. The sequestered mitochondrion is breaking down. ×37 725

for autophagic vacuoles in other tissues (Fedorko & Cohn 1968), in mature muscle the Golgi apparatus is rare and confined to the perinuclear regions, and is therefore not ideally situated to participate in a generalized cellular reaction. The T system and SR do not have this logistic drawback because they both ramify thoughout the fibre and at no point are they more than 1 μm or so distant from any part of the muscle cell. Honeycomb structures which are derived from the T system (Schotland 1970) are sometimes seen in continuity with the membranes of the autophagic vacuoles (Fig. 3.47) (Engel 1970a, Markesbery et al 1977) and it has been shown that the exogenous electron-dense tracer horseradish peroxidase can diffuse into the vacuoles (MacDonald & Engel 1970). These two pieces of evidence indicate clearly that the contents of the autophagic vacuoles, in these cases at least, are circumscribed by the membranes of a dilated T system. However, it has not been established that the T tubule membranes actively surround and isolate the contents. It is quite possible that material is broken down in autophagic vacuoles separately from the T system and is subsequently extruded into the T system which serves as a route to the extracellular space.

There is also a certain amount of evidence for involvement of the SR in autophagic vacuole membrane formation. MacDonald & Engel (1970) observed SR tubules abutting against, and in some places apparently fusing with, the external membranes of small vacuoles. In these laboratories we have seen double membranes of the SR (identifiable by their continuity with the terminal cisternae of the triads) surrounding mitochondria and portions of the cytoplasm in both human biopsy material and experimental animal material (Cullen & Bindoff, unpublished observations). Christie & Stoward (1977), in a study of dystrophic hamster muscle, have shown how, theoretically, the membranes of the SR could form the membranes of the autophagic vacuoles. The SR is in some ways the most likely of the alternative membrane sources because not only is it the muscle equivalent of the smooth endoplasmic reticulum which has been most widely implicated in isolation membrane formation (Ericsson 1969), but there is also some histochemical and biochemical evidence that the SR is the source of lysosomal enzymes in

muscle (Christie & Stoward 1977, Bird et al 1980, Decker et al 1980). The possibility of the SR being involved in autophagic vacuole formation is not excluded by the evidence that the T system is involved in certain conditions if, as discussed above, the debris is discharged into the transverse tubules after digestion in the autophagic vacuoles.

It is still not clear which parts of the muscle cell are digested in autophagic vacuoles and, in particular, whether myofibrillar material can be broken down or turned over in this way. To our knowledge there is no good morphological evidence of whole myofilaments being sequestered into autophagic vacuoles, but this does not rule out the possibility that disassociated contractile protein molecules (not resolvable in conventional electron microscopy of sectioned material) might be broken down in cytoplasm. As the myofibrils represent about 80% of the mass of a muscle, the problem of how they are degraded remains an important question to be resolved.

Vacuolar degeneration

Vacuolation of muscle fibres is one of the common histological changes encountered in biopsy and necropsy material (Figs 3.32, 3.33, 3.34, 3.35). It is useful for practical purposes to subdivide vacuolar change into the categories outlined below.

Dilatation of the sarcotubular system

The marked vacuolation of muscle fibres which occurs in the familial forms of hypo- and hyperkalaemic periodic paralysis results principally from dilatation of the terminal cisternae of the sarcoplasmic reticulum (Fig. 3.32). Dilatation of the SR and T system also occurs in acquired forms of hypokalaemia which, when of sufficient severity, may lead to a vacuolar myopathy. The vacuoles in these situations are usually empty, being fluid-cotaining during life, but may at times contain PAS-positive material in hypokalaemic periodic paralysis (Engel 1966b).

Autophagic vacuolation

The vacuoles seen with the light microscope represent membrane-bound areas of autodigestion

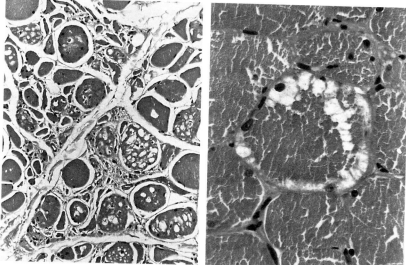

Fig. 3.32

Fig. 3.33

Fig. 3.32 Vacuolar degeneration in a case of hypokalaemic periodic paralysis. There is extensive vacuolation of the myofibres. H&E, ×440

Fig. 3.33 A vacuolated myofibre in a patient with a progressive limb-girdle syndrome. H&E, ×450

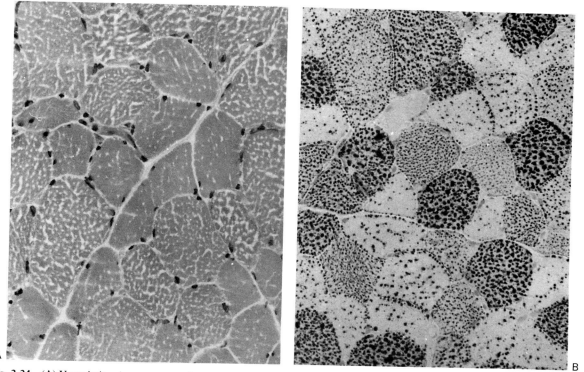

A

B

Fig. 3.34 (A) Vacuolation due to storage of neutral lipid. H&E, ×238. (B) Neutral lipid storage in the same patient as in (A). Oil Red O. ×238

of the muscle fibre (see Autophagy, above). Autophagic vacuoles are to be distinguished from the 'rimmed vacuoles' which are not bounded by membranes and are seen characteristically in oculopharyngeal dystrophy and inclusion body myositis (Dubowitz & Brooke 1973).

Storage vacuoles

Excessive accumulation of neutral lipid or glycogen gives rise to characteristic patterns of vacuolation of muscle fibres so that the nature of the storage substance can often be deduced in advance of histochemical confirmation. Moderate degrees of neutral lipid storage give rise to small, spherical vacuoles (Fig. 3.34) which are evenly distributed throughout the fibre. Type 1 fibres are often more severely affected than type 2 fibres. Unless lipid storage is severe, the size of individual vacuoles rarely exceeds 1–2 μm, their uniform size and shape distinguishing them from the much larger size and uneven profile of glycogen storage vacuoles.

In infantile Pompe's disease (acid maltase deficiency) severe glycogenosis may render the cytoarchitecture of individual fibres virtually unrecognizable because of extensive vacuolation. In glycogenoses of late onset, storage of glycogen may result in the formation of irregular clefts between myofibrils and in subsarcolemmal accumulation. This pattern of storage is characteristic of glycogenosis due to defects of cytosolic enzymes such as myophosphorylase. In contrast the glycogen storage in acid maltase deficiency is intralysosomal, and in late-onset forms of the disorder, individual membrane-bound vacuoles may measure 10–20 μm in diameter (Fig. 3.35).

REACTIONS OF MUSCLE FIBRE COMPONENTS

Basal lamina

The basal lamina (BL) (lamina densa) forms the external, 30–50 nm, coating of the muscle fibre. A thin electron-lucent layer (lamina lucida) be-

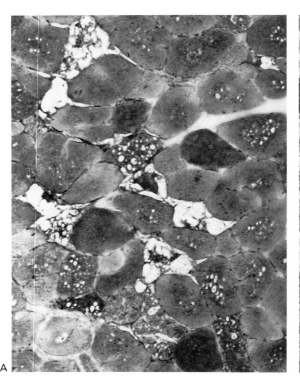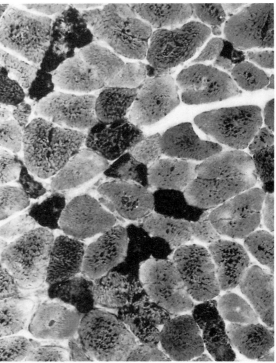

Fig. 3.35 (A) Vacuolation due to glycogen storage in late-onset glycogenosis type 2. Periodic acid-Schiff. ×133. (B) Serial section to (A) in which glycogen has been retained by celloidinization. Periodic acid–Schiff. ×133

tween the BL and plasma membrane has also been described, although there is evidence that this might be a fixation artefact (Goldberg 1986). On the outside of the BL is a thin coating of collagen fibrils (lamina reticularis) which is very sparsely developed in healthy muscle. The composite of all three layers is sometimes termed the basement membrane. The basement membrane, together with the plasma membrane, constitutes the sarcolemma, first described by Bowman (1840).

The BL is secreted by the cells it surrounds. Although the precise composition can vary from place to place in the same lamina, all basal laminae contain type IV collagen along with proteoglycans (mainly heparin sulphates) and the glycoproteins laminin and entactin. The detailed molecular organization of the BL is still uncertain. The proteoglycan molecules appear to lie on either side of the type IV collagen. The laminin is thought to be located mainly on the plasma membrane side of the BL while fibronectin helps to bind the matrix molecules and cells or myofibres on the opposite side.

As well as serving a structural role, basal laminae can, depending on their situation, determine cell polarity, influence cell metabolism, organize the proteins in adjacent plasma membranes, induce cell differentiation and serve as specific routes for cell migration (see below). In contrast to the plasma membrane, the BL seems resistant to many noxious agents which bring about injury or death of a muscle fibre. Thus, in necrotic fibres, when the plasma membrane is invariably lost or damaged, the basal lamina usually remains as a so-called *sarcolemmal tube* (Allbrook 1962, Price et al 1964) (Fig. 3.36). The tube can however be penetrated by phagocytes involved in removing the myofibre debris (Fig. 3.37). Any subsequent regeneration of the necrotic fibre appears to take place within the sarcolemmal tube, the basal lamina being likened to scaffolding in the subsequent rebuilding of the fibre (Schochet & Lampert 1978).

The sheath of BL that surrounds the muscle fibre extends through the synaptic cleft at the neuromuscular junction. Constituents of the synaptic portion of the BL are involved in organizing differentiation when neuromuscular junctions regenerate following damage to adult muscle. This was shown by removing the cellular components of the neuromuscular junction in ways that spared the BL, and then allowing either axons or myofibres to regenerate. When axons regenerated, they made nearly all of their contacts with BL sheaths at the original synaptic sites and differentiated into nerve terminals (Sanes et al 1978, Glicksman & Sanes 1983). Thus, components of the BL are able to guide re-innervation of original synaptic sites and organize the differentiation of axons into nerve terminals at those sites. Conversely, when myotubes regenerated within BL sheaths in the absence of axons or Schwann cells, they accumulated acetylcholine receptors, and formed junctional folds in precise apposition to the original synaptic sites on the BL (Burden et al 1979, Slater & Allen 1985). Thus BL can trigger postsynaptic as well as presynaptic differentiation during regeneration.

In an attempt to identify the specific triggering components of the BL, Hunter et al (1989) generated antibodies that selectively stained synaptic sites on the BL. They identified one synaptic antigen, involved in the formation and stabilization of synapses, as a homologue of laminin. Because its distribution is restricted to the synapses they have termed this protein s-laminin.

Several groups have similarly searched for BL components that might account for its postsynaptic organizing abilities. McMahan and his colleagues showed that material extracted from *Torpedo* electric organs could induce clustering of acetylcholine receptors on cultured chick myotubes. This protein has been termed agrin (Nitkin et al 1987). McMahan and his colleagues have proposed that agrin-like molecules in the synaptic BL induce receptor clustering during muscle regeneration and perhaps also during embryonic synaptogenesis.

In pathological muscle the most common change seen in the basal lamina is the formation of the extensive folds, skeins and tubes already described. Another non-specific change is thickening of the basal lamina from its normal 30–50 nm up to 500 nm, for example in dystrophia myotonica (Mair & Tomé 1972), rheumatoid arthritis (Wroblewski & Nordemar 1975) and intermittent claudication (Teräväinen & Makitie 1977). Duance et al (1980) have demonstrated far more

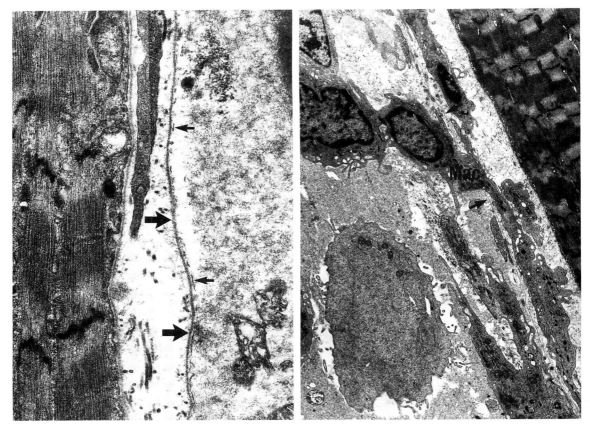

Fig. 3.36 Part of two myofibres in a case of polymyositis. The right-hand fibre is necrotic and has a fragmented plasma membrane (small arrow). The basal lamina (large arrow) remains. ×16 725

Fig. 3.37 Part of a necrotic fibre in a case of polymyositis. Note the elongated macrophage (Mac) passing through the basal lamina (arrows). ×4652

intense fluorescent antibody labelling for basal lamina types IV and V collagen around the smaller muscle fibres in Duchenne muscular dystrophy when compared with controls, and they have speculated about whether this reflects a thickening of the basal lamina or a more extensive infolding of the basal lamina coincident with myofibrillar loss. The cause, the mechanism and the effect of basal lamina thickening in diseased muscle is not known.

The plasma membrane

The involvement of the plasma membrane in several vital functions of the muscle cell (ionic regulation, transmitter reception, action potential propagation, endocytosis and exocytosis) underlines its great importance to the well-being of the cell. Despite this, our understanding of the plasma membrane in diseased muscle is limited in comparison with that of other muscle constituents largely because of the technical difficulties involved in isolating and purifying it.

Like other cell membranes, the muscle plasma membrane consists of a proteolipid bilayer comprised of neutral lipid, phospholipids, and cholesterol esters and cholesterol. Apart from the proteins which contribute to its intrinsic structure the plasma membrane also contains a number of proteins serving a range of specialized functions these include the acetylcholine receptor and other receptor molecules, transport channels for a range of ionic species, ATPases associated with metabolically driven ionic pumps, and transport proteins for glucose and amino acids.

In the healthy myofibre the plasma membrane is a complex structure with ramifications to the fibre interior (the transverse tubular system) and connections with the myofibrils. The plasma membrane is attached to the underlying myofibrils at the Z line by intermediate filaments of desmin which also link adjacent myofibrils at the Z line and appear to function in the mechanical integration of the fibre components during the contraction–relaxation cycle (Lazarides & Hubbard 1978, Lazarides 1980). It is this attachment that causes the plasma membrane to be thrown into prominent folds during strong contractions.

Internal to the plasma membrane are numerous small vesicles, approximately 80–100 nm in diameter, termed caveolae (Fig. 3.38A). The caveolae are continuous with the plasma membrane and open to the extracellular space, as revealed by experiments using electron-dense tracers (Franzini-Armstrong 1973). The function of the caveolae is as yet unknown. Their position and size suggest that they may be analogous to pinocytotic vesicles (for example of endothelial cells, Fig. 3.38A) but there is no evidence of pinocytosis being a widespread phenomenon in healthy mature muscle, in contrast to pathological muscle (see below). Their greater concentration opposite the I band (Fig. 3.38A) suggests that they may act as membrane sinks taking up the 'slack' when the

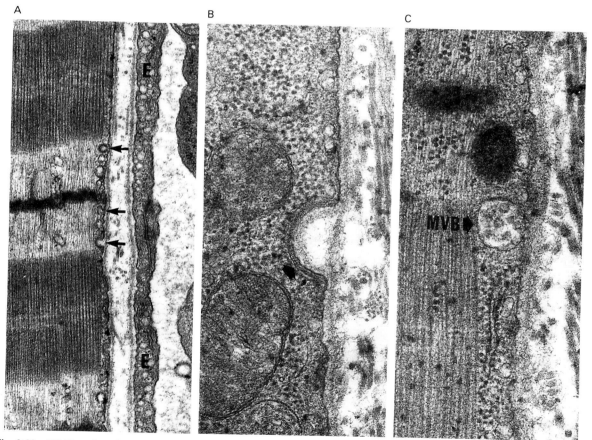

Fig. 3.38 (A) The edge of a normal myofibre showing caveolae (arrows) contiguous with the plasma membrane and grouped mostly opposite the I band. Note the similarity in size of the caveolae and the pinocytotic vesicles in the endothelial cells (E). ×27 665. (B) A coated vesicle opening to the surface of a muscle fibre from a patient with spinal muscular atrophy. Note the lattice-like coat (arrowed) on the cytoplasmic side of the membrane. ×50 300. (C) A multivescicular body (MVB) situated at the periphery of a muscle fibre from the same patient from whom (B) was taken. ×50 300

sarcomeres shorten. However in a study using frog muscle, Dulhunty & Franzini-Armstrong (1975) have shown that at sarcomere lengths less than 3.0 μm (i.e. at most physiological lengths) 'excess' membrane is taken up as folds in the plasma membrane. At the non-physiological length of about 8 μm all the caveolae are open and the fibres rupture with further stretch.

It is likely that some of the caveolae are an integral part of the T system as the T tubules often open to the outside through them, and the tubules develop from caveolae-like vesicles in embryonic muscle (Ezerman & Ishikawa 1967). The caveolae may also have a metabolic role in increasing the effective surface of the fibre (by 70% in frog sartorius; Dulhunty & Franzini-Armstrong 1975).

The coated pit is another class of plasma membrane-linked vesicle occasionally seen in mature muscle but more conspicuous in immature and diseased muscle (Fig. 3.38B). They are characterized by the lattice-like coat on the cytoplasmic side of the membrane. It has been shown that certain membrane proteins are excluded from coated pits and that they thus serve as molecular filters pinching off lipid vesicles containing a limited number of specific proteins into the cell (Bretscher et al 1980). They are thought to act as intracellular carriers sorting and transporting lipids and proteins between their site of synthesis (the rough endoplasmic reticulum), the Golgi apparatus and the plasma membrane (Rothman & Fine 1980).

The involvement of the plasma membrane in membrane turnover and renewal also explains the frequent observation, in pathological muscle, of lysosomes situated immediately adjacent to it. When lysosome contents are exocytosed, the lysosomal membrane becomes incorporated into the cell membrane. Figure 3.38C shows a multivesicular body (a class of lysosome involved in membrane turnover) at the edge of a fibre from a patient with spinal muscular atrophy.

Investigations of the role of the plasma membrane in muscle disease have been largely biochemical, electrophysiological or electronmicroscopical. Because of the limitations of resolution in sectioned material, it is not possible to detect subtle changes in the plasma membrane in diseased muscle by conventional transmission electron microscopy of ultrathin sections. Loss, fenestration or vesiculation of the membrane can be seen (Fig. 3.36), but changes in the component phospholipid and protein configurations cannot be picked out. Since the first edition of this book was written, however, considerable advances have been made in the technique of freeze–fracture which allows an en face view of the internal organization of the membrane. Three main features of the membrane have been examined in normal and dystrophic tissue: intramembranous particles (IMPs), orthogonal arrays and caveolae (Yoshioka & Okuda 1977, Schotland et al 1981, Bonilla et al 1982, Wakayama et al 1984, 1989). The only feature about which there seems to be agreement between different laboratories is that there is a significant diminution of orthogonal arrays in DMD, from a median of about $13.2/\mu m^2$ in the controls, to almost none. Wakayama et al (1989) have also counted orthogonal arrays in early stage amyotrophic lateral sclerosis where they found a similar range to controls, and in the *mdx* mouse where the reduction was not as severe as in DMD. Thus the extent of loss of orthogonal arrays does not seem to parallel the loss of dystrophin (see below).

The membrane theory of dystrophy

Perhaps the most widely acknowledged hypothesis concerning the aetiology of Duchenne muscular dystrophy is the membrane theory, which states simply that the basic genetic defect lies in one of the components of the plasma membrane. The membrane theory was initially proposed following the discovery of increased aldolase activity in the serum of boys with Duchenne muscular dystrophy (Dreyfus et al 1954, Zierler 1958). This finding, together with subsequent findings of raised serum levels of creatine kinase and other muscle enzymes, remained until recently one of the strongest sources of evidence for a membrane lesion. It is generally assumed that the enzymes escape from necrotic fibres, that is, those that are already breaking down, so it is surprising that their release into the serum must be selective as other enzymes more abundant in muscle than, for example, creatine kinase (including some such as adenylate kinase of much smaller molecular weight) are not detected in the serum. If the enzymes are emanating from already necrotic fibres, the case for a primary membrane lesion is weakened, because the lesion could easily be the secondary result of necrosis initiated at other locations. However, if it could be shown that the enzymes were leaking through the plasma membrane of living non-necrotic fibres, the argument for a membrane lesion would be far stronger. This task is made more difficult by the fact that fibre necrosis in Duchenne muscular dystrophy can be segmental, with a structurally normal area of a fibre immediately adjacent to a necrotic zone (see for example Fig. 1 in Cullen & Mastaglia 1980).

Evidence of a different kind for a membrane lesion came from the ultrastructural observation of a localized loss of membrane which has been described and clearly illustrated by several workers (Mokri & Engel 1975, Schmalbruch 1975; Carpenter & Karpati 1979; Cullen & Mastaglia 1980). What was surprising was that the loss of plasma membrane was sometimes observed in areas in which the myofibrillar structure was normal (Carpenter & Karpati 1979; Cullen & Mastaglia 1980), when one might have expected the (presumed) entry of extracellular ions to bring about contraction or disassembly of the myofibrils. These unusual observations could not, however, be taken as firm evidence that a membrane lesion is the primary event, because the loss could have been caused by events in the fibre at some distance from the area sectioned and where necrotic changes had already begun.

The membrane theory has been frequently linked with a picture of 'calcium damage' (Wrogeman & Pena 1976, Oberc & Engel 1977, Bodensteiner & Engel 1978, Duncan 1978). Cullen & Fulthorpe (1975) pointed out, on purely morphological grounds, that an increased sarcoplasmic calcium ion level might explain some of the morphological changes seen in dystrophic muscle. At the time we thought it might be linked with the reported defective calcium accumulation by the sarcoplasmic reticulum in dystrophic muscle, for which there was good evidence (Takagi et al 1973, Peter & Worsfold 1969, Samaha & Gergely 1969, Wood et al 1978). This possibility has been generally overtaken by the alternative of a calcium leakage via a plasma membrane lesion down the calcium concentration gradient. There is little doubt that the morphological changes seen in the myofibrils in dystrophic muscle could be caused by a raised free calcium ion level, and there is likewise little doubt that loss of the plasma membrane, as often observed, would facilitate an increased calcium level, but there is still no incontrovertible evidence that calcium entry is part of the primary sequence of events in fibre breakdown. Similarly the question of whether the membrane lesion is a primary or secondary event has been the main uncertainty in the membrane theory.

Dystrophin and the membrane theory

After approximately a decade in which no great advances were made in understanding the molecular background to the membrane hypothesis, the last few years have seen a great resurgence of interest following the identification of the protein which is quantitatively severely reduced or qualitatively altered in Duchenne (DMD) and Becker muscular dystrophy (BMD). This protein has been termed dystrophin (Hoffman et al 1987a).

This rapid step forward has been made possible by the application of 'reverse genetics' to the study of the Xp21 dystrophies. This approach takes advantage of modern advances in genetic techniques that allow the responsible gene to be mapped to a particular part of the chromosome, and then cloned and analysed without any prior knowledge of its identify or function. Koenig et al (1987) were the first to succeed in isolating a series of cDNA clones corresponding to the entire 14 kb DMD gene transcript. The interested reader is referred to several reviews which describe the cloning of the DMD gene (Brown and Hoffman 1988, Worton & Burghes 1988, Ray 1988, Hoffman & Kunkel 1989). The DMD gene is now believed to consist of 65 exons distributed over approximately 2500 kb of the human X chromosome, by far the largest genetic locus characterized to date. Knowing the complete cDNA sequence (Koenig et al 1988) it was possible to predict the amino acid sequence of the protein product (dystrophin) of the gene.

Perhaps the greatest significance of this to the

muscle pathologist is that knowledge of the cDNA and amino acid sequence data has allowed the generation of antibodies directed against fusion proteins and synthetic peptides, corresponding to discrete regions of the dystrophin molecule. The antibodies can in turn be used at both light and electron microscopic levels to examine the subcellular localization and tissue distribution of dystrophin.

The first localization reports suggested that dystrophin was primarily situated at the triad and in particular at the junctional T tubule membrane (Hoffman et al 1987b, Knudson et al 1988). However, subsequent immunocytochemical studies showed that the protein is most abundant at the outer edge of the muscle fibres (Arahata et al 1988, Zubrzycka-Gaarn et al 1988, Bonilla et al 1988, Nicholson et al 1989, 1990).

Figure 3.39 shows immunoperoxidase labelling of dystrophin in normal human quadriceps muscle. The labelling is clearly concentrated at the peri-

phery of the fibre. In the muscle of patients with DMD, dystrophin may be completely absent or may be expressed in only a few fibres (often less than 0.1% of the total fibre population) (Fig. 3.40). In BMD patients, the majority of muscle fibres show immunolabelling for dystrophin, though considerable inter- and intra-fibre variation in labelling intensity is a hallmark of the BMD phenotype (Fig. 3.41). An 'outlier' group of patients of mild DMD/severe BMD phenotype show characteristically very weak or absent labelling for dystrophin in all muscle fibres (Nicholson et al 1990). The muscle of manifesting DMD carriers (Fig. 3.42) consists typically of a mosaic of dystrophin-positive and dystrophin-negative fibres due to random X-inactivation (Lyonization) (Arahata et al 1989).

The first ultrastructural localization was carried out on mouse muscle using a polyclonal antibody raised against a fusion protein which contained a 30 kDa peptide sequence from the rod domain of

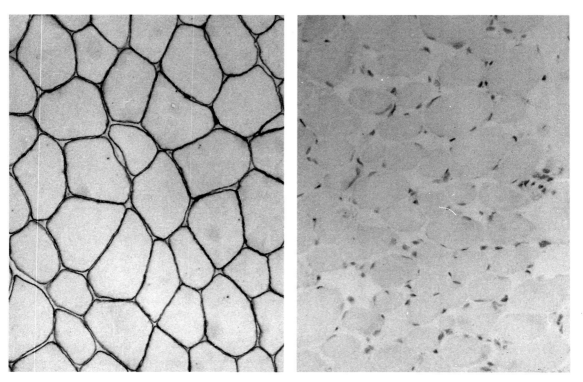

Fig. 3.39 Dystrophin immunolabelling in normal human skeletal muscle. Indirect peroxidase. ×237

Fig. 3.40 Absence of immunolabelling for dystrophin in Duchenne muscular dystrophy. Indirect peroxidase. ×237

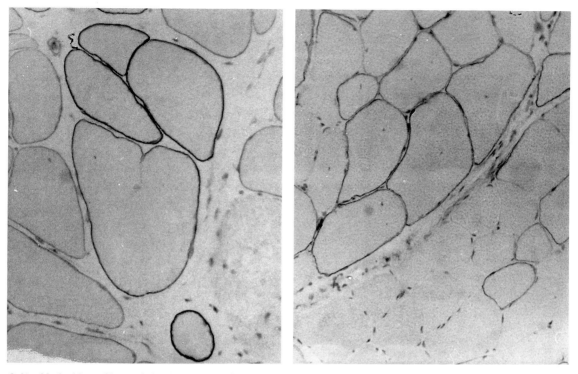

Fig. 3.41   Marked inter-fibre variation in intensity of dystrophin immunolabelling in Becker muscular dystrophy. Indirect peroxidase. ×238

Fig. 3.42   Mosaic of dystrophin-positive and dystrophin-negative fibres in manifesting carrier of Duchenne muscular dystrophy. Indirect peroxidase. ×238

dystrophin (Watkins et al 1988). These authors reported a concentration of label in a zone immediately internal to the plasma membrane and also suggested that there was some labelling of the T-system. In our own laboratories we have carried out a similar study but on human muscle and using a monoclonal antibody (Dy4/6D3) raised against the same fusion protein (Cullen et al 1990). As in the mouse the label was most concentrated immediately internal to the plasma membrane of the muscle fibres (Fig. 3.43). We found very little, however, associated with the tubules of the T-system. Careful measurement of the position of the labelling sites showed that they were most concentrated approximately 15 nm internal to the cytoplasmic face of the plasma membrane. Measurement of the sideways spacing of the labelling sites in a plane parallel to the plane of the plasma membrane showed the commonest nearest neighbour distance to be about 120 nm, close to

the estimated length of the rod domain of 125 nm (Koenig et al 1988). The same spacing was found in both longitudinal and transverse sections of the muscles implying that dystrophin forms an interconnecting lattice that does not have a strong axial component (longitudinal or transverse) in its organization.

We have recently repeated the above study using a polyclonal antibody raised against the last 17 amino acids of the C-terminus of the dystrophin molecule (kindly donated by the late Dr E. Zubrzycka-Gaarn, University of Toronto). The nearest neighbour distance was very similar to that found for Dy4/6D3 but the position of the label relative to the membrane was altered, with the main concentration of label lying over the membrane itself (Fig. 3.44). This implies that the C-terminus of dystrophin is inserted in the plasma membrane. This finding has to be considered preliminary and has yet to be confirmed. Work is

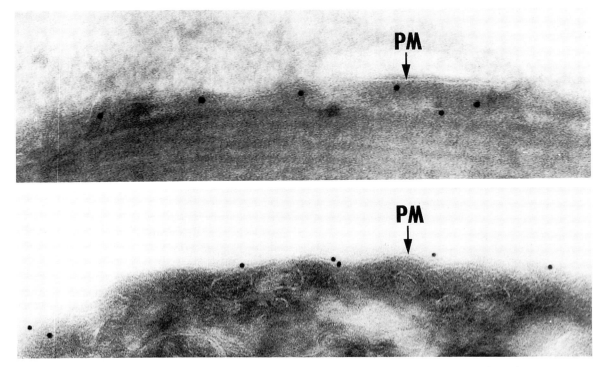

Fig. 3.43 An example of 10 nm gold immunolabelling using a monoclonal antibody (Dy4/6D3) raised against a fusion protein containing a 30 kDa protein sequence from the rod domain of dystrophin. The labelling sites are mostly immediately internal to the plasma membrane (PM). ×175 000

Fig. 3.44 Gold immunolabelling of human muscle using a polyclonal antibody (P1460) raised against the last 17 amino acids of the C-terminus of the dystrophin molecule PM = plasma membrane. ×160 000

advancing rapidly in this field and subsequent studies should allow a complete picture of how dystrophin is arranged on the membrane to be visualized in the near future.

The various studies which have shown that dystrophin is associated with the plasma membrane and moreover that it is severely reduced quantitatively and/or qualitatively in DMD (and to a variable extent in BMD) together suggest that it is important in the normal functioning of the membrane. In fact the membrane theory can be updated to one in which the initial lesion (in DMD and BMD) is consequent upon a quantitative or qualitative alteration in the normal complement of dystrophin. However, until we understand what the normal role of dystrophin is, this more specific restatement hardly advances our understanding of the disease at the cellular level.

Suggestions for the normal function of dystro-

phin have largely fallen into one of two categories: either that it is part of a link between the cytoskeleton and plasma membrane providing elasticity to the membrane during normal contractile activity, or that it provides a structural framework for the position of ion channels, receptors or other integral proteins in the plasma membrane. However, good evidence for any one role is unfortunately still lacking.

Any role which is identified has to take into account the fact that the muscles of the *mdx* mouse (which lack dystrophin) can perform normally. It has been suggested that in the mouse, a related protein, yet unidentified, can substitute for dystrophin (Worton & Gillard 1990). It must also be recognized that, even in DMD, many muscle fibres appear to function normally at least temporarily in the absence or near absence of dystrophin. This could imply that there might be a secondary factor which interacts with the lack of dystrophin to make its absence critical to the physiological integrity of the plasma membrane. Possible candidates for this secondary factor may lie within the muscle fibre or outside it, that is, intrinsic muscle proteins or perhaps components of fibrous connective tissue. A significant difference between DMD and the *mdx* myopathy is the presence of severe fibrous connective tissue increase in the former but not the latter (Carnwath & Shotton 1987, Cullen & Jaros 1988). In DMD the interface between the muscle fibre and connective tissue can be so close that pseudomyotendinous junctions can form (Schmalbruch 1984, Watkins & Cullen 1985) and the gross increase in fibrous connective tissue in this condition may be an important factor influencing the capacity of the muscle fibre population to cope with dystrophin absence or decrease.

In summary, the identification of dystrophin and the finding that it is very closely associated with the plasma membrane, has provided a molecular basis for the membrane hypothesis of DMD. However, until more is learnt about the exact role of dystrophin in the muscle cell we are still some way from an accurate understanding of the aetiology of the disease.

The membrane systems

T system

In human muscle the transverse tubular system or T system can usually be distinguished from the sarcoplasmic reticulum (SR), with which it closely associates at the triads, by its less electron-dense contents (Figs. 3.8, 3.45, 3.46). In healthy muscle the lumina of the T tubules, which are continuous with the extracellular space, are in fact empty. In diseased muscle they are sometimes dilated and contain debris which has been exocytosed or extruded from inside the fibre (Fig. 3.29).

Two types of changes to the T system are very common in pathological muscle; changes in orientation and structure at the triad, and proliferation to form honeycomb or labyrinthine structures. In healthy muscle the triads run transversely across the fibres at the A-I band juntion, two per sarcomere length, but in diseased muscle the tubules

often become twisted so that the triads run longitudinally between the myofibrils (Fig. 3.8). This is particularly common in conditions producing denervation and atrophy of the fibres. At the same time there is often duplication of the tubules and the adherent SR cisternae, so that more complex multiple associations of T system and SR build up (Figs 3.8, 3.45).

Honeycomb structures were first described, in denervated rat muscle, by Pellegrino & Franzini (1963). They take the form of more-or-less regular three-dimensional interconnecting arrays of tubules which vary in size from <1.0 μm in diameter (Figs 3.23, 3.46) up to 10 μm or larger (Fig. 3.47). Honeycomb structures are often connected to vacuoles of the T system, and their intercommunication with the T tubules has been demonstrated by tracer experiments (Schotland 1970). They have been described in many conditions, including neurogenic atrophy (Shafiq et al 1967b), myotonic dystrophy (Schroder & Adams 1968, Schotland 1970), muscular dystrophy (Fardeau 1970), polymyositis (Chou 1969, Mastaglia & Walton 1971a), periodic paralysis (MacDonald et al 1968, Engel 1970b), acid maltase deficiency (Engel & Dale 1968), reducing-body myopathy (Neville 1973), hypothyroidism (Afifi et al 1974), rhabdomyoma (Cornog & Gonatas 1967), trichinosis (Ribas-Mujal & Rivera-Pomar 1968), chloroquine myopathy (Fardeau 1970), myoglobinuria (Schutta et al 1969), Cushing's syndrome (Jerusalem 1970), alcoholic neuropathy (Tomé & Mair 1970), distal myopathy (Markesbery et al 1977) and perhexiline maleate-induced polyneuropathy (Fardeau et al 1979). They have also been observed in experimental myopathies (MacDonald & Engel 1970, Reznik 1973) and in cultured muscle (Ishikawa 1968) and are also often seen in regenerating fibres. Their significance is unknown.

Sarcoplasmic reticulum

As with the T system, the main morphological changes seen in the sarcoplasmic reticulum (SR) in diseased muscle are dilatation and proliferation. Dilatation of the SR has been described in Duchenne muscular dystrophy (Fig. 3.48) (Cullen & Fulthorpe 1975, Oberc & Engel 1977) and appears to be consistently one of the earliest

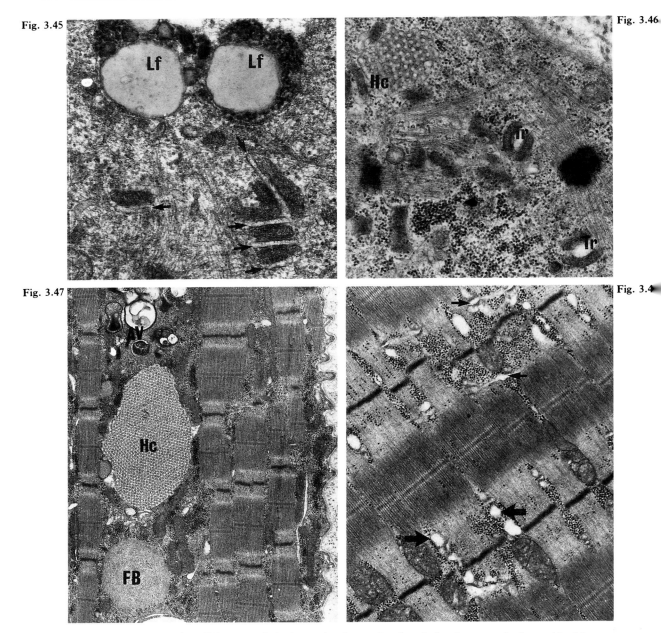

Fig. 3.45   A complex association of T system tubules (arrows) and sarcoplasmic reticulum in a case of polymyositis. Lf = lipofuscin granules. ×40 360

Fig. 3.46   Part of an atrophic myofibre in a case of Werdnig-Hoffmann disease showing a honeycomb structure (Hc) and prominent triads (Tr). Z = Z lines. ×32 360

Fig. 3.47   Part of a muscle fibre in a case of polymyositis containing a large honeycomb structure (Hc), a filamentous body (FB) and autophagic vacuoles (AV). ×9332

Fig. 3.48   Dilated sarcoplasmic reticulum (large arrows) in a case of Duchenne muscular dystrophy. There is also some localized dilation of the T system (small arrow) but the rest of the muscle ultrastructure appears normal. ×14 968

changes seen in this disease. Dilatation of the SR has also been reported in cases of chronic alcoholism (Rubin et al 1976), distal myopathy (Markesbery et al 1977), myopathy with hyperaldosteronism (Gallai 1977), myotonic dystrophy (Casanova & Jerusalem 1979), perhexiline maleate-induced polyneuropathy (Fardeau et al 1979), and in a myopathy due to triosephosphate deficiency (Bardosi et al 1990). When muscle fibres are experimentally overloaded with calcium by incubation with an anticholinesterase there is marked dilatation of the SR (Leonard & Salpeter 1979), and Somlyo and her colleagues (1981) have shown directly, by X-ray microanalysis, that dilatation of the SR is associated with calcium overloading.

Proliferation of the SR can be localized at the

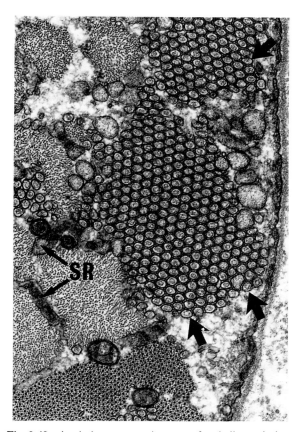

Fig. 3.49 A tubular aggregate in a case of periodic paralysis. The tubules (arrows), approximately 70 nm in diameter, are hexagonally packed and double walled. SR = sarcoplasmic reticulum. ×35 000

triads (Fig. 3.45) or it can result in the formation of extensive tubular aggregates. On morphological criteria alone there seem to be at least three types of aggregate described in the literature. Each consists of collections of parallel tubules 60–80 nm in diameter. In the first type, the tubules contain intraluminal coaxial inner tubules; in the second, tubules have a granular core, and in the third the tubules have filaments, approximately 10 nm in diameter, attached around their outer edge. The evidence for derivation from the SR, that is continuity of the membranes with SR membranes, is strongest for the first type (Fig. 3.49). They are seen most often in cases of periodic paralysis (Bradley 1969, Engel et al 1970, Meyers et al 1972) but have also been associated with alcoholic myopathy (Chui et al 1975) and myotonia (Schröder & Becker 1972). They are often confined to type 2 fibres and are of unknown significance.

Myofibrils

Z-line streaming

Z-line streaming is perhaps the commonest alteration in myofibril structure seen in diseased muscle. At its simplest, it appears as an extension of the electron-dense component of the Z line into the adjacent I band (Fig. 3.50, 3.51). More commonly, the Z line material extends throughout the length of the sarcomere and into neighbouring sarcomeres (Fig. 3.51) and at its most severe, zones of Z-line streaming can occupy large areas of fibre (Fig. 3.52). A certain amount of Z-line streaming can be detected in normal muscle, especially where there is a 'mismatch' between the Z lines of adjacent myofibrils. Fischman and his colleagues (1973) studied the extent of Z-line streaming in 30 control subjects and tentatively concluded that, if Z-line streaming covers more than four sarcomere lengths in four adjacent myofibrils in more than 2% of fibres, it should be considered to be outside normal limits.

The significance of Z-line streaming and what it represents is poorly understood. Z lines wider than normal are seen in regenerating fibres (Fischman 1986); in certain circumstances, therefore, streaming may be part of sarcomere growth and turnover. Figure 3.53 shows an area of streaming in which two sarcomeres may be being differentiated, as suggested by the indistinct presence of two M lines (arrows). It has been suggested that new sarcomere formation normally begins at the Z line (Auber 1969, Goldspink 1971) but evidence of this as it occurs has proved difficult to obtain. There is little doubt, on the other hand, that Z-line streaming is a major component of myofibrillar damage in many pathological conditions. It has been described in a wide variety of neuromuscular diseases including muscular dystrophy (Milhorat et al 1966, Fardeau 1970), myotonic dystrophy (Klinkerfuss 1967, Casanova & Jerusalem 1979), polymyositis (Mastaglia & Walton 1971a, Sato et al 1971), neurogenic atrophy (Schotland 1969, Kobarsky et al 1973), distal myopathy (Markesbery et al 1977) and Parkinson's disease (Ahlqvist et al 1975). It is most marked where there is target-fibre formation (see below). Unlike the situation with rod-body formation, there are as yet no biochemical data on the identification of the proteins involved in streaming.

Fischman and his colleagues (1973) pointed out that, rather than being an inert rigid structure, the Z line is probably the most labile part of the myofibrils. With this in mind, it is likely that several phenomena which appear similar and fall under the same general classification of Z-line streaming, in fact represent different processes; for example, the streaming involved in sarcomerogenesis probably bears no relation to that involved in myofibril breakdown, except in its morphological appearance.

Rod-body formation

Rods originating from the Z line were first described in a congenital non-progressive disease of skeletal muscle by Shy and his colleagues (1963) who termed the disease nemaline myopathy. Z-line (nemaline) rods are highly electron-dense, usually about the width of a myofibril and up to 6–7 μm in length. They are more clearly defined than streaming Z lines and do not impinge on the A bands. Thin filaments run parallel to the longitudinal axis of the rods and connect with the thin filaments of the adjacent I bands (Fig. 3.54). Perpendicular to the longitudinal filaments is a transverse periodicity with a spacing of 20–25 nm. In transverse section the rods contain a square array of filaments in a basket-weave pattern comparable with that of the Z-line transverse lattice.

Since the original description of nemaline myopathy, many other cases have been reported (Gonatas 1966, Engel & Gomez 1967, Fardeau 1969, Karpati et al 1971, Nonaka et al 1989). However, it has become apparent that rod formation is not disease-specific, as rods have also been seen in muscular dystrophy (Fardeau 1970), centronuclear myopathy (Schochet et al 1972), central core disease (Neville 1973), rhabdomyomas (Wyatt et al 1970), polymyositis (Cape et al 1970, Mair & Tomé 1972), distal myopathy (Markesbery et al 1977) cricopharyngeal dysphagia (Hanna & Henderson 1980), mitochondrial myopathies (Kornfeld 1980) and ovine muscular dystrophy (Richards & Passmore 1989). Shafiq and his colleagues (1969) described rods in experimentally

---

Fig. 3.50 Z–line streaming (asterisk) and myofibril splitting (arrows) in a case of muscular dystrophy. Both these phenomena occur to a limited extent in normal muscle. The interlinking of the myofibrils shows that they cannot act independently and individually. ×8074

Fig. 3.51 Z-line streaming (asterisks) and membrane whorl formation (arrow) in a case of hypokalaemic periodic paralysis. ×10 286

Fig. 3.52 Widespread Z-line streaming (asterisks) in emetine-induced myopathy in the rat. ×2990. (From Bindoff & Cullen 1978, with permission of Elsevier North-Holland Biomedical Press)

Fig. 3.53 Localized Z-line streaming in a case of polymyositis. Note the suggestion of new M-line development (arrows) which implies that sarcomerogenesis may be taking place. ×9180

Fig. 3.54 Part of a rod body in a case of nemaline myopathy. Note the longitudinal filaments and the transverse periodicity (arrows). The longitudinal filaments attach to the thin filaments of the adjacent I band. Z = Z line. ×44 240

Fig. 3.50

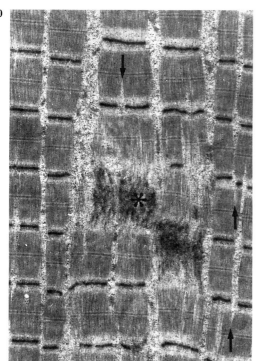

Fig. 3.51

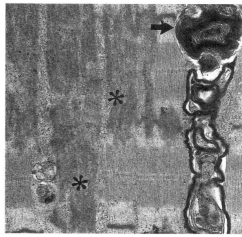
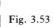

Fig. 3.52

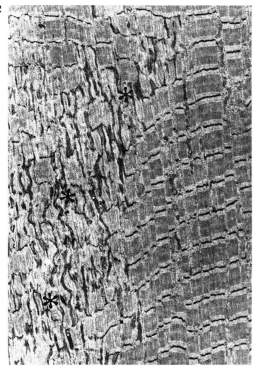

Fig. 3.53

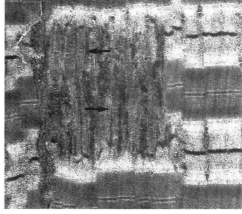

Fig. 3.54

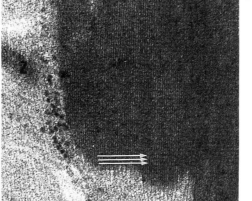

tenotomized rat soleus muscle. They have also been found in intrafusal fibres (Shafiq et al 1967c) and within myonuclei (Jenis et al 1969).

Biochemical and immunocytochemical work has clarified the composition of the rods. When teased myofibres containing rods were treated with Ca^{2+}-activated neutral protease (CAP), the dense material was removed from the rods leaving the backbone of longitudinal filaments (Yamaguchi et al 1978). Because of the specificity of CAP in removing α-actinin from Z lines (Dayton et al 1976) and because antibodies to α-actinin bind to intact rods (Schollmeyer et al 1974) it seemed highly likely that some at least of the material removed was α-actinin. This has been confirmed in an indirect immunofluorescence study using specific antibodies to actin, α-actinin, tropomyosin and desmin (Jockusch et al 1980). Only anti-α-actinin reacted strongly with the nemaline rods. Anti-desmin reacted peripherally with the rods, suggesting that desmin is located at the margins of the rods reminiscent of its marginal location at the Z lines. Yamaguchi and his colleagues (1978) also investigated the constitution of the longitudinal filaments of the rods by allowing the CAP-treated rods to react with heavy meromyosin. The filaments became decorated in an actin-like way with heavy meromyosin arrow heads. Neither Yamaguchi nor Jockusch and their respective colleagues found that anti-actin stained the rods, but suggest that this may be due to an inability of the antibody to penetrate the rods. These results do not exclude the possibility that tropomyosin may be associated with actin in the longitudinal filaments as in the myofibril I band.

In a more recent study Hashimoto et al (1989) carried out an immunochemical analysis of α-actinin in nemaline myopathy after two-dimensional electrophoresis. They looked at labelling of control Z-line and nemaline material using a monoclonal antibody and found only a quantitative abnormality. In general, the recent biochemical work seems to confirm the earlier suggestions that the rods can be considered as replicating Z-line lattices or lateral polymers of the Z-line subunits (MacDonald & Engel 1971, Stromer et al 1976).

Z-line and I-band loss

Z-line loss, sometimes accompanied by loss of the I band, has been described in several conditions including central core disease (Gonatas et al 1965), myotonic dystrophy (Johnson 1969), denervation atrophy (Johnson 1969) and prune belly syndrome (Afifi 1972). Z-line loss is a prominent feature of ischaemic muscle (Karpati et al 1974, Mastaglia et al 1974, Makitie & Teräväinen 1977). Loss of both Z line and I bands was seen in plasmocid-poisoned rat muscle (Price et al 1962) and in rat muscle undergoing degeneration after free grafting (Hansen-Smith & Carlson 1979). In these laboratories we have observed Z-line and I band loss in an aminocaproic acid-induced myopathy, in polymyositis and in an experimentally induced hamster myositis (Cullen & Fulthorpe 1982). Figure 3.55 shows part of a muscle fibre from a polymyositis patient from which the Z lines and I bands have completely disappeared, leaving the individual A bands virtually intact. Although the section of the I filaments normally in the I band is lost, the section in the overlap region is still present.

There is evidence that Z-line loss in necrotic fibres may be due to the action of a calcium-activated proteinase (CAP) which quickly extracts Z-lines *in vitro* (Busch et al 1972). It has been proposed moreover that CAP may be involved in the normal turnover of myofilaments (Dayton et al 1975) but this has been questioned because the

Fig. 3.55 Part of a myofibre in a case of polymyositis in which the Z lines and I bands have been lost. Although the portion of the I filaments in the I bands has been lost, the portion in the A band is still present. ×21 260

Fig. 3.56 Part of a myofibre in a case of dermatomyositis in which the A bands are absent. There is a small number of individual A filaments (arrows). The triads (Tr) are prominent and are in the correct position for this muscle. N = N line. ×14 140

Fig. 3.57 Partial loss of the A band from a myofibre in a case of polymyositis. At the bottom of the area illustrated the A bands appear complete but at the top there is an almost total absence of A filaments. ×9885

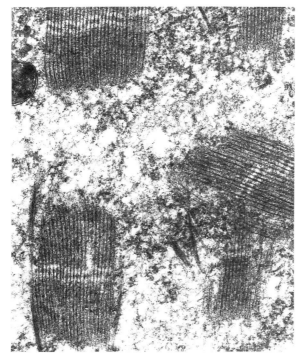

Fig. 3.55

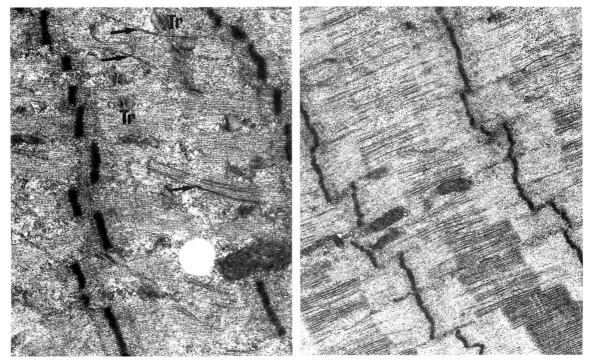

Fig. 3.56

Fig. 3.57

physiological concentration of free calcium ions in the muscle cell is several orders lower than that needed for optimal activity of CAP (see Cellular Mechanisms of Atrophy p 126). This is not the case, however, in necrotic muscle where the plasma membrane is breached and calcium ion levels rise to external concentrations. Thus breakage of the myofibrils at the Z line, perhaps CAP-induced, could be part of a self-destruct mechanism conferring advantage by making the diseased tissue easily accessible for phagocytosis and removal and thereby facilitating regeneration of the tissue (Cullen & Fulthorpe 1982). In those conditions in which we have observed Z-line loss, we have also seen widespread phagocytosis of the A bands by macrophages. Phagocytosis of A bands after Z-line loss has also been reported in ischaemic rabbit muscle (Reznik 1973) and may be a commoner event than hitherto suspected.

A-band loss

Loss of the A band is a rare occurrence in neuromuscular disease. To the authors' knowledge only nine cases have been reported in the literature. Carpenter and his colleagues (1976) observed A-band loss in two cases of childhood dermatomyositis, two cases of adult dermatomyositis and in myopathy associated with thrombotic thombocytopenic purpura. It has also been seen in two cases of congenital myopathy (Yarom & Shapira 1977, Fidzianska et al 1981), in a case of polyradiculopathy (Yarom & Reches 1980) and in a patient suffering from severe hypoxia, shock and acidosis (Sher et al 1979). Selective thick-filament loss has been produced experimentally by tenotomy of rat soleus muscle (Karpati et al 1972) and has also been reported in dystrophic mouse muscle (Cullen & Jaros 1988). The two examples illustrated here were from patients with dermatomyositis (Fig. 3.56) and polymyositis (Fig. 3.57) respectively. In the former, some of the fibres showed a complete absence of A-filaments but, more typically, isolated filaments were still present (Fig. 3.56). In both cases areas of A-filament absence graded into normal areas (Fig. 3.57). The I bands and Z lines were of normal dimensions and the N line was prominent in some fibres (Fig. 3.56). The T tubules and triads were in the normal position at the junction of the I band and (ghost) A band (Figs. 3.56, 3.57). Mitochondria appeared to be normal.

It is difficult to speculate about the cause of the selective A-filament absence. We cannot even distinguish whether the filaments were at one time present and were subsequently lost, or whether they were never assembled. Clearly, the fibres will not contract normally in their absence, but surprisingly there is little evidence of stretching or tearing of the myofibrils. At the moment A-band loss remains an unexplained phenomenon.

Hypercontraction and disassembly

Hypercontraction of the myofibrils is one of the commonest observations in diseased muscle. It is non-specific and can also be produced by artefactual damage to the muscle fibre, so its occurrence must be interpreted with care. When the hypercontraction is artefactual, the affected fibres tend to be grouped together at the periphery of a biopsy, where damage due to handling is greatest. However, the only reliable criterion of true pathological change is the presence of phagocytic cells within the hypercontracted fibre (Cullen et al 1979). Unfortunately, by this stage, changes to the fibre are widespread and clues to the original cause of the hypercontraction are difficult to recognize.

The regions of hypercontraction may be very localized (Fig. 3.58) or widespread. In Figure 3.58, four sarcomeres of one myofibril have contracted into a space of about 2 μm. There is nearby membrane proliferation, perhaps associated with the hypercontraction. Although hypercontraction is a non-specific change, it is particularly characteristic of Duchenne muscular dystrophy where it is thought to be a stage in the death of the muscle fibres (Cullen & Fulthorpe 1975). As hypercontraction can be caused by mechanical damage to muscle fibres in contact with calcium-containing media (Karpati & Carpenter 1982) it seems likely that it is initiated in vivo by a massive, perhaps rapid, influx of calcium from the extracellular fluid which overwhelms the buffering capacity of the sarcoplasmic reticulum and mitochondria.

A second common non-specific observation in

diseased muscle is for the myofibrils to disassemble and to be taken up by phagocytic cells without previous hypercontraction. In this case the fibre volume is occupied by a near-homogeneous mass of short filaments (Fig. 3.59). The banding pattern is lost and the filaments are randomly orientated with no side-to-side alignment. The filaments mostly have the diameter of I filaments, but it is conceivable that there are fragments of dissociated A filaments among them. The mechanism of myofibril disassembly is not understood. Dayton et al (1975) have proposed that CAP may promote disassembly by digesting out Z lines, M lines, C proteins, tropomyosin and troponins T and I from the myofibrils and thus allowing the filaments to fragment. If CAP is involved, an explanation has then to be sought as to why some necrotic fibres have the above appearance, while in others the A bands remain intact (Fig. 3.55).

Minicores, central cores and target fibres

Focal areas of disruption involving a single or a few adjoining sarcomeres are commonly found in a variety of disorders and their significance is uncertain. In a number of children with a congenital myopathy this was found to be the principal change in the muscle fibres and the terms multicore and minicore disease were applied (Engel et al 1971). Typically there is Z-line streaming and loss of mitochondria, SR and glycogen within the minicores (Swash & Schwartz 1981, Pagès et al 1985).

More extensive disorganization of the myofibrils and a clear loss of oxidative enzyme activity (Fig. 3.60) is found in central cores and in target fibres. Central cores were first described by Shy & Magee (1956). Ultrastructurally they display a variable amount of myofibril disorganization (Figs. 3.61, 3.62); Z-line streaming is common (Palmucci et al 1978) and there may be extensive rod formation (Bethlem et al 1978); there is also marked reduction or absence of mitochondria and a lack of intermediate filaments (Thornell et al 1983). There is however an increase in the relative amounts of sarcoplasmic reticulum and T-system (Hayashi et al 1989).

Neville & Brooke (1973) subdivided central cores into structured and unstructured types

according to whether the cross-striations and myofibrillar ATPase staining were retained or lost. However, both types of core have been reported in the same biopsy (Telerman-Toppet et al 1973, Isaacs et al 1975) although Neville (1979) considers this to be unusual. Sewry (1985) has pointed out that some cores can have both structured and unstructured features.

Target fibres are found in denervating conditions, after re-innervation, and in some myopathies including familial periodic paralysis and polymyositis. Within such fibres, a central zone of marked myofibrillar disorganization is separated from an outer zone of normal myofibrils by an intermediate zone in which the degree of myofibrillar disarray is relatively mild (Engel 1961). Within the central zone there is disruption of the myofibril pattern, spreading of Z-band material, loss of mitochondria and disorganisation of the SR (Schotland 1969). Autophagic vacuoles and honeycomb structures have also been observed in the target centres with mitochondrial disintegration in the intermediate area (Mrak et al 1982). In so-called targetoid fibres, which may be found in both myopathic and neurogenic conditions, the intermediate zone is lacking (Dubowitz & Brooke 1973, Dubowitz 1985).

The cause and significance of central cores and target fibres is equivocal. Whether core and target formation are manifestations of the same process is not clear (Schmitt & Volk 1975). Both are found in type 1 fibres and lack mitochondria in their central zones. The main difference should be the lack of an intermediate zone to the central cores, but a clear-cut distinction is hard to maintain (Palmucci et al 1978). Target fibres are generally interpreted as indicators of recent denervation (Kobarsky et al 1973) or of long-standing incomplete denervation (Tomonaga & Sluga 1969), or of re-innervation (Dubowitz 1967).

Cytoplasmic bodies

Cytoplasmic bodies are structures of variable size, usually round or oval in profile, having a dense core and an outer layer of radially arranged filaments (Figs. 3.63, 3.64) which in some cases connect with adjoining myofibrils. The dense core contains tightly packed randomly arranged filaments. Its biochemical nature is unknown but it is sometimes linked to an adjoining Z-line. The radiating filaments resemble actin although a case has been reported in which they contained desmin (Osborn & Goebel 1983). The factors bringing about the formation of cytoplasmic bodies are unknown. They are associated with localized disruption of the myofibre fine structure but are non-specific in their occurrence. The conditions in which they have been reported include muscular

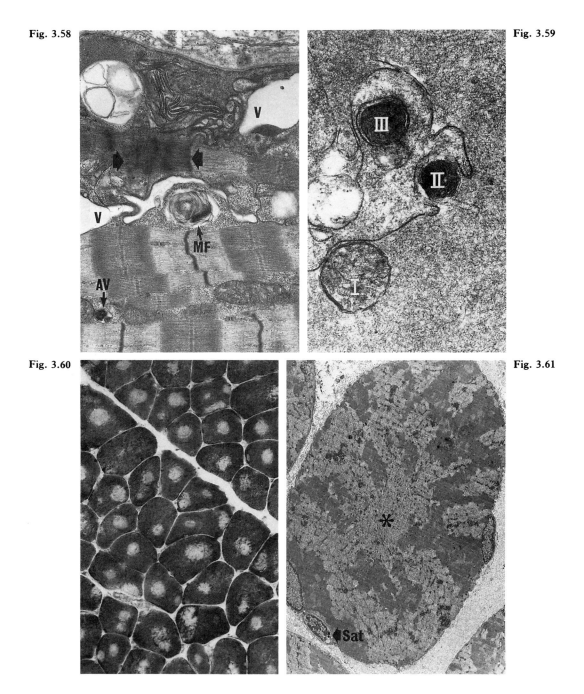

Fig. 3.58

Fig. 3.59

Fig. 3.60

Fig. 3.61

dystrophy (MacDonald & Engel 1969), myotonic dystrophy (Schröder & Adams 1968), inflammatory myopathies (Yunis & Samaha 1971), periodic paralysis (Howes et al 1966, MacDonald et al 1968), mitochondrial myopathies (Hudgson et al 1972), inclusion-body myositis (Carpenter et al 1978) and perhexiline maleate-induced neuromyopathy (Fardeau et al 1979). Although they seem to be non-specific in their occurrence they are the major change in an unusual form of chronic progressive neuromyopathy which has been termed 'cytoplasmic body neuromyopathy' (Jerusalem et al 1979).

Filamentous bodies

Filamentous bodies consist of tightly packed masses of thin 6 nm actin-like filaments (Fig. 3.47). They are frequently subsarcolemmal in location but can lie deeper in the fibres (Fig. 3.47). Like the cytoplasmic bodies, they are non-specific in distribution, and of unknown significance. Conditions in which they have been seen include muscular dystrophy (Hurwitz et al 1967), hypokalaemic (Odor et al 1967) and hyperkalaemic periodic paralysis (MacDonald et al 1968), intermittent claudication (Teräväinen & Makitie 1977) and perhexiline maleate-induced polyneuropathy (Fardeau et al 1979). They have also been described in normal human muscle (Shafiq et al 1966, Schmalbruch 1968) and in the bat cricothyroid muscle (Revel 1962).

An unusual filamentous body is illustrated in figure 3.65 and is similar to a type described by Thornell et al (1983). The filaments are 10 nm wide and are straighter than in other filamentous bodies. Intermediate 10 nm filaments in muscle are composed of desmin (= skeletin) (Lazarides 1980); this structure, therefore, should probably be regarded as quite a different species of filamentous body from that described above.

Concentric laminated bodies

Concentric laminated bodies are found principally in type 2 fibres (Payne & Curless 1976) and are hollow cylindrical structures of characteristic form (Fig. 3.66). Concentric laminae, approximately 7 nm thick with a centre-to-centre spacing of 8.5 nm, make up the walls of the cylinders. The laminae consist of parallel double bands approximately 12 nm deep running circumferentially and projecting about 7 nm at the outside edge with a repeat of 16 nm (Fig. 3.66 inset). There may be up to 25 laminae to each cylinder. The origin of concentric laminated bodies is obscure. Luft et al (1962) considered that they arise from mitochondria, while Toga et al (1970) and Payne & Curless (1976) thought that they derive from myofilaments. Engel and Banker (1986) show concentric laminated bodies apparently attached to myofibril A-bands. However, their subunit dimensions suggest that they are not composed of any of the well-known muscle filaments. Moreover, they are also found in tissues other than muscle (Policard et al 1961, Gambetti et al 1969), so attempts at derivation from any of the well-known muscle components may be naive. The sorts of conditions in which concentric laminated bodies are found offer no clues to their origin. They were first described in hypermetabolism of non-thyroid origin (Luft et al 1962) and subsequently in many other conditions, including neurogenic atrophy (Thiebaut et al 1963, Tomé & Mair 1970),

---

Fig. 3.58 Localized hypercontraction (arrows) in a case of facioscapulohumeral dystrophy. There is considerable membrane proliferation and vacuolation (V) in the affected area. MF = myelin figure. Av = autophagic vacuole. ×10 700

Fig. 3.59 Part of a necrotic fibre in muscular dystrophy in which the myofibrils are reduced to a near-homogeneous pool of filaments and fragments of filaments. The portion of macrophage shown appears to be actively engaged in ingesting muscle mitochondria (successive steps, I, II and III). ×30 000

Fig. 3.60 Central core disease. One or more central or eccentric cores showing loss of enzyme activity are present in all fibres. NADH tetrazolium reductase. ×160

Fig. 3.61 A myofibre from a patient with central core disease showing the loss of normal myofibrillar structure in its centre (asterisk). Sat = satellite cell. ×2000

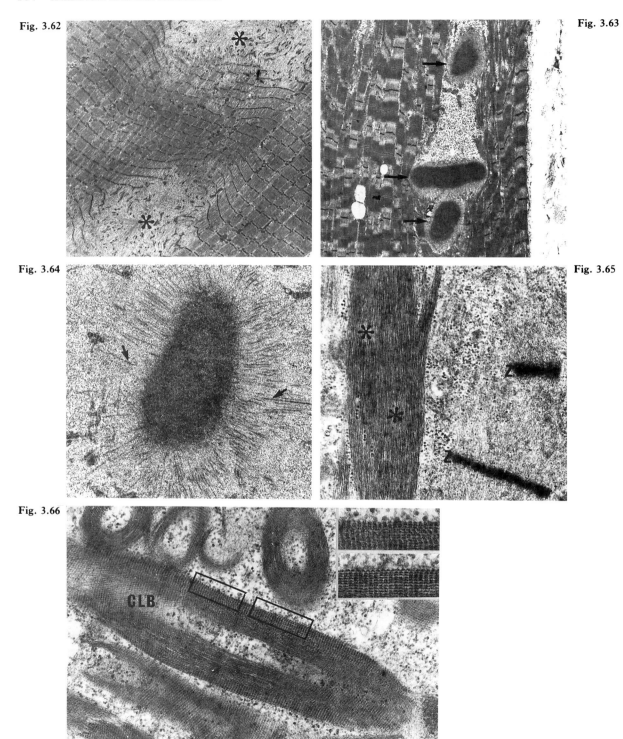

Fig. 3.62

Fig. 3.63

Fig. 3.64

Fig. 3.65

Fig. 3.66

nemaline myopathy (Shafiq et al 1967a), hypothyroid myopathy (Bergouignan et al 1967),
glycogenosis (Engel & Dale 1968), central core
disease (Dubowitz & Roy 1970), infantile neuro-
axonal dystrophy (Toga et al 1970), acromegaly
(Mastaglia 1973), spinal muscular atrophy
(Ketelsen 1975), cerebral hypotonia (Payne &
Curless 1976), McArdle's disease (Korenyi-Both et
al 1977), polymyositis (Cullen et al 1979) and
hairy-cell leukaemia (Rosner & Golomb 1980).

Ringbinden and sarcoplasmic masses

Ringbinden or ring fibres are fibres in which one
or more myofibrils are circumferentially orientated
in the transverse axis of the muscle fibre rather
than having their normal longitudinal orientation
(Fig. 3.67). The disorientated myofibrils may be
situated in the immediate subsarcolemmal region
or, in some instances, are separated from the
sarcolemma by a zone of sarcoplasm containing
disorganized myofilaments, myonuclei and other
organelles. Such peripheral areas are referred to as
sarcoplasmic masses. These changes are non-
specific, being encountered in a variety of
situations including myotonic dystrophy, Becker
dystrophy, hypothyroid myopathy and the limb-
girdle syndrome.

The nucleus

Changes in the nuclei are sometimes found in
fibres that otherwise appear morphologically
normal (Figs. 3.68A, B) but are more usually seen
in necrotic or sublethally injured fibres (Fig.
3.68C). The nuclei can become pyknotic and highly
electron-dense (Fig. 3.68C) or, in contrast, can
become enlarged (Fig. 3.68A). The chromatin
may be dispersed (Fig. 3.68A) or may take up
unusual configurations (Fig. 3.69A).

Filamentous aggregates are sometimes seen
within the nuclei of diseased muscle fibres. The
filaments are of several types. We have observed
thin, 6 nm, actin-like filaments (Fig. 3.69B) and

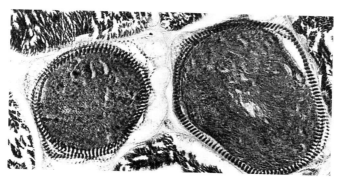

Fig. 3.67 Two ringbinden in a case of hypothyroid myopathy. PTAH-stained. ×430

Fig. 3.62 Part of two cores (asterisks) in a myofibre from a patient with spinal muscular atrophy. Note the loss of striations within the cores. ×1847

Fig. 3.63 Three cytoplasmic bodies (arrowed) in a muscle fibre in a case of myotonic dystrophy. Note the area of disruption around the bodies. ×3650

Fig. 3.64 A cytoplasmic body at higher magnification. Note that in this case both thick (arrows) and thin filaments radiate from the dense central core. From a patient with myotonic dystrophy. ×10 286

Fig. 3.65 An aggregation of 10 nm filaments (asterisks) in a case of dermatomyositis. Z = Z-line. ×24 332

Fig. 3.66 Part of a group of concentric laminated bodies (CLB) in a case of polymyositis. The insets show that the laminae are not composed of membranes nor of individually resolvable filaments. ×32 074. Inset ×74 102

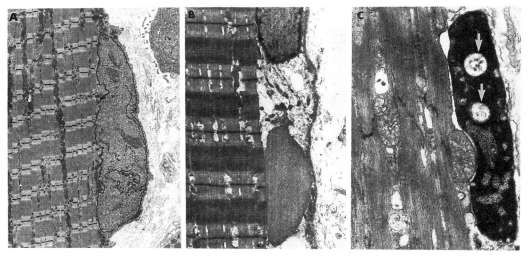

Fig. 3.68 (A) An exceptionally large (~20 μm in length) nucleus with abnormal filamentous and membranous contents in a case of myotonic dystrophy. The muscle fibre appears normal in other respects. ×2726. (B) Part of a muscle fibre from a case of polymyositis. The upper nucleus is normal in appearance but the contents of the lower one have been replaced by a filamentous mass. ×4544. (C) A pyknotic nucleus at the edge of a fibre in a case of Duchenne muscular dystrophy. The two 'vesicles' are surrounded by double membranes and are probably pseudoinclusions (arrows). ×10 565

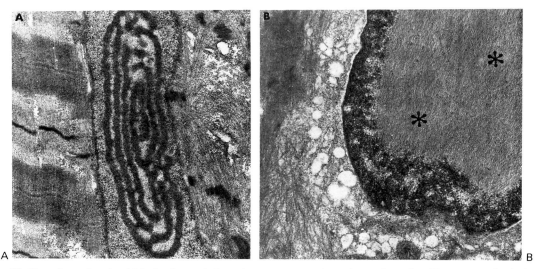

Fig. 3.69 (A) Part of a nucleus in which the chromatin has taken up an unusual annular configuration. From a case of spinal muscular atrophy. ×11 360. (B) Part of a myonucleus which is largely filled by thin 6 nm filaments (asterisks). From a patient with polymyositis. ×13 632

thick, 25 nm filaments (Fig. 3.70). Aggregations of filaments have been described by other authors in polymyositis (Chou 1973), inclusion-body myositis (Schochet & McCormick 1973) and in a Duchenne muscular dystrophy carrier (Ionasescu et al 1975). Tomé & Fardeau (1980) describe tubular filaments approximately 8.5 nm in diameter in the myonuclei in cases of oculopharyngeal muscular dystrophy and 16–18 nm tubular filaments have been described in reducing body myopathy (Carpenter et al 1985) and inclusion body myositis (Tomé and Fardeau 1986). The nucleus illustrated in Figure 3.71, from a patient with polymyositis, contains filaments but

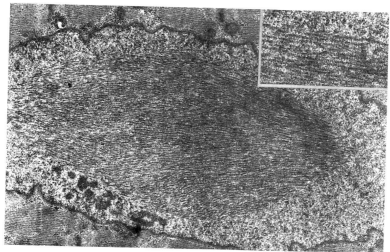

Fig. 3.70 A filamentous mass in a myonucleus in a case of dermatomyositis. The inset shows that the filaments are approximately 25 nm in diameter and are not hollow or tubular. ×14 768. Inset ×34 080

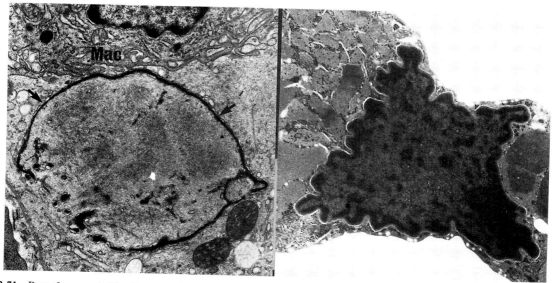

Fig. 3.71 Part of a necrotic fibre in a case of polymyositis in which the nucleus is reduced to an electron-dense envelope (arrows) that is open to the cell cytoplasm. Mac = macrophage. ×11 690

Fig. 3.72 An abnormally crenellated nucleus in a case of nemaline myopathy. ×6662

they are of sarcoplasmic origin. The nuclear contents have been completely lost and replaced by sarcoplasm. In this example the space between the nuclear membranes contains a layer of very electron-dense material of indeterminate origin.

The myonuclei of diseased muscle fibres often become extremely irregular in shape (Fig. 3.72)

and deep invaginations of the nuclear membrane can give rise to the appearance of 'pseudo-inclusions' within the nucleus (Fig. 3.68C). These are distinguishable from real inclusions by having a double nuclear membrane and nuclear pores. Irregularly shaped nuclei are a non-specific abnormality and have been described in polymyositis (Mastaglia & Walton 1971a), distal myopathy (Markesbery et al 1977), inclusion-body myositis (Carpenter et al 1978) dystrophia myotonica (Tomé & Fardeau 1986) and in myopathy due to a triosephosphate isomerase deficiency (Bardosi et al 1990).

Localization of some or all of the nuclei in a central or near-central position in a muscle fibre is usually taken as an indication that regeneration of the fibre has occurred, following earlier necrosis. Why the nuclei do not move to the periphery of the fibre, as they do during normal myogenesis, is not understood, although it seems likely that differences in mechanical constraints imposed by the myofibrils may influence the movement (Cullen & Mastaglia 1982, Tomé & Fardeau 1986). Central nuclei are a common feature of certain diseases. They are particularly abundant in myotonic dystrophy and are often arranged in characteristic chains. Centronuclear or 'myotubular' myopathy was first described by Spiro and his colleagues (1966), who attributed the presence of a large proportion of fibres with central nuclei to an arrested morphological development at the myotube stage. Fibres with central nuclei in 'centronuclear myopathy' cannot be regarded as 'myotubes' except in a broad morphological sense since they are histochemically differentiated fibres, generally type 1 in metabolic profile, whereas true myotubes show '2C' histochemical characteristics. Sarnat (1990) has demonstrated the persistence of fetal cytoskeletal proteins (vimentin and desmin) in muscle fibres in cases of neonatal centronuclear myopathy and has postulated that this is responsible for the persisting central position of nuclei in this disorder.

An unusual feature of muscle, consequent upon its syncytial nature, is that in any one diseased fibre there can be both normal and abnormal nuclei. Figure 3.68B shows part of a fibre from a patient with polymyositis. The upper nucleus is morphologically entirely normal but the lower one is completely filled with thin filaments. The fine structure of the fibre appears to be normal, apart from the possible loss of some subsarcolemmal mitochondria. This implies that muscle fibres can survive with less than their normal complement of viable nuclei. Moreover, we might speculate that there is a threshold proportion of normal nuclei

below which a fibre will die. Assuming that each nucleus has a domain or sphere of influence, this may go some way to explaining why muscle fibre breakdown can be segmental or discontinuous in its distribution.

Mitochondrial abnormalities

Morphological mitochondrial abnormalities are most frequently associated with defects of the respiratory chain, which is located on the inner mitochondrial membrane. Deficiencies of major enzyme systems of the mitochondrial matrix, including acyl-CoA dehydrogenases and electron transfer flavoprotein (ETF) dehydrogenase result in varying degrees of lipid storage (see Ch. 11) but morphological lesions in the mitochondria themselves are a relatively minor feature.

'Ragged-red' fibres (Olson et al 1972) are muscle fibres with prominent sub-sarcolemmal accumulations of abnormal mitochondria (Fig. 3.73A). Ultrastructural studies may reveal a variety of abnormalities, including paracrystalline inclusions and malformations of the membranes of mitochondrial cristae (see Ch. 10). This type of abnormality is characteristic of the myopathy associated with Kearns–Sayre syndrome and the more restricted syndrome of chronic progressive external ophthalmoplegia (CPEO). These disorders are frequently associated with defects of the mitochondrial genome; complexes I, III, IV and V of the respiratory chain may be involved since all have at least one protein subunit coded on mitochondrial DNA (mtDNA). Defects of the mitochondrial genome give rise to heteroplasmy of the muscle fibre population. Some muscle fibres may contain predominantly normal mitochondria, whereas other fibres in which abnormal mtDNA predominates may contain mainly defective mitochondria. This causes a mosaic of normal and respiration deficient fibres, which can be detected using a histochemical 'marker' of the respiratory chain, such as cytochrome oxidase (Fig. 3.73). The majority of mitochondrial proteins, however, are coded on nuclear DNA and defects of the nuclear genome are expressed in all fibres of the muscle population.

Not all respiratory chain defects give rise to morphological mitochondrial abnormalities. For

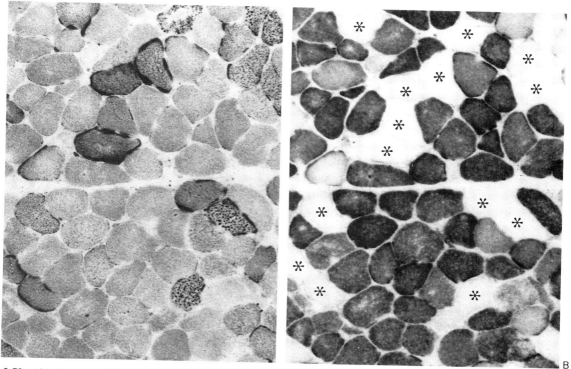

Fig. 3.73 (A) 'Ragged-red' fibres in mitochondrial myopathy (Kearns–Sayre syndrome). Succinate dehydrogenase. ×142. (B) Serial section to (A) showing that 'ragged-red' fibres are cytochrome oxidase-deficient (asterisks). Cytochrome oxidase. ×142

example, muscle biopsies from patients with Leigh's disease (subacute necrotising encephalomyelopathy) associated with severe complex IV deficiency are generally morphologically normal. Even where complex IV (cytochrome oxidase) deficiency is total, as in the fatal infantile myopathy which occurs with the de Toni–Fanconi–Debre syndrome (Fig. 3.74), morphological abnormalities detectable at light microscope level are seen only in scattered fibres, though ultrastructural abnormalities are more widespread.

Whereas 'ragged-red' fibres are almost always associated with definite defects of mitochondrial metabolism, other severe abnormalities of mitochondrial distribution have not, as yet, been shown to be due to any specific underlying defect. In particular 'floccular' or 'lobulated' fibres (Fig. 3.75) are common in some late-onset neuromuscular syndromes, especially those of facioscapulohumeral (FSH) or scapuloperoneal type. Such abnormalities may merely reflect a general derangement of muscle organelles due, possibly, to defective regeneration or reinnervation; the constituent mitochondria of these aggregations rarely show any ultrastructural abnormalities (Fig. 3.76).

Pleomorphic mitochondria are found in some patients with lactic acidosis and proximal myopathy (Fig. 3.77). A variety of paracrystalline inclusions have also been reported (described in detail in Ch. 10). Electron-dense granules, sometimes seen in normal mitochondria, may be particularly large and prominent in certain myopathies such as acid maltase deficiency (Engel & Dale 1968) and hypothyroid myopathy (Fig. 3.78). Mitochondrial vacuolation is usually due to suboptimal fixation of muscle tissue and is only infrequently of pathological significance. The low amplitude swelling which has been described in other tissues and which results from separation of the inner and outer membranes, has also been described in chloroquine neuromyopathy (Fig. 3.79) (Mastaglia

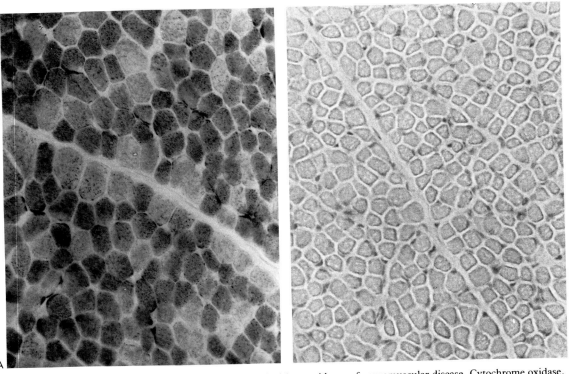

Fig. 3.74 (A) Normal cytochrome oxidase activity in a child with no evidence of neuromuscular disease. Cytochrome oxidase. ×285. (B) Total absence of cytochrome oxidase activity in an infant with De Toni–Fanconi–Debré syndrome. Cytochrome oxidase with methyl green (nuclear) counterstain. ×428

et al 1977). Bizarrely structured mitochondria are also sometimes seen in other neuromuscular syndromes. For example, in the myofibre illustrated in Figure 3.80, from a patient with a polyneuropathy of unknown aetiology, some of the mitochondria are extremely large, many contain electron-dense material and the cristae are abnormally shaped.

Lysosomes

Examination of normal muscle under the electron microscope reveals few structures which are recognizable as lysosomes, apart from a variable amount of lipofuscin which is considered to represent the residue of lysosomal action. In diseased muscle, in contrast, all the organelles normally recognized as being part of the lysosomal system can be found. These include autophagic vacuoles (Figs 3.30, 3.31), membrane whorls (Fig. 3.51), multivesicular bodies (Fig. 3.38C), myelin figures (Fig. 3.58), residual bodies (Fig. 3.29) and lipofuscin granules (Figs 3.45, 3.81). Ideally, the identification of these organelles as secondary lysosomes should be based on rigorous electron-cytochemical procedures but this has proved difficult for muscle. However, Bird and his colleagues (1986) have succeeded in carrying out electron-cytochemical demonstration of the activity of cathepsins B and D and have clearly identified lysosomes in the muscle of vitamin E-deficient guinea-pigs. Similarly, Decker et al (1980) have carried out immunocytochemical labelling of cardiac myocytes using a peroxidase-conjugated antibody to cathepsin D. They found reaction product in secondary lysosomes such as autophagic vacuoles, dense bodies and residual bodies, and also in elements of the sarcoplasmic reticulum.

The identification of primary lysosomes (the membrane-bound packages of lysosomal enzymes without cell debris) is difficult. By analogy with other tissues we might speculate that the sort of organelle illustrated in Figure 3.82 is a primary lysosome (Cullen & Pluskal 1977) but positive

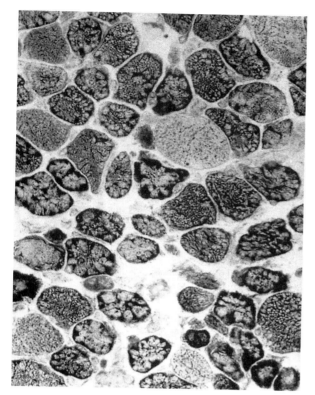

Fig. 3.75 Floccular distribution of mitochondria in a patient with facioscapulohumeral muscular dystrophy. Succinate dehydrogenase. ×150

proof is lacking. The extreme rarity or apparent lack of primary lysosomes in skeletal muscle led some authors to suggest that muscle does not have a conventional lysosomal system and that the lysosomal enzymes are contained in specialized parts of the sarcotubular system (Hudgson & Pearce 1969, Christie & Stoward 1977). This suggestion is based on the positive reactions for acid phosphatase (using Gomori's lead phosphate technique) localized in the cisternae of the sarcoplasmic reticulum and the transverse tubules. It is likely that the sarcoplasmic reticulum provides the isolating membranes of the autophagic vacuoles (see section on autophagy) so it is not unreasonable that it should also be the source of lysosomal enzymes. For a summary of the evidence for an origin of primary lysosomes in the sarcoplasmic reticulum, the reader is referred to a review by Bird & Roisen (1986).

Apart from Pompe's disease (Fig. 3.83), where a lysosomal enzyme, acid maltase, is deficient, the role of lysosomes in muscle disease is most prominent in those conditions where there is severe atrophy of the fibres. Examples of conditions in which lysosomes are prominent include chloroquine myopathy (Humphrey & Rewcastle 1963, Garcin et al 1964), acute polymyositis (Rose et al 1967), colchicine myopathy (Markand & D'Agostino 1971), preclinical muscular dystrophy (Hudgson et al 1967), myotonic dystrophy (Mair & Tomé 1972), juvenile Batten's disease (Carpenter et al 1972), distal myopathy (Markesbery et al 1977), cytochrome c oxidase deficiency (Nonaka et al 1988), a myopathy due to triosephosphate isomerase deficiency (Bardosi et al 1990), germanium myopathy (Higuchi et al 1989), and inclusion-body myositis (Carpenter et al 1978). The contents of the lysosomes are usually heterogeneous. Mitochondria, glycogen and lipid can sometimes be distinguished but much of the material is frequently unidentifiable (Fig. 3.29). Lipofuscin, demonstrable using the histochemical Schmorl reaction, is present in increasing amounts in the muscles of older patients. Batten's disease, associated with lysosomal accumulation of ceroid and lipofuscin pigments is primarily due to abnormal processing of subunit c of the mitochondrial ATP synthase complex which is also found sequestered in lysosomes (Medd et al 1991). Lipofuscin and ceroid pigment also accumulate in muscle fibres in chronic vitamin E deficiency (Neville et al 1983). Myofibrillar material has not yet been discovered in muscle lysosomes (see action on atrophy) and whether lysosomes are involved in myofibril breakdown is still not known.

Golgi apparatus

The Golgi apparatus is usually inconspicuous in normal mature skeletal muscle but can occasionally be seen near a nucleus or at the periphery of a fibre. It consists of a stack of flattened cisternae, each stack having two distinct sides; a usually convex 'cis' or forming face and a usually concave 'trans' or maturing face (Fig. 3.84).

Golgi membrane systems are most commonly seen in immature regenerating fibres where they are involved in the modification and packaging of proteins synthesized in the rough endoplasmic reticulum. Relatively little is known about their

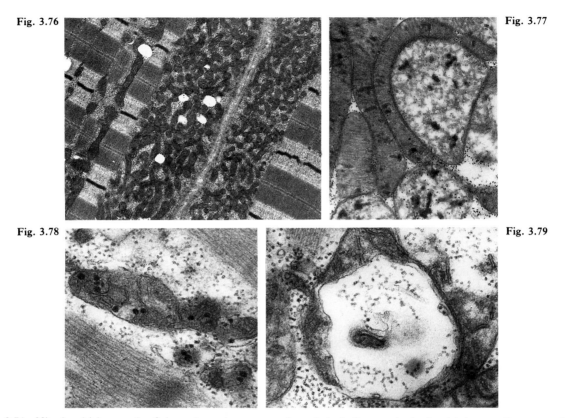

Fig. 3.76   Mitochondrial myopathy. Subsarcolemmal aggregates of morphologically normal mitochondria in two adjacent muscle fibres. ×7000

Fig. 3.77   Pleomorphic mitochondria in a case of mitochondrial myopathy. ×24 000

Fig. 3.78   Mitochondria containing electron-dense calcific granules in a case of hypothyroid myopathy. ×30 000. (Reproduced from Mastaglia & Hudgson (1981) with kind permission of Churchill Livingstone)

Fig. 3.79   Intramitochondrial vacuole containing glycogen granules and membranous debris in a case of chloroquine neuromyopathy. ×36 700

reactions in disease states but membranes derived from the Golgi apparatus are thought to contribute to the formation of autophagic vacuoles in certain situations such as acid maltase deficiency (Engel & Dale 1968) and chloroquine myopathy (Engel & MacDonald 1970).

Other changes

A number of other distinctive structures of uncertain origin have been identified in muscle fibres with the electron microscope (Papadimitriou & Mastaglia 1982).

Tubular aggregates

These are collections of parallel tubules 60–80 nm in diameter, usually found at the edges of type 2 fibres but also occasionally in type 1 fibres. They have distinctive histochemical properties showing an intense reaction in sections for NADH-TR (Fig. 3.85) but lacking α-glycerophosphate dehydrogenase and succinate dehydrogenase. They are found in a range of unrelated and experimental conditions (Banker 1986), the only definite disease connection apparently being with periodic paralysis (Bradley 1969, Meyers et al 1972,

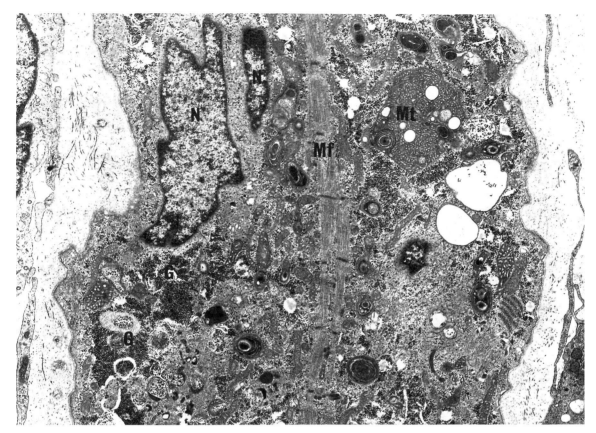

Fig. 3.80 A highly atrophic fibre in a patient having a polyneuropathy of unknown aetiology. The myofibrils (Mf) occupy a very small part of the fibre. The nucleus (N) is very irregular in shape. Most of the mitochondria are extremely abnormal in structure and one (Mt) is very large. There are large accumulations of glycogen (G). ×7545

Rosenberg et al 1985, Roullet et al 1985) (see Ch. 9). The ultrastructure of the tubular aggregates (Fig. 3.86) is described in the section dealing with changes to the sarcoplasmic reticulum (p. 153).

Fingerprint bodies

These structures appear to consist of lamellae, approximately 30 nm apart, with a characteristic saw-tooth-like configuration arranged in curvilinear patterns. They are non-specific, having been described in benign congenital myopathy (Engel et al 1972), dystrophia myotonica (Tomé & Fardeau 1973), oculopharyngeal muscular dystrophy (Julien et al 1974) and Marfan's syndrome (Jadro-Santel et al 1980). Their origin is obscure.

Zebra bodies or leptomeres

These are filamentous structures with light bands alternating with thinner darker bands with a repeat of about 150 nm (Fig. 3.87). They are found at normal myotendinous junctions, in normal extraocular muscle and in intrafusal muscle fibres as well as in diseased muscle. They were a frequent finding in a patient with an unusual form of slowly progressive congenital myopathy (Lake & Wilson 1975) and we have also observed them in a case of hypothyroid myopathy.

Cylindrical spirals

These bodies have been reported in a variety of conditions during the last 10 or so years (Carpenter et al 1979, Bove et al 1980, McDougall et al 1980, Sahashi et al 1982, Gibbels et al 1983, Danon et al 1989). With the light microscope they are seen as heteromorphic subsarcolemmal clusters that stain

red with the modified Gomori trichrome tech nique. The clusters can be 30 μm wide and up t 300 μm long. With the electron microscope the have the appearance of cylindrical structures mad

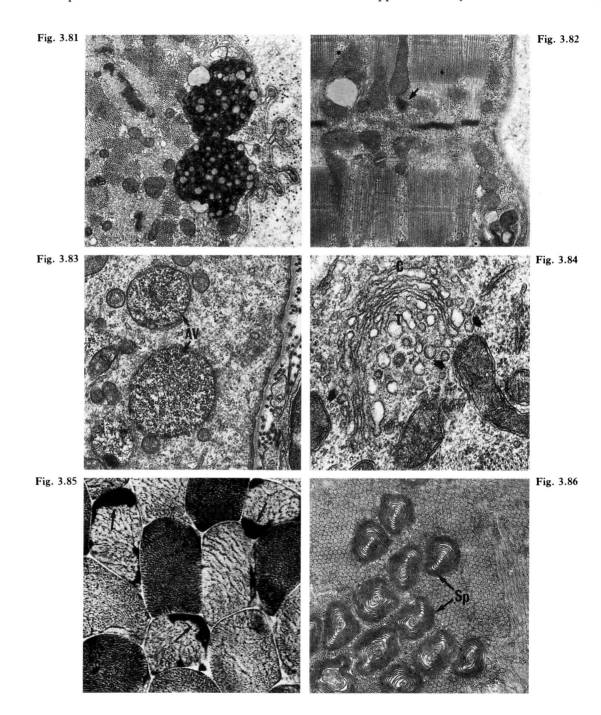

Fig. 3.81

Fig. 3.82

Fig. 3.83

Fig. 3.84

Fig. 3.85

Fig. 3.86

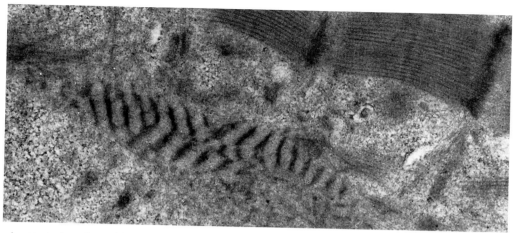

Fig. 3.87 A zebra body at the periphery of a muscle fibre in a case of hypothyroid myopathy. ×30 300

up of paired membranes in a spiral arrangement often with a core of glycogen (Fig. 3.86). Their origin is uncertain but they have sometimes been reported to be associated with tubular aggregates (Danon et al 1989 and Fig. 3.86) so it is possible that they are derived from membranes of the sarcoplasmic reticulum.

Curvilinear bodies

These are identical to the curvilinear bodies found in cerebral glial and nerve cells in neuronal ceroid-lipofuscinosis (Rapola & Haltia 1973). They are typically membrane-bound, having a characteristic appearance which is suggestive of an anastomosing tubular structure. They have been observed in chloroquine myopathy and are commonly found in

close association with lipofuscin bodies (Mastaglia et al 1977, Neville et al 1979).

CONCLUSION

It has been shown that skeletal muscle displays a wide range of pathological reactions. Some, such as atrophy, hypertrophy, autophagy and various forms of degeneration and necrosis, are fundamentally the same as in other tissues, although their expression in muscle is modified by the unique multinucleated state of the muscle fibres and their other functional and structural peculiarities. Although the pathological changes seen in muscle fibres with the light and electron microscope are quite varied, the number of basic reactions is nevertheless fairly limited and, as will

Fig. 3.81 Two lipofuscin granules at the periphery of a muscle fibre in a biopsy from a patient with spinal muscular atrophy ×10 000

Fig. 3.82 Part of a myofibre in a case of spinal muscular atrophy. The small dark body with the halo (arrowed) meets the usual morphological criteria for a primary lysosome. ×14 000

Fig. 3.83 Glycogen accumulation in autophagic vacuoles (AV) in Pompe's disease. ×24 000

Fig. 3.84 Golgi apparatus in an immature myofibre showing cis (C) and trans (T) faces with Golgi vesicles (arrows) being shed at the periphery. ×39 000

Fig. 3.85 Tubular aggregates in a case of periodic paralysis. An NADH–tetrazolium reductase preparation showing densely stained aggregates at the periphery of several type 2 fibres (arrows). ×408

Fig. 3.86 Spiral membrane bodies (Sp) associated with tubular aggregates in a case of periodic paralysis. ×16 700

be seen in subsequent chapters, few if any of these changes are specific to individual disease states. Nevertheless, recognition of certain combinations of histological changes is of value in the diagnostic evaluation of biopsy or necropsy material. The recognition of patterns of histological changes will often provide an important clue to the nature of the injurious influence on the muscle and will allow conclusions to be reached regarding the natural history of the disorder. Thus, the finding of multiple foci of regenerating fibres at a similar stage of development in a muscle would point to a single monophasic metabolic or toxic insult occurring at some defined period beforehand. On the other hand, the finding of disseminated lesions of different ages would point to a more chronic progressive pathological process.

While observations on human material have added to our understanding of the pathological reactions of muscle, the contribution of such studies has been relatively restricted because of the limited possibilities for serial observations during the course of a disease process. It is for this reason that studies in the experimental animal have been important. Such studies have allowed the sequential changes following defined forms of muscle injury to be documented carefully and have greatly enhanced our understanding of the pathological reactions of muscle as a tissue and of the natural history of muscle injury and repair.

The variety of techniques for looking at pathological reactions is rapidly expanding as a direct consequence of the advances being made in the molecular biology of muscle disease. In a review written two years ago (Cullen et al 1988) we predicted that new analytical techniques, and in particular immunolabelling, would transform our view of muscle in the succeeding five years. That process is now well under way and, as we have tried to show, is beginning to bear fruit.

REFERENCES

Adams R D, Denny-Brown D, Pearson C M 1962 Diseases of muscle: a study in pathology, 2nd edn. Hoeber, New York
Afifi A K 1972 The myopathology of the prune belly syndrome. Journal of the Neurological Sciences 15: 153
Afifi A K, Najar S S, Mire-Salman J, Bergman R A 1974 The myopathology of the Kocher–Debré–Semelaigne syndrome: electromyography, light- and electron-microscopic study. Journal of the Neurological Sciences 22: 445
Ahlqvist G, Landin S, Wroblewski R 1975 Ultrastructure of skeletal muscle in patients with Parkinson's disease and upper motor lesions. Laboratory Investigation 32: 673
Allbrook D 1962 An electron miscroscopic study of regenerating skeletal muscle. Journal of Anatomy 96: 137
Arahata K, Ishiura S, Ishiguro T et al 1988 Immunostaining of skeletal and cardiac muscle cell surface membrane with antibody against Duchenne muscular dystrophy peptide. Nature 33: 861
Arahata K, Ishihara T, Kamakura K et al 1989 Mosaic expression of dystrophin in symptomatic carriers of Duchenne's muscular dystrophy. New England Journal of Medicine 320: 138
Argov Z, Gardner-Medwin D, Johnson M A, Mastaglia F L 1980a Congenital myotonic dystrophy. Fibre type abnormalities in two cases. Archives of Neurology (Chicago) 37: 693
Argov Z, Gardner-Medwin D, Johnson M A, Mastaglia F L 1980b Fibre type disproportion in hypotonic infants. Neuropathology and Applied Neurobiology 6(1): 78
Astrom K E, Adams R D 1988 Pathological changes in disorders of skeletal muscle. In: Walton J N (ed) Disorders of voluntary muscle, 5th edn. Churchill Livingstone, Edinburgh, p 153

Auber J 1969 La myofibrillogenese du muscle strie. I. Insectes. Journal of Microscopy 8: 197
Banker B Q 1986 The congenital myopathies. In: Engel A G, Banker B Q (eds) Myology. McGraw-Hill, New York, p 1527
Bardosi A, Eber S W, Hendrys M, Pekran A 1990 Myopathy with altered mitochondria due to a triosephosphate isomerase (TPI) deficiency. Acta Neuropathologica 79: 397
Bergouignan M, Vital C, Bataille J M 1967 Les Myopathies hypothyroidiennes. Aspects cliniques et histopathologiques. Presse Médicale 75: 1551
Bethlem J, Arts W F, Dingemans K P 1978 Common origin of rods, cores, miniature cores, and total loss of cross-striations. Archives of Neurology (Chicago) 35: 555
Bindoff L, Cullen M J 1978 Experimental (−) emetine myopathy. Ultrastructural and morphometric observations. Journal of the Neurological Sciences 39: 1
Bird J W C, Roison F J 1986 Lysosomes in muscle: developmental aspects, enzyme activities and role in protein turnover. In: Engel A G, Banker B Q (eds) Myology. McGraw-Hill, New York, p 745
Bird J W C, Carter J H, Triemer R E, Brooks R M, Spanier A M 1980 Proteinases in cardiac and skeletal muscle. Federation Proceedings 39: 20
Bischoff R 1979 Tissue culture studies on the origin of myogenic cells during muscle regeneration in the rat. In: Mauro A (ed) Muscle regeneration. Raven Press, New York, p 13
Bodensteiner J P, Engel A G 1978 Intracellular calcium accumulation in Duchenne dystrophy and other myopathies: a study of 567 000 fibers in 114 biopsies. Neurology (Minneapolis) 28: 439
Bonilla E, Schotland D L, Wakayama Y 1982 Freeze–fracture

studies in human muscular dystrophy. In: Schotland D L (ed) Disorders of the motor unit. John Wiley, New York, p 475

Bonilla E, Samitt C E , Miranda A F et al 1988 Duchenne muscular dystrophy: deficiency of dystrophin at the muscle cell surface. Cell 54: 447

Borg K, Solders G, Borg J, Edstrom L, Kristensson K 1989 Neurogenic involvement in distal myopathy (Welander). Histochemical and morphological observations on muscle and nerve biopsies. Journal of the Neurological Sciences 91: 53

Bove K E, Iannaccone S T, Hilton P K, Samaha F, 1980 Cylindrical spirals in a familial neuromuscular disorder. Annals of Neurology 7: 550

Bowman W 1840 On the minute structure and movements of voluntary muscle. Philosophical Transactions of the Royal Society of London 130: 457

Bradley W G 1969 Ultrastructural changes in adynamia episodica hereditaria and normokalaemic familial periodic paralysis. Brain 92: 379

Bretscher M S, Thomson J N, Pearse B M F 1980 Coated pits act as molecular filters. Proceedings of the National Academy of Sciences 77: 4156

Brooke M H, Engel W K 1969a The histographic analysis of human muscle biopsies with regard to fiber types. I. Adult male and female. Neurology (Minneapolis) 19: 221

Brooke M H, Engel W K 1969b The histographic analysis of human muscle biopsies with regard to fiber types. IV. Children's biopsies. Neurology (Minneapolis) 19: 591

Brooke M H, Engel W K 1969c The histographic analysis of human muscle biopsies with regard to fiber types II Diseases of the upper and lower motor neurons. Neurology (Minneapolis) 19: 378

Brown R H, Hoffman E P 1988 Molecular biology of Duchenne muscular dystrophy. Trends in Neuroscience 11: 480

Burden S J, Sargent P B, McMahan U J 1979 Acetylcholine receptors in regenerating muscle accumulate at original synaptic site in the absence of the nerve. Journal of Cell Biology 82: 412

Busch W A, Stromer M H, Goll D E, Suzuki A 1972 Ca^{2+}-specific removal of Z lines from rabbit skeletal muscle. Journal of Cell Biology 52: 367

Campion D R 1984 The muscle satellite cell: a review. International Review of Cytology 87: 225

Cape C A, Johnson W W, Pitner S E 1970 Nemaline structures in polymyositis: a non-specific pathological reaction of skeletal muscle. Neurology (Minneapolis) 20: 494

Carlson B M 1970 Regeneration of the rat gastrocnemius muscle from sibling and non-sibling muscle fragments. American Journal of Anatomy 128(1): 21

Carnwath J W, Shotton D M 1987 Muscular dystrophy in the mdx mouse: histopathology of the soleus and extensor digitorum longus muscles. Journal of Neurological Sciences 80: 39

Carpenter S, Karpati G 1979 Duchenne muscular dystrophy. Plasma membrane loss initiates muscle cell necrosis unless it is repaired. Brain 102: 147

Carpenter S, Karpati G, Andermann F 1972 Specific involvement of muscle, nerve and skin in late infantile and juvenile amaurotic idiocy. Neurology (Minneapolis) 22: 170

Carpenter S, Karpati G, Rothman S, Walters H 1976 The childhood type of dermatomyositis. Neurology (Minneapolis) 26: 952

Carpenter S, Karpati G, Heller I, Eisen A 1978 Inclusion body myositis: a distinct variety of idiopathic inflammatory myopathy. Neurology (Minneapolis) 28: 8

Carpenter S, Karpati G, Robitaille Y, Melmed C 1979 Cylindrical spirals in human skeletal muscle. Muscle and Nerve 2: 282

Carpenter S, Karpati G, Holland P 1985 New observations in reducing body myopathy. Neurology (Cleveland) 35: 818

Casanova G, Jerusalem F 1979 Myopathology of myotonic dystrophy. A morphometric study. Acta Neuropathologica 45: 231

Chou S M 1969 Megaconial mitochondria in a case of chronic polymyositis. Acta Neuropathologica 12: 68

Chou S M 1973 Prospects of viral etiology in polymyositis. In: Kakulas B A (ed) Clinical studies in myology, part 2. Excerpta Medica, Amsterdam, p 17

Christie K N, Stoward P J 1977 A cytochemical study of acid phosphatases in dystrophic hamster muscle. Journal of Ultrastructure Research 58: 219

Chui L A, Nenstein H, Munsat T L 1975 Tubular aggregates in subclinical alcoholic myopathy. American Journal of Neurology 25: 405

Cornog J L, Gonatas N K 1967 Ultrastructure of rhabdomyoma. Journal of Ultrastructure Research 20: 443

Cullen M J, Fulthorpe J J 1975 Stages in fibre breakdown in Duchenne muscular dystrophy. An electron miscroscopic study. Journal of the Neurological Sciences 24: 179

Cullen M J, Fulthorpe J J 1982 Phagocytosis of the A band following Z line and I band loss. Its significance in skeletal muscle breakdown. Journal of Pathology 138: 129

Cullen M J, Jaros E 1988 Ultrastructure of the skeletal muscle of the X chromosome-linked dystrophic (mdx) mouse. Comparison with Duchenne muscular dystrophy. Acta Neuropathologica 77: 69

Cullen M J, Mastaglia F L 1980 Morphological changes in dystrophic muscle. British Medical Bulletin 36: 145

Cullen M J, Mastaglia F L 1982 Pathological reactions of skeletal muscle. In: Mastaglia F L, Walton J N (eds) Skeletal muscle pathology, 1st. Edn. Churchill Livingstone, Edinburgh.

Cullen M J, Pluskal M G 1977 Early changes in the ultrastructure of denervated rat skeletal muscle. Experimental Neurology 56: 115

Cullen M J, Appleyard S T, Bindoff L 1979 Morphological aspects of muscle breakdown and lysosomal activation. Annals of the New York Academy of Sciences 317: 440

Cullen M J, Hudgson P, Mastaglia F L 1988 Ultrastructural studies of diseased muscle. In: Walton J N (ed) Disorders of voluntary muscle, 5th edn. Churchill Livingstone, Edinburgh, p 284

Cullen M J, Walsh J, Nicholson L V B, Harris J B 1990 Ultrastructural localization of dystrophin in human muscle using gold immunolabelling. Proceedings of the Royal Society of London, B 240: 197

Danon M J, Carpenter S, Harati Y 1989 Muscle pain associated with tubular aggregates and structures resembling cylindrical spirals. Muscle and Nerve 12: 265

Dayton W R, Goll D E, Stromer M H, Reville W J, Zeece M G, Robson R M 1975 Some properties of a Ca^{2+}-activated protease that may be involved in myofibrillar protein turnover. In: Reich E, Rifkin D B, Shaw E (eds) Proteases and biological control. Cold Spring Harbor Laboratory, Cold Spring Harbor, New York, p 551

Dayton W R, Reville W J, Goll D E, Stromer M H 1976 A Ca^{2+}-activated protease possibly involved in myofibrillar protein turnover. Partial characterization of the purified enzyme. Biochemistry 15: 2159

Dayton W R, Schollmeyer J V, Lepley R A, Cortes L R 1981 A

calcium-activated protease possibly involved in myofibrillar protein turnover. Isolation of a low-calcium-requiring form of the protease. Biochimica Biophysica Acta 659: 48

Decker R S, Decker M, Poole A R 1980 The distribution of lysosomal cathepsin D in cardiac myocytes. Journal of Histochemistry and Cytochemistry 28: 231

Dreyfus J C, Schapira G, Schapira F 1954 Biochemical study of muscle in progressive muscular dystrophy. Journal of Clinical Investigation 33: 794

Duance V C, Restall D J, Beard H, Bourne F J, Bailey A J 1977 The location of three collagen types in skeletal muscle. FEBS Letters 79: 248

Duance V C, Black C M, Dubowitz V, Hughes G R V, Bailey A J 1980 Polymyositis — an immunofluorescence study on the distribution of collagen types. Muscle and Nerve 3: 487

Dubowitz V 1967 Pathology of experimentally reinnervated skeletal muscle. Journal of Neurology, Neurosurgery and Psychiatry 30: 99

Dubowitz V 1985 Muscle biopsy. A practical approach. Bailliere Tindall, London

Dubowitz V, Brooke M H 1973 Muscle biopsy: a modern approach. W B Saunders, Philadelphia

Dubowitz V, Roy S 1970 Central core disease of muscle: clinical, histochemical and electron miscroscopic studies of an affected mother and child. Brain 93: 133

Dulhunty A F, Franzini-Armstrong C 1975 The relative contributions of the folds and caveolae to the surface membrane of frog skeletal muscle fibres at different sarcomere lengths. Journal of Physiology 250: 513

Duncan C J 1978 Role of intracellular calcium in promoting muscle change: a strategy for controlling the dystrophic condition. Experientia 34: 1531

Edström L, Thornell L–E, Eriksson A 1980 A new type of hereditary distal myopathy with characteristic sarcoplasmic bodies and intermediate (skeletin) filaments. Journal of the Neurological Sciences 47: 171

Engel W K 1961 Muscle target fibres. A newly recognised sign of denervation. Nature 191: 389

Engel A G 1966a Thyrotoxic and corticosteroid-induced myopathies. Mayo Clinic Proceedings 41: 785

Engel A G 1966b Electron microscopic observations in primary hypokalemic and thyrotoxic periodic paralyses. Mayo Clinic Proceedings 41: 797

Engel A G 1970a Evolution and content of vacuoles in primary hypokalemic periodic paralysis. Mayo Clinic Proceedings 45: 774

Engel A G 1970b Acid maltase deficiency in adults: studies in four cases of a syndrome which may mimic muscular dystrophy or other myopathies. Brain 93: 559

Engel A G 1973 Vacuolar myopathies: multiple etiologies and segmental structural studies. In: Pearson C M, Mostofi F K (eds) The striated muscle. Williams and Wilkins, Baltimore, p 301

Engel A G, Banker B Q 1986 Ultrastructural changes in diseased muscle. In: Engel A G, Banker B Q (eds) Myology. McGraw-Hill, New York, p 909

Engel A G, Dale A J D 1968 Autophagic glycogenosis of late onset with mitochondrial abnormalities: light and electron microscopic observations. Mayo Clinic Proceedings. 43: 233

Engel A G, Gomez M R 1967 Nemaline (Z disc) myopathy: observations on the origin, structure and solubility properties of the nemaline structures. Journal of Neuropathology and Experimental Neurology 26: 601

Engel A G, MacDonald R D 1970 Ultrastructural reactions in muscle disease and their light-microscopic correlates. In:

Walton J N, Canal N, Scarlato G (eds) Muscle diseases. Excerpta Medica, Amsterdam

Engel W K, Brooke M H, Nelson P G 1966 Histochemical studies of denervated and tenotomized cat muscle: illustrating difficulties in relating experimental animal conditions to human neuromuscular diseases. Annals of the New York Academy of Sciences 138: 160

Engel W K, Gold G N, Karpati G 1968 Type I fibre hypotrophy and central nuclei. Archives of Neurology (Chicago) 18: 435

Engel A G, Gomez M R, Groover R V 1971 Multicore disease. A recently recognised congenital myopathy associated with multifocal degeneration of muscle fibers. Mayo Clinic Proceedings 46: 666

Engel W K, Bishop D W, Cunningham G G 1970 Tubular aggregates in type II muscle fibres: ultrastructural and histochemical correlation. Journal of Ultrastructure Research 31: 507

Engel A G, Angelini C, Gomez M R 1972 Fingerprint body myopathy. Mayo Clinic Proceedings 47: 377

Ericsson J L E 1969 Mechanisms of cellular autophagy. In: Dingel J T, Fell H B (eds) Lysosomes in biology and pathology, vol 2. North-Holland, Amsterdam, p 345

Ezerman E B, Ishikawa H 1967 Differentiation of the sarcoplasmic reticulum and T-system in developing chick skeletal muscle in vitro. Journal of Cell Biology 35: 405

Fardeau M 1969, Étude d'une nouvelle observation de nemaline myopathy. II Données ultrastructurales. Acta Neuropathologica 13: 250

Fardeau M 1970 Ultrastructural lesions in progressive muscular dystrophies. A critical review of their specificities. In: Walton J N, Canal N, Scarlato G (eds) Muscle diseases. International congress series no. 199, Excerpta Medica, Amsterdam, p 98

Fardeau M, Tomé F M S, Simon P 1979 Muscle and nerve changes induced by perhexiline maleate in man and mice. Muscle and Nerve 2: 24

Farkas-Bargeton E, Aicardi J, Arsenio-Nunes M L, Wehrle R 1978 Delay in the maturation of muscle fibers in infants with congenital hypotonia. Journal of the Neurological Sciences 39: 17

Fedorko M E, Cohn Z A 1968 Autophagic vacuoles produced in vitro. II. Studies on the mechanism of formation of autophagic vacuoles produced by chloroquine. Journal of Cell Biology 38: 392

Fidzianska A 1976 Morphological differences between the atrophied small muscle fibres in amyotrophic lateral sclerosis and Werdnig-Hoffman disease. Acta Neuropathologica 17: 234

Fidzianska A, Badurska B, Ryniewicz B, Dembek I 1981 'Cap disease': new congenital myopathy. Neurology (Minneapolis) 31: 1113

Fischman D A 1986 Myofibrillogenesis and the morphogenesis of skeletal muscle. In: Engel A G, Banker B Q (eds) Myology. McGraw-Hill, New York, p 5

Fischman D A, Meltzer H Y, Poppei R W 1973 The ultrastructure of human skeletal muscle: variations from archetypal morphology. In: Pearson C M, Mostofi F K (eds) The striated muscle. Williams and Wilkins, Baltimore, p 58

Franzini-Armstrong C 1973 Membranous systems in muscle fibres. In: Bourne G H (ed) The structure and function of muscle, 2nd edn, vol 2. Academic Press, New York, p 532

Furuno K, Goldberg A L 1986 The activation of protein degradation in muscle by calcium or muscle injury does not involve a lysosomal mechanism. Biochemical Journal 237: 859

Gallai M 1977 Myopathy with hyperaldosteronism — an electron-microscopic study. Journal of the Neurological Sciences 32: 337

Gambetti P, Mellman W J, Gonatas N K 1969 Familial spongy degeneration of the central nervous system (van Bogaert-Bertrand disease). An ultrastructural study. Acta Neuropathologica 12: 103

Garcin R, Rondot P, Fardeau M 1964 Sur les accidents neuromusculaires et en particular sur une 'myopathie vacuolaire' observé au cours d'un traitement prolongé par la chloroquine. Revue Neurologique 111: 177

Gibbels E, Henke U, Schädlich H J, Haupt W F, Fiehn W 1983 Cylindrical spirals in skeletal muscle: a further observation with clinical, morphological and biochemical analysis. Muscle and Nerve 6: 646

Glicksman M A, Sanes J R 1983 Differentiation of motor nerve terminals in the absence of muscle fibres. Journal of Neurocytology 12: 661

Goldberg M 1986 Is the lamina lucida of the basement membrane a fixation artefact? European Journal of Cell Biology 42: 365

Goldspink G 1971 Changes in striated muscle fibres during contraction and growth with particular reference to myofibril splitting. Journal of Cell Science 9: 123

Goldspink D 1972 Postembryonic growth and differentiation of striated muscle. In: Bourne G H (ed) Structure and function of muscle, vol 1. Academic Press, New York and London, p 179

Goll D E, Okitani A, Dayton W R, Reville W J 1978 A Ca^{2+}-activated protease in myofibrillar protein turnover. In: Segal H L, Doyle P J (eds) Protein turnover and lysosomal function. Academic Press, New York, p 587

Gonatas N K 1966 The fine structure of the rod-like bodies in nemaline myopathy and their relation to the Z-discs. Journal of Neuropathology and Experimental Neurology 25: 409

Gonatas N K, Perez M C, Shy G M, Evangelista I 1965 Central 'core' disease of skeletal muscle. Ultrastructural and cytochemical observations in two cases. American Journal of Pathology 47: 503

Guarnieri G, Toigo G, Situlin R, Del Bianco M A, Crapesi L 1989 Cathepsin B and D activity in human skeletal muscle in disease states. In: Proteases in Health and Disease, Academic Press, p 243

Hanna W, Henderson R D 1980 Nemaline rods in cricopharyngeal dysphagia. American Journal of Clinical Pathology 74: 186

Hansen-Smith F M, Carlson B M 1979 Cellular responses to free grafting of the extensor digitorum longus muscle of the rat. Journal of the Neurological Sciences 41: 149

Hashimoto K, Shimizu T, Nonaka I, Mannen T 1989 Immunochemical analysis of α-actinin of nemaline myopathy after two-dimensional electrophoresis. Journal of Neurological Sciences 93: 199

Hay E 1971 Skeletal muscle regeneration. New England Journal of Medicine 284: 1033

Hayashi K, Miller R G, Brownell A K W 1989 Central core disease: ultrastructure of the sarcoplasmic reticulum and T-tubules. Muscle and Nerve 12: 95

Higuchi I, Izumo S, Kuriyama M et al 1989 Germanium myopathy: clinical and experimental pathological studies. Acta Neuropathologica 79: 300

Hoffman E P, Kunkel L M 1989 Dystrophin abnormalities in Duchenne/Becker muscular dystrophy. Neuron 2: 1019

Hoffman E P, Brown R H, Kunkel L M 1987a Dystrophin: the protein product of the Duchenne muscular dystrophy locus. Cell 51: 919

Hoffman E P, Knudson C M, Campbell K P, Kunkel L M 1987b Subcellular fractionation of dystrophin to the triads of skeletal muscle. Nature, London 330: 754

Holtzman E 1976 Lysosomes: a survey, Springer-Verlag, Vienna

Howes E L, Price H M, Pearson C M, Blumberg J M 1966 Hypokalemic periodic paralysis. Electron miscroscopic changes in the sarcoplasm. Neurology (Minneapolis) 16: 242

Hsu L, Trupin G L, Roisen F J 1979 The role of satellite cells and myonuclei during myogenesis in vitro. In: Mauro A (ed) Muscle regeneration. Raven Press, New York, p 115

Hudgson P, Pearce G W 1969 Ultramicroscopic studies of diseased muscle. In: Walton J N (ed) Disorders of voluntary muscle. Churchill, London, p 277

Hudgson P, Pearce G W, Walton J N 1967 Pre-clinical muscular dystrophy: histopathological changes observed on muscle biopsy. Brain 90: 565

Hudgson P, Bradley W G, Jenkinson M 1972 Familial 'mitochondrial' myopathy associated with disordered oxidative metabolism in muscle fibre. Journal of the Neurological Sciences 16: 343

Humphrey J G, Rewcastle N B 1963 Vacuolar myopathy. A clinical and electron microscopic study. Transactions of the American Neurological Association 88: 225

Hunter D D, Shah V, Merlie J P, Sanes J R 1989 A laminin-like adhesive protein concentrated in the synaptic cleft of the neuromuscular junction. Nature 338: 229

Hurwitz L J, Carson N A, Allen I V, Fannin T F, Lyttle J A, Neill D W 1967 Clinical, biochemical and histopathological findings in a family with muscular dystrophy. Brain 90: 799

Ionasescu V, Radu H, Nicolescu P 1975 Identification of Duchenne muscular dystrophy carriers. Archives of Pathology 99: 436

Isaacs H, Heffron J J A, Badenhorst M 1975 Central core disease: a correlated genetic, histochemical, ultramicroscopic and biochemical study. Journal of Neurology, Neurosurgery and Psychiatry 38: 1177

Ishikawa H 1968 Formation of elaborate networks of T-tubules — reference to T-system formation. Journal of Cell Biology 38: 51

Jadro-Santel D, Grcević N, Dogan S, Franjić J, Benc H 1980 Centronuclear myopathy with type 1 fibre hypotrophy and 'fingerprint' inclusions associated with Marfan's syndrome Journal of Neurological Sciences 45: 43

Jenis E H, Lindquist R R, Lister R C 1969 New congenital myopathy with crystalline intranuclear inclusions. Archives of Neurology (Chicago) 20: 281

Jennekens F G I, Tomlinson B E, Walton J N 1971 Data of the distribution of fibre types in five human limb muscles. Journal of the Neurological Sciences 14: 245

Jerusalem F 1970 Biptische befunde des T-systems and tubuläre strukturkomplexe bei neoplastischer cortisonmyopathie. Acta Neuropathologica 14: 338

Jerusalem F, Ludin H, Bischoff A, Hartmann G 1979 Cytoplasmic body neuromyopathy presenting as respiratory failure and weight loss. Journal of the Neurological Sciences 41: 1

Jockusch B M, Veldman H, Griffiths G W, van Oost B A, Jennekens F G I 1980 Immunofluorescence microscopy of a myopathy. α-actinin is a major constituent of nemaline rods. Experimental Cell Research 127: 409

Johnson A G 1969 Alterations of the Z-lines and I-band

myofilaments in human skeletal muscle. Acta Neuropathologica 12: 218

Johnson M A, Fulthorpe J J, Hudgson P 1973a Lipid storage myopathy. A clinicopathologically recognizable entity. Acta Neuropathologica (Berlin) 24: 97

Johnson M A, Polgar J, Weightman D, Appleton D 1973b Data on the distribution of fibre types in 36 human muscles. An autopsy study. Journal of the Neurological Sciences 18: 111

Julien J, Vital C L, Vallat J M, Vallat M, Le Blanc M 1974 Oculopharyngeal muscular dystrophy—a case with abnormal mitochondria and 'fingerprint' inclusions. Journal of the Neurological Sciences 21: 165

Kakulas B A 1975 Experimental muscle diseases. In: Jasmin G, Cantin M (eds) Methods and achievements in experimental pathology, vol 7. Karger, Basel, p 109

Karpati G 1979 The principles of skeletal muscle histochemistry in neuromuscular diseases. In: Vinken P J, Bruyn G W (eds) Diseases of muscle. Handbook of Clinical Neurology, vol 40. North-Holland, Amsterdam, p 1

Karpati G, Carpenter S 1982 Micropuncture lesions of skeletal muscle cells: a new experimental model for the study of muscle cell damage, repair and regeneration. In: Schotland D L (ed) Disorders of the motor unit. John Wiley, New York, p 517

Karpati G, Carpenter S, Andermann F 1971 A new concept of childhood nemaline myopathy. Archives of Neurology (Chicago) 24: 291

Karpati G, Carpenter S, Eisen A A 1972 Experimental core-like lesions and nemaline rods. Archives of Neurology (Chicago) 27: 237

Karpati G, Carpenter S, Melmed C, Eisen A 1974 Experimental ischemic myopathy. Journal of the Neurological Sciences 23: 129

Katz B 1961 The termination of the afferent nerve fibre in the muscle spindle of the frog. Proceedings of the Royal Society of London B 243: 221

Kelly F J, McGrath J A, Goldspink D F, Cullen M J 1986 A morphological/biochemical study of the actions of corticosteroids on rat skeletal muscle. Muscle and Nerve 9: 1

Ketelsen U-P 1975 On the ultrastructure of the atrophic muscle cell. Pathology Europe 10: 73

Kinoshita M, Kawasaki K 1976 Myotubular (centronuclear) myopathy. Advances in Neurological Science 20: 48

Klinkerfuss G H 1967 An electron microscopic study of myotonic dystrophy. Archives of Neurology (Chicago) 16: 181

Knudson C M, Hoffman E P, Kahl S D, Kundel L M, Campbell K P 1988 Characterization of dystrophin in skeletal muscle triads. Journal of Biological Chemistry 263: 8480

Kobarsky J, Schochet S S Jr, McCormick W F 1973 The significance of target fibres: a clinicopathological review of 100 patients with neurogenic atrophy. American Journal of Clinical Pathology 59: 790

Koenig M, Hoffman E P, Bertelson C J, Monaco A P, Feener C, Kunkel L M 1987 Complete cloning of the Duchenne muscular dystrophy (DMD) cDNA and preliminary genomic organization of the DMD gene in normal and affected individuals. Cell 50: 509

Koenig M, Monaco A P, Kunkel L M 1988 The complete sequence of dystrophin predicts a rod-shaped cytoskeletal protein. Cell 53: 219

Konigsberg U R, Lipton B Y, Konigsberg I R 1975 The regenerative response of single mature muscle fibers isolated in vitro. Developmental Biology 45: 260

Korenyi-Both A, Smith B H, Baruah J K 1977 McArdle's syndrome. Fine structural changes in muscle. Acta Neuropathologica 40: 11

Kornfeld M 1980 Mixed nemaline-mitochondrial 'myopathy'. Acta Neuropathologica 51: 185

Lake B D, Wilson J 1975 Zebra body myopathy. Clinical, histochemical and ultrastructural studies. Journal of the Neurological Sciences 24: 437

Lazarides E 1980 Intermediate filaments as mechanical integrators of cellular space. Nature 283: 249

Lazarides E, Hubbard B D 1978 Desmin filaments-a new cytoskeletal structure in muscle cells. Trends in Neurosciences 1: 149

Leonard J P, Salpeter M M 1979 Agonist-induced myopathy at the neuromuscular junction is mediated by calcium. Journal of Cell Biology 82: 811

Lester J M, Silber D I, Cohen M H, Hirsch R P, Bradley W G, Brenner J F 1983 The codispersion index for the measurement of fiber type distribution patterns. Muscle and Nerve 6: 581

Luft R, Ikkos D, Palmieri G, Ernster L, Afzelius B 1962 A case of severe hypermetabolism of non-thyroid origin with a defect in the maintenance of mitochondrial respiratory control; a correlated clinical, biochemical and morphological study. Journal of Clinical Investigation 41: 1776

MacDonald R D, Engel A G 1969 The cytoplasmic body: another structureal anomaly of the Z disc. Acta Neuropathologica 14: 99

MacDonald R D, Engel A G 1970 Experimental chloroquine myopathy. Journal of Neuropathology and Experimental Neurology 29: 479

MacDonald R D, Engel A G 1971 Observations on organizations of Z-disc components and on rod-bodies of Z-disc origin. Journal of Cell Biology 48: 431

MacDonald R D, Rewcastle N B, Humphrey J G 1968 Myopathy of hypokalemic periodic paralysis. Archives of Neurology (Chicago) 20: 565

McDougall J, Wiles C M, Edwards R H T 1980 Spiral membrane cylinders in the skeletal muscle of a patient with melorheostosis. Neuropathology and Applied Neurobiology 6: 69

Mair W G P, Tomé F M S 1972 Atlas of the ultrastructure of diseased human muscle. Churchill, London

Makitie J, Teräväinen H 1977 Ultrastructure of striated muscle of the rat after temporary ischemia. Acta Neuropathologica (Berlin) 37: 237

Markand O N, D'Agostino A N 1971 Ultrastructural changes in skeletal muscle induced by colchicine. Archives of Neurology (Chicago) 24: 72

Markesbery W R, Griggs R C, Herr B 1977 Distal myopathy: electron microscopic and histochemical studies. Neurology (Minneapolis) 27: 727

Mastaglia F L 1970 Pathogenesis of human myopathies. MD Thesis, University of Western Australia

Mastaglia F L 1973 Pathological changes in skeletal muscle in acromegaly. Acta Neuropathologica 14: 273

Mastaglia F L, Argov Z 1981 Drug-induced neuromuscular disorders in man. In: Walton J N (ed) Disorders of voluntary muscle, 4th edn. Churchill Livingstone, Edinburgh

Mastaglia F L, Hudgson P 1981 Ultrastructural studies of diseased muscle. In: Walton J N (ed) Disorders of voluntary muscle, 4th edn. Churchill Livingstone, Edinburgh

Mastaglia F L, Walton J N 1971a An ultrastructural study of skeletal muscle in polymyositis. Journal of the Neurological Sciences 12: 473

Mastaglia F L, Walton J N 1971b Histological and histochemical changes in skeletal muscle from cases of chronic juvenile and early adult spinal muscular atrophy (the Kugelberg–Welander syndrome). Journal of the Neurological Sciences 12: 15

Mastaglia F L, Dawkins R L, Papadimitriou J M 1975 Morphological changes in skeletal muscle after transplantation: a light- and electron-microscopic study of the initial phases of degeneration and regeneration. Journal of the Neurological Sciences 25: 227

Mastaglia F L, Papadimitriou J M, Dawkins R L, Beveridge B 1977 Vacuolar myopathy associated with chloroquine, lupus erythematosus and thymoma. Journal of the Neurological Sciences 34: 315

Mauro A 1961 Satellite cells of skeletal muscle fibres. Journal of Biophysical and Biochemical Cytology 9: 493

Mawatari S, Takagi A, Rowland L 1974 Adenyl cyclase in normal and pathologic human muscle. Archives of Neurology (Chicago) 30: 96

Medd S M, Fearnley I M, Walker J E, Palmer D N, Jolly R D 1991 Lysosomal storage of a mitochondrial protein in Batten's disease (ceroid lipofuscinosis) In: Gorrod J W, Albano O, Ferrari E, Papa S (eds) Molecular basis of neurological disorders and their treatment. Chapman and Hall, London

Meyers K R, Gilden D H, Rinaldi C F 1972 Periodic muscle weakness, normokalemia and tubular aggregates. Neurology (Minneapolis) 22: 269

Milhorat A T, Shafiq S A, Goldstone L 1966 Changes in muscle structure in dystrophic patients, carriers and normal siblings seen by electron microscopy: correlation with levels of serum creatine phosphokinase (CPK). Annals of the New York Academy of Sciences 138: 246

Millward D J 1980 Protein degradation in muscle and liver. In: Neuberger A, Vandeenen L L M (eds) Comprehensive biochemistry, vol 19B. Elsevier, Amsterdam, p 77

Mokri B, Engel A G 1975 Duchenne dystrophy: electron microscopic findings pointing to a basic or early abnormality in the plasma membrane of the muscle fibre. Neurology (Minneapolis) 24: 1111

Mortimore G E, Schworer C M 1977 Induction of autophagy by aminoacid deprivation. Nature 270: 73

Mrak R E, Saito A, Evans O B, Fleischer S 1982 Autophagic degradation in human skeletal muscle target fibers. Muscle and Nerve 5: 745

Neville H W E 1973 Ultrastructural changes in muscle disease. In: Dubowitz V, Brooke M H (eds) Muscle biopsy: a modern approach, W. B. Saunders, Philadelphia, p 383

Neville H E 1979 Ultrastructural changes in diseases of human muscle. In: Vinken P J, Bruyn G W (eds) Handbook of Clinical Neurology, vol 40. North Holland, Amsterdam, p 63

Neville H E, Brooke M H 1973 Central core fibres: structured and unstructured. In: Kakulas B (ed) Basic research in myology. Excerpta Medica, Amsterdam, p 497

Neville H E, Maunder-Sewry C A, McDougall J, Sewell R J, Dubowitz V 1979 Chloroquine-induced cytosomes with curvilinear profiles in muscle. Muscle and Nerve 2: 376

Neville H E, Ringel S P, Guggenheim M A, Wehling C A, Starcevich J M 1983 Ultrastructural and histochemical abnormalities of skeletal muscle in patients with chronic vitamin E deficiency. Neurology (Minneapolis) 33: 483

Nicholson L V B, Davison K, Johnson M A et al 1989 Dystrophin in skeletal muscle. II. Immunoreactivity in patients with Xp21 muscular dystrophy. Journal of the Neurological Sciences 94: 137

Nicholson L V B, Johnson M A, Gardner-Medwin D, Bhattacharya S, Harris J B 1990 Heterogeneity of dystrophin expression in patients with Duchenne and Becker muscular dystrophy. Acta Neuropathologica 80: 239

Nitkin R M, Smith M A, Magill C, Fallon J R, Yao Y-M M, Wallace B G, McMahan U J 1987 Identification of agrin, a synaptic organizing protein from Torpedo electric organ. Journal of Cell Biology 105: 2471

Nonaka I, Sugita H 1980 Muscle pathology in Duchenne dystrophy — with particular reference to 'opaque fibers'. Advances in Neurological Science 24(4): 727

Nonaka I, Sunohara N, Satoyoshi E, Teerasawa K, Yonemoto K 1985 Autosomal recessive distal muscular dystrophy: a comparative study with distal myopathy with rimmed vacuole formation. Annals of Neurology 17: 51

Nonaka I, Koga Y, Shikura K et al 1988 Muscle pathology in cytochrome c oxidase deficiency. Acta Neuropathologica 77: 152

Nonaka I, Ishiura S, Arahata K, Ishibashi-Ueda H, Maruyama T, Ii K 1989 Progression in nemaline myopathy. Acta Neuropathologica 78: 484

Oberc M A, Engel W K 1977 Ultrastructural localization of calcium in normal and abnormal skeletal muscle. Laboratory Investigation 36: 566

Odor D L, Patel A N, Pearce L A 1967 Familial hypokalemic periodic paralysis with permanent myopathy. A clinical and ultrastructural study. Journal of Neuropathology and Experimental Neurology 26: 98

Olson W, Engel W K, Walsh G O, Einaugler R 1972 Oculocraniosomatic neuromuscular disease with 'ragged-red' fibers. Archives of Neurology 26: 193

Osborn M, Goebel H H 1983 The cytoplasmic bodies in a congenital myopathy can be stained with antibodies to desmin, the muscle-specific intermediate filament protein. Acta Neuropathologica 62: 149

Pagès M, Echenne B, Pages A M, Dimeglio A, Sires A 1985 Multicore disease and Marfan's syndrome: a case report. European Neurology 24: 170

Palmucci L, Bertolotto A, Monga G, Andizzone G, Schiffer D 1978 Histochemical and ultrastructural findings in a case of centronuclear myopathy. European Neurology 17: 327

Panegyres P K, Papadimitriou J M, Hollingsworth P N, Armstrong J A, Kakulas B A 1990 Vesicular changes in the myopathies of AIDS. Ultrastructural observations and their relationship to zidovudine treatment. Journal of Neurology, Neurosurgery and Psychiatry 53: 649

Papadimitriou J M, Mastaglia F L 1982 Ultrastructural changes in muscle fibres in disease. Journal of Submicroscopic Cytology 14: 525

Payne C M, Curless R G 1976 Concentric laminated bodies — ultrastructural demonstration of fibre type specificity. Journal of the Neurological Sciences 29: 311

Pellegrino C, Franzini C 1963 An electron microscopic study of denervation atrophy in red and white skeletal muscle fibres. Journal of Cell Biology 17: 327

Peter J B, Worsfold M 1969 Muscular dystrophy and other myopathies: sarcotubular vesicles in early disease. Biochemical Medicine 2: 364

Pfeifer U 1978 Inhibition by insulin of the formation of autophagic vacuoles in rat liver. A morphometric approach to the kinetics of intracellular degradation by autophagy. Journal of Cell Biology 78: 152

Policard A, Collet A, Martin J C, Pregermain S 1961 Etudes inframicroscopique sur les processes d'alvéolite. Presse Médicale 69: 1709

Price D C, Pearson C M 1962 Selective actin filament and Z-band degeneration induced by plasmocid: an electron microscope study. Laboratory Investigation 11: 549

Price H M, Howes E L, Blumberg J M 1964 Ultrastructural alterations in skeletal muscle fibres injured by cold. II. Cells of the sarcolemmal tube: observations on discontinuous regeneration and myofibril formation. Laboratory Investigation 13: 1279

Prince F P, Hikida R S, Hagerman F C 1977 Muscle fiber types in women athletes and non-athletes. Pflügers Archive 371: 161

Rapola J Haltia M 1973 Cytoplasmic inclusions in the vermiform appendix and skeletal muscle in two types of so-called ceroid-lipofuscinosis: Brain 96: 833

Ray P N 1988 Duchenne muscular dystrophy: from gene mapping to the protein product. In: Disorders of the developing nervous system: Changing views on their origins, diagnosis and treatments. Alan Liss, New York, p 195

Reger J R, Craig A S 1968 Studies on the fine structure of muscle fibres and associated satellite cells in hypertrophic human deltoid muscles. Anatomical Record 162: 483

Revel J P 1962 The sarcoplasmic reticulum of the bat cricothyroid muscle. Journal of Cell Biology 12: 571

Rewcastle N B, Humphrey J G 1965 Vacuolar myopathy: clinical, histochemical and microscopic study. Archives of Neurology (Chicago) 12: 570

Reznik M 1972 Electron microscopy and histochemistry of regenerating skeletal muscle. Neurology (India) 10: 71

Reznik M 1973 Current concepts of skeletal muscle regeneration. In: Pearson C M, Mostofi F K (eds) The striated muscle. Williams and Wilkins, Baltimore, p 185

Ribas-Mujal D, Rivera-Pomar J M 1968 Biological significance of the early structural alterations in skeletal muscle fibers infected by Trichinella spiralis. Virchow Archiv 345: 154

Richards R B, Passmore I K 1989 Ultrastructural changes in skeletal muscle in ovine muscular dystrophy. Acta Neuropathologica 79: 168

Rose A L, Walton J N, Pearce G W 1967 Polymyositis: an ultramicroscopic study of muscle biopsy material. Journal of the Neurological Sciences 5: 457

Rosenberg N L, Neville H E, Ringel S P 1985 Tubular aggregates. Their association with neuromuscular diseases, including the syndrome of myalgias/cramps. Archives of Neurology 42: 973

Rosner M C, Golomb H M 1980 Ribosome-lamella complex in hairy cell leukemia. Ultrastructure and distribution. Laboratory Investigation 42: 236

Rothman J E, Fine R E 1980 Coated vesicles transport newly synthesized membrane glycoproteins from endoplasmic reticulum to plasma membrane in two successive stages. Proceedings of the National Academy of Sciences 77: 780

Roullet E, Fardeau M, Collin H, Marteau R 1985 Myopathie avec agrégates tubulaires. Étude clinique biologique et histologique de deux cas. Revue Neurologique 141: 655

Rowland J B, Mastaglia F L, Hainsworth D, Kakulas B A 1969 Clinical and pathological aspects of a fatal case of Mulga (*Pseudechis australis*) snakebite. Medical Journal of Australia 1: 226

Rubin E, Katz A M, Lieber C S, Stein E P, Purzkin S 1976 Muscle damage produced by chronic alcohol consumption. American Journal of Pathology 83: 499

Sahashi K, Mizuno Y, Ibi T, Sobue G 1982 A case of mitochondrial myopathy with cylindrical spirals. Clinical Neurology (Tokyo) 22: 244

Saltin B, Nazar K, Costil D L, Stein E, Jansson E, Essen B, Gollnick P 1976 The nature of the training response; peripheral and central adaptations to one-legged exercise. Acta Physiologica Scandinavica 96: 289

Samaha F J, Gergely J 1969 Biochemical abnormalities of the sarcoplasmic reticulum in muscular dystrophy. New England Journal of Medicine 280: 184

Sanes J R, Marshall L M, McMahan U K 1978 Reinnervation of muscle fiber basal lamina after removal of muscle fibers. Journal of Cell Biology 78: 176

Santa T 1969 Fine structure of the human skeletal muscle in myopathy. Archives of Neurology (Chicago) 20: 479

Sarnat H 1990 Myotubular myopathy: arrest of morphogenesis of myofibres associated with persistence of fetal vimentin and desmin. Canadian Journal of Neurological Sciences 17: 109

Sarnat H B, Silbert S W 1976 Maturational arrest of fetal muscle in neonatal myotonic dystrophy. Archives of Neurology (Chicago) 33: 466

Sato T, Wilkes D L, Peters H A, Reese H H, Chou S M 1971 Chronic polymyositis and myxovirus-like inclusions. Archives of Neurology (Chicago) 24: 409

Schiaffino S, Hanzlikova V 1972 Studies on the effect of denervation in developing muscle. II. The lysosomal system. Journal of Ultrastructure Research 39: 1

Schmalbruch H 1968 Lyse und Regeneration von Fibrillen in der normalen menschlichen Skelettmuskulatur. Virchows Archiv fur pathologischen Anatomie und Physiologie 344: 159

Schmalbruch H 1975 Segmental fibre breakdown and defects of the plasmalemma in diseased human muscles. Acta Neuropathologica 33: 129

Schmalbruch H 1984 Regenerated muscle fibre in Duchenne muscular dystrophy: a serial section study. Neurology (Cleveland) 34: 60

Schmitt H, Volk B 1975 The relationship between target, targetoid, and targetoid/core fibers in severe neurogenic muscular atrophy. Journal of Neurology 210: 167

Schochet S S, Lampert P W 1978 Diagnostic electron microscopy of skeletal muscle. In: Trump B F, Jones R T (eds) Diagnostic electron microscopy. John Wiley, New York, p 209

Schochet S S, McCormick W F 1973 Polymyositis with intranuclear inclusions. Archives of Neurology (Chicago) 28: 280

Schochet S S, Zellweger H, Ionasescu V, McCormick W F 1972 Centronuclear myopathy: disease entity or a syndrome? Journal of the Neurological Sciences 16: 215

Schollmeyer J V, Goll D, Stromer M H, Dayton W, Singh I, Robson R M 1974 Studies on the composition of the Z disk. Journal of Cell Biology 63: 303

Schotland D L 1969 An electron microscopic study of target fibers, target-like fibers and related abnormalities in human muscle. Journal of Neuropathology and Experimental Neurology 28: 214

Schotland D L 1970 An electron microscopic investigation of myotonic dystrophy. Journal of Neuropathology and Experimental Neurology 29: 241

Schotland D L, Bonilla E, Wakayama Y 1981 Application of freeze–fracture technique to the study of human neuromuscular disease. Muscle and Nerve 3: 21

Schröder J M, Adams R D 1968 The ultrastructural morphology of the muscle fiber in myotonic dystrophy. Acta Neuropathologica 10: 128

Schröder J M, Becker P E 1972 Anomalien des T-systems and der sarkoplasmatischen Reticulums bei der Myotonie, paramyotonie und Adynamie. Virchows Archiv fur pathologischen Anatomie und Physiologie 357: 319

Schutta H S, Kelly A M, Zacks S I 1969 Necrosis and regeneration of muscle in paroxysmal and idiopathic myoglobinuria: electron miscroscopic observations. Brain 92: 191

Schwartz W N, Bird J W C 1977 Degradation of myofibrillar proteins by cathepsins B and D. Biochemical Journal 167: 811

Schwartz M S, Sargent M, Swash M 1976 Longitudinal fibre splitting in neurogenic muscle disorders — its relation to the pathogenesis of 'myopathic' change. Brain 99: 617

Sewry C A 1985 Ultrastructural changes in diseased muscle. In: Dubowitz V, Muscle Biopsy. A practical approach. Baillière Tindall, London, p 129

Shafiq S A, Gorycki M A, Goldstone L, Milhorat A T 1966 Fine structure of fiber types in normal human muscle. Anatomical Record 156: 283

Shafiq S A, Milhorat A T, Goldstone M A 1967a An electron microscopic study of muscle degeneration and vascular changes in polymyositis. Journal of Pathology and Bacteriology 94: 139

Shafiq S A, Milhorat A T, Gorycki M A 1967b Fine structure of human muscle in neurogenic atrophy. Neurology (Minneapolis) 17: 934

Shafiq S A, Dubowitz V, Peterson H De C, Milhorat A T 1967c Nemaline myopathy: a report of a fatal case with histochemical and light microscopic studies. Brain 90: 817

Shafiq S A, Gorycki M A, Asiedu S A, Milhorat A T 1969 Tenotomy. Effects on the fine structure of the soleus of the rat. Archives of Neurology (Chicago) 20: 625

Sher J H, Shafiq S A, Schutta H S 1979 Acute myopathy with selective lysis of myosin filaments. Neurology (Minneapolis) 29: 100

Shy G M, Magee K R 1956 A new congenital non-progressive myopathy. Brain 81: 461

Shy G M, Engel W K, Somers J E, Wanko T 1963 Nemaline myopathy. A new congenital myopathy. Brain 86: 793

Slater C R, Allen E G 1985 Acetycholine receptor distribution on regenerating mammalian muscle fibers at sites of mature and developing nerve-muscle junctions. Journal of Physiology (Paris) 80: 238

Snow M H 1973 Metabolic activity during the degenerative and early regenerative stages of minced skeletal muscle. Anatomical Record 176: 185

Snow M H 1977 Myogenic cell formation in regenerating rat skeletal muscle injured by mincing. II. An autoradiographic study. Anatomical Record 188: 201

Snow M H 1978 An autoradiographic study of satellite cell differentiation into regenerating myotubes following transplantation of muscles in young rats. Cell and Tissue Research 186: 535

Somlyo A V, Gonzalez-Serratos H, Shuman H, McClennan G, Somlyo A P 1981 Calcium release and ionic changes in the sarcoplasmic reticulum of tetanized muscle — an electron probe study. Journal of Cell Biology 90: 577

Song S K, Shimada N, Anderson P J 1963 Orthogonal diameters in the analysis of muscle fibre size and form. Nature 200: 1220

Spiro A J, Shy G M, Gonatas N K 1966 Myotubular myopathy. Persistence of fetal muscle in an adolescent boy. Archives of Neurology (Chicago) 14: 1

Staron R S, Hikida R S, Murray T F, Hagerman F C, Hagerman M T 1989 Lipid depletion and repletion in skeletal muscle following a marathon. Journal of the Neurological Sciences 94: 29

Stromer M H, Tabatabai L B, Robson R M, Goll D E, Zeece M G 1976 Nemaline myopathy, an integrated study: selective extraction. Experimental Neurology 50: 402

Swash M, Schwartz M S 1981 Familial multicore disease with focal loss of cross-striations and ophthalmoplegia. Journal of the Neurological Sciences 52: 1

Swash M, Schwartz M S, Sargeant M K 1978 Pathogenesis of longitudinal splitting of muscle fibres in neurogenic disorders and in polymyositis. Neuropathology and Applied Neurobiology 4: 99

Takagi A, Schotland D L, Rowland L P 1973 Sarcoplasmic reticulum in Duchenne muscular dystrophy. Archives of Neurology (Chicago) 28: 380

Telerman-Toppet N, Gerrard J M, Coers C 1973 Central core disease: a study of clinically unaffected muscle. Journal of the Neurological Sciences 19: 207

Teräväinen H, Makitie J 1977 Striated muscle ultrastructure in intermittent claudication. Archives of Pathology and Laboratory Medicine 101: 230

Thiebaut F, Gruner J E, Isch F, Isch-Treussard C 1963 Corrélations cliniques, electriques et histologiques en pathologie amusculaire. Revue neurologique 108: 575

Thornell L E, Eriksson A, Edström L 1983 Intermediate filaments in human myopathies. In: Dowben R M, Shay J W (eds) Cell and muscle motility, vol 4. Plenum, New York, p 85

Toga M, Berard-Badier M, Gambarelli D, Pinsard N 1970 Ultrastructure des lésions neuromusculaires dans un cas de dystrophie neuroaxonale infantile ou maladie de Seitelberger. Communication to IIme Journées Internationales de Pathologie Neuromusculaire, Marseille

Tomé FMS, Fardeau M 1973 'Fingerprint inclusions' in muscle fibres in dystrophia myotonica. Acta Neuropathologica 24: 62

Tomé F M S, Fardeau M Nuclear inclusions in oculopharyngeal dystrophy. Acta Neuropathologica 49: 85

Tomé F M S, Fardeau M 1986 Nuclear changes in muscle disorders. Methods and achievements in experimental pathology 12: 261

Tomé F M S, Mair W G P 1970 Electron microscopical and histochemical studies of muscle in a case of a neuropathy with target fibres and laminar cytoplasmic structures. Proceedings of the 6th International Congress of Neuropathology, Masson, Paris, p 1070

Tomonaga M, Sluga E 1969 Zur ultrastruktur der 'target-fasern'. Virchows Archiv für pathologischen Anatomie und Physiologie 348: 89

Trupin G L, Hsu L 1979 The identification of myogenic cells in regenerating skeletal muscle. Developmental Biology 68: 72

Vracko R, Benditt E P 1972 Basal lamina: the scaffold for orderly cell replacement. Observations on regeneration of injured skeletal muscle fibers and capillaries. Journal of Cell Biology 55: 406

Wakayama Y, Okayasu H, Shibuya S, Kumagai T 1984 Duchenne dystrophy: reduced density of orthogonal array sub unit particles in muscle plasma membrane. Neurology (Cleveland) 34: 313

Wakayama Y, Jimi T, Misngi N, Kumagai T, Miyake S, Shibuya S, Miike T 1989 Dystrophin immunostaining and freeze fracture studies of muscles of patients with early stage amyotrophic lateral sclerosis and Duchenne muscular dystrophy. Journal of the Neurological Sciences 91: 191

Watkins S C, Cullen M J 1985 Histochemical fibre typing and ultrastructure of the small fibres in Duchenne muscular dystrophy. Neuropathology and Applied Neurobiology 11: 447

Watkins S C, Hoffman E P, Slayter H S, Kunkel L M 1988 Immunoelectron microscopic localization of dystrophin in myofibers. Nature 333: 863

Webster C, Silverstein L, Hays A P, Blau H M 1988 Fast muscle fibers are preferentially affected in Duchenne muscular dystrophy. Cell 52: 503

Wood D S, Sorenson M M, Eastwood A B, Charash W E, Reuben J P 1978 Duchenne dystrophy: abnormal generation of tension and Ca regulation in single skinned fibers. Neurology (Minneapolis) 28: 447

Worton R G, Burghes A H M 1988 Molecular genetics of Duchenne and Becker muscular dystrophy. International Review of Neurobiology 29: 1

Worton R G, Gillard E F 1990 Duchenne muscular dystrophy. In: Brosius J, Fremeau R (eds) Molecular genetic approaches to neuropsychiatric disease. Academic Press, San Diego (in press)

Wroblewski R, Nordemar R 1975 Ultrastructural and histochemical studies of muscle in rheumatoid arthritis.

Scandinavian Journal of Rheumatology 4: 197

Wrogeman K, Pena S D J 1976 Mitochondrial calcium overload: a general mechanism for cell necrosis in muscle diseases. Lancet i: 672

Wyatt R B, Schochet S S, McCormick W F 1970 Rhabdomyoma: light and electron microscopic study of a case with intranuclear inclusions. Archives of Otalaryngology 92: 32

Yamaguchi M, Robson R M, Stromer M H, Dahl D S, Oda T 1978 Actin filaments form the backbone of nemaline myopathy rods. Nature 271: 265

Yarom R, Reches A 1980 Thick filament degeneration in a case of acute quadriplegia. Journal of the Neurological Sciences 45: 13

Yarom R, Shapira Y 1977 Myosin degeneration in a congenital myopathy. Archives of Neurology (Chicago) 34: 114

Yoshioka M, Okuda R 1977 Human skeletal muscle fibers in normal and pathological states: freeze–etch observations. Journal of Electronmicroscopy (Tokyo) 26: 103

Yunis E J, Samaha F J 1971 Inclusion body myositis. Laboratory Investigation 25: 240

Zeece M G, Katoh K 1989 Cathepsin D and its effects on myofibrillar proteins: a review. Journal of Food Biochemistry 13: 157

Zierler K L 1958 Muscle membrane as a dynamic structure and its permeability to aldolase. Annals of the New York Academy of Sciences 75: 227

Zubrzycka-Gaarn E E, Bulman D E, et al 1988 The Duchenne muscular dystrophy gene product is localized in sarcolemma of human skeletal muscle. Nature 333: 466

4. Immunopathology of muscle

Robert P. Lisak

INTRODUCTION

Abnormalities of the immune system are an important cause or contributing factor to diseases of skeletal muscle. In some instances immune mechanisms are directly involved in the production of pathological changes and/or changes in function in muscle and at the neuromuscular junction. Abnormalities in immunoregulation and in genetic control of the immune system are important in the pathogenesis and aetiology of these disorders since they result from persistence of what would ordinarily be a normal immunological mechanism or the perversion of a normal immune mechanism so that it becomes directed against self-antigens. In addition, changes in immune system function such as the development of broad-based or polyclonal immunodeficiency involving one or more arms of the immune system may lead to immune-mediated disorders or infections that affect skeletal muscle or the neuromuscular junction. Such immune deficiency may result from hereditary or congenital diseases or may often be acquired through drug therapy, other therapeutic interventions, or as a result of infections of the immune system itself.

The immune system is an extremely complex system consisting of multiple bone marrow-derived cell types which interact in a series of regulatory circuits; some of these are stimulatory and others inhibit or down-regulate immune functions. In addition, the immune system as a whole and its component parts interact in multiple ways with other organ systems and tissues both influencing those other tissues and systems and being in turn influenced by them. Indeed, only the nervous system is more complex. Our increased under-

standing of the normal functions of the immune system has enabled us to develop a better understanding of certain diseases of the neuromuscular junction and skeletal muscle. However, it is this complexity that has prevented us from answering many of the questions about these disorders.

IMMUNOPATHOLOGICAL REACTIONS

The immune system is capable of a great variety of immunological reactions which are designed to protect the host from both external and internal threats. However, at times these reactions may become harmful by being directed at self-antigens (autoimmunity), by being excessive, or prolonged (Coombs & Gell 1968). On other occasions immune-mediated injury to the organism occurs as part of a normal protective immune response, such as an attempt to eliminate an infectious agent that concomitantly causes a small amount of damage to the cells or tissue harbouring the agent (e.g. a small granulomatous lesion from healed tuberculosis or histoplasmosis), or major clinically significant damage to an organ (e.g. the liver in schistosomiasis) or critical cells (e.g. certain viral encephalitides). Therefore, when these immune reactions become harmful to the host they are generally termed immunopathological. The reasons that some of these harmful reactions occur, persist or recur relate to abnormalities in immunological control which in turn are heavily influenced by multiple genes involved in the immune system (see below) as well as by environmental factors.

When immunopathological reactions were first classified, our view of the immune system, and of its interactions with other organ systems, was simpler. Thus, the original four types of immuno-pathological reactions have been expanded and/or subclassifications of the original four mechanisms have been defined (Lisak 1988). One such scheme is presented in Table 4.1.

It is important to point out that one or more mechanisms may be involved in any immuno-pathologically mediated disease. Moreover, more than one antigen might be the target of an immunological autoimmune response in the development of a clinical-pathological entity.

IMMUNOREGULATION AND MECHANISMS OF MAINTAINING TOLERANCE

The presence of an autoimmune disease or per-sistence of any immunopathological reaction is abnormal and suggests that there has been a failure in one or more parts of the very elaborate regula-tory mechanisms and interactions that are part of a normal immune response. Such a failure in immunoregulation would be causative or per-missive for the immunopathological reaction since the reactions themselves are not inherently abnormal. There are several possible mechanisms that may be involved in preventing a true auto-immune reaction, and there is evidence to support each of these and data to refute each of these theories as well. Among the possible mechanisms preventing the emergence of an antibody (B-cell) or cell-mediated (T-cell) autoimmune reaction are: (i) clonal deletion (or abortion) (Burnet 1959); (ii) suppressor T-cells (antigen-specific or non-specific suppressor T-cells) (Miller & Schwartz 1982); (iii) sequestration of self antigens; (iv) idiotype net-works (Jerne 1974); and (v) antigen-induced antigen-specific tolerance or anergy (Nossal 1983, Cohen & Epstein 1978, Feldman et al 1985). More than one explanation for the loss of tolerance and

Table 4.1 Immunopathological reactions

Immunopathologic mechanism	Normal function	Diseases
Reaginic	Killing of parasites	Anaphylaxis, allergic respiratory diseases
Antibody to self-antigens		
Direct cytotoxic	Extracellular infections	EAMG; MG; certain haemolytic anaemias
Alteration of membranes and cell receptors	Infections	
(a) sequestration via cell surface activation		Certain haemolytic anemias; ITP
(b) block of ligand binding		EAMG, MG, diabetes and acanthocytosis secondary to antibodies to insulin receptor
(c) receptor or membrane component down-regulation		EAMG; MG; LEMS
(d) receptor stimulation		Autoimmune hyperthyroidism; anti-insulin receptor antibodies
Immune complex deposition	Antigen clearance	Serum sickness; SLE nephritis, rare haemolytic anaemias, some drug thrombocytopenias, PAN, childhood DM
Cell-mediated reactions		
T-cell-mediated		
(a) delayed hypersensitivity	Infections with obligate intracellular organisms, fungi	EAE, EAN, ADEM*
(b) T-cell cytotoxic	(?) Tumour necrosis, infections-viral (intracellular organisms)	Certain forms of hepatitis, GVH, allograft rejection
ADCC	(?) Infections, tumour destruction, killing of multicellular organisms (parasites)	Allograft rejection
NK-cell reactions	(?) tumour destruction, infections	??

EAMG: experimental autoimmune myasthenia gravis; MG: myasthenia gravis; LEMS: Lambert–Eaton myasthenic syndrome; ITP: idiopathic thrombocytopenic purpura; EAE: experimental allergic encephalomyelitis; EAN: experimental allergic neuritis; Childhood DM: childhood onset dermatomyositis; ADEM: acute disseminated encephalomyelitis; GVH: graft-versus-host reaction; SLE: systemic lupus erythematosus; PAN: polyartertitis nodosa; ADCC:antibody-dependent cell-mediated cytotoxicity; NK: natural killer cell.
* Highly likely.

the emergence of an immunopathological reaction may be correct.

1. It was originally proposed (Burnet 1959) that antigens that are 'seen' by the immune system during lymphocyte ontogeny were not viewed as foreign and that the immune system could not therefore react to these self-antigens. This tolerance resulted from actual deletion or inactivation of these autoreactive clones. It is quite clear, however, that normal subjects frequently have low-titre autoantibodies to some self-antigens and can be shown to have autoantibody-producing cells for some autoantigens. Moreover, T-cells have been recovered from normal individuals that are specific for autoantigens. Many of these antigens are known to produce autoimmune diseases when used to sensitize experimental animals (Burns et al 1983). Autoantigen-specific T-cell lines and clones passively transfer the appropriate autoimmune disease to naive experimental animals.

2. Suppressor cells found among one or more subpopulations of T-lymphocytes can be shown to suppress the immune response of other T-cells and B-cells. If these cells fail to function, are deficient in number, or if there is excessive antigen-specific or antigen-non-specific help that is not in turn suppressed, self-reactive T- and/or B-cells could emerge. B-cells that produce auto-antibodies (primarily IgM and some IgG) are a part of the normal repertoire early in life and failure to suppress these may lead to antibody-mediated autoimmune disease. Expansion of an autoimmune B-cell clone secondary to somatic mutation with failure to suppress or eliminate these cells would also lead to an antibody-mediated autoimmune disease.

3. Jerne (1974) suggested that the immune system is controlled in part by interactions between antibody molecules in which an antibody reactive to an antigen (an idiotype) could itself normally be an antigen for another antibody molecule (an anti-idiotype antibody or anti-antibody). This so-called idiotypic network in which each immunoglobulin molecule can itself react with another immunoglobulin would help maintain balance in the immune system. A failure in this network, either because of the lack of a protective antibody (Zanetti 1985) or if the anti-idiotypic antibody reacts to a so-called internal image of the antigen-binding site which allows it to react with the self-antigen, could lead to an unchecked autoimmune response. It has also been reported that T- and B-cells themselves are also influenced by such idiotypic networks. While there is a good deal of evidence to support the concept of the idiotypic network, especially in experimental protocols, there is evidence that there are limits to this network and it may only become operative when immunoglobulin-producing cells are activated (Bona & Pernis 1984).

4. If an autoantigen is sequestrated from the developing immune system, or the immune system is exposed to such an antigen in the absence of major histocompatibility complex (MHC) antigens, the immune system may not recognize the antigen as 'self' (Cowing 1985). If exposed to the antigen later, especially in the context of MHC antigens, an autoimmune response to the 'new' antigen might result. Another possible scenario is that an immune response is induced by exposure to an exogenous substance which is antigenically similar to one of the host's own components. An immune response to this foreign substance would give rise to autoreactive clones and a subsequent autoimmune response may result. This is called molecular mimicry (Oldstone et al 1986).

5. The exposure of antigen-specific cells, in this case autoantigen-specific cells to the autoantigen, in the absence of MHC molecules, results in tolerance or anergy of these antigen-specific cells.

IMMUNOGENETICS

The immune response is strongly influenced by multiple allelic systems which together control immune responsiveness and undoubtedly have a major role in the development or lack of development of immunopathological reactions. These genes are important in both the normal and abnormal immune response of the organism. Perhaps the best known and most widely studied are the several alleles of the major histocompatibility complex (MHC). MHC molecules control the interactions of cells of the immune system. The reaction of a T-cell with a given antigen requires co-recognition of the antigen with MHC type I molecules (HLA A,B, C) for a cytotoxic T-cell and type II molecules (HLA-DR and DQ, often called Ia in humans) for a helper T-cell. These MHC molecules are highly polymorphic and it is quite clear that there are yet many more of these molecules to be discovered and characterized (Hansen & Sachs 1989, Robinson & Kindt 1989). Several other important genes map to the region of the MHC including those coding for components of the complement system (Alper 1981).

A second level of control is exercised by the genes that code for the protein chains of the T-cell receptor molecule itself (Acuto & Reinherz 1985, Hedrick 1989). Each mature T-cell has a receptor that recognizes its specific antigen and the chains of the receptor are controlled by different genes.

The heavy and light chains of individual immunoglobulin molecules are also controlled by different genes. For both the T-cell receptor and immunoglobulin, somatic recombinations of multiple gene segments result in the formation of a functional gene which codes for the variable and constant regions of the protein chains (Leder 1983, Tonegawa 1983).

The importance of these genes in determining the response of the immune system to specific antigens explains the intense interest in determining associations of various immunological diseases with MHC types, Gm allotypes and, more recently, with genes controlling the T-cell receptor. The increased familial incidence of certain immunopathologically mediated diseases and the higher association of a familial tendency towards immunopathologically mediated diseases in general may be in large part explained by the influence of these multiple allelic systems. The importance and complexity of each of these systems in controlling the normal and abnormal immune response may also explain why simple single-gene explanations have not provided an answer as to the reason why some patients get certain immunological diseases.

IMMUNODEFICIENCY

Failure of one or more components of the immune system is considered as immunodeficiency. This may be secondary or primary in nature and may vary from severe, leading to death, to asymptomatic — such as is seen in many individuals who have very low levels of IgA. Antigen-specific cells such as B- and T-cells may be involved separately or together. Accessory cells or cells that are not involved in antigen-specific responses, such as monocyte/macrophages or other phagocytic cells (PMNs), may be deficient in number or function. Genetically determined defects in proteins of the complement system can also result in immunodeficiency and have been reported in association with autoimmune/immunopathological disorders. In infection with human immunodeficiency virus (HIV) the immunodeficiency that ultimately results from infection of $CD4^+$ cells leads to additional opportunistic infections with other microorganisms and an increased incidence of tumours as is also seen with other severe inherited or acquired immunodeficiencies. Early in the course of infection however, there may actually be a broad-based polyclonal increase in immune function including autoantibodies and immunopathologically mediated disorders.

ANTIGENS OF SKELETAL MUSCLE AND THE NEUROMUSCULAR JUNCTION

Potentially almost any protein, lipid or carbohydrate determinant found on the surface, within the cytoplasm or within the nucleus of skeletal muscle fibres could be antigenic. The same can be said for the nerve terminal side of the neuromuscular junction. Indeed, antisera and monoclonal antibodies are routinely produced experimentally as probes to study the structure and function of muscle, nerve and the neuromuscular junction. Of interest in discussions of autoimmunity and immunopathologically mediated disorders are those which are antigenic targets in immunological diseases, either induced or naturally occurring.

The serum from patients with myasthenia gravis has been reported to produce a variety of patterns of immunofluorescent staining when incubated with skeletal muscle (Fig. 4.1). The serum of some patients reacts with more than one antigen and that of others with one antigen only based on the immunocytological pattern (Penn et al 1971, Lisak & Barchi 1982, Williams & Lennon 1986,

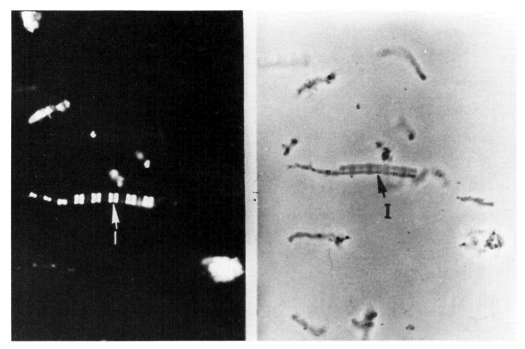

Fig. 4.1 Immunofluorescent demonstration of antistriational antibodies in the serum of a patient with myasthaenia gravis. Skeletal muscle fibres are incubated with a dilution of the patient's serum and then with fluorescein isothiocyanate (FITC)-labelled rabbit antibody to human immunoglobulins. The left panel is viewed with fluorescent optics and the right panel with light optics. The 'I' band (arrow) is labelled with this particular serum. (Courtesy of Dr Donald Schotland)

Zimmerman & Weiss 1987). Myosin, actin and other proteins have also been shown to react with some of these sera. Aarli and his colleagues (Aarli et al 1981) have reported that sera from a large number of patients with myasthenia gravis and thymoma react with a citric acid extract of muscle. More recently he has reported that many of these patients' sera react with titin, a protein with a very high molecular weight (>500 kDa) (Aarli, personal communication).

A second group of antigens of importance are those of the MHC. Although early data suggested that transplantation antigens could be found on normal muscle it is now clear that if they are present in the normal situation they are present in very low levels (Isenberg et al 1986, Karpati et al 1988, McDouall et al 1989, Honda & Rostami 1989). Class II MHC antigens are not found on normal muscles and are restricted in distribution in the normal state to B-cells and some cells of the monocyte/macrophage lineage. Immunocytological studies of normal muscle using monoclonal anti-

bodies directed at non-polymorphic determinants of class I and class II MHC antigens show some low level of activity which is basically limited to non-muscle elements. Recently Honda and Rostami (1989) have reported that rat myoblasts cultured in the absence of neuronal influence show class I but not class II MHC antigens. Hohlfeld and Engel (1990) have likewise detected MHC class I but not class II on human myoblasts. As the rat cells mature into multinucleated myotubes class I expression is lost. Incubation of these class I-negative myotubes with supernatants from cultures of activated inflammatory cells and interferon could induce class I expression on these fibres. Thus such fibres could be the target of a cytotoxic T-cell-specific autoimmune or anti-viral reaction in which a viral antigen is seen by viral antigen-specific cytotoxic T-cells in the presence of MHC class I antigens. Of interest is that at least in vitro treatment of the myoblast cultures with anti-MHC class I antibodies inhibited the maturation of the myoblasts into myotubes suggesting

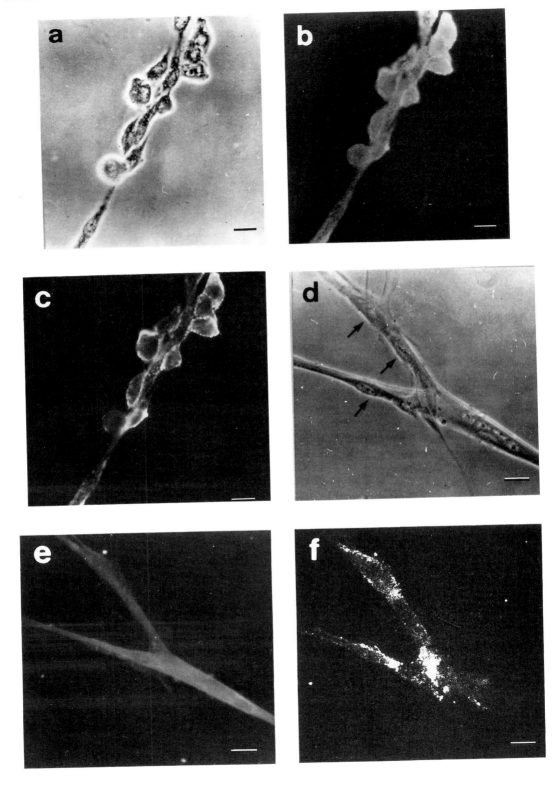

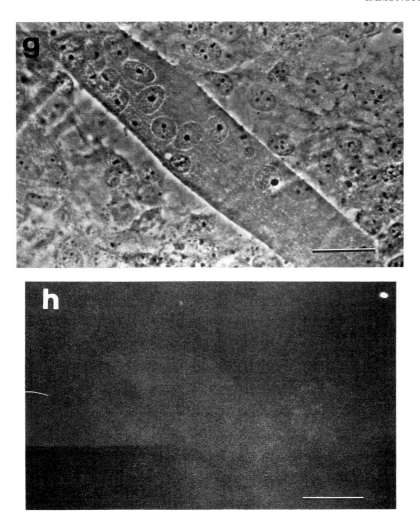

Fig. 4.2 Immunofluorescent staining of embryonic rat muscle cultures at different stages of myogenesis with rhodamine-conjugated anti-skeletal muscle myosin antibody (MY-32) and FITC-conjugated anti-rat class I antibody (OX18). (a–c) Cluster of myoblasts aligned for fusion, 2-day culture. (a) Phase-contrast. (b and c) Stained with MY-32(b) and OX18(c), viewed with rhodamine and FITC optics, respectively. (d–f) Myoblasts (arrows) apposed to a young myotube, 3-day culture. (d) Phase-contrast. (e and f) Stained with MY-32 (e) and OX18(f). Class I antigens were expressed on the myoblasts but were undetectable on the surface of a newly formed myotube. (g and h) Multinucleate myotube, 10-day culture. (g) Phase-contrast. (h) Negative OX18 staining. Bars = 30 μm. (From Honda & Rostami 1989)

that there was an important physiological developmental function to MHC class I in this system (Fig. 4.2, 4.3). Induction of MHC class I can be seen in regeneration after muscle necrosis (Fig. 4.4) even when the necrosis is not induced by an immune reaction; however, it may be the effect of soluble substances secreted by the phagocytic/inflammatory cells near the necrotic muscle fibres. Honda and Rostami (1989) were unable to induce

MHC class II antigens on rat myotubes with γ-interferon, whereas Hohlfeld and Engel (1990) were able to induce MHC class II molecules on human myoblasts. The reasons for this difference are as yet not known. All of this will need to be kept in mind when considering muscle transplantation as a potential form of therapy for degenerative muscle disorders.

The nicotinic acetylcholine receptor at the post-

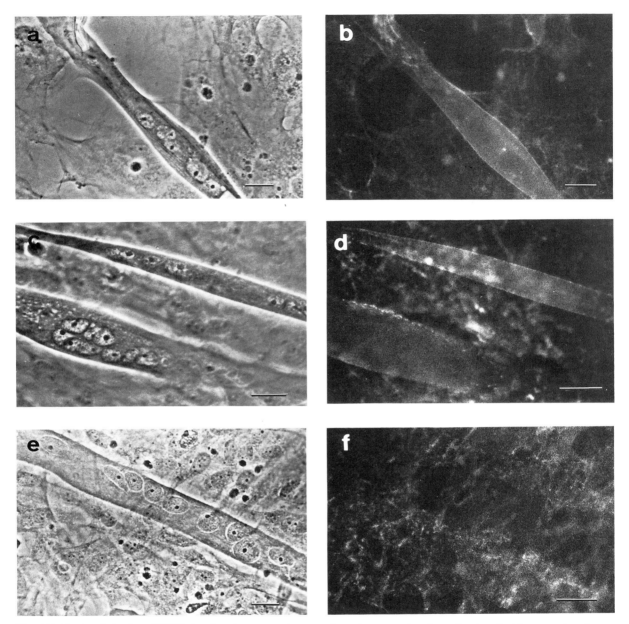

Fig. 4.3 In vitro induction of MHC class I antigen expression on embyronic rat muscle cultures incubated with supernatant from con A-activated spleen cells or rat recombinant IFN-γ. (a) Phase-contrast view of the culture treated with 25% con A supernatant for 3 days. (b) The same field stained with anti-class I antibody OX18. (c and d) Phase-contrast and OX18 staining with fluorescein optics, respectively. The cells were incubated with IFN-γ at 100 units/ml for 24 h. (e and f) Phase-contrast and fluorescein (anti-rat Ia antibody, OX6) optics, respectively. The culture was incubated with IFN-γ at 100 units/ml for 5 days. Note negative staining for class II MHC antigens on the multinucleate myotube. Flat, irregular-shaped cells (presumably fibroblasts) were stained with OX18 (b and c) and OX6 (f) antibodies. Bars = 20 μm. (From Honda & Rostami 1989)

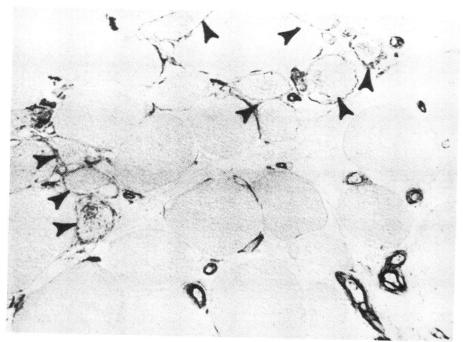

Fig. 4.4 Presence of class I MHC antigens on muscle in Duchenne muscular dystrophy. Monoclonal antibody to MHC class I is demonstrated (employing biotinylated anti-mouse IgG and vector ABC avidin–peroxidase complex) binding to sarcolemma and sarcoplasmic reticulum of regenerating fibres (arrowheads) and blood vessels. Non-regenerating fibres do not bear MHC class I molecules. ×280. (From Karpati et al 1988)

synaptic muscle membrane is the most carefully studied muscle antigen since it is the target of an immune response in myasthenia gravis and in experimental autoimmune myasthenia gravis. The junctional receptor consists of five peptide chains in the configuration $\alpha_2\beta\epsilon\delta$ (Conti-Tronconi & Raftery 1983, Changeux et al 1984, Mishina et al 1984). Extra-junctional receptor has a substitution of a γ chain for the ϵ chain. The genes have been isolated and sequenced, and the protein has been synthesized for mouse and human AChR. There is a considerable amount of sequence homology between the four types of peptide chains. The sequences for the α chain are known for several species, including man. The protein has an extracellular transmembrane and an intra-cytoplasmic portion. There is one ligand binding site on each α-chain. The protein itself is an ion channel which changes its configuration upon interaction with the ligand (ACh) to allow entry of sodium and exit of potassium ions. There is no involvement of a second messenger (Schwartz

1985). Antibodies to all the peptide chains have been reported in the serum of patients with myasthenia gravis. In patients with myasthenia gravis, in animals with experimental autoimmune myasthenia gravis and when monoclonal antibodies to AChR are raised in rodents, much of the antibody response is directed against sequences of the chain (Lennon & Lambert 1980, Tzartos & Lindstrom 1980, Tzartos et al 1982, Ashizawa & Appel 1985, Vincent et al 1987). Using inhibition of human myasthenic serum binding to AChR by monoclonal antibodies it has been suggested that much of the antibody response is to a region of the α-chain which has been called the major immunogenic region (MIR) (Tzartos et al 1982). Monoclonal antibodies specific for this region are particularly effective in passively transferring a chronic neuromuscular block to naive animals. Monoclonal antibodies to the ligand (ACh or α-bungarotoxin) binding site transfer a rapidly evolving neuromuscular block in avian species (Gomez & Richman 1983). Recently, however, the concept of an MIR for patients has been challenged (Lennon & Griesman 1989). It has also been hypothesized that some patients with acquired autoimmune myasthenia gravis whose serum does not react to AChR might have an antibody response to an as yet uncharacterized component of the post-synaptic membrane (Mossman et al 1985). Data has now been presented suggesting that some of these 'antibody-negative' patients with myasthenia as well as some antibody-positive myasthenics have an IgM antibody directed at a portion of the AChR within the channel itself (Yamamoto et al 1990).

Serum from some patients with polymyositis and dermatomyositis as well as patients with the collagen-vascular (connective tissue) diseases have antibodies to several different nuclear and cytoplasmic components of muscle and other cells. Some of these have now been well characterized. Whether these antibodies could be pathogenic, since they are not directed at cell surface components, or whether they are markers of disease is not known (Lisak 1988). These are discussed later in this chapter and outlined in Table 4.2.

It has also been possible to immunize animals to peripheral nerve and nerve terminals and obtain antibodies to presynaptic components, but these sensitized animals fail to develop disease reproducibly. However, it is now clear that serum of patients with the Lambert–Eaton myasthenic syndrome, with or without associated small cell carcinoma, have an antibody to a presynaptic component and on the basis of physiological studies

the antigen of Lambert–Eaton syndrome has been identified as a voltage-gated calcium channel (Vincent et al 1989). Whether different patients have antibodies to different epitopes of the channel is not as yet known (Lennon & Lambert 1990). The channel is also present on small cell (oat cell) tumours and it has been suggested that these tumours arise from cells of neural crest origin.

DISEASES OF MUSCLE AND NEUROMUSCULAR JUNCTION: IMMUNOPATHOLOGY AND IMMUNOLOGY

Polymyositis

There is a large number of disorders associated with inflammation of skeletal muscle; these disorders are therefore classified as 'inflammatory myopathies'. Some of these, such as parasitic infections, are of known aetiology, and certainly the immune system is involved in the host defense and perhaps contributes to the tissue damage in these disorders. Others, such as granulomatous diseases — especially sarcoid — are of unknown aetiology. For this chapter, however, the discussion will be limited to a group of inflammatory disorders of unknown aetiology with certain clinical and laboratory similarities which are termed polymyositis and dermatomyositis. For many years some authors have insisted on splitting rather than lumping these two syndromes because of differences in certain clinical and pathological

Table 4.2 Antinuclear and related antibodies in inflammatory myopathies

Antibody	Disease subset	Antigen
PM-1	60–70% PM; some childhood DM	Unknown
Jo-1	30–40% of PM; 60–70% with pulmonary fibrosis	Histidyl-tRNA synthetase
Mi	Seen in some DM	Cathodic non-histone protein
Ku	PM with features of scleroderma	Acidic nuclear proteins (80 and 70 kDa)
PM-Scl	PM with features of scleroderma	Nucleus/nucleolar
PL-7	PM	Threonyl-tRNA synthetase
RNP	Mixed connective tissue disease; some SLE	Small nuclear ribonuclear protein
Sm	SLE	Small nuclear ribonuclear protein
Ro	Sjogren's; some SLE, some PM; mothers of infants with congenital heart block	Small cytoplasmic ribonuclear proteins (60 and 52 kDa)
La	Sjogren's; some SLE	Small cytoplasmic ribonuclear protein involved in termination of RNA polymerase transcription (48 kDa)
ds-DNA	Active SLE	Native DNA

Reviewed in Lisak (1988), Dawkins & Garlepp (1988), Zweiman & Lisak (1990) and Moore & Lisak (1990).

features. Current immunological research supports the concept of 'splitting', and, indeed, defining further subcategories within polymyositis and dermatomyositis may well be justified.

Animal models

There have been numerous attempts in the past to develop and use experimental models for polymyositis, generally immune or virally mediated. There now are two reasonably well-established models of immune pathogenesis for polymyositis. Graft-versus-host reactions employing grafts of muscle have resulted in an inflammatory myopathy which is eventually characterized by inflammatory lesions and necrosis in which mononuclear cells predominate (Mastaglia et al 1975, Kakulas 1988). It is of interest that graft-verus-host disease is associated with a polymyositis-like syndrome in humans (Anderson et al 1982, Reyer et al 1983). The other experimental model is experimental allergic myositis. For several years it was not clear that such a disorder could be reliably produced, especially in rats where adjuvant arthritis interfered with interpretation of both clinical and histological changes. It is now clear that an experimental allergic (autoimmune) myositis (EAM) can be produced in several species (Lisak 1988, Kakulas 1988). The nature of the target antigen(s) is (are) not certain, and the relative roles of humoral (antibody) and cell-mediated mechanisms are still to be elucidated. Serial studies of cell subpopulations in muscle of these animals as well as the use of passive transfer with cell-lines and clones may provide important information about the pathogenesis of EAM. To date, published studies of passive transfer have not used such cell preparations, and the ability to transfer disease passively with a mixed population of cells, including cells that can either make antibodies or help cells of the recipient animal make antibodies, is not of itself sufficient evidence to prove that EAM is a T-cell (delayed hypersensitivity or cytotoxic) disorder, although this seems highly likely.

There is also interest in the possible role of viruses in the pathogenesis of polymyositis, either as an infection of muscle leading to cell destruction, by evoking an immune response which also damages the muscle cell (the immune system sees the viral antigen in the context of MHC), or perhaps as a trigger to an autoimmune (molecular mimicry, including triggering via anti-idiotypic network, polyclonal stimulation of a susceptible immune system, induction of neoantigen) or immune complex deposition disorder (Denman 1988). Acute infectious necrotizing myopathies have been reported in humans in association with RNA and DNA viruses. In addition the description of chronic inflammatory changes in muscle of some patients with HIV infection has added further credence to the possible role of viruses in the development of polymyositis. There are reports of induction of muscle necrosis or an acute myositis as well as a more chronic syndrome which more closely resembles the clinical and pathological features of polymyositis. In addition, in a sub-human primate model of HIV infection (simian AIDS; SAIDS), 50% of experimentally infected monkeys develop clinical, pathological and laboratory evidence of polymyositis (Dalakas et al 1986). Of interest is that virus seems to be localized to the inflammatory cells rather than to muscle fibres, using immunofluorescence.

Immunopathological mechanisms in polymyositis

As described in detail elsewhere in this volume, one of the hallmarks of the lesion in polymyositis is the presence of inflammatory cells, predominately lymphocytes and macrophages. The cells are found both in a perivascular and endomysial pattern and it has been suggested that the endomysial pattern is more closely associated with polymyositis than with dermatomyositis. With the exception of eosinophilic polymyositis, a disorder most frequently seen as part of the hypereosinophilic syndrome (Layzer et al 1977), there are no pathological features to suggest that polymyositis is a reaginic-mediated immune disorder. There have been multiple studies to explore the possibility that antibodies to muscle components are causative in polymyositis. While there have been some reports of such antibodies this has not been uniformly described and the presence of immunoglobulin and complement components at the site of necrotic muscle is equally compatible with immune complex deposition (Whitaker 1982,

Behan & Behan 1985, Mastaglia & Ojeda 1985, Lisak 1988).

There is an interesting series of antibodies reported in various subgroups of patients with polymyositis and dermatomyositis which have varying degrees of specificity for these disorders, but the target antigens are not surface antigens. In addition, antibodies to some of these cytoplasmic and nuclear antigens are found in other disorders. However, there are two of potential aetiological/pathogenic interest, Jo-1 and PL-7. These antibodies react with histidyl-tRNA synthetase and threonyl-tRNA synthetase respectively. If these antibodies could gain access to the intact cells abnormalities in cell function might be expected to occur. The antibodies might also represent a virus-triggered or -mediated disease with the elevated titres being to a shared epitope between host and virus (molecular mimicry) (Lisak 1988).

Patients with polymyositis have been reported to have elevated levels of circulating immune complexes in their serum, similar to those with dermatomyositis (Behan et al 1982). The nature of the antigen or antigens is not known. However, the pathology of polymyositis and most of the immunohistological evidence does not support a major role for deposition of immune complexes in vessels within muscle especially in comparision to juvenile dermatomyositis.

There is excellent indirect evidence that cell-mediated mechanisms are of paramount importance in the pathogenesis of many cases of polymyositis. The strongest evidence is the recent immunohistological analysis of muscle biopsies undertaken by several groups. The predominant infiltrating cell is the T-cell and both presumptive cytotoxic T-cells (CD8$^+$) and delayed hypersensitivity T-cells (CD4$^+$) cells, as well as macrophages, are present (Rowe et al 1981, Giorno et al 1984, Arahata & Engel 1984, Engel & Arahata 1984, Olsson et al 1985, Arahata & Engel 1986). There is also immunohistological evidence that these infiltrating cells are activated (Giorno et al 1984, Olsson et al 1985, Isenberg et al 1986, Nennesmo et al 1989). Cells likely to mediate NK or ADCC reactions do not seem to be prominent, nor are there many B-cells located in the lesions. There is some controversy over whether the predominant cell is the CD8$^+$ or CD4$^+$ cell, and the implica-

tions over which is the predominant or more important initial cell are not trivial since the former implies a T-cell-specific cytotoxic reaction and the latter a classic delayed hypersensitivity reaction — with the CD8$^+$ cell then being a secondary pathogenic cell, a non-specific cell or even representing the presence of CD8$^+$ suppressor cells. Unfortunately, one cannot do frequent serial biopsy studies in patients with adequate sampling. It has been shown that the nature of the infiltrating cell subsets in experimental allergic encephalomyelitis and neuritis varies over time as the lesions evolve. The work of Engel and his colleagues strongly supports a primary role for the CD8$^+$ cells (Figs 4.5, 4.6). The predominance of class I MHC molecules in the muscle of patients with polymyositis (Appleyard et al 1985, Karpati et al 1988, McDouall et al 1989) is also compatible with this hypothesis (Figs 4.7, 4.8).

The results of in vitro studies to demonstrate T-cell-specific muscle-specific and disease-specific myotoxicity are controversial (Lisak 1988). Only one study of in vitro cytotoxicity to muscle used MHC-matched muscle as a target for cytotoxic reactions (the patient's own muscle) (Johnson et al 1972) and only one employed other cell types as controls for non-specific cytotoxicity (Currie et al 1971). Recently, T-lines were obtained from a single patient with adult-onset dermatomyositis. The CD4$^+$ line from this single subject was said to show HLA-restricted in vitro proliferation to human muscle but non-MHC myotoxicity (to rat muscle), and the CD8$^+$ line was not toxic for rat muscle with respect to proliferation (rat muscle cells would not be expected to have the appropriate human MHC I required for a CD8$^+$ cell cytotoxic reaction) and non-HLA restricted proliferative response to muscle with respect to proliferation (Rosenschein et al 1987). These are preliminary results and further studies are required including studies to explain the CD4$^+$ myotoxicity. Studies demonstrating enhanced in vitro proliferative responses to muscle and muscle constituents have not yielded consistent results. A putative target antigen has not been identified as yet. It is possible that the cell-mediated immune reaction is directed at a viral antigen in muscle present as a result of a clinical or subclinical infection. There is indirect evidence for this possibility based on clinical

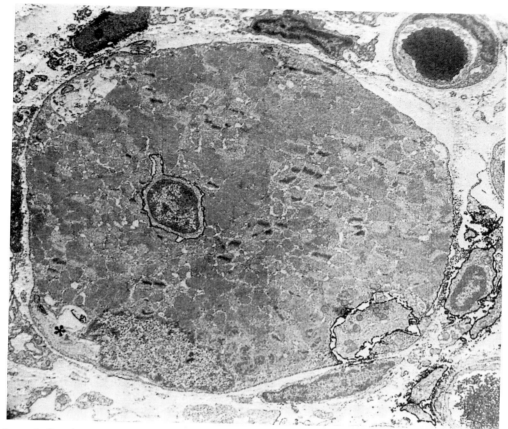

Fig. 4.5 A muscle fibre from a patient with polymyositis demonstrating a deeply placed invading CD8$^+$ cell as well as surrounding CD8$^+$ cells ×6000. (From Arahata & Engel 1986)

syndromes such as acute myositis seen in association with certain viral infections, what seems to be a viral myositis in certain immunodeficient patients, animal models, serological studies and, more recently, findings with molecular biological probes. Inclusion body myositis is discussed elsewhere in this volume. Some have interpreted the inclusions as being of viral origin, and one group has claimed that mumps virus is the aetiological agent on the basis of immunological staining techniques. The former must be considered theory and the latter has not been confirmed by other workers in the field. In addition there are both clinical and histological differences between inclusion body myositis and the more usual idiopathic polymyositis or polymyositis associated with collagen vascular diseases.

There are no studies to support an NK or ADCC reaction as being primary in polymyositis. Indeed, most immunohistological studies have not shown significant numbers of NK cells in muscle biopsies. Since ADCC reactions can be demonstrated across MHC and species barriers it is quite feasible to study the possibility that there are antibodies in the serum of patients with inflammatory myopathies capable of mediating an ADCC reaction against muscle.

Abnormalities of immunoregulation

There have been few studies of immunoregulation in patients with polymyositis and dermatomyositis. Two groups have reported a decrease in the frequency of CD8$^+$ T-cells in the blood of patients with these disorders (Behan et al 1983, Lisak et al 1984) but others have not (Iyer et al 1983). A

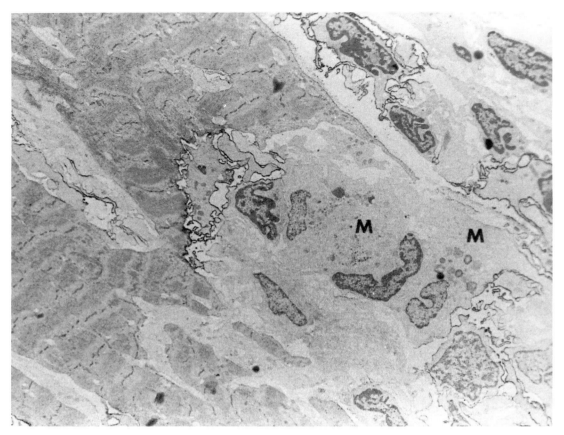

Fig. 4.6 Advanced muscle fibre invasion in polymyositis. The fibre shows honeycomb cavities containing CD8$^+$ and CD8$^-$ cells as well as large invading cells which are macrophages (M). ×4400. (From Arahata & Engel 1986)

polyclonal increase in serum immunoglobulins has been reported but this has not been a universal finding (Lisak 1988). There is some evidence of increase in polyclonal B-cell activity based on the study of the frequency of spontaneous immuno-globulin-secreting cells (Lisak, Levinson, Zweiman, unpublished observations). There have also been a few functional studies demonstrating in vitro abnormalities of suppressor function (Mastaglia & Ojeda 1985) as well as a reduced in vitro response of lymphocytes to a T-cell mitogen (Behan & Behan 1985) in patients with inflammatory myopathies.

Dermatomyositis

In dealing with dermatomyositis it may be useful to consider the childhood variety as a different entity from the adult form on the basis of both clinical, histological and immunological data. The adult form may be divided into cases seen in association with a remote solid neoplasm, the unusual patient with an another classic collagen vascular disease and the more common idiopathic variety. These last subdivisions are based on the results of testing for the associated disorder or clinical identification of the associated disorder (neoplasm or other collagen vascular disease) but not on any demonstrated difference in the clinical or histological presentation, other than perhaps age (within the adult range) and sex of the patient.

Animal models

There are really no satisfactory experimental animal models, immune or viral induced, for dermatomyositis. There are several naturally occurring and experimental disorders that have

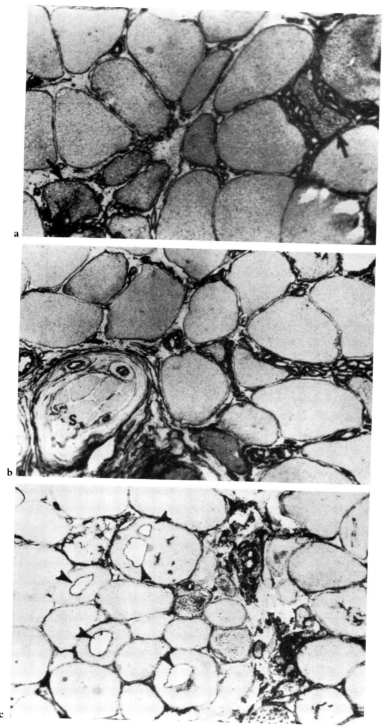

Fig. 4.7 MHC class I molecule expression in polymyositis. Staining with antibody to MHC class I on sarcolemma and in sarcoplasm of fibres being invaded by inflammatory cells in (arrows) (a); lack of MHC class I on intrafusal fibres in (b); and MHC class I molecules (arrow heads) in vacuolar spaces (presumably dilated T tubules) in (c). ×314 in (a) and (b), and ×196 in (c). (From Karpati et al 1988)

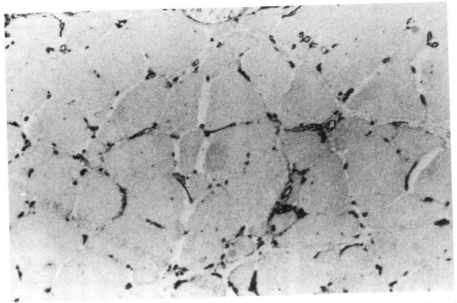

Fig. 4.8 Lack of MHC class II molecules on muscle fibres in polymyositis. MHC class II is limited to blood vessels and inflammatory cells. ×245. (From Karpati et al 1988)

been suggested to be useful models for polymositis but even here most of these infections or nutritional lesions do not really provide a useful model or analogue of polymyositis. None of these resemble dermatomyositis. While there have been reports of naturally occuring polymyositis in dogs and the experimental disorder experimental allergic myositis has been used as a model of polymyositis (see above) there are none in either category that resemble dermatomyositis, certainly none that reproduce the vasculitic picture seen in the classical juvenile form.

Immunopathogenic mechanisms in dermatomyositis

There are no studies addressing reaginic immune mechanisms in dermatomyositis, and, as in polymyositis, little about the pathological lesions to suggest that such mechanisms might play a prominent role in this disorder. There have been reports of antibodies to muscle on the basis of immunofluorescent staining but much of this appears to be non-specific and cannot be considered strong evidence for an antibody-mediated immune mechanism (Lisak 1988, Kakulas 1988). In addition, there have been reports of antibodies

to nuclear constituents in some patients with dermatomyositis — including anti-PM-1 in some childhood dermatomyositis patients (occurs in 60–70% of polymyositis patients) and anti-Mi (Behan & Behan 1985, Lisak 1988).

There is very strong indirect evidence for deposition of immune complexes in vessels and on and around some muscle fibres in patients with childhood dermatomyositis (Whitaker 1982, Lisak 1988). Deposition of immunoglobulin and C3 were seen in muscle biopsies of childhood dermatomyositis patients (Whitaker & Engel 1972). Moreover it has been shown that complement activation occurs in these lesions since the C5b–9 membrane attack (activation) neoantigen can be demonstrated (Fig 4.9). These findings are not part of polymyositis. There is the reported tendency for slightly more prominent perivascular location of inflammatory cells in dermatomyositis in comparison to more prominent endomysial location of these cells in polymyositis as noted earlier. Most recently, Emslie-Smith and Engel (1990) have demonstrated focal capillary depletion, reduced capillary density and the presence of the complement membrane attack complex in muscle biopsies of adult onset dermatomyositis patients.

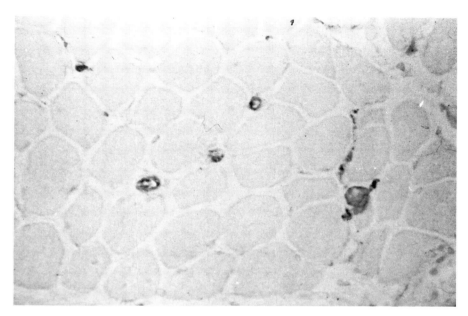

Fig. 4.9   Muscle biopsy from a patient with childhood dermatomyositis demonstrating C5b–9 membrane attack complex neoantigen deposited in vessel walls. (From Kissel et al 1986)

It therefore seems likely that there are similar immunopathogenic mechanisms involved in childhood- and adult-onset dermatomyositis. Elevated levels of circulating immune complexes have been reported in patients with dermatomyositis and polymyositis.

Cell-mediated mechanisms have been investigated in dermatomyositis generally as part of studies of both polymyositis and dermatomyositis (see previous discussion). Indeed the 'lumping' of all inflammatory myopathies together in many studies confuses the issue since, as discussed, they may well result from different pathogenic mechanisms and thus cancel out differences from controls that would be evident if compared to controls as separate entities. With these caveats there is no strong evidence that either juvenile (childhood) or adult dermatomyositis results from a T-cell-mediated reaction. Studies of T-cell subsets and distribution of MHC antigens on muscle fibres and other cells within muscle are less suggestive of a cytotoxic T-cell reaction in juvenile dermatomyositis than is present (see above) in classical polymyositis. It is possible that some cases of adult onset are the result of an immune complex deposition whereas others may be the result of a T-cell-mediated reaction to an antigen present in muscle.

Abnormalities of immunoregulation

Most studies of abnormal immunoregulation have combined polymyositis and dermatomyositis patients. Therefore, one can re-state what was noted earlier, i.e, there is some indirect evidence in a few — but not all — studies of abnormal levels and function of suppressor cells in the blood of some patients with inflammatory myopathies.

Myasthenia gravis

Myasthenia gravis is now the prototypic autoimmune antibody-mediated disorder involving the nervous system. There has been a tremendous increase in our knowledge about the immunopathogenesis of myasthenia gravis, the nature of the target antigen, immunogenetic factors and even progress in understanding abnormalities of immunoregulation that may be responsible or at least permissive for the emergence of the autoantibodies that mediate this disease (Lisak in press).

Animal models

In no autoimmune disorder has an animal model been as important in leading to the understanding of the naturally occurring human disorder as it has been in myasthenia gravis. Indeed, the induction of the animal model, experimental auotimmune myasthenia gravis (EAMG), by Patrick and Lindstrom (1973) by sensitization of rabbits with nicotinic AChR from electric fish, can really be considered the beginning of the modern era of investigation of the immunology of myasthenia gravis. The lesions that are found at the end-plate in animals actively immunized with AChR, like those in patients with myasthenia gravis, are essentially acellular (few or no inflammatory cells) (Sahashi et al 1978, Lisak and Barchi 1982, Lisak 1988) although an acute form associated with inflammatory cells at the end-plate occurs in a few species (Engel et al 1976a, b). These cells seem to represent a response to an antibody-mediated complement activation immunological process (Lennon et al 1978). These animals later develop a more classical non-inflammatory cell-associated chronic myasthenia gravis.

Active induction of EAMG has also been accomplished by immunizing animals with antibodies directed against an agonist of ACh or with the agonist (Bis Q). The production of EAMG and anti-AChR by these methods seems to be through the idiotype network and illustrates the potential harmful (disease induction) effects of this system (Wasserman et al 1982, Cleveland et al 1983). Also of interest in relation to anti-idiotype network induction of disease and to molecular mimicry is the induction of an EAMG-like syndrome in mice in response to an anti-dextran antibody (Dwyer et al 1986). Sequence homology between portions of the α-chain of AChR and certain Gram-negative bacterial proteins (Stephansson et al 1984) and herpes simplex virus (Schwimmbeck et al 1989) have been reported using monoclonal antibodies raised to AChR and sera from some patients with myasthenia gravis, respectively. Protective effects (inhibition of induction of EAMG) have also been reported using antibodies raised to anti-AChR (Souroujon et al 1986). A curious effect is the capacity of a monoclonal antibody to a monoclonal antibody to AChR to inhibit the development of

EAMG although the anti-idiotypic antibody is not directed against any of the predominant idiotypes in the serum of mice with EAMG (Agius et al 1985). EAMG has also served as a useful model to examine other models of treatment and prevention of myasthenia gravis.

Monoclonal antibodies have been used to determine which epitopes on AChR may be important in the development of EAMG and, by implication, as well as by antibody-blocking experiments using these monoclonal antibodies and human sera, which epitopes are important in human MG. One region of the chain has been called the major immunogenic region (MIR), but recently questions have been raised as to whether there is an MIR in human MG. Passive transfer experiments in rodents have demonstrated differences in the capacity of different monoclonal antibodies to transfer passively disease to naive recipients. It is of interest that antibodies to the ligand (ACh or α-bungarotoxin)-binding site do not effectively transfer chronic neuromuscular block but are capable of transferring a rapidly evolving, severe block to birds. A cellular response to antibody-mediated end-plate damage may be involved in this immunopathological reaction.

Immunopathogenic mechanisms

Several antibody-associated mechanisms seem to be involved in the production of the abnormalities at the motor end-plate by anti-AChR antibodies with the resultant defect in neuromuscular transmission (Engel 1984, Ashizawa & Appel 1985, Levinson et al 1987a). Each of these has in common that they lead to a decrease in available AChR to interact with the normal amounts of ACh released from the presynaptic nerve terminals in MG. Those mechanisms thought to play a significant role in human MG include: (i) activation of complement cascade by anti-AChR binding to AChR with resulting production of membrane destruction (pathological changes as well as deposition of IgG, C3, C9 and the C5b−9 activation neoantigen at the membrane have been described) (Fig 4.10); (ii) antigen-specific down-regulation of AChR by anti-AChR by cross-linking of epitopes on adjacent AChR molecules by the bivalent IgG antibody

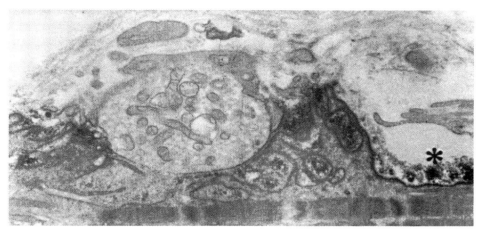

Fig. 4.10 Deposition of C9 at the neuromuscular junction in myasthenia gravis. C9 is demonstrated on debris in the synaptic space, over short segments of the junctional folds and on material to the right of the folds as well as on the surface of the muscle fibres and between layers of the basal lamina (asterisk). ×15 300. (From Sahashi et al 1980)

molecule (this can be produced in vitro and in experimental animals in vivo) (Kao and Drachman 1977, Appel et al 1977); and (iii) blocking of the ligand binding site by anti-AChR antibodies that are directed at epitopes at or near the ligand binding site. The original demonstration that sera from patients with MG had anti-AChR antibodies was based on the blocking of α-bungarotoxin binding to AChR (Almon et al 1974). However, the relative importance of such antibodies is not clear since they can be demonstrated in only 30% of patients with MG using competitive binding assays (Keesey et al 1976, Lennon 1976, Lindstrom et al 1976, Whiting et al 1983, Sterz et al 1986). However, newer assays employing a human tumour cell line that bears AChR (Pachner 1989) and the demonstration of a rapidly evolving neuro-muscular block in birds passively administered monoclonal antibody to the ligand binding site (Gomez & Richman 1983) raises the possibility that antibodies to the ligand-binding site of AChR may be important in some patients with MG at certain stages of their disease.

It should be pointed out that more than one antibody-mediated mechanism is likely to be involved in any patient at any time. Patients have antibodies to AChR that are polyclonal and can be found in all four subclasses of IgG and rarely IgM (reviewed in Lisak & Barchi 1982) and thus these antibodies will have different biological effects.

Patients have antibodies to different epitopes on different peptide chains and some of these may have no biological consequence. Anti-AChR antibodies that are capable of cross-linking (a complement-independent reaction) must combine with the identical epitope on adjacent molecules and not on the same AChR molecule in order to have this particular biological effect (Conti-Tronconi et al 1982). In addition, there are important factors involved in neuromuscular transmission that are non-immunological and that have clinically significant effects in any neuro-muscular junction where the physiological safety factor for transmission is already abnormal from any immunological or non-immunological patholo-gical or pathophysiological defect. The lack of clinical correlation with the overall titre of anti-AChR and severity of disease may be understood by keeping all of these factors in mind.

Abnormalities of immunoregulation

There is evidence for abnormalities of immuno-regulation, both broad-based and AChR-specific, in patients with myasthenia gravis (Lisak et al 1985, Levinson et al 1985, 1987a, Lisak 1988). Among the studies supporting broad-based 'polyclonal' defects in immunoregulation are: (i) a high incidence of autoantibodies to non-muscle antigens (Penn et al 1971); (ii) increased association of other immunopathological disorders in patients with myasthenia gravis (Simpson 1960); (iii) decrease in the percentage of circulating CD8[+] T-cells in some studies (Skolnik et al 1982); (iv) increase in the percentage of blood B-cells that bear the CD5 antigen similar to what has been reported in rheumatoid arthritis, Sjogren's syndrome, recovery from bone marrow transplantation, and insulin-dependent diabetes mellitus and autoimmune mice (these cells synthesize autoantibodies of IgM and IgG isotypes) (Ragheb & Lisak 1990); (v) increased frequency of IgG-secreting cells in suspensions of blood and thymus mononuclear cells (Levinson et al 1985, 1987a); (vi) mitogen stimulated thymic cells from the thymus secrete predominantly IgG whereas blood cells from the same myasthenics secrete equal amounts of IgG and IgM (Levinson et al 1987b); (vii) abnormal thymus histology (germinal centre hyperplasia and/or thymoma) (Castleman 1966) in immunohistological studies of the 'hyperplastic' thymuses demonstrating changes of a reactive lymph node (Kornstein et al 1984); (viii) the thymus contains a significant number of B-cells in comparison to control thymuses by the criteria of the CD20 marker (Durelli et al 1990) and many of these CD20 B-cells do not bear surface IgM differing from blood B-cells (Zweiman et al 1989); (ix) thymic cells of patients with germinal centre follicular hyperplasia stimulate an autologous mixed leukocyte reaction by blood cells whereas thymoma cells and cells of cardiac surgery controls do not (Abdou et al 1974).

Abnormalities related to AChR include: (i) elevated titres to AChR are found in myasthenia and rarely borderline or minimally elevated levels in other disorders (Almon et al 1974, Appel et al 1975, Bender et al 1975, Lindstrom 1977, Lisak & Barchi 1982); (ii) myasthenic serum IgG, but not other sera, passively transfers a myasthenic block to recipient animals (Toyka et al 1975); (iii) peripheral blood mononuclear cell cultures from myasthenics, but not normals, secrete anti-AChR in vitro both without and with stimulation by a polyclonal T-cell-dependent B-cell activator (Lisak et al 1985); (iv) removal of CD8[+] suppressor T-cells from the cultures of normal individuals does not result in the in vitro production of anti-AChR but does result in an increase in production of IgG whereas in identical experiments performed with blood cells of patients with MG there was an increase in synthesized anti-AChR in parallel with an increase in the polyclonal immunoglobulin response (Lisak et al 1987); (v) peripheral blood cells proliferate in vitro in response to AChR to a greater degree than those of control subjects (Abramsky et al 1975, Richman et al 1976) and T-cell lines specific for AChR can be obtained from blood of patients with myasthenia (Hohlfeld et al 1984, 1986) (it is not clear whether there are certain epitopes of AChR that are recognized specifically by cells of myasthenics (Hohlfeld et al 1988, Harcourt et al 1989, Protti et al 1990), whether there is a higher frequency of AChR specific T-cells in the blood or thymus of myasthenics or whether AChR-specific T-cells are in a different subpopulation in myasthenia in comparison to controls); (vi) thymic cells of patients with myasthenia synthesize anti-AChR (Vincent et al 1978), often in large amounts and often without in vitro polyclonal stimulation (Newsom-Davis et al 1981, Fujii et al 1984, Lisak et al 1986), whereas thymic cells of controls do not; and (vii) one group has reported that thymic T-cells from patients with myasthenia specifically enhance anti-AChR synthesis by blood cells of myasthenics (Newsom-Davis et al 1981).

Lambert–Eaton myasthenic syndrome

Patients with Lambert–Eaton myasthenic syndrome (LEMS) have a presynaptic disorder of neuromuscular transmission which also involves the autonomic nervous system. Its frequent association with small cell (oat cell) carcinoma of the lung (55–75%) led to the theory that it was due to a substance, presumably a peptide, secreted by these tumour cells, which are known to secrete several peptides, some of which have hormonal properties. It is now clear that the Lambert–Eaton myasthenic syndrome, whether occurring in association with small cell carcinoma or idiopathic, is an autoimmune antibody-mediated disease directed against one or more epitopes of the voltage-gated calcium channels associated with transmitter release (Newsom-Davis 1985, Vincent et al 1989, Sher et al 1989, Lennon & Lambert 1990).

Animal models

Although it is now clear that one or more epitopes of presynaptic voltage-gated calcium channels are the antigenic targets for the autoimmune antibody response in LEMS, the antigen has not been identified or isolated and therefore at this time there is no model of active induction or passive transfer with cells or serum from experimental animals to naive recipient animals. However, physiological and pathological abnormalities typical of LEMS have been passively transferred to immunosuppressed mice with serum IgG from patients with LEMS (Fukunaga et al 1983, Newsom-Davis 1985).

Immunopathogenic mechanisms in LEMS

The evidence for a primary role of an immuno-pathological reaction affecting presynaptic structures in patients with LEMS is based on the ability to reproduce both the electrophysiological defect characteristic of LEMS and the anatomical abnormalities in the number and appearance of presynaptic active zones described in patients with LEMS (Fukunaga et al 1982) in immunosuppressed mice given IgG from patients with LEMS (Lang et al 1981, Fukunaga et al 1983, Engel et al 1987). As described earlier, one or more components of a presynaptic voltage-gated calcium channel seem to be the antigenic target of an antibody-mediated non-complement-dependent modulation of the antigen which leads to a decrease in the calcium-dependent quantal release of ACh. To date there is no evidence to support other antibody or cell-mediated immunopathological mechanisms as being of major importance in this disorder.

Abnormalities of immunoregulation in LEMS

LEMS occurs in two settings either in association with small cell carcinoma (almost invariably of pulmonary origin) or in the absence of carcinoma but in patients who seem to have an increased incidence of other autoantibodies and immuno-logically mediated diseases (Lennon et al 1982, O'Neil et al 1988). As in myasthenia gravis, this raises the issue of more broadly based deficits in immunoregulation. Patients with LEMS in asso-

ciation with small cell carcinoma of the lung tend to have a decrease in the frequency of CD8[+] lymphocytes (Robb et al 1985). Although there are no familial cases of LEMS reported to my knowledge, there is evidence that immunoregulatory genes may play a role in who develops LEMS, both the idiopathic- and small-cell-carcinoma-associated types. There is an increased frequency of HLA-B8 among patients with LEMS when compared to a normal control population both in idiopathic- or small-cell-carcinoma-associated cases, although the increase in comparison to controls is greater for the idiopathic LEMS group. There is an increase in the incidence of the IgG heavy-chain allotype marker Gm1(2) in patients with small cell carcinoma and LEMS but not in other patients with small cell carcinoma, suggesting that there is a genetically influenced abnormality in regulation of the immune response which, in part, determines which patients with small cell carcinoma develop LEMS (Willcox et al 1985, Lisak 1988). It is equally likely that other alleles of the MHC, immunoglobulin and the T-cell receptor determine which patients with small cell carcinoma develop immune responses to other shared or cross-reacting small cell tumour/neural antigens and develop other immunologically mediated disorders of the PNS and CNS (Lisak in press).

The target antigen or antigens in both groups of patients with LEMS would seem to be one or more components of a presynaptic voltage-gated calcium channel (Wray et al 1987, Kim 1987, Login et al 1987, Vincent et al 1989). As described earlier, there is now ample evidence that the small cell tumours have antigenic determinants similar or identical to those neurons (Tischler et al 1977). Recently a radioimmunoassay has been established by at least two groups employing ω-conotoxin (a calcium-channel toxin derived from the fish-eating snail *Conus geographus*) bound to an extract of small cell tumour line (Sher et al 1989, Lennon & Lambert 1990). Serum from patients with LEMS but not other disorders (with the exception of a few patients with other PNS complications of small cell carcinoma) show elevated titres to calcium-channel antigen using this assay. Patients with LEMS associated with small cell carcinoma seem to have a higher incidence of significantly elevated titres than the patients with the idiopathic variety, although patients with LEMS of either type may be 'antibody-negative by RIA'. Why patients with idiopathic LEMS should develop antibodies to voltage-gated calcium channels is not known, but a role for genetically influenced, disease-permissive abnormalities in immuno-regulation is probably important.

Myopathies associated with HIV infection

Patients infected with HIV have prominent neuro-logical involvement of the central nervous system even in the absence of neurological disorders that occur as the result of opportunistic infections associated with the severe state of acquired immunodeficiency. In addition both an acute (Guillain–Barré syndrome) and chronic inflam-matory demyelinating neuropathy occur early in the course of HIV infection, and other types of neuropathies have been reported in the latter stages of HIV infection as well. Clinical myopathy in such patients, however, has been reported, but it is very uncommon — although, as noted earlier in this chapter, a simian retrovirus similar to HIV causes clinical and pathological changes in 50% of monkeys infected with that retrovirus. The virus can infect muscle cultures and replicate in myotubes without causing any apparent cellular cytotoxic changes, but the simian virus seems to involve the invading inflammatory cells in the in vivo model and in the few patients with HIV there was a similar localization of the HIV virus.

REFERENCES

Aarli J A, Lefvert A K, Tonder O 1981 Thymoma specific antibodies in the sera from patients with myasthenia gravis demonstrated by indirect hemagglutination. Journal of Neuroimmunology 1: 421

Abdou N I, Lisak R P, Zweiman B, Abrahamsohn I, Penn A S 1974 The thymus in myasthenia gravis. Evidence for altered cell populations. New England Journal of Medicine 291: 1271

Abramsky O, Aharanov A, Webb C, Fuchs S 1975 Cellular immune response to acetylcholine receptor-rich fraction in patients with myasthenia gravis. Clinical and Experimental Immunology 19: 11

Acuto O, Reinherz E L 1985 The human T-cell receptor. New England Journal of Medicine 312: 1100

Agius M A, Geannopoulos C G, Richman D P 1985 Antiidiotypic modification of the immune response in experimental autoimmune myasthenia gravis. Society for Neuroscience 11: 139

Almon R R, Andrew C G, Appel S H 1974 Serum globulin in myasthenia gravis: inhibition of α-bungarotoxin binding to acetylcholine receptors. Science 186: 55

Alper C A 1981 Complement and the MHC. In: Dorf M E (ed) The role of the major histocompatability complex in immunobiology. Garland Press, New York, p 173

Anderson B A, Young V, Kean W F, Ludwin S K, Galbraith P R, Anastassiades T P 1982 Polymyositis in chronic graft versus host disease. Archives of Neurology 39: 188

Appel S H, Almon R R, Levy N R 1975 Acetylcholine receptor antibodies in myasthenia gravis. New England Journal of Medicine 293: 760

Appel S H, Anwyl R, McAdams M W, Elias S 1977 Accelerated degradation of acetylcholine receptor from cultured rat myotubes with myasthenia gravis sera and globulins. Proceedings of the National Academy of Sciences of the USA 74: 2130

Appleyard S T, Dunn M J, Dubowitz V, Rose M L 1985 Increased expression of HLA ABC class I antigens by muscle fibers in Duchenne muscular dystrophy, inflammatory myopathy, and other neuromuscular disorders. Lancet i: 367

Arahata K, Engel A G 1984 Monoclonal antibody analysis of mononuclear cells in myopathies. 1. Quantitation of subsets according to diagnosis and sites of accumulation and demonstrations and counts of muscle fibers invaded by T-cells. Annals of Neurology 16: 198

Arahata K, Engel A G 1986 Monoclonal antibody analysis of mononuclear cells in myopathies. III. Immunoelectron microscopic aspects of cell-mediated muscle fibre injury. Annals of Neurology 19: 112

Ashizawa T, Appel S A 1985 Immunopathologic events at the endplate in myasthenia gravis. Springer Seminars in Immunopathology 8: 177

Behan W M H, Behan P O 1985 Immunologic features of polymyositis. Springer Seminars in Immunopathology 8: 267

Behan W M H, Barkas T, Behan P O 1982 Detection of immune complexes in polymyositis. Acta Neurologica Scandinavica 65: 320

Behan W M H, Behan P O, Micklem H S, Durward W F 1983 Lymphocyte subset analysis in polymyositis. British Medical Journal 287: 181

Bender A N, Ringel S P, Engel W K, Daniels M P, Vogel Z 1975 Myasthenia gravis: a serum factor blocking acetylcholine receptors of the human neuromuscular junction. Lancet i: 607

Bona C A, Pernis B 1984 Idiotype networks. In: Paul W E (ed) Fundamental immunology, 1st Edn. Raven Press, New York, p 577

Burnet F M 1959 The clonal selection theory of acquired immunity. Cambridge University Press, New York

Burns J B, Rosenzweig A, Zweiman B, Lisak R P 1983 Isolation of myelin basic protein-reactive T-cell lines from normal human blood. Cellular Immunology 81: 435

Castleman B 1966 The pathology of the thymus gland in myasthenia gravis. Annals of the New York Academy of Sciences 135: 496

Changeux J P, Devilliers-Thiery A, Chemoulli P 1984 Acetylcholine receptor: an allosteric protein. Science 115: 1335

Cleveland W L, Wasserman N H, Sarangarajan R, Penn A S, Erlanger B F 1983 Monoclonal antibodies to the acetylcholine receptor by a normally functioning auto-anti-idiotypic mechanism. Nature 305: 56

Cohen M, Epstein R 1978 T-cell inhibition of humoral responsiveness. II. Theory on the role of restrictive recognition in immune regulation. Cellular Immunology 39: 125

Conti-Tronconi B M, Raftery M A 1983 Structure of electric organ and mammalian acetylcholine receptor molecules. Advances in Cellular Neurobiology 4: 105

Conti-Tronconi B M, Gotti C M, Hunkapeller M W, Raftery M A 1982 Mammalian muscle acetylcholine receptor: a supramolecular structure formed by four related proteins. Science 218: 1227

Coombs R R A, Gell P G H 1968 Classification of allergic reactions responsible for clinical hypersensitivity and disease. In: Gell P G H, Coombs, R R A (eds) Clinical aspects of immunity. F A Davis, Philadelphia, p 575

Cowing C 1985 Does T-cell restriction to Ia limit the need for self-tolerance? Immunology Today 6: 72

Currie S, Saunders M, Knowles M, Brown A E 1971 Immunologic aspects of polymyositis. The in vitro activity of lymphocytes with muscle antigen and with mouse cultures. Quarterly Journal of Medicine 60: 63

Dalakas M C, London W T, Gravell M, Sever J L 1986 Polymyositis in an immunodeficiency induced by a type D retrovirus. Neurology 36: 569

Dawkins R L, Garlepp M J 1988 Immunopathology of polymyositis and dermatomyositis. In: Dalakas M C (ed) Polymyositis and dermatomyositis. Butterworths, Boston, p 85

Denman A M 1988 Viral etiology of polymyositis/dermatomyositis. In: Dalakas M C (ed) Polymyositis and dermatomyositis. Butterworth, Boston, p 97

Durelli L, Massazza U, Poccardi G et al 1990 Increased thymocyte differentiation in myasthenia gravis: a dual-color immunofluorescence phenotypic analysis. Annals of Neurology 27: 174

Dwyer D S, Vakil M, Kearney J F 1986 Idiotypic network connectivity and a possible cause of myasthenia gravis. Journal of Experimental Medicine 164: 1310

Emslie-Smith A, Engel A G 1990 Microvascular changes in early and advanced dermatomyositis: a quantitative study. Annals of Neurology 27: 343

Engel A G 1984 Myasthenia gravis and myasthenic syndromes. Annals of Neurology 16: 519

Engel A G, Arahata K 1984 Monoclonal antibody analysis of mononuclear cells in myopathies. II. Phenotypes of autoinvasive cells in polymyositis and inclusion body myositis. Annals of Neurology 16: 209

Engel A G, Tsujihata M, Lambert E H, Lindstrom J M, Lennon V A 1976a Experimental autoimmune myasthenia gravis: a sequential and quantitative study of the neuromuscular ultrastructure and electrophysiologic correlations. Journal of Neuropathology and Experimental Neurology 35: 569

Engel A G, Tsujihata M, Lindstrom J N, Lennon V A 1976b The motor endplate in myasthenia gravis and in experimental autoimmune myasthenia gravis: a quantitative ultrastructural study. Annals of the New York Academy of Sciences 274: 60

Engel A G, Fukuoka T, Lang B, Newsom-Davis J, Vincent A, Wray D 1987 Lambert–Eaton myasthenic syndrome IgG: early morphologic effects and immunolocalization at the motor endplate. Annals of the New York Academy of Sciences 505: 333

Feldman M, Zanders E D, Lamb J R 1985 Tolerance in T-cell clones. Immunology Today 6: 58

Fujii Y, Monden Y, Nakahara K, Hashimoto J, Kawashima Y 1984 Antibody to acetylcholine receptor in myasthenia gravis: production by lymphocytes from thymus or thymoma. Neurology 34: 1182

Fukunaga H, Engel A G, Osame M, Lambert E H 1982 Paucity and disorganization of presynaptic membrane active zones in the Lambert Eaton myasthenic syndrome. Muscle and Nerve 5: 686

Fukunaga H, Engel A G, Lang B, Newsom-Davis J, Vincent A 1983 Passive transfer of Lambert–Eaton myasthenic syndrome with IgG from man to mouse depletes the presynaptic membrane active zones. Proceedings of the National Academy of Sciences of the USA 80: 7636

Giorno R, Barden M T, Kohler P F, Ringel S P 1984 Immunohistochemical characterization of the mononuclear cells infiltrating muscle of patients with inflammatory and noninflammatory myopathies. Immunology and Immunopathology 30: 405

Gomez C M, Richman D P 1983 Anti-acetylcholine receptor antibodies directed against the α-bungarotoxin binding site induce a unique form of experimental myasthenia. Proceeding of the National Academy of Sciences of the USA 80: 4089

Hansen T H, Sachs D H 1989 The major histocompatibility complex. In: Paul W E (ed) Fundamental immunology, 2nd edn. Raven Press, New York, p 445

Harcourt G C, Somner N, Rothbard J, Willcox H N A, Newsom-Davis J 1989 A juxta-membrane epitope on the human acetylcholine receptor recognized by T-cells in myasthenia gravis. Journal of Clinical Investigation 82: 1295

Hedrick S M 1989 T lymphocyte receptors. In: Paul W E (ed) Fundamental immunology, 2nd edn. Raven Press, New York, p 291

Hohlfeld R, Engel A G 1990 Induction of HLA-DR expression on human myoblasts with interferon-gamma. American Journal of Pathology 136: 503

Hohlfeld H, Toyka K V, Heininger V, Grosse-Wilde H, Kalis I 1984 Autoimmune human T lymphocytes specific for acetylcholine receptor. Nature 340: 244

Hohlfeld R, Kalis I, Kohleisen B, Heininger K, Conti-Tronconi B, Toyka K V 1986 Myasthenia gravis: stimulation of anti-receptor autoantibody production by autoreactive T-cell lines. Neurology 36: 618

Hohlfeld R, Toyka K V, Miner L L, Walgrave S L, Conti-Tronconi B M 1988 Amphipathic segment of the nicotinic receptor alpha subunit contains epitopes recognized by T lymphocytes in myasthenia gravis. Journal of Clinical Investigation 81: 657

Honda H, Rostami A 1989 Expression of major histocompatibility complex class I antigens in rat muscle cultures: the possible developmental role in myogenesis. Proceedings of the National Academy of Science of the USA 86: 7007

Isenberg D A, Rowe M, Shearer M, Novick D, Beverley P C L 1986 Localization of interferons and interleukin 2 in polymyositis and muscular dystrophy. Clinical and Experimental Immunology 63: 450

Iyer V, Lawton A R, Fenichel G M 1983 T-cell subsets in polymyositis. Annals of Neurology 13: 452

Jerne N K 1974 Towards a network theory of the immune system. Annals of the Immunologic Institute Pasteur (Paris) 125: 373

Johnson R L, Fink C W, Ziff M 1972 Lymphotoxin formation by lymphocytes and muscle in polymyositis. Journal of Clinical Investigation 51: 2435

Kakulas B A 1988 Animal models of polymyositis and dermatomyositis. In: Dalakas M C (ed) Polymyositis and dermatomyositis. Butterworths, Boston p 133

Kao I, Drachman D B 1977 Myasthenic immunoglobulin accelerates acetylcholine receptor degredation. Science 274: 244

Karpati G, Pouliot Y, Carpenter S 1988 Expression of immunoreactive skeletal muscles. Annals of Neurology 23: 64

Keesey J, Sharkh I, Wolfgram F, Chao L-P 1976 Studies on the ability of acetylcholine receptors to bind alpha-bungarotoxin after exposure to myasthenic serum. Annals of the New York Academy of Sciences 274: 244

Kim Y I 1987 Lambert–Eaton myasthenic syndrome: evidence for calcium channel blockade. Annals of the New York Academy of Sciences 505: 377

Kissel J T, Mendell J R, Tammohan K W 1986 Microvascular deposition of complement membrane attack complex in dermatomyositis. New England Journal of Medicine 314: 329

Kornstein M J, Brooks J J, Anderson A O, Levinson A I, Lisak R P, Zweiman B 1984 The immunohistology of the thymus in myasthenia gravis. American Journal of Pathology 117: 184

Lang B, Newsom-Davis J, Vincent A, Murray N 1981 Autoimmune aetiology for myasthenic (Eaton–Lambert) syndrome. Lancet ii: 24

Layzer R B, Shearn M A, Satya-Murti S 1977 Eosinophilic polymyositis. Annals of Neurology 1: 65

Leder P 1983 Genetics of Immunoglobulin production. In: Dixon F J, Fisher D W, (eds) The biology of immunologic disease. Sinauer Associates, p 3

Lennon V A 1976 Immunology of the acetylcholine receptor. Immunologic Communications 5: 323

Lennon V A, Griesman G E 1989 Evidence against acetylcholine receptor having a main immunogenic region as target for autoantibodies in myasthenia gravis. Neurology 39: 1069

Lennon V A, Lambert E H 1980 Myasthenia gravis induced by monoclonal antibodies to acetylcholine receptors. Nature 285: 238

Lennon V A, Lambert E H 1990 Autoantibodies bind solubilized calcium channel ω-conotoxin complexes from small cell lung carcinoma: a diagnostic aid for Lambert–Eaton myasthenic syndrome. Proceedings of the Mayo Clinic 64: 1490

Lennon V A, Seybold M E, Lindstrom J M, Cochrane C, Ulevitch R 1978 Role of complement in the pathogenesis of experimental autoimmune myasthenia gravis. Journal of Experimental Medicine 147: 973

Lennon V A, Lambert E H, Whittingham S, Fairbanks V 1982 Autoimmunity in the Lambert–Eaton syndrome. Muscle and Nerve 5: S21

Levinson A I, Lisak R P, Zweiman B, Kornstein M 1985 Phenotypic and functional analysis of lymphocytes in myasthenia gravis. Springer Seminars in Immunopathology 8: 209

Levinson A I, Zweiman B, Lisak R P 1987a Immunopathogenesis and treatment of myasthenia gravis. Journal of Clinical Immunology 7: 187

Levinson A I, Zweiman B, Lisak R P 1987b Isotype restriction of thymic B-cell immunoglobulin synthesis in myasthenia gravis. Annals of the New York Academy of Science 505: 701

Lindstrom J M 1977 An assay for antibodies to human acetylcholine receptor in serum from patients with myasthenia gravis. Clinical Immunology and Immunopathology 7: 36

Lindstrom J M, Seybold M E, Lennon V A, Whitingham S 1976 Experimental autoimmune myasthenia gravis and myasthenia gravis: biochemical and immunochemical aspects. Annals of the New York Academy of Sciences 274: 254

Lisak R P 1988 The immunology of neuromuscular disease. In: Walton J N (ed) Disorders of voluntary muscle, 5th edn. Churchill Livingstone, Edinburgh, p 345

Lisak R P (in press) Myasthenia gravis, myasthenic syndromes and experimental myasthenia gravis. In: Greenstein J (ed) Neuroimmunology. Telford Press, Caldwell, NJ

Lisak R P, Barchi R L 1982 Myasthenia gravis. W B Saunders, Philadelphia

Lisak R P, Zweiman B, Skolnik P, Guerro F 1984 Circulating T-cell subsets in inflammatory myopathies. Neurology 34 (suppl 1): 191

Lisak R P, Levinson A I, Zweiman B 1985 Autoimmune aspects of myasthenia gravis. In: Cruse J M, Lewis R E, (eds) Organ based autoimmune diseases. Karger, Basel, p 65

Lisak R P, Levinson A I, Zweiman B, Kornstein M J 1986 Antibodies to acetylcholine receptor and tetanus toxoid: in vitro synthesis by thymic lymphocytes. Journal of Immunology 137: 1221

Lisak R P, Levinson AI, Zweiman B, Kornstein M J 1987 In vitro synthesis of IgG and antibodies to AChR by peripheral blood and thymic lymphocytes. Annals of the New York Academy of Sciences 505: 39

Login I S, Kim Y I, Judd A M, Spaneglo B L, MacLeod 1987 Immunoglobulins of Lambert–Eaton myasthenic syndrome inhibit rat pituitary hormone release. Annals of Neurology 22: 610

MacDouall R M, Dunn M J, Dubowitz V 1989 Expression of class I and class II MHC antigens in neuromuscular diseases. Journal of the Neurological Sciences 89: 213

Mastaglia F L, Ojeda V J 1985 Inflammatory myopathies. Annals of Neurology 17: 215, 317

Mastaglia F L, Papadimitriou J M, Dawkins R L 1975 Mechanisms of cell-mediated myotoxicity: morphological observations in muscle grafts and in muscle exposed to sensitized spleen cells in vivo. Journal of the Neurological Sciences 25: 269

Miller K B, Schwartz R S 1982 Autoimmunity and suppressor T lymphocytes. Advances in Internal Medicine 160: 27, 281

Mishina M, Kurosaki T, Tobimatsu T et al 1984 Expression of functional acetylcholine receptor from cloned cDNAs. Nature 307: 604

Moore P M, Lisak R P 1990 Multiple sclerosis and Sjogren's syndrome: a problem in diagnosis or in definition of two disorders of unknown etiology? Annals of Neurology 27: 585

Mossman S, Vincent A, Newsom-Davis J 1985 Myasthenia gravis without acetylcholine-receptor antibody; a distinct entity. Lancet i: 116

Nennesmo I, Olsson T, Ljungdahl A, Kristensson, van der Meide P H 1989 Interferon-gamma-like immunoreactivity and T-cell expression in rat skeletal muscle. Brain Research 504: 306

Newsom-Davis J 1985 Lambert–Eaton myasthenic syndrome. Springer Seminars in Immunopathology 8: 129

Newsom-Davis J, Willcox N, Calder L 1981 Thymus cells in myasthenia gravis selectively enhance production of anti-acetylcholine receptor antibody by autologous blood lymphocytes. New England Journal of Medicine 305: 1313

Nossal G J V 1983 Cellular mechanisms of immunologic tolerance. In: Paul W E, Fathman C G, Metzger H (eds) Annual review of immunology. Annual Reviews, Palo Alto, p 33

Oldstone M B A, Schwimmbeck P, Dryberg T, Fujinami R 1986 Mimicry by virus of host molecules: implications for autoimmune disease. Progress in Immunology 6: 787

Olsson T, Henriksson K G, Klareskog L, Forsum U 1985 HLA-DR expression, T lymphocyte phenotypes, OKM1 and OKT9 reactive cells in inflammatory myopathy. Muscle and Nerve 8: 419

O'Neill J H, Murray J M, Newsom-Davis J 1988 The Lambert–Eaton myasthenic syndrome: a review of 50 cases. Brain 111: 577

Pachner A R 1989 Anti-acetylcholine receptor antibodies block bungarotoxin binding to native human acetylcholine receptor on the surface of TE 671 cells. Neurology 39: 1057

Patrick J, Lindstrom J 1973 Autoimmune response to acetylcholine receptor. Science 180: 871

Penn A S, Schotland D L, Rowland L P 1971 Immunology of muscle disease. Research Publication of the Association for Research in Nervous and Mental Diseases 49: 215

Protti M P, Manfredi A A, Straub C, Howard J F Jr, Conti-Tronconi B 1990 CD4+ T cell response to the human acetylcholine receptor α subunit in myasthenia gravis. A study with synthetic peptides. Journal of Immunology 144: 1276

Ragheb S, Lisak R P 1990 The frequency of CD5+ B lymphocytes in the peripheral blood of patients with myasthenia gravis. Neurology 40: 1120

Reyer M G, Noronha P, Thomas W, Hereda R 1983 Myositis of graft versus host disease. Neurology 33: 1222

Richman D P, Patrick J, Arnason B G W 1976 Cellular immunity in myasthenia gravis: response to purified acetylcholine receptor and autologous thymocytes. New England Journal of Medicine 294: 694

Robb S A, Bowley T J, Willcox N, Newsom-Davis 1985 Circulating T-cell subsets in the Lambert–Eaton syndrome. Journal of Neurology, Neurosurgery and Psychiatry 48: 501

Robinson M A, Kindt T J, 1989 Major histocompatibility antigens and genes. In: Paul W E (ed) Fundamental immunology, 2nd edn. Raven Press, New York, p 489

Rosenschein U, Radnay J, Shoham D, Shainberg A, Klajman A, Rozenszajn L A 1987 Human muscle-derived tissue specific, myocytotoxic T cell lines in dermatomyositis. Clinical and Experimental Immunology 67: 309

Rowe D J, Isenberg D A, McDougall J, Beverley P C L 1981 Characterization of polymyositis using monoclonal antibodies to human leukocyte antigen. Clinical and Experimental Immunology 45: 290

Sahashi K, Engel A G, Lindstrom J M, Lambert E H, Lennon V A 1978 Ultrastructural localization of immune complexes (IgG and C3d) at the endplate in experimental autoimmune myasthenia gravis. Neurology 29: 291

Schwartz JH, 1985 Molecular aspects of postsynaptic receptors. In: Kandel E R, Schwartz J H (eds) Principles of neural science, 2nd edn. Elsevier, New York, p 159

Schwimmbeck P L, Dryberg T, Drachman D B, Oldstone M B A 1989 Molecular mimicry and myasthenia gravis. An autoantigenic site of the acetylcholine receptor α-subunit that has biologic activity and reacts immunochemically with herpes simplex virus. Journal of Clinical Investigation 84: 1174

Sher E, Gotti C, Canal N, Scoppetta C, Piccolol G, Evoli A, Clementi F 1989 Specificity of calcium channel autoantibodies in Lambert–Eaton myasthenic syndrome. Lancet ii: 640

Simpson J A 1960 Myasthenia gravis: a new hypothesis. Scottish Medical Journal 5: 419

Skolnik P R, Lisak R P, Zweiman B 1982 Monoclonal antibody analysis of blood T cell subsets in myasthenia gravis. Annals of Neurology 11: 170

Souroujon M C, Pachner A R, Fuchs S 1986 The treatment of passively transferred experimental myasthenia with anti-idiotypic antibodies. Neurology 36: 622

Stephansson K, Dieperink M E, Richman D P, Gomez C M, Marton L S, 1984 Sharing of antigenic determinants between the nicotinic acetylcholine receptor and proteins in Escherichia coli, Proteus vulgaris, and Klebsiella pneumoniae. New England Journal of Medicine 312: 221

Sterz R, Hohfeld R, Rajki K, Kaul M, Heininger K, Peper K, Toyka K V 1986 Effector mechanisms in myasthenia gravis. Muscle and Nerve 9: 306

Tischler A S, Dichter M, Beales M 1977 Electrical excitability of oat cell carcinoma. Journal of Pathology 122: 153

Tonegawa S 1983 Somatic generation of antibody diversity. Nature 302: 575

Toyka K V, Drachman D B, Pestronk A, Kao I 1975 Myasthenia gravis: passive transfer from mouse. Science 190: 397

Tzartos S, Lindstrom J M 1980 Monoclonal antibodies used to prove acetylcholine receptor structure: localization of the main immunogenic region and detection of similarities between subunits. Proceeding of the National Academy of Sciences of the USA 77: 755

Tzartos S, Seybold M E, Lindstrom J M 1982 Specificity of antibodies to acetylcholine receptors in sera from myasthenia gravis patients measured by monoclonal antibodies. Proceedings of the National Academy of Sciences of the USA 79: 188

Vincent A, Scadding G K, Thomas H C, Newsom-Davis J 1978 In vitro synthesis of anti-acetylcholine receptor antibody by thymic lymphocytes in myasthenia gravis. Lancet i: 305

Vincent A, Whiting P J, Schluep M et al 1987 Antibody heterogeneity and specificity in myasthenia gravis. Annals of the New York Academy of Sciences 505: 106

Vincent A, Lang B, Newsom-Davis J 1989 Autoimmunity to the voltage-gated calcium channel underlies the Lambert–Eaton myasthenic syndrome, a paraneoplastic disorder. Trends in Neurosciences 12: 17

Wasserman N H, Penn A S, Freimuth P I et al 1982 Anti-idiotypic route to anti-acetylcholine receptor antibodies and experimental myasthenia gravis. Proceedings of the National Academy of Sciences of the USA 79: 4810

Whitaker J N, 1982 Inflammatory myopathy: a review of etiologic and pathogenic factors. Muscle and Nerve 5: 573

Whitaker J N, Engel W K 1972 Vascular deposits of immunoglobulin and complement in idiopathic inflammatory myopathy. New England Journal of Medicine 286: 333

Whiting P J, Vincent A, Newsom-Davis J 1983 Acetylcholine receptor antibody characteristics in myasthenia gravis. Fractionation of alpha-bungarotoxin binding site antibodies and their relationship to IgG subclasses. Journal of Neuroimmunology 5: 1

Willcox N A, Demaine A G, Newsom-Davis J, Welsh K I, Robb S A, Spirfo S G 1985 Increased frequency of IgG heavy chain marker G1m(2) and of HLA-B8 in Lambert–Eaton myasthenic syndrome with and without associated lung carcinoma. Human Immunology 14: 29

Williams C L, Lennon V A 1986 Thymic B lymphocyte clones from patients with myasthenia gravis secrete monoclonal striational autoantibodies reacting with myosin, alpha actinin or actin. Journal of Experimental Medicine 164: 1043

Wray D W, Peers C, Lang B, Lande S, Newsom-Davis J 1987 Interference with calcium channels by Lambert–Eaton myasthenic syndrome antibody. Annals of the New York Academy of Sciences 505: 368

Yamamoto Y, Ciulla T, Lang B, Vincent A, Newsom-Davis J 1990 Anticetylcholine receptor (AChR) antibody negative plasma from myasthenia gravis (MG) patients reduces 22Na+ through AChR channels. Neurology 40 (suppl 1): 185

Zanetti M 1985 The idiotype network in autoimmune processes. Immunology Today 6: 299

Zimmerman C W, Weiss G 1987 Antibodies not directed against the acetylcholine receptor in myasthenia gravis. An immunoblot study. Journal of Neuroimmunology 16: 225

Zweiman B, Lisak R P 1990 Autoantibodies, autoimmunity and immune complexes. In: Henry J (ed) Clinical diagnosis and management by laboratory methods, 18th edn. W B Saunders, Philadelphia

Zweiman B, Levinson A I, Lisak R P 1989 Phenotypic characteristics of thymic B lymphocytes in myasthenia gravis. Journal of Clinical Immunology 9: 942

5. Developmental disorders of muscle

Harvey B. Sarnat

INTRODUCTION

Developmental disorders of muscle are conditions in which striated muscle fails to develop, or to mature normally, because of altered embryological mechanisms, abnormal innervation or neural induction of muscle, or intrinsic metabolic errors which interfere with the maturation process. Some congenital myopathies may be viewed as developmental disorders if the premise is accepted that their pathogenesis involves distorted or arrested stages of fetal muscle fibre maturation. Progressive diseases altering mature muscle fibres are excluded.

EFFECTS OF OSSEOUS AGENESIS ON SKELETAL MUSCLE

Agenesis of particular bones results from genetically determined traits or exogeneously induced malformations of the fetus. Two groups of these congenital bony anomalies may be distinguished, each of which has a different effect upon the development of the skeletal muscles of the extremities. This difference is related to whether the osseous agenesis involves the vertebral column or long bones of the limbs.

Agenesis of the axial skeleton

Agenesis of sacral, lumbar, or even thoracic and cervical vertebral segments in the embryo may result in congenital contractures of the extremities, or arthrogryposis, but the long bones of the limbs are well formed (Sarnat et al 1976b, 1979). Teratogenic chemicals, including trypan blue and

streptonigrin, induce sacral agenesis in embryonic rats (Warkany & Takacs 1965). Lumbosacral agenesis in man is most commonly associated with maternal diabetes mellitus (Rusnak & Driscoll 1965, Passarge & Lenz 1966, Szalay 1975). Rumpless fowls are produced by injecting incubating eggs with insulin, but some strains of chickens are more susceptible, suggesting a genetic factor in addition to a possible teratogenic effect of insulin (Landauer 1945). An autosomal recessive trait for sacrococcygeal agenesis is found in a strain of laboratory mice (Frye et al 1964).

Aplasia or hypoplasia of skeletal muscle in the lower extremities of patients with lumbosacral agenesis is not progressive and may be attributed to three factors. The most important mechanism appears to be primary aplasia of muscle derived from embryonic myotomes at the same segmental levels as the absent vertebral bodies (Sarnat et al 1976a). Both bone and muscle are mesodermal structures and the same genetic or teratogenic factors may affect both. The subcutaneous space between skin and bone in the leg may be completely filled with fat, or small remnants of histologically normal muscle may remain, just as hypoplastic vertebral structures may be partly formed in the spine (Sarnat et al 1976a, Fig. 5.1). A second factor in the pathogenesis of deficient skeletal muscle in sacral agenesis is neuropathy caused by entrapment of ventral nerve roots, similar to the condition associated with meningomyelocele. A third factor, of uncertain importance, in malformation of the sacral spinal cord in some cases. This anomaly consists of displacement of motor neurones or fusion of the ventral horns. The complete or partial absence of muscle in

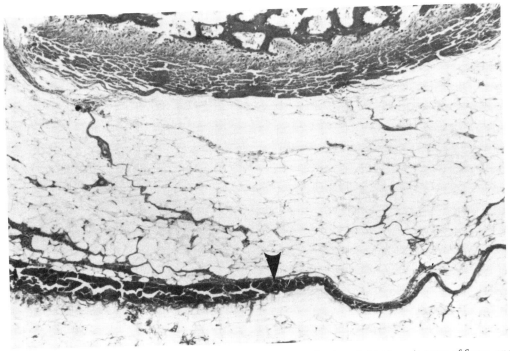

Fig. 5.1 Section of posterior calf of neonate with fatal lumbosacral agenesis. Portion of tibial bone is at top of figure, and fat replaces muscle except for a thin ribbon of soleus (arrowhead) composed of muscle fibres and a dense band of collagen. Primary amyoplasia. Picro-Mallory stain, × 32

sacral agenesis usually results in arthrogryposis from lack of antagonistic muscle balance and impaired joint movement in utero.

Agenesis of appendicular bones

Hypoplastic limbs or congenital absence of extremities may be due to hereditary epiphyseal dysplasias, as in achondroplasia, to known teratogenic drugs, such as thalidomide, or may represent sporadic congenital anomalies of unknown aetiology. In phocomelia, the long bones of the extremities fail to develop, and the hands may be imperfectly formed and attached at the shoulders. In amelia, the trunk, neck, and head are normally developed, but the extremities and usually the scapulae are totally absent. Less extreme variations include the absence of a single bone, such as the ulna, with the radius formed. In Sprengel's deformity, hypoplasia and upward displacement of the scapula result in a limited range of motion and shoulder girdle weakness. In these disorders, deformities of involved joints and contractures

may appear at birth as a result of mechanical factors.

Skeletal muscles of the extremities fail to differentiate from embryonic truncal myomeres if the long bones and other structures of the limbs fail to develop. In amelia or complete failure of limb buds to develop in man, it has been known for many years that the ventral horn motor neurones of the corresponding spinal segments are greatly reduced in number (Curtis & Helmholz 1911). This influence of the developing limb upon the number of surviving motor neurones is the result of an abnormally high rate of cell death in the spinal cord when immature motor neurones are unable to match with peripheral targets. Although the life of spinal motor neurones is unaffected by the peripheral field during early stages of neuronal differentiation, the establishment of peripheral connections is critical to their further survival. Amputation of developing limb buds of amphibians and birds results in a predictable reduction in the number of fetal motor neurones that survive to maturity (Hughes & Tschumi 1958, Prestige

1967, Lamb 1974). The earlier the limb bud is removed, the shorter the latent period before the motor neurones begin to degenerate (Prestige 1967). In contrast, the grafting of extra limbs in amphibians causes an increase in the total number of maturing motor neurones of the corresponding spinal cord segment (Hamburger 1934, Bueker 1945, Hollyday & Mendell 1976). Polydactyly in the chick and the mouse is also associated with hyperplasia of motor neurones in spinal segments supplying the extra digits (Tsang 1939, Baumann & Landauer 1943). Other factors influencing the number of embryonic motor neurones reaching maturity include hormones, growth factors, nutrients within the developing nervous system, temperature, and general nutrition (Jacobson 1978).

In extremities shortened or deformed because of defective long bones, the associated skeletal muscle may be small in bulk and is shortened because of a reduced number of sarcomeres and decreased sarcomere length. In postnatal growth, increase in skeletal muscle length results from the serial addition of sarcomeres (Williams & Goldspink 1971). The ability to add or delete sarcomeres is retained in the adult by immobilizing muscle in the lengthened or shortened position (Tabary et al 1972, Williams & Goldspink 1973). The addition of new sarcomeres in chronically stretched muscle allows the length of each sarcomere to be restored to optimal; the stretching due to bone growth is probably the necessary stimulus for normal postnatal increase in the number of sarcomeres (Williams & Goldspink 1978). However, young mammalian muscle does not respond to the stresses of immobilization by the addition of sarcomeres, as does adult muscle. Despite the added stretch stimulus of bone growth, immobilization in either extension or flexion results in a markedly decreased number of sarcomeres and a reduced length of muscle fascicles; the length of individual repeating sarcomeres is adjusted to attain maximum tension in the immobilized position, and may involve a lengthening of the tendon to achieve optimal sarcomere length (Crawford 1973, Williams & Goldspink 1978). Thus, the short muscles in the extremities of patients with phocomelia and other disorders of limb development are not replaced by fat and connective tissue as with vertebral agenesis, but rather consist of a decreased total number of sarcomeres with altered sarcomere length to achieve maximal tension. If the limb is relatively immobile, disuse atrophy, predominantly of type 2 fibres, occurs as an additional physiological reaction. Tenotomized muscle, by contrast, shortens due to a sustained reduction in sarcomere length, and central core lesions eventually develop in the fibres (Baker & Hall-Craggs 1980).

EFFECTS OF PERINATAL MYOPATHY ON OTHER BODY STRUCTURES

Undescended testes

In the male fetus, the testicles descend from the abdominal cavity into the scrotum during the eighth month of gestation. They are pulled down by the gubernaculum testis (Fig. 5.2). This thick cord contains both smooth and striated muscle. It extends from the skin of the embryonic groin forming the scrotum, through the inguinal canal, to the body and epididymis of the testis. The descent is partly under hormonal control, presumably affecting the smooth muscle component. Infants symptomatic at birth with diseases of striated muscle causing generalized weakness often have undescended testes, because of involvement of the striated muscle fibres of the gubernaculum. Cryptorchidism occurs both in neurogenic diseases, such as Werdnig–Hoffmann disease, and in myopathic disorders, such as neonatal myotonic dystrophy.

Prune-belly syndrome

Congenital absence of the rectus abdominis muscles as an isolated muscular anomaly is associated with hydronephrosis, probably resulting from deficient intra-abdominal pressure. Other urinary tract and renal anomalies may also be present. Most infants are male and have cryptorchidism, but the gubernaculum has not been studied in this syndrome to determine if it, too, is congenitally absent.

Hypoplasia of lungs

Amyoplasia of the diaphragm, resulting from phrenic nerve agenesis or bilateral diaphragmatic eventration, results in pulmonary hypoplasia and

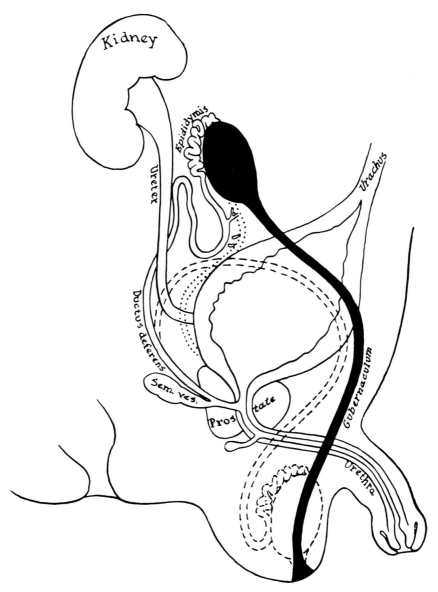

Fig. 5.2 The gubernaculum testis is a cord composed of a solid cylinder of smooth muscle surrounded by a sheath of striated muscle, that pulls the testis from the anterior abdominal wall into the scrotum in late fetal life. Neuromuscular diseases that begin in utero and are symptomatic at birth are often associated with undescended testicles because of weakness of the gubernaculum. (From Sarnat & Sarnat 1983, reproduced with permission.)

remodelling of the pulmonary circulation causing persistent pulmonary hypertension (Areechon & Reid 1963, Kitagawa et al 1971, Goldstein & Reid 1980).

Dysmorphism

Agenesis of single limbs may be attributed to amniotic bands interfering with limb bud development in the upper extremity before 28 days' gestation (Higginbottom et al 1979). Other limb abnormalities, including amputations and ring constrictions, also occur in utero from early amniotic rupture and entanglement of the fetus by strands of amnion (Jones et al 1974, Higginbottom et al 1979).

Failure of normal development of distal appendicular muscles may result in malformation of the hands and feet. In addition, there are congenital contractures of associated joints, the wrists and ankles and often hypoplasia of fingers, clinodactyly, abnormal position of the thumb, and distorted palmar creases and dermatoglyphics. Such dysmorphic features are particularly frequent in neurogenic diseases involving fetal muscle (Darwish et al 1981, Fig. 5.3).

Weakness of muscles of the head and jaw such as the temporalis, of the pharynx and palate, and of the face, contribute to abnormal moulding of the head and palate. Dolichocephaly and high arched palate are particularly common clinical features of some congenital myopathies such as nemaline rod disease and congenital muscle fibre type disproportion. Facial weakness prenatally results in the characteristic inverted V-shaped upper lip of some neonates with myotonic dystrophy, similar to the facies seen in the affected older child. By contrast, the characteristic facies of patients with Down's syndrome (trisomy 21) are due to extra slips of platysma muscle at the corners of the mouth and anomalous bands of muscle attached to the orbicularis oculi muscles (Bersu 1980).

Congenital dislocated hips

This condition is a common consequence of weakness or hypotonia of muscles of the hip girdle, regardless of whether the underlying disease is a progressive muscular dystrophy or spinal muscular atrophy, or a non-progressive condition such as 'benign congenital hypotonia' or congenital muscle fibre type disproportion.

ARTHROGRYPOSIS

Infants born with limbs fixed in abnormal postures and lacking the full range of motion have been recognized since Otto's description in 1841. In 1905, Rosenkranz introduced the term 'arthrogryposis', which means 'curved joint'. It was expanded by Stern in 1923 to 'arthrogryposis multiplex congenita' (AMC), a name which has given rise to considerable confusion because it was accepted for many years as a single disease entity.

AMC is a heterogeneous disorder, but is not a constant feature of any disease of either neurogenic or myopathic origin. Even among monozygotic twins, only one of the pair may be involved (Brandt 1947, Hillman & Johnson 1952, Kite 1955, Pedreira & Long 1971), or both infants may have contractures (Lipton & Morgenstern 1955).

Most infants with AMC have spinal muscular atrophy (Brandt 1947, Kanof et al 1956, Fowler 1959, Byers & Banker 1961, Drachman & Banker 1961, Swinyard & Mogora 1962, Smith et al 1963, Vestermark 1966, Amick et al 1967). However, only 5 of 52 cases of Werdnig–Hoffmann disease had arthrogryposis (Byers & Banker 1961). Multiple congenital contractures occur regularly in other diseases associated with deficiency or degeneration of spinal motor neurones at birth, such as the Pena–Shokeir syndrome (Hageman et al 1987) and the Marden–Walker syndrome (Sees et al 1990). AMC was found in 19 of 61 cases diagnosed as Möbius' syndrome, presumably because of congenital deficiency of motor neurones in the spinal cord as well as the brainstem (Henderson 1939), but this diagnosis is often made incorrectly. Contractures have not been found in infants with perinatal poliomyelitis (Pugh & Dudgeon 1954, Grossiord et al 1958). Cases of infants with AMC and lesions of spinal motor roots or peripheral nerves, such as neurofibromas, are also known (Moore 1941, Hooshmand et al 1971), and the association of lumbosacral meningomyeloceles with talipes deformities and other contractures in the lower limbs is well recognized (Dodge 1960).

AMC is associated with a variety of cerebral lesions and malformations of the brain (Ek 1958, Fowler 1959, Sandbank & Cohen 1964, Fowler & Manson 1973), but dystrophic lesions in muscle are found in some (Fowler & Manson 1973). A syndrome of hydranencephaly and AMC occurs in calves (Whittem 1957), and hereditary AMC in sheep is also known (Roberts 1929).

Among the human myopathies, AMC is more common in neonatal myotonic dystrophy than in any other congenital muscle disease (Sarnat et al 1976b). It is also a common feature of congenital muscle fibre type disproportion (Brooke 1973). Contractures may occur in other myopathies in the neonatal period, but were reported in neonatal myasthenia gravis only once, in an infant of a myasthenic mother (Holmes et al 1980). Amyo-

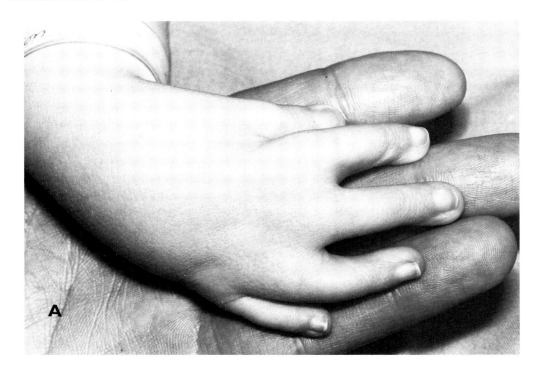

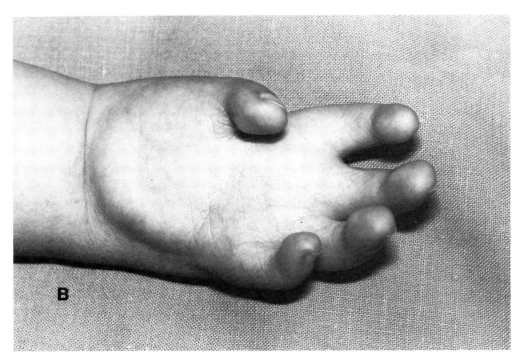

Fig. 5.3 (A) Dorsal surface of right hand and (B) palmar surface of left hand of infant with spinal muscular atrophy. Poor development of muscles of forearm and hands in utero is associated with malformation of hand and fingers

plasia, as associated with agenesis of the lower spine, consistently results in AMC of the lower limbs (Sarnat et al 1976a).

The type of contracture, flexor or extensor, is related to the in utero posture of the fetus which lacks active movement of joints because of weakness. Drachman & Coulombre (1962) produced AMC in chicks by infusing D-tubocurarine into incubating eggs, thus producing the effect of denervation by neuromuscular blockade. In every case, the fixed posture of the joints of the legs, wings and neck corresponded to the position of the embryo within the shell. Such joint deformities are a function of the duration of paralysis, chick embryos immobilized for 24 hours do not develop contractures, but after 48 hours, arthrogryposis develops (Oppenheim et al 1978). The probable reason that most infants with Werdnig–Hoffmann disease are merely hypotonic and weak without contractures is that the time of most rapid progression of the disease occurs after birth, when the infant lies fully extended most of the time. Infants with Potter syndrome associated with oligohydramnios and limitation of fetal movement often have contractures at birth (Thomas & Smith 1974). The suggestion that talipes deformities and even some forms of arthrogryposis might result from excessive intrauterine pressure associated with a reduced volume of amniotic fluid has been proposed by several authors (Rosenkranz 1905, Browne 1936, Friedlander et al 1968).

AMC is not necessarily the result of weakness alone in all cases. Daentl et al (1974) reported a family without clinical weakness despite AMC and lesions in muscle. Contractures may also develop postnatally in congenital muscular dystrophies (Short 1963), probably because of progressive fibrosis of muscle.

Proliferation of connective tissue is suspected to be a primary mechanism in the development of AMC in some cases, such as Marfan's syndrome (Hecht & Beals 1972) and other diseases of connective tissue (McKusick 1956). Histopathological evidence suggests that an increase in connective tissue precedes muscle fibre degeneration in some cases (Hariga et al 1963), and an increased rate of collagen synthesis, measured by the rate of amino acid incorporation, has been shown in vitro in muscle from two patients with idiopathic AMC

(Ionasescu et al 1970). The muscle biopsies of those infants revealed several abnormal findings, including scattered immature fibres. The amount of connective tissue proliferation in the muscles of neonates with myotonic dystrophy or with Werdnig–Hoffmann disease is insufficient to account for the contractures.

Viral myositis may be the cause of AMC in some infants. Coxsackie A2 virus produces severe AMC in chicks by causing an intense inflammatory reaction in the muscles of embryos, resulting in total paralysis in 48 hours and almost complete replacement of muscle by fat and connective tissue within 4 days, before the. time of hatching (Drachman et al 1976).

Contractures of the extremities are common in some chromosomal disorders, especially trisomies 13 and 18. Characteristic flexion deformities of the fingers are due to displacement of the tendons of extensor digitorum and digiti minimi; an absence of some muscles and duplication of other muscles account for additional contractures (Ramirez-Castro & Bersu 1978, Pettersen 1979). Histological and histochemical study of extensor and flexor muscles associated with contractures in neonates dying with trisomy 18 does not show abnormalities.

DISORDERS OF MUSCLE MATURATION

Some neonatal myopathies are characterized pathologically by immature muscle fibres, mostly fetal myotubes, beyond the time when they are normally present. Whether small muscle fibres with central nuclei in early infancy are actually arrested in maturation, delayed in development, or are morphologically altered fibres which merely resemble myotubes remains an issue for debate.

Some investigators object to the use of the term 'myotube' in any reference other than to the myofibre normally seen at 8 to 15 weeks' gestation in the human embryo. Despite the lack of semantic purity, it is useful to designate muscle fibres as 'myotubes' in some pathological conditions of early infancy, if sufficient morphological similarity to true fetal myotubes suggests that maturational delay is the likely mechanism. Use of the term myotube requires one to identify some features detectable only by histochemistry and electron microscopy, and the term should not be applied

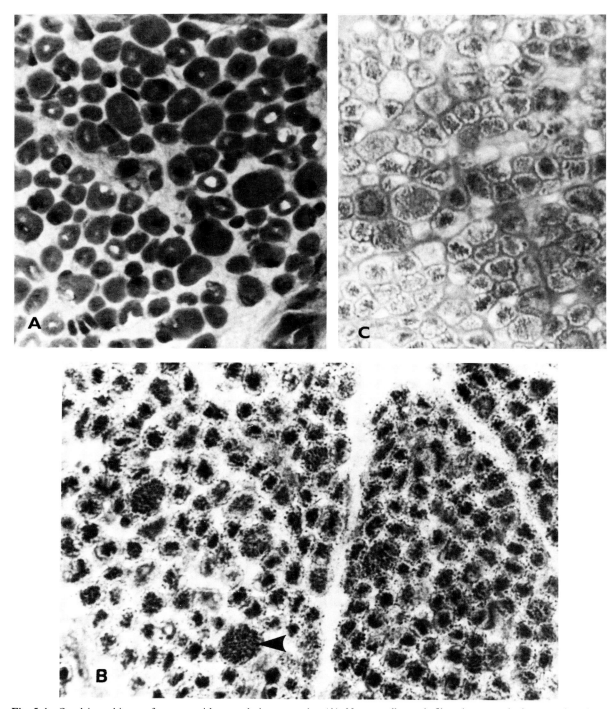

Fig. 5.4 Quadriceps biopsy of neonate with myotubular myopathy. (A) Many small muscle fibres have a vesicular central nucleus or a central clear zone at levels between nuclei (H&E). (B) Oxidative enzymatic activity is concentrated in central clear zones of muscle fibres and in subsarcolemmal regions, as in fetal myotubes. A few mature fibres have uniform sarcoplasmic distribution of diformazan products (arrowhead) (NADH–TR). (C) Glycogen has a similar distribution in most fibres, as in fetal myotubes (PAS). × 320

indiscriminately to any muscle fibre with internal nuclei; the secondary migration of peripheral sarcolemmal nuclei to an internal position between myofibrils is a non-specific myopathic feature of many acquired myopathies of later life.

The following criteria are proposed for application of the term 'myotube' to muscle fibres in the biopsy of neonates or young infants (Fig. 5.4).

1. Muscle fibre diameter should not exceed 15 μm. Most measure 5–8 μm.

2. In cross-section, each fibre has either a single central nucleus or a central pale or clear zone, as seen with haematoxylin–eosin or trichrome stains. In longitudinal section, a single row of unevenly spaced nuclei occupies the centre of the muscle fibre and peripheral nuclei are not found in the same fibre. Cross-striations are distinct only in the myofibrils forming the peripheral rim or tube; the cytoplasm in the centre of the muscle fibre, between nuclei, appears pale and amorphous with haematoxylin–eosin or trichrome, and striations are not identified in this zone. The distance between nuclei varies from one to three nuclear diameters, which is greater than that found in true myotubes of embryos.

3. Nuclei are large and vesicular, slightly elongated, and have a prominent nucleolus. With the haematoxylin stain, the chromatin appears less densely concentrated than in mature sarcolemmal nuclei.

4. With incubation for activity of nicotinamide adenine dinucleotide tetrazolium reductase (NADH–TR) or succinic dehydrogenase (SDH), cross-sections disclose that the centres of fibres cut at levels between nuclei have intense enzymatic activity; the activity within the rim of myofibrils is sparse, and another thin zone of activity is concentrated in the subsarcolemmal region. Type 1 and 2 muscle fibres cannot be distinguished.

5. The periodic acid–Schiff (PAS) reaction reveals a pattern similar to that of NADH–TR. Glycogen is concentrated in the centre of the fibre between the nuclei, and is completely digested by diastase. Clear centres of muscle fibres in cross-section that do not stain with PAS correspond to nuclei.

6. The oil red O stain is positive for lipid in the centre of the fibre between nuclei.

7. Phosphorylase activity is greatest in the centre of the fibre between nuclei. Fibre types are indistinguishable.

8. Myofibrillar adenosine triphosphatase (ATPase) activity is confined to the peripheral rim of myofibrils; the centres of fibres are unstained, regardless of whether the section is at the level of a nucleus or between nuclei. One difference between true myotubes of embryos, and fibres called myotubes in myotubular myopathy or neonatal myotonic dystrophy, is that embryonic myotubes are histochemically undifferentiated; in pathological 'myotubes', fibre types are not distinguished with oxidative or glycolytic enzymatic activity, but ATPase does show differentiation, including reversibility of inhibition by pre-incubation at low and high pH ranges. This differentiation may be complete or incomplete.

9. Electron microscopy reveals that organelles, particularly mitochondria, and glycogen, are concentrated in the centre of fibres between nuclei, rather than being evenly distributed in the sarcoplasm between myofibrils. Mitochondria have cristae. Nuclei may have convoluted membranes. The transverse tubular system may maintain an immature longitudinal orientation in the muscle fibre instead of the perpendicular position of mature transverse tubules.

10. Immunoreactivity for vimentin and desmin is positive, resembling true fetal myotubes (see *Myotubular myopathy*, below).

Maturational arrest of muscle in early stages of development

In the newborn rat, 90% of soleus muscle fibres are still myotubes. Sciatic neurotomy at birth arrests further development and the myotubes persist without histochemical differentiation into fibre types (Engel & Karpati 1968). In the adult rat, denervation retards or prevents the structural, metabolic and functional differentiation of regenerating muscle fibres (Carlson & Gutmann 1976). The normal transformation of type 2 muscle fibres to type 1, the result of changing physiological properties of motor neurones from phasic to tonic (Kugelberg 1976), is arrested or delayed after damage to the nerve (Karpati & Engel 1967). Abnormal or impaired innervation in fetal life, therefore, may be postulated as one cause of maturational arrest in neonates with neuromuscular disease. This factor probably accounts for the scattered myotubes in muscle biopsies of infants with Werdnig–Hoffmann disease (Fidziańska 1976) and with congenital neuropathies, except those attributable to trauma sustained during delivery.

Peripheral nerve involvement in myotonic dystrophy is described (Panayiotopoulos & Scarpalezos 1977), but this disease is believed to be primarily a myopathy. There are many reports of abnormal sarcolemmal membrane structure and function in myotonic dystrophy. These data suggest another mechanism of maturational arrest of fetal muscle in the neonatal form of this disease: the innervation is normal, but the abnormal muscle membrane does not respond to trophic induction by the motor neurone (Sarnat & Silbert 1976).

Myotonia may be induced in neonatal as well as adult rats by the administration of hypocholesterolaemic drugs, but whether this phenomenon is related to myotonic dystrophy is not known, and these drugs do not cause maturational delay of skeletal muscle when administered perinatally (Ramsey et al 1978).

Muscle regeneration

Regenerating muscle after traumatic injury to mature muscle fibres also bears many similarities to developing fetal muscle, including the formation of myotubes (Allam 1979).

Myotubular myopathy

This term has generated considerable controversy because of its explicit implication of maturational arrest of fetal myotubes. It is probably best reserved to characterize a congenital centronuclear myopathy with clinical expression at birth. Affected infants exhibit reduced muscle bulk, generalized hypotonia and weakness, and involvement of pharyngeal and respiratory muscles. Most cases are inherited as an X-linked recessive trait (van Wijngaarden et al 1969, Barth et al 1975, Palmucci et al 1988), but autosomal dominant (Torres et al 1985) and autosomal recessive (Sher et al 1967,

Radu et al 1977, Martin et al 1977) forms are also described.

The resemblance to fetal myotubes is based upon the cyto-architecture of myofibres, consisting of a central row of spaced nuclei and intervening cytoplasm in which the mitochondria, glycogen particles, and oxidative enzymatic activities are concentrated (Fig. 5.4). Many authors have questioned this interpretation (Sher et al 1967, Munsat et al 1969). Munsat et al (1969) demonstrated mature rather than fetal myoglobin in the muscle of affected infants, similar to their findings in the full-term neonate. A prospective study comparing muscle from fetuses of 8–16 weeks' gestation, full-term and preterm neonates, and infants with myotubular myopathy showed many histochemical and ultrastructural features of normal maturation in myotubular myopathy: complete histochemical differentiation of fibre types with myofibrillar ATPase; registry of Z-bands between adjacent myofibrils; formation of triads and perpendicular orientation relative to the long axis of the myofibre; condensation of nuclear chromatin and nucleoli; and a well-formed fascicular organization of the muscle, with perimysium, muscle spindles, mature blood vessels, myelinated intramuscular nerves, and well-formed motor end-plates (Sarnat 1990). In addition, the number, morphology and cytoplasmic distribution of RNA in motor neurones was normal. Other features common in true fetal muscle, such as frequent mitoses of presumptive myoblasts, programmed cell death of scattered myotubes, and extrajunctional acetylcholine receptors, are absent or rare in both full-term neonatal muscle and in myotubular myopathy.

One feature of neonatal myotubular myopathy that does resemble fetal muscle, however, is a persistence of high concentrations of vimentin and desmin (Sarnat 1990; Fig. 5.5). These intermediate filament proteins may contribute to the apparent arrest in morphogenesis of myofibres by retaining nuclei and mitochondria in immature central positions, their normal place in fetal myotubes. They are present in high concentration in fetal myotubes, but diminish with maturation so that vimentin normally disappears entirely by term and desmin is reduced to extremely low concentrations (Bennett et al 1979). Muscle biopsies from mothers of affected infants show strong immunoreactivity for vimentin and desmin in scattered small myofibres (Sarnat 1990). In other conditions, desmin but not vimentin is increased in myotonic muscular dystrophy and in some atrophic fibres in infantile spinal muscular atrophy, and both proteins may be increased in regenerating myofibres (Sarnat, unpublished observations).

Some authors have suggested lesions of peripheral nerve as a cause of myotubular myopathy, but the evidence for a neurogenic mechanism is meagre and inconclusive. If persistent vimentin and desmin are indeed the pathogenetic basis of the disease, the genetic factors are complex. Not only are several modes of inheritance demonstrated, but the gene locus for vimentin is linked to chromosome 10 (10p13) and that for desmin is localized to chromosome 2 (2q35), rather than to the X-chromosome (Quax et al 1985, Ferrari et al 1987, Viegas-Péquignot et al 1989). The defective gene in X-linked myotubular myopathy has now been linked to the Xq28 locus (Thomas et al 1990, Darnfors et al 1990).

Neonatal myotonic muscular dystrophy

The severely involved neonate is nearly always the offspring of an affected mother, despite autosomal dominant inheritance in which either parent may transmit the usual form of the disease (Dyken & Harper 1973, Harper 1975). Only a minority of infants with myotonic dystrophy are already symptomatic at birth. The severe neonatal disease is unrelated to the severity of the maternal disease (Sarnat et al 1976b). Its characteristic clinical pattern includes severe generalized muscle weakness involving respiratory and pharyngeal muscles, arthrogryposis, hypotonia, facial weakness and an inverted V-shaped upper lip (Bell & Smith 1972, Dyken & Harper 1973, Aicardi et al 1974, Sarnat et al 1976b). Smooth muscle, particularly of the gastrointestinal tract, is also frequently involved (Sarnat et al 1976b, Lenard et al 1977). The muscle biopsy shows delayed or arrested maturation in all stages of development (Karpati et al 1973, Farkas-Bargeton et al 1974, Sarnat & Silbert 1976). Myotubes are most readily recognized, but electron microscopy also reveals many primitive myoblasts and excessive numbers of satellite cells.

Muscle fibres more mature than myotubes, with peripheral sarcolemmal nuclei, but incompletely differentiated histochemically, are also found, and scattered fibres appear fully mature. The involvement is variable among different muscles in the same patient: the largest number of immature fibres are in those muscles associated with joint contractures, the diaphragm, and the pharynx (Sarnat & Silbert 1976). By contrast with the findings in the muscle biopsy of the older child or adult, muscle fibre necrosis, endomysial fibrosis, and such cytoarchitectural changes as split fibres and striated annulets are not found. Atrophy predominantly of type 1 muscle fibres may be seen in early infancy in muscles not severely affected by maturational delay (Argov et al 1984).

Muscle biopsy performed in the neonatal period in infants with myotubular myopathy and neonatal myotonic dystrophy may show changes which are difficult to distinguish but, in the latter, a greater variety of fibres arrested in different stages of development is seen.

Maturational delay of muscle in late stages of development

Intrauterine growth retardation and chronic systemic illness

Skeletal muscle fibres become histochemically differentiated between 20 and 30 weeks' gestation in man. At the end of this period, the normal mosaic pattern of types 1 and 2 muscle fibres of approximately equal number is seen (Dubowitz 1966). Type 2 fibre subtypes are distinguished with ATPase stains during the final three months of gestation, and at term, about 15–20% of fibres are still classified as undifferentiated (Farkas-Bargeton et al 1977, Colling-Saltin 1978). Early in the period of 20–30 weeks' gestation about 10% of muscle fibres, the 'Wohlfart b-fibres', are larger than the rest and have histochemical properties of type 1 fibres; the remaining 90% of 'Wohlfart a-fibres' are of type 2 (Wohlfart 1937, Fenichel 1963, Dubowitz 1966). Wohlfart b-fibres are evenly distributed in the muscle fascicles and not grouped. Additional type 2 fibres become converted to type 1 as maturation proceeds. A few scattered large type 1 fibres resembling Wohlfart

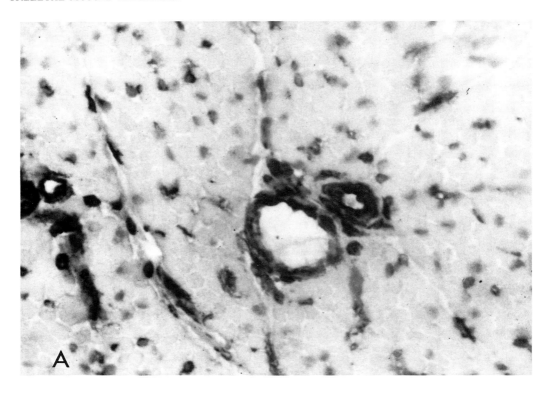

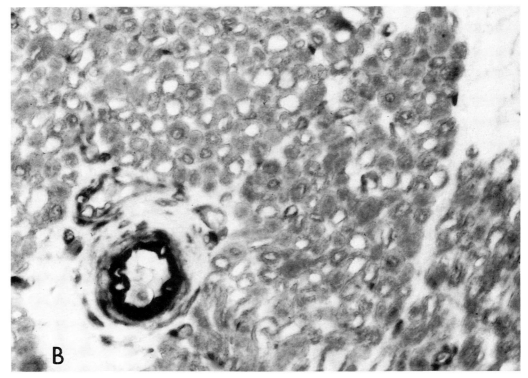

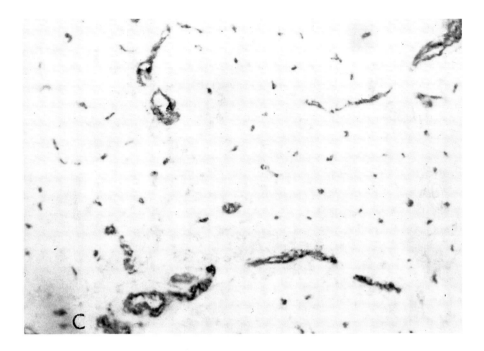

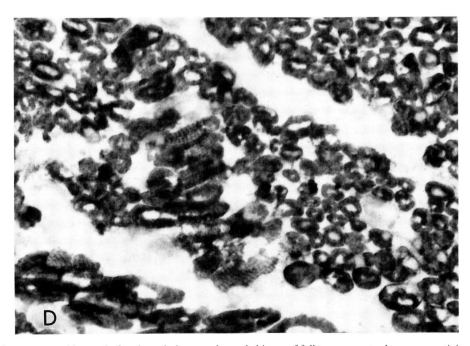

Fig. 5.5 (A) Immunoperoxidase stain for vimentin in normal muscle biopsy of full-term neonate shows no reactivity of myofibres, though endothelial cells of small blood vessels are stained. (B) Myotube-like muscle fibres in neonatal X-linked myotubular myopathy show strong immunoreactivity for vimentin. (C) Immunoperoxidase stain for desmin in normal muscle biopsy of full-term neonate shows no staining of striated myofibres; smooth muscle of vascular walls is strongly reactive. (D) Strong immunoreactivity to anti-desmin antibodies is seen in myofibres of neonate with X-linked myotubular myopathy. A and B ×460, C and D ×400

b-fibres are still encountered in the muscle biopsy of normal full-term neonates, but they are rare (Wohlfart 1937, Fenichel 1963, Dubowitz 1966, Colling-Saltin 1978). They are proportionately more numerous in premature infants, although they are not found in all muscles at any time of gestation (Colling-Saltin 1978).

Infants who have suffered intrauterine growth retardation and are small for gestational age have an increased number of Wohlfart b-fibres at birth. This type of mildly delayed muscle maturation also occurs in young infants who have chronic systemic stress or illness, and is not evidence of specific neuromuscular disease. Examples include premature infants with chronic respiratory distress or nutritional deficiencies. It might also be expected to occur in some endocrinopathies at birth, particularly cretinism (Mastaglia et al 1988), although the pathological and histochemical muscular findings in cretins at birth are incompletely documented. In this regard, it may be relevant that high doses of thyroxine administered to metamorphosing amphibians result in precocious cytodifferentiation and death of spinal motor neurones (Reynolds 1963), while the antithyroid drug thiourea prevents normal embryonic cell death in the spinal cord of tadpoles (Prestige 1965).

Protein-calorie malnutrition

Muscular changes seen postnatally in children with protein-calorie malnutrition consist of generalized smallness of individual muscle fibres, excessive variation in fibre size, grouped atrophy in places, and poor differentiation of histochemical fibre types (Dastur et al 1979). Sarcolemmal nuclei retain their peripheral position in the muscle fibre and are not increased in number; myopathic cytoarchitectural alterations are not seen by light microscopy, but the electron microscope reveals focal degenerative changes in myofibrils and loss of mitochondria and other sarcoplasmic constituents. Regenerating muscle fibres and fetal-type myotubes are also seen in infancy. These changes indicate not only retarded development and atrophy of previously formed muscle fibres but also degeneration of some fibres followed by regeneration (Dastur et al 1979). Some of these changes in muscle may be due to

the effects of malnutrition on growth and conduction velocity of myelinated nerve in man and other mammals (Sima 1974, Sima & Jankowska 1975, Dastur et al 1977).

Abnormal growth of histochemical type 1 muscle fibres

In the adult, muscle fibres of histochemical type 2 (physiological fast-twitch fibres) undergo disuse atrophy and work hypertrophy more readily than type 1 fibres. In the developing fetus, however, type 1 fibres alter their size in a predictable manner under specific circumstances.

Hypoplasia of type 1 muscle fibres

Several non-progressive congenital myopathies of uncertain relationship to one another are characterized by a common pathological finding of uniformly small type 1 fibres, and normal or mildly enlarged type 2 fibres.

Congenital muscle fibre type disproportion (CMFTD)

This term was originally used to describe a series of 14 patients, ranging in age from infancy to adolescence, with congenital non-progressive hypotonia, mild weakness, and variable congenital contractures, dislocated hips, and minor skeletal deformities (Brooke 1973). Intelligence was normal and chromosomes were also normal in number and morphology.

The muscle biopsies from these cases revealed a uniformly small size of all type 1 fibres, which otherwise appeared morphologically mature, and normal size or mild hypertrophy of type 2 fibres. Subtype 2b fibres were the largest in size. In the majority of cases, 'disproportion' not only involves the size of muscle fibres of each type, but also the relative numbers of fibres of each type, the small type 1 fibres being more numerous than the type 2 fibres (Fig. 5.6). Neurogenic type grouping does not occur and no myopathic features or degenerative changes are found. The characteristic muscle biopsy findings of CMFTD are already present at birth (Fardeau et al 1975, Sarnat 1978).

Hypothesis. Congenital muscle fibre type disproportion may be due to an abnormally high rate of embryonic cell death among spinal motor

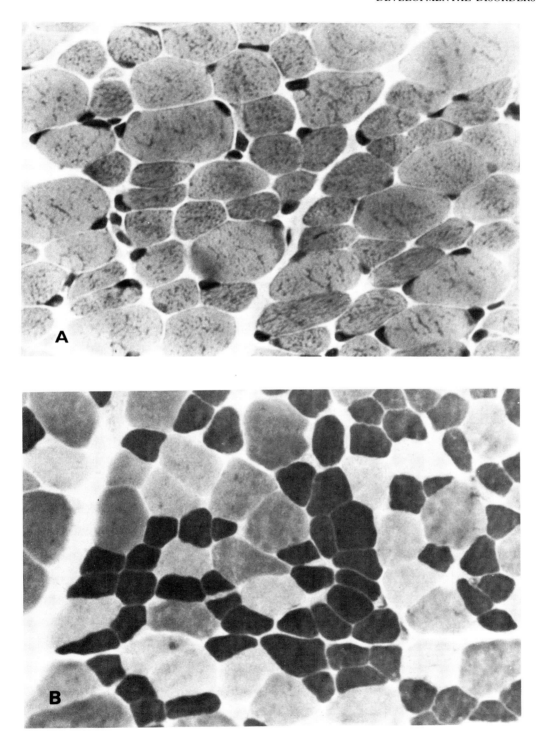

Fig. 5.6   CMFTD in 13-month-old infant with Krabbe's disease. Small fibres are uniformly of type 1, are more numerous than large type 2 fibres, and are both grouped and scattered in distribution. (A) Modified Gomori trichrome stain. (B) Myofibrillar ATPase pH 4.7; × 320

neuroblasts early in gestation. Each surviving motor neurone attempts to induce growth in its larger number of muscle fibres by increasing its rate of electrical discharge. This continuous stimulation results in maturation of the giant motor unit and induction of histochemical type 1 muscle fibres, but the large size of the motor unit prevents individual muscle fibres from achieving a normal diameter.

A large overproduction of neuroblasts in the early stages of embryogenesis is followed by programmed degeneration of some neuroblasts. Some motor neurones are already in an advanced stage of differentiation while production of new motor neurones by mitosis of germinal cells is still in progress. In the chick embryo, the first motor axons contact anterior truncal muscles at 3.5 days' incubation, and reach proximal limb muscles on day 5, normal cell death in the ventral horn of the spinal cord is maximal at 4.5 days, and mitosis of motor neuronal precursors persists until day 8 (Fujita 1963, 1965, Wechsler 1966 a,b). Neuronal cell death in the ventral horn of the spinal cord is not related to the shift from the primitive pattern of polyneuronal innervation of embryonic muscle fibres to single neuronal innervation (Oppenheim & Majors-Willard 1978). This change is accomplished by the retraction of collateral axons.

As species-specific examples of the balance between the production of excess neuroblasts and subsequent elimination by cell death of those that do not successfully match, beavers have six times as many neurones in their mature mesencephalic trigeminal nucleus as do hamsters, although it is likely that both species produce an approximately equal surplus of neuroblasts. Turtles have few thoracic muscle fibres, and consequently require very few thoracic spinal motor neurones; the evolutionary process has reduced the total number of surviving ventral motor neuroblasts generated, to levels well below those of other reptiles (Katz & Lasek 1978). The embryological process thus influences evolution as much as the converse is true, and ontogenesis and phylogenesis are intimately related developmental programmes for each species. While relative smallness of type 1 muscle fibres is not representative of any known stage in the normal ontogenesis of human muscle, it is the

normal adult condition in some mammals, such as rodents (Fig. 5.7). CMFTD may thus represent a neuromuscular developmental disorder of phylogenetic–ontogenetic interaction. Quantitative studies of motor neurones in idiopathic CMFTD have not been performed; it is not usually a lethal disease. Peculiar facies, in addition to facial weakness and other minor dysmorphic features, often occur in children with idiopathic CMFTD, although chromosomal analysis is normal (Brooke 1973). These clinical features are consistent with a putative brief disturbance in early embryogenesis involving a generation of motor neuroblasts in spinal cord and brain stem and the morphogenesis of facial structures. Such an insult may be acquired or genetically determined.

The occurrence of CMFTD in Krabbe's disease suggests a neurogenic aetiology (Martin et al 1976, Dehkharghani et al 1981, Fig. 5.6), since segmental demyelination, fibrosis, and axonal degeneration in peripheral nerves are characteristic of this leukodystrophy of early infancy (Hogan et al 1969). The deficient enzyme in Krabbe's disease, galactocerebroside β-galactosidase, is not known to participate directly in the metabolism of muscle.

The ability of fully mature motor neurones to sustain abnormally large motor units is well shown by the re-innervation phenomenon of histochemical type grouping in muscles of adult patients with motor neurone disease or motor neuropathy. Although the individual muscle fibres of these large adult motor units are not uniformly small as in CMFTD, often a greater-than-normal variability of muscle fibre diameter persists within the group and some fibres remain atrophic. Thus, even a mature motor neurone cannot exert uniform trophic control in an excessively large motor unit.

A minority of motor neurones may innervate a relatively smaller number of muscle fibres, and these are the only motor units capable of differentiating into type 2. The large size of type 2 muscle fibres in CMFTD is more pronounced in older infants and children than in neonates and probably represents compensatory hypertrophy in other normal-sized motor units. Because the maximum diameter of a muscle fibre is inversely proportional to the square root of its metabolic rate, type 2

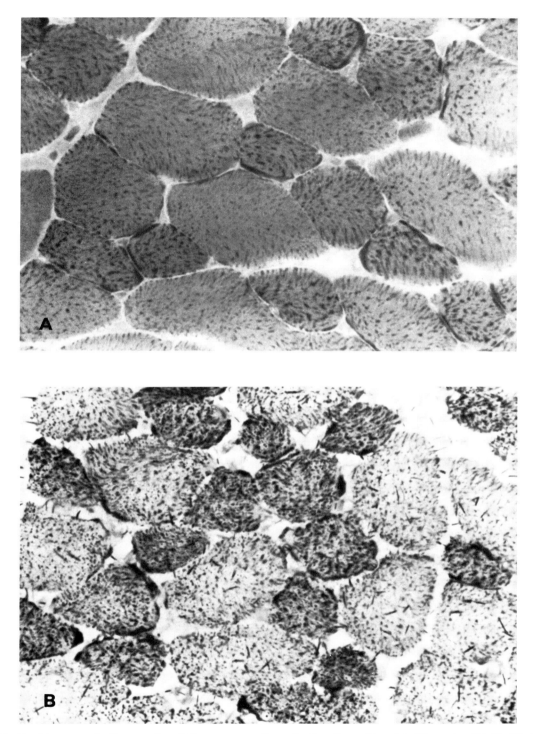

Fig. 5.7 Quadriceps muscle of mouse. Type 1 fibres are normally smaller than those of type 2 in this species. (A) Modified Gomori trichrome stain. (B) NADH–TR; × 320

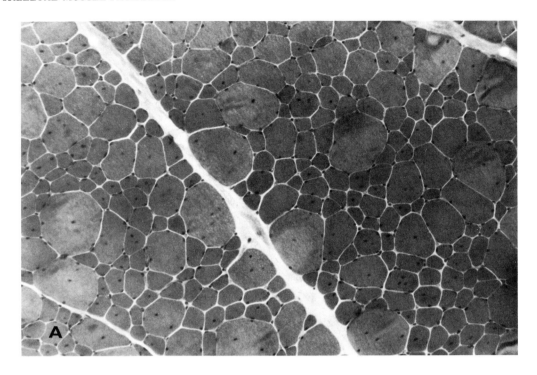

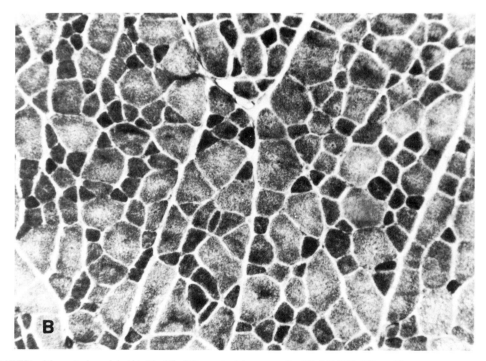

Fig. 5.8   CMFTD with central nuclei. (A) Modified Gomori trichrome stain. (B) NADH–TR; × 80

muscle fibres more easily attain a larger diameter than type 1 fibres with physical work because of their lower metabolic rate; experimental surgically induced imbalance of antagonistic muscles in animals and isometric training in human weight-lifters lead to well-maintained enlargement of type 2 fibres (James 1979).

In some congenital neuromuscular diseases of a developmental or non-progressive type, all or nearly all muscle fibres are differentiated histo-chemically as type 1, and type 2 fibres fail to develop or are sparse. This condition is found in some centronuclear myopathies (Palmucci et al 1978a), central core disease (Dubowitz & Roy 1970, Palmucci et al 1978b), and in some families with nemaline rod disease (Fukuhara et al 1978).

CMFTD with central nuclei. In a congenital myopathy which has been described by several authors, CMFTD is accompanied by central nuclei in many muscle fibres of both histochemical types (Engel et al 1968, Bethlem et al 1969, Karpati et al 1970, Sarnat 1979, Bergen et al 1980, Fig. 5.8). These features are not only present in the neonate, but persist in childhood and adult life. Involved children are generally weaker than those with CMFTD alone, and many have ptosis, ophthal-moplegia and facial weakness, uncommon features of simple CMFTD. Whether the central nuclei represent maturational arrest of fetal myotubes is not certain, and the relationship of central nuclei and of CMFTD to each other and to the matura-tion process in these cases is also unknown.

CMFTD with nemaline rods. Nemaline rods are inclusion-like accumulations of Z-band material which are unevenly distributed in the muscles of some children with non-progressive congenital myopathies, and which also occur in other diseases and under experimental conditions of tenotomy. A characteristic clinical pattern is associated with 'nemaline rod disease', similar to that of CMFTD. Furthermore, type 1 muscle fibre predominance and smallness of type I fibres is found, in addition to nemaline rods, in the muscle biopsy of many such patients (Gonatas et al 1966, Bender & Willner 1978, Fukuhara et al 1978). This asso-ciation suggests that CMFTD may actually be the primary developmental disorder, and the nemaline rods a secondary reaction of muscle.

Type 1 fibre hypertrophy

By contrast with hypoplasia of type 1 muscle fibres in CMFTD, one of the distinguishing features of the muscle biopsy in acute infantile spinal muscular atrophy (Werdnig–Hoffmann disease) is the presence of hypertrophic muscle fibres, almost all of type 1 as defined by the myofibrillar ATPase stain. They are mostly grouped, unlike the evenly scattered distribution of fetal Wohlfart b-fibres. This pattern of grouped giant type 1 muscle fibres is not found in other neuropathies or spinal muscular atrophies in which clinical symptoms are delayed until after early infancy.

The pathological findings in the muscles of patients with Werdnig–Hoffmann disease are already present at birth (Sarnat 1978) and persist indefinitely even into adult life in those few who survive. The pathological findings are character-istic, but not pathognomonic for this disease, because similar features occur in other less common disorders of perinatal motor neurone function. Congenital cervical spinal atrophy is a sporadic disorder involving muscle wasting and contractures of the upper limbs at birth. The lower limbs are normal, except for overactive knee jerks and ankle clonus. The disorder is associated with a segmental reduction in density of the spinal cord in the lower cervical region as determined by computerized tomography, and biopsy of affected muscles reveals focal replacement by fat and other findings characteristic of Werdnig–Hoffmann disease, including groups of hypertrophic type 1 muscle fibres within fascicles of mixed atrophic fibres (Darwish et al 1981). It would appear, therefore, that denervation of muscle in late fetal life, of any aetiology, may result in grouped giant fibres of histochemical type 1.

The trophic influence of nerve on muscle and neuronal imposition on muscle fibres of their contractile and metabolic characteristics may be related to the pattern of impulse activity of the motor neurone without invoking the participation of hypothetical neurotrophic substances (Kugelberg 1976, Salmons & Sréter 1976). The giant fibres in Werdnig–Hoffmann disease and other perinatal denervating diseases probably represent as yet uninvolved motor units undergoing compensatory hypertrophy. Their conversion to type 1 supports the concept that a continuous rapid rate of discharge of motor neurones induces growth of immature muscle fibres. Thus, a high rate of neural stimulation of perinatal muscle may result in muscle fibre hypertrophy if the motor unit is relatively small, as in Werdnig–Hoffmann disease, or fibre hypoplasia if the motor unit is large as here speculated in CMFTD. In both cases, the stimulation induces histochemical type 1 characteristics in the muscle fibres.

Spinal muscular atrophy as a developmental disorder of motor neurones

From a developmental perspective, it has been suggested that Werdnig–Hoffmann disease may be a failure of arrest of the embryonic process of programmed cell death of excess motor neuroblasts, so that an initially normal ontogenetic process becomes pathological by continuing beyond the time when it should have ceased (Hanson 1984, Sarnat et al 1989). Programmed death of spinal motor neuroblasts occurs subsequent to the cessation of mitotic proliferation (Hamburger 1975, Hollyday & Hamburger 1977, Oppenheim & Majors-Willard 1978, Nurcombe et al 1981). Morphological differences between degenerating nerve cells in spinal muscular atrophy and fetal motor neuroblasts are probably related to the greater number of cytoplasmic membranous organelles in the more mature nerve cells, and the higher concentration of lyosomal autolytic enzymes in immature nerve cells. The factors that arrest physiological programmed cell death in the embryo are incompletely known, but a failure to match with target muscle fibres is probably not as important as once thought because degeneration often occurs before axonal sprouting and synaptic contact normally occur.

One aspect of cell death that may be important is a sudden arrest of RNA transcription that results in inability of the cell to synthesize proteins, including enzymes essential to metabolism. In the wobbler mouse, RNA content is reduced and RNA synthesis is abnormal in neurones before morphological changes are detected by light microscopy (Murakami et al 1981). In human motor neurone disease (amyotrophic lateral sclerosis of adults), the RNA content of motor neurones is reduced (Davidson & Hartmann 1981). In Werdnig–Hoffmann disease, RNA histofluorescence after staining with acridine orange disappears seemingly abruptly and totally from motor neurones, unlike the sequential changes that are seen with impairment of RNA synthesis due to ischaemic/hypoxic insults in the perinatal period (Sarnat et al 1989).

DEVELOPMENTAL LESIONS OF THE BRAIN AND MUSCLE MATURATION

Less is known about the effects of suprasegmental lesions on the developing motor unit than about the effects of perinatal denervation of muscle. Cerebral malformations may profoundly affect muscle tone and functional control in the postnatal period, but dysplasias of the brain may also interfere with muscle development by altering the discharge pattern of spinal motor neurones. The histochemical differentiation of myofibres would be the aspect of muscle development most adversely affected by abnormal patterns of upper motor neurone discharge because the formation of fibre types is almost entirely determined by innervation.

Case reports have described abnormal histochemical patterns of fibre types in the muscles of infants with various cerebral dysgeneses associated clinically with muscular hypotonia (Fenichel 1967,

Fig. 5.9 Muscle biopsies of vastus lateralis from two infants (A) 9 months, and (B) 4 months of age, with generalized muscular hypotonia, mild weakness, and developmental delay. Both infants were shown by computed tomography to have cerebellar hypoplasia involving the vermis and both cerebellar hemispheres. The infant in (B) also had partial callosal agenesis. Muscle biopsies show more than 80% predominance of type I myofibres without cyto-architectural alterations, degenerative changes, or neurogenic grouping of type II fibres. The infant in (B) shows classical CMFTD with disparate fibre growth as well as type predominance (compare with Fig. 5.6). These abnormal patterns of histochemical differentiation probably reflect altered suprasegmental (i.e. upper motor neurone) influences on the developing motor unit. Myofibrillar ATPase pre-incubated at pH 4.3. ×210

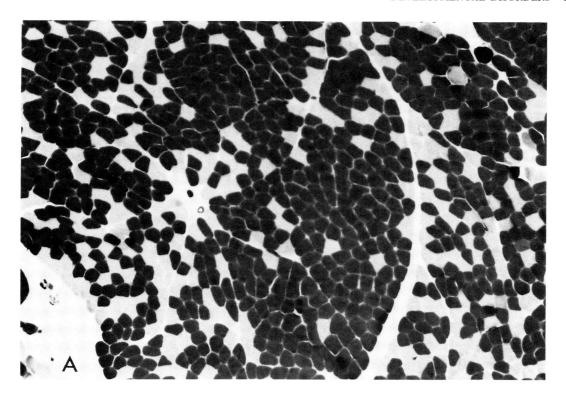

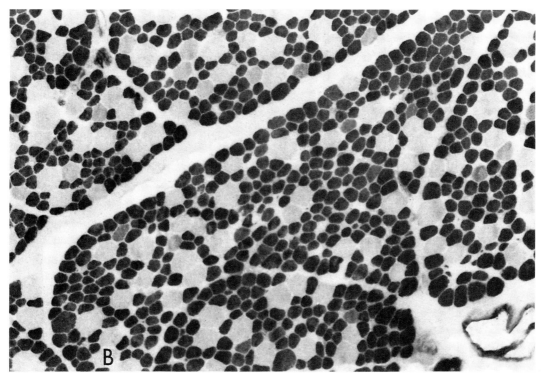

Curless et al 1978, Farkas-Bargeton et al 1978, Argov et al 1984). A systematic survey of the state of histochemical development of muscle in infants with a variety of cerebral and cerebellar dysplasias, confirmed by imaging studies during life or by postmortem examination, was performed in 27 patients (Sarnat 1985, 1986). Cases in which the brain was severely hypoplastic, and no motor pathways descended to the spinal cord, were associated with no abnormalities of differentiation, distribution, or ratios of histochemical fibre types or subtypes, showing that the motor unit can develop normally in the absence of suprasegmental influences. Supratentorial cerebral malformations, including severe forms such as holoprosencephaly or lissencephaly, and milder forms such as callosal agenesis or focal dysplasias of cortical lamination, also were not expressed as aberrations in the histochemical development of muscle. By contrast, cerebellar hypoplasia and brainstem dysgeneses profoundly influenced muscle development. Several patterns of abnormal histochemical differentiation were seen: (i) delayed or incomplete maturation; (ii) type predominance of more than 80% of either type I or II myofibres, more commonly type I; (iii) classical congenital muscle fibre-type disproportion, involving hypoplasia as well as predominance of type I myofibres and hypertrophy of type II fibres (Fig. 5.9). Cytoarchitectural alterations of myofibres, central nuclei, nemaline rods or abnormal inclusions, and degenerative changes were not found.

The period of histochemical differentiation of muscle is 20 to 28 weeks' gestation. During this time, numerous bulbospinal pathways are acquiring myelin and forming terminal axonal ramifications and synapses within the spinal cord. These descending motor pathways, such as the vestibulospinal, reticulospinal, tectospinal, rubrospinal, and olivospinal tracts, are capable of altering the rate and pattern of discharges of spinal motor neurones, hence influencing the growth and histochemical differentiation of muscle fibres. By contrast, the corticospinal tract has few synaptic connections and has not yet even begun its myelination cycle during this same period. It is not therefore surprising that supratentorial lesions fail to affect neuromuscular development while infratentorial lesions may severely alter the histochemical differentiation of muscle. The cerebellum projects no direct 'cerebellospinal tract' in humans, and most of its output ascends to the thalamus to be relayed to the cerebral motor cortex and to mediate cerebellar influence via the corticospinal tract. However, some efferent cerebellar fibres also project to the vestibular nuclei, reticular formation, and red nucleus, relayed by the deep cerebellar nuclei or as direct projections of Purkinje cell axons. It is probably these nonthalamic cerebellar connections that influence neuromuscular maturation.

From a clinical perspective, human cerebellar hypoplasia is consistently associated with generalized muscular hypotonia and developmental delay in infancy, and often with depressed tendon stretch reflexes (Sarnat & Alcalá 1980). One mechanism is decreased fusimotor activity leading to diminished muscle spindle function (Gilman 1969), but other mechanisms may also be involved. A precise correlation between the type of histochemical aberration in muscle and anatomical localization of the cerebellar and bulbospinal lesions is not yet available.

In most forms of muscular dystrophy, the ratio of fibre types is altered or, in the case of myotonic dystrophy, there is a selective atrophy of type I myofibres. While these minor changes are difficult to interpret in the presence of primary myopathy, the possibility remains that suprasegmental influences from the brain may play a role in the pathogenesis of the composite lesions of muscle. Cerebral disease in Duchenne muscular dystrophy and other dystrophies is expressed through learning disabilities and mental retardation; mild ventriculomegaly is often demonstrated by imaging. Minor neuropathological lesions are frequently found at autopsy (Rosman & Kakulas 1966, Rosman & Rebeiz 1967, Dubowitz & Crome 1969, Rosman 1970). Congenital muscular dystrophies of both the Fukuyama and non-Fukuyama types are often associated with frank cerebral malformations (Fowler & Manson 1973, Krijgsman et al 1980, Fukuyama et al 1981, McMenamin et al 1982, Egger et al 1983, Goebel et al 1983). Cerebellar dysfunction may contribute to the myopathology in muscular dystrophies, whether cerebellar lesions are morphologically demonstrable or not.

REFERENCES

Aicardi J, Conti D, Goutières F 1974 Les formes néo-natales de la dystrophie myotonique de Steinert. Journal of the Neurological Sciences 22: 149

Allam Ali M 1979 Myotube formation in skeletal muscle regeneration. Journal of Anatomy 128: 553

Amick, L D, Johnson W W, Smith H L 1967 Electromyographic and histopathologic correlations in arthrogryposis. Archives of Neurology (Chicago) 16: 512

Areechon W, Reid L 1963 Hypoplasia of lung with congenital diaphragmatic hernia. British Medical Journal 1: 230

Argov Z, Gardner-Medwin D, Johnson M A, Mastaglia F L 1984 Patterns of muscle fiber-type disproportion in hypotonic infants. Archives of Neurology 41: 53

Baker J H, Hall–Craggs E C B 1980 Changes in sarcomere length following tenotomy in the rat. Muscle and Nerve 3: 413

Barth P G, Van Wijngaarden G K, Bethlem J 1975 X-linked myotubular myopathy with fatal neonatal asphyxia. Neurology (Minneapolis) 25: 531

Baumann L, Landauer W 1943 Polydactyly and anterior horn cells in fowl. Journal of Comparative Neurology 79: 153

Bell D B, Smith D W 1972 Myotonic dystrophy in the neonate. Journal of Pediatrics 81: 83

Bender A N, Willner J P 1978 Nemaline (rod) myopathy. The need for histochemical evaluation of affected families. Annals of Neurology 4: 37

Bennett G S, Fellini S A, Toyama Y et al 1979 Redistribution of intermediate filament subunits during skeletal myogenesis and maturation in vitro. Journal of Cell Biology 82: 577

Bergen B J, Carry M P, Wilson W B, Barden M T, Ringel S P 1980 Centronuclear myopathy: Extraocular and limb-muscle findings in an adult. Muscle and Nerve 3: 165

Bersu E T 1980 Anatomical analysis of the developmental effects of aneuploidy in man: the Down syndrome. American Journal of Medical Genetics 5: 399

Bethlem J, Van Wijngaarden G K, Meijer A E F H 1969 Neuromuscular disease with type I fiber atrophy, central nuclei, and myotube-like structures. Neurology (Minneapolis) 19: 705

Brandt S 1947 A case of arthrogryposis multiplex congenita anatomically appearing as a foetal spinal muscular atrophy. Acta Paediatrica 34: 365

Brooke M H 1973 Congenital fiber type dysproportion. In: Kakulas B A (ed) Clinical studies in myology, part 2. Excerpta Medica, Amsterdam, p 147

Browne D 1936 Congenital deformities of mechanical origin. Proceedings of the Royal Society of Medicine 29: 1409

Bueker E D 1945 Hyperplastic changes in the nervous system of a frog (Rana) as associated with multiple functional limbs. Anatomical Record 93: 323

Byers R K, Banker B Q 1961 Infantile muscular atrophy. Archives of Neurology (Chicago) 5: 140

Carlson B M, Gutmann E 1976 Contractile and histochemical properties of sliced muscle grafts regenerating in normal and denervated rat limbs. Experimental Neurology 50: 319

Colling-Saltin A-S 1978 Enzyme histochemistry on skeletal muscle of the human foetus. Journal of the Neurological Sciences 39: 169

Crawford G N C 1973 The growth of striated muscle immobilized in extension. Journal of Anatomy 114: 165

Curless R G, Nelson M G, Brimmer F 1978 Histological patterns of muscle in infants with developmental brain abnormalities. Developmental Medicine and Child Neurology 20: 159

Curtis A H, Helmholz H F 1911 A study of the anterior horn cells of an abrachius and their relation to the development of the extremities. Journal of Comparative Neurology 21: 323

Daentl D L, Berg B O, Layzer R B, Epstein C J 1974 A new familial arthrogryopsis without weakness. Neurology (Minneapolis) 24: 55

Darnfors C, Borje Larsson H E, Oldfors A, Kyllerman M, Gustavson K-H, Bjursell G, Wahlström J 1990 X-linked myotubular myopathy. A linkage study. Clinical Genetics 37: 335

Darwish H, Sarnat H B, Archer C, Brownell K, Kotagal S 1981 Congenital cervical spinal atrophy. Muscle and Nerve 4: 106

Dastur D K, Dewan A, Manghani D K, Udani P M 1977 Quantitative histology of nerve in normal children and in children with protein-calorie malnutrition. Neuropathology and Applied Neurobiology 3: 405

Dastur D K, Daver S M, Manghani D K 1979 Changes in muscle in human malnutrition; with an emphasis on the fine structure in protein-calorie malnutrition. Progress in Neuropathology 4: 299

Davidson T J, Hartmann H A 1981 RNA content and volume of motor neurons in amyotrophic lateral sclerosis. Journal of Neuropathology and Experimental Neurology 40: 187

Dehkharghani F, Sarnat H B, Brewster M A, Roth S I 1981 Congenital muscle fibre type disproportion in Krabbe's leukodystrophy. Archives of Neurology (Chicago) 38: 585

Dodge P R 1960 Congenital neuromuscular disorders. Proceedings of the Association for Research in Nervous and Mental Diseases 38: 479

Drachman D B, Banker B Q 1961 Arthrogryposis multiplex congenita. Case due to disease of the anterior horn cells. Archives of Neurology (Chicago) 5: 77

Drachman D B, Coulombre A J 1962 Experimental clubfoot and arthrogryposis multiplex congenita. Lancet 2: 523

Drachman D B, Weiner L P, Price D L, Chase J 1976 Experimental arthrogryposis caused by viral myopathy. Archives of Neurology (Chicago) 33: 362

Dubowitz V 1966 Histochemistry. Enzyme histochemistry of developing human muscle. Nature 211: 884

Dubowitz V, Crome L 1969 The central nervous system in Duchenne muscular dystrophy. Brain 92: 805

Dubowitz V, Roy S 1970 Central core disease of muscle: clinical, histochemical and electron microscopic studies of an affected mother and child. Brain 93: 133

Dyken P R, Harper P S 1973 Congenital dystrophia myotonica. Neurology (Minneapolis) 23: 465

Egger J, Kendall B E, Erdohazi M, Lake B D, Wilson J, Brett E M 1983 Involvement of the central nervous system in congenital muscular dystrophies. Developmental Medicine and Child Neurology 25: 32

Ek J I 1958 Cerebral lesions in arthrogryposis multiplex congenita. Acta Paediatrica 47: 302

Engel W K, Karpati G 1968 Impaired skeletal muscle maturation following neonatal neurectomy. Developmental Biology 17: 713

Engel W K, Gold G N, Karpati G 1968 Type I fiber hypotrophy and central nuclei. Archives of Neurology (Chicago) 18: 435

Fardeau M, Harpey J P, Caille B, Lafourcade J 1975 Hypotonies néo-natales avec disproportion congénitale des differents types de fibre musculaire et petitesse relative des fibres de type I. Archives Françaises de Pédiatrie 32: 901

Farkas-Bargeton E, Tomé F M S, Fardeau M, Arsénio-Nunes M L, Dreyfus P, Diebler M F 1974 Histochemical and ultrastructural study of muscle biopsies in three cases of dystrophia myotonica in the newborn child. Journal of the Neurological Sciences 21: 273

Farkas-Bargeton E, Diebler M F, Arsénio-Nunes M L, Wehrlé R, Rosenberg B 1977 Etude de la maturation histochimique, quantitative et ultrastructurale du muscle foetal humaine. Journal of the Neurological Sciences 31: 245

Farkas-Bargeton E, Aicardi J, Arsénio-Nunes M L et al 1978 Delay in the maturation of muscle fibres in infants with congenital hypotonia. Journal of the Neurological Sciences 39: 17

Fenichel G M 1963 The B fibre of human skeletal muscle. Neurology (Minneapolis) 13: 219

Fenichel G M 1967 Abnormalities of skeletal muscle maturation in brain damaged children: a histochemical study. Developmental Medicine and Child Neurology 9: 419

Ferrari S, Cannizzaro L A, Battini R, Huebner K, Baserga R 1987 Coding sequence and growth regulation of the human vimentin gene. Molecular and Cell Biology 6: 3614

Fidziańska A 1976 Morphologic differences between the atrophied small muscle fibres in amyotrophic lateral sclerosis and Werdnig–Hoffmann disease. Acta Neuropathologica (Berlin) 34: 321

Fowler M 1959 A case of arthrogryposis multiplex congenita with lesions in the nervous system. Archives of Disease in Childhood 34: 505

Fowler M, Manson J I 1973 Congenital muscular dystrophy with malformation of the central nervous system. In: Kakulas B A (ed) Clinical studies in myology, part 2. Excerpta Medica, Amsterdam, p 192

Friedlander H L, Westin G W, Wood W L Jr 1968 Arthrogryposis multiplex congenita. Journal of Bone and Joint Surgery 50A: 89–112

Frye F L, McFarland L Z, Enright J B 1964 Sacrococcygeal agenesis in Swiss mice. Cornell Veterinarian 54: 487

Fujita S 1963 The matrix cell and cytogenesis in the developing central nervous system. Journal of Comparative Neurology 120: 37

Fujita S 1965 The matrix cell and histogenesis of the nervous system. Laval Medicine 36: 125

Fukuhara N, Yuasa T, Tadao T, Kushiro S, Takasawa N 1978 Nemaline myopathy: histological, histochemical and ultrastructural studies. Acta Neuropathologica (Berlin) 42: 33

Fukuyama Y, Osawa M, Suzuki H 1981 Congenital progressive muscular dystrophy of the Fukuyama type. Clinical, genetic, and pathological considerations. Brain and Development (Tokyo) 3: 1

Gilman S 1969 The mechanism of cerebellar hypotonia: an experimental study in the monkey. Brain 92: 621

Goebel H H, Fidziańska A, Lenard H G, Osse G, Hori A 1983 A morphological study of non-Japanese congenital muscular dystrophy associated with cerebral lesions. Brain and Development (Tokyo) 5: 292

Goldstein J D, Reid L M 1980 Pulmonary hypoplasia resulting from phrenic nerve agenesis and diaphragmatic amyoplasia. Journal of Pediatrics 97: 282

Gonatas N K, Shy G M, Godfrey E H 1966 Nemaline myopathy: the origin of nemaline structures. New England Journal of Medicine 274: 535

Grossiord A, Held P, Begzadian-Khatchatrian V, Raverdy-Nozal E 1958 Trois cas d'arthrogryposis multiplex congenita. Revue neurologique 98: 263

Hageman G, Willemse J, van Ketel B A, Barth P G, Lindout D 1987 The heterogeneity of the Pena–Shokeir syndrome. Neuropediatrics 18: 45

Hamburger V 1934 The effects of wing bud extirpation on the development of the central nervous system in chick embryos. Journal of Experimental Zoology 68: 449

Hamburger V 1975 Cell death in the development of the lateral column of the chick embryo. Journal of Comparative Neurology 160: 535

Hanson P A 1984 Research strategies in infantile spinal muscular atrophy. In: Gamstorp I, Sarnat H B (eds) Progressive spinal muscular atrophies. Raven Press, New York, p 209

Hariga J, Lowenthal A, Guazzi G C 1963 Nosological place and correlations of arthrogryposis 'restricto'. Acta Neurologica Belgica 63: 766

Harper P S 1975 Congenital myotonic dystrophy in Britain. I Clinical aspects. Archives of Disease in Childhood 50: 505

Hecht F, Beals R K 1972 'New' syndrome of congenital contractural arachnodactyly originally described by Marfan in 1896. Pediatrics 49: 574

Henderson J L 1939 The congenital facial diplegia syndrome: Clinical features, pathology, and aetiology. Brain 62: 381

Higginbottom M C, Jones K L, Hall B D, Smith D W 1979 The amniotic band disruption complex: timing of amniotic rupture and variable spectra of consequent defects. Journal of Pediatrics 95: 544

Hillman J W, Johnson J T H 1952 Arthrogryposis multiplex congenita in twins. Journal of Bone and Joint Surgery 34A: 211

Hogan G R, Gutmann L, Chou S M 1969 The peripheral neuropathy of Krabbe's (globoid) leukodystrophy. Neurology (Minneapolis) 19: 1094

Hollyday M, Hamburger V 1977 An autoradiographic study of the formation of the lateral motor column in the chick embryo. Brain Research 132: 311

Hollyday M, Mendell L M 1976 Analysis of moving supernumerary limbs of Xenopus laevis. Experimental Neurology 51: 316

Holmes L B, Driscoll S G, Bradley W G 1980 Contractures in a new born infant of a mother with myasthenia gravis. Journal of Pediatrics 96: 1067

Hooshmand H, Martinez A J, Rosenblum W I 1971 Arthrogryposis multiplex congenita. Simultaneous involvement of peripheral nerve and skeletal muscle. Archives of Neurology (Chicago) 24: 561

Hughes A F, Tschumi P-A 1958 The factors controlling the development of the dorsal root ganglia and ventral horn in Xenopus laevis. Journal of Anatomy 92: 498

Ionasescu V, Zellweger H, Filer L J, Jr, Conway T W 1970 Increased collagen synthesis in arthrogryposis multiplex congenita. Archives of Neurology (Chicago) 23: 128

Jacobson M 1978 Developmental neurobiology 2nd ed. Plenum Press, New York

James N T 1979 Studies on the responses of different types of muscle fibre during surgically induced compensatory hypertrophy. Journal of Anatomy 129: 769

Jones K L, Smith D W, Hall B D, Hall J G, Ebbin A J, Massoud H, Golbus M S 1974 A pattern of craniofacial and limb defects secondary to aberrant tissue bands. Journal of Pediatrics 84: 90

Kanof A, Aronson S M, Volk B W 1956 Arthrogryposis. Pediatrics 17: 532

Karpati G, Engel W K 1967 Neuronal trophic function. A new aspect demonstrated histochemically in developing soleus muscle. Archives of Neurology (Chicago) 17: 542

Karpati G, Carpenter S, Nelson R F 1970 Type I muscle fiber atrophy and central nuclei. Journal of the Neurological Sciences 10: 489

Karpati G, Carpenter S, Watters G V 1973 Infantile myotonic dystrophy. Histochemical and electron microscopic features in skeletal muscle. Neurology (Minneapolis) 23: 1066

Katz M J, Lasek R J 1978 Evolution of the nervous system: Role of ontogenetic mechanisms in the evolution of matching populations. Proceedings of the National Academy of Sciences of the United States of America 75: 1349

Kitagawa M, Hislop A, Boyden E A, Reid L 1971 Lung hypoplasia in congenital diaphragmatic hernia — a quantitative study of airway, artery, and alveolar development. British Journal of Surgery 58: 342

Kite J H 1955 Arthrogryposis multiplex congenita: review of 54 cases. Southern Medical Journal 48: 1141

Krijgsman J B, Barth P G, Stam F C, Slooff J L, Jaspar H H J 1980 Congenital muscular dystrophy and cerebral dysgenesis in a Dutch family. Neuropädiatrie 11: 108

Kugelberg E 1976 Adaptive transformation of rat soleus motor units during growth. Histochemistry and contraction speed. Journal of the Neurological Sciences 27: 269

Lamb A H 1974 The timing of the earliest motor innervation in the hind limb bud in the Xenopus tadpole. Brain Research 67: 527

Landauer W 1945 Rumplessness of chicken embryos produced by the injection of insulin and other chemicals. Journal of Experimental Zoology 98: 65

Lenard H G, Goebel H H, Weigel W 1977 Smooth muscle involvement in congenital myotonic dystrophy. Neuropädiatrie 8: 42

Lipton E L, Morgenstern S H 1955 Arthrogryposis multiplex congenita in identical twins. American Journal of Diseases of Children 98: 233

McKusick V A 1956 Heritable disorders of connective tissue. Journal of Chronic Diseases 3: 360

McMenamin J B, Becker L E, Murphy E G 1982 Fukuyama-type congenital muscular dystrophy. Journal of Pediatrics 101: 580

Martin J J, Clara R, Ceuterick C, Joris C 1976 Is congenital fibre type disproportion a true myopathy? Acta Neurologica Belgica 76: 335

Martin J J, Ceuterick J, Joris C et al 1977 Myopathie centro-nucléaire. Acta Neurologica Belgica 77: 285

Mastaglia F L, Sarnat H B, Ojeda V J, Kakulas B A 1988 Myopathies associated with hypothyroidism: a review based upon 13 cases. Australian and New Zealand Journal of Medicine 18: 799

Moore B H 1941 Some orthopedic relationships of neurofibromatosis. Journal of Bone and Joint Surgery 23: 109

Munsat T L, Thompson L R, Coleman R F 1969 Centronuclear ('myotubular') myopathy. Archives of Neurology 20: 120

Murakami T, Mastaglia F L, Mann D M A, Bradley W G 1981 Abnormal RNA metabolism in spinal motor neurons in the wobbler mouse. Muscle and Nerve 4: 407

Nurcombe V, McGrath P A, Bennett M R 1981 Postnatal death of motor neurons during the development of the brachial spinal cord of the rat. Neuroscience Letters 27: 249

Oppenheim R W, Majors-Willard C 1978 Neuronal cell death in the brachial spinal cord of the chick is unrelated to the loss of polyneuronal innervation in wing muscle. Brain Research 154: 148

Oppenheim R W, Pittman R, Gray M, Maderdrut J L 1978 Embryonic behavior, hatching and neuromuscular development in the chick following a transient reduction of spontaneous motility and sensory input by neuromuscular blocking agents. Journal of Comparative Neurology 179: 619

Palmucci L, Bertolotto A, Monga G, Ardizzone G, Schiffer D 1978a Histochemical and ultrastructural findings in a case of centronuclear myopathy. European Neurology 17: 327

Palmucci L, Schiffer D, Monga G, de Marchi M 1978b Central core disease: histochemical and ultrastructural study of muscle biopsies of father and daughter. Journal of Neurology 218: 55

Palmucci L, De Angelis S, Leone M et al 1988 Centronuclear myopathy: type of inheritance and clinical pattern in 268 cases. Clinical Neuropathology 7: 194

Panayiotopoulos C P, Scarpalezos S 1977 Dystrophia myotonica. A model of combined neural and myopathic muscle atrophy. Journal of the Neurological Sciences 31: 261

Passarge E, Lenz W 1966 Syndrome of caudal regression in infants of diabetic mothers: observations of further cases. Pediatrics 37: 672

Pedreira F A, Long R E 1971 Arthrogryposis multiplex congenita in one of identical twins. American Journal of Diseases of Children 121: 64

Pettersen J C 1979 Anatomical studies of a boy trisomic for the distal portion of 13q. American Journal of Medical Genetics 4: 383

Prestige M C 1965 Cell turnover in the spinal ganglia of Xenopus laevis tadpoles. Journal of Embryology and Experimental Morphology 13: 63

Prestige M C 1967 The control of cell number in the lumbar ventral horns during the development of Xenopus laevis tadpoles. Journal of Embryology and Experimental Morphology 18: 359

Pugh R C B, Dudgeon J A 1954 Fatal neonatal poliomyelitis. Archives of Disease in Childhood 29: 381

Quax W, Meera Khan P, Quax-Jeuken Y, Bloemendal H 1985 The human desmin and vimentin genes are located on different chromosomes. Gene 38: 189

Radu H, Killyen I, Ionescu V, et al 1977 Myotubular (centronuclear) (neuro-) myopathy. I. Clinical, genetical and morphological studies. European Neurology 15: 285

Ramirez-Castro J L, Bersu E T 1978 Anatomical analysis of the developmental effects of aneuploidy in man — the 18-trisomy syndrome II. Anomalies of the upper and lower limbs. American Journal of Medical Genetics 2: 285

Ramsey R B, McGarry J, Fischer V W, Sarnat H B 1978 Alteration of developing and adult rat muscle membranes by zuclomiphene and other hypocholesterolemic agents. Acta Neuropathologica (Berlin) 44: 15

Reynolds W A 1963 The effect of thyroxine upon the initial formation of the lateral motor column and differentiation of motor neurons in Rana pipiens. Journal of Experimental Zoology 153: 237

Roberts J A F 1929 The inheritance of a lethal muscle contracture in sheep. Journal of Genetics 21: 57

Rosenkranz E 1905 Ueber kongenitale Kontraturen der oberen Extremitaten. Zeitschrift für Orthopädie und Chirurgie: 14: 52

Rosman N P 1970 The cerebral defect and myopathy in Duchenne muscular dystrophy. Neurology 20: 329

Rosman N P, Kakulas B A 1966 Mental deficiency associated with muscular dystrophy. A neuropathological study. Brain 89: 769

Rosman N P, Rebeiz J J 1967 The cerebral defect and myopathy in myotonic dystrophy. Neurology 17: 1106

Rusnak S L, Driscoll S G 1965 Congenital spinal anomalies in infants of diabetic mothers. Pediatrics 35: 989

Salmons S, Sréter F A 1976 Significance of impulse activity in the transformation of skeletal muscle type. Nature 263: 30

Sandbank U, Cohen L 1964 Arthrogryposis multiplex congenita with tuberous sclerosis. Journal of Pediatrics 64: 571

Sarnat H B 1978 Diagnostic value of the muscle biopsy in the neonatal period. American Journal of Diseases of Children 132: 782

Sarnat H B 1979 Neuromuscular disorders in the neonatal period. In: Korobkein R, Guilleminault C (eds) Advances in perinatal neurology, Volume 1. Spectrum Publications, New York, pp 153

Sarnat H B 1985 Le cerveau influence-t-il le développement musculaire du foetus humain? Mise en évidence de 21 cas. Canadian Journal of Neurological Sciences 12: 111

Sarnat H B 1986 Cerebral dysgeneses and their influence on fetal muscle development. Brain and Development (Tokyo) 8: 495

Sarnat H B 1990 Myotubular myopathy: arrest of morphogenesis of myofibres associated with persistence of fetal vimentin and desmin. Canadian Journal of Neurological Sciences 17: 109

Sarnat H B, Alcalá H 1980 Human cerebellar hypoplasia: a syndrome of diverse causes. Archives of Neurology 37: 300

Sarnat H B, Silbert S W 1976 Maturational arrest of fetal muscle in neonatal myotonic dystrophy. A pathologic study of four cases. Archives of Neurology (Chicago) 33: 466

Sarnat H B, Case M E, Graviss R 1976a Sacral agenesis. Neurologic and neuropathologic features. Neurology (Minneapolis) 26: 1124

Sarnat H B, O'Connor T, Byrne P A 1976b Clinical effects of myotonic dystrophy on pregnancy and the neonate. Archives of Neurology 33: 459

Sarnat H B, Sarnat M S 1983 Disorders of muscle in the newborn. In: Moss A J, Stern L (eds) Pediatrics update, 4th edn. Elsevier North-Holland, New York, p 211

Sarnat H B, Jacob P, Jiménez C 1989 Atrophie spinale musculaire: l'évanouissement de la fluorescence à l'ARN des neurones moteurs en dégénérescence. Une étude à l'acridine-orange. Revue Neurologique (Paris) 145: 305

Sees J N, Towfighi J, Robins B 1990 Marden-Walker syndrome: neuropathologic findings in two siblings. Pediatric Pathology 10: 807

Sher J H, Rimalovski A B, Athanassiades T J et al 1967 Familial centronuclear myopathy: a clinical and pathological study. Neurology 17: 727

Short J K 1963 Congenital muscular dystrophy. Neurology (Minneapolis) 13: 526

Sima A 1974 Studies on fibre size in developing sciatic nerve and spinal roots in normal, undernourished and rehabilitated rats. Acta physiologica scandinavica (Suppl) 406: 1

Sima A, Jankowska E 1975 Sensory nerve conduction velocity as correlated to fibre size in experimental undernutrition in the rat. Neuropathology and Applied Neurobiology 1: 31

Smith E M, Bender I F, Stover C N 1963 Lower motor neuron deficit in arthrogryposis. Archives of Neurology (Chicago) 8: 97

Stern W G 1923 Arthrogryposis multiplex congenita. Journal of the American Medical Association 81: 1507

Swinyard C A, Mogora A 1962 Multiple congenital contractures (arthrogryposis). An electromyographic study. Archives of Physical Medicine and Rehabilitation 43: 36

Szalay G C 1975 Comments on diabetic embryopathy syndrome. Pediatrics 55: 446

Tabary J C, Tabary C, Tardieu C, Tardieu G, Goldspink G 1972 Physiological and structural changes in the cat's soleus muscle due to immobilization at different lengths by plaster casts. Journal of Physiology 224: 231

Thomas I T, Smith D W 1974 Oligohydramnios, cause of the nonrenal features of Potter's syndrome, including pulmonary hypoplasia. Journal of Pediatrics 84: 811

Thomas N S, Williams H, Cole G, Robert K, Clarke A et al 1990 X-linked neonatal centronuclear/myotubular myopathy: evidence for linkage to Xq28 DNA marker loci. Journal of Medical Genetics 27: 284

Torres C F, Griggs T C, Goetz J P 1985 Severe neonatal centronuclear myopathy with autosomal dominant inheritance. Archives of Neurology 42: 1011

Tsang Y 1939 Ventral horn cells and polydactyly in mice. Journal of Comparative Neurology 70: 1

van Wijngaarden G K, Fleury P, Meyer A E F H 1969 Familial 'myotubular' myopathy. Neurology (Minneapolis) 19: 901

Vestermark B 1966 Arthrogryposis multiplex congenita. A case of neurogenic origin. Acta paediatrica scandinavica 55: 177

Viegas-Péquignot E, Lin L Z, Dutrillaux B, Apiou F, Paulin D 1989 Assignment of human desmin gene to band 2q35 by nonradioactive in situ hybridization. Human Genetics 83: 33

Warkany J, Takacs E 1965 Congenital malformations in rats from streptonigrin. Archives of Pathology 79: 65

Wechsler W 1966a Elektronenmikroskopischer Beitrag zur Histogenese des Weissen Substanz des Rückenmarks von Hühnerembryonen. Zeitschrift für Zellforschung und mikroskopische Anatomie 74: 232

Wechsler W 1966b Elektronenmikroskopischer Beitrag zur Nervenzelldifferenzierung und Histogenese der grauen Substanz der Rückenmarks von Huhnerembryonen. Zeitschrift für Zellforschung und mikroskopische Anatomie 74: 401

Whittem J H 1957 Congenital abnormalities in calves: arthrogryposis and hydranencephaly. Journal of Pathology and Bacteriology 73: 375

Williams P E, Goldspink G 1971 Longitudinal growth of striated muscle fibres. Journal of Cell Science 9: 751

Williams P E, Goldspink G 1973 The effect of immobilization on the longitudinal growth of striated muscle fibres. Journal of Anatomy 116: 45

Williams P E, Goldspink G 1978 Changes in sarcomere length and physiologic properties in immobilized muscle. Journal of Anatomy 127: 459

Wohlfart G 1937 Über das Vorkommen verschiedener Arten von Muskelfasern in der Skelettmuskulatur des Menschen und einiger Säugetiere. Acta psychiatrica neurologica scandinavica. Suppl. 12

6. Congenital myopathies

Michel Fardeau

INTRODUCTION AND HISTORY

The description of central core disease by Shy & Magee in 1956 heralded the beginning of the modern era of muscle pathology. For the first time, a specific structural abnormality of the muscle fibres was reported in a genetically determined muscular disorder. This report introduced the first of a series of previously undescribed muscular conditions, now commonly known as the congenital myopathies.

This report also shed new light on the confused nosological field of the hypotonias and muscular disorders occurring in early childhood (Greenfield et al 1958). Three papers (Werdnig 1891, Hoffmann 1893, 1900) had clearly identified a familial condition characterized by severe hypotonia, diffuse muscular atrophy and weakness leading to death in less than 2 years due to a progressive disappearance of the anterior horn cells. In contrast with these descriptions, Oppenheim (1900) briefly reported under the title of 'myatonia' a series of patients who were extremely hypotonic at birth, but who subsequently improved and survived. Lastly, in 1903, Batten described three cases of what he suggested were 'infantile myopathies'; he considered that Oppenheim's description concerned a 'simple atrophic type' of these myopathies.

The concept of 'myatonia', later called 'amyotonia congenita' (Collier & Wilson 1908), was extensively adopted in the first decades of the century. Greenfield & Stern (1927) opposed this terminology. From an analysis of 25 cases, reported as amyotonia congenita in spite of their unfavourable evolution, these authors showed that all these cases except one (not classified) could be classified

in the group of infantile spinal muscular atrophies, as identified by Werdnig and by Hoffmann.

Despite this critical analysis, cases of infantile hypotonia with a relatively favourable course were subsequently reported in the literature under different headings. Members of a family initially examined by Batten (1915), in which six out of 13 siblings were followed over a 50-year period, were described in three different reports (Turner 1940, 1949, Turner & Lees 1962). Krabbe (1947) reported cases of non-progressive muscle weakness and atrophy which he termed 'universal muscular hypoplasia'. Brandt (1950), who analysed 297 cases from the literature, found that 20 of them showed clinical improvement not compatible with Werdnig–Hoffmann disease, and considered that amyotonia congenita was a 'symptom complex' rather than a specific entity. In 1956, Walton reviewed 115 cases of amyotonia congenita observed in London paediatric and neurological hospitals, and identified 17 patients who gradually improved, eight of them recovering completely and nine incompletely. In view of the 'unfortunate connotation' acquired by the term 'amyotonia congenita', Walton preferred the label 'benign congenital hypotonia' for such cases.

Thus the stage was set for the recognition of a group of congenital non-progressive myopathies. In accordance with Walton's prediction that the application of new morphological techniques to the examination of muscle biopsies would allow more categories to be defined in this field, a number of new entities were identified after the description of central core disease. These displayed somewhat similar clinical but distinct morphological features, e.g. nemaline myopathy (Shy et al 1963), myotubular myopathy (Spiro et al 1966), and multicore disease (Engel & Gomez 1966).

The concept of congenital myopathies was gradually extended to include a number of clinical conditions with distinctive structural abnormalities of intracellular organelles, e.g. 'megaconial' and 'pleoconial' mitochondrial myopathies (Shy & Gonatas 1964, Shy et al 1966). It also became clear that in a number of hypotonic conditions in children there were striking histochemical changes in the muscle without any ultrastructural abnormality in the muscle fibres (Brooke & Engel 1969). In addition, several cases were reported with a very severe clinical course (Engel et al 1968, van Wijngaarden et al 1969) which were clearly progressive (Brooke & Neville 1972).

Following the report of Afifi et al (1965), certain observers emphasized the possible occurrence of different structural abnormalities in the same patient or family, and two reports stressed the non-specific character of the structural changes found in the congenital myopathies (Engel & MacDonald 1970, Fardeau 1970). The experience of many research groups in this field made it increasingly clear that certain cases were difficult to identify other than by the coining of new exotic names.

In due course, the intensive development of histochemical techniques for the investigation of muscle biopsies (Engel 1962, 1965), together with the understanding of the organization and significance of the different muscle fibre types (Engel 1966), led W. K. Engel to emphasize the possible selectivity of the structural changes for one fibre type, together with the frequent modification of the histochemical pattern of muscle tissue, and to propose a neurogenic influence in the pathophysiology of these congenital muscular disorders. The term 'congenital myopathies' then became somewhat controversial and was replaced by less evocative terminologies by some authors (Engel 1971, Brooke 1977, Brooke et al 1979), but was maintained by others (Bethlem 1970, Dubowitz and Brooke 1973, Bender 1979, Dubowitz 1980).

These developments over the past few years have ushered in a new period in the study of congenital myopathies and several critical reviews have appeared (Fardeau et al 1978, Brooke et al 1979).

In the absence of biochemical or experimental data which might help to resolve the controversy, the analysis in this chapter endeavours successively to explore: (i) The nosology of the congenital myopathies as defined by their structural abnormalities. (ii) Some related disorders, including certain structurally undefined conditions and the different congenital muscular 'dystrophies'; mitochondrial myopathies which were initially included in this group should now be considered apart, their biochemical and genetic mechanism being now elucidated at a molecular level. (iii) Some unresolved problems, relating to the specificity of the structural changes: i.e. whether the structural changes described are an essential factor in these diseases, the relationship of the different congenital myopathies to each other, and their presumed pathophysiological mechanisms.

THE NOSOLOGY OF THE CONGENITAL MYOPATHIES

Central core disease

In 1956, Shy & Magee reported a new muscular disorder in which almost every muscle fibre exhibited a well-defined round azurophilic central core after trichrome staining and which contrasted with the normal red colour of the periphery. The disorder was also intriguing because of the congenital onset and the non-progressive nature of the muscular weakness. The disease affected five people (four male and one female) in the same family over three generations. In a subsequent paper, Greenfield et al (1958) coined the term 'central core disease' for this newly recognized disorder. Its description was of major importance, as this was the first time that a structural abnormality of the muscle fibre was considered to be 'primary' in skeletal muscle pathology. There was no evidence of necrosis, regeneration or interstitial changes.

Over 50 cases of this condition have been described in detail since the original report (Bethlem & Posthumus Meyjes 1960, Engel et al 1961, Gonatas et al 1965, Dubowitz & Platts 1965, Bethlem et al 1966, Mittelbach & Pongraz 1968, Dubowitz & Roy 1970, Mrozek et al 1970, de

Giacomo et al 1971, Armstrong et al 1971, Bethlem et al 1971, Jean et al 1971, Morgan-Hughes et al 1973, Telerman-Toppet et al 1973, Pascual-Castroviejo et al 1974, Ramsey & Hensinger 1975, Isaacs et al 1975, Saper & Itabashi 1976, Tanabe et al 1976, Radu et al 1977, Cohen et al 1978, Palmucci et al 1978, Eng et al 1978, Patterson et al 1979, Kar et al 1980, Byrne et al 1982, Shuaib et al 1987). To these should be added a number of cases included in less detailed reports (Neville & Brooke 1973, Brooke 1977, Fardeau et al 1978).

Most of the reported cases have exhibited a clinical pattern very similar to that of the original cases described by Shy & Magee (1956). The muscular weakness is manifest in early childhood; marked hypotonia is rarely noted (Bethlem et al 1971, case 1), but motor milestones are usually slightly delayed. A breech presentation at birth has been mentioned in several reports (Engel et al 1961, Gonatas et al 1966, Mrozek et al 1970, Armstrong et al 1971, Cohen et al 1978). The muscle weakness predominates in the lower extremities. Proximal muscles are usually more involved than distal, but foot-drop may occur (Isaacs et al 1975). Severe handicap is exceptional (Bethlem et al 1971, case 2, Cohen et al 1978). The facial, sternomastoid and trapezius muscles may be slightly affected, but there is never any involvement of extraocular muscles.

Skeletal and joint deformities are frequent, in particular hip dislocation (Gonatas et al 1965, Armstrong et al 1971, Ramsey & Hensinger 1975, Radu et al 1977, Palmucci et al 1978, Eng et al 1978). Tendon reflexes are sometimes diminished or absent. There is no fasciculation or myotonia. The heart has generally been considered to be normal, apart from one case (Mittelbach & Pongraz 1968). Intelligence is normal. The condition is non-progressive and most patients remain active throughout their lives. Some improvement has even been noted with age or after intensive rehabilitation in some cases (Mrozek et al 1970).

Unusual features have been mentioned in a few reports. These include focal wasting of the shoulder girdle (Dubowitz & Platts 1965), severe weakness in facioscapulohumeral distribution (Bethlem et al 1971, case 2) and unilateral foot deformity of late onset (Telerman-Toppet et al

1973). More intriguing was the occurrence of painless muscle stiffness after exercise, and increased by ischaemia, noted in one family by Bethlem et al (1966), and in another case by Morgan-Hughes et al (1973). Of major interest is the association with malignant hyperthermia after general anaesthesia with halothane and succinylcholine in some cases. This was first noted in a family at risk by Denborough et al (1973), and confirmed by two subsequent reports (Isaacs et al 1975, Eng et al 1978), in which central core disease was diagnosed only after an episode of hyperthermia. Susceptibility to malignant hyperthermia was demonstrated in a series of 11 patients by Shuaib et al (1987) suggesting that all patients with central core disease should be considered at risk. This view has received strong support from recent work suggesting that the gene locus for central core disease is on chromosome 19q and is linked to that of malignant hyperthermia (Kausch et al 1990).

The electromyogram (EMG) in this disease is usually considered to be normal or 'myopathic'. Motor conduction velocities are normal. Single fibre electromyography has given conflicting results for motor unit fibre density, which has been found to be normal (Engel & Warmolts 1973), or increased (Cruz-Martinez et al (1979). Serum levels of creatine kinase and other muscle enzymes are very seldom elevated (Eng et al 1978, Palmucci et al 1978, Patterson et al 1979).

Histopathology. As with the other congenital myopathies, muscle biopsy is necessary to make the diagnosis with certainty; histochemistry and electron microscopy should be employed. Core lesions may indeed be overlooked in paraffin sections stained with haematoxylin and eosin. The results of trichrome staining are sometimes disappointing. In contrast, after histochemical staining of cryostat sections, the cores show up clearly. With most oxidative enzyme preparations (Fig. 6.1A), the core appears as a well-defined rounded unstained zone, occupying a large area of the muscle fibre and is sometimes surrounded by a thin dense rim. As initially noted by Dubowitz & Pearse (1960), the cores appear as light zones with the PAS and phosphorylase reactions. They are often more difficult to detect with the myofibrillar ATPase reaction, which may be slightly weaker in

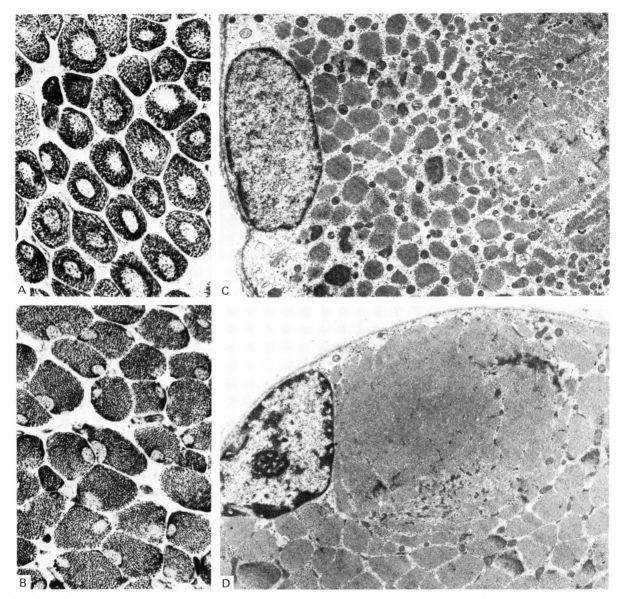

Fig. 6.1 Central core disease. (A) Cryostat section; NADH–tetrazolium reductase; ×135. Well-defined central cores in almost every muscle fibre. (B) Cryostat section. NADH–tetrazolium reductase; ×135. Eccentric cores in every muscle fibre. (C) Electron micrograph; ×6200. Same case as (A). Abnormal packing of myofilaments in the core region. Numerous mitochondrial profiles around the core. Progressive increase of myofibrillar size from the core to the periphery of the fibre. (D) Electron micrograph; ×7400. Same case as (B). Sharp edges of the core region, in contact with the periphery of the muscle fibre. Streaming of Z lines in the core

the core, but without a clear delineation from the remainder of the muscle fibre.

The cores were typically described as 'central', running the whole length of the muscle fibre (Engel et al 1961). They are, however, often found (Fig. 6.1B) in an eccentric position (Bethlem et al 1966, Morgan-Hughes et al 1973). Several cores, up to five, may be present in some hypertrophic fibres. In some biopsies, core limits are not sharply defined.

Apart from the cores, there are few other changes in muscle fibres. Variability in fibre size, some hypertrophic fibres, and an increase in the number of internal nuclei may be found. Necrosis and regeneration are absent, and interstitial fibrosis is usually not prominent.

Cores can be readily recognized in semi-thin sections of epoxy-embedded material. Electron microscopy shows that they are zones in which the myofilaments are densely packed and not segregated into distinct myofibrils (Fig. 6.1C,D). Inter-myofibrillary spaces, mitochondria, sarcotubular profiles, glycogen and lipids are absent in these areas, in keeping with their cytochemical features. Only the T-tubule system may remain visible within the cores (Gonatas et al 1965).

The filamentary architecture of the core is somewhat variable. The sarcomeric striation may be preserved and is in register, but sarcomeres in the core are slightly shorter than those of the peripheral myofibrils, the ratio between thick and thin filaments is altered, and the Z lines often have a zig-zag appearance. Such cores were described as 'structured' by Neville & Brooke (1973). In 'unstructured' cores, sarcomeric organization is disrupted, myofilaments are in complete disarray, and long 'streams' of Z material are seen. In some cases (Gonatas et al 1965), Z lines are completely absent. The differentiation into 'structured' and 'unstructured' cores is purely descriptive, and does not justify division into pathological subgroups. 'Unstructured' and 'structured' cores may co-exist in the same biopsy, and 'unstructured' areas may occur in otherwise 'structured' cores.

Core limits are typically abrupt, without any limiting membrane, as noted in the early study by Seitelberger et al (1961). The myofibrils running along the cores are often smaller in diameter than at the fibre periphery. The core is often surrounded by a slight accumulation of mitochondria and reticular triads and distorted reticular profiles and T-tubules are also visible within the core (Hayashi et al 1989). When the core is unstructured its limits are less clearly defined, with an intermediary zone of disorganized myofibrils. The overall structure is then very close to that described in target fibres (Resnick & Engel 1966) although targets do not extend throughout the length of the fibre. The peripheral part of the 'cored' muscle fibre is usually normal. However, it is not uncommon to find small foci of myofibrillar disruption suggestive of 'minicore' lesions at some distance from the core.

Scattered atrophic fibres containing a few filamentary bundles at their periphery, with Z-band widening suggestive of rod formation, are also occasionally found (Telerman-Toppet et al 1973, Isaacs et al 1975). Association with clusters of rods which have sometimes been found in the same patient (Afifi et al 1965, Karpati et al 1971, Kulakowski et al 1973) or within the same fibres (personal observations) will be examined later in this chapter.

The incidence of the cores varies from one case to another. As pointed out by Telerman-Toppet et al (1973), the reduction in number of the type 2 fibres often seems proportional to the prominence of core formation in type 1 fibres. In fact, numerous biopsies displaying a type 1 uniformity show cores in almost 100% of the fibres. When the normal fibre type mosaic is present, only a few cores are visible. Core frequency may vary in the same patient from one muscle to another, and in the same family from one member to another. There is no clear correlation between the frequency of the cores and the clinical severity of the disease (Bethlem et al 1971, Palmucci et al 1978). In some families the biopsies reveal major changes in the parents, and minor changes in the children. This suggests that the structural changes, as well as the histochemical changes, evolve slowly throughout life. This hypothesis was supported by the follow-up study of a child whose biopsy showed 3% of cored fibres at the age of 4 years, and universal involvement with lack of fibre differentiation at 16 years of age (Dubowitz & Roy 1970, Dubowitz 1980). Conversely, cores may be lacking in some affected members of a family. Morgan-Hughes et al (1973) reported a family in which the mother had typical cores but her two sons showed only a marked type 1 predominance in their biopsies.

The innervation pattern has been studied in a few biopsies. The motor innervation ratio was found to be higher than normal in two cases (1.43: Telerman-Toppet et al 1973, 1.32: Isaacs et al 1975), and normal in another case (Bethlem et al

1966). End-plate structure showed no significant change in cored fibres and extra-junctional acetylcholine receptors were not present (Ringel et al 1976). Intrafusal fibres were found to be normal (Radu et al 1977). Immunocytochemical staining for the desmin network has shown that the cores are sharply delimited (Thornell et al 1983).

With regard to biochemical changes, a marked reduction in phosphorylase activity was found by Engel et al (1961). Isaacs et al (1975) found normal phosphorylase activity, but reductions in both Ca^{2+}-dependent ATPase activity and Ca^{2+} uptake by the sarcoplasmic reticulum in two cases. These reductions may be related to the scarcity of type 2 fibres observed in these cases. The same explanation can be applied to the findings of Kar et al (1980), of a fructose 1-6 diphosphatase deficiency associated with atypical cores in a case of congenital non-progressive myopathy; however, the enzymatic activity was about 15% lower than in other biopsies showing type 1 fibre predominance.

Genetics. Most of the cases reported are sporadic. An autosomal dominant transmission was demonstrated in several families in which several generations could be studied (Shy & Magee 1956, Gonatas et al 1965, Bethlem et al 1966, Dubowitz & Roy 1970, Isaacs et al 1975, Ramsey & Hensinger 1975, Eng et al 1978, Palmucci et al 1978, Byrne et al 1982). In a large Australian kindred (Haan et al 1990) linkage studies localized the gene at 19q 12–q13:2. A few reports have raised the possibility of an autosomal recessive transmission (Dubowitz & Platts 1965, Armstrong et al 1971, Bethlem et al 1971). The possibility of a non-genetic environmental mechanism was suggested by the involvement of only one of two identical twins in one family (Cohen et al 1978) but the data in this report have been criticised (Banker 1986).

Nemaline myopathy

In 1963, two papers published almost simultaneously drew attention to a new type of structural congenital myopathy. Myriads of minute rod-shaped granules were present in most of the muscle fibres. Even if their description as 'myogranules' by Conen et al (1963) was closer to their real structure, the attractive name proposed by Shy et al (1963) has been more widely used in the literature. The term 'nemaline myopathy' refers to the thread-like undulations produced in the muscle fibres by the accumulation of granules. When the electron microscope allowed clear definition of these structures, many authors after Engel & Resnick (1966) preferred the name 'rod myopathy', or 'congenital rod disease' (Dahl & Klutzow 1974).

Conen et al (1963) described a single sporadic case. In the report by Shy et al (1963) the familial incidence was apparent, as four members in two generations exhibited floppiness at birth, with delayed motor development. Since the two original reports, about 100 cases have been described in detail (Engel et al 1964, Afifi et al 1965, Price et al 1965, Spiro & Kennedy 1965, Gonatas et al 1966, Hopkins et al 1966, Engel & Gomez 1967, Hudgson et al 1967, Kolin 1967, Shafiq et al 1967, Martin & Reniers 1968, Heffernan et al 1968, Nakao et al 1968, Fulthorpe et al 1969, Badurska et al 1970, Battin et al 1972, Karpati et al 1971, Kuitunen et al 1972, Radu & Ionescu 1972, Caulet et al 1973, Danowski et al 1973, Kamieniecka 1973, Neustein 1973, Dahl & Klutzow 1974, Kinoshita & Satoyoshi 1974, Groslambert et al 1976, Bender & Willner 1978, Dubowitz 1978, Fukuhara et al 1978, McComb et al 1979, Gillies et al 1979, Norton et al 1983, Tsujihata et al 1983, Schmalbruch et al 1987, Martinez & Lake 1987, Berezin et al 1988, Wallgren-Pettersson et al 1988, Shahar et al 1988, Nonaka et al 1989, Voirin et al 1990, Ishibashi-Ueda et al 1990). To this list should be added some less detailed reports of cases (Yuasa et al 1977, Arts et al 1978). Our own experience is based on 12 cases, three of which have been previously documented (Fardeau 1969, Caille et al 1971, Kulakowski et al 1973).

At birth, the hypotonia is often marked, with generalized muscle weakness. Respiratory, sucking and swallowing difficulties may be severe. Recurrent pneumonia may occur as a result of gastro-oesophageal reflux (Berezin et al 1988). Contractures of the limbs and deformities of the feet may exist. Curiously, intrauterine mobility is rarely felt to be reduced (Neustein 1973, McComb et al 1979). Cardiac involvement has been reported (Ishibashi-Ueda et al 1990). When severe, this neo-natal hypotonia often leads to a fatal outcome

(Gillies et al 1979, Schmalbruch et al 1987, Martinez & Lake 1987) but not always (Voirin et al 1990).

During childhood, the clinical features are characteristic: diffuse muscle thinness and weakness, particularly in proximal segments of the limbs, and of the spinal and abdominal muscles. However, the strength in the limbs is frequently noted to be better than the muscle bulk would lead one to suppose (Brooke 1977). It is noticeable that the patient described in Ford's textbook (Ford 1960) as a typical example of Krabbe's universal muscular hypoplasia was subsequently demonstrated to have a nemaline myopathy (Hopkins et al 1966). Skeletal abnormalities such as scoliosis are common. Contractures of the fingers (Bender & Willner 1978) and simian palmar creases (Peterson & Munsat 1969) may also be present, but are unusual. The face often looks elongated, with an open mouth. The palate is usually highly arched. The voice is often high-pitched. The tongue may be slightly atrophic (Fukuhara et al 1978). Extraocular movements are normal. Cardiac abnormalities are observed in rare cases (Gonatas et al 1966, Hudgson et al 1967). With the years, the muscle weakness does not usually progress, and may be compatible with a reasonable degree of activity. The prognosis can, however, be altered by the severity of respiratory and pharyngeal involvement. It has been estimated that about one in five patients die in the first six years of life (Kulakowski et al 1973, Neustein 1973, Shahar et al 1988).

In adult life the condition may present in different ways. There may be a mild diffuse muscle weakness dating from childhood (Hopkins et al 1966), or the condition may be virtually asymptomatic and may be discovered almost by chance in some cases (Engel 1970, Brooke 1977, Arts et al 1978). In contrast, a few cases have a severe and progressive muscle deficit (Engel 1966, Engel & Resnick 1966, Heffernan et al 1968, Kamieniecka 1973, Groslambert et al 1976, Brownell et al 1978, Harati et al 1987). Ptosis was noted in two cases (Kuitunen et al 1972, Groslambert et al 1976) and diaphragmatic paralysis in one (Harati et al 1987). Nemaline myopathy may also present in adults as a severe cardiomyopathy (Meier et al 1984, Stoessl et al 1985). Classification of this subgroup of late-onset cases as a distinct nosological entity was initially suggested by W. K. Engel & Resnick (1966) and A. G. Engel (1966), but its inclusion in the nemaline myopathy group was favoured by others such as Heffernan et al (1968). The histopathological findings in such cases may differ from those in the majority of cases of nemaline myopathy in that rods may be present in atrophic fibres only and also because of the frequency of inflammatory changes.

Serum enzyme levels are generally normal. In three cases (Danowski et al 1973) a distinct β-globulin peak was found, attributable to an increase in the C_3 component of serum complement. Late-onset forms may be associated with monoclonal gammopathies (Engel et al 1966, 1975). In most reports the EMG has been considered to be normal or myopathic. In a few cases, a neuropathic pattern was suggested by the presence of fibrillations, high-amplitude potentials or a reduced number of motor units (Hopkins et al 1966, Fulthorpe et al 1969, Radu & Ionescu 1972, Neustein 1973, Kinoshita & Satoyoshi 1974) or a higher fibre density than normal (Wallgren-Pettersson et al 1989) which was attributed to an active degenerative/regenerative process. Motor conduction velocities were always normal.

Histopathology. Here again, muscle biopsy is the only means of certain diagnosis. Lesions may easily be overlooked on paraffin-embedded, haematoxylin and eosin stained material; the rods may become apparent only on phase contrast examination or after PTAH staining. On cryostat sections, they stain brightly with the modified Gomori trichrome technique (Engel & Cunningham 1963), forming red clusters against the purple-green background of the muscle fibre (Fig. 6.2A). The rods do not stain with the routine histochemical techniques, and in ATPase preparations they appear as transparent defects (Fig. 6.2B). Specific reactions have shown that rods contain tyrosine and tryptophan (Jenis et al 1969).

Electron microscopy reveals characteristic features of the rods. In longitudinal section, their electron density is similar to that of the Z lines (Fig. 6.2D) (Engel 1967). They are elongated, oblong or roughly rectangular. Their length varies and may reach 5 μm. In transverse section, their shape is irregularly polygonal with a lobulated

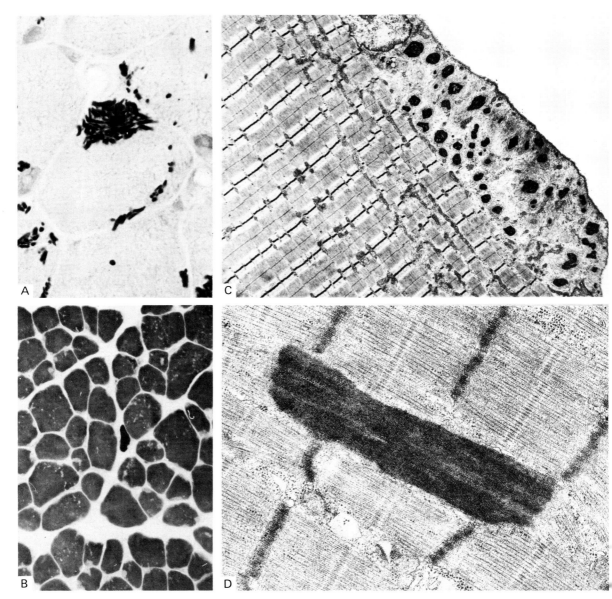

Fig. 6.2 Nemaline myopathy. (A) Cryostat section. Gomori's trichrome; ×1020. Accumulation of fuchsinophilic rodlets at the periphery of the muscle fibres. (B) Cryostat section, myofibrillar ATPase reaction; ×170. Marked type 1 predominance. The rods appear as unstained dots in the muscle fibres. (C) Electron micrograph; ×5100. Collection of rods at the periphery of the muscle fibre. Beneath, integrity of the myofibrillar architecture. (D) Electron micrograph; ×29 325. Typical aspect of a rod, with a 14 nm transverse periodicity

interior sometimes containing tubular structures (Fardeau 1969). Their diameter varies from 0.2 to 1 μm, and is not very different from that of the myofibrils. Thin filaments are continuous with the edges of the rods. Continuity between the rods and the Z lines of the adjacent sarcomeres is often seen.

Fine analysis of rod structure gives further evidence of their close relationship with the normal Z lines (Price et al 1965). When sectioned parallel to their longitudinal axes, rods exhibit a filamentary structure with a double striation: one parallel to the long axis of the rods, with a mean periodicity of 12 nm, the other perpendicular to their long axis, with a periodicity varying from 14 to 20 nm, which is constant within short segments of the same rod, and varies mainly with the angle between the long axis of the rod and the section. Transverse lines are not straight, but are formed by slightly zig-zagging thin filaments. Extraction by glycerination (Goldstein et al 1980) clearly shows a 38 nm periodicity along the axis of the rod, as in normal Z lines. In transverse section, a quadratic network with an 8–10 nm mesh shows up after osmic and aldehyde–osmic fixation. Extraction at low ionic strength yields a different lattice with 16.7 nm spacing, similar to that of Z discs treated in the same way. All these observations demonstrate the presence of a highly ordered filament lattice similar to that of the native Z lines, the rod appearing to be a 'lateral polymer' of the Z line (Stromer et al 1976).

Nevertheless, rods and Z lines display slight differences in morphology (Gonatas 1966, Fardeau 1969) and in solubility (Engel & Gomez 1967). These differences have not, however, been reflected in biochemical studies of the rods. Electrophoretic analysis of rod extracts has not shown any new or unknown proteins (Stromer et al 1976). Immunofluorescence techniques have demonstrated the presence of the 10S component of α-actinin (Sugita et al 1974), and actin (Yamaguchi et al 1978) in the rods. These proteins are normally present in the Z lines. The accumulation of α-actinin was shown to be restricted to muscle tissue (Jennekens et al 1983), but α-actinin isovariants were indistinguishable from those of control muscles (Hashimoto et al 1989).

In general, rods are found only in the cytoplasm. They frequently form aggregates at the periphery (Fig. 6.2C) or in the centre of the muscle fibre. When isolated within a myofibril, they may take the place of a sarcomere. At the periphery their orientation is fairly variable and they are surrounded by randomly disposed bundles of thin filaments. In the centre of the muscle fibre, they are usually arranged longitudinally, or slightly obliquely, in an area of myofibrillar disorganization. The boundaries between these areas and those containing normal myofibrillar structures are usually sharp. In the borderline areas, small dense spindle-shaped widenings of the Z lines may be encountered, and may represent the beginning of rod formation. They are more abundant near the myotendinous junction, where they may be found normally (Mair & Tomé 1972a).

In two cases, rods have been found in muscle nuclei (Jenis et al 1969, Engel & Oberc 1975). Prominent nuclear inclusions were present in the case described by Jenis et al (1969), in which the sarcoplasmic crystals were smaller than the nuclear ones. The authors suggested that this case might be a variant of nemaline myopathy.

Three points should also be emphasized from the ultrastructural study of nemaline myopathy:

1. There is usually a contrast between the accumulation of rods and the minor changes in the other cellular components of muscle fibres.
2. There is no clear correlation, in many cases (Nienhuis et al 1967, Dahl & Klutzow 1974, Arts et al 1978, Karpati et al 1971), between the severity of the weakness and the degree of rod accumulation, suggesting that the weakness is not related to the nemaline bodies, which may indicate nothing more than the site of the basic abnormality (Banker 1986); focal myofibrillar degeneration and increase in lysosomal enzymes may be more readily correlated with the muscle weakness (Nonaka et al 1989).
3. Smooth-muscle fibres do not show typical rods (Shafiq et al 1967).

The histochemical pattern of the muscle biopsy was altered in nearly all the reported cases. Type 1 fibre predominance was noted in the original cases and has been observed in most of the others (Fig. 6.2B). Type 1 predominance may vary from one fascicle to another (Neustein 1973, Bender & Willner 1978) and may be associated with a type 2B fibre deficiency (Shinomura & Nonaka 1989). There is never any grouping of the few type 2 fibres. The mean diameter of the type 1 fibres, as well as type 2A fibres (Dahl & Klutzow 1974) is relatively small in comparison with normal controls. In a few cases (Engel et al 1964, Gonatas et al 1966, Caille et al 1971, Radu & Ionescu 1972, Kinoshita & Satoyoshi 1974), the histochemical pattern is different. The type 1 predominance is less marked and there is a size disproportion between type 1 and type 2 fibres. Type 1 fibres are uniformly small and type 2 fibres are normal, or even larger than normal. Some studies of myosin light chains showed either a pure 'slow' pattern (Volpe et al 1981, Stuhlfauth et al 1983) or 'hybrid' patterns (Fardeau et al 1978).

It is also noticeable, as pointed out early by Engel et al (1964), that the rods selectively involve the type 1 fibres. Defects are seldom apparent in type 2 fibres. Only occasionally (Dahl & Klutzow 1974, Kinoshita & Satoyoshi 1974) are a few rods present in type 2A fibres.

The intrafusal muscle fibres are normally differentiated. The presence of rods within spindle muscle fibres is still debatable. Some authors thought that they found sparse rods in a few intrafusal muscle fibres (Shafiq et al 1967, Martin & Reniers 1968, Dahl & Klutzow 1974, Fukuhara et al 1978). However, Jenis et al (1969) found no rods in 15 spindles and Karpati et al (1971) found none in nine serially sectioned spindles.

The motor innervation pattern was found to be subnormal or normal in some cases (Coërs et al 1976). Some end-plates, incidentally found in biopsies, were considered to be normal (Heffernan et al 1968, Fardeau 1969, Karpati et al 1971). Extra-junctional ACh receptors were not demonstrated (Ringel et al 1976). In a number (255) of neuromuscular junctions found in three biopsies, Fukuhara et al (1978) noted a decrease in the number and depth of the secondary synaptic clefts, although they found no axonal degeneration or denervation. The authors did not think that these changes were fully explained by the type 1 fibre predominance in these biopsies.

Similarly, a few necropsy samples of peripheral nerves and spinal cords from such cases showed no obvious abnormality (Shafiq et al 1967, Caille et al 1971, Kulakowski et al 1973, McComb et al 1979). Robertson et al (1978) reported that morphometric analysis revealed a reduction in size without any decrease in the number of the motor neurones. A paucity of anterior horn cells was also found in the mid-cervical spinal cord, in keeping with the histological changes in the sternomastoid muscle in this case (Dahl & Klutzow 1974).

Genetics. An autosomal dominant pattern was

suggested in the original paper by Shy et al (1963). In two other families, the presence of affected parents in more than one generation was demonstrated histologically (Spiro & Kennedy 1965, Hopkins et al 1966). Arts et al (1978) reported the pedigree of a family with six affected subjects in three generations. The dominant mode of inheritance, with a reduced penetrance, seems to be involved in the majority of the families studied (Kondo and Yuasa 1980). However, a dominant pattern of inheritance does not explain the preponderance of female cases in the literature. Possible explanations of this include semi-lethal involvement of the male, sex influence on dominance, and sex-linked dominance.

Several other cases were reported in which more than one sib was affected and the parents were clinically normal. In two such families, Arts et al (1978) found a few rods in a small number of muscle fibres in the biopsies of both parents. These findings suggested an autosomal recessive pattern of inheritance, and Arts et al (1978) postulated that genetic heterogeneity exists in nemaline myopathy. In particular, the severe neonatal forms of the disease are often considered as belonging to this autosomal recessive group.

Centronuclear myopathies

In 1966, Spiro et al wrote a report with a new title in the field of congenital myopathies, *viz. Myotubular myopathy*, with an intriguing subtitle, *Persistence of fetal muscle in an adolescent boy*. The 12-year-old boy in question had neurological disturbances from birth, and a bilateral subdural haematoma was removed at 6 months of age. At the time when he was admitted for operation, a ptosis was noticed. He walked at 17 months, but never ran well. Progressive generalized weakness and wasting developed insidiously with bilateral foot-drop and increased lordosis. The deep tendon reflexes were absent. Two gastrocnemius muscle biopsies showed, respectively, 85% and 45% of centrally located nuclei. Around the nuclei there was a small area devoid of enzymatic activity. Very limited changes were seen on electron microscopy. The muscle fibres were thought to resemble myotubes, suggesting arrest of fetal development at the cellular level. No other muscle disorders were found in the boy's family. The two teenage sisters, described soon after by Sher et al (1967), were remarkably similar to the original case. The clinically normal mother of the two girls was found to have 29% central muscle nuclei in her biopsy. As the term 'myotubular myopathy' had been criticized (Banker 1986) the term 'centro-nuclear myopathy' was proposed for this new entity.

Since these two reports, more than 100 cases have been published, morphologically defined by the high frequency of central nuclei. Important differences exist from one case to another, and the homogeneity of the group was soon questioned (van Wijngaarden et al 1969, Bradley et al 1970).

Subdivisions were proposed, according to different criteria (Bradley et al 1970, Harriman & Haleem 1972, Brooke et al 1979) such as age of onset, clinical severity, presence or absence of ocular signs, histochemical patterns and mode of inheritance. However, because of the non-specificity of the morphological lesions, the variability of clinical expression within the same family, and the large number of sporadic cases, it is still impossible to make precise distinctions between different subentities within this group. Nevertheless, perusal of the literature indicates that there are three groups of cases with features differing from the original description: cases of late onset, cases with type 1 fibre atrophy in the muscle biopsy, and cases of severe neonatal hypotonia in male infants. Only in the latter group is there clinical and genetic homogeneity, and this is nowadays referred to as X-linked myotubular myopathy.

Early-onset centronuclear myopathies

A series of cases similar to the three original cases has been reported (Munsat 1967, Coleman et al 1968, Kinoshita & Cadman 1968, Badurska et al 1969, Bethlem et al 1970, Bradley et al 1970, Headington et al 1975 (case 2), Hawkes & Absolon 1975, Martin et al 1977, Palmucci et al 1978, PeBenito et al 1978, Serratrice et al 1978, Jadros-Santel et al 1980, Moosa & Dawood 1987).

These cases are characterized clinically by a marked neonatal hypotonia, relatively slight delay in motor development, diffuse muscle weakness

with easy fatiguability, scapular winging and waddling gait, severe involvement of the flexors of the feet, bilateral facial and masticatory weakness, external ocular muscle involvement with drooping of the eyelids and the voice is sometimes affected. The tongue is normal. There is generalized areflexia, without myotonia or fasciculation. EEG dysrhythmias are frequent with seizures in some cases (Munsat et al 1969, PeBenito et al 1978). The serum CK level is slightly raised, or normal, and the electromyogram is usually considered to be myopathic.

There are very few clinical variations in this group: they include association with a marfanoid syndrome (Jadros-Šantel et al 1980), abnormal mental development (Badurska et al 1969) or psychosis (Bradley et al 1970), lens opacities (Hawkes & Absolon 1975) and the presence of a cardiomyopathy (Verheist et al 1976). In a few cases, the electromyogram shows fibrillation (Bethlem et al 1968, Headington et al 1975) or positive sharp waves and myotonic bursts (Coleman et al 1967, Hawkes & Absolon 1975).

The general course of the disease is slowly progressive, and the patients may be severely disabled in their early thirties (Bethlem et al 1968, Palmucci et al 1978) or may even die (Campbell et al 1969, Bradley et al 1970). Some patients who are severely affected in early childhood may nevertheless progress slowly, or remain relatively static (Bill et al 1979, Jadros-Šantel et al 1980).

Histopathology. In the muscle biopsies, centralization of myonuclei may be seen in 25–95% of the muscle fibres. The nuclei are disposed in long rows in longitudinal section. It is important to note that the central location of the nuclei is, in itself, an insufficient description of the abnormal architecture of the muscle fibre. In fact, the number of subsarcolemmal nuclei is reduced (Badurska et al 1969, Bradley et al 1970); the central nucleus is usually single in transverse section (Fig. 6.3A); there is a small area of myofibril-free sarcoplasm around the nucleus, with occasional small empty vacuoles; there is frequently a radial disposition of the intermyo-fibrillary network around the central nucleus (Fig. 6.3B) (Headington et al 1975, Serratrice et al 1978); splitting of hypertrophic fibres may occur; there are no necrotic or regenerative changes, and

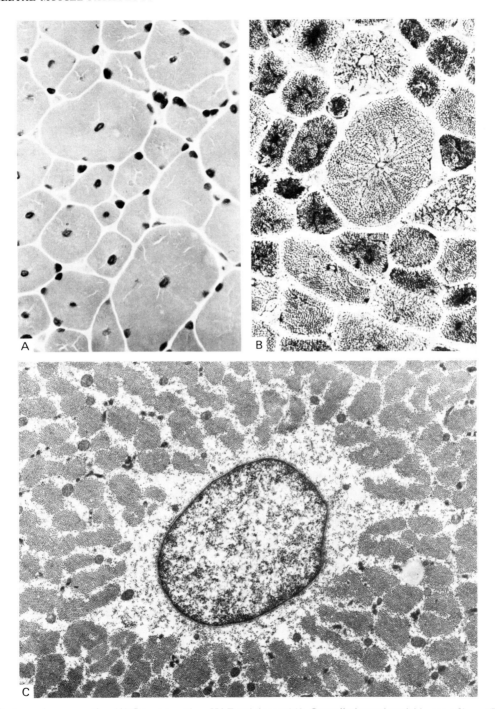

Fig. 6.3   Centronuclear myopathy. (A) Cryostat section, H&E staining; ×160. Centrally-located nuclei in most fibres. (B) Cryostat section. NADH–tetrazolium reductase; ×160. Radial disposition of the intermyofibrillary network in the large fibres. (C) Electron micrograph; ×14 000. A small area devoid of organelles surrounds the centrally located nucleus.

only a slight increase of endomysial connective tissue. Both muscle fibre types are equally affected. The muscle fibre changes are usually widespread, being found in a number of muscles, including the diaphragm and intercostal muscles, at post mortem (Munsat et al 1969, Bradley et al 1970).

Electron microscopy shows that there is no change in nuclear morphology (Fig. 6.3C); there is an accumulation of mitochondria, Golgi or sarcoplasmic reticular profiles at the nuclear poles; the myofibrillar architecture reflects a gradient in size from the core to the periphery of the muscle fibre; foci of myofibrillar disorganization are rare and limited; vacuoles are frequent, but lipid droplets, myelin bodies and fingerprint inclusions are rarely noticed (Jadros-Šantel et al 1980).

The size of the muscle fibres and the absence of ribosomes and microtubules are clear differences from normal myotubes; the general architecture of the fibre and the paucity of degenerative changes also clearly distinguish centronuclear myopathy from other conditions in which internal nuclei are frequent, such as neurogenic atrophies or myotonic dystrophies.

The histochemical pattern is modified in all cases. Type 1 predominance is found in most cases sometimes leading to type 1 uniformity (Palmucci et al 1978). There is often a tendency to type 1 atrophy (or smallness), sometimes with a net difference between type 1 and type 2 mean fibre diameters.

An autosomal recessive transmission pattern was initially proposed by Sher et al (1967) and was retained by others (Banker 1986). The number of sporadic cases may indirectly support this hypothesis. However, an alternative explanation would be an autosomal dominant gene with variable expression, as suggested by Schochet et al (1972) and by Dubowitz (1980).

Late-onset centronuclear myopathies

In some cases the muscular weakness is apparent only in adults or even in elderly patients (Bethlem et al 1970, Vital et al 1970, Harriman & Haleem 1972, McLeod et al 1972, Schochet et al 1972, Headington et al 1975, Pongratz et al 1975, Goulon et al 1976, Pepin et al 1976 , Bergen et al

1980 Edström et al 1982). In most of these reported patients, muscular wasting and weakness involved predominantly trunk and limb-girdle muscles, without any ocular symptoms. Very rarely, the facial muscles are involved (Serratrice et al 1987). Apparent hypertrophy was noted in the calves by Harriman & Haleem (1972), and more diffusely in another case (Pepin et al 1976). Generalized areflexia was common. However, limited, even asymmetrical, external ocular involvement was present in a few cases (Vital et al 1970, McLeod et al, case III$_6$, 1972, Pongratz et al 1975, Bergen et al 1980). The condition usually followed a slowly progressing downhill course, and patients were sometimes confined to a wheelchair by the fifth decade (Vital et al 1970).

Histopathology. The structural changes in muscle fibres are similar to those described in the early-onset form of the myopathy. The central nuclei are present with the same frequency in both fibre types. A gradient in myofibrillar size from the centre of the fibre to the periphery is frequent (Headington et al 1975, Goulon et al 1976, Pepin et al 1976). Vacuoles, splitting, annular fibrils, and sarcoplasmic masses are perhaps more frequently observed in these late-onset cases. The innervation pattern was strikingly well preserved in limb (Harriman & Haleem 1972) as well as in extraocular muscle samples (Bergen et al 1980). Numerous 'passing-by' myotendinous junctions have been noted (Goulon et al 1976).

No clear-cut clinical or morphological differences therefore distinguish the late-onset and early-onset types of centronuclear myopathy. In the former, however, a dominant mode of inheritance is more often clearly demonstrated. McLeod et al (1972) reported a family in which 16 members over five generations were affected. The dominant mode is compatible with the observations reported by Schochet et al (1972), Mortier et al (1975), Pepin et al (1976), Bergen et al (1980), Edström et al (1982) and Reske-Nielsen et al (1987).

Centronuclear myopathy with type 1 fibre atrophy

In some cases, the selective type 1 fibre hypotrophy or atrophy has been so striking that it has featured in the title of the reports (Engel et al

1968, Bethlem et al 1970, Karpati et al 1970, Radu et al 1974, Inokuchi et al 1975, Coquet et al 1976, Dubowitz 1980).

The initial report of this condition by Engel et al (1968) concerned a severely hypotonic child with diffuse muscle weakness but without any ocular or facial weakness, who died at the age of 18 months of pulmonary infection. Virtually all the type 1 fibres were small and hypotrophic, and virtually all had central nuclei. Similar changes were found in various muscles at necropsy.

There is no clinical homogeneity in the papers which followed this report. The cases reported by Bethlem et al (1970), Karpati et al (1970) and Inokuchi et al (1975) showed a common clinical pattern of a benign congenital myopathy, with no extraocular muscle involvement. However, in another case there was limitation of the ocular movements (Radu et al 1974).

Histopathology. In the cases studied by Karpati et al (1970), Inokuchi et al (1975), Radu et al (1974) and Dubowitz (1980) only type 1 fibres had centrally located nuclei. In contrast, in the case described by Bethlem et al (1970), both fibre types were affected. Electron microscopic examination showed no remarkable changes in the case described by Karpati et al (1970), but focal myofibrillar alterations were found by Inokuchi et al (1975), and large areas of myofibrillar disorganization were present in the large type 2 fibres in two instances (Radu et al 1974, Coquet et al 1976).

Two of the above cases were familial. A dominant mode of transmission was suggested in the paper by Karpati et al (1970) and an autosomal recessive mode with expression in carriers in the cases presented by Radu et al (1974).

All these findings argue against the classification of a particular entity, or even of a subgroup of centronuclear myopathies. Consequently, cases with type 1 atrophy should be re-assigned to the other groups of congenital myopathies.

X-linked myotubular myopathy

Two large unrelated families have been reported in the Netherlands (van Wijngaarden et al 1969, Barth et al 1975). There was a 25% mortality of affected male children in the first family, and a 100% mortality in the second. A diminution of fetal movement and hydramnios were often noted.

Death from respiratory failure was frequent in the first hours or days of life. Only a few of the affected children were able to overcome these early difficulties and to show a slow improvement in their motor condition. Ptosis, limitation of eye movements, and Achilles tendon contractures were then observed. In two cases, the clinical course was compatible with an active life.

Since these two reports, a few other cases have been documented (Fardeau et al 1978, Askanas et al 1979, Ambler et al 1984) with a rapid and poor prognosis. In the case observed by Dubowitz (1980) there was some improvement in motor function after a year.

Histopathology. The histological picture consists of a uniform myotubular pattern with only rare large fibres (Fig. 6.4A). The oxidative enzyme activities in the centre of the fibres, surrounded by a clear halo, produce a characteristic mosaic appearance in muscle sections (Fig. 6.4B). Myofibrillar ATPase reactions give the reverse pattern, with a clear central zone surrounded by a peripheral rim. Electron microscopy shows a rim of myofilaments, poorly segregated into myofibrillar bundles, surrounding a central nucleus or an accumulation of mitochondria and reticular profiles (Fig. 6.4C, D). The ultrastructural pattern is also striking because of the very few satellite cells (Fardeau et al 1978), contrasting with the growth potential of the muscle in tissue culture (Askanas et al 1979). Necropsy examinations showed the abnormalities in all muscles, and a normal number and appearance of anterior horn cells in the spinal cord.

In most of the cases mentioned (van Wijngaarden et al 1969, Barth et al 1975, Askanas et al 1979) the pedigrees favoured an X-linked pattern of inheritance. All the sporadic cases were males. It is notable that, in the families studied, biopsies from female carriers often exhibited some myotubes or small type 1 fibres scattered among normal myofibres. A study of two families in which several female carriers were identified by muscle biopsy revealed linkage to the Xq 28 locus (Thomas et al 1987). This finding needs to be confirmed by study of other families.

Multicore disease

The name 'multicore disease' was proposed by

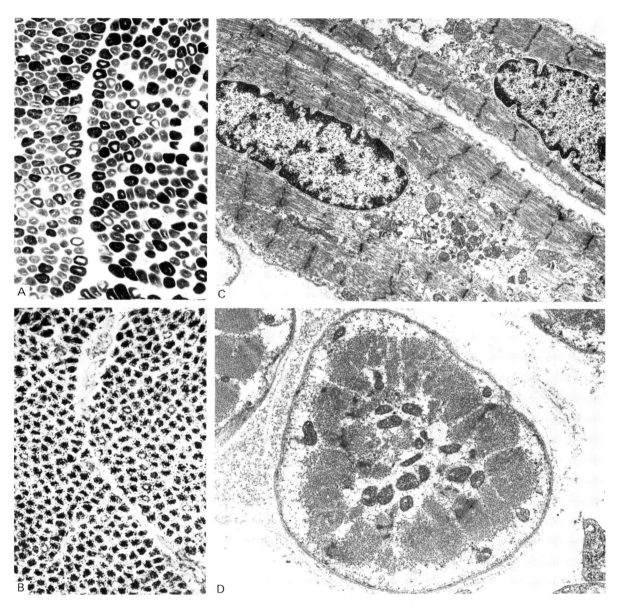

Fig. 6.4 Severe neonatal centronuclear myopathy. (A) Cryostat section. Myofibrillar ATPase reaction; ×135. Numerous fibres resembling myotubes; normal type-differentiation of the myofibres. (B) Cryostat section. NADH–tetrazolium reductase; ×135. Concentration of the oxidative activities in the centre of all the myofibres. (C) Electron micrograph, longitudinal section; ×8630. Accumulation of mitochondrial, reticular and Golgi profiles near the poles of central nuclei. (D) Electron micrograph, transverse section; ×10 460. Myofilaments forming a compact rim around the mitochondria located in the centre of the myofibre

Engel et al (1971) to denote a new congenital non-progressive myopathy, in which multifocal degeneration of the muscle fibres was found. The first of the two cases described in this report had been briefly reported five years earlier under a purely descriptive title (A. Engel & Gomez 1966). At about the same time, W. K. Engel (1967b) included in a general review the description of a patient with non-progressive muscle weakness from birth, and numerous foci in the muscle fibres where the normal striations were lost, a condition he termed 'segmental striatal loss'. Simultaneously, Schotland (1967) briefly presented the case of a child with a congenital muscular disorder and numerous 'target-like' lesions within the muscle fibres; a detailed description was included in a further paper (Schotland 1969). The authors of these three publications themselves agree that their cases were closely related. Since then, more than 30 cases have been reported under various titles including multicore disease (Mukoyama et al 1973, Bonnette et al 1974, Heffner et al 1976, Taratuto et al 1978, Brownell 1979, Dubowitz 1979, Vanneste & Stam 1982, Shuaib et al 1988), minicore disease (Currie et al 1974, Paljarvi et al 1987), myopathy with minicores (Lake et al 1977, Ricoy et al 1980), multicores with focal loss of cross-striations (Swash & Schwartz 1981), focal loss of cross striations (van Wijngaarden et al 1977) and multiminicore disease (Fardeau 1987, Ben Hamida et al 1987)—all with similar structural changes. The time which elapsed between presentation of the cases and their publication, and the variety of the eponyms used to denote this condition, reflect the difficulty in clearly delineating this new entity. Moreover, the 'minicore' lesion does not represent a specific change (see Banker 1986), and, as in the other congenital myopathies, it is only the frequency of the lesion which identifies this disease.

Clinically, most of these cases shared the usual pattern of a benign congenital myopathy: floppiness at birth, delayed motor development, and a generalized reduction in muscle bulk. Often the upper limbs were more involved than the lower, and global facial weakness was observed. Skeletal deformities were frequent (Heffner et al 1976, De Lumley et al 1976, Ricoy et al 1980, Fitzsimons & Tyer 1980). Contractures may exist (Schotland 1969, Engel et al, case 2, 1971) torticollis (Heffner et al 1976), rigid spine (Ben Hamida et al 1987). Tendon reflexes were generally reduced or absent. In some cases there was extraocular muscle involvement as evidenced by ptosis (Engel et al, case 2), limitation of eye movement (Schotland 1969, van Wijngaarden et al 1977) or even total ophthalmoplegia (Mukoyama et al 1973, Swash & Schwartz 1981). Cardiac abnormalities are sometimes present and include congenital defects (Engel et al 1971) or cardiac hypertrophy (De Lumley et al 1976). Most cases exhibit a nonprogressive course. However, progressive worsening may occur both in early-onset (Schotland 1969, van Wijngaarden et al 1977, Shuaib et al 1988) and late-onset cases (Bonnette et al 1974).

As in the other congenital myopathies, the serum CK and the EMG do not contribute to the diagnosis, which is made on the muscle biopsy alone.

Histopathology. On longitudinally sectioned material, numerous foci are visible where the normal cross-striations of the myofibrils are blurred. These foci are roughly fusiform, but may vary in size and shape; their long axis is often perpendicular to the long axis of the fibre, and they tend to occur very close to the blood vessels (Bethlem et al 1978, Bender 1979). Vesicular nuclei are frequent in and around these lesions (Engel 1967a, Schotland 1967). In transversely sectioned material the lesions may have three concentric zones, as seen in target fibres, but these are often difficult to see in paraffin-embedded material.

When stained by histochemical techniques, muscle fibres show numerous small foci of decreased oxidative enzyme, ATPase and phosphorylase activities, and glycogen content (Fig. 6.5A). There is always a 5–15% increase in internally located nuclei. However, the diagnosis may be difficult to establish before the examination of epoxy-embedded material. With light or phase-contrast microscopic examination of semi-thin sections, the foci look like a coalescence of multiple minute lesions (Engel et al 1971) with disruption of the normal sarcomeric pattern (Fig. 6.5C). Electron microscopy shows that the lesions are small areas of sarcomeric disintegration (Fig. 6.5D), with Z-band zig-zagging and streaming (Tanimura et al 1974), running over 2–6 sarcomeres, with sharp limits from the adjoining normal sarcomeres. The smaller lesions resemble 'dislocation' defects in the normal striational pattern (Fardeau et al 1977).

The foci are devoid of mitochondria. Engel et al (1971) noted that the areas with a reduced mitochondrial population are larger and more numerous than those with decreased ATPase activity or myofibrillar disorganization. Collections of sarco-

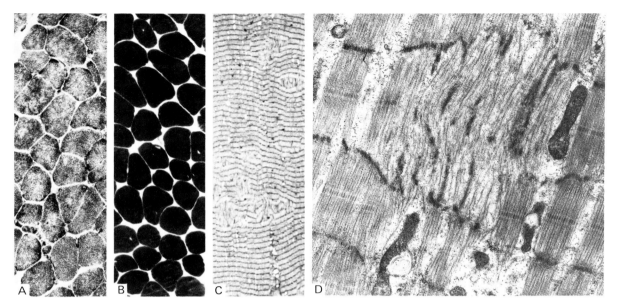

Fig. 6.5 Multicore disease. (A) Cryostat section, NADH–tetrazolium reaction; ×135. Small defects and irregularities in the intermyofibrillar network of the muscle fibres. (B) Cryostat section. Myofibrillar ATPase reaction after pre-incubation at pH 4.35; ×135. Type 1 fibre uniformity. (C) Thick section of epoxy-embedded material; ×340. Several foci of disruption in the myofibrillar striations. (D) Electron micrograph, longitudinal section; ×14 875. Small focus of sarcomeric disorganization, with streaming of Z-line material

tubular profiles are sometimes intermingled with irregularly arranged myofibrils. Vesicular nuclei, with prominent nucleoli, are often noted in the neighbourhood of the lesions.

The histochemical pattern is always modified. All cases exhibit a marked type 1 fibre predominance (Fig. 6.5B), with no grouping of the few type 2 fibres. Type 1 fibres are usually smaller in diameter than normal, while the type 2 fibres may be hypertrophic (Bonnette et al 1974). The minicores are present in type 2 as well as in type 1 fibres.

The motor innervation has been studied in a few cases. In one instance, nerve axons and end-plates were considered to be normal (Engel et al 1971). In the case described by van Wijngaarden (1977) there was poor ramification of the motor arborizations, which was thought to reflect immaturity of the motor nerve endings.

Evidence of the familial character of multicore disease is provided in a few reports (Heffner et al 1976, Lake et al 1977, Ricoy et al 1980). Many cases are sporadic. An autosomal recessive trans-

mission of the myopathy is suggested by the characteristics of the families studied by van Wijngaarden et al (1977) and by Bethlem et al (1978). Autosomal dominant inheritance has been reported or suggested in other families (Brownell 1979, Bender 1979, Swash & Schwartz 1981, Vanneste & Stam 1982, Paljarvi et al 1987.)

Congenital myopathies with intracytoplasmic inclusion bodies

Fingerprint body myopathy

In 1972 Engel et al reported the case of a 5-year-old girl with congenital non-progressive weakness, whose muscle biopsy contained numerous inclusion bodies which resembled fingerprints in their ultrastructural characteristics. Since this report, five other cases have been proposed for classification in the same category: a woman of 55 years (Gordon et al 1974), two half-brothers, 13 months and 12 years of age respectively at the time of the biopsy (Fardeau et al 1976), and the twins reported by

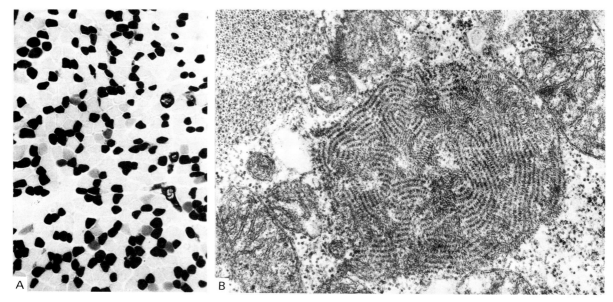

Fig. 6.6 Fingerprint body myopathy. (A) Cryostat section. Myofibrillar ATPase reaction after pre-incubation at pH 4.65; ×135. Normal spatial distribution of the muscle fibre types. Relative smallness of the type 1 fibres. (B) Electron micrograph, transverse section; × 36 380. One of the numerous fingerprint bodies, mainly present at the periphery of the muscle fibres

Curless et al (1978). All cases had exhibited weakness and hypotonia since birth. The condition was considered to be non-progressive or very slowly progressive. The EMG was considered to be normal or myopathic. The serum CK level was normal or slightly raised.

Histopathology. The biopsies were remarkable for their numerous sarcoplasmic inclusions with a fingerprint appearance. These bodies were generally oval, 0.5–7 μm long, and up to 4 μm wide. They were situated at the periphery of the muscle fibres, often near the nuclear poles. They were formed by convoluted lamellae lying 30–32 nm apart (Fig. 6.6B), each lamella displaying sawtooth-like densities 6 nm wide, 16 nm high, spaced out at intervals of 14–16 nm on the lamella. The inclusions were sometimes surrounded by poorly defined amorphous material (Engel et al 1972, Fardeau et al 1976).

Judging by the width of the Z lines in the muscle fibres, the inclusions were present mainly in type 1 fibres. Glycerination, digestion with RNAase or α-amylase and selective extraction of myofibrillar components did not modify the structure of the fingerprint bodies (Engel et al 1972). Other ultrastructural changes included myofibrillar disorganization or focal disruption, but these were considered to be minor.

The histochemical pattern was different in each of these cases. Marked type 1 predominance was found in three (Engel et al 1972, Gordon et al 1974, Fardeau et al 1976, case 1); type 1 smallness was evident in one case (Engel et al 1972) and less marked in another (Fardeau et al 1976, case 1) (Fig. 6.6A).

When A. G. Engel et al presented their observations in 1972, they had not observed similar inclusions in any other condition. Since then, however, fingerprint inclusions have been found in myotonic dystrophy (Tomé & Fardeau 1973), dermatomyositis, oculopharyngeal dystrophy, distal myopathy, and in many other different conditions (Sengel & Stoebner 1974), and are clearly non-specific. Nevertheless, the familial incidence of the changes observed in some cases (Fardeau et al 1976, Curless 1978) favours the view that fingerprint body myopathy may represent a distinct entity.

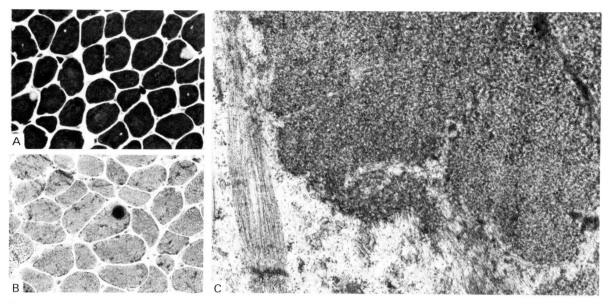

Fig. 6.7 Reducing body myopathy. (A) Cryostat section. Myofibrillar ATPase reaction; ×135. Two unstained inclusion bodies are visible. (B) Cryostat section. Menadione-linked α-glycerophosphate dehydrogenase. ×135. Strong positivity of the inclusion body. (C) Electron micrograph; ×28 475. Portion of an inclusion body, showing its loosely defined granular appearance and the presence of bundles of thin filaments at its pole

Reducing body myopathy

In 1972 Brooke & Neville reported two unrelated cases in which muscle biopsy revealed numerous unusual intracytoplasmic bodies which reduced tetrazolium salts without the addition of a substrate. The first was a floppy baby, who developed wasting and contractures of both proximal and distal muscles, a mild bilateral ptosis and facial weakness, and who died of respiratory failure. The second child, also abnormally floppy at birth, died at the age of 9 months following rapidly progressive diffuse muscle weakness. Both children were mentally normal, had normal or subnormal serum levels of CK and polyphasic potentials in the EMG.

Histopathology. Besides an increased variability in muscle fibre size, the muscle biopsies were remarkable because of the presence of numerous rounded bodies, frequently close to the subsarcolemmal nuclei, non-reactive for oxidative and ATPase reactions (Fig. 6.7A), stained intensely by the direct NBT-menadione method (Fig. 6.7B), and specific reactions for sulphydryl groups, as well as with PAS and gallocyanin. Electron microscopy showed that the bodies were not membrane-limited and consisted of a matrix of closely packed ill-defined particles, 12–16 nm in diameter, with holes of various shapes containing glycogen, mitochondria, sarcoplasmic reticulum, and sometimes long strands of fibrillar material (Fig. 6.7C).

Since the report by Brooke & Neville (1972), similar reducing activity has been demonstrated in inclusion bodies in five other cases (Tomé & Fardeau 1975, Dubowitz 1980, Hübner & Pongratz 1981, Oh et al 1983, Carpenter et al 1985). The clinical pictures of the 14-year-old boy studied by Tomé & Fardeau (1975) and of the 4-year-old-boy studied by Oh et al (1983) were less severe than in the original cases. In the muscle biopsy, inclusion bodies were infrequent, there was marked type 1 fibre predominance, and ultrastructurally the relationship between the bodies and thin filament bundles was often very close. In the adult case reported by Sahgal & Sahgal (1977) with a scapulo-peroneal distribution, the numerous subsarcolemmal bodies in type 1 fibres were positive for sulphydryl groups, but were however different from reducing bodies in their cytochemical characteristics and ultrastructural appearance. Another case was mentioned by Dubowitz & Brooke (1973) in a 4.5-year-old infant in whom a viral origin was suspected on serological grounds. The 7-year-old girl studied by Carpenter et al had an asymmetrical, progressive weakness predominating in the upper limbs. Reducing masses were abundant and had characteristic cytochemical features. Ultrastructural studies showed that they were mainly formed by tubular filaments 17 nm in diameter. Biochemical studies detected abnormal amounts of two proteins, 62 and 53 kDa. Despite the limited number of cases reported to date, the unique characteristics of these inclusion bodies strongly support the individuality of this disease.

Congenital (neuro) myopathy with cytoplasmic bodies, spheroid bodies or myofibrillar inclusions

Different reports have emphasized the frequency of filamentous inclusions similar to the intrasarcoplasmic inclusions commonly known as 'cytoplasmic bodies' (Nakashima et al 1970, Kinoshita et al 1975c, Clark et al 1978, Goebel et al 1978b, Jerusalem et al 1979, Wolburg et al 1982, Patel et al 1983, Fardeau 1987, Chapon et al 1989, Mizuno et al 1989).

In a few cases (Fardeau 1987, Mizuno et al 1989), there was severe infantile hypotonia with limb and respiratory muscle weakness requiring early mechanical ventilation. In most cases a severe progressive respiratory insufficiency was also the predominant feature, but developed at a later age (Kinoshita et al 1975c, Jerusalem et al 1979, Patel et al 1983) or even later (Chapon et al 1989). Other cases (Nakashima et al 1970, Clark et al 1978, Goebel et al 1978b, Wolburg et al 1982) had a more benign clinical picture, with marked fatiguability, pain and slowly developing muscle atrophy beginning during adolescence. In the cases studied by Jerusalem et al (1979) and Goebel et al (1978b), there was clinical and electrical evidence of neurogenic muscle involvement. A similar case, of severe limb and respiratory muscular weakness in a young child, is currently under investigation in our laboratory.

Histopathology. In the muscle biopsies, the inclusions were displayed as clear spheroidal

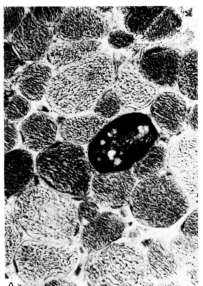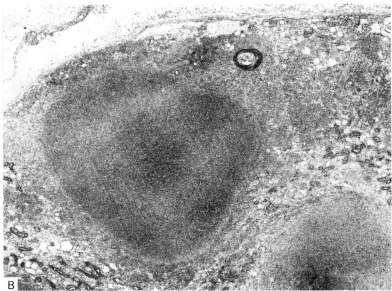

Fig. 6.8 Cytoplasmic body myopathy. (A) Cryostat section. NADH–tetrazolium reaction; ×135. Several unstained areas are visible in a muscle fibre. (B) Electron micrograph, ×9860. Fine filamentous structure of the inclusion bodies, surrounded by numerous mitochondrial and reticular profiles

defects by most of the cytochemical reactions (Fig. 6.8A); they stained red–purple with Gomori trichrome and were surrounded by a clear halo. The periphery of the bodies, or sometimes the inclusions themselves, are labelled by desmin antibodies (Osborn & Goebel 1983). Electron microscopy (Fig. 6.8B) showed that these rounded bodies have a dense core formed by fine filaments, 12–15 nm in diameter (Goebel et al 1978b), arranged like a ball of twine, surrounded by a halo with disarrayed filaments, glycogen and mitochondria. These inclusion bodies are often stacked along small segments of the fibres and are linked by areas of Z-band streaming (Jerusalem et al 1979, Goebel et al 1978b).

In contrast with the cytoplasmic bodies, which preferentially affect type 2 muscle fibres (MacDonald & Engel 1969) spheroid bodies are observed only in type 1 fibres (Clark et al 1978, Goebel et al 1978b, Jerusalem et al 1979). There has been type 1 predominance in most of the cases reported.

This group seems to be genetically heterogeneous. In three of these reports (Clark et al 1978, Goebel et al 1978b, Chapon et al 1989) an autosomal dominant inheritance was clearly established. In one report (Patel et al 1983), an autosomal recessive inheritance was postulated. Other cases were sporadic.

Miscellaneous — congenital myopathies reported in single patients or families

Several other morphologically distinct congenital myopathies have been described but so far only in single cases or families.

Familial myopathy with probable lysis of myofibrils in type 1 fibres. A brother and sister with marked hypotonia from birth, a steppage gait and thin muscles, whose biopsies showed similar morphological features, were reported by Cancilla et al (1971). The type 1 fibres were uniformly small and showed homogeneous peripheral areas which were stained by oxidative reactions but stained intensely by the ATPase reaction. Electron microscopy showed that these areas consisted of a uniform, finely granular matrix which contained nuclei and other organelles. The central myofibrils showed focal alteration at the interface between

the two different zones of the fibre. The absence of a family history of muscle disease suggested autosomal recessive inheritance. The case described by Sahgal & Sahgal (1977) had some morphological similarities to those observed by Cancilla et al (1971). The biopsies from two familial cases, brother and sister (Fardeau, personal observations) with severe infantile hypotonia and progressive weakness, could also belong to the same group.

Sarcotubular myopathy. Jerusalem et al (1973b) reported two brothers, aged 15 and 11 years, of a Hittite colony and consanguineous parentage. These boys had been suffering from a non-progressive, moderately severe diffuse muscle weakness since infancy, with normal mental development. The EMG was myopathic. Serum enzyme activities were increased in the older sib and normal in the younger.

Four biopsies showed a curious vacuolar myopathy with a myriad of small empty spaces, more so in type 2 fibres (20–30%) than in the type 1 fibres (4%). There was no type 1 predominance. Electron microscopy showed that the vacuoles were attributed to dilatation and coalescence of sarcotubular profiles, with a minimum of other structural changes. Morphometrically there was a significant increase in reticular profiles. The segmental distribution of the vacuoles along the muscle fibres remains unexplained. Except for similar pathological data seen in one adult by S. Carpenter, briefly mentioned as an addendum to the original paper, no other case has been reported to date.

Zebra body myopathy. A boy of 15 years, weak from birth, with generalized muscle wasting was considered by Lake & Wilson (1975) as 'provisionally' justifying a separate identification. In addition to the large variation in fibre diameter, vacuolation, fibre splitting and increased endomysial connective tissue in the muscle biopsy sections, electron microscopy showed frequent 'zebra bodies' in the muscle fibres, as well as numerous rod-like bodies. A second case (Reyes et al 1987) has been reported in a 4-day old baby, with congenital hypotonia and a favourable course, in which the zebra bodies were also associated with a number of other filamentary changes. It should be emphasized that leptofibrils (zebra bodies) are normal components of the fibres in

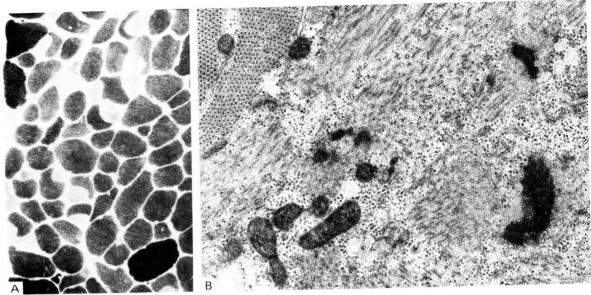

Fig. 6.9 Non-classified congenital myopathy. (A) Cryostat section, myofibrillar ATPase reaction; ×135. Clear-cut crescents at the periphery of numerous type 1 fibres. (B) Electron micrograph; ×25 500. Portion of a peripheral crescent filled with disarrayed filamentous bundles and slightly enlarged Z bands

some muscles (Mair & Tomé 1972a, b) and are frequent in the vicinity of myotendinous junctions or around areas of abnormal vacuolation of muscle fibres.

Trilaminar muscle fibre disease. The curious appearance of the muscle fibres suggested to Ringel et al (1977) the possibility that this was a new congenital myopathy. On cryostat sections stained by the NADH–TR reaction, the muscle fibres showed three concentric zones, the inner and outer being densely stained. Electron microscopy indicated packed mitochondria in the centre, myofibrillary bundles in the middle zone and disarranged filaments in the periphery of the muscle fibres. The child had marked rigidity, weakness with little spontaneous movement, and a high CK level, at birth.

Others. It should be emphasized that many cases are still difficult or impossible to classify according to present criteria, mainly cases presenting with severe neonatal hypotonia. For instance, a few cases were reported with a segmental absence of myosin ATPase activity (Yarom & Shapira 1977). Another case was reported (Fidzianska et al 1981) as 'Cap disease'

because of the presence of clear-cut peripheral crescents in the muscle fibres. A similar case also showed (Fardeau et al 1978) disarrayed bundles of myofilaments and enlarged Z-bands within the peripheral zones (Fig. 6.9A, B) which stained strongly positive with the NADH–TR, PAS and phosphorylase reactions, and negative with the ATPase reaction. Whether these cases represent new, well-individualized congenital myopathies, or morphological variants of diseases previously described, is still difficult to assess.

SOME RELATED DISORDERS, AS YET IMPRECISELY DEFINED

Congenital fibre type disproportion

This entity was recognized as a result of a review by Brooke & Engel (1969) of a series of children's biopsies which were grouped according to changes in fibre size. One group, comprising 10 children with non-progressive weakness, had type 1 fibres which were significantly (more than 12%) smaller than type 2 fibres. A similar pattern was noted by Farkas-Bargeton et al (1968) and by Caille et al

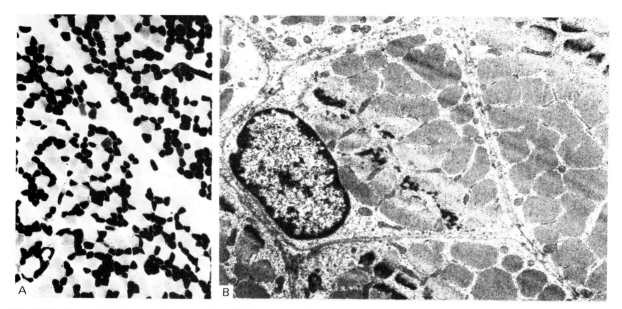

Fig. 6.10 Congenital fibre type disproportion. (A) Cryostat section. Myofibrillar ATPase reaction after pre-incubation at pH 4.65; ×135. Relative smallness of the type 1 fibres. Almost all the type 2 fibres are of type 2A. Homogeneity in size of both muscle fibre types. (B) Electron micrograph, transverse section; ×5850. Normal appearance of the small fibres

(1971) in severely hypotonic children. After studying 12 additional cases, Brooke (1973) suggested the label 'congenital fibre type disproportion' (CFTD) for this group, the common features being a fairly uniform clinical picture, a possible familial incidence and a relatively good prognosis. Furthermore, the singularity of the histochemical pattern provided some clue to the pathophysiology, the small size of the type 1 fibres possibly being related to changes in the reflex control of motor activity (Brooke & Williamson 1969). Since Brooke's series, a few further reports have adopted the same designation (Dubowitz & Brooke 1973, Fardeau et al 1975, Kinoshita et al 1975a, Lenard & Goebel 1975, Serratrice et al 1975, Martin et al 1976, Curless & Nelson 1977, Cavanagh et al 1979, Eisler & Wilson 1978, Clancy et al 1980, Sulaiman et al 1983, ter Laak et al 1981, Argov et al, 1984, Glick et al 1984, Jaffé et al 1988). Meanwhile, however, a growing controversy has developed about the limits of this entity, and the value of maintaining such a framework has been contested by its promoters themselves (Spiro et al 1977, Fardeau et al 1978, Brooke et al 1979, Cavanagh et al 1979).

The cases described in the early reports and in a few subsequent ones were relatively homogeneous from the clinical viewpoint (Farkas-Bargeton et al 1968, Brooke 1973, Fardeau et al 1975, Kinoshita et al 1975a, Serratrice et al 1975, Curless & Nelson 1977). The children were more or less severely hypotonic at birth, with a long thin face, open mouth and high-arched palate. The muscle weakness was diffuse. The children were generally of short stature and low body weight with frequent skeletal abnormalities; about half the cases had a congenital hip dislocation. Contractures of various muscles were frequent; deep tendon reflexes were weak or absent. Mental development was normal. The delay in attaining motor milestones was variable and in some cases a kyphoscoliosis developed when the children grew older. Respiratory problems were confined to the first two years of life. After this the general condition remained stationary, or even tended to improve with the years. The serum CPK level was usually normal, and the EMG was normal or myopathic.

Histopathology. On cryostat sections (Fig. 6.10A), the type 1 fibres were smaller than the type 2 fibres, which were often slightly hypertrophic (Farkas-Bargeton et al 1968, Fardeau et al 1975). On histograms of the muscle fibres, the lesser diameters of the type 1 and type 2 fibres formed two sharply defined peaks; the coefficient of variability (Dubowitz & Brooke 1973) was low for both types (<250). Cases with wider variability in fibre size should be discarded from the CFTD group (Martin et al 1976). Type 1 predominance, often with type 2B deficiency, was usual in this condition. The structure of the fibres appeared to be normal; in some cases, there was a slight increase in centrally located nuclei. On electron microscopy, the most significant finding was the normal architecture of the muscle fibres (Fig. 6.10). The absence of abnormal folding of the basement lamina around the smallest fibres suggested a hypotrophic rather than an atrophic process.

The familial incidence suggested in the original series (Brooke 1973) has been confirmed by other reports (Fardeau et al 1975, Kinoshita et al 1975a, Curless & Nelson 1977, Eisler & Wilson 1978, Jaffé et al 1988). However, some reports have suggested widening the group, because certain cases displayed an unusual severity, with respiratory insufficiency (Lenard & Goebel 1975) or even death (Spiro et al 1977, Cavanagh et al 1979). In cases mentioned in two other reports there was a bizarre rigidity of the neck and spine, with flexion contractures of knees and elbows (Seay et al 1977, Goebel et al 1978a). In addition, electrophysiological studies showed fibrillation and complex high-amplitude potentials, while the ultrastructure of the small fibres was notable for large sectors of sarcomeric disarray (Lenard & Goebel 1975).

These cases render the limits of the CFTD group uncertain and raise the question of the specificity of the histological features. In addition, it must be emphasized that a similar disproportion in fibre size may be found in various other conditions, particularly in neurogenic disorders (Brooke & Engel 1969, Martin et al 1976). In the case reported by Bethlem et al (1969) a disproportion in fibre type size coexisted with some myotubes, the EMG showed numerous fibrillation potentials at rest, and the brother of the propositus presented a typical picture of peroneal muscular atrophy. Similarly, a type 1 atrophy may be found in several myogenic processes during childhood,

such as congenital myotonic dystrophy (Farkas-Bargeton et al 1974), or the infantile variety of facioscapulohumeral dystrophy. One of the original cases of CFTD was subsequently shown to have such a dystrophy (Brooke et al 1979). One of the first reported familial cases (Fardeau et al 1975) was found to be suffering, years later, from a hypertrophic polyneuropathy.

As already pointed out in this chapter, a disproportion in fibre size, with small type 1 fibres, may be encountered in most of the other congenital myopathies including nemaline myopathy (Engel et al 1964, Radu & Ionescu 1972, Dahl & Klutzow 1974, Kinoshita & Satoyoshi 1974), centronuclear myopathies (Meyers et al 1974, Inokuchi et al 1975), and fingerprint myopathy (Fardeau et al 1976). Myotubular myopathy may be observed in one member of a family, and CFTD in another (Kinoshita et al 1975a). Several cases initially reported as CFTD showed rods in their muscle biopsies (Caille et al 1971, case 2, Brooke 1973, Kinoshita et al 1975a), or a high percentage of central nuclei (Brooke 1973), or moth-eaten and whorled fibres (Dubowitz & Brooke 1973). It therefore seems likely that the histological picture of CFTD represents a 'mixed bag' of cases (Fardeau et al 1978, Dubowitz 1980, Brooke et al 1979) and is not in itself a sufficient criterion to characterize a subgroup of the congenital myopathies. Nevertheless, it remains certain that a 'pure' size disproportion is highly suggestive of congenital myopathy, and that there are numerous cases of benign congenital hypotonia in which CFTD is the only histological abnormality.

Congenital hypotonia with type 1 fibre predominance

In their less restrictive category of 'benign congenital hypotonias', Engel & Warmolts (1973) emphasized the frequency of a marked type 1 fibre predominance, with or without small type 2 fibres, in familial or sporadic cases. In several children with mild weakness, skeletal deformities kyphoscoliosis and decreased deep tendon reflexes, Brooke (1977) found the same pattern. Dubowitz (1980) considered this 'congenital type 1 fibre predominance' to be an entity comparable to congenital fibre type disproportion. Of 50 cases fulfilling the clinical criteria of the congenital

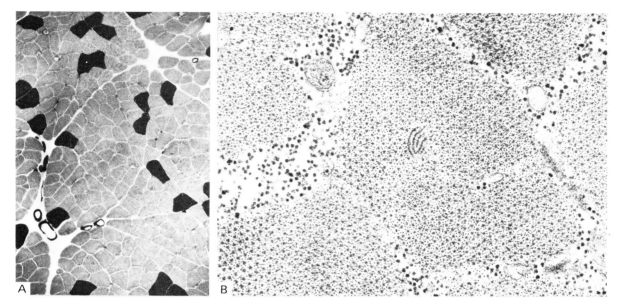

Fig. 6.11 Benign congenital myopathy with type 1 predominance. (A) Cryostat section, myofibrillar ATPase reaction; ×135. Marked type 1 fibre predominance. (B) Electron micrograph, transverse section; ×42 500. Small 'fingerprint' structure in the centre of a myofibril

myopathies, five exhibited 'pure' type 1 predominance (Fardeau et al 1978). Such a case has been studied in detail (Pellegrini et al 1985, Biral et al 1987).

In such cases, the type 1 fibre predominance was marked (over 60%) and was the only significant abnormality. Fibrosis, necrosis, internal nuclei or abnormal fibre-size variability were absent. However it should be noted that very few of these cases underwent thorough electron-microscopic investigation. In our experience, minimal changes of the myofibrillar architecture of the fibre such as small fingerprint structures or focal disruptions of the Z bands were not rare (Fig. 6.11A, B).

It is also noteworthy that a similar histochemical pattern has been reported on several occasions (Morgan-Hughes et al 1973, Bethlem et al 1978, Pou-Serradell et al 1980) in members of families in which more typical cases of congenital myopathy were found. It is conceivable that most of these cases with type 1 fibre predominance should be included within different groups of congenital myopathies. Some of them are indeed familial (Dubowitz 1980).

Nevertheless, it should be stressed that these cases may be difficult to distinguish from the mild, slowly-evolving forms of infantile spinal muscular atrophy. The distinction rests mainly on clinical and electromyographic grounds. The diagnosis of congenital hypotonia with type 1 fibre predominance should therefore imply the absence of any sign of a denervation–re-innervation process.

Congenital hypotonia with delayed maturation of muscle fibres

In two out of eight biopsies of hypotonic children studied before the 20th day of life, Farkas-Bargeton et al (1978) noticed several points indicating a delayed maturation of the extrafusal muscle fibres: type 2 fibre predominance (more than 80%) with an abnormal proportion of type 2 fibre subtypes, the presence of numerous large type 1 fibres (the 'B' fibres described by Wohlfart 1937) and sub-sarcolemmal haloes devoid of any oxidative activity on cryostat sections. These haloes were found to be devoid of mitochondria and myofibrils on electron microscopy.

These features were reminiscent of those observed in the severe neonatal forms of myotonic dystrophy, in which consistent peripheral haloes, frequent myotubes and a very high percentage of satellite cells were found (Farkas-Bargeton et al 1974, Sarnat & Silbert 1976). They were, however, much less pronounced in cases of neonatal hypotonia than in myotonic dystrophy.

Congenital hypotonia with small type 2 fibres

Relatively small type 2 fibres may be observed in congenital hypotonia secondary to cerebral lesions, whatever their mechanism (Fenichel 1967). However, reduced type 2 fibre size may be found in some children presenting the clinical features of benign congenital myopathy and in the absence of any sign of CNS involvement. Type 2 fibre smallness may be accompanied by type 1 fibre predominance, by a slight increase in the number of internal nuclei (Scelsi et al 1976), or by rod accumulation in type 1 fibres (Engel & Warmolts 1971) and was considered as a type 2 muscle fibre hypoplasia (Yoshioka et al 1987). Some of these cases should certainly be included in the group of congenital myopathies. However, such a histochemical pattern (type 1 predominance, type 2 smallness or atrophy) should first raise the possibility of a metabolic disorder in the lipid or respiratory chain pathways.

Minimal change myopathy

Dubowitz (1978) proposed the term of 'minimal change myopathy' for two cases with significant clinical manifestations but only minor abnormalities on muscle histology.

Some other cases have been reported (Nonaka et al 1983, Jong et al 1987) in which there was an increased number of type IIc muscle fibres, suggesting a maturational defect and a defect of neural influence upon the developing muscles.

Benign congenital hypotonia

The term 'benign congenital hypotonia' (BCH), introduced by Walton (1956) in place of the well-worn label 'amyotonia congenita', referred purely to a clinical syndrome: the early appearance of hypotonia with a non-progressive or improving course. In the classification proposed by Walton (1957), this syndrome was distinguished, not only from the infantile spinal muscular atrophies, but also from symptomatic hypotonias secondary to cerebral, nutritional, metabolic or skeletal disorders.

Most of the structurally defined congenital myopathies described after this classification was proposed may in fact mimic this syndrome. A more restrictive definition of BCH therefore emerged after the discovery of these myopathies. Engel & Warmolts (1973) maintained the designation BCH when the congenital hypotonia 'cannot be attributed to another specific disease after detailed histochemical, electromyographic and biochemical tests are done'. Brooke (1977) considered that 'stringent criteria should be applied to this diagnosis, all clinical, biochemical, electromyographic and histological tests being normal, except the abnormal tone'. Similarly, Dubowitz (1980) reserved the term of BCH for a 'residuum of cases with no apparent underlying muscle weakness, intellectual retardation or associated disease'. He mentioned, however, that a number of cases which he originally designated as BCH, subsequently turned out to be examples of the Prader-Willi syndrome.

Consequently, according to current criteria, BCH cannot be diagnosed without a morphologically normal muscle biopsy.

The congenital muscular dystrophies

Congenital muscular dystrophy (CMD)

Since the presentation by Batten (1903) of three early infantile types of myopathy to the Neurological Society of the United Kingdom, a number of cases with symptoms usually present at birth, a variable clinical course and dystrophic muscle-pathology have been recorded in the literature under the heading of congenital muscular dystrophy (CMD), a term first proposed by Howard (1908). A review of the literature may give the impression that this is a relatively rare disease. The reality is quite different. Rospide et al (1972) considered that CMD constituted 16% of childhood muscle dystrophies; Donner et al (1975) estimated that it comprised 9% of all the neuro-muscular disorders seen in a paediatric hospital, and 35% of cases with clinical signs of myopathy.

Because of the lack of detailed histological data, most of the early reports of CMD are extremely difficult to authenticate. Only a few had verification post mortem, showing the integrity of the central and peripheral nervous system. Before 1940, only the case reported by Haushalter (1920) was well documented. The most interesting data were contributed by the record of the family successively studied by Batten (1915), Turner (1940, 1949) and Turner & Lees (1962). Six of 13 sibs were affected and markedly hypotonic during childhood. Two died early and the four who survived, improved clinically and learned to walk at about five years of age. When examined in their sixth decade, three of them were healthy and had enjoyed an active life. One died from rheumatic carditis, and the necropsy by Greenfield (see Turner 1949) revealed myopathic changes in the muscles without any abnormalities of the central or peripheral nervous system.

Other isolated cases with verification post mortem have been published (Levesque et al 1956, Short 1963, Wharton 1965). Of special interest were those reported by Banker et al (1957), Greenfield et al (1958), and Pearson & Fowler (1963), with a clinical picture of arthrogryposis multiplex congenita (AMC). A number of Japanese patients with severe central nervous system involvement were studied by Fukuyama et al (1960) and will be discussed separately.

More recently, several small series of cases have been reported (Vassella et al 1967, Zellweger et al 1967a, b, Rotthauwe et al 1969, Lücking & Otto 1971, Rospide et al 1972, Raju et al 1973, Donner et al 1975, Jones et al 1979, Lazaro et al 1979, Serratrice et al 1980, McMenamin et al 1982) in which detailed histochemical and ultrastructural data were obtained. In some of these reports (Zellweger et al 1967a, b, Nonaka & Chou 1979) subclassification of CMD into benign and severe forms was proposed. This seems confusing, because of the large overlap between these two categories, because of the identity of the patho-logical findings, and because of the difficulty in distinguishing CMD from the other muscular dystrophies (Banker 1986, Fenichel 1988).

Clinically, generalized muscular involvement is usually present at birth. Reduced fetal movements during pregnancy are frequently noted. Contractures of various muscles and joint abnormalities may be evident at birth, producing an arthrogrypotic picture. In other cases, the contractures tend to develop a little later, affecting preferentially the neck muscles (Jones et al 1979, Serratrice et al 1980) and the flexors of the fingers, as in the family studied by Turner (Turner 1940, 1949, Turner & Lees 1962). Muscular atrophy and weakness are symmetrical and predominate in proximal muscles. Hypertrophy is never noted, neither are ptosis or ophthalmoplegia. The tendon reflexes are often depressed or absent. Mental development is normal but the EEG is abnormal in a few cases (Zellweger et al 1967a,b, Rotthauwe et al 1969, Lücking & Otto 1971, Donner et al 1975) without any clinical seizures. Cardiac abnormalities are rare, except in the Arab family studied by Lebenthal et al (1970), which may well have been suffering from a condition other than CMD.

There is great variability in the clinical severity and evolution of the condition. Some patients died within the first weeks or months of life (Levesque et al 1956, Banker et al 1957, Wharton 1965). In other cases the condition remained stationary although the patient was severely disabled (Pearson & Fowler 1963, Serratrice et al 1980). A number of patients may be able to walk without support, and are able to lead an independent life, if the development of kyphoscoliosis or respiratory problems do not interfere. Serum CK levels tend to be high in the early phases of the disease, and to fall into the normal range at a later stage. The EMG usually shows a 'myopathic' pattern. Motor conduction velocities are normal.

Histopathology. Histopathological muscle changes are as a rule very striking. There is a marked reduction in the number of muscle fibres and a considerable increase in interstitial connective and adipose tissue. The size of the muscle fibres varies widely (Fig. 6.12A). Fibre necrosis is uncommon, except in the very early stages, and

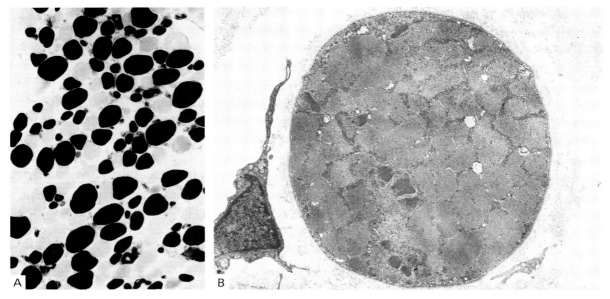

Fig. 6.12 Congenital muscular dystrophy. (A) Cryostat section. Myofibrillar ATPase after preincubation at pH 4.65; ×135. Variability in size of both fibre types. Marked increase in size of the endomysial spaces. (B) Electron micrograph, transverse section; ×7055. A small rounded muscle fibre is surrounded by collagen fibres and fibroblastic processes

there are no remarkable changes in internal structure of the muscle fibres, except for a few central nuclei, myofibrillar whorls or annular fibrils. Regenerative activity is strikingly absent (Afifi et al 1969).

Electron-microscopic findings (Gubbay et al 1966, Afifi et al 1969, Ketelsen et al 1971, Otto & Lücking 1971) are quite variable. Disarray of myofibrils, Z-line spreading, vacuolated sarco-plasmic reticulum and dilated mitochondria have repeatedly been found. In many cases the structure of the small fibres is not altered (Fig. 6.12B). Probably of greater relevance are the abundance and location of the collagen fibrils close to the sarcolemma (Afifi et al 1969). The very small satellite cells which have an inactive appearance (Fardeau et al 1978) may be related to the impaired capacity of muscle fibres to grow and regenerate. This led Fidzianska et al (1982) to propose that some disorder of collagen synthesis was basic to this myopathy. However, no qualitative changes in the different collagens was demonstrated by immunocytochemical studies (Hantaï et al, 1985). A few motor end-plates examined (Afifi et al 1969, Fardeau et al 1978) were considered to be normal.

All histochemical fibre types are affected (Fig. 6.12A). There is never any type-grouping. Type 1 predominance has been found in several cases. There is almost always a discrepancy between the severity of the pathological changes in muscle and the degree of motor disability. As emphasized by Dubowitz (1980), the biopsy can never be used as a means of assessing prognosis in CMD.

Most of the cases are sporadic. However, several sets of affected siblings have been reported (McMenamin et al 1982) suggesting an autosomal recessive transmission.

Congenital muscular dystrophy with central nervous system involvement (Fukuyama disease, FCMD)

In 1960, Fukuyama et al reported a peculiar condition in 15 Japanese children with diffuse muscle wasting, joint contractures, mental re-tardation and, frequently, convulsive disorders. Subsequently, a number of similar cases were found in Japan, and 192 cases were identified in 1976 (Nonaka & Chou 1979).

This condition has several features in common with the other congenital dystrophies. It is recognized at birth or in early infancy. Muscle weakness and hypotonia are diffuse. Contractures affect mainly the hip and knee joints. Muscle atrophy and contractures evolve slowly. More characteristic features are the prominent facial weakness, giving an expressionless face, and the occasional mild pseudohypertrophy of the calf muscles. The most distinctive feature of the condition is the severity of central nervous system involvement. Intellectual development is markedly impaired (IQ <50). Grand mal convulsions occur in half the cases, and ventricular enlargement and hypoplasia of the cerebellar vermis can be shown by computed tomography. Motor development is considerably impaired and only a few children are able to walk unassisted for some years. The average life span is 8–10 years.

The serum CK level rises markedly during the early stages of the disease, and subsequently returns to the normal range. The EMG shows a myopathic pattern. Motor conduction velocities are slightly delayed in most cases, but remain unchanged throughout the course of the disease.

Histopathology. Histological changes in muscle (Nonaka et al 1972) include variation in muscle fibre diameters, frequent necrotic fibres, fibres with central nuclei, occasional regenerating fibres, dense proliferation of the interstitial connective tissue and thickening of blood vessel walls. Mild inflammatory infiltrates may be found in the interstitial spaces and around the blood vessels. Both fibre types are affected; type IIc fibres are frequent (Nonaka et al 1982). Electron microscopy shows non-specific myofibrillar alterations, marked fibrosis and an increased number of satellite cells.

More than 10 cases submitted to neuropathological examination were reported in Japan (Nonaka & Chou 1979). Diffuse micropolygyria is a constant finding in the cerebral cortex, being predominant in the temporal and occipital lobes, with fusion of the thickened leptomeninges. The cerebellum is almost always also affected and hydrocephalus may occur. There is no demyelination and spinal cord neurones are well preserved.

The condition is transmitted as an autosomal recessive trait with no sex preference, a high incidence of consanguinity, and a high frequency of affected sibs with a segregation ratio close to 25%. The existence of FCMD outside Japan is

still controversial, except for some patients born from Japanese parents in Canada (McMenamin et al 1982) or in the United States (Olney & Miller 1983). A few possible cases of CMD with cerebral or cerebro-ocular involvement have been reported, but their identity with the Japanese cases is open to question (Fowler & Manson 1973, Nonaka & Chou 1979, Dubowitz 1980, Goebel et al 1983, Heggie et al 1987, Federico et al 1988, Leyten et al 1989, Streib & Lucking 1989, Topaloglu et al 1990).

Rigid spine syndrome

This term was introduced by Dubowitz (1973) to highlight the main element of a muscular disorder in a 13-year-old boy, disabled by a non-painful progressive limitation of flexion of the neck and trunk. Since this description, about 30 cases have been reported under this designation, although the nosological position of this syndrome is still debated (Dunn 1976, Seay et al 1977, Goto et al 1979, Mussini et al 1981, Echenne et al 1983, Serratrice et al 1984, Poewe et al 1985, Ishimoto et al 1986, Tardieu et al 1986, Vanneste et al 1988, Merlini et al 1989.)

The onset is usually around 6–7 years of age. Boys seem to be more often affected than girls. Weakness of the girdle muscles is mild. Muscle contractures cause flexion of the elbows and equinus deformity of the feet. The attitude of the patients is rather stereotyped, with hyperextension of the neck and the trunk often tilted forward. Tendon reflexes are decreased. The course of the disease is very slowly progressive, with development of a scoliosis, worsening of the contractures, and in some cases deterioration of respiratory function (Merlini et al 1989). Cardiac abnormalities have been reported in several cases (Mussini et al 1981, Poewe et al 1985). Serum CK is slightly increased, the EMG findings are usually considered to be myopathic.

The biopsy studies reveal non-specific features, with variation in muscle fibre diameter, occasional degenerative changes, and a marked increase of endomysial and perimysial connective tissue, especially in the axial muscles. Variations in fibre type ratio have been documented in some cases. Most cases are sporadic, and familial occurrence is rare (Echenne et al 1983). Even if the natural history of this syndrome is peculiar, the non-specific histological and biological features explain the difficulties of defining precisely the boundaries of this syndrome, and in distinguishing it from other muscle disorders such as Emery–Dreifuss muscular dystrophy and the group of congenital muscular dystrophies, in which the syndrome is often included (Banker 1986).

Ullrich's syndrome

The contrast between the severe contractures of the proximal joints and the marked hyperflexibility of distal joints was considered as sufficiently peculiar for this condition to be individualized as a subtype within the group of CMD. Two boys were reported by Ullrich (1930) as having a congenital atonic-sclerotic muscular dystrophy (Stoeber 1939, Gött and Josten 1954, Furukawa and Toyokura 1977, Nonaka et al 1981, De Paillette et al 1989, Santoro et al 1989). There are no other histopathological or biological distinctive features from other types of CMD. The evolution appears to be stationary or very slowly progressive. Only future genetic research will determine whether this syndrome should be separately identified within CMD.

SOME UNRESOLVED PROBLEMS

Specificity of the structural changes in muscle fibres

The various structural changes in the congenital myopathies, such as cores, rods, and the different types of inclusion body, were all initially considered to be specific or at least conspicuous abnormalities. Later, however, the non-specificity of the ultrastructural changes was underlined in two presentations (Engel & MacDonald 1970, Fardeau 1970). Rods similar to those observed in nemaline myopathy have been seen in many other conditions, for instance in individuals without known muscle disorders (Schmalbruch 1968, Meltzer et al 1973, 1976), especially in the vicinity of the myotendinous junctions (Mair & Tomé 1972a), in extraocular (Mair & Tomé 1972b) and in cardiac muscles (Fawcett 1968, Munnel &

Getty 1968, Côté et al 1970). Collections of rods have been found in various pathological states including rhabdomyoma (Cornog & Gonatas 1967), hypothyroid myopathy (Fardeau 1970), polymyositis (Cape et al 1970), acute alcoholic myopathy (Martinez et al 1973), spinal progressive muscular atrophy (Konno et al 1987) and HIV infection (Dalakas et al 1987). Focal disruptions in myofibrillar structure similar to those observed in multicore disease can be seen in any type of dystrophic, inflammatory, endocrine or toxic muscular process (Engel et al 1971, Pellissier et al 1979). Moreover, fingerprint bodies have been detected in various pathological conditions (Tomé & Fardeau 1973, Sengel & Stoebner 1974) and in extra-ocular muscles (Radnot 1974) as well as in normal fetal muscle (Ambler et al 1987). Cytoplasmic bodies have been reported in a variety of diseases (Mair & Tomé 1972b), and only reducing bodies have not to date been detected in acquired muscular disorders.

The definition of particular varieties of congenital myopathy cannot usually be based upon a simple specific morphological finding unless it is a very peculiar and ubiquitous pathological change — e.g. the cores in central core disease. The similarities between cores and target fibres, which are observed mainly in the neurogenic atrophies (Resnick & Engel 1967, De Coster et al 1976) have been stressed repeatedly. Cores differ from targets in their length, by their degree of demarcation and by their multiplicity within the same fibre. This point is also of importance in the definition of the centronuclear myopathies. As already emphasized, the central position of the muscle nuclei goes hand in hand with a reduction in the number of subsarcolemmal nuclei and frequently with a radial disposition of the inter-myofibrillary spaces around the central nuclei.

In general, the recognition of each muscular disorder requires an overall appreciation of a set of pathological features, including: (i) the frequency of the structural anomaly concerned — i.e. the proportion of muscle fibres affected; (ii) its predominance over any other changes present in muscle fibres; (iii) its degree of selectivity for one fibre type. It is indeed remarkable that in most cases of congenital myopathy, large numbers of cores, rods, mini-cores and other changes may be present in muscle fibres which display no atrophy or other 'secondary' changes, and almost exclusively affect type 1 fibres. Similarly, fingerprint or cytoplasmic bodies in the congenital myopathies of which they are the morphological determinant are not only frequent and selective for type 1 fibres, but are often present in otherwise unaffected muscle fibres.

Relationship between the different congenital myopathies

Afifi et al (1965) reported a family with both central core disease and nemaline myopathy. The daughter's biopsy showed cores in every muscle fibre while the mother's biopsy displayed cores, as well as collections of rods in the subsarcolemmal areas of muscle fibres. Both had a non-progressive myopathy. The pedigree showed dominant transmission of the trait. The authors suggested 'that nemaline myopathy and central core disease may be different manifestations of one disease process'.

Since this description, the association of different structural changes characteristic of congenital myopathy in the same patient, or in the same

family, has been observed relatively frequently. For instance, Karpati et al (1971) and Kulakowski et al (1973) reported cases in which core lesions were present in the diaphragm, while collections of rods were present in the other skeletal muscles. The association of cores and rods was also noted by Telerman-Toppet et al (1973), Issacs et al (1975), and Bethlem et al (1978 — families A and E). Two of our own cases fall into this category (Fardeau et al 1978). As in the original case reported by Afifi et al (1965), the rods were mostly situated at the periphery of the fibres and had no connection with the core region. However rods may also be present in the central portions of the muscle fibres in rare cases (Fig. 6.13) (Engel & Warmolts 1973). An association between cores and minicores, or focal loss of cross-striations, has also been reported in several instances (Bethlem et al 1978 — families B and F; Fardeau et al 1978).

Another previously noted association links the central situation of nuclei, the focal areas of myofibrillar disorganization and a disproportion in size between type 1 and type 2 fibres with relative atrophy of the type 1 fibres (Fig. 6.14) (Karpati et al 1970, Radu et al 1974, Inokuchi et al 1975,

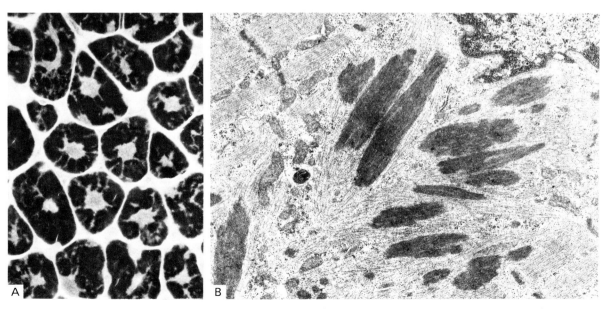

Fig. 6.13 Nemaline myopathy with central localization of rods. (A) Cryostat section. Myofibrillar ATPase reaction after preincubation at pH 4.35; ×340. Type 1 fibre uniformity. Central unstained areas due to accumulation of rods. (B) Electron micrograph, logitudinal section; ×14 025. Numerous rods located in the centre of a myofibre

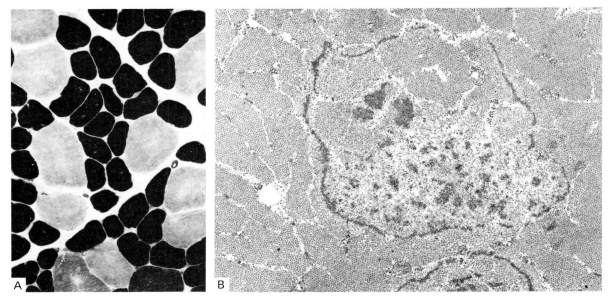

Fig. 6.14 Congenital myopathy with central nuclei, type 1 atrophy and 'minicores'. (A) Cryostat section. Myofibrillar ATPase reaction after preincubation at pH 4.65; ×135. Smallness and predominance of type 1 fibres. Some internal nuclei are seen as small unstained dots. (B) Electron micrograph, transverse section; ×17 340. Small foci of myofibrillar disorganization, encircled by a thin rim of spreading Z material

Coquet et al 1976, Fardeau et al 1978, Dubowitz 1980).

The frequency of all these associations strongly suggests some kinship between the different structural congenital myopathies. Viewed through a clinician's eye, their similarities are sometimes so great that 'one has the eerie feeling of looking at a family album' (Brooke et al 1979). However, it is also clear that variations exist in the severity of the disease and its symptomatology (e.g. extraocular muscle involvement), and different patterns of inheritance are clearly demonstrated by some pedigrees.

Taking all these points into account, certain relationships may exist between some of the main congenital myopathies, for instance between the benign congenital myopathies with cores, rods, cores plus rods, and some of the cases with type 1 predominance or fibre type disproportion. An autosomal dominant mode of inheritance with variable expression is alleged in many of these cases.

In addition, some cases classified as multicore disease or 'centronuclear myopathy with type 1 atrophy' may be closely related in view of the frequency of extraocular muscle involvement and their autosomal recessive mode of transmission.

The cases classified as centronuclear myopathy, with early or late onset, still raise the possibility of one (dominantly inherited) or two (dominant and autosomal recessive) diseases. The specificity of the severe neonatal form of myotubular myopathy which shows X-linked transmission is now well established, even if based on a very limited number of cases.

As for the different congenital myopathies defined by the presence of inclusion bodies, the number of cases reported is obviously too limited to allow any conclusion to be drawn about their mutual relationship. The non-specificity of the inclusion bodies, their possible rarity and the underlying histochemical changes still make their autonomy questionable. The only exception is reducing body myopathy, due to the specific morphological and cytochemical characteristics of the inclusions present in this condition.

'Essentiality' of the structural changes in muscle fibres

Three points noted in the analysis of all types of congenital myopathy allow a more basic question to be raised, concerning the 'essentiality' of the structural changes in muscle fibres in permitting definition of these myopathies:

1. The variability in intensity of structural changes, not only from one case to another but from one muscle to another in the same patient (Telerman-Toppet et al 1973).
2. The variability and possible absence of structural changes in affected members of the same family (Morgan-Hughes et al 1973).
3. The absence of correlation between the frequency of morphological alterations in muscle fibres and the severity and progression of muscle weakness (Bethlem et al 1971).

Two additional puzzling questions were posed by Telerman-Toppet et al (1973). First, when only a small proportion of the type 1 fibres exhibit structural abnormalities, does this necessarily mean that the other type 1 fibres are normal? Secondly when, as in most of the congenital myopathies, the type 2 fibres do not show any structural changes, what is the explanation of their reduction in number? In other words, should the structural changes in the muscle fibres be considered as only epiphenomena in these myopathies?

The answer to this question must necessarily be cautious. The cores, rods, central nuclei and other changes are organized in a remarkable structural design in the muscle fibre. But it is still not clear how close this relationship is, and what the threshold is for the structural expression of the biochemical abnormality which may be involved either in the synthesis and spatial organization of the filamentary proteins, or in the control of Z-band width and structure, or in the migration of the muscle nuclei.

Another aspect of the questionable 'essentiality' of the structural changes concerns their relationship to the modification of the histochemical muscle pattern. In most of the reported cases this pattern is greatly modified by type 1 fibre predominance, or relative type 1 fibre smallness, or much more rarely type 2 fibre smallness.

These histochemical changes are often the only morphological expression of the disease, although careful ultrastructural study of such cases often shows minimal changes in myofibrillar or cytoplasmic architecture (Fardeau et al 1975, 1977). It is important to note that the reverse is not true: that the distinctive structural expressions of the congenital myopathies never occur without a modification of the histochemical pattern in the muscle. These considerations may imply that the histochemical changes are more closely connected with the genetic abnormality than are the structural changes in muscle fibres. This possibility prompted Engel (1962, 1965, 1970) to put forward a neurogenic theory in opposition to the more academic myogenic concept of the congenital myopathies.

Pathophysiology of congenital myopathies

The early manifestation of these diseases, their frequent lack of progression, the presence of structural changes in muscle fibres, their selectivity for one muscle fibre type and the change in the histochemical pattern of affected muscles, are all suggestive of a unique underlying pathophysiological mechanism. Two main possibilities have been considered.

Impairment of the normal maturation process of muscle fibres

A 'block' in the early development of the muscle fibres was first considered in the second case report of central core disease (Engel et al 1961). The possibility that this block caused only the centre of the fibre to be a core region was considered, and different possibilities for the formation of multicored fibres were proposed. After the recognition of the myotubular myopathies a similar hypothesis was put forward (Spiro et al 1966) which suggested that a 'block' might occur in the normal process of nuclear migration to the subsarcolemmal region. This hypothesis was reinforced by the study of cases of congenital hypotonia exhibiting disproportion in the fibre type size (Farkas-Bargeton et al 1968, Caille et al

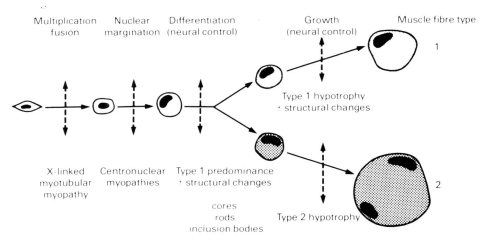

Fig. 6.15 Operational diagram of the pathophysiology of the congenital myopathies. The different developmental phases of the myofibres are schematically separated. Structural and histochemical changes characteristic of the congenital myopathies may be related to impairment of these phases. However, the mechanism responsible is not fully understood. X-linked myotubular myopathy may be due to an abnormally small pool of myoblastic cells, but there is also lack of margination of the nuclei and reduced growth of the myofibre. In the centronuclear myopathies, margination of most of the muscle nuclei is impaired, myofibre growth is reduced, but fibre type differentiation is also often abnormal. In core and rod myopathies, the structural changes roughly follow the abnormal shift towards type 1 fibre predominance. Type 1 fibre growth impairment, with or without structural changes of the myofibre, may be caused by functional, segmental (?), motor neuronal changes. Impairment of type 2 fibre growth is mainly due to a supraspinal nervous dysfunction; structural changes of the myofibres are exceptional in this latter case

1971, Brooke 1973, Fardeau et al 1975, Bender & Bender 1977). The absence of myofibrillar disorganization and of folding of the basal lamina of the muscle fibres was suggestive of a hypotrophic rather than an atrophic process in muscle fibres.

Various studies of the normal embryogenesis of human muscles (Fenichel 1966, Kamieniecka 1968, Farkas-Bargeton et al 1977, Korenyi-Both & Marosan 1979) lend support to this hypothesis, by showing patterns similar to those encountered in some of the congenital hypotonias.

Extension of this block hypothesis to the early stages of myogenesis may be advanced by the ultrastructural study of the X-linked neonatal form of myotubular myopathy (Fardeau et al 1978). The ratio of satellite cell nuclei to myonuclei was very low (<4%) compared with matched controls (8–14%) and the neonatal forms of myotonic dystrophy (20–30%), in which the morphology of the muscle fibres is very close to that of myotubular myopathy. These findings suggest some impairment in the normal capacities of multiplication or fusion of myoblastic cells.

However, this theory of a maturational defect in muscle fibres was subject to various criticisms based on the differences between normal myotubes and the fibres observed in the centronuclear myopathies, the differences between the histochemical pattern in maturing muscle and in these myopathies. This theory could not account easily for the accumulation of rods, the distribution of minicores, or the presence of inclusion bodies. Moreover, little is known as yet about the molecular basis of the relevant events in myogenesis, such as the margination of muscle nuclei and the spatial arrangement of filamentary proteins.

Abnormal neural control of muscle fibre differentiation and growth

As already mentioned, this hypothesis arose from the discovery of the histochemical changes in fibre type distribution and in the remarkable selectivity of the structural abnormalities, particularly for the type 1 fibres. It was developed in several papers by W. K. Engel and coworkers (Engel 1967b, 1970, 1971, Engel & Warmolts 1973). The idea was also supported by the morphological resemblance between cores and target or targetoid fibres. Similarly, differential involvement of intrafusal and extrafusal muscle fibres was noted on several occasions (Karpati et al 1971).

As the cytochemical properties of the muscle fibres have been amply demonstrated to be under neural control, different experimental models have been proposed in order to reproduce the structural changes and histochemical patterns of the congenital myopathies. For instance, denervation at birth in rats impaired skeletal muscle maturation, the hypotrophic type 2 fibres retaining their myotubular characteristics (Engel & Karpati 1968, Karpati & Engel 1968, Shafiq et al 1972).

However, the experimental models also emphasize the complexity of the mechanisms concerned (Engel et al 1966). Core-like lesions and nemaline rods can be produced experimentally by tenotomy (Resnick et al 1968, Shafiq et al 1969), but only if neuronal activation of the muscle fibres is maintained (Karpati et al 1972). As has already been pointed out, there is no consistent evidence of pathological involvement of motor neurones. Most of the necropsy studies of the spinal cord have shown normal findings (Engel et al 1968, Meyers et al 1974, Caille et al 1971), although Dahl & Klutzow (1974) found a reduced number of anterior horn cells in the cervical region. End-plate morphology and the motor innervation ratio were subnormal or normal (Coërs et al 1976). The distribution of the different molecular forms of acetylcholinesterase was not altered (Fardeau et al 1978), and there was no spread of extrajunctional cholinergic receptors (Ringel et al 1977).

All these considerations led Engel & Warmolts (1973) to postulate a 'functional' defect of the muscle fibre innervation, connected for instance with hypothetical 'trophic-maturing' or 'trophic-sustaining' factors, originating from type 1 motor neurones, and possibly accompanied by a more complete defect in type 2 motor neurones, causing the complete disappearance of the type 2 muscle fibres. Any analysis of these neural influences on muscle fibre differentiation is still largely conjectural.

CONCLUSION

On the basis of all these arguments, an operational diagram may be proposed which takes account of the different steps in muscle fibre differentiation, and their possible deviations (Fig. 6.15). Its only merit is to provide an overall view of the pathophysiology of the congenital myopathies. However, this diagram will no doubt have to be altered or replaced following the accumulation of new data, a longer follow-up of the cases reported and a greater insight into the processes of muscle fibre differentiation.

ACKNOWLEDGEMENTS

I am indebted to Mrs J. Godet-Guillain, Dr F. M. S. Tomé, Mrs M. Chevallay, H. Collin and Miss J. Reix for their assistance in the study of the muscle biopsies on which this chapter is based, to Miss A. Rouche for preparing the photographs and to Mrs V. Ortega for typing the manuscript.

We are grateful to the following publishers and editors for their permission to reproduce illustrations previously published:

Doin: Archives Françaises de Pédiatrie (Figs. 6.2A, B, D)
Masson: Revue Neurologique (Fig. 4.3c)
Springer International: Acta neuropathologica (Figs 6.2C and 6.8C)
Excerpta Medica: Neurology ICS No. 434 (Figs 6.5D & 6.15)
Current Topics in Nerve and Muscle Research ICS No. 455 (Figs. 6.4B, 6.4D, 6.10).

REFERENCES

Afifi A K, Smith J W, Zellweger H 1965 Congenital non-progressive myopathy. Central core disease and nemaline myopathy in one family. Neurology (Minneapolis) 15: 371
Afifi A K, Zellweger H, McCormick W F, Mergner W 1969 Congenital muscular dystrophy: light and electron microscopic observations. Journal of Neurology, Neurosurgery and Psychiatry 32: 273
Ambler M W, Neave C, Tutschka B G, Pueschel S M, Orson J M, Singer D B 1984 X-linked chromosome recessive myotubular myopathy. 1. Clinical and pathological findings in a family. Human Pathology 15: 566
Ambler M W, Neave C, Entwistle R 1987 Fingerprint inclusions in normal fetal muscle. Acta neuropathologica (Berlin) 73: 185
Argov Z, Gardner-Medwin D, Johnson M A, Mastaglia F L 1984 Patterns of muscle fibre-type disproportion in hypotonic infants. Archives of Neurology (Chicago) 41: 53
Armstrong R M, Koenigsberger R, Mellinger J, Lovelace R E 1971 Central core disease with congenital hip dislocation. Neurology (Minneapolis) 21: 369
Arts W F, Bethlem, J, Dingemans K P, Eriksson A W 1978 Investigations on the inheritance of nemaline myopathy. Archives of Neurology (Chicago) 35: 72
Askanas V, Engel W K, Reddy N B, Barth P G, Bethlem J,

Krauss D R et al 1979 X-linked recessive congenital muscle fibre hypotrophy with central nuclei. Abnormalities of growth and adenylate cyclase in muscle tissue cultures. Archives of Neurology (Chicago) 36: 604

Badurska B, Fidzianska A, Kamienecka Z, Prot J, Strugalska H 1969 Myotubular myopathy. Journal of the Neurological Sciences 8: 563

Badurska B, Fidzianska A, Jedrzejowska H 1970 Nemaline myopathy. Neuropathologia polska 8: 389

Banker B Q 1986 Congenital Muscular Dystrophy. In: Engel A G, Banker B Q (eds) Myology. McGraw-Hill Book Co, New York, p 1367

Banker B Q, Victor M, Adams R D 1957 Arthrogryposis multiplex due to congenital muscular dystrophy. Brain 80: 319

Barth P G, Van Wijngaarden G K, Bethlem J 1975 X-linked myotubular myopathy with fatal neonatal asphyxia. Neurology (Minneapolis) 25: 531

Batten F E 1903 Three cases of myopathy, infantile type. Brain 26: 147

Batten F E 1915 Myopathy. Simple atrophic type. Proceedings of the Royal Society of Medicine (Neurology Section) 8: 69

Battin J, Vital C, Vallat J M, Fontan D 1972 Une nouvelle myopathie non-progressive à transmission dominante autosomique: la myopathie nemaline. Nouvelle Presse Médicale 1: 1097

Bender A N 1979 Congenital myopathies. In: Vinken P J, Bruyn G W (eds) Handbook of clinical neurology. North Holland Publ. Co, Amsterdam, vol 41, p 1

Bender A N, Bender M B 1977 Muscle fibre hypotrophy with intact neuromuscular junctions. Neurology (Minneapolis) 27: 206

Bender A N, Willner J P 1978 Nemaline (rod) myopathy: the need for histochemical evaluation of affected families. Annals of Neurology 4: 37

Ben Hamida M, Hentati F, Ben Hamida C 1987 A case of multiminicore disease with rigid spine syndrome. Revue Neurologique (Paris) 143: 284

Berezin S, Newman L J, Schwarz S M, Spiro A J 1988 Gastro-oesophageal reflux associated with nemaline myopathy of infancy. Pediatrics 81: 111

Bergen B J, Carry M P, Wilson W B, Barden M T, Ringel S P 1980 Centronuclear myopathy: extra-ocular and limb-muscle findings in an adult. Muscle & Nerve 3: 165

Bethlem J 1970 Muscle Pathology. Introduction and atlas. North Holland Pub. Co, Amsterdam–London

Bethlem J, Posthumus Meyjes F E 1960 Congenital, non-progressive central core disease of Shy & Magee. Psychiatria, Neurologia, Neurochirurgia 63: 246

Bethlem J, Van Gool J, Hülsmann W C, Meijer A E F H 1966 Familial non-progressive myopathy with muscle cramps after exercise. A new disease associated with cores in the muscle fibres. Brain 89: 569

Bethlem J, Meijer A E F H, Schellens J P M, Vroom J J 1968 Centronuclear myopathy. European Neurology 1: 325

Bethlem J, Van Wijngaarden G K, Meijer A E F H, Hülsmann W C 1969 Neuromuscular disease with type 1 fibre atrophy, central nuclei and myotube-like structures. Neurology (Minneapolis) 19: 705

Bethlem J, Van Wijngaarden G K, Mumenthaler M, Meijer A E F H 1970 Centronuclear myopathy with type 1 atrophy and 'myotubes'. Archives of Neurology (Chicago) 23: 70

Bethlem J, Van Wijngarden G K, Meijer A E F H, Fleury P 1971 Observations on central core disease. Journal of the Neurological Sciences 14: 293

Bethlem J, Arts W F, Dingemans K P 1978 Common origin of rods, cores, miniature cores and focal loss of cross-striations. Archives of Neurology (Chicago) 35: 555

Bill P L A, Cole G, Proctor N S F 1979 Centronuclear myopathy. Journal of Neurology, Neurosurgery and Psychiatry 42: 548

Biral D, Damiani E, Scarpini E, Bet L, Bresolin N, Moggio M, Pellegrini G, Barbieri S, Scarlato G 1987 Biochemical and immunologic studies in a case of congenital myopathy with unusual morphologic features. Neurology 37: 1658

Bonnette H, Roelofs R, Olson W H 1974 Multicore disease: report of a case with onset in middle age. Neurology (Minneapolis) 24: 1039

Bradley W G, Price D L K, Watanabe C K 1970 Familial centronuclear myopathy. Journal of Neurology, Neurosurgery and Psychiatry 33: 687

Brandt S 1950 Werdnig-Hoffman's infantile progressive muscular atrophy. Munksgaard, Copenhägen

Brooke M H 1973 Congenital fibre type disproportion. In: Kakulas B A (ed) Clinical studies in myology, Proceedings of 2nd International Congress on Muscle Diseases, Perth, Australia 1971, ICS no. 295 Excerpta Medica, Amsterdam, part 2, p 147

Brooke M H 1977 A clinician's view of neuromuscular diseases. Williams & Wilkins Co, Baltimore

Brooke M H, Engel W K 1969 The histographic analysis of human muscle biopsies with regard to fibre types IV. Children's biopsies. Neurology (Minneapolis) 19: 591

Brooke M H, Neville H E 1972 Reducing body myopathy. Neurology (Minneapolis) 22: 829

Brooke M H, Williamson T 1969 An adult case of the type 1 muscle fibre hypotrophy: an abnormality of monosynaptic reflex functions. Neurology (Minneapolis) 19: 280

Brooke M H, Carroll J E, Ringel S P 1979 Congenital hypotonia revisited. Muscle & Nerve 2: 84

Brownell A K W 1979 Familial multicore disease. Annales of Neurology 6: 155

Brownell A K W, Gilbert J J, Garcia B, Wenkebach G F, Lam A K S 1978 Adult-onset nemaline myopathy. Neurology 28: 1306

Buscaino G A, de Giacomo P, Mazzarella L 1970 Two cases of so-called 'mitochondrial myopathy': preliminary report. In: Walton J N, Canal N, Scarlato G, (eds) Muscle diseases. Excerpta Medica, Amsterdam, p 112

Byrne E, Blumbergs P C, Hallpike J F 1982 Central core disease: study of a family with five affected generations. Journal of the Neurological Sciences 53: 77

Caille B, Fardeau M, Harpey J P, Lafourcade J 1971 Hypotonie congénitale avec atteinte sélective des fibres musculaires de type 1. Archives Françaises de Pédiatrie 28: 205

Campbell M J, Rebeiz J J, Walton J N 1969 Myotubular, centronuclear or pericentronuclear myopathy. Journal of the Neurological Sciences 8: 425

Cancilla P A, Kalyanaraman K, Verity M A, Munsat T, Pearson C M 1971 Familial myopathy with probable lysis of myofibrils in type 1 fibres. Neurology (Minneapolis) 21: 579

Cape C A, Johnson W W, Pitner S E 1970 Nemaline structures in polymyositis. A non-specific pathological reaction of skeletal muscles. Neurology (Minneapolis) 20: 494

Carpenter S K, Karpati G 1984 Pathology of skeletal muscle. Churchill Livingstone, New York

Carpenter S, Karpati G, Holland P 1985 New observations in reducing body myopathy. Neurology 35: 818

Caulet F, Petit J, Pluot M 1973 Myopathie à inclusions en

bâtonnets (nemaline myopathy). Annales d'Anatomie Pathologique 18: 437

Cavanagh N P C, Lake B D, McMenamin P 1979 Congenital fibre type disproportion myopathy; a histological diagnosis with an uncertain clinical outlook. Archives of Disease in Childhood 54: 735

Chapon F, Viader F, Fardeau M, Tomé F, Daluzeau N, Berthelin C, Thenint J P, Lechevalier B 1989 Myopathie familiale avec inclusions de type 'corps cytoplasmiques' (ou sphéroïdes) révélée par une insuffisance respiratoire. Revue Neurologique (Paris) 145: 460

Clancy R R, Kelts K A, Oehlert J W 1980 Clinical variability in congenital fiber type disproportion. Journal of the Neurological Sciences 46: 257

Clark J R, di Agostino A N, Wilson J, Brooks R R, Cole G C 1978 Autosomal dominant myofibrillar inclusion body myopathy. Clinical, histologic, histochemical and ultrastructural characteristics. Neurology (Minneapolis) 28: 399

Coërs C, Telerman-Toppet N, Gerard J M, Szliwowski H, Bethlem J, Wijngaarden G K Van 1976 Changes in motor innervation and histochemical pattern of muscle fibres in some congenital myopathies. Neurology (Minneapolis) 26: 1046

Cohen M E, Duffner P K, Heffner R 1978 Central core disease in one of identical twins. Journal of Neurology, Neurosurgery and Psychiatry 41: 659

Coleman R F, Nienhuis A W, Brown W J, Munsat T L, Pearson C M 1967 New myopathy with mitochondrial enzyme hyperactivity. Journal of the American Medical Association 199: 624

Coleman R F, Thomson L R, Nienhuis A W, Munsat T L, Pearson C M 1968 Histochemical investigation of 'myotubular' myopathy. Archives of Pathology 86: 365

Collier J, Wilson S A K 1908 Amyotonia congenita. Brain 31: 1

Conen P E, Murphy E G, Donohue W L 1963 Light and electron microscopic studies of 'myogranules' in a child with hypotonia and muscle weakness. Canadian Medical Association Journal 89: 983

Coquet M, Vital C, Hemunstre J P, Hedreville A M 1976 Un cas de myopathie congénitale associant une hypotrophie des fibres de type 1, des centralisations nucléaires et une atteinte myofibrillaire localisée. Archives d'Anatomie et de Cytologie Pathologique 24: 275

Cornog J L Jr, Gonatas N K 1967 Ultrastructure of rhabdomyoma. Journal of Ultrastructure Research 20: 433

Côté G, Mohiuddin S M, Roy P E 1970 Occurrence of Z-band widening in human atrial cells. Experimental Molecular Pathology 13: 307

Cruz Martinez A, Ferrer M T, Lopez-Terradas J M, Pascual-Castroviejo I, Mingo P 1979 Single fibre electromyography in central core disease. Journal of Neurology, Neurosurgery and Psychiatry 42: 662

Curless R G, Nelson M B 1977 Congenital fibre type disproportion in identical twins. Annals of Neurology 2: 455

Curless K G, Payne C M, Brimmer F M 1978 Fingerprint body myopathy: a report of twins. Developmental Medicine in Child Neurology 20: 793

Currie S, Noronha M, Harriman D 1974 'Minicore' disease. In: Abstracts of papers presented at the 3rd International Congress of Muscle Diseases (Newcastle upon Tyne 1974). Excerpta Medica, Amsterdam, ICS no. 334, p 12

Dahl D S, Klutzow F W 1974 Congenital rod disease. Further evidence of innervational abnormalities as the basis for the clinicopathologic features. Journal of the Neurological Sciences 23: 371

Dalakas M C, Pezeshpour G H, Flaherty M 1987 Progressive nemaline (rod) myopathy associated with HIV infection. New England Journal of Medicine 317: 1602

Danowski T S, Fisher E R, Wald N, Vester J W, Zawadzki Z A 1973 Rod myopathy: beta-globulin peak and increased complement. Metabolism 22: 597

De Coster W, De Reuck J, Vander Eecken H 1976 The target phenomenon in human muscle. A comparative light microscopic, histochemical and electron microscopic study. Acta neuropathologica (Berlin) 34: 329

De Giacomo P, Mazzarella L, Buscaino G A 1971 Central core disease. Clinical, histochemical and electron microscopical studies on a case. In: Serratrice G, Roux H (eds) Actualités de pathologie neuro-musculaire. L'Expansion Scientifique Française, Paris, p 325

De Lumley L, Vallat J M, Catanzano G 1976 Etude clinique et ultrastructurale d'un cas de myopathie congénitale à foyers multiples. La Semaine des Hôpitaux de Paris 52: 733

Denborough M A, Dennett X, Anderson R McD 1973 Central core disease and malignant hyperthermia. British Medical Journal 1: 272

De Paillette L, Aicardi J, Goutières F 1989 Ullrich's congenital atonic sclerotic muscular dystrophy. A case report. Journal of Neurology 236: 108

Di Donato S, Cornelio F, Balastrini M R, Bertagnolio B, Peluchetti D 1978 Mitochondria-lipid-glycogen myopathy, hyperlactacidemia and carnitine deficiency. Neurology (Minneapolis) 28: 1110

Di Mauro S, Mendell J R, Sahenk Z, Bacham D, Scarpa A, Scofield R M 1980 Fatal infantile mitochondrial myopathy and renal dysfunction due to cytochrome-c-oxidase deficiency. Neurology (Minneapolis) 30: 795

Donner M, Rapola J, Somer H 1975 congenital muscular dystrophy: a clinicopathological and follow-up study of 15 patients. Neuropädiatrie 6: 239

Dubowitz V 1973 Rigid spine syndrome: a muscle syndrome in search of a name. Proceedings of the Royal Society of Medicine 66: 219

Dubowitz V 1978 Muscle disorders in childhood. W B Saunders, Philadelphia

Dubowitz V 1980 The floppy infant, 2nd edn. Clinics in developmental medicine no. 76 London SIMP with Heinemann Medical, Lippincott, Philadelphia

Dubowitz V, Brooke M 1973 Muscle biopsy: a modern approach. W B Saunders, London, Philadelphia, Toronto

Dubowitz V, Pearse A G E 1960 Oxidative enzymes and phosphorylase in central core disease of muscle. Preliminary communication. Lancet 2: 23

Dubowitz V, Platts M 1965 Central core disease of muscle with focal wasting. Journal of Neurology, Neurosurgery and Psychiatry 28: 432

Dubowitz V, Roy S 1970 Central core disease of muscle: clinical, histochemical and electron microscopic studies of an affected mother and child. Brain 93: 133

Dunn H G 1976 The rigid spine syndrome (Dubowitz). Canadian Journal of Neurological Sciences 3: 155

Echenne B, Astruc J, Brunel D, Pagès M, Baldet P K, Martinazzo G 1983 Congenital muscular dystrophy and rigid spine syndrome. Neuropediatrics 14: 97

Edström L, Wroblewski R, Mair W G P 1982 Genuine myotubular myopathy. Muscle and Nerve 5: 604

Eisler T, Wilson J H (1978) Muscle fibre-type disproportion. Report of a family with symptomatic and asymptomatic members. Archives of Neurology 35: 823

Eng G D, Epstein B S, Engel W K, McKay D W, McKay R

1978 Malignant hyperthermia and central core disease in a child with congenital dislocating hips. Archives of Neurology (Chicago) 35: 189

Engel W K 1962 The essentiality of histo- and cytochemical studies of skeletal muscle in the investigation of neuromuscular disease. Neurology (Minneapolis) 12: 778

Engel W K 1965 Muscle biopsy. In: Engel W K (ed) Current concepts of myopathies. Lippincott, Philadelphia & Montreal, p 80

Engel A G 1966 Late-onset rod myopathy (a new syndrome?) Light and electron microscopic observations in two cases. Mayo Clinic Proceedings 41: 713

Engel A G 1967 Pathological reactions of the Z-disk. In: Milhorat A T (ed) Exploratory concepts in muscular dystrophy and related disorders. Excerpta Medica, Amsterdam, ICS no. 147, p 398

Engel W K 1966 Histochemistry of neuromuscular diseases. Significance of muscle fibre types. Neuromuscular diseases. In: Proceedings of the VIIIth International Congress of Neurology, Vienna. Amsterdam, vol II, p 67

Engel W K 1967a Muscle biopsies in neuromuscular diseases. Pediatric Clinics of North America 14: 963

Engel W K 1967b A critique of congenital myopathies and other disorders. In: A T Milhorat (ed) Exploratory concepts in muscular dystrophy and related disorders. Excerpta Medica Foundation, Amsterdam, ICS no. 147, p 27

Engel W K 1970 Selective and non-selective susceptibility of muscle fibre types A new approach to human neuromuscular diseases. Archives of Neurology (Chicago) 22: 97

Engel W K 1971 Classification of neuromuscular disorders. Birth defects: original article series, vol VII, no. 2, p 18

Engel A G, Angelini C 1973 Carnitine deficiency of human skeletal muscle with associated lipid storage myopathy: a new syndrome. Science 179: 899

Engel W K, Cunningham G C 1963 Rapid examination of muscle tissue. An improved trichrome method for rapid diagnosis of muscle biopsy fresh frozen sections. Neurology (Minneapolis) 13: 919

Engel A G, Gomez M R 1966 Congenital myopathy associated with multifocal degeneration of muscle fibres. Transactions of the American Neurological Association 91: 222

Engel A G, Gomez M R 1967 Nemaline (Z-disk) myopathy: observations on the origin, structure and solubility properties of the nemaline structures. Journal of Neuropathology and Experimental Neurology 26: 601

Engel W K, Karpati G 1968 Impaired skeletal muscle maturation following neonatal neurectomy. Developmental Biology 17: 713

Engel A G, MacDonald R D 1970 Ultrastructural reactions in muscle disease and their light-microscopic correlates. Walton J N, Canal N, Scarlato G (eds) Muscle diseases. Excerpta Medica, Amsterdam, ICS no. 199, p 71

Engel W K, Oberc M A 1975 Abundant nuclear rods in adult-onset rod disease. Journal of Neuropathology and Experimental Neurology 34: 119

Engel W K, Resnick J S 1966 Late-onset rod myopathy: a newly recognized, acquired and progressive disease. Neurology (Minneapolis) 16: 308

Engel W K, Warmolts J R 1971 New concepts on the possible role of motoneuron abnormalities in neuromuscular diseases not usually considered neurogenic. In: Serratrice G, Roux H (eds) Advances in neuromuscular diseases. L'Expansion Scientique Française, Paris, p 19

Engel W K, Warmolts J R 1973 The motor unit — diseases affecting it in toto or in partio. In: Desmedt J E (ed) New

developments in EMG and clinical neurophysiology. Karger, Basel, vol 1, p 141

Engel W K, Foster J B, Hughes B P, Huxley H E, Mahler R 1961 Central core disease — an investigation of a rare muscle cell abnormality. Brain 84: 167

Engel W K, Wanko T, Fenichel G M 1964 Nemaline myopathy. A second case. Archives of Neurology (Chicago) 11: 22

Engel W K, Brooke M H, Nelson P G 1966 Histochemical studies of denervated or tenotomized cat muscle: illustrating difficulties in relating experimental animal conditions to human neuromuscular diseases. Annals of the New York Academy of Sciences 138: 160

Engel W K, Gold G N, Karpati G 1968 Type 1 fibre hypotrophy and central nuclei. A rare congenital muscle abnormality with a possible experimental model. Archives of Neurology (Chicago) 18: 435

Engel A G, Gomez M R, Groover R V 1971 Multicore disease: a recently recognized congenital myopathy associated with multifocal degeneration of muscle fibres. Mayo Clinic Proceedings 46: 666

Engel A G, Angelini C, Gomez M R 1972 Fingerprint body myopathy. Mayo Clinic Proceedings 47: 377

Fardeau M 1969 Etude d'une nouvelle observation de 'nemaline myopathy' II. Données ultrastructurales. Acta neuropathologica (Berlin) 13: 250

Fardeau M 1970 Ultrastructural lesions in progressive muscular dystrophies. A critical study of their specificity. In: Walton J N, Canal N, Scarlato G (eds) Muscle diseases. Excerpta Medica, Amsterdam, ICS no. 199, p 98

Fardeau M 1987 Some orthodox and non-orthodox considerations on congenital myopathies. In: Ellingson R J, Murray N M F, Halliday A M (eds) The London symposia. Elsevier, Amsterdam (EEG suppl. 39) p 85

Fardeau M, Harpey J P, Caille B, Lafourcade J 1975 Hypotonies néo-natales avec disproportion congénitale des différents types de fibre musculaire, et petitesse relative des fibres de type 1. Démonstration du caractère familial de cette nouvelle entité. Archives Françaises de Pédiatrie 32: 901

Fardeau M, Tomé F M S, Derambure S 1976 Familial fingerprint body myopathy. Archives of Neurology (Chicago) 33: 724

Fardeau M, Godet-Guillain J, Tomé F M S, Dreyfus P, Billard C 1977 Difficulties and limits in the classification of congenital myopathies. In: Subirana (ed) Neurology. Proceedings of the XIth World Congress of Neurology, Amsterdam, Excerpta Medica, ICS no. 434, p 144

Fardeau M, Godet-Guillain J, Tomé F M S, Carson S, Whalen R G 1978 Congenital neuromuscular disorders: a critical review. In: Aguayo A J, Karpati G (eds) Current topics in nerve and muscle research. Excerpta Media, Amsterdam and Oxford, p 164

Fardeau M, Tomé F M S, Rolland J C 1981 Congenital neuromuscular disorder with predominant mitochondrial changes in type 2 muscle fibres.Acta neuropathologica (Berlin), suppl. VII, p 279

Farkas-Bargeton E, Aicardi J, Chevrie J J, Thieffry S 1968 Apport des techniques histo-enzymologiques à l'étude des hypotonies congénitales. Revue Neurologique 119: 513

Farkas-Bargeton E, Tomé F M S, Fardeau M, Arsenio-Nunès M L, Dreyfus P, Diebler M F 1974 Histochemical and ultrastructural study of muscle biopsies in 3 cases of dystrophia myotonica in the newborn child. Journal of the Neurological Sciences 21: 273

Farkas-Bargeton E, Diebler M F, Arsenio-Nunès M L, Wehrlé

R, Rosenberg B 1977 Etude de la maturation histochimique quantitative et ultrastructurale du muscle foetal humain. Journal of the Neurological Sciences 31: 245

Farkas-Bargeton E, Aicardi J, Arsenio-Nunès L, Wehrlé R 1978 Delay in the maturation of muscle fibres in infants with congenital hypotonia. Journal of the Neurological Sciences 39: 17

Fawcett D W 1968 The sporadic occurrence in cardiac muscle of anomalous Z-bands, exhibiting a periodic structure suggestive of tropomyosin. Journal of Cell Biology 36: 266

Federico A, Dotti M T, Malandrini A, Guazzi G C, Hayek G, Simonati A, Rizzuto N, Toti P 1988 Cerebro-ocular dysplasia and muscular dystrophy: report of two cases. Neuropediatrics 19: 109

Fenichel G M 1966 A histochemical study of developing human skeletal muscle. Neurology (Minneapolis) 16: 741

Fenichel G M 1967 Abnormalities of skeletal muscle maturation in brain-damaged children: a histochemical study. Developmental Medicine and Child Neurology 9: 419

Fenichel G M 1988 Congenital muscular dystrophies. Neurologica Clinica 6: 519

Fidzianska A, Badurska B, Ryniewicz B, Dembek I 1981 'Cap disease': new congenital myopathy. Neurology 31: 113

Fidzianska A, Goebel H H, Lenard H G, Heckmann C 1982 Congenital muscular dystrophy (CMD). A collagen formative disease? Journal of Neurological Sciences 55: 79

Fitzsimons R B, Tyer H D D 1980 A study of a myopathy presenting as idiopathic scoliosis: multicore disease or mitochondrial myopathy? Journal of Neurological Sciences 46: 33

Ford F R 1960 Diseases of the nervous system in infancy, childhood and adolescence, 4th edn. C C Thomas, Springfield, Illinois, p 1259

Fowler M, Manson J I 1973 Congenital muscular dystrophy with malformation of central nervous system. In: Kakulas B A (ed) Clinical study of myology. Excerpta Medica, Amsterdam, p 192

Fukuhara N, Yusa T, Tsusubaki T, Kushiro S, Takasawa N 1978 Nemaline myopathy — histological, histochemical and ultrastructural studies. Acta neuropathologica (Berlin) 42: 33

Fukuyama Y, Segawa M 1974 Genetic-clinical studies of congenital muscular dystrophy. Japanese Journal of Human Genetics 19: 42

Fukuyama Y, Kawazura M, Haruna H 1960 A peculiar form of congenital progressive muscular dystrophy. Report of 15 cases. Paediatria Universitatis Tokyo 4: 5

Fulthorpe J J, Gardner-Medwin D, Hudgson P, Walton J N 1969 Nemaline myopathy. Neurology (Minneapolis) 19: 735

Furukawa T K, Toyokura Y 1977 Congenital, hypotonic-sclerotic muscular dystrophy. Journal of Medical Genetics 14: 426

Gillies C, Raye J, Vasan U, Hart W E, Goldblatt P J 1979 Nemaline (rod) myopathy: a possible cause of rapid fatal, infantile myotonia. Archives of Pathology and Laboratory Medicine 103: 1

Glick B, Shapira Y, Stern A, Blank A, Rosenmann E 1984 Congenital muscle fiber-type disproportion myopathy: a follow-up study of twenty cases. Annals of Neurology 16: 405

Goebel H H, Lenard H G, Goerke W, Kunze K 1978a Fibre type dispoportion in the rigid spine syndrome. Neuropädiatrie 8: 467

Goebel H H, Muller J, Gillen H W, Merritt A D 1978b Autosomal dominant 'spheroid body myopathy'. Muscle & Nerve 1: 14

Goebel H, Fidzianska A, Lenard H, Osse G, Hori A 1983 A morphological study of non-Japanese congenital muscular-dystrophy associated with cerebral lesions. Brain Development (Tokyo) 5: 292

Goldstein M A, Stromer M H, Schroeter J P, Sass R L 1980 Optical reconstruction of nemaline rods. Experimental Neurology 70: 83

Gonatas N K 1966 The fine structure of the rod-like bodies in nemaline myopathy and their relation to the Z-discs. Journal of Neuropathology and Experimental Neurology 25: 409

Gonatas N K, Perez M C, Shy G M, Evangelista I 1965 Central 'core' disease of skeletal muscle. Ultrastructural and cytochemical observations in two cases. American Journal of Pathology 47: 503

Gonatas N K, Shy G M, Godfrey E H 1966 Nemaline myopathy: the origin of nemaline structures. New England Journal of Medicine 274: 535

Gordon A S, Rewcastle N B, Humphrey J G, Stewart G M 1974 Chronic benign congenital myopathy: fingerprint body type. Canadian Journal of Neurological Sciences 1: 106

Goto I, Nagasaka S, Nagara H, Kuroiwa Y 1979 Rigid spine syndrome: clinical and histological problems. Journal of Neurology 226: 143

Gött H, Josten E A 1954 Beitrag fur Kongenitalen atonisch-sclerotischen Muskeldystrophy (Typ Ullrich). Zeitschrift für Kinderheilkunde 75: 105

Goulon M, Fardeau M, Got C, Babinet P, Manko E 1976 Myopathie centro-nucléaire d'expression clinique tardive. Etude clinique, histologique et ultrastructurale d'une nouvelle observation. Revue Neurologique (Paris) 132: 275

Greenfield J G, Stern R O 1927 The anatomical identity of the Werdnig-Hoffmann and Oppenheim forms of infantile muscular atrophy. Brain 50: 652

Greenfield J G, Cornman T, Shy G M 1958 The prognostic value of the muscle biopsy in the floppy infant. Brain 81: 461

Groslambert R, Stoebner P, Pollak P, Perret J 1976 Myopathie à bâtonnets d'expression clinique tardive. Etude clinique et données des examens en microscopie électronique. A propos d'une observation. Lyon Médical 236: 779

Gubbay S S, Walton J N, Pearce G W 1966 Clinical and pathological study of a case of congenital muscular dystrophy. Journal of Neurology, Neurosurgery and Psychiatry 29: 500

Haan E A, Freemantle C J, McCure J A, Friend K L, Mulley J C 1990 Assignment of the gene for central core disease to chromosome 19. Human Genetics 86: 187–190

Hackett T N, Bray P F, Ziter F A, Nyhan W L, Creer K M 1973 A metabolic myopathy associated with chronic lactic acidemia, growth failure and nerve deafness. Journal of Pediatrics 83: 426

Hantaï D, Labat-Fobert J, Grimaud J A, Fardeau M 1985 Fibronectin, laminin, type I, III and IV collagens in Duchenne's muscular dystrophy, congenital muscular dystrophies and congenital myopathies: an immunocyto-chemical study. Connective Tissue Research 13: 273

Harati Y, Niakan E, Bloom K, Casar G 1987 Adult-onset nemaline myopathy presenting as diaphragmatic paralysis. Journal of Neurology, Neurosurgery and Psychiatry 50: 108

Harriman D G F, Haleem M A 1972 Centronuclear myopathy in old age. Journal of Pathology 108: 237

Hashimoto K, Shimizu T, Nonaka I, Mannen T 1989 Immunochemical analysis of alpha-actinin of nemaline myopathy after two-dimensional electrophoresis. Journal of Neurological Sciences 93: 199

Haushalter P 1920 Sur la myotonie congénitale (maladie d'Oppenheim). Archives de Médecine des Enfants 23: 133

Hawkes C H, Absolon M J 1975 Myotubular myopathy associated with cataract and electrical myotonia. Journal of Neurology, Neurosurgery and Psychiatry 38: 761

Hayashi K, Miller R G, Brownell A K 1989 Central core disease: ultrastructure of the sarcoplasmic reticulum and T-tubules. Muscle and Nerve 12: 95

Headington J Y, McNamara J O, Brownell A K 1975 Centronuclear myopathy. Histochemistry and electron microscopy. Report of two cases. Archives of Pathology 99: 16

Heffernan L P, Rewcastle N B, Humphrey J G 1968 The spectrum of rod myopathies. Archives of Neurology (Chicago) 18: 529

Heffner R, Cohen M, Duffner P, Daigler G 1976 Multicore disease in twins. Journal of Neurology, Neurosurgery and Psychiatry 39: 602

Heggie P, Grossniklaus H E, Roessmann U, Chou S M, Cruse R P 1987 Cerebro-ocular dysplasia — muscular dystrophy syndrome. Archives of Ophthalmology 105: 520

Hoffmann J 1893 Über chronische spinale Muskelatrophie im Kindesalter auf familiäres Basis. Deutsche Zeitschrift für Nervenkrankheiten 3: 427

Hoffmann J 1900 Uber die hereditäre progressive spinale Muskelatrophie im Kindesalter. Münchener Medizinische Wochenschrift 47: 1649

Hopkins I J, Lindsey J R, Ford F R 1966 Nemaline myopathy. A long-term clinicopathologic study of affected mother and daughter. Brain 89: 299

Howard R 1908 A case of congenital defect of the muscular system (dystrophia muscularis congenita) and its association with congenital talipes equino-varus. Proceedings of the Royal Society of Medicine 1: 157

Hübner G, Pongratz D 1981 Granularkörpermyopathie (reducing body myopathy): Beitrag zur feinstruktur und klassifiezerung. Virchows Archiv (Pathology-Anatomy) 392: 87

Hudson P, Gardner-Medwin D, Fulthorpe J J, Walton J N 1967 Nemaline myopathy. Neurology (Minneapolis) 17: 1125

Hülsmann W C, Bethlem J, Meijer A E F H, Fleury P, Schellens J P M 1967 Myopathy with abnormal structure and function of muscle mitochondria. Journal of Neurology, Neurosurgery and Psychiatry 30: 519

Inokuchi T, Umezaki H, Santa T 1975 A case of type 1 muscle fibre hypotrophy and internal nuclei. Journal of Neurology, Neurosurgery and Psychiatry 38: 475

Isaacs H, Heffron J J A, Badenhorst M 1975 Central core disease. A correlated genetic, histochemical, ultrastructural and biochemical study. Journal of Neurology, Neurosurgery and Psychiatry 38: 1177

Ishibashi-Ueda, Imakita M, Yutani C, Takahashi S, Yazawa K, Kamiya T, Nonaka I 1990 Congenital nemaline myopathy with dilated cardiomyopathy: an autopsy study. Human Pathology 21: 77

Ishimoto S, Goto I, Yamada T 1986 The rigid spine syndrome and Emery-Dreifuss muscular dystrophy: clinical and histological problems. Muscle and Nerve 9: 255

Jadros-Santel D, Grčevic N, Dogan S, Franjič J, Benc H 1980 Centronuclear myopathy with type 1 fibre hypotrophy and 'fingerprint' inclusions associated with Marfan's Syndrome. Journal of the Neurological Sciences 45: 43

Jaffé M, Shapira J, Borochowitz Z 1988 Familial congenital fiber type disproportion (CFTD) with an autosomal recessive inheritance. Clinics in Genetics 33: 33

Jean R, Bonnet H, Pages A, Cadilhac J, Baldet P, Dumas R 1971 Myopathie congénitale non-progressive avec axe central (central core disease). Archives Françaises de Pédiatrie 28: 65

Jenis E A, Lindquist R R, Lester R C 1969 New congenital myopathy with crystalline intranuclear inclusions. Archives of Neurology (Chicago) 20: 281

Jennekens F G I, Roord J J, Veldman H, Willemse J, Jockusch B M 1983 Congenital nemaline myopathy: 1. Defective organization of alpha-actinin is restricted to muscle. Muscle and Nerve 6: 61

Jerusalem F, Angelini C, Engel A G, Groover R V 1973a Mitochondria-lipid-glycogen (MLG) disease of muscle. A morphologically regressive congenital myopathy. Archives of Neurology (Chicago) 29: 162

Jerusalem F, Engel A G, Gomez M R 1973b Sarcotubular myopathy. A newly recognized, benign, congenital, familial muscle disease. Neurology (Minneapolis) 23: 897

Jerusalem F, Ludin H, Bischoff A, Hartmann G 1979 Cytoplasmic body neuromyopathy presenting as respiratory failure and weight loss. Journal of the Neurological Sciences 41: 1

Jones R, Khan R, Hughes S, Dubowitz V 1979 Congenital muscular dystrophy: the importance of early diagnosis and orthopaedic management in the long-term prognosis. Journal of Bone and Joint Surgery 61B: 13

Jong Y J, Shishikura K, Aoyama M et al 1987 Non-specific congenital myopathy (minimal change myopathy). A case report. Brain Development 9: 61

Kamieniecka Z 1968 The stages of development of human foetal muscles with reference to some muscular diseases. Journal of the Neurological Sciences 7: 319

Kamieniecka Z 1973 Late-onset myopathy with rodlike particles. Acta neurologica scandinavica 49: 547

Kar N C, Pearson C M, Verity M A 1980 Muscle fructose-1-6-diphosphatase deficiency associated with an atypical central core disease. Journal of the Neurological Sciences 48: 243

Karpati G, Engel W K 1968 Correlative histochemical study of skeletal muscle after suprasegmental denervation, peripheral nerve section and skeletal fixation. Neurology (Minneapolis) 18: 681

Karpati G, Carpenter S, Nelson R F 1970 Type 1 muscle fibre atrophy and central nuclei. A rare familial neuromuscular disease. Journal of the Neurological Sciences 10: 489

Karpati G, Carpenter S, Andermann F 1971 A new concept of childhood nemaline myopathy. Archives of Neurology (Chicago) 24: 291

Karpati G, Carpenter S, Eisen A A 1972 Experimental core-like lesions and nemaline rods. A correlative morphological and physiological study. Archives of Neurology (Chicago) 27: 237

Karpati G, Carpenter, S, Engel A G, Watters G V, Allen J, Rothman S et al 1975 The syndrome of systemic carnitine deficiency. Clinical, morphologic, biochemical and pathophysiologic features. Neurology (Minneapolis) 25: 16

Kausch K, Grimm T, Janka M, Lehmann-Horn F, Wieringa B, Müller C R 1990 Evidence for linkage of the central core disease locus to chromosome 19q. Journal of the Neurological Sciences 98 (suppl.): 549

Kearns T P, Sayre G P 1958 Retinitis pigmentosa, external ophthalmoplegia and complete heart block. Archives of Ophthalmology 60: 280

Ketelsen U P, Freund-Mölbert E, Beckmann R 1971 Klinische und ultrastrukturelle Befunde bei kongenitaler Muskeldystrophie. Monatsschrift für Kinderheilkunde 119: 586

Kinoshita M, Cadman T E 1968 Myotubular myopathy. Archives of Neurology (Chicago) 18: 265

Kinoshita M, Satoyoshi E 1974 Type 1 fibre atrophy and nemaline bodies. Archives of Neurology (Chicago) 31: 423

Kinoshita M, Satoyoshi E, Kumagai M 1975a Familial type 1 fibre atrophy. Journal of the Neurological Sciences 25: 11

Kinoshita M, Satoyoshi E, Matsuo N 1975b 'Myotubular myopathy' and 'type 1 fibre atrophy' in a family. Journal of the Neurological Sciences 26: 575

Kinoshita M, Satoyoshi E, Suzuki Y 1975c A typical myopathy with myofibrillar aggregates. Archives of Neurology (Chicago) 32: 417

Kolin I 1967 Nemaline myopathy: a fatal case. American Journal of Diseases of Children 114: 95

Kondo K, Yuasa T 1980 Genetics of congenital nemaline myopathy. Muscle and Nerve 3: 308

Konno H, Iwasaki Y, Yamamoto T, Inosaka T 1987 Nemaline bodies in spinal progressive muscular atrophy. An autopsy case. Acta Neuropathologica (Berlin) 74: 84

Korenyi-Both A, Marosan G 1979 Patterns of neuromuscular disease as related to stages of normal embryogenesis in voluntary muscle. American Journal of Pathology 95: 359

Krabbe K H 1947 Kongenit generaliseret muskelaplasi. Nordisk Medicin 35: 1756

Krijsmann J B, Barth P G, Stam F C, Sloof J L, Jaspar H H J 1980 Congenital muscle dystrophy and cerebral dysgenesis in a dutch family. Neuropädiatrie 108: 120

Kuitunen P, Rapola J, Noponen A L, Donner M 1972 Nemaline myopathy. Acta paediatrica scandinavica 61: 353

Kulakowski S, Flament-Durand J, Malaisse-Lagae F, Chevallay M, Fardeau M 1973 Myopathie à bâtonnets ('nemaline myopathy'). Archives Françaises de Pédiatrie 30: 505

Lake B D, Wilson J 1975 Zebra body myopathy. Clinical, histochemical and ultrastructural studies. Journal of the Neurological Sciences 24: 437

Lake B D, Cavanagh N, Wilson J 1977 Myopathy with minicores in siblings. Neuropathology and Applied Neurobiology 3: 159

Lapresle J, Fardeau M, Godet-Guillain J 1972 Myopathie distale et congénitale, avec hypertrophie des mollets. Présence d'anomalies mitochondriales à la biopsie musculaire. Journal of the Neurological Sciences 17: 87

Lazaro R P, Fenichel G M, Kilroy A W 1979 Congenital muscular dystrophy: case reports and reappraisal. Muscle & Nerve 2: 349

Lebenthal E, Shocket S B, Adam A, Seelenfrund M, Fried A, Najenson T et al 1970 Arthrogryposis multiplex congenita; 23 cases in an Arab kindred. Pediatrics 46: 891

Lenard H G, Goebel H H 1975 Congenital fibre type disproportion. Neuropädiatrie 6: 220

Levesque J, Lepage F, Boes Willwald M, Gruner J 1956 Deux cas de dystrophie musculaire familiale congénitale simulant une maladie de Werdnig-Hoffmann-Oppenheim. Archives Françaises de Pédiatrie 13: 202

Leyten Q H, Gabreels F S, Renier W O, ter Laak H J, Sengers R C, Mullaart R A 1989 Congenital muscular dystrophy. Journal of Pediatry 115: 214

Lüking T, Otto H F 1971 Kongenitale Muskeldystrophie. Zeitschrift für Kinder-heilkunde 110: 59

Luft R, Ikkos D, Palmieri G, Ernster L, Afzelius B 1962 A case of severe hypermetabolism of non-thyroid origin with a defect in the maintenance of mitochondrial respiratory control: a correlated clinical, biochemical and morphological study. Journal of Clinical Investigation 41: 1776

McComb R D, Markesbury W R, O'Connor W N 1979 Fatal neonatal nemaline myopathy with multiple congenital anomalies. Journal of Pediatrics 94: 47

MacDonald R D, Engel A G 1969 The cytoplasmic body — another structural anomaly of the Z disk. Acta neuropathologica (Berlin) 14: 99

McLeod J G, Baker W de, Lethlean A K, Shorey C D 1972 Centronuclear myopathy with autosomal dominant inheritance. Journal of the Neurological Sciences 15: 375

McMenamin J B, Becker L E, Murphy E G 1982 Congenital muscular dystrophy: a clinicopathologic report of 24 cases. Journal of Pediatry 100: 692

Mair W G P, Tomé F M S 1972a The ultrastructure of the adult and developing human myotendinous junction. Acta neuropathologica (Berlin) 21: 239

Mair W G P, Tomé F M S 1972a Atlas of the ultrastructure of diseased human muscle. Churchill Livingstone, Edinburgh & London

Martin L, Reniers J 1968 Nemaline myopathy. I. Histochemical study. Acta neuropathologica (Berlin) 11: 282

Martin J J, Clara R, Centerick C, Joris C 1976 Is congenital fibre type disproportion a true myopathy? Acta neurologica belgica 76: 335

Martin J J, Centerick C, Joris C, Martens C 1977 Myopathie centro-nucléaire. Acta neurologica belgica 77: 285

Martinez B A, Lake B D 1987 Childhood nemaline myopathy. A review of clinical presentation in relation to prognosis. Developmental Medicine and Child Neurology 29: 815

Martinez A J, Hooshmand H, Faris A A 1973 Acute alcoholic myopathy. Enzyme histochemistry and electron microscopic findings. Journal of the Neurological Sciences 20: 245

Meier C, Voellmy W, Gertsch M, Zimmermann A, Geissbühler J 1984 Nemaline myopathy appearing in adults as cardiomyopathy. Archives of Neurology 41: 443

Meltzer H Y, McBride E, Popei R W 1973 Rod (nemaline) bodies in the skeletal muscle of an acute schizophrenic patient. Neurology (Minneapolis) 23: 769

Meltzer H Y, Kunel R W, Click J 1976 Incidence of Z-band streaming and myofibrillar disruptions in skeletal muscle from healthy young people. Neurology (Minneapolis) 26: 853

Merlini L, Granata C, Ballestrazzi A, Marini M L 1989 Rigid spine syndrome and rigid spine sign in myopathies. Journal of Child Neurology 4: 274

Meyers K R, Golomb H M, Hansen J L, McKusick V A 1974 Familial neuromuscular disease with myotubes. Clinical Genetics 5: 327

Mittelbach F, Pongratz D 1968 Klinische, histologische und histochemische Untersuchungen über einen Fall von Central Core Disease (Zentralfibrillen Myopathie). Deutsche Zeitschrift für Nervenheilkunde 194: 232

Mizuno Y, Nakamura Y, Komiya K 1989 The spectrum of cytoplasmic body myopathy: report of a congenital severe case. Brain Development 11: 20

Moosa A, Dawood A A 1987 Centronuclear myopathy in black African children-report of 4 cases. Neuropediatrics 18: 213

Morgan-Hughes J A, Brett E M, Lake B D, Tomé F M S 1973 Central core disease or not? Observations on a family with a non-progressive myopathy. Brain 96: 527

Mortier W, Michaelis E, Becker J, Ferhard L 1975 Centronucleäre Myopathie mit autosomal dominantem Erbgang. Human genetik 27: 199

Mrozek K, Strugalska M, Fidzianska A 1970 A sporadic case of central core disease. Journal of the Neurological Sciences 10: 339

Mukoyama M, Matsuoka Y, Kato H, Sobue I 1973 Multicore disease. Clinical Neurology (Tokyo) 13: 221

Munnel J F, Getty R 1968 Canine myocardial Z-disk alterations resembling those of nemaline myopathy. Laboratory Investigation 19: 303

Munsat T L 1967 In: UCLA Interdepartmental Conference: skeletal muscle. Annals of Internal Medicine 67: 643

Munsat T L, Thompson L R, Coleman R F 1969 Centronuclear ('myotubular') myopathy. Archives of Neurology (Chicago) 20: 120

Mussini J M, Gray F, Hauw J J, Piette A M, Prost A 1981 Rigid spine syndrome: histological examinations of male and female cases. Acta Neuropathologica (Suppl. VII) 331

Nakao K, Tomonaga M, Muro T, Kot S, Mozai T 1968 A case of congenital myopathy with special findings in its biopsied muscle: 'nemaline myopathy'. Clinical neurology (Tokyo) 8: 404

Nakashima N, Tamura Z, Okamoto S, Goto H 1970 Inclusion bodies in human neuromuscular disorder. Archives of Neurology 22: 270

Neustein H B 1973 Nemaline myopathy, a family study with three autopsied cases. Archives of Pathology 96: 192

Neville H E, Brooke M H 1973 Central core fibres: structured and unstructured. In: Kakulas B A (ed) Basic research in myology. Excerpta Medica, Amsterdam, p 497

Nienhuis A W, Coleman R F, Brown J W, Munsat T L, Pearson C M 1967 Nemaline myopathy, a histopathological and histochemical study. American Journal of Clinical Pathology 48: 1

Nonaka I, Chou S 1979 Congenital muscular dystrophy. In: Vinken P J, Bruyn G W (eds) Handbook of clinical neurology. North-Holland Publ. Co, Amsterdam, vol 41, p 27

Nonaka I, Miyoshino S, Miike T, Ueno T, Usuku G 1972 An electron microscopical study of the muscle in congenital muscular dystrophy. Kumamoto Medical Journal 25: 68

Nonaka I, Une Y, Ishihara T, Miyoshino S, Nakashima T, Sugita H 1981 A clinical and histological study of Ullrich's disease (congenital atonic-sclerotic muscular dystrophy). Neuropediatrics 12: 197

Nonaka I, Sugita H, Takada K, Kumagai K 1982 Muscle histochemistry in congenital muscular dystrophy with central nervous system involvement. Muscle and Nerve 5: 102

Nonaka I, Nakamura Y, Tojo M, Sugita H, Ishikawa T, Awaya A, Sugiyama N 1983 Congenital myopathies without specific features (minimal change myopathy). Neuropediatrics 14: 237

Nonaka I, Ishiura S, Arahata K, Ishibashi-Ueda H, Maruyama T, Ii K 1989 Progression in nemaline myopathy. Acta Neuropathologica (Berlin) 78: 484

Norton P, Ellison P, Sulaiman A R, Harb J 1983 Nemaline myopathy in the neo-nate. Neurology 33: 351

Oh S J, Wilson E R, Alexander E B 1983 A benign form of reducing body myopathy. Muscle and Nerve 6: 278

Olney R K, Miller R G 1983 Inflammatory infiltration in Fukuyama type congenital muscular dystrophy. Muscle and Nerve 6: 75

Olson W, Engel W K, Walsh G O, Einaugler R 1972 Oculocraniosomatic neuromuscular disease with 'ragged-red' fibres. Archives of Neurology (Chicago) 26: 193

Oppenheim H 1900 Ueber allgemeine und localisierte Atonie der Muskulatur (Myatonie) im frühen Kindesalter. Monatsschrift für Psychiatrie und Neurologie 8: 232

Osborn M, Goebel H H 1983 The cytoplasmic bodies in a congenital myopathy can be stained with antibodies to desmin, the muscle specific intermediate filament protein. Acta Neuropathologica (Berlin) 62: 149

Otto H F, Lücking Th 1971 Congenitale Muskel dystrophie. Licht- und elektron-mikroskopische Befunde. Virchows Archiv- Abt A: Pathol Anat. 352: 324

Paljarvi L, Kalimo H, Lang H, Savontaus M-AL, Sonninen V 1987 Minicore myopathy with dominant inheritance. Journal of Neurological Sciences 77: 11

Palmucci L, Bertolotto A, Monga G, Ardizzone G, Schiffer D 1978a Histochemical and ultrastructural findings in a case of centronuclear myopathy. European Neurology 7: 327

Palmucci L, Schiffer D, Monga G, Mollo F, de Marchi M 1978b Central core disease: histochemical and ultrastructural study of muscle biopsies of father and daughter. Journal of Neurology 218: 55

Pascual-Castroviejo I, Gutierrez M, Rodriguez Costa T, Lopez M V, Ricoy J M, Morales M C 1974 Central core disease: presentacíon de 4 casos y revision de la literatura. Anales Españoles de Pediatria 7: 524

Patel H, Berry K, MacLeod P, Dunn H G 1983 Cytoplasmic body myopathy: report on a family and review of the literature. Journal of Neurological Sciences 60: 281

Patterson V H, Hill T R, Fletcher P J, Heron J R 1979 Central core disease: clinical and pathological evidence of a progression within a family. Brain 102: 581

Pearson C M, Fowler W G 1963 Hereditary non-progressive muscular dystrophy inducing arthrogryposis syndrome. Brain 86: 75

PeBenito R, Sher J H, Cracco J B 1978 Centronuclear myopathy: clinical and pathologic features. Clinical Pediatrics 17: 259

Pellegrini G, Barbieri S, Moggio M 1985 A case of congenital neuromuscular disease with uniform type I fibers, abnormal mitochondrial network and jagged Z-line. Neuropediatrics 16: 162

Pellissier J F, De Barsy T, Faugere M C, Rebuffel P 1979 Type III glycogenosis with multicore structures. Muscle & Nerve 2: 124

Pepe F A 1966 Some aspects of the structural organisation of the myofibrils as revealed by antibody-staining methods. Journal of Cell Biology 28: 505

Pepin B, Mikol J, Goldstein B, Haguenau M, Godlewski S 1976 Forme familiale de myopathie centronucléaire de l'adulte. Revue Neurologique 132: 845

Peterson D I, Munsat T 1969 The clinical presentation of nemaline myopathy. Bulletin of the Los Angeles Neurological Societies 34: 39

Poewe W, Willeit H, Sluga E, Mayr U 1985 The rigid spine syndrome — a myopathy of uncertain nosological position. Journal of Neurology, Neurosurgery and Psychiatry 48: 887

Pongratz D, Heuser M, Mittelbach F, Struppler A 1975 Die sogenannte congenitale centronucleäre Myopathie — eine primäre Neuropathie? Acta neuropathologica (Berlin) 32: 9

Pou-Serradell A, Aguilar M, Soler L, Ferrer I 1980 Myopathie congénitale bénigne avec prépondérance des fibres de type I, et rares 'cores' chez la mère asymptomatique. Revue Neurologique 136: 853

Price H M, Gordon G B, Pearson C M, Munsat T L, Blumberg J M 1965 New evidence for excessive accumulation of Z-band material in nemaline myopathy. Proceedings of the National Academy of Sciences of the United States of America 54: 1398

Radnot M 1974 'Fingerprint' einschlüsse in M. orbicularis oculi. Ophthalmologica 168: 282

Radu H, Ionescu V 1972 Nemaline (neuro) myopathy. Rod-like bodies and type I fibre atrophy in a case of congenital hypotonia with denervation. Journal of the Neurological Sciences 17: 53

Radu H, Ionescu V, Radu A, Paler V, Rosu A M, Marian A 1974 Hypotrophic type 1 muscle fibres with central nuclei, and central myofibrillar lysis preferentially involving type 2 fibres. European Neurology 11: 108

Radu H, Rosu-Serbu A M, Ionescu V, Radu A 1977 Focal abnormalities in mitochondrial distribution in muscle. Two atypical cases of so-called 'central core disease'. Acta neuropathologica (Berlin) 39: 25

Raju T M K, Deshpande D H, Desai A D Congenital muscular dystrophy. In: Kakulas B A (ed) Clinical studies in myology. Excerpta Medica, Amsterdam, p 502

Ramsey P L, Hensinger R N 1975 Congenital dislocation of the hip associated with central core disease. Journal of Bone and Joint Surgery 57A: 648

Reske-Nielsen E, Hein-Sorensen O, Vorre P 1987 Familial centronuclear myopathy: a clinical and pathological study. Acta Neurologica Scandinavica 76: 115

Resnick J S, Engel W K 1967 Target fibres: structural and cytochemical characteristics and their relationship to neurogenic muscular disease and fibre types. In: Exploratory concepts in muscular dystrophy and related disorders. Excerpta Medica, NY, Harriman, ICS 147, p 255

Resnick J S, Engel W K, Nelson P G 1968 Changes in the Z-disk of skeletal muscle induced by tenotomy. Neurology (Minneapolis) 18: 737

Reyes M G, Goldbarg H, Fresco K, Bouffard A 1987 A zebra-body myopathy: a second case of ultrastructurally distinct congenital myopathy. Journal of Child Neurology 2: 307

Ricoy J R, Cabello A, Goizueta G 1980 Myopathy with multiple minicores. Report of two siblings. Journal of the Neurological Sciences 48: 81

Ringel S P, Bender A N, Engel W K 1976 Extrajunctional acetylcholine receptors. Alterations in human and experimental neuromuscular diseases. Archives of Neurology (Chicago) 33: 751

Ringel S P, Neville H E, Duster M C, Carroll J E 1977 A new congenital neuromuscular disease with trilaminar fibres. Neurology (Minneapolis) 27: 347

Robertson W C, Kawamura Y, Dyck P J 1978 Morphometric study of motoneurons in congenital nemaline myopathy and Werdnig-Hoffmann disease. Neurology (Minneapolis) 28: 1057

Rospide H A D, Vincent O, Gaudin E S, Scarbino R, Medici M 1972 Distrofia muscular congenita pura. Acta neurologica latino americana 18: 20

Rotthauwe H W, Kowalewski S, Mumenthaler M 1969 Kongenitale Muskeldystrophie. Zeitschrift für Kinderheilkunde 106: 131

Sahgal V, Sahgal S 1977 A new congenital myopathy. A morphological, cytochemical and histochemical study. Acta neuropathologica (Berlin) 37: 225

Santoro L, Marmo C, Gasparo-Rippa P, Toscano A, Sadile F, Barbieri F 1989 A new case of Ullrich's disease. Clinical Neuropathology 8: 69.

Saper J R, Itabashi H H 1976 Central core disease: a congenital myopathy. Diseases of the Nervous System 37: 225

Sarnat H B, Silbert S W 1976 Maturational arrest of foetal muscle in neonatal myotonic dystrophy. Archives of Neurology (Chicago) 33: 466

Scelsi R, Lanzi G, Nespoli L, Poggi P 1976 Congenital non-progressive myopathy with type 2 fibre atrophy and internal nuclei. European Neurology 14: 285

Schellens J P M, Ossentjuk E 1969 Mitochondrial ultrastructure with crystalloid inclusions in an unusual type of human myopathy. Virchows Archiv, Abt. B, Zellpathologie 4: 21

Schmalbruch H 1968 Lyse und regeneration von Fibrillen in der normalen menschlichen skelettmuskulatur. Virchows Archiv für Pathologische Anatomie und Physiologie 344: 159

Schmalbruch H, Kamienecka Z, Arroe M 1987 Early fatal nemaline myopathy: case report and review. Developmental Medicine in Child Neurology 29: 800

Schochet S S, Zellweger H, Ionescu V, McCormick W F 1972 Centronuclear myopathy: disease entity or a syndrome? Light and electron-microscopic study of two cases and review of the literature. Journal of Neurological Sciences 16: 215

Schotland D L 1967 Congenital myopathy with target fibres. Transactions of the American Neurological Association 92: 107

Schotland D L 1969 An electron microscopic study of target fibres, target-like fibres and related abnormalities in human muscle. Journal of Neuropathology and Experimental Neurology 28: 214

Schotland D L, Di Mauro S, Bonilla E, Scarpa A, Lee C P 1976 Neuromuscular disorder associated with a defect in mitochondrial energy supply. Archives of Neurology (Chicago) 33: 475

Seay A R, Ziter F A, Petajan J H 1977 Rigid spine syndrome. A type 1 myopathy. Archives of Neurology (Chicago) 34: 119

Seitelberger F, Wanko T, Gavin M A 1961 The muscle fibre in central core disease. Histochemical and electron microscopic observations. Acta neuropathologica (Berlin) 1: 223

Sengel A, Stoebner P 1974 Une inclusion musculaire atypique rare: les corps en 'empreinte digitale' ou 'fingerprint bodies'. Acta neuropathologica (Berlin) 27: 61

Sengers R C A, ter Haar B G A, Trisbels J M F, Willems J L, Daniels O, Stadhouders A M 1975 Congenital cataract and mitochondrial myopathy of skeletal and heart muscle associated with lactic acidosis after exercise. Journal of Pediatrics 86: 873

Serratrice G, Pellissier J F, Gastaut J L, Pouget J 1975 Myopathie congénitale avec hypotrophie sélective des fibres de type 1. Revue Neurologique 131: 813

Serratrice G, Pellissier J F, Faugère M C, Gastaut J L 1978 Centronuclear myopathy: possible central nervous system origin. Muscle & Nerve 1: 62

Serratrice G, Cros D, Pellissier J F, Gastaut J L, Pouget J 1980 Dystrophie musculaire congénitale. Revue Neurologique 136: 445

Serratrice G, Pellissier J F, Pouget J, Gastaut J L 1984 Le syndrome de la colonne vertébrale rigide et ses frontières nosologiques. Presse Médicale 13: 115

Serratrice G, Pellissier J F, Bes A K, Arne-Bes M C 1987 Centronuclear myopathy in adults. A facio-scapulo-peroneal case. Revue Neurologique, Paris, 143: 693

Shafiq S A, Dubowitz V, Peterson H de C, Milhorat A T 1967 Nemaline myopathy: report of a fatal case, with histochemical and electron microscopic studies. Brain 90: 817

Shafiq S A, Gorycki M A, Asiedu S A, Milhorat A T 1969 Tenotomy: Effect on the fine structure of the soleus of the rat. Archives of Neurology (Chicago) 20: 625

Shafiq S A, Asediu S A, Milhorat A T 1972 Effect of neonatal neurectomy on differentiation of fibre types in rat skeletal muscle. Experimental Neurology 35: 529

Shahar E, Tervo R C, Murphy E G 1988 Heterogeneity of nemaline myopathy. A follow-up study of 13 cases. Pediatric Neurosciences 14: 236

Shapira Y, Cederbaum S D, Cancilla P A, Nielsen D, Lippe B M 1975 Familial poliodystrophy, mitochondrial myopathy, and lactate acidemia. Neurology (Minneapolis) 25: 614

Sher J H, Rimalovski A B, Athanassiades T J, Aronson S M 1967 Familial centronuclear myopathy: a clinical and pathological study. Neurology (Minneapolis) 17: 727

Shinomura C, Nonaka I 1989 Nemaline myopathy: comparative muscle histochemistry in the severe neo-natal, moderate congenital, and adult-onset forms. Pediatric Neurology 5: 25

Short J K 1963 Congenital muscular dystrophy. A case report with autopsy findings. Neurology (Minneapolis) 13: 526

Shuaib A, Paasuke R T, Brownell K W 1987 Central core disease. Clinical features in 13 patients. Medicine 66: 389

Shuaib A, Martin J M, Mitchell L B, Brownell A K 1988 Multicore myopathy: not always a benign entity. Canadian Journal of Neurological Sciences 15: 10

Shy G M, Gonatas N K 1964 Human myopathy with giant abnormal mitochondria. Science 145: 493

Shy G M, Magee K R 1956 A new congenital non-progressive myopathy. Brain 79: 610

Shy G M, Engel W K, Somers J E, Wanko T 1963 Nemaline myopathy: a new congenital myopathy. Brain 86: 793

Shy G M, Gonatas N K, Perez M 1966 Two childhood myopathies with abnormal mitochondria. I. Megaconial myopathy. II. Pleoconial myopathy. Brain 89: 133

Spiro A J, Kennedy C 1965 Hereditary occurrence of nemaline myopathy. Archives of Neurology (Chicago) 13: 155

Spiro A J, Shy G M, Gonatas N K 1966 Myotubular myopathy. Persistence of fetal muscle in an adolescent boy. Archives of Neurology (Chicago) 14: 1

Spiro A J, Prineas J W, Moore C L 1970 A new mitochondrial myopathy in a patient with salt craving. Archives of Neurology (Chicago) 22: 259

Spiro A J, Horoupian D S, Snyder D R 1977 Biopsy and autopsy studies of congenital muscle fibre type disproportion: a broadening concept. Neurology (Minneapolis) 27: 405

Sreter F A, Aström K E, Romanul F C A, Young R R, Roydenjones H Jr 1976 Characteristics of myosin in nemaline myopathy. Journal of the Neurological Sciences 27: 99

Stoeber E 1939 Uber atonisch-sklerotische Muskeldystrophie (typ Ullrich). Zeitschrift für Kinderheilkunde 60: 279

Stoessl A J, Hahn A F, Malott D, Jones D T, Silver M D 1985 Nemaline myopathy with associated cardiomyopathy. Archives of Neurology 42: 1084

Streib E W, Lucking C H 1989 Congenital muscular dystrophy with leukoencephalopathy. European Neurology 29: 211

Stromer M H, Tabatabai L B, Robson R M, Goll D E, Zeece M G 1976 Nemaline myopathy, an integrated study: selective extraction. Experimental Neurology 50: 402

Stuhlfauth I, Jennekens F G I, Willemse J K, Jockusch B M (1983) Congenital nemaline myopathy: II. Quantitative

changes in alpha-actinin and myosin in skeletal muscle. Muscle and Nerve 6: 69

Sugita H, Masaki T, Ebashi S, Pearson C M 1974 Staining of the nemaline rod by fluorescent antibody against 10S-actinin. Proceedings of the Japan Academy 50: 237

Sulaiman A R, Swick H M, Kinder D S 1983 Congenital fibre type disproportion with unusual clinico-pathologic manifestations. Journal of Neurology, Neurosurgery and Psychiatry 46: 175

Swash M, Schwartz M S 1981 Familial multicore disease with focal loss of cross striations and ophthalmoplegia. Journal of Neurological Sciences 52: 1

Tanabe H, Ito K, Yamane K, Tabuchi Y, Nozawa T, Kumano K 1976 Central core disease: a clinical, histochemical and electron microscopic study on 2 cases with scoliosis, the first two cases in Japan. Advances in Neurological Sciences 20: 458

Tanimura R, Suzuki H, Yokota J, Segawa M, Fukuyama Y 1974 Multicore myopathy. A case of congenital non-progressive myopathy associated with 'multicore' changes of muscle fibres. Clinical Neurology 14: 613

Taratuto A L, Sfaello Z M, Rezzonico C, Morales R C 1978 Multicore disease. Report of a case with lack of fibre type differentiation. Neuropaediatrie 9: 285

Tardieu M, Schovart D, Metral S, Landrieu P 1986 Syndrome de la colonne raide — aspect d'hypotrophie et prédominance des fibres musculaires de type I. Archives Françaises de Pédiatrie 43: 115

Tarlow M J, Lake B D, Lloyd J K 1973 Chronic lactic acidosis in association with myopathy. Archives of Disease in Childhood 48: 489

Telerman-Toppet N, Gérard J M, Coërs C 1973 Central core disease: a study of clinically unaffected muscle. Journal of the Neurological Sciences 19: 207

ter Laak H J, Jaspar H H J, Gabreels F J M, Breuer T J M, Sengers R C A, Joosten E M G, Stadhouders A M, Gabreels-Festen A A W M 1981 Congenital fibre type disproportion: a morphometric study (4 cases). Clinics in Neurology and Neurosurgery 83: 67

Thomas N S T, Sarfarazi M, Roberts K, Williams H, Cole G, Liechti-Gallati S, Harper P S 1987 X-linked myotubular myopathy (MTMI): evidence for linkage to Xq28 DNA markers. Cytogenetics and Cell Genetics 46: 704

Thornell L E, Eriksson A, Edström L 1983 Intermediate filaments in human myopathies. In: Bowden R M, Shay J W (eds) Cell and muscle motility. Plenum Publishing Co, 4: 85

Tomé F M S, Fardeau M 1973 'Fingerprint inclusions' in muscle fibres in dystrophia myotonica. Acta neuropathologica (Berlin) 24: 62

Tomé F M S, Fardeau M 1975 Congenital myopathy with 'reducing bodies' in muscle fibres. Acta neuropathologica (Berlin) 31: 207

Topaloglu H, Yalaz K, Kale G, Ergin M 1990 Congenital muscular dystrophy with cerebral involvement. Report of a case of 'occidental type of cerebromuscular dystrophy'. Neuropediatrics 21: 53

Tsujihata M, Shimomura C, Yoshimura T, Sato A, Ogawa T, Tsuji Y, Nagataki S K, Matsuo T 1983 Fatal neonatal nemaline myopathy: a case report. Journal of Neurology, Neurosurgery and Psychiatry 46: 856

Turner J W A 1940 The relationship between amyotonia congenita and congenital myopathy. Brain 63: 163

Turner J W A 1949 On amyotonia congenita. Brain 72: 25

Turner J W A, Lees F 1962 Congenital myopathy. A fifty-year follow-up. Brain 85: 732

Ullrich O 1930 Kongenitale, atonisch-sklerotische muskeldystrophie, ein weiterer Typus der heredodegenerativen erkrankungen des neuromuskularen systems. Zeitschrift für die Gesante Neurologie und Psychiatrie 126: 171

van Biervhet J P A M, Bruinvis L, Ketting D, De Bree P K, van der Heiden C, Wadman S, Willems J L, Bookelman H, van Haelst U, Monnens L A H 1977 Hereditary mitochondrial myopathy with lactic acidemia, a De Toni–Fanconi–Debré Syndrome, and a defective respiratory chain in voluntary striated muscles. Pediatric Research 11: 1088

Vanneste J A L, Stam F C 1982 Autosomal dominant multicore disease. Journal of Neurology, Neurosurgery and Psychiatry 45: 360

Vanneste J A, Augustijn P B, Stam P C 1988 The rigid spine syndrome in two sisters. Journal of Neurology, Neurosurgery and Psychiatry 51: 131

van Wijngaarden G K, Bethlem J, Meijer A E F H, Hulsmann W C, Feltkamp C 1967 Skeletal muscle disease with abnormal mitochondria. Brain 90: 577

van Wijngaarden G K, Fleury P, Bethlem J, Meijer A E F M 1969 Familial 'myotubular' myopathy. Neurology (Minneapolis) 19: 901

van Wijngaarden G K, Bethlem J, Dingemans K P, Coërs C, Telerman-Toppet N, Gérard J M 1977 Familial focal loss of striations. Journal of Neurology 216: 163

Vassella F, Mumenthaler M, Rossi E, Moser H, Weisman U 1967 Die Kongenitale Muskeldystrophie. Deutsche Zeitschrift für Nervenheilkunde 190: 349

Verheist W, Brucher J M, Goddeeris P, Lauweryns J, de Geest H 1976 Familial centronuclear myopathy associated with cardiomyopathy. British Heart 38: 504

Vital C, Vallat J M, Martin F, Le Blanc M, Bergouignan M 1970 Etude clinique et ultrastructurale d'un cas de myopathie centronucléaire ('myotubular myopathy') de l'adulte. Revue Neurologique 123: 117

Voirin J, Bonte J B, Laloum D, Chapon F 1990 Myopathie à bâtonnets de découverte néo-natale et d'évolution favorable. Archives Françaises de Pédiatrie 47: 201

Volpe P, Damiani E, Margreth A, Pellegrini G, Scarlato G 1981 Fast to slow change of myosin in nemaline myopathy: electrophoretic and immunologic evidence. Neurology (Minneapolis) 32: 37

Wallgren-Pettersson C 1989 Congenital nemaline myopathy — a clinical follow-up of twelve patients. Journal of Neurological Sciences 89: 1

Wallgren-Pettersson C, Rapola J, Donner M 1988 Pathology of congenital nemaline myopathy. A follow-up study. Journal of Neurological Sciences 83: 243

Wallgren-Pettersson C, Sainio K, Salmi T 1989 Electromyography in congenital nemaline myopathy. Muscle and Nerve 12: 587

Walton J N 1956 Amyotonia congenita. A follow-up study. Lancet 1: 1023

Walton J N 1957 The limp child. Journal of Neurology, Neurosurgery and Psychiatry 20: 144

Werdnig G 1891 Zwei frühinfantile hereditäre Fälle von progressiver Muskelatropic unter dem Bilde der Dystrophie, uber auf neurotischer Grundlage. Archiv für Psychiatrie 22: 437

Wharton B A 1965 An unusual variety of muscular dystrophy. Lancet 1: 248

Wohlfart G 1937 Uber das Vorkommen verschiedener Arten von Muskelfasern in der Skelett muskulatur des Menschen und einiger Saügetieren. Acta psychiatrica et neurologica scandinavica Supplt. 12: 1

Wolburg H, Schlote W, Langohr H D, Peiffer J, Reiher K H, Heckl R W 1982 Slowly progressive congenital myopathy with cytoplasmic bodies. Clinical Neuropathology 1: 55

Yamaguchi M, Robson R M, Stromer M H, Dahl D S, Oda T 1978 Actin filaments form the backbone of nemaline myopathy rods. Nature 271: 265

Yarom R, Shapira Y 1977 Myosin degeneration in a congenital myopathy. Archives of Neurology 34: 114

Yoshioka M, Kuroki S, Ohkura K, Itagaki Y, Saida K 1987 Congenital myopathy with type II muscle fiber hypoplasia. Neurology 37: 860

Yuasa T, Fukuhara N, Ohoshima F, Tsubaki T, Kushiro S 1977 Nemaline myopathy. Clinical and histologic studies of five cases from three families. Clinical Neurology 17: 38

Zellweger H, Afifi A, McCormick W F, Mergner W 1967a Severe congenital muscular dystrophy. American Journal of Diseases of Children 114: 591

Zellweger H, Afifi A, McCormick W F, Mergner W 1967b Benign congenital muscular dystrophy. A special form of congenital hypotonia. Clinical Pediatrics 6: 655

7. The muscular dystrophies

Henning Schmalbruch

INTRODUCTION

The term muscular dystrophy covers a group of genetically determined disorders which cause progressive weakness and wasting of the skeletal muscles and in which there is assumed to be a primary defect in the muscle cell. Some forms cause death after 15–20 years, while in others life expectancy may be normal, but the patient becomes progressively disabled. No curative treatment for these muscle disorders is at present available. The diagnosis cannot be established solely on the basis of morphological changes, but histology can help to decide whether the patient has a neuromuscular disorder at all, and whether the disorder is of myogenic origin. Moreover, histology can exclude inflammatory processes and other myopathies with specific features, for example 'mitochondrial' myopathies, other metabolic myopathies and various forms of congenital myopathy.

CLASSIFICATION OF THE MUSCULAR DYSTROPHIES

X-linked muscular dystrophies

Duchenne and Becker type

Duchenne muscular dystrophy becomes symptomatic in early childhood and causes death usually at the end of the second or during the third decade. Proximal limb muscles are affected first, whereas distal muscles may undergo compensatory hypertrophy. Later these muscles also become weak, but may retain their volume because fat cells proliferate ('pseudohypertrophy'). In a number of patients the cardiac muscle is affected

as well, but clinically manifest cardiomyopathy is rare. Muscle enzymes are lost from skeletal muscle and accumulate in the serum, elevation of the serum creatine kinase (CK) activity being an important diagnostic finding.

The disease affects males, while females are carriers and are rarely affected clinically ('manifesting carriers') (Barkhans & Gilchrist 1989). Data on the incidence in different ethnic populations range from 186 to 326 cases per million male births (1 in 5400 to 1 in 3100) (Thompson 1986), the commonly accepted average incidence being 1 in 3500 male births (Emery 1987). The prevalence in the total population is about 50 cases per million. Roughly one-tenth of patients show a milder course and are classified as having the more benign Becker type of dystrophy (Becker & Kiener 1955, Becker 1964). Useful clinical criteria for distinguishing Duchenne and Becker dystrophy are as follows: diagnosis before or after the age of 7 years; wheelchair-dependent or not by the age of 15 years; death before or after the age of 30 years. The serum CK activity in Becker dystrophy may be as high as in Duchenne dystrophy during childhood but tends to decrease later. There is also considerable heterogeneity within the group of patients with Duchenne dystrophy, some patients having to be classified as 'atypical' (Spiegler et al 1987) or 'outliers' (Brooke et al 1989).

About 30% of Duchenne cases are sporadic (Caskey et al 1980, Yasuda & Kondo 1980, Williams et al 1983); this agrees with Haldane's (1935) estimation that the number of new mutations must be responsible for one-third of the affected male patients. If mutations occur in male and female gametes at the same rate, and if carriers and non-carriers produce the same number of surviving children, one-third of the mothers of patients are non-carriers. This implies that, even with optimal genetic counselling, one-third of Duchenne births are not predictable and therefore not preventible.

Girls sometimes present with a similar clinical and myopathological picture to that seen in boys with Duchenne dystrophy. Some of these female patients probably have autosomal recessive limb-girdle dystrophy (see below). Other cases occur in families with unequivocally X-linked dystrophy. The disorder may be expressed in females in the following situations:

1. Turner's syndrome (X0) (Walton & Gardner-Medwin 1981)
2. When the father is an affected male and the mother is a carrier. Duchenne patients may reproduce (Thompson 1978), but no affected child of a Duchenne patient has been reported.
3. Manifesting carriers. The intact X-chromosome and the X-chromosome carrying the disease in carriers are randomly inactivated but, in rare cases, the defective chromosome may be active in the majority of myonuclei. The disorder in these patients tends to be mild, but occasionally it may be as severe as in boys (Meola et al 1986).
4. When there is a structural abnormality of the X-chromosome (X-autosome translocations).

The disease gene for Duchenne and Becker dystrophy is on the short arm (p) of the X-chromosome in band 21 (Xp21). About half of the patients have various gene deletions in this band, while the remainder probably have point mutations or deletions which cannot be detected with current methods. Attempts to relate the size, site or type of gene deletion to the clinical course have given conflicting results (Medori et al 1989, Baumbach et al 1989). The clinical course may vary even in patients from the same family who presumably share the same gene defect. This suggests that factors other than the gene defect itself may have some effect in determining the clinical severity of the disease (Fischbeck 1989). The product of the disease gene is a large cytoskeletal protein molecule ('dystrophin') which is absent in skeletal muscle fibres of Duchenne patients and reduced in Becker patients (see page 311). Manifesting carriers show a mosaic pattern of dystrophin expression in their muscle fibres (Arahata et al 1989).

Very rarely, Duchenne patients are susceptible to malignant hyperthermia. We have seen a boy who survived a severe attack at the age of 3 years and was afterwards found to have typical Duchenne dystrophy; the mother had a positive halothane test. On the other hand, a muscle biopsy taken after an attack of malignant hyperthermia may show pronounced myopathic changes. Together with the chronic elevation of serum CK present in most patients susceptible to malignant hyperthermia, this may lead to the erroneous diagnosis of muscular dystrophy.

Emery–Dreifuss dystrophy

This disorder is characterized by onset during the first decade, scapulohumeroperoneal distribution of weakness and wasting, early contractures of elbow and ankle joints, cardiopathy with conduction block in most patients and long survival (Emery & Dreifuss 1966, Rotthauwe et al 1972, Thomas et al 1972, Mawatari & Katayama 1973, Rowland et al 1979, Hara et al 1987). The sequence in which the different muscle groups are affected varies in the different kinships studied; whether they represent different diseases is unknown. According to the pattern in which the muscles are affected, the patients may be classified as having the 'scapuloperoneal syndrome'. This term, however, also covers disorders of neurogenic origin, and there are also cases with a myogenic form of the scapuloperoneal syndrome which is not X-linked. The myopathic nature of Emery–Dreifuss dystrophy has been proven in a careful autopsy study (Hara et al 1987).

X-linked myopathy with excessive autophagy

Kalimo et al (1988) described a Finnish family in which five males had a mild proximal myopathy with X-linked inheritance. The onset was in early childhood, serum CK activity was markedly elevated, and life expectancy was normal. There was no evidence of cardiac involvement and the muscle fibres showed strikingly pronounced autophagocytosis. The authors referred to a second family studied in England by Dubowitz and Sewry (unpublished). The nosological status of this disorder remains obscure.

Limb–girdle muscular dystrophy

This term describes a group of different disorders, and some authors prefer the term limb–girdle syndrome. The classical form (Leyden–Möbius) starts in the second or third decade of life and causes death or disability after 15–20 years. Pelvifemoral muscles are initially involved. A scapulohumeral form has been distinguished with onset in childhood or early adult life. Inheritance is as an autosomal recessive trait. Many cases are sporadic. The prevalence in the total population is about 20 cases per million (Becker & Lenz 1955).

A distinctly different form which resembles Duchenne dystrophy is limb–girdle dystrophy of childhood. It is found mainly in populations with many consanguineous marriages (e.g. the Amish people: Jackson & Strehler 1968; in Tunisia: Ben Hamida et al 1983; and in the Sudan: Salih et al 1983). The inheritance is autosomal recessive as in the classical Leyden–Möbius form. Many female patients with the Duchenne phenotype may in fact have this limb–girdle dystrophy of childhood.

In addition, several families with benign autosomal dominant myopathy with onset at birth or early childhood and normal life expectancy have been reported (Bethlem & van Wijngaarden 1976, Arts et al 1978, Fenichel et al 1982, Schmalbruch et al 1987, Mohire et al 1988). The distribution of muscle weakness is humeropelvic or humeropelvicoperoneal. Heel cord shortening, torticollis and joint contractures are frequently observed. Serum CK activity is mildly elevated (up to 10 times normal), and the muscle biopsy shows changes typical of muscular dystrophy. In some families cardiac conduction block occurs (Fenichel et al 1982). Whether or not all of these patients have the same disease is unknown, and whether they should be classified as having autosomal dominant limb–girdle dystrophy, congenital dystrophy, or even autosomal dominant Emery–Dreifuss dystrophy, appears to be a matter of semantics.

Still another group of patients has late-onset limb–girdle dystrophy. However, few familial cases with autosomal dominant inheritance have been reported (e.g. Gilchrist et al 1988), and most cases are sporadic. Many sporadic patients presenting in this way will in fact turn out to have some alternative disorder such as polymyositis, or an endocrine or metabolic myopathy.

Facioscapulohumeral dystrophy (Landouzy–Dejerine)

This is inherited as a dominant trait with onset during childhood or in early adult life. The shoulder–girdle or facial muscles are affected first, and in most patients the disease also involves the anterior tibial muscles. The life expectancy is usually close to normal. Abortive cases with little progression are frequent, but in some families the disease may be as devastating as Duchenne muscular dystrophy leading to death before the age of 20 years (Bailey et al 1986). Some patients present with sensorineural hearing loss and may rarely also have an exudative retinopathy (Coats' syndrome) (Wulff et al 1982, Taylor et al 1982, Bailey et al 1986). The prevalence is about one-tenth that of limb–girdle dystrophy (Becker & Lenz 1955). It is a matter of debate whether a separate scapuloperoneal syndrome exists, or whether this is a variety of facioscapulohumeral or Emery–Dreifuss dystrophy (see Thomas et al 1975).

The differential diagnosis is difficult. Of 17 patients suspected of having facioscapulohumeral dystrophy in one study, the diagnosis proved to be correct in only seven (van Wijngaarden & Bethlem 1973). Patients with congenital myopathies, mitochondrial myopathy, polymyositis, or myasthenia gravis may have a similar distribution of muscular weakness and wasting.

Distal myopathy

This is an inhomogeneous group of disorders and not all patients with 'distal myopathy' will prove to have a myogenic disorder. Numerous familial cases with autosomal dominant inheritance, later onset, and very slow progression have been reported from Scandinavia by Welander (1951), Dahlgaard (1960), Tarkkanen & Klemetti (1973), and Edström (1975) (Welander myopathy). Two kinships showing similar clinical features have been observed in the United States (Markesbery et al 1974) and in Germany (Bachmann & Wagner 1980). Early-onset cases with dominant inheritance have been described by Magee & De Jong (1965), van der Does de Willebois et al (1968) and Bautista et al (1978). Congenital myopathies may have a preferentially distal distribution of weakness as well, and some patients classified as having distal myopathy probably suffer from a neurogenic disorder or from polymyositis. There is evidence, even in Swedish patients, that the disorder may in reality be neurogenic (Stålberg & Ekstedt 1969, Thornell et al 1984, Borg et al 1987, 1989). Walton & Gardner-Medwin (1981) stress that patients with confirmed distal myopathy have become increasingly rare as diagnostic methods have improved.

Two other forms of distal myopathy characterized by autosomal recessive inheritance, onset in early adulthood and more rapid progression than in the Welander type occur predominantly in Japan. 'Autosomal recessive distal muscular dystrophy' (Miyoshi et al 1986) affects the gastrocnemius and not the peroneal muscles. Serum CK activity is elevated, and biopsies show muscle fibre necrosis. 'Distal myopathy with rimmed vacuole formation' (Nonaka et al 1981a, Kumamoto et al 1982, Mizusawa et al 1987a,b, Sunohara et al 1989) affects mainly the peroneal muscles; serum CK activity is normal or only slightly elevated, and muscle biopsies show atrophic fibres with autophagocytotic vacuoles but no necrosis (Nonaka et al 1985). Kuhn & Schröder (1981) in Germany reported two siblings with a distal myopathy resembling the Miyoshi type. Markesbery et al (1977) in the United States observed two sporadic cases with features of both Japanese forms: serum CK activity was high (20–100 times normal), ankle dorsiflexors and plantarflexors were equally mildly affected, and muscle biopsies showed pronounced formation of autophagocytotic vacuoles. (For a comparison of the different forms, see Miyoshi et al (1986) and Sunohara et al (1989).)

Ocular myopathies

Chronic progressive external ophthalmoplegia (CPEO) (von Graefe 1866, Kiloh & Nevin 1951) may be part of a syndrome characterized by generalized mitochondrial myopathy, retinitis pigmentosa, cardiac conduction block, hearing loss, defects of the central and peripheral nervous system, small stature and endocrine dysfunction ('oculocraniosomatic syndrome', 'ophthalmoplegia plus', or Kearns–Sayre syndrome) (Kearns & Sayre 1958, Drachman 1968, Olson et al 1972). The completeness of the syndrome varies, even within the same family (see Kamieniecka & Schmalbruch 1980), and it is not clear whether the different phenotypes in unrelated patients represent one or several nosological entities. Ophthalmoplegia may be due to the myopathy but it may also be of neurogenic origin because the central nervous system is often affected in mitochondrial myopathies.

It is not known whether, in addition to ophthalmoplegia-plus, an isolated ocular dystrophy exists. In a thesis reviewing all published cases with chronic external ophthalmoplegia, Bastiaensen (1978) reported that many patients classified as having 'pure' ocular myopathy or dystrophy have additional features of the ophthalmoplegia-plus syndrome, as do some of their relatives. He concluded that patients classified as having ocular dystrophy in reality suffer from a less complete form of ophthalmoplegia-plus. Kamieniecka & Sjö (1984) observed 13 patients, all females aged 55 to 75 years, with ptosis, ophthalmoplegia and mild proximal myopathy. With one exception, all cases were sporadic, and muscle biopsies showed abnormal mitochondria. Most of these patients had been suspected of having myasthenia gravis.

Oculopharyngeal dystrophy

This disorder was first observed in French Canada (Taylor 1915, Victor et al 1962, Little & Perl 1982) but later also in other countries (see Murphy & Drachman 1968, Bastiaensen 1978, Vita et al 1983). The disease is dominantly inherited with variable expressivity, a late onset usually after the age of 40 years, and a slow progression. Ptosis and dysphagia are the key symptoms; the latter may become severe enough to cause malnutrition which was formerly often the cause of death in such patients. The facial and limb–girdle muscles may also be affected. Dubowitz & Brooke (1973) described a patient with 'pure' ocular myopathy whose mother had oculopharyngeal dystrophy.

Other diseases may produce a similar clinical picture. In a Japanese family with familial spinal muscular atrophy, seven members had ophthalmoplegia and dysphagia, while one patient presented with an isolated oculopharyngeal syndrome (Matsunaga et al 1973). In four other Japanese families a late-onset oculopharyngeal myopathy with additional involvement of the distal limb muscles was observed ('oculopharyngeal distal myopathy', Satoyoshi & Kinoshita 1977) and a similar syndrome has also been reported in Melanesians (Scrimgeour and Mastaglia 1984). Ptosis and ophthalmoplegia may occasionally also occur in facioscapulohumeral muscular dystrophy but are usually preceded by involvement of other muscle groups. Dysphagia may occur in polymyositis, in the oculocraniosomatic syndrome and also in the late stages of myotonic dystrophy. In oculopharyngeal dystrophy it is always one of the first symptoms.

Myotonic dystrophy

This is a dominantly inherited multisystem disorder characterized by myotonia, myopathic muscular weakness and wasting, cataracts, gonadal atrophy, frontal alopecia, cardiac lesions and mental defect. The condition is dealt with in greater detail in Ch. 8.

THE BIOLOGICAL INTERPRETATION OF THE HISTOPATHOLOGICAL CHANGES IN MUSCULAR DYSTROPHY

The approach to the histopathology of diseased muscles is usually descriptive: changes observed consistently in a certain clinical condition come to be attributed to this condition and are then used as diagnostic criteria. Before the histopathology of the different forms of muscular dystrophy is described, I wish to define, predominantly on the basis of animal experiments, which of the histological features indicate or are the sequelae of necrosis and regeneration, or of degeneration and atrophy. The virtue of a biological interpretation of the morphology of dystrophic muscle is that a developmental order of abnormalities is established

and that the search for pathogenetic factors can concentrate on 'primary', that is, early, changes.

Necrosis and breakdown of muscle fibres

It is generally agreed that a dead muscle fibre can be identified by the fact that it is invaded by phagocytes digesting the remaining cell debris (see Figs 7.6, 7.11, 7.12). From cross-sections it is impossible to decide whether necrosis affects the entire fibre or only a segment. In many instances the length of the muscle fibre (up to 10 cm) and the large number of nuclei within it (30–50/mm fibre length) ensure that viable fragments of the fibre survive. They are sealed off by plasma membranes and, under favourable conditions, the gap produced by segmental necrosis is closed by fusing myoblasts derived from satellite cells (Church 1970).

Animal experiments and observations on diseased human muscle fibres suggest that at least two cellular mechanisms may lead to necrosis.

1. Localized defects of the plasma membrane and swelling of the sarcoplasmic reticulum initiate a segmental contracture with shortening and swelling of the muscle fibre, which may otherwise appear intact. During the initial phase, mitochondria appear normal. Experimentally, this type of necrosis is produced by physical injury and can follow intramuscular injection of detergents or local anaesthetics. In man, it is found shortly after acute attacks of myoglobinuria or malignant hyperthermia, and in Duchenne dystrophy (Schmalbruch 1973, 1975, Cullen & Fulthorpe 1975, Mokri & Engel 1975, Bradley & Fulthorpe 1978). The late stage of contracture is identical to the 'waxy degeneration' described by Zenker (1864) in typhoid fever (Figs 7.1, 7.2).

2. Myeloid bodies and autophagic vacuoles are formed inside muscle fibres and undergo exocytosis. In some fibres this leads to segmental necrosis, which is not initiated by membrane defects. Autophagocytosis with subsequent fibre necrosis is produced in rats by drugs such as chloroquine or chlorphentermine (MacDonald & Engel 1970, Drenckhahn & Lüllmann–Rauch 1976, 1979, Schmalbruch 1980) and may also be found in chronically denervated muscles. It does

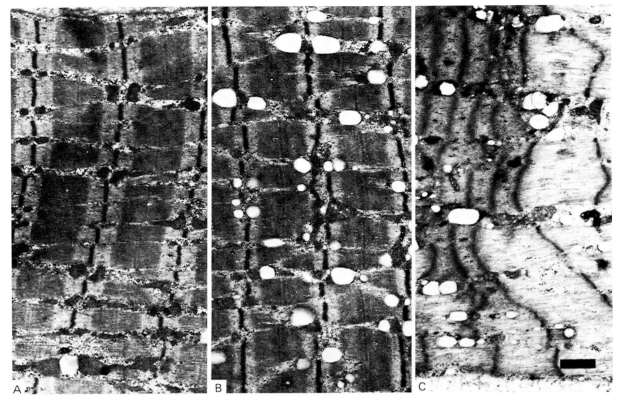

Fig. 7.1 Segmental fibre contracture in a 2-year-old boy with Duchenne dystrophy. EM; bar = 1 μm. (A) Normal fibre. (B) Early stage of contracture with swelling of the sarcoplasmic reticulum and moderate shortening of sarcomeres. (C) Excessive shortening of some sarcomeres and disruption of adjacent sarcomeres

not occur in Duchenne dystrophy, at least not in young patients from whom biopsies are usually obtained.

The final stages of both processes are identical; the plasma membrane of the muscle fibre vanishes within the necrotic segment, and myofilaments disintegrate into a fine granular substance which is kept together solely by the persisting basal lamina (Milhorat et al 1966). The fibre is then invaded by phagocytes. Satellite cells within necrotic fibre segments are intact. It is not known how excessive autophagocytosis and exocytosis lead to segmental necrosis of the muscle fibre. For fibres with defects of the plasma membrane, it has been suggested that calcium entering the sarcoplasm from the extracellular space acts as the 'molecular assassin' (Engel 1979). Segmentally hypercontracted fibres appear dense (hyaline fibres) (Fig. 7.2A) and stain

intensely with almost all histochemical stains, either because the enzyme concentration in the shortened fibre segment is high, or because the disintegrating myofilaments physically bind the reaction product.

Necrotic muscle fibres in idiopathic myoglobinuria and occasionally in inflammatory myopathies may contain IgG and the necrotic process may be the result of an antigen–antibody reaction. This is not the case in the muscular dystrophies. However, in all necrotic fibres in various disorders including Duchenne dystrophy the end-products of the complement pathways (classical or alternative) C3 and the membrane attack complex of complement (MAC) (C5b–9) are present. C3b and C5a, which are cleavage products of C3 and C5, attract neutrophils and macrophages and induce and facilitate phagocytosis (Engel & Biesecker 1982, Cornelio & Dones

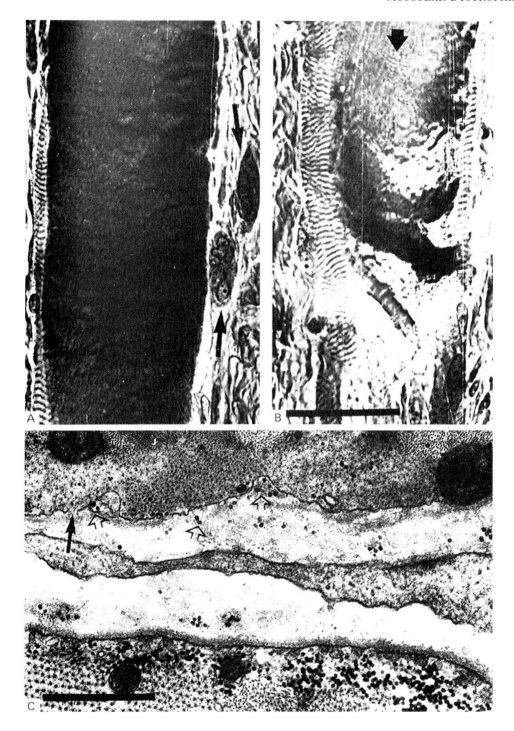

Fig. 7.2   (A,B) Fourteen-year-old girl with Duchenne-like dystrophy. Segmentally contracted fibres with new myotubes at the periphery. The myotubes have normal cross striations. In (A) myoballs (arrows); in (B) short sarcomeres within the contracted segment (arrow). Plastic sections, P-phenylenediamine, phase contrast; bar = 50 μm. (C) Ten-year-old boy with Duchenne dystrophy. Cross section of two fibres. The fibre below shows a normal sarcolemma; in the upper fibre there is a focal deficiency in the plasma membrane (arrow) and glycogen granules are present in the extracellular space (open arrows). EM; bar = 1 μm

1984). Complement activation in necrotic muscle fibres may be a secondary process induced by altered cell membranes.

In acutely injured rat muscles, necrotic fibre material is phagocytosed within 2–4 days, provided the blood supply remains intact. In view of the fact that the total duration of even the most progressive form of muscular dystrophy exceeds 10 years, it is no surprise that in a small biopsy sample relatively few fibres are encountered while being in the state of 'necrosis'.

Hypercontracted fibres may occur in normal biopsies which have been treated unsuitably. These artefacts are found almost exclusively at the periphery of the specimen. Contraction clots formed in vivo are invaded by phagocytes (Cullen & Fulthorpe 1975, Schmalbruch 1975); occasionally, thin myotubes with normal sarcomere spacing appear within the shortened fibre segment (Fig. 7.2A,B).

In Duchenne dystrophy defects of the plasma membrane occur not only in areas of segmental contracture, but also in fibres which are otherwise normal in appearance. These defects may be repaired before irreversible damage is done. Small defects are often not seen in the plane of sectioning but may be marked by the presence of glycogen granules in the extracellular space (Fig. 7.2C). Membrane defects are probably the cause of the increase in serum enzymes.

Sequelae of regeneration

In diseased muscles, regenerating fibres are identified by their basophilia indicating enhanced protein synthesis related to myofibrillogenesis (Mastaglia

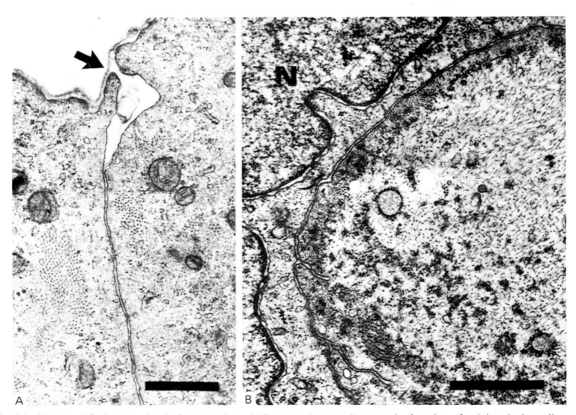

Fig. 7.3 Narrow clefts between developing myotubes. (A) Regenerating rat soleus muscle, four days after injury by hot saline. Two myotubes separated by a membrane-bound cleft within the persisting basal lamina tube of a necrotic fibre (arrow). EM; bar = 1 μm. (B) Seven-year-old boy with Duchenne dystrophy. Two myotubes within a common basal lamina. Myofilaments are sparse. N = nucleus. EM; bar = 1 μm

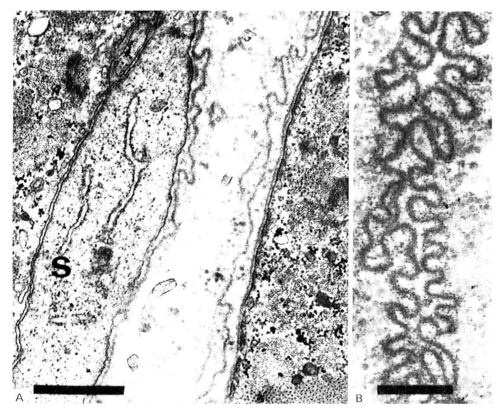

Fig. 7.4 Fourteen-year-old girl with Duchenne-like dystrophy. (A) Two regenerated fibres enclosed by the folded basal laminae of the necrotic fibres. The fibre on the right has already formed a new basal lamina attached to its plasma membrane. S = satellite cell. EM; bar = 1 μm. (B) Empty basal lamina tube of a lost fibre. EM; bar = 0.5 μm

et al 1970). In regenerating rat muscles, new fibres are basophilic during the first week only, whereas sequelae of regeneration may persist for several months or even permanently (Duchen et al 1974, Schmalbruch 1976b).

After fibre necrosis, satellite cells proliferate while phagocytosis is taking place (Fig. 7.6); they then fuse to form myotubes which remain enclosed by the persisting basal lamina of the lost fibre. One old basal lamina tube usually contains several myotubes separated by narrow gaps of about 20 nm (Fig. 7.3). In rat muscles, this stage is reached 4–5 days after an acute lesion. The young fibres form their own basal laminae, but the original basal laminae persist for weeks. Thus the basal laminae of regenerated fibres may appear to be reduplicated (Fig. 7.4A). The fibres within the same basal lamina either fuse laterally, often

incompletely, or begin to detach and the gaps between them become wider. Because the 20 nm gaps are not visible by light microscopy, separation of young myofibres may suggest that a cleft is formed within a large fibre that is undergoing longitudinal fission. If regeneration fails completely, the site of a lost fibre is marked by the collapsed and empty basal lamina tube (Fig. 7.4B). Failure of regeneration will lead to a progressive loss of muscle fibres.

When the cluster of young fibres grows, adjacent meshes of the endomysium in which regeneration is less advanced condense to form fibrous sheaths around this cluster of regenerated fibres. Often the fibres of a cluster remain moulded to each other, probably because the enclosing fibrous sheath prevents further separation. Although the formation of several fibres within a common basal lamina resembles fetal myogenesis, focal regeneration in an already existing endomysium rarely restores the normal muscle architecture but produces 'myopathic' changes: the fibres vary in diameter more than normal; many do not mature fully and retain internal nuclei; groups of fibres are enclosed by fibrous sheaths, and incomplete lateral fusion and detachment produces branched fibres and the impression of fibre 'splitting' (Figs. 7.5, 7.7, 7.8).

The successive development of myopathic changes after acute fibre necrosis has been observed not only in mouse (Duchen et al 1974) and rat muscles (Schmalbruch 1976b, 1977) but also in human muscle after an attack of paroxysmal myoglobinuria (Schmalbruch 1979).

Repeated cycles of necrosis and the formation of clusters of new fibres increasingly dissociate muscle fibres and endomysium and lead to 'fibrosis' (Fig. 7.8). This process is comparable to the development of pseudolobular hepatic cirrhosis. It is possible, but not proven, that the dissociation of parenchyma and stroma in muscle, as in liver, has a self-enhancing effect on the disease.

Fibre 'splitting' is not always a consequence of necrosis; satellite cells attached to damaged but surviving fibres may be induced to proliferate and fuse and to form short striated myotubes which remain adjacent to a large mature fibre (Fig. 7.9A). These 'satellite elements' are not innervated.

Young muscle cells that are not innervated and not subjected to stretch, acquire an ellipsoid shape and lose their cross-striations (Figs. 7.2A, 7.9B). Electron micrographs show myofilaments with the hexagonal array of thick and thin filaments, but no ordered myofibrils. Multinucleated muscle cells of this type are produced in tissue culture when fusing myoblasts are prevented from adhering to a surface. They have been termed 'myoballs' (Fischbach & Lass 1978). Myoballs are regularly found in regenerating muscles; in cross sections they may be mistaken for atrophic fibres (Fig. 7.9C).

Ringbinden are myofibrils running obliquely or transversely in relation to the longitudinal axis of the muscle fibre. These myofibrils probably deviate from their normal course because during myofibrillogenesis the fibre has been subjected to stretch deviating from the long axis of the fibre. Ringbinden are normally found in muscles which do not span two points of the skeleton (e.g. the tongue and pharyngeal muscles). They also occur after muscle regeneration (Duchen et al 1974) and are particularly abundant in regenerated minced muscles (personal observation). When an intact muscle fibre is cultured, it undergoes necrosis and its satellite cells form young fibres which grow in a spiral (Bischoff 1979). In diseased human muscles, ringbinden may consist of a few myofilaments or of mature-looking myofibrils complete with T-tubules and sarcoplasmic reticulum.

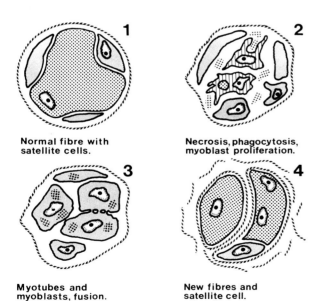

Normal fibre with satellite cells.

Necrosis, phagocytosis, myoblast proliferation.

Myotubes and myoblasts, fusion.

New fibres and satellite cell. Fibre "splitting", central nucleus reduplication of basal lamina.

Fig. 7.5 Scheme to illustrate the formation of new fibres within the basal lamina tube of a necrotic fibre. The number of satellite cells in (1) is exaggerated. Incomplete lateral fusion in (3) produces branching ('split') muscle fibres

Degeneration of muscle fibres

The term 'degeneration' originally described only those regressive alterations of a living cell that were reversible and did not inevitably lead to necrosis; as soon as degenerative changes inevitably caused necrosis, the process was called 'necrobiosis' (Virchow 1862). When it became clear that the morphological methods available

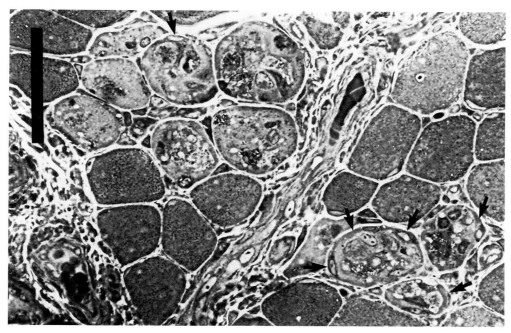

Fig. 7.6 Brachial biceps muscle of a 5-year-old boy with Duchenne dystrophy. Two groups of necrotic fibres invaded by phagocytes. Myoblasts are proliferating on the inner face of the old sarcolemma (arrows) (see Fig. 7.5). The connective tissue is increased. One central nucleus is visible (upper left corner). Plastic section, *p*-phenylenediamine, phase contrast; bar = 50 μm

were too crude to distinguish between degenerative and necrobiotic changes, the term 'degeneration' was used more indiscriminately. Nevertheless, in view of the wealth of information accumulated from electron-microscopic studies and tissue culture, the original definition has now regained its meaning and usefulness. For the sake of clarity, the terms degeneration and necrosis should not be confused. According to a modern definition, degeneration describes 'the morphological changes resulting from non-lethal injury to cells' whereas 'necrosis is the sum of the morphological changes caused by progressive degradative action of enzymes on the lethally injured cell' (Robbins 1974).

The best investigated degenerative change of muscle is that caused by denervation. The muscle fibre atrophies, the cross-striations become irregular, and Z lines show streaming. The fibre may survive as a living cell for months or even years, and may recover if it is re-innervated. In cross-sections the sarcolemma is scalloped and appears redundant (Fig. 7.10A). The following criteria distinguish atrophic fibres from thin regenerating fibres. Atrophic fibres are surrounded by a single leaflet of basal lamina material which runs parallel to the plasma membrane (Fig. 7.10A), whereas regenerating fibres are often enclosed by an extra leaflet formed by the folded residua of the basal lamina of the original necrotic fibre (Figs. 7.4A, 7.5). Denervated fibres are often band-like or angulated in cross-sections and usually appear dense because the relative amount of sarcoplasm is small; immature fibres are mostly round and appear light because they contain abundant sarcoplasm (Figs. 7.10B, 7.13). In denervated fibres, the nuclei are dense and usually situated beneath the sarcolemma; in immature fibres they appear vesicular, contain prominent nucleoli, and are often internally placed (Figs. 7.6, 7.11, 7.13). In a cross-section, atrophic fibres may show clusters of normal-looking or pyknotic nuclei. The primary cause of a neuromuscular disorder is often difficult to determine because denervation also activates satellite cells that may form new fibres; in myopathic muscles, too, regenerating fibres may fail to become innervated and finally develop features resembling those of denervated fibres.

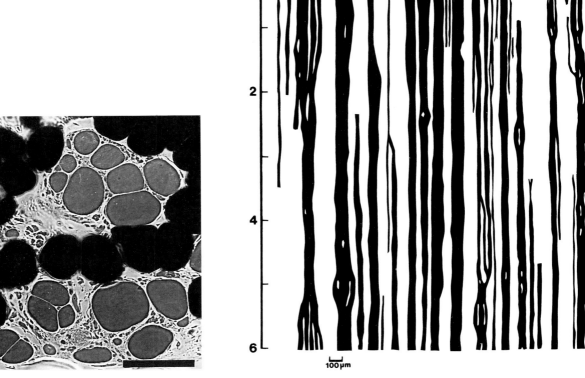

Fig. 7.7 Brachial biceps muscle of an eight-year-old boy with Duchenne dystrophy. (A) Cross section of a group of muscle fibres intermingled with fat cells (black). Plastic section, *p*-phenylenediamine, phase contrast; bar = 100 μm. (B) Longitudinal reconstruction of the muscle fibres shown in (A) from 1200 serial sections 5 μm thick. The fibres branch repeatedly and vary in cross-sectional area along their length. Several fibres or fibre branches end blind within the endomysium. It is not known whether the end-plate region is below or above the fibre segments studied, but it is obvious that, in any case, some of the thin fibres do not pass through the end-plate region and hence are not innervated. (With permission, from Schmalbruch 1984)

A degenerative change which differs from common denervation atrophy is seen in toxic myopathies caused by chloroquine or chlorphentermine (MacDonald & Engel 1970, Drenckhahn & Lüllmann-Rauch 1976, 1979, Schmalbruch 1980). Myeloid bodies appear within the sarcoplasm and, together with mitochondria, within autophagic vacuoles, which eventually undergo exocytosis. This type of degeneration may result in segmental necrosis of the muscle fibres with invasion of phagocytes and subsequent regeneration. Continued administration of chloroquine produces histopathological chaos, somewhat reminiscent of the picture seen in muscular dystrophy.

Autophagic vacuoles and myelin bodies often occur in oculopharyngeal dystrophy (Fig. 7.18); they are regularly found in an autosomal recessive form of distal myopathy (see page 286) and in inclusion body myositis. Also, chronically denervated muscles show autophagocytosis, which may eventually lead to muscle fibre necrosis. This explains why necrosis and sequelae of regeneration also occur to some extent in neurogenic disorders.

Myopathic changes and regeneration

The crucial issue in the biological interpretation of 'myogenic' lesions is the role of regeneration and the mechanism causing fibre 'splitting'. The fact that myopathic changes follow regeneration rather than degeneration stresses the importance of fibre

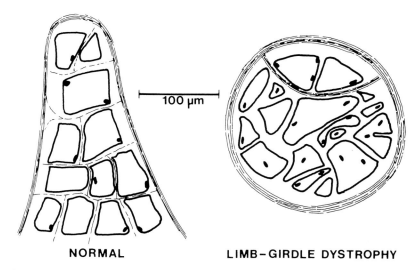

Fig. 7.8 Contours of muscle fibres, localization of myonuclei and array of connective tissue in a normal brachial biceps muscle and in the biceps muscle from a patient with limb–girdle dystrophy. The 'nodular' appearance of the fascicle in the dystrophic muscle is due to focal regeneration

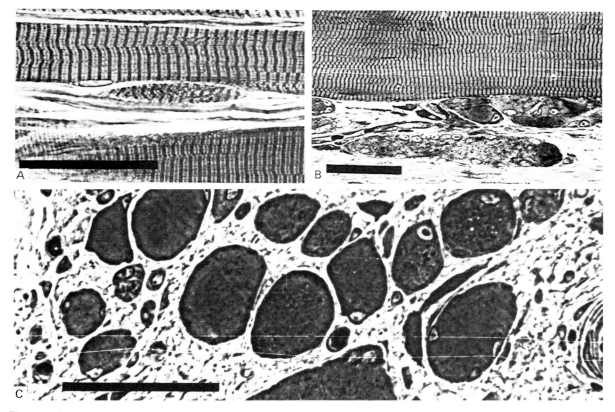

Fig. 7.9 Satellite elements and myoballs ('myogenic giant cells'). (A) Ten-year old boy with Duchenne dystrophy. A short satellite element (see Fig. 7.7) between normal-appearing fibres. Plastic section, *p*-phenylenediamine, phase contrast; bar = 50 μm. (B,C) Thirty-five-year-old woman with limb–girdle dystrophy. The longitudinal section shows multinuclear muscle cells ('myoballs') adjacent to an almost normal fibre. In cross-section, the myoballs resemble atrophic fibres. Plastic section, *p*-phenylenediamine, phase contrast; bars = 50 μm

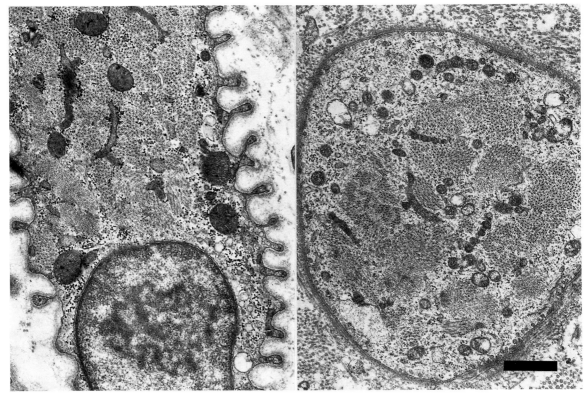

Fig. 7.10 Atrophic and immature fibres. (A) Sixty-year-old woman with a chronic polyradiculopathy. Typical long-term denervated fibre with redundant sarcolemma, densely-packed myofilaments and normal myonucleus. (B) Forty-nine-year-old man with limb–girdle dystrophy. Young myotube with few myofibrils and copious sarcoplasm. The cross-sectional profile is almost circular. EM; bar = 1 μm

necrosis, at least in those forms of muscular dystrophy that during the initial phase do not show degeneration in the strict sense. The interpretation of fibre 'splitting' given above (Schmalbruch 1976a,b, 1977, 1979, 1985) is in keeping with observations in overloaded rat muscles (James 1973), in individually cultured muscle fibres (Bischoff 1975), in several forms of toxic myopathy in the rat (Drenckhahn & Lüllmann-Rauch 1979) and with the generally accepted mechanism of fetal myogenesis (Kelly & Zacks 1969). It is, however, at variance with the traditional neuropathological interpretation (see Schwartz et al 1976) which maintains that mature muscle fibres can divide and that the central migration of subsarcolemmal myonuclei precedes the division of muscle fibres. Swash & Schwartz (1977) assume that, in myopathic and neurogenic lesions, some

muscle fibres hypertrophy and split to compensate for lost or inactive muscle fibres, and that this produces myopathic changes. No cytological evidence for the central migration of myonuclei and the division of muscle fibres has ever been presented, nor is it clear where the nuclei of the new fibres might come from, because myonuclei are postmitotic and do not divide.

THE HISTOPATHOLOGICAL CHANGES IN DIFFERENT FORMS OF MUSCULAR DYSTROPHY

Duchenne and Becker dystrophy

In *Duchenne dystrophy* (Figs. 7.11, 7.12) the scatter of fibre diameters is increased. The mean fibre diameter in very young patients may be greater

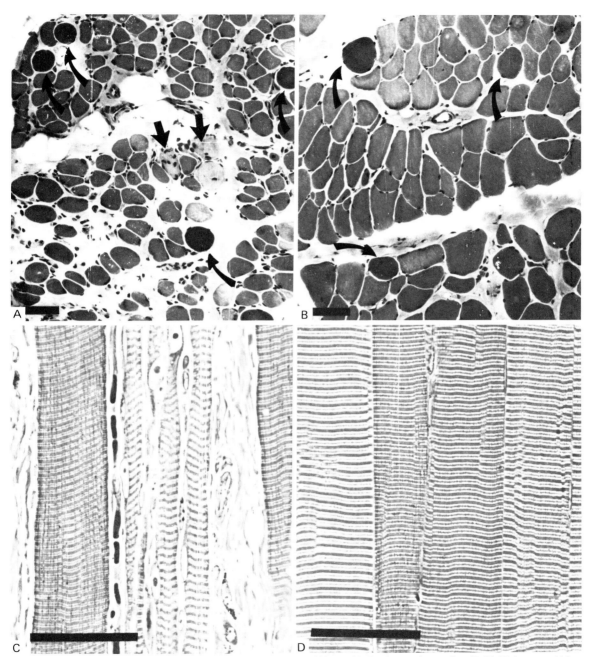

Fig. 7.11 Duchenne and Becker-type dystrophy. (A,C) Eight-year old boy with Duchenne dystrophy. (B,D) Eight-year-old boy with Becker-type dystrophy. (A,B) The scatter of fibre diameters is increased in both micrographs. In (A) necrotic fibres with phagocytes (arrows) and segmentally contractured fibres (curved arrows) are present; in (B) only segmentally contractured fibres (curved arrows) are shown; phagocytosis was seen in other parts of the biopsy. The architecture of the endomysium is changed more in (A) than it is in (B). 'Split' fibres are scarce in (A) but prominent in (B). Fat cells are present only in (A). (C,D) Intact sarcomeres in both micrographs, no Z-streaming or other degenerative changes. In (C), three young fibres with poorly aligned sarcomeres and large vesicular nuclei with prominent nucleoli are visible. (A,B) Frozen section, H&E; (C,D): plastic section, *p*-phenylenediamine, phase contrast, bars = 50 μm

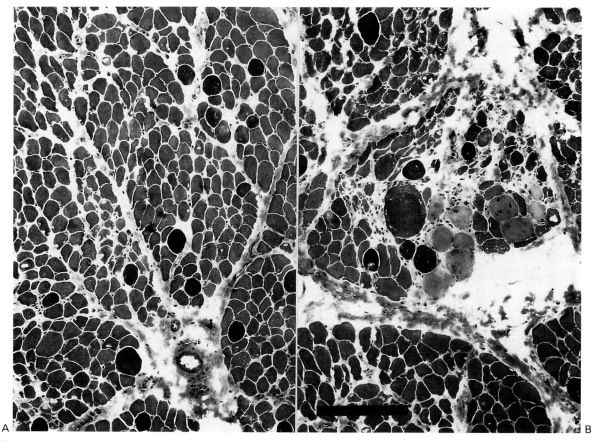

Fig. 7.12 Typical low-power micrographs of a biopsy from a 5-year-old boy with Duchenne muscular dystrophy. The muscle fibres vary in diameter and the amount of connective tissue is only moderately increased. The empty spaces in (B) are fat cells. Hyaline fibres (contractured fibre segments) (dark) are often larger than normal fibres, but they may also be of normal size. One hyaline fibre in (B) measures almost 100 μm in diameter. Several necrotic fibres with phagocytes in (B). Frozen section, H&E; bar = 200 μm

than normal, but it becomes smaller than normal as the disease progresses. Internal nuclei are more frequent than normal, but not very abundant. Necrotic fibres containing macrophages and some lymphocytes (usually T-lymphocytes (Engel & Arahata 1984)) are present in almost all biopsies. The necrotic fibres in cross-sections may appear singly or in small groups (Figs. 7.6, 7.12). Grouping of necrotic fibres probably reflects the fact that the fibres branch extensively (Fig. 7.7), and that all branches of a fibre are undergoing necrosis at the same time (Engel 1986). The occasional grouping of necrotic fibres has been misinterpreted in the past as indicating that Duchenne

dystrophy is due to functional impairment of the blood supply.

Most cross-sections through necrotic fibres do not show phagocytes. These necrotic fibres, which often but not always are larger than the adjacent fibres, and sometimes even larger than normal, are round and appear dense (opaque or hyaline fibres). Such cross-sectional profiles are almost pathognomonic for early Duchenne dystrophy. The affected fibres stain intensely with almost all enzyme histochemical procedures, and the interfibrillar network may be prominent, incomplete or absent. The reaction for calcium and for various complement components is positive (Bodensteiner & Engel

1978, Engel & Biesecker 1982, Cornelio & Dones 1984). Opaque fibres are locally contracted (Schmalbruch 1973, 1975, Mokri & Engel 1975, Lotz & Engel 1987) and are undergoing segmental necrosis (Figs. 7.1, 7.2, 7.11, 7.12). In sections stained with haematoxylin and eosin their incidence is underestimated because this stain may show a normal or near-normal appearance.

Electron micrographs reveal that dense fibre segments lack a plasma membrane and are enclosed by a basal lamina only (Milhorat et al 1966). In adjacent segments of the same fibre, sarcomere spacing is usually normal but the plasma membrane may show small focal defects (Mokri & Engel 1975, Schmalbruch 1975, Carpenter and Karpati 1979) through which glycogen granules are lost into the interstitial space (Fig. 7.2C). The sarcoplasmic reticulum is distended, whereas T-tubules and mitochondria appear normal (Fig. 7.1).

Segmental necrosis of muscle fibres activates satellite cells to form myoblasts. In Duchenne muscles they are two to three times more frequent than in normal muscles (Wakayama et al 1979). Satellite cells at the periphery of the basal lamina fuse to form young myofibres which may be seen among the necrotic material (Figs. 7.2a,b, 7.6). Thin myotubes apparently without tendon attachment and innervation often are only a few millimetres long, or, as satellite elements or myoballs, are even shorter (Figs. 7.2A, 7.8A). The gaps between the viable stumps of a segmentally necrotic fibre may be bridged by one or several strands of fusing myoblasts. Some of these strands connect only to one fibre stump and end blindly. After repeated cycles of necrosis and regeneration, many fibres branch and reunite; they vary in diameter, and many new myotubes end blindly and are presumably neither innervated nor attached to the tendons (Schmalbruch 1984) (Fig. 7.7). The functional value of such fibres is therefore questionable. Eventually regeneration fails. As the disease progresses, cross-sections show groups of fibres enclosed by sheaths of fibrous tissue and the normal fascicular architecture of the muscle is lost; an increasing number of fat cells appear between muscle fibres. The origin of the fat cells is unknown.

About 15% of the muscle fibres are of type 2C.

Interestingly, in serial sections, histochemical reactions characteristic for 2C fibres may be present in segments of a fibre which in other parts is either a type 1 or type 2 fibre. Type 2C fibres are immature and probably regenerating; the segmental staining pattern indicates repair of mature fibres that have undergone necrosis. There is no consistent change in the ratio of type 1 to type 2 fibres in Duchenne dystrophy (Nonaka et al 1981b).

The mean cross-sectional area of muscle fibres served by one capillary is normal (Jerusalem et al 1974a); in advanced cases the microvascular network is reduced and muscle fibres are separated from capillaries by fibrous tissue capsules (Lipton 1979). Single necrotic endothelial cells may be found in the late stages of dystrophy. The basal lamina of capillaries is occasionally reduplicated (Jerusalem et al 1974a, Koehler 1977, Lipton 1979), indicating that endothelial cells have undergone necrosis and regeneration.

The neuromuscular junctions of adjacent fibres are longitudinally dispersed over a distance of about 10 mm compared with 0.5 mm in normal muscle. The degree of branching of subterminal axons is normal, as is the morphology of terminal axons. Numerous nerve endings are 'unemployed' and end freely within the connective tissue (Cöers & Telerman-Toppet 1977). The number of postjunctional folds is smaller than normal, and the size of the postsynaptic area may exceed that of the terminal axon (Jerusalem et al 1974b, Harriman 1976).

The histopathological findings in *Becker dystrophy* vary (Fig. 7.11B). In scarcely or moderately affected muscles the changes resemble those in Duchenne dystrophy, except that each stage is reached at a later age. Hypercontracted fibre segments, necrotic fibres containing phagocytes (Markand et al 1969), and defects of the plasma membrane are found. In more advanced cases, the picture differs from that in Duchenne dystrophy as internal nuclei and 'split' fibres become more prominent (Ringel et al 1977, Bradley et al 1978, Kuhn et al 1979). Bradley et al (1978) also noted angulated fibres which, they assumed, indicated denervation. In several reports, small inflammatory infiltrates have been mentioned. However, the distinction between groups of phagocytes engaged in phagocytosis and perivascular infiltrates of lymphocytes and plasma cells is not always clear.

'At-risk' fetuses and preclinical Duchenne dystrophy

Investigations of fetuses suspected of being affected by Duchenne dystrophy, and of children during the preclinical stages of the disease, are rare. Several histological studies of fetuses (Emery 1977, Vassilopoulos & Emery 1977, Mahoney et al 1977) gave inconclusive results because of poor preservation of the muscle tissue. Hypercontracted fibre segments, distended sarcoplasmic reticulum and breaks of the plasma membrane were found. These changes might indicate prenatal breakdown of muscle fibres, but they may also be preparation artefacts. Measurement of the CK activity in placental blood samples is not reliable in deciding whether or not a fetus is affected; DNA linkage analysis is now the most reliable procedure for prenatal diagnosis (Rowland 1988). However, in future studies of aborted fetuses it will be possible to establish the diagnosis by testing for dystrophin (see page 311) by means of electrophoresis of muscle tissue (Western blot) (Patel et al 1988).

In three Duchenne patients aged 8 weeks, 12 months and 2 years, who were not yet clinically affected, Hudgson et al (1967) found gross histopathological abnormalities including hyaline fibres, fibre necrosis, regeneration and fibrosis. The serum CK activity was high in all three patients. In a boy 2½ weeks of age, the serum CK level was high, but the only abnormality in a biopsy was the presence of hyaline fibres; at the age of 3 years the child was still clinically normal, but a biopsy then showed changes typical of Duchenne dystrophy. In another boy studied at the age of 2 months, manifest histopathological changes were present (Bradley et al 1972).

Engel (1986) performed an electron microscopic study of muscle tissue from an 18-day-old boy with Duchenne dystrophy. Most muscle fibres appeared normal, but there were also hypercontracted fibres. Minimally affected fibres showed small plasma membrane defects, dilated sarcoplasmic reticulum, and a few degenerating mitochondria.

Carriers

Duchenne dystrophy is an X-chromosomal disorder which affects males. Statistically, the one defective X-chromosome in females will be active in half of the individual's nuclei. Because myofibres are syncytia derived from numerous mononucleated myoblasts, each myofibre in a female carrier will be a mosaic of normal and 'dystrophic' myonuclei. Only a few definite carriers show clear histopathological changes in muscle such as increased numbers of internal nuclei, increased scatter of fibre diameters, and segmentally hypercontracted and necrotic fibres. Muscle biopsy is therefore helpful in establishing the carrier state in only a few cases. Very few carriers (5–10%) develop a clinically manifest myopathy (Moser & Emery 1974, Barkhaus & Gilchrist 1989). Determination of serum CK activity under standard conditions has been until recently the most popular method for carrier detection. Detection rates of up to 80% have been reported (see Lane et al 1979, Walton & Gardner-Medwin 1981). Pedigree analysis and DNA linkage studies are now established procedures which, however, require that enough individuals of a kinship are available for testing. Since the identification of the coding sequence of the Duchenne gene and its gene product (dystrophin), the use of cloned dystrophin–cDNA probes has provided a more direct and powerful method for determination of carrier status and for the prenatal diagnosis of the disease (Darras et al 1988). Immunohistochemical studies in manifesting carriers have shown a mosaic pattern of dystrophin expression in muscle fibres (Arahata et al 1989) but, as yet, it is not known how useful such studies will be in confirming carrier status in clinically normal females.

The histogenesis of Duchenne dystrophy

Experimental necrosis of muscle fibres produced in animals gives rise to focal and often incomplete regeneration, resulting in myopathic changes (see p. 294). Increased scatter of muscle fibre diameters, internal nuclei, fibre branching, fibrosis with dissociation of muscle fibres and endomysium, and fibrous capsules around blood vessels in dystrophic muscles are sequelae of regeneration following segmental necrosis rather than of degeneration, atrophy or hypertrophy of previously normal mature fibres. The progressive deterioration of the muscle is due to repeated cycles of necrosis and regeneration, with decreasing efficiency of regeneration. Whether the inefficiency of regeneration reflects exhaustion of the proliferative capacity of the satellite cells, an increasing rate of necrosis, or impairment of regeneration because of fibrotic transformation of the muscle, is not known. Clusters of young fibres enclosed by fibrous sheaths are often poorly supplied by capillaries. Secondary impairment of the capillary supply of individual fibres is possibly one reason why more and more fibres undergo necrosis before maturing (Lipton 1979).

This hypothesis for the histogenesis of Duchenne and Becker dystrophy implies that they are necrotizing myopathies and that thin fibres are not atrophic. In very advanced cases, however, truly atrophic fibres may be found. Lack of innervation of immature fibres has been demonstrated by staining for extrajunctional acetylcholine receptors (Ringel et al 1976). Although the scatter of end-plates increases in dystrophic muscles, they remain concentrated in the middle of the muscle belly (Cöers & Telerman-Toppet 1977) and the branches of the motor axons do not reach all new fibres, which may be short and may not pass through the end-plate zone. Lack of innervation of immature fibres is one explanation for the electrophysiological finding of denervation changes in the electromyogram (Lang & Partanen 1976), the other possible cause being the functional isolation of viable parts of muscle fibres by segmental necrosis (Desmedt & Borenstein 1975). In Duchenne dystrophy, isolated fibre segments may be re-innervated by peripheral sprouts of motor nerve fibres (Desmedt & Borenstein 1973, 1976), but this is debatable (Cöers & Telerman-Toppet 1977).

Emery–Dreifuss muscular dystrophy

The histological picture resembles that seen in Becker dystrophy. As in Becker dystrophy, changes suggestive of a neurogenic process may be found. The most prominent features are random variation in fibre size, fibre branching, many internal nuclei, and fat infiltration. In a patient who died at the age of 50 from cardiac complications, Hara et al (1987) found pronounced fatty replacement of muscle fibres, particularly in the trapezius, brachial triceps, peroneal and anterior tibial muscles. The fibre composition of the motor nerves and the ventral roots was normal, and there was no evidence of motor neurone loss.

Limb–girdle muscular dystrophy

The histological picture depends on the stage of the disease. The mildest changes which suggest that the patient has a myopathy are a slightly increased scatter of fibre diameter and an increased number of internal nuclei. Branching of fibres is another abnormality that may occur at an early stage. When the muscle is more severely affected, more fibres appear to be 'split', the scatter of fibre diameters increases, and internal nuclei are more abundant. The diameter of fibres in cross-sections may exceed 200 μm or may be less than 10 μm; many small myofibres may not be identifiable as muscle cells under the light microscope. Groups of large and thin fibres are moulded together and enclosed by fibrous capsules which become more prominent as the disease progresses. Dense, hypercontracted fibre segments (hyaline fibres) and necrotic fibres containing phagocytes are often, but not always, encountered (Figs. 7.13–7.15); in individual patients the finding of necrotic fibres appears to be related to the rate of progression of the disease (Fig. 7.15). Light microscopy may also show clusters of small fibres lacking cross-striations (Fig. 7.9). Electron microscopy shows that these are very short fibres filled with disorganized myofilaments. These fibres correspond to 'myoballs' (or 'myogenic giant cells') and are presumably neither innervated nor connected to the tendon. Ringbinden are commonly found in severely affected muscles.

Histochemistry shows various non-specific abnormalities. In large fibres the distribution of mitochondria may be uneven; central areas may contain few, if any, mitochondria and may not stain for mitochondrial enzymes. In other cases, multiple foci lack reactivity for mitochondrial enzymes — 'moth-eaten' fibres (Fig. 7.13D). Also 'lobulated' fibres showing a peripheral rim of mitochondria with strands of mitochondria

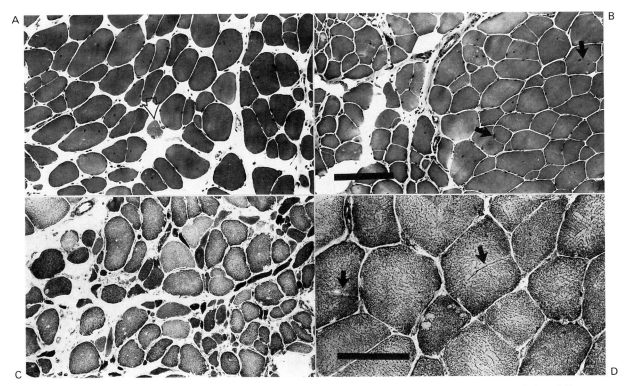

Fig. 7.13 Different parts of the biopsy from a 30-year-old woman with limb-girdle dystrophy. (A,B) Large variation of fibre diameters, branching ('split') fibres (arrow), central nuclei. One immature fibre is seen in (A) (open arrow). (C,D) Staining for a mitochondrial enzyme shows dark and light fibres; this staining pattern does not correspond to the fibre types seen in sections stained for ATPase. Many small regenerated fibres react intensely because the density of mitochondria is high. Two narrow clefts (see Fig. 7.16) (arrows) and a moth-eaten fibre are seen in (B). (A,B) Frozen sections, H&E; (C,D) frozen sections, reacted for NADH; bars = 200 μm (A–C) and 100 μm (D)

extending into the centre of the fibre are some-times seen and may be prominent in some cases (Fig. 7.14).

The fibre type distribution and the sizes of different histochemical fibre types vary between different biopsies and are of little diagnostic value. Fibres separated by a narrow cleft are often branches of the same fibre and therefore stain identically for metabolic enzymes and ATPase whereas if they were independent cells their staining properties might differ.

In 'split' fibres the clefts between fibres in cross-sections may be of two types: ~0.5 μm wide and bordered by two plasma membranes, each covered by a basal lamina, or 20 nm wide and bordered by plasma membranes alone. In cross-sections, both types of cleft may be complete or incomplete. Myonuclei are often found close to the plasma membranes bordering a cleft and sometimes lie, together with a strand of mito-chondria, in continuation of a blind-ending cleft. These myonuclei and mitochondria were originally subsarcolemmal and now mark the site of lateral fusion of young fibres. Light microscopy does not usually reveal the clefts 20 nm wide, but occa-sionally they can be identified as faint lines trans-versing large fibres (Figs. 7.15, 7.16). Satellite cells are frequently seen on fibres divided by clefts and are often situated at the openings of a cleft.

Limb–girdle muscular dystrophy in males may be indistinguishable clinically and histologi-cally from Becker dystrophy if there are no affected relatives. Duchenne dystrophy differs histopatho-logically from limb–girdle dystrophy, whereas the early stages of Becker dystrophy resemble Duchenne dystrophy. In each of the three forms,

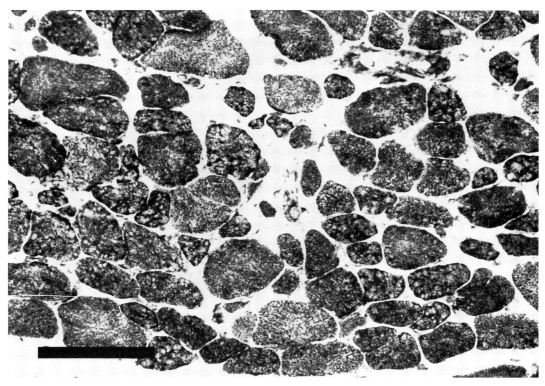

Fig. 7.14 Medial vastus muscle of a 50-year-old woman with limb–girdle dystrophy. Numerous 'lobulated' muscle fibres. Frozen section, stained for LDH; bar = 100 μm

hypercontracted fibre segments and necrosis occur and in each the serum CK activity is raised, least so in limb–girdle dystrophy. In none of the three forms do denervated or atrophic fibres occur during the early stages. Denervated atrophic fibres, though rare, may be found in the late stages, indicating failure of innervation of regenerated fibres.

Severe autosomal recessive limb–girdle dystrophy in children is histologically indistinguishable from Duchenne dystrophy. However, type 1 fibre preponderance has been reported in some cases (Salih et al 1983, Ben Hamida et al 1983). It may occasionally be difficult to differentiate Becker or limb–girdle dystrophy on the one hand and pseudodystrophic juvenile spinal muscular atrophy (Kugelberg–Welander disease) on the other. Histochemical fibre type preponderance in some fascicles, random variability in fibre diameters and hypertrophic fibres may be found in any of these diseases. Excessive fibre hyper-

trophy is more suggestive of Kugelberg–Welander disease, and fibre type grouping excludes a myopathy. However, fibre type preponderance may mimic type grouping, and it is essential for the diagnosis of type grouping to ensure that there are groups of both fibre types. Electromyography and testing for dystrophin are essential to establish the diagnosis in such cases.

Several families with autosomal dominant limb–girdle dystrophy with onset in early childhood and little if any progression have been described (page 285). Muscle biopsies in these cases often show pronounced myopathic changes (Fig. 7.17) with some features of both Duchenne and limb–girdle dystrophy.

Facioscapulohumeral dystrophy

In most cases the biopsy shows only moderate signs of myopathy such as an increased scatter of fibre diameters and an increase in the number of

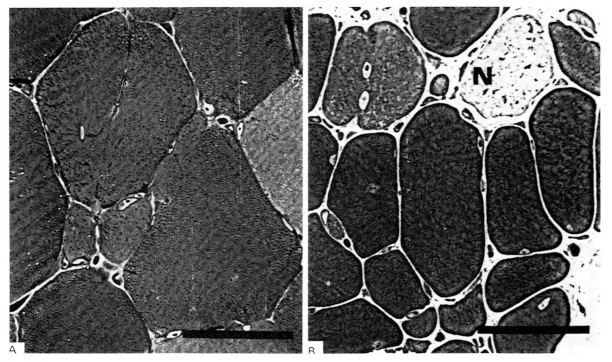

Fig. 7.15

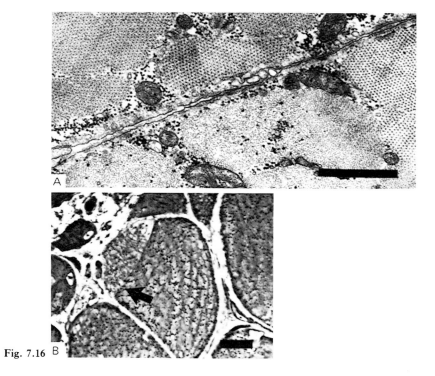

Fig. 7.16

internal nuclei. Fibre necrosis and hyaline fibres are sparse. Branching fibres may be present but are far less prominent than in limb–girdle dystrophy. Fibrosis is pronounced in severely affected muscles. In addition to these changes, which may also be present in other forms of dystrophy, thin angulated fibres and small inflammatory infiltrates are also often found. The angulated fibres differ from denervated fibres in that they do not stain intensely for mitochondrial enzymes (Dubowitz & Brooke 1973). In a patient with familial facioscapulohumeral dystrophy with moderately severe histopathological changes, these thin fibres were found to have normal cross-striations, the sarcolemma was folded, and in places the basal lamina formed pouches as if the fibre had retracted. This suggested that the fibres were atrophic, although this was probably not attributable to denervation. The moderately increased levels of muscle enzymes in serum and the occasional observation of hyaline and necrotic fibres suggest that facioscapulohumeral dystrophy is a necrotizing myopathy with a low rate of necrosis. However, this does not explain the peculiar atrophic fibres found in this condition.

Histochemistry shows a normal pattern of fibre types. Moth-eaten fibres are less frequent than in limb–girdle dystrophy. Bethlem et al (1973) found that 'lobulated' fibres, with a prominent rim of mitochondria that extends in short strands between the myofibrils, are particularly frequent in facioscapulohumeral dystrophy although not specific for this condition.

In 6 of 21 patients with facioscapulo-humeral dystrophy the muscle biopsy showed non-specific changes only (Buchthal & Kamieniecka 1982). Wulff et al (1982) observed a patient with facioscapulohumeral dystrophy and Coats' syndrome who, in three biopsies over a period of 13 years, consistently showed evidence of an inflammatory myopathy which did not respond to steroids.

Some patients with a facioscapulohumeral syndrome may in fact have polymyositis or a neurogenic disorder. In a family with several members affected with a facioscapulohumeral syndrome, Hudgson et al (1972) found a mitochondrial myopathy which would not have been diagnosed without histochemical and electron microscopic examination of muscle tissue.

Distal myopathy

Few muscle biopsies from patients with the classical Welander form of distal myopathy have been studied by histochemistry and electron microscopy (Markesbery et al 1974, 1977). Two patients, 76 and 68 years old, who belonged to the same kinship, were investigated during the terminal phase of the disease and at autopsy. Distal limb muscles consisted of fat and fibrous tissue with a few small muscle fibres, some of them angulated. In proximal muscles, necrotic fibres, often containing phagocytes, were found. Internal nuclei were frequent. Inflammatory infiltrates were absent. In both patients the heart muscle showed interstitial fibrosis. In one patient, loss of myelin in the spinal cord and in some ventral roots was observed. A third, moderately affected member of the same kinship was studied at the age of 48 years. A biopsy from the biceps brachii contained numerous necrotic fibres with phagocytes; the scatter of fibre diameters was increased and internal nuclei were frequent. Fibrosis was not severe. Histochemistry showed a tendency to fibre type grouping. Two sporadic cases (age 27 years, onset at the age of 20 years) showed essentially the same changes, and in one of the sporadic cases angulated fibres were also

---

Fig. 7.15 Limb–girdle dystrophy. Representative areas of the biopsies from the brachial biceps muscles of a 61-year-old (A) and a 50-year-old man (B). In both cases, affected relatives were known. One patient (A) was only moderately affected although the total duration of the disease was 35 years, and serum CK was at the upper limit of normal. The other patient (B) was severely affected; the duration was 15 years and the serum CK was three times the normal level. The scatter of fibre diameters was increased and hypertrophic fibres, internal nuclei, and fibre 'splitting' were present in both. In (B), one necrotic fibre is seen (N); the biopsy from the first patient (A) did not contain necrotic fibres. Plastic sections, p-phenylenediamine, phase contrast; bars = 50 μm

Fig. 7.16 Thirty-three-year-old man with limb–girdle dystrophy. Electron- and light-microscopical serial sections; bars 1 and 10 μm respectively. The arrow in (B) marks the area shown in (A). Narrow gap between two fibres bordered by plasma membranes ('splitting'), (see Figs 7.3, 7.5)

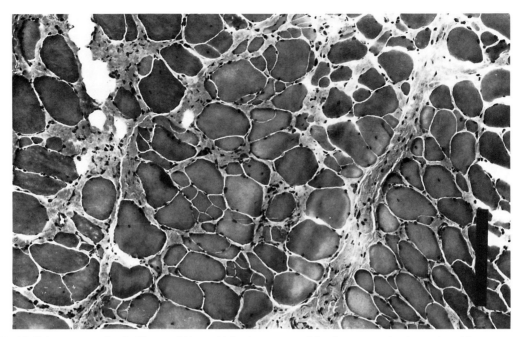

Fig. 7.17 Medial vastus muscle of a 13-year-old boy with benign autosomal dominant muscular dystrophy with humeropelvicoperoneal distribution of weakness (Schmalbruch et al 1987). Several members of the family, including the 80-year-old grandmother of the patient, are affected; all patients are ambulatory. The disease starts in early childhood and might be classified either as dominant limb–girdle dystrophy or as congenital dystrophy. The section shows pronounced histopathological changes which partly resemble Duchenne dystrophy and partly limb–girdle dystrophy. The biopsy also contained necrotic fibres (not shown) and the serum CK was 10 times the upper limit of normal. Frozen section, H&E; bar = 200 μm

present. The serum CK level was high in both sporadic cases but was normal or only slightly raised in the familial cases.

Electron microscopy revealed small defects in the plasma membrane even in fibre regions which did not appear necrotic, and reduplication of the basal lamina. Intact myotubes were present within necrotic segments of muscle fibres. Repeated undulations of the sarcolemma were occasionally seen in fibres that were angulated and appeared atrophic. In the familial cases, numerous fibres showed Z-band streaming and 'sarcoplasmic masses' (i.e. peripheral fibre regions containing randomly oriented myofilaments associated with mitochondria, glycogen granules and lipofuscin bodies). The most striking finding in all patients was the presence of large intracellular membrane-bound vacuoles which contained myeloid bodies, glycogen granules and membrane remnants and resembled autophagic vacuoles with signs of exocytosis.

The high incidence of necrotic fibres in proximal muscles, and the high level of CK activity

in the two sporadic cases indicate that these two patients had a necrotizing myopathy. The normal or almost normal serum CK activity in the familial cases is probably due to the slow course or the late stage of the disease. Nevertheless, the combination of atrophy and necrosis distinguishes distal myopathy from Duchenne and limb–girdle dystrophy. Large autophagic vacuoles do not occur in Duchenne dystrophy, while in limb–girdle dystrophy they are found only in the most severely affected muscles.

Autophagic vacuoles ('rimmed vacuoles') containing myeloid bodies are claimed to be typical for 'distal myopathy with rimmed vacuole formation', an autosomal recessive form of distal myopathy observed in Japanese patients. The vacuoles react strongly for acid phosphatase. Necrotic muscle fibres are lacking. Satellite cell numbers are normal and there are no signs of muscle fibre regeneration (Nonaka et al 1981a, 1985); this may account for the poor prognosis as to daily life (Sunohara et al 1989). In contrast, the histopathology of 'autosomal recessive distal muscular dystrophy' (Miyoshi et al 1986), also described in Japanese patients, resembles that of Duchenne and Becker dystrophy although progression is slow. Proximal limb muscles show hypercontracted fibres, phagocytosis, pronounced regeneration and numerous type 2C fibres. Rimmed vacuoles are not seen. The gastrocnemius muscle is most severely affected and is eventually replaced by fibrous and adipose tissue. The number of satellite cells is increased by a factor of 4 (Nonaka et al 1985).

While there is convincing evidence that these two disorders are different, the pathognomonic role of autophagocytosis may be questioned. Vacuoles containing myeloid bodies have been observed in American (Markesbery et al 1977) and Swedish (Thornell et al 1984) patients with the classical Welander form. Autophagocytosis occurs in other disorders as well, and is most prominent in inclusion body myositis. Inclusion body myositis and 'distal myopathy with rimmed vacuoles' may be histologically indistinguishable; even intranuclear filaments which are a prerequesite for diagnosing inclusion body myositis have been found in 'distal myopathy with rimmed vacuoles' (Sunohara et al 1989).

Ocular myopathies

An unknown number of disorders are covered by this term. The best-defined form genetically is that of oculopharyngeal dystrophy. Biopsies from extraocular muscles show fibrosis, increased scatter of fibre diameters and fibre loss. In proximal limb muscles, small angulated fibres which stain histochemically like denervated fibres, and fibres with vacuoles are present. Dubowitz & Brooke (1973) consider that these vacuoles are a prerequisite for the diagnosis. Internal nuclei are increased in number but are not usually abundant. Moth-eaten fibres are frequently encountered. Necrotic fibres and signs of regeneration are absent, and the serum level of CK activity is normal or, at most, at the upper limit of normal. A biopsy from the vastus muscle of a severely affected patient from a Swedish kinship with six affected members in two generations showed many angulated fibres reminiscent of denervation. Large vacuoles were found both in atrophic and normal-sized fibres (Fig. 7.18).

Tomé & Fardeau (1980) found intranuclear filaments 8.5 nm in diameter in biopsy specimens from several patients with oculopharyngeal dystrophy and consider this change to be specific. This has been confirmed by others (see Tomé & Fardeau 1986). Dr Tomé also found one such nucleus in the biopsy of our Swedish patient (Fig. 7.19). However, the incidence of affected nuclei in this patient must have been extremely small, and, even if the filaments are

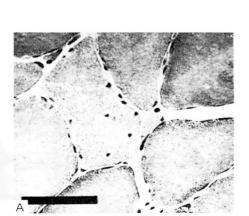
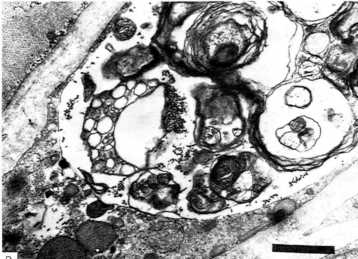

Fig. 7.18 Oculopharyngeal dystrophy in a 65-year-old woman of Swedish origin. The rimmed vacuole in (A) corresponds to an autophagic vacuole (B). (A) Frozen section, Gomori trichrome stain; bar = 50 μm; (B) EM; bar = 1 μm

specific, one can hardly exclude the diagnosis if no affected nuclei are found.

Another disorder causing ptosis and ophthalmoplegia which is possibly of myogenic origin is the ophthalmoplegia-plus syndrome, an abortive form of the oculocraniosomatic syndrome. This disease is characterized by a 'mitochondrial' myopathy and is described elsewhere (see Ch. 10).

Muscles from patients with pure ocular myopathy or dystrophy have been studied by routine methods only. The changes in extraocular muscles are non-specific. These muscles normally are most inhomogeneous with respect to fibre size and fibre types and differ from skeletal muscles (Schmalbruch 1985). Normal data for human material at different ages do not exist, and the histopathological criteria for myopathy or dener-

vation which are established for skeletal muscles are of little help. Many fibres of normal extra-ocular muscles resemble 'ragged-red fibres' and it is therefore difficult to make a diagnosis of a mitochondrial myopathy purely on the basis of histochemical findings.

Myotonic dystrophy

See Ch. 8

THE HISTOPATHOLOGICAL CLASSIFICATION OF MUSCULAR DYSTROPHIES

The different forms of muscular dystrophy have been established according to clinical criteria. On

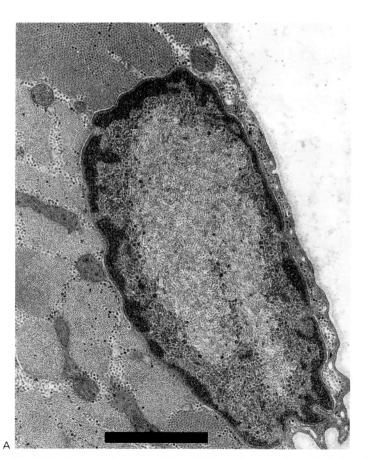
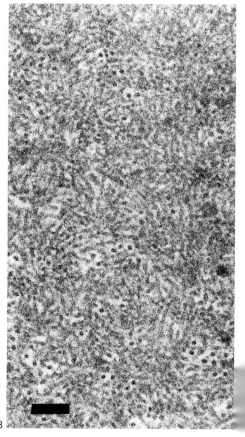

Fig. 7.19 Same specimen as in Figure 7.18. (A) A myonucleus with hollow filaments which are shown at higher magnification in (B). These filaments are assumed to be specific for oculopharyngeal dystrophy. EM; bars = 1 μm (A) and 0.1 μm (B). (Micrographs courtesy of Dr Tomé, INSERM, Paris)

the basis of the histological changes described, the muscular dystrophies may be classified into three main groups:

1. Primarily necrotizing myopathies characterized mainly by the non-specific sequelae of regeneration.

2. Necrotizing myopathies with morphological features that cannot be explained by necrosis and the sequelae of regeneration alone.

3. Myopathies which rarely, if ever, show signs of necrosis and regeneration.

Duchenne, Becker, Emery-Dreifuss and limb–girdle dystrophies are all necrotizing myopathies. Also 'autosomal recessive distal muscular dystrophy' (Miyoshi et al 1986) probably belongs to this group. Segmental necrosis is regularly found, and the level of CK activity in serum is increased, probably reflecting the extent of necrosis. Other changes can be explained, and can be reproduced in animal experiments, by focal necrosis followed by regeneration. Sequelae of regeneration are most prominent in advanced Becker dystrophy and in limb–girdle dystrophy.

Necrotic fibres may be found and the serum CK level is often moderately increased in facioscapulohumeral dystrophy and in the Welander type of distal myopathy. Nevertheless, atrophic fibres in both disorders indicate that these are not exclusively necrotizing myopathies. It is debatable whether fibre atrophy indicates that the motor neurone is affected. Autophagocytosis is pronounced in 'distal myopathy with rimmed vacuoles' and also in oculopharyngeal dystrophy. The process destroys the muscle fibres but not by means of segmental necrosis and the serum CK activity is normal or only mildly elevated.

Skeletal muscles from patients with the ophthalmoplegia-plus syndrome show the same intramitochondrial crystalloids which are present in the oculocraniosomatic syndrome; both are probably different expressions of the same disease. It is not known whether 'pure' ocular myopathy also belongs to this group. No recent cases have been studied by electron microscopy.

This attempt at a morphological classification is based predominantly on changes in muscles that are barely or moderately affected, because 'end-stage muscle disease' is similar in appearance whatever the cause. Those patients who have degenerative changes other than necrosis are the most difficult to classify.

THE DIAGNOSTIC APPROACH

Although the histological changes differ in the various forms of muscular dystrophy, it is rarely possible to classify a patient solely on the basis of these changes. Analysis of the biopsy specimen shows whether signs of necrosis, regeneration, or degeneration and atrophy prevail. The results have then to be related to the clinical picture and the case history.

Predominance of the sequelae of regeneration with discrete or no signs of necrosis indicates either that the process is long-lasting and slow, or that the muscle is recovering from an acute attack of fibre necrosis. A short history excludes muscular dystrophy. Predominance of atrophic and degenerative changes excludes Duchenne and limb–girdle dystrophy and, if ocular and facial symptoms are lacking, other forms of muscular dystrophy also, except distal myopathy.

In practically all biopsies from patients with myopathy the scatter of fibre diameters is greater than normal and the number of internal nuclei is increased. In normal human muscles the standard deviation of the mean diameter of muscle fibres never exceeds 20% of the mean value, and the number of fibres with internal nuclei in a cross-section is, at most, 1% (Kamieniecka, unpublished observations). The same maximum incidence of internal nuclei is given by Mastaglia et al (1969), whereas Dubowitz & Brooke (1973) accept up to 4% of fibres with internal nuclei as normal. The incidence of nuclei, and thus also of internal nuclei in cross-sections, depends on the thickness of the section and on the degree of shortening during fixation or freezing. Shortening also affects the diameter of the muscle fibres. This is a serious problem with needle biopsies because it is impossible to standardize the sarcomere length of the muscle fibres.

In most myogenic disorders the histogram of fibre diameters is unimodal and almost symmetrical, whereas in neurogenic disorders a bimodal or skew distribution is found (Reniers et al 1970). In advanced myotonic dystrophy, however, the distribution may be bimodal if type-2 hypertrophy and type-1 atrophy are pronounced (see Ch. 8). In Duchenne dystrophy one has to be aware of cross-sections through contracted and swollen fibre segments, which should not be mistaken for hypertrophic fibres. Data for fibre diameters in normal muscles of children have been reported by Oertel (1988); published data for normal adult muscles are reviewed in Schmalbruch (1985).

Whether fibrosis, fat cells, and architectural abnormalities of muscle fibres are present depends on the stage at which the biopsy is taken rather than on the particular type of dystrophy. However, some features are almost diagnostic for certain forms of dystrophy. Hypercontracted and swollen fibre segments in young males characterize Duchenne and Becker dystrophy, but also occur shortly after attacks of malignant hyperthermia, paroxysmal myoglobinuria, or acute alcoholic myopathy. Chains of internal nuclei with few other changes, or in combination with ring-binden, or in a muscle in which type 1 fibres are distinctly smaller than type 2 fibres, are suggestive of myotonic dystrophy. Cross-sections often look as if nuclei have been scattered from a salt-cellar on to the section. Excessive fibre branching is usually seen in limb–girdle dystrophy, but the same change may occur during the regenerative phase after acute muscle necrosis. Numerous thin angulated fibres suggest a neurogenic disorder rather than a myopathy; if a neuropathy is excluded by electrophysiological studies, facioscapulo-humeral or oculopharyngeal dystrophy should be considered. For oculopharyngeal dystrophy, large autophagocytotic vacuoles in otherwise normal-looking fibres are characteristic, but probably not diagnostic. These vacuoles stain blue with haematoxylin and red with the Gomori trichrome stain, at least at their periphery ('rimmed vacuoles'; Dubowitz & Brooke 1973). Very pronounced autophagocytosis occurs in some forms of distal myopathy, in some toxic myopathies (e.g. chloroquine myopathy), in inclusion body myositis, and occasionally in chronic progressive neuropathies. Ragged-red fibres identified by the Gomori trichrome stain or by staining for mitochondrial enzymes should make one suspect the ophthalmoplegia-plus syndrome.

'End-stage' muscles contain numerous fat cells and a large amount of connective tissue. Only a few muscle fibres are left, and these may show signs of denervation, necrosis or regeneration. To establish a diagnosis from such biopsies is difficult or impossible because denervated fibres may be regenerated fibres which have not been reinnervated or necrosis may be secondary to denervation.

In most laboratories, biopsies from patients who clinically do not fit one of the established forms of muscular dystrophy are encountered; the muscle, however, shows changes compatible with muscular dystrophy, and electrophysiological studies have excluded a neuropathy. After a carcinomatous myopathy or an endocrine myopathy have been excluded, three possibilities remain. First, the patient may be an atypical case of one of the established forms of dystrophy; secondly, the patient may have a form of chronic polymyositis, inflammatory infiltrates being absent or inconspicuous; thirdly, the patient may have a hitherto unknown type of myopathy. The diagnostic decision then has to be made on clinical grounds alone.

The situation with Duchenne and Becker dystrophy will probably change in the future (Gutmann & Fischbeck 1989) and muscle biopsies for histological examination alone in most cases may become obsolete. In about half of the patients DNA analysis discloses a gene deletion; this test can be done on a blood sample. If the disease in a family is found to be due to a deletion, prenatal diagnosis is possible with 100% certainty. If no deletion is found, or if the technique is not available, it is possible to demonstrate lack of dystrophin by the Western blot technique. This can be done on a small fragment of muscle tissue obtained by needle biopsy. However, immunohistochemistry is reported to be more sensitive than Western blotting (Gutmann & Fischbeck 1989) and there may still be some patients who will need an open surgical biopsy. It is tempting to perform immunohistochemical staining for dystrophin on needle biopsy specimens as well. However, given the harsh treatment of muscle tissue in many laboratories, this could cause confusion. Even in proper biopsies of non-fibrotic control muscles, the reaction varies considerably in different parts of a section. Different degrees of stretch, ice-crystal artefacts, and varying section thickness probably account for such inconsistencies. It may be dangerous to diagnose Duchenne dystrophy if the few fibre fragments in a needle biopsy of a fibrotic muscle do not react. The author has already learned of one case in which falsely negative dystrophin immunohistochemistry resulted in inappropriate genetic counselling.

CLUES TO THE PATHOGENESIS OF DUCHENNE AND BECKER DYSTROPHY

Recently the cellular defect in muscle fibres in Duchenne dystrophy has been characterized. The full coding sequence of the disease gene (Koenig et al 1987) and its gene product (Hoffman et al 1987a, Lev et al 1987) have been identified. The gene is in band 21 of the short arm of the X-chromosome and is 2000 kilobase pairs long, the coding sequence comprising 14 kilobases. The gene product, dystrophin, is a large (427-kDa, 3685-amino acid) rod-shaped (150 nm long) cytoskeletal protein which is expressed in myotubes and muscle fibres, both in culture and in vivo, in cardiac and smooth muscle and in the brain (Koenig et al 1988).

Dystrophin is present at low abundance in normal muscle and absent in skeletal muscles from boys with Duchenne dystrophy. Abnormal abundance or abnormal molecular weight of dystrophin was found in boys with Becker dystrophy (Hoffman et al 1987a, 1988, Patel et al 1988). Dystrophin was lacking in the muscles of four of six male fetuses aborted because they were at a high risk of having Duchenne dystrophy. The muscles from 16 patients with other forms of myopathy all contained normal amounts of dystrophin (Patel et al 1988).

With respect to amino acid sequence and also immunologically, dystrophin is related to the cytoskeletal proteins spectrin, non-muscle α-actinin, and a fast-twitch isoform of myofibrillar α-actinin (Hammonds 1987, Baron et al 1987, Davison & Critchley 1988, Hoffman et al 1989). All these proteins are rod-shaped but contain non-rodlike domains which are believed to form non-covalent interactions with other proteins, thus forming a linkage between bound proteins at each end of the central rod domain. α-Actinin binds F-actin via the N-terminal domain (Mimura & Asano 1986, 1987). Since there is considerable sequence homology shared between the non-rod-like terminal domains of cytoskeletal α-actinin and dystrophin (Hammonds 1987, Davison & Critchley 1988, Hoffman et al 1989), one might speculate that dystrophin also binds to F-actin. Dystrophin was originally localized to the triadic junctions (Hoffman et al 1987b, Knudson et al 1988), but immunohistochemistry and cytochemistry have now demonstrated that it is localized beneath the sarcolemma. Muscle fibres from patients with Duchenne dystrophy do not stain with antibodies against dystrophin; in Becker patients, only some fibres show spotty staining (Arahata et al 1988, Bonilla et al 1988, Zubrzycka-Gaarn et al 1988, Watkins et al 1988) (Fig. 7.20).

The characteristics of the dystrophin molecule and its localization close to the plasma membrane of the muscle fibre suggest that it maintains the mechanical stability of the cell membrane and connects the cytoskeleton of the fibre and probably also the Z-discs to the cell membrane. The dystrophin molecule possibly binds to spectrin as well. Spectrin links cytoplasmic actin to the cell membrane (Branton et al 1981, Repasky et al 1982). Segmental necrosis in Duchenne dystrophy starts with plasma membrane breaks (Mokri & Engel 1975, Schmalbruch 1975), and it appears reasonable to propose that lack of dystrophin reduces the mechanical stability of the membrane. Membrane breaks may result from contraction-induced strains on the membrane. There exists experimental evidence that eccentric contractions in normal animal and human muscles may damage the plasma membrane (Fridén 1983, Newham et al 1983a,b, McCully & Faulkner 1985, Maughan et al 1989). ('Eccentric contraction' means that the contracting muscle is stretched; this occurs when the muscle is inadvertently overloaded, but also when it is used to brake a movement.) Edwards et al (1984) hypothesize that muscular dystrophy affects predominantly proximal limb muscles because these muscles, more than others, are subjected to eccentric contractions during daily life. The progression of muscular 'dystrophy' in hamsters and mice can be prevented by immobilization (Karpati et al 1982, 1983, Loermans & Wirtz 1983, Wirtz et al 1986).

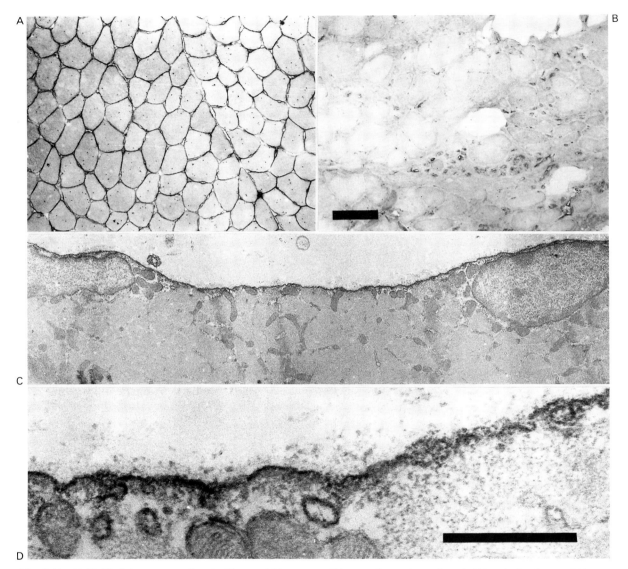

Fig. 7.20 (A,B) Medial vastus muscles of a 15-year-old boy susceptible to malignant hyperthermia (A) and of a 15-year-old boy with Duchenne muscular dystrophy with large gene deletion (B). Immunohistochemical reaction for dystrophin. Distinct staining of the surface of the muscle fibres is seen in (A) but not in (B). (B) was intentionally over-reacted and shows high background; the dark spots in the interstitial space indicate endogeneous peroxidase activity. (C,D) Muscle fibre of the soleus muscle of rat. Immunocytochemical staining for dystrophin. The reaction product is localized beneath the sarcolemma. (A,B) Frozen sections, indirect immunohistochemistry, HRP-labelling; bar = 100 μm. (C, D) EM, pre-embedding indirect immunocytochemistry, HRP-labelling, bars = 5 μm (C) and 0.5 μm (D). (The antibody (D10) against a fusion protein containing a fragment of the human dystrophin molecule was a gift of Dr Hoffmann, Boston. (C,D) Courtesy of Dr Bornemann, Department of Neuropathology, University of Mainz, FRG)

Karpati & Carpenter (1986) stress that thin muscle fibres are less susceptible to necrosis than thick fibres, possibly because the surface-to-volume ratio increases with decreasing fibre size, and they suggest that compensatory fibre hypertrophy is

detrimental in dystrophic muscles. Wirtz et al (1986) were able to prevent permanently the development of the dystrophic process by transiently immobilizing the muscles shortly after birth. This indicates that, at least in the mouse, the muscles are more susceptible to damage during the early period of growth.

The identification of dystrophin is a major step towards the understanding of Duchenne and Becker dystrophy, and testing for dystrophin in a small muscle sample by means of electrophoresis represents a diagnostic procedure which eventually may replace diagnostic muscle biopsies in Duchenne patients (Rowland 1988). The presumed role of dystrophin in the muscle fibre is in agreement with the 'membrane hypothesis' as based on morphological studies. This supports the notion that segmental fibre necrosis is the basic pathological event and that 'myopathic' or 'dystrophic' changes are nothing more than non-specific signs of imperfect regeneration (Schmalbruch 1979). The muscle fibres do not undergo 'degeneration' due to faulty or incomplete 'nutrition' ('dystrophy'). Theories based on an abnormal lipid structure of the membranes of myoblasts, myofibres, erythrocytes or lymphocytes and also the 'vascular hypothesis' and the 'neurogenic hypothesis' (for references, see first edition of this book) have all become obsolete. Most animal models of hereditary muscular 'dystrophy' have suffered the same fate. Only the X-linked muscular dystrophies in the mouse (mdx-mouse; Bulfield et al 1984), and in dogs (CXMD; Cooper et al 1988, Valentine et al 1988), are, like Duchenne dystrophy, characterized by lack of dystrophin (Hoffman et al 1987c).

The mdx-mouse shows most interesting features. The muscle fibres undergo necrosis and regenerate as in Duchenne dystrophy, but the disease shows little clinical progression (Torres & Duchen 1987, Cullen & Jaros 1988). The disease in dogs is a true phenotypic copy of Duchenne dystrophy. The cellular mechanism which in mice prevents muscle wasting even in the absence of dystrophin is obscure. One might speculate that other cytoskeletal proteins are produced in excess to compensate for the lack of dystrophin, or that the regenerative capacity of the muscle can counterbalance the loss of muscle fibres; it is also possible that in mice the stress which is imposed on the muscles during positive or negative accelerations, and which depends on the inertia of the limbs, is too small to cause permanent fibre damage. The fact that the disorder in the mdx-mouse is non-progressive, although the cellular defect is the same as in Duchenne dystrophy, may contribute to the development of a rational treatment for Duchenne patients. In this context, the rare non-progressive forms of muscular dystrophy in man (Fig. 7.17) are also of interest.

ACKNOWLEDGEMENTS

I wish to thank Mrs M Bjærg for technical help, and Dr Z. Kamieniecka for numerous discussions and for permission to photograph some of her preparations. My own work was supported by the Danish Medical Research Council and the Foundation for the Progress of Experimental Neurology.

REFERENCES

Arahata K, Ishiura S, Ishiguro T et al 1988 Immunostaining of skeletal and cardiac muscle surface membrane with antibody against Duchenne muscular dystrophy peptide. Nature 333: 861

Arahata K, Ishihara T, Kamakura K et al 1989 Mosaic expression of dystrophin in symptomatic carriers of Duchenne's muscular dystrophy. New England Journal of Medicine 320: 138

Arts W F, Bethlem J, Volkers W S 1978 Further investigations on benign myopathy with autosomal dominant inheritance. Journal of Neurology 217: 201

Bachmann H, Wagner A 1980 Myopathia distalis tarda hereditaria. Ergebnisse einer genealogischen, klinischen, klinisch-chemischen und elektromyographischen Familienuntersuchung. Psychiatrie, Neurologie und medizinische Psychologie 32: 20

Bailey R O, Marzulo D C, Hans M B 1986 Infantile facioscapulohumeral muscular dystrophy: new observations. Acta Neurologica Scandinavica 74: 51

Barkhaus P E, Gilchrist J M 1989 Duchenne muscular dystrophy manifesting carriers. Archives of Neurology 46: 673

Baron M D, Davison M D, Jones P, Critchley D R 1987 The sequence of chick alpha-actinin reveals homologies to spectrin and calmodulin. Journal of Biological Chemistry 262: 17 623

Bastiaensen L A K 1978 Chronic progressive external ophthalmoplegia. Stafleu Publishers, Alphen a/d Rhyn-Netherlands

Baumbach L L, Chamberlain J S, Ward P A, Farwell N J, Caskey C T 1989 Molecular and clinical correlations of deletions leading to Duchenne and Becker muscular dystrophies. Neurology 39: 465

Bautista J, Rafel E, Castilla J M, Alberca R 1978 Hereditary distal myopathy with onset in early infancy. Observation of a family. Journal of the Neurological Sciences 37: 149

Becker P E 1964 Myopathien. In: Becker P E (ed) Humangenetik. Ein kurzes Handbuch, vol 3. Georg Thieme, Stuttgart

Becker P E, Kiener F 1955 Eine neue X-chromosomale Muskeldystrophie. Archiv für Psychiatrie und Nervenkrankheiten 193: 427

Becker P E, Lenz F 1955 Zur Schätzung der Mutationstrate bei Muskeldystrophien. Zeitschrift für menschliche Vererbungs- und Konstitutionslehre 33: 42

Ben Hamida M, Fardeau M, Attia N 1983 Severe childhood muscular dystrophy affecting both sexes and frequent in Tunisia. Muscle and Nerve 6: 469

Bethlem J, van Wijngaarden G K 1976 Benign myopathy, with autosomal dominant inheritance. A report on three pedigrees. Brain 99: 91

Bethlem J, van Wijngaarden G K, De Jong J 1973 The incidence of lobulated fibres in the faciocapsulo-humeral type of muscular dystrophy and the limb–girdle syndrome. Journal of the Neurological Sciences 18: 351

Bischoff R 1975 Regeneration of single skeletal muscle fibers in vitro. Anatomical Record 182: 215

Bischoff R 1979 Tissue culture studies on the origin of myogenic cells during muscle regeneration in the rat. In: Mauro A (ed) Muscle regeneration. Raven Press, New York, p 13

Bodensteiner J B, Engel A G 1978 Intracellular calcium accumulation in Duchenne dystrophy and other myopathies: a study of 567 000 muscle fibers in 114 biopsies. Neurology (Minneapolis) 28: 439

Bonilla E, Samitt C E, Miranda A F et al 1988 Duchenne muscular dystrophy. Deficiency of dystrophin at the muscle cell surface. Cell 54: 447

Borg K, Borg J, Lindblom U 1987 Sensory involvement in distal myopathy (Welander). Journal of the Neurological Sciences 80: 323

Borg K, Solders G, Edström L, Kristensson K 1989 Neurogenic involvement in distal myopathy (Welander). Histochemical and morphological observations on muscle and nerve biopsies. Journal of the Neurological Sciences 91: 53

Bradley W G, Fulthorpe J J 1978 Studies of sarcolemmal integrity in myopathic muscle. Neurology (Minneapolis) 28: 670

Bradley W G, Hudgson P, Larson P F, Papapetropoulos T A, Jenkison M 1972 Structural changes in the early stages of Duchenne muscular dystrophy. Journal of Neurology, Neurosurgery and Psychiatry 35: 451

Bradley W G, Jones M Z, Fawcett P R W 1978 Becker-type muscular dystrophy. Muscle and Nerve 1: 111

Branton D, Cohen C M, Tyler J 1981 Interaction of cytoskeletal proteins on the human erythrocyte membrane. Cell 24: 24

Brooke M H, Fenichel G M, Griggs R C et al 1989 Duchenne muscular dystrophy: patterns of clinical progression and effects of supportive therapy. Neurology 39: 475

Buchthal F, Kamieniecka Z 1982 The diagnostic yield of quantified electromyography and qualified muscle biopsy in neuromuscular disorders. Muscle and Nerve 5: 265

Bulfield G, Siller W G, Wight P A L, Moore K J 1984 X chromosome-linked muscular dystrophy (mdx) in the mouse. Proceedings of the National Academy of Sciences of the United States of America 81: 1189

Carpenter S, Karpati G 1979 Duchenne muscular dystrophy. Plasma membrane loss initiates muscle cell necrosis unless it is repaired. Brain 102: 147

Caskey C T, Nussbaum R L, Cohan L C, Pollack L 1980 Sporadic occurrence of Duchenne muscular dystrophy: evidence for new mutation. Clinical Genetics 18: 329

Church J C T 1970 Cell quantitation in regenerating bat web muscle. In: Mauro A, Shafiq S A, Milhorat A T (eds) Regeneration of striated muscle, and myogenesis. Excerpta Medica, Amsterdam, p 101

Coërs C, Telerman-Toppet N 1977 Morphological changes of motor units in Duchenne's muscular dystrophy. Archives of Neurology (Chicago) 34: 396

Cooper B J, Winand N J, Stedman H et al 1988 The homologue of the Duchenne locus is defective in X-linked muscular dystrophy of dogs. Nature 334: 154

Cornelio F, Dones I 1984 Muscle fiber degeneration and necrosis in muscular dystrophy and other muscle diseases: cytochemical and immunocytochemical data. Annals of Neurology 16: 694

Cullen M J, Fulthorpe J J 1975 Stages in fibre breakdown in Duchenne muscular dystrophy. Journal of the Neurological Sciences 24: 179

Cullen M J, Jaros E 1988 Ultrastructure of the skeletal muscle in the X chromosome-linked dystrophic (mdx) mouse. Comparison with Duchenne muscular dystrophy. Acta Neuropathologica (Berlin) 77: 69

Dahlgaard E 1960 Myopathia distalis tarda hereditaria. Acta Psychiatrica et Neurologica Scandinavica 35: 440

Darras B T, Koenig M, Kunkel L M, Francke U 1988 Direct method for prenatal diagnosis and carrier detection in Duchenne/Becker muscular dystrophy using the entire dystrophin cDNA. American Journal of Medical Genetics 29: 713

Davison M D, Critchley D R 1988 Alpha-actinins and the DMD protein contain spectrin-like repeats. Cell 52: 159

Desmedt J E, Borenstein S 1973 Collateral innervation of muscle fibres by motor axons of dystrophic motor units. Nature 246: 500

Desmedt J E, Borenstein S 1975 Relationship of spontaneous fibrillation potentials to muscle fibre segmentation in human muscular dystrophy. Nature 258: 531

Desmedt J E, Borenstein S 1976 Regeneration in Duchenne muscular dystrophy. Electromyographic evidence. Archives of Neurology (Chicago) 33: 642

Drachman D A 1968 Ophthalmoplegia plus. The neurodegenerative disorders associated with progressive external ophthalmoplegia. Archives of Neurology (Chicago) 18: 654

Drenckhahn D, Lüllmann–Rauch R 1976 Myopathy in rats treated with chlorphentermine or iprindole. Virchows Archiv, B Cell Pathology 20: 343

Drenckhahn D, Lüllmann–Rauch R 1979 Experimental myopathy induced by amphiphilic cationic compounds including several psychotropic drugs. Neuroscience 4: 549

Dubowitz V, Brooke M H 1973 Muscle biopsy: a modern approach. Saunders, Philadelphia

Duchen L W, Excell B J, Patel R, Smith B 1974 Changes in motor end-plates resulting from muscle fibre necrosis and regeneration. A light and electron microscopic study of the effects of the depolarizing fraction (cardiotoxin) of Dendroaspis jamesoni venom. Journal of the Neurological Sciences 21: 391

Edström L 1975 Histochemical and histopathological changes in skeletal muscle in late-onset hereditary distal myopathy (Welander). Journal of the Neurological Sciences 26: 147

Edwards R H T, Newham D J, Jones D A, Chapman S J 1984 Role of mechanical damage in pathogenesis of proximal myopathy in man. Lancet i: 548

Emery A E H 1977 Muscle histology and creatine kinase levels in the foetus in Duchenne muscular dystrophy. Nature 266: 472

Emery A E H 1987 Duchenne muscular dystrophy. Oxford monographs on medical genetics, no. 15. University Press, Oxford

Emery A E H, Dreifuss F E 1966 Unusual type of benign X-linked muscular dystrophy. Journal of Neurology, Neurosurgery and Psychiatry 29: 338

Engel W K 1979 Dagen des Oordeels. Pathokinetic mechanisms and molecular messengers (a dramatic view). Archives of Neurology (Chicago) 36: 329

Engel A G 1986 Duchenne dystrophy. In: Engel A G, Banker B Q (eds) Myology. Basic and clinical, vol 2. McGraw-Hill, New York, p 1185

Engel A G, Arahata K 1984 Monoclonal antibody analysis of mononuclear cells in myopathies: II. Phenotypes of autoinvasive cells in polymyositis and inclusion body myositis. Annals of Neurology 16: 209

Engel A G, Biesecker G 1982 Complement activation in muscle fiber necrosis: demonstration of the membrane attack complex of complement in necrotic fibers. Annals of Neurology 12: 289

Fenichel G M, Sul Y C, Kilory A W, Blouin R 1982 An autosomal-dominant dystrophy with humeropelvic distribution and cardiomyopathy. Neurology 32: 1399

Fischbach G D, Lass Y 1978 Acetylcholine noise in cultured chick myoballs: a voltage clamp analysis. Journal of Physiology 280: 515

Fischbeck K H 1989 The difference between Duchenne and Becker dystrophies. Neurology 39: 584

Fridén J 1983 Exercise-induced muscle soreness. Umeå University Medical Dissertations. New Series no. 105. Umeå

Gilchrist J M, Perick-Vance M, Silverman L, Roses A D 1988 Clinical and genetic investigation in autosomal dominant limb–girdle muscular dystrophy. Neurology 38: 5

Gutmann D H, Fischbeck K H 1989 Molecular biology of Duchenne and Becker's muscular dystrophy: clinical applications. Annals of Neurology 26: 189

Haldane J B S 1935 The rate of spontaneous mutation of a human gene. Journal of Genetics 31: 317

Hammonds R G 1987 Protein sequence of DMD gene is related to actin-binding domain of alpha-actinin. Cell 51: 1

Hara H, Nagara H, Mawatari S, Kondo A, Sato H 1987 Emery–Dreifuss muscular dystrophy. An autopsy case. Journal of the Neurological Sciences 79: 23

Harriman D G F 1976 A comparison of the fine structure of motor end-plates in Duchenne dystrophy and in human neurogenic diseases. Journal of the Neurological Sciences 28: 233

Hoffman E P, Brown R H, Kunkel L M 1987a Dystrophin: the protein product of the Duchenne muscular dystrophy locus. Cell 51: 919

Hoffman E P, Knudson C M, Campbell K P, Kunkel L M 1987b Subcellular fractionation of dystrophin to the triads of skeletal muscle. Nature 330: 754

Hoffman E P, Monaco A P, Feener C C, Kunkel L M 1987c Conservation of the Duchenne muscular dystrophy gene in mice and humans. Science 238: 347

Hoffman E P, Fischbeck K H, Brown R H et al 1988 Characterization of dystrophin in muscle-biopsy specimens from patients with Duchenne's or Becker's muscular dystrophy. New England Journal of Medicine 318: 1363

Hoffman E P, Watkins S C, Slayter H S, Kunkel L M 1989 Detection of a specific isoform of alpha-actinin with antisera directed against dystrophin. Journal of Cell Biology 108: 503

Hudgson P, Pearce G W, Walton J N 1967 Pre-clinical muscular dystrophy: histopathological changes observed on muscle biopsy. Brain 90: 565

Hudgson P, Bradley W G, Jenkison M 1972 Familial 'mitochondrial' myopathy. A myopathy associated with disordered oxidative metabolism in muscle fibres. 1. Clinical, electrophysiological and pathological findings. Journal of the Neurological Sciences 16: 343

Jackson C E, Strehler D A 1968 Limb–girdle muscular dystrophy: clinical manifestations and detection of preclinical disease. Pediatrics 41: 495

James N T 1973 Compensatory hypertrophy in the extensor digitorum longus muscle of the rat. Journal of Anatomy 116: 57

Jerusalem F, Engel A G, Gomez M R 1974a Duchenne dystrophy. I. Morphometric study of the muscle microvasculature. Brain 97: 115

Jerusalem F, Engel A G, Gomez M R 1974b Duchenne dystrophy. II. Morphometric study of motor end-plate fine structure. Brain 97: 123

Kalimo H, Savontaus M-L, Lang H, Paljärvi L, Sonninen V, Dean P B, Katevuo K, Salminen A 1988 X-linked myopathy with excessive autophagy: a new hereditary muscle disease. Annals of Neurology 23: 258

Kamieniecka Z, Schmalbruch H 1980 Neuromuscular disorders with abnormal muscle mitochondria. International Review of Cytology 65: 321

Kamieniecka Z, Sjö O 1984 Mitochondrial myopathy as a cause of ptosis and ophthalmoplegia in elderly females. Acta Ophthalmologica 62: 401

Karpati G, Carpenter S 1986 Small-caliber skeletal muscle fibers do not suffer deleterious consequences of dystrophic gene expression. American Journal of Medical Genetics 25: 653

Karpati G, Carpenter S, Prescott S 1982 Prevention of skeletal muscle fiber necrosis in hamster dystrophy. Muscle and Nerve 5: 369

Karpati G, Armani M, Carpenter S, Prescott S 1983 Re-innervation is followed by necrosis in previously denervated skeletal muscles of dystrophic hamsters. Experimental Neurology 82: 358

Kearns T P, Sayre G P 1958 Retinitis pigmentosa, external ophthalmoplegia and complete heart block. Archives of Ophthalmology 60: 280

Kelly A M, Zacks S I 1969 The histogenesis of rat intercostal muscle. Journal of Cell Biology 42: 135

Kiloh L G, Nevin S 1951 Progressive dystrophy of external ocular muscles (ocular myopathy). Brain 74: 115

Knudson C M, Hoffman E P, Kahl S D, Kunkel L M, Campbell K P 1988 Evidence for the association of dystrophin with the transverse tubular system in skeletal muscle. Journal of Biological Chemistry 263: 8480

Koehler J 1977 Blood vessel structure in Duchenne muscular dystrophy. I. Light and electron microscopic observations in resting muscle. Neurology (Minneapolis) 27: 861

Koenig M, Hoffman E P, Bertelson C J, Monaco A P, Feener C, Kunkel L M 1987 Complete cloning of the Duchenne muscular dystrophy (DMD) cDNA and preliminary genomic organization of the DMD gene in normal and affected individuals. Cell 50: 509

Koenig M, Monaco A P, Kunkel L M 1988 The complete sequence of dystrophin predicts a rod-shaped cytoskeletal protein. Cell 53: 219

Kuhn E, Schröder J M 1981 A new type of distal myopathy in two brothers. Journal of Neurology 226: 181

Kuhn E, Fiehn W, Schröder J M, Assmus H, Wagner A 1979 Early myocardial disease and cramping myalgia in Becker-type muscular dystrophy: a kindred. Neurology (Minneapolis) 29: 1144

Kumamoto T, Fukuhara N, Nagashima M, Kanda T, Wakabayashi M 1982 Distal myopathy. Histochemical and ultrastructural studies. Archives of Neurology 39: 367

Lane R J M, Maskrey P, Nicholson G A et al 1979 An evaluation of some carrier detection techniques in Duchenne muscular dystrophy. Journal of the Neurological Sciences 43: 377

Lang A H, Partanen V S J 1976 'Satellite potentials' and the duration of motor unit potentials in normal, neuropathic and myopathic muscles. Journal of the Neurological Sciences 27: 513

Lipton B H 1979 Skeletal muscle regeneration in muscular dystrophy. In: Mauro A (ed) Muscle regeneration. Raven Press, New York, p 31

Lev A A, Feener C C, Kunkel L M, Brown R H 1987 Expression of the Duchenne's muscular dystrophy gene in cultured muscle cells. Journal of Biological Chemistry 262: 15 817

Little B W, Perl D P 1982 Oculopharyngeal muscular dystrophy. An autopsied case from the French-Canadian kindred. Journal of the Neurological Sciences 53: 148

Loermans H, Wirtz P 1983 Inhibition of the expression of pathology in dystrophic mouse leg muscles by immobilization. British Journal of Experimental Pathology 64: 225

Lotz B P, Engel A G 1987 Are hypercontracted muscle fibers artifacts and do they cause rupture of the plasma membrane? Neurology 37: 1466

McCully K K, Faulkner J A 1985 Injury to skeletal muscle fibers of mice following lengthening contractions. Journal of Applied Physiology 59: 119

MacDonald R D, Engel A G 1970 Experimental chloroquine myopathy. Journal of Neuropathology and Experimental Neurology 29: 479

Magee K R, De Jong R N 1965 Hereditary distal myopathy with onset in infancy. Archives of Neurology (Chicago) 13: 387

Mahoney M J, Haseltine F P, Hobbins J C, Banker B Q, Caskey C T, Golbus M S 1977 Prenatal diagnosis of Duchenne's muscular dystrophy. New England Journal of Medicine 297: 968

Markand O N, North R R, D'Agostino A N, Daly D D 1969 Benign sex-linked muscular dystrophy. Clinical and pathological features. Neurology (Minneapolis) 19: 617

Markesbery W R, Griggs R C, Leach R P, Lapham L W 1974 Late onset hereditary distal myopathy. Neurology (Minneapolis) 24: 127

Markesbery W R, Griggs R C, Herr B 1977 Distal myopathy: electron microscopic and histochemical studies. Neurology (Minneapolis) 27: 727

Mastaglia F L, Papadimitriou J M, Kakulas B A 1969 Restricted forms of muscular dystrophy: a study of 11 cases. Proceedings of the Australian Association of Neurologists 6: 107

Mastaglia F L, Papadimitriou J M, Kakulas B A 1970 Regeneration of muscle in Duchenne muscular dystrophy: an electron microscope study. Journal of the Neurological Sciences 11: 425

Matsunaga M, Inokuchi T, Onishi A, Kuroiwa Y 1973 Oculopharyngeal involvement in familial neurogenic muscular atrophy. Journal of Neurology, Neurosurgery and Psychiatry 36: 104

Maughan R J, Donnelly A E, Gleeson M, Whiting P H, Walker K A, Clough P J 1989 Delayed-onset muscle damage and lipid peroxidation in man after a downhill run. Muscle and Nerve 12: 332

Mawatari S, Katayama K 1973 Scapuloperoneal muscular atrophy with cardiopathy. An X-linked recessive trait. Archives of Neurology (Chicago) 28: 55

Medori R, Brooke M H, Waterston R H 1989 Genetic abnormalities in Duchenne and Becker dystrophies: clinical correlations. Neurology 39: 461

Meola G, Scarpini E, Velicogna M, Scarlato G, Larizza L, Fuhrman Conti A 1986 Cytogenetic analysis and muscle differentiation in a girl with severe muscular dystrophy. Journal of Neurology 233: 168

Milhorat A T, Shafiq S A, Goldstone L 1966 Changes in muscle structure in dystrophic patients, carriers and normal siblings seen by electron microscopy; correlation with levels of serum creatinephosphokinase (CPK). Annals of the New York Academy of Sciences 138: 246

Mimura N, Asano A 1986 Isolation and characterization of a conserved actin-binding domain from rat hepatic actinogelin, rat skeletal muscle, and chicken gizzard alpha-actinins. Journal of Biological Chemistry 261: 10 680

Mimura N, Asano A 1987 Further characterization of a conserved actin-binding 27-kDa fragment of actinogelin and alpha-actinins and mapping of their binding sites on the actin molecule by chemical cross-linking. Journal of Biological Chemistry 262: 4717

Miyoshi K, Kawai H, Iwasa M, Kusaka K, Nishino H 1986 Autosomal recessive distal muscular dystrophy as a new type of progressive muscular dystrophy. Seventeen cases in eight families including an autopsied case. Brain 109: 31

Mizusawa H, Kurisaki H, Takatsu M, Inoue K, Mannen T, Toyokura Y, Nakanishi T 1987a Rimmed vacuolar distal myopathy: a clinical, electrophysiological, histopathological and computed tomographic study of seven cases. Journal of Neurology 234: 129

Mizusawa H, Kurisaki H, Takatsu M, Inoue K, Mannen T, Toyokura Y, Nakanishi T 1987b Rimmed vacuolar distal myopathy. An ultrastructural study. Journal of Neurology 234: 137

Mohire M D, Tandan R, Fries T J, Little B W, Pendlebury W W, Bradley W G 1988 Early-onset benign autosomal dominant limb–girdle myopathy with contractures (Bethlem myopathy). Neurology 38: 573

Mokri B, Engel A G 1975 Duchenne dystrophy: electron microscopic findings pointing to a basic or early abnormality in the plasma membrane of the muscle fiber. Neurology (Minneapolis) 25: 1111

Moser H, Emery A E H 1974 The manifesting carrier in Duchenne muscular dystrophy. Clinical Genetics 5: 271

Murphy S F, Drachman D B 1968 The oculopharyngeal syndrome. Journal of the American Medical Association 203: 1003

Newham D J, McPhail G, Mills K R, Edwards R H T 1983a Ultrastructural changes after concentric and eccentric contractions of human muscle. Journal of the Neurological Sciences 61: 109

Newham D J, Jones D A, Edwards R H T 1983b Large delayed plasma creatine kinase changes after stepping exercise. Muscle and Nerve 6: 380

Nonaka I, Sunohara N, Ishiura S, Satoyoshi E 1981a Familial

distal myopathy with rimmed vacuole and lamellar (myeloid) body formation. Journal of the Neurological Sciences 51: 141

Nonaka I, Takagi A, Sugita H 1981b The significance of type 2C muscle fibers in Duchenne muscular dystrophy. Muscle and Nerve 4: 326

Nonaka I, Sunohara N, Satoyoshi E, Terasawa K, Yonemoto K 1985 Autosomal recessive distal muscular dystrophy: a comparative study with distal myopathy with rimmed vacuole formation. Annals of Neurology 17: 51

Oertel G 1988 Morphometric analysis of normal skeletal muscles in infancy, childhood and adolescence. An autopsy study. Journal of the Neurological Sciences 88: 303

Olson W, Engel W K, Walsh G O, Einaugler R 1972 Oculocraniosomatic neuromuscular disease with 'ragged-red' fibers. Histochemical and ultrastructural changes in limb muscles of a group of patients with idiopathic progressive external ophthalmoplegia. Archives of Neurology (Chicago) 26: 193

Patel K, Voit T, Dunn M J, Strong P N, Dubowitz V 1988 Dystrophin and nebulin in the muscular dystrophies. Journal of the Neurological Sciences 87: 315

Reniers J, Martin L, Joris C 1970 Histochemical and quantitative analysis of muscle biopsies. Journal of the Neurological Sciences 10: 349

Repasky E A, Granger B L, Lazarides E 1982 Widespread occurrence of avian spectrin in non erythroid cells. Cell 29: 821

Ringel S P, Bender A N, Engel W K 1976 Extrajunctional acetylcholine receptors. Alterations in human and experimental neuromuscular diseases. Archives of Neurology (Chicago) 33: 751

Ringel S P, Carroll J E, Schold S C 1977 The spectrum of mild X-linked recessive muscular dystrophy. Archives of Neurology (Chicago) 34: 408

Robbins S L 1974 Pathologic basis of disease. Saunders, Philadelphia

Rotthauwe H W, Mortier W, Beyer H 1972 Neuer Typ einer recessiv X-chromosomal vererbten Muskeldystrophie: Scapulo-humero-distale Muskeldystrophie mit frühzeitigen Kontrakturen und Herzrhythmusstörungen. Humangenetik 16: 181

Rowland L P 1988 Dystrophin. A triumph of reverse genetics and the end of the beginning. New England Journal of Medicine 318: 1392

Rowland L P, Fetell M, Olarte M, Hays A, Singh N, Wanat F E 1979 Emery–Dreifuss muscular dystrophy. Annals of Neurology 5: 111

Salih M A M, Omer M I A, Bayoumi R A, Karrar O, Johnson M 1983 Severe autosomal recessive muscular dystrophy in an extended Sudanese kindred. Developmental Medicine and Child Neurology 25: 43

Satoyoshi E, Kinoshita M 1977 Oculopharyngodistal myopathy. Report of four families. Archives of Neurology (Chicago) 34: 89

Schmalbruch H 1973 Contracture knots in normal and diseased muscle fibres. Brain 96: 637

Schmalbruch H 1975 Segmental fibre breakdown and defects of the plasmalemma in diseased human muscles. Acta neuropathologica (Berlin) 33: 129

Schmalbruch H 1976a Muscle fibre splitting and regeneration in diseased human muscle. Neuropathology and Applied Neurobiology 2: 3

Schmalbruch H 1976b The morphology of regeneration of skeletal muscles in the rat. Tissue and Cell 8: 673

Schmalbruch H 1977 Regeneration of soleus muscles of rat

autografted in toto as studied by electron microscopy. Cell and Tissue Research 177: 159

Schmalbruch H 1979 Manifestations of regeneration in myopathic muscles. In: Mauro A (ed) Muscle regeneration. Raven Press, New York, p 201

Schmalbruch H 1980 The early changes in experimental myopathy induced by chloroquine and chlorphentermine. Journal of Neuropathology and Experimental Neurology 39: 65

Schmalbruch H 1984 Regenerated muscle fibers in Duchenne muscular dystrophy: a serial section study. Neurology 34: 60

Schmalbruch H 1985 Skeletal muscle. Springer, Berlin

Schmalbruch H, Kamieniecka Z, Fuglsang-Frederiksen A, Trojaborg W 1987 Benign congenital muscular dystrophy with autosomal dominant heredity: problems of classification. Journal of Neurology 234: 146

Schwartz M S, Sargeant M, Swash M 1976 Longitudinal fibre splitting in neurogenic muscular disorders — its relation to the pathogenesis of 'myopathic' change. Brain 99: 617

Scrimgeour E M, Mastaglia F L 1984 Oculopharyngeal and distal myopathy. A case study from Papua New Guinea. American Journal of Medical Genetics 17: 763

Spiegler A W J, Hausmanowa-Petrusewicz I, Borkowska J, Herrmann F H 1987 Atypical form of X-linked proximal pseudohypertrophic muscular dystrophy. Journal of Neurology 234: 163

Stålberg E, Ekstedt J 1969 Signs of neuropathy in distal hereditary myopathy (Welander). Electroencephalography and Clinical Neurophysiology 26: 343

Sunohara N, Nonaka I, Kamei N, Satoyoshi E 1989 Distal myopathy with rimmed vacuole formation. A follow-up study. Brain 112: 65

Swash M, Schwartz M S 1977 Implications of longitudinal muscle fibre splitting in neurogenic and myopathic disorders. Journal of Neurology, Neurosurgery and Psychiatry 40: 1152

Tarkkanen A, Klemetti A 1973 Hereditary senile cataracts in distal late hereditary myopathy (myopathia distalis tarda hereditaria). Ophthalmologica 166: 441

Taylor E W 1915 Progressive vagus-glossopharyngeal paralysis with ptosis. A contribution to the group of family diseases. Journal of Nervous and Mental Disease 42: 129

Taylor D A, Carroll J E, Smith M E, Johnson M O, Johnston G P, Brooke M H 1982 Facioscapulohumeral dystrophy associated with hearing loss and Coats' syndrome. Annals of Neurology 12: 395

Thomas P K, Calne D B, Elliott C F 1972 X-linked scapuloperoneal syndrome. Journal of Neurology, Neurosurgery, and Psychiatry 35: 208

Thomas P K, Schott G D, Morgan-Hughes J A 1975 Adult onset scapuloperoneal myopathy. Journal of Neurology, Neurosurgery and Psychiatry 38: 1008

Thompson C E 1978 Reproduction in Duchenne dystrophy. Neurology 28: 1045

Thompson M W 1986 The genetic transmission of muscle diseases. In: Engel A G, Banker B Q (eds) Myology, basic and clinical, vol 1. McGraw-Hill, New York, p 1151

Thornell L-E, Edström L, Billeter R, Butler-Browne G S, Kjörell U, Whalen R G 1984 Muscle fibre type composition in distal myopathy (Welander). An analysis with enzyme- and immuno-histochemical, gel-electrophoretic and ultrastructural techniques. Journal of the Neurological Sciences 65: 269

Tomé F M S, Fardeau M 1980 Nuclear inclusions in

oculopharyngeal dystrophy. Acta neuropathologica (Berlin) 49: 85

Tomé F M S, Fardeau M 1986 Nuclear changes in muscle disorders. In; Jasmin G, Simard R (eds) Methods and achievements in experimental pathology, vol 12. Karger, Basel, p 261

Torres L F B, Duchen L W 1987 The mutant mdx: inherited myopathy in the mouse: morphological studies of nerves, muscles and end-plates. Brain 110: 269

Valentine B A, Cooper B J, De Lahunta A, O'Quinn R, Blue J T 1988 Canine X-linked muscular dystrophy. An animal model of Duchenne muscular dystrophy: clinical studies. Journal of the Neurological Sciences 88: 69

van der Does de Willebois A E M, Meijer A E F H, Simons A J R, Bethlem J 1968 Distal myopathy with onset in early infancy. Neurology (Minneapolis) 18: 383

van Wijngaarden G K, Bethlem J 1973 The facioscapulo-humeral syndrome. In: Kakulas B A (ed) Clinical studies in myology, Proceedings of the Second International Congress on Muscle Diseases, part 2. Excerpta Medica, Amsterdam, p 498

Vassilopoulos D, Emery A E H 1977 Muscle nuclear changes in fetuses at risk for Duchenne muscular dystrophy. Journal of Medical Genetics 14: 13

Victor M, Hayes R, Adams R D 1962 Oculopharyngeal muscular dystrophy. A familial disease of late life characterized by dysphagia and progressive ptosis of the eyelids. New England Journal of Medicine 267: 1267

Virchow R 1862 Vorlesungen über Pathologie. Erster Band: Die Cellularpathologie in ihrer Begründung auf physiologische und pathologische Gewebelehre. Dritte, neubearbeitete und vermehrte Auflage. Hirschwald, Berlin, p 297

Vita G, Dattola R, Santoro M, Messina C 1983 Familial oculopharyngeal muscular dystrophy with distal spread. Journal of Neurology 230: 57

von Graefe A 1866 Bemerkungen über doppelseitige Augenmuskellähmungen basilaren Ursprungs. Albrecht von Graefes Archiv für Klinische und Experimentelle Ophthalmologie 12: 265

Wakayama Y, Schotland D L, Bonilla E, Orecchio E 1979 Quantitative ultrastructural study of muscle satellite cells in Duchenne dystrophy. Neurology (Minneapolis) 29: 401

Walton J N, Gardner-Medwin D 1981 Progressive muscular dystrophy and the myotonic disorders. In: Walton J N (ed) Disorders of voluntary muscle, 4th edn. Churchill Livingstone, Edinburgh, p 481

Watkins S C, Hoffman E P, Slayter H S, Kunkel L M 1988 Immunoelectron microscopic localization of dystrophin in myofibres. Nature 333: 863

Welander L 1951 Myopathia distalis tarda hereditaria. Acta Medica Scandinavica 141 (suppl) 265: 1

Williams W R, Thompson M W, Morton N E 1983 Complex segregation analysis and computer-assisted genetic risk assessment for Duchenne muscular dystrophy. American Journal of Medical Genetics 14: 315

Wirtz P, Loermans H, Wallinga-de Jonge W 1986 Long-term functional improvement of dystrophic mouse leg muscles upon early immobilization. British Journal of Experimental Pathology 67: 201

Wulff J D, Lin J T, Kepes J J 1982 Inflammatory facioscapulohumeral muscular dystrophy and Coats' syndrome. Annals of Neurology 12: 398

Yasuda N, Kondo K 1980 No sex difference in mutation rates of Duchenne muscular dystrophy. Journal of Medical Genetics 17: 106

Zenker A 1864 Über die Veränderungen der willkührlichen Muskeln im Typhus abdominalis. Vogel, Leipzig

Zubrzycka-Gaarn E E, Bulman D E, Karpati G et al 1988 The Duchenne muscular dystrophy gene product is localized in sarcolemma of human skeletal muscle. Nature 333: 466

8. Myotonic disorders

Ikuya Nonaka   Eijiro Satoyoshi

INTRODUCTION

Myotonia is the phenomenon of delayed relaxation of muscle after strong voluntary contraction or mechanical or electrical stimulation. This phenomenon is believed to result from abnormal excitability of sarcolemmal, transverse tubular and sarcoplasmic reticular membranes due to a variety of mechanisms. The phenomenon cannot be reduced by blockade of peripheral nerve or of the neuromuscular junction. Myotonia is recognizable in various hereditary disorders and in some acquired conditions as shown in Table 8.1 (Harper 1986).

MYOTONIC DYSTROPHY (MYOTONIA DYSTROPHICA)

Myotonic dystrophy is the most common of the myotonic disorders, estimates of its prevalence ranging from 2.4 to 5.5 per 100 000 (Harper 1986). The clinical characteristics of this disorder including weakness of facial muscles, atrophy of the sternomastoid and limb muscles, and a slow relaxation of certain muscles after contraction (myotonia) had been described under various names in the early 1900s. Steinert (1909) and Batten and Gibb (1909) gave independent descriptions of patients who shared the common clinical symptoms, and suggested that the condition was a distinct clinical entity. The disease follows an autosomal dominant pattern of inheritance, and recent linkage analyses have assigned the locus to the long arm of chromosome 19 (Eiberg et al 1983, Shaw et al 1985, Hulsebos et al 1986, Brunner et al 1989, Korneluk et al 1989), though the precise

Table 8.1 The myotonic disorders

Hereditary	
Myotonic dystrophy	Autosomal dominant
Myotonia congenita	
Thomsen's disease	Autosomal dominant
Recessive (Becker) type	Autosomal recessive
With painful cramps	Autosomal dominant
Paramyotonia congenita	Autosomal dominant
Periodic paralysis	
Hypokalaemic	Autosomal dominant
Normo/hyperkalaemic (adynamia episodica)	Autosomal dominant
Chondrodystrophic myotonia (Schwartz–Jampel syndrome)	Autosomal recessive
Acquired	
Drug-induced	
Associated with malignancy	

From Harper (1986), with permission.

gene locus and the gene products have not as yet been identified.

In addition to the muscle symptoms of myotonia and weakness, there is also involvement of smooth muscle, cardiac muscle, central nervous and endocrine systems, the eye, bone, skin, respiratory organs, immune and haemopoietic systems. The topographic distribution of muscle weakness differs from that in the other muscular dystrophies. Facial muscle weakness (myopathic facies) and ptosis are frequently present for years before the diagnosis of myotonic dystrophy is made. Preferential neck (sternomastoid) muscle involvement sparing the posterior neck muscles is a characteristic and useful distinguishing feature in the differential diagnosis from facioscapulohumeral muscular dystrophy (Roses et al 1979, Harper 1986).

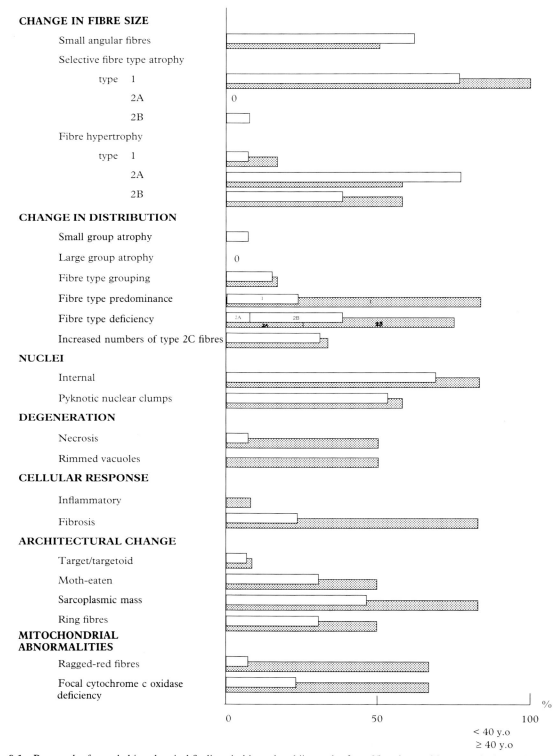

Fig. 8.1 Bar graph of muscle histochemical findings in biceps brachii muscles from 25 patients with myotonic dystrophy (13 patients less than 40 years of age and 12 over 40 years)

Muscle pathology

In all patients with the clinical characteristics of myotonic dystrophy, the biopsied muscles exhibit abnormal pathological findings with the exception of some in the very early stages with no muscle weakness in whom muscle morphology may be normal (Åström & Adams 1982). Since the onset of the disease and the degree of muscle involvement differ from patient to patient, the myopathological abnormalities do not necessarily correlate with age or duration of the disease. However, most patients have developed muscle weakness by 40 years of age when the muscle changes become evident. There is a good correlation between muscle weakness and morphological alterations in muscle rather than the severity of myotonia (Wohlfart 1951, Pongratz et al 1979, Grimby et al 1988). Therefore, our 25 patients (Fig. 8.1) were divided into two groups, the first consisting of 13 patients less than 40 years of age and the second comprising 12 patients over the age of 40 years, to determine how the muscle pathology advances.

Although topographic differences in muscle pathology and histochemistry are important because certain muscles such as the levator palpebrae, orbicularis oculi, masseter, perioral muscles, pharyngeal and sternomastoid muscles are preferentially involved, muscle biopsy study provides little information about the severity of the disease. Pongratz et al (1979) recommended the biceps brachii muscle for the site of muscle biopsy, because type 1 fibre atrophy, which is thought to be an early morphological sign of the disease, could be demonstrated only in proximal muscles, such as the biceps, whereas the tibialis anterior muscle showed a slight atrophy of both fibre types. In our patients, all specimens were obtained from the left biceps brachii muscle.

Changes in fibre size

From the early stages of the disease, the most common finding is an excessive variation in the calibre of muscle fibres which ranged from 10 to 150 μm in one study (Adams & Rebeiz 1966) and from 7 to 195 μm in another (Engel & Brooke 1966). Scattered small angulated fibres which are usually stained darkly with the non-specific esterase stain are also found (Fig. 8.2A). Although these fibres have similar histochemical characteristics to those seen in neurogenic atrophy, they are nearly always type 1 fibres and probably do not result from a denervating process.

Even in the early stages of the disease, when there is no muscle weakness, there is variation in type 1 and 2 fibre sizes, usually with type 1 fibre atrophy (Fig. 8.2A–D) (Brooke & Engel 1969, Dubowitz 1973, 1987, Pongratz et al 1979, Casanova & Jerusalem 1979). In rare instances there is atrophy of both fibre types. Type 1, 2A and 2B fibres are distributed in a normal mosaic pattern in less affected muscles, except for some biopsies in which type 2B fibres are deficient (Fig. 8.2C, D). Hypertrophy of either type 2A or 2B fibres, or both, can be recognizable from the early stages (Fig. 8.2C, D). Type 1 fibre hypertrophy is exceptional. Although atrophic type 1 fibres are occasionally aggregated, there is no grouping of atrophic fibres of the type seen in denervated muscles.

Fibre type grouping, including some fascicles consisting entirely of type 1 fibres may occur (Fig. 8.2E) but there is no type 2 fibre grouping.

Since type 1 fibres are preferentially involved from the early stages in this disorder, one might expect to see type 2 fibre predominance in the advanced stages of the disease. Contrary to expectations, type 1 fibres become predominant with decreased numbers of type 2A and 2B fibres with age (Borg et al 1987) (Fig. 8.2F). In most patients over 40 years of age, type 1 fibres predominate, usually comprising more than 70%; in three of our patients more than 90% of fibres were of type 1. To explain this contradictory result, one must consider the possibility of an active transformation from type 2 to type 1 fibres (Borg et al 1987, Grimby et al 1988). Therefore, it seems that type 1 fibres transformed from type 2 fibres in this disorder are not normal type 1 fibres either structurally or histochemically (Borg et al 1987). An increased number of undifferentiated type 2C fibres (up to 19%) supports the contention of an active fibre type transformation (Grimby et al 1988).

The type 2C fibres are undifferentiated fibres which may subsequently differentiate into type 1, 2A or 2B fibres (Brooke et al 1971). They are seen

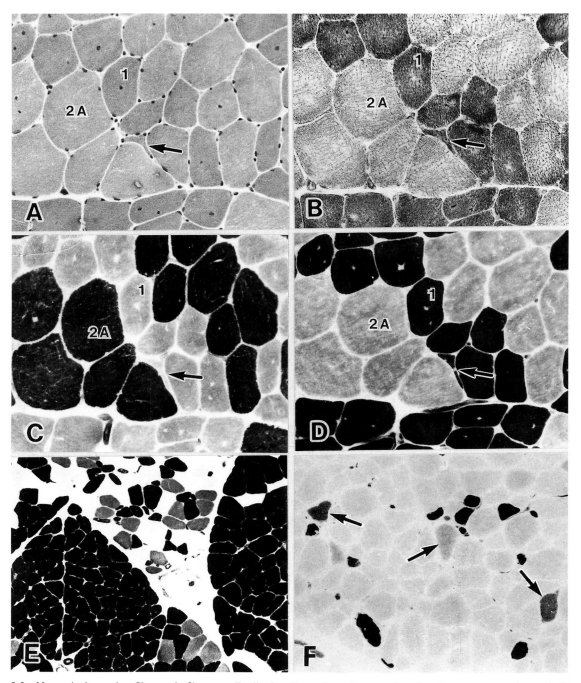

Fig. 8.2 Myotonic dystrophy. Changes in fibre type distribution. From the early stage when there is no muscle weakness (A–D), there is a variation in fibre size with scattered small angular fibres (arrow), type 1 (1) fibre atrophy and type 2A (2A) fibre hypertrophy. Type 2B fibre deficiency, as commonly seen in the advanced stage, is already recognizable. The centrally placed nuclei are predominantly seen in type 1 fibres. Fibre type grouping, consisting of type 1 fibres (E), and fibre type predominance (F) can be seen in the advanced stages. Type 2C fibres (arrow) are increased in number. Fourteen-year-old male (A–D); 63-year-old male (E); 41-year-old male (F). A, H&E; B, NADH–TR; C, routine ATPase; D, ATPase with pre-incubation at pH 4.6; E, same at pH 4.2, F, routine ATPase. A–D (serial sections) ×190, E ×65, F ×110

in fetal muscle, diseased or injured muscle with active fibre necrosis and regeneration (Nonaka et al 1981a), or in denervation when there is an active re-innervating process whereby muscle fibres are transformed from one fibre type to another via type 2C fibres: type 1 → 2C → 2; or type 2 → 2C → 1 (Brooke et al 1971). As there is little muscle fibre necrosis and little evidence of a demyelinating process in intramuscular nerves in myotonic dystrophy, it is likely that a large number of type 2C fibres in this disorder represent type 2 fibres which are undergoing transformation to type 1 fibres. Abnormal electrical stimuli (myotonia) and/or an abnormal neural influence on muscle fibres may be responsible for the fibre type transformation. A progressive decrease of type 2B fibres and a concomitant increase of type 2A and type 1 fibres were also well demonstrated in an experimentally induced myotonia in the rat (Salviati et al 1986).

Type 2B fibre deficiency in myotonic dystrophy may also result from transformation of type 2B to 2A fibres as has been suggested in myotonia congenita and paramyotonia congenita (Heene 1986). In conclusion, in myotonic dystrophy, type 2B fibres appear to be transformed into type 2A fibres, which are subsequently transformed into type 1 fibres resulting in marked type 1 fibre predominance.

Nuclear changes

The finding of increased numbers of 'internally placed nuclei' or 'central nuclei' is a striking finding in myotonic dystrophy (Adie & Greenfield 1923, Wohlfart 1951, Adams & Rebeiz 1966, Åström & Adams 1982). In the early stages, the central nuclei are seen predominantly in atrophic type 1 fibres when examined in cross-section (Fig. 8.3A). The myonuclei increase in number as the disease progresses; multiple centrally placed nuclei appear in almost all type 1 and 2 fibres. The nuclei are larger than normal and hyperchromatic with occasional prominent nucleoli. On longitudinal section, they are often arranged end-to-end in long rows which may extend over many sarcomeres (nuclear chains) (Fig. 8.3B). The centrally placed nuclei are usually not euchromatic but are found to contain large amounts of hetero-

chromatin on electron microscopy (Fig. 8.3C). The nuclear membrane is irregularly indented. The perinuclear zone is occasionally devoid of myofibrils where glycogen particles, ribosomes, proliferated sarcotubular structures and lipofuscin granules are present. In cross-sections, the myofibrils around centrally placed nuclei may be radially orientated as seen in myotubular myopathy.

The morphogenesis of an increased number of myonuclei, which are frequently present in the central portion of the sarcoplasm remains unknown. Central nuclei are found in diseased muscles in which active muscle fibre regeneration is occurring after fibre necrosis as in the progressive muscular dystrophies and polymyositis. The central nuclei in myotonic dystrophy are increased in number from the early stages of the disease when no necrotic and regenerating process is evident. Accordingly the central nuclei in myotonic dystrophy are not the result of fibre necrosis and regeneration. Although the central nuclei in myotubular (centronuclear) myopathy are mostly single nuclei in fibres in cross-section, the ultrastructural findings are very similar to those seen in myotonic dystrophy. Since the myonuclei are not capable of division, an increased number of myonuclei is thought to be supplied from satellite cells located between the sarcolemma and basal lamina (Vassilopoulos & Lumb 1980). Although no statistical analysis of satellite cell populations in biopsied muscles from patients with myotonic dystrophy has been attempted, there are 3.3 times as many satellite cells per myofibre nucleus in myotonic mice than in controls (Schimmelpfeng et al 1987).

When the fibres with increased numbers of nuclei undergo atrophy, the atrophic fibres come to be filled with nuclei forming 'pyknotic nuclear clumps' (Fig. 8.3A). The ultrastructural features of these nuclei are similar to those of centrally placed nuclei (Fig. 8.6B). The myofibrils in such atrophic fibres are disorganized and decreased in number (Fig. 8.6B).

Degenerative changes

Muscle fibre necrosis is less frequent in myotonic dystrophy than in the other progressive muscular

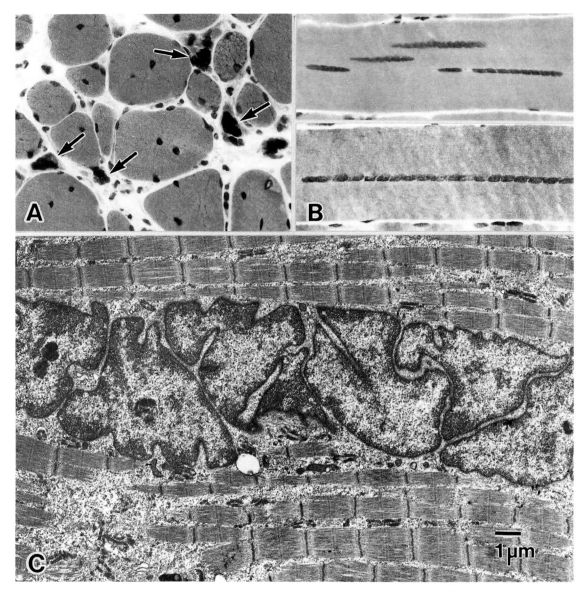

Fig. 8.3   Myotonic dystrophy. Nuclear changes. In addition to marked variation in fibre size and mild interstitial fibrosis, the myonuclei are increased in number with numerous internally placed nuclei and pyknotic nuclear clumps (arrow) (A). They are arranged in long rows placed end-to-end in longitudinal section (B), and are irregular in shape with marked indentation (C). Forty-seven-year-old male. A, B, H&E; A ×450, B, ×400, C, electron micrograph

Fig. 8.4   Myotonic dystrophy. Degenerative changes. In the advanced stage there appear some necrotic fibres undergoing phagocytosis (asterisk) in which myofibrillar detail has disappeared and organelles are aggregated (NF)(B). There is no relationship between sarcoplasmic mass formation (SM) and the necrotic process. Focal myofibrillar degeneration followed by an autophagic phenomenon forming occasional rimmed vacuoles (C,D) is an additional degenerative process inducing muscle fibre atrophy and fibre loss (E). Note empty sarcolemmal tubes (arrowheads) and numerous autophagic vacuoles (arrow) (E), and cytoplasmic bodies (arrows) (D). Forty-six-year-old female (A–D); 52-year-old female (E). A, C; H&E, D, modified Gomori trichrome. A ×190, C, D (serial sections) ×500; B, E, electron micrographs

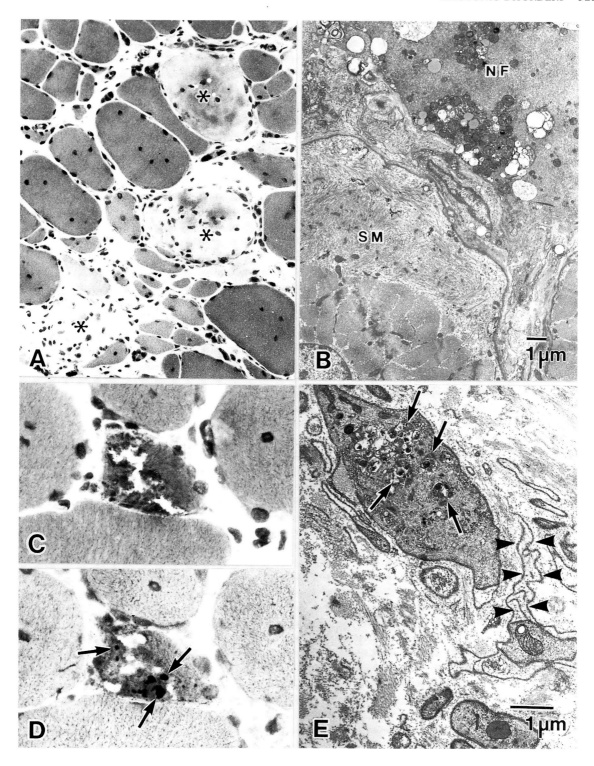

dystrophies. Fibre necrosis with occasional phagocytosis followed by regeneration becomes slightly more prominent in the advanced stages of the disease (Fig. 8.4A, B). The necrotic fibres are scattered, not in groups as in other muscular dystrophies and polymyositis. Fibre necrosis is segmentally distributed in a single fibre (Silver et al 1983), similar to that seen in Duchenne muscular dystrophy (Cullen & Fulthorpe 1975, Schmalbruch 1975).

Focal myofibrillar degeneration is a striking finding in myotonic dystrophy, predominantly in atrophic fibres. The degenerated material is then digested by lysosomal vacuoles, which subsequently form myelin (myeloid) bodies. The areas with such active autophagic phenomena are demonstrated as rimmed vacuoles on frozen sections (Fig. 8.4C, D) (Fukuhara et al 1980, Nonaka et al 1981b). The vacuoles are rimmed by fine granules which are basophilic with haematoxylin and eosin, and purple red in colour with the modified Gomori trichrome stain. Increased acid phosphatase activity in most atrophic fibres also suggests an activated state of lysosomes. Numerous autophagic vacuoles can be seen in degenerated atrophic fibres on electron microscopy (Fig. 8.4E). The end-products are either converted into lipofuscin granules or extruded on to the sarcolemmal surface (Åström & Adams 1979, 1982). A marked increase in lipofuscin granules in muscle fibres from the early stages of disease suggests that focal myofibrillar degeneration is taking place. The extrusion to the surface may disrupt the continuity of the muscle fibres resulting in a fibre which is split, serrated or subdivided where connective tissue and capillaries seem to invade into the surface indentation (Wohlfart 1951, Samaha et al 1967, Schröder and Adams 1968, Schröder & Becker 1972, Casanova & Jerusalem 1979, Åström & Adams 1982).

Cellular response

Inflammatory cell infiltration is exceptional and mild and probably represents a reactive phenomenon to fibre necrosis. As the disease progresses, a large proportion of the total fibre population is lost and replaced by densely proliferated connective tissue and fat cells. When the muscle fibre has completely disappeared, remnants of basal lamina (empty sarcolemmal tubes) are scattered in the fibrotic areas (Fig. 8.4E) (Wechsler & Hager 1961). The small blood vessels surrounded by connective tissue are reduced in internal diameter and their lumens are narrowed (Åström & Adams 1982).

Architectural changes

Disorganized intermyofibrillar networks demonstrated on oxidative enzyme stains are seen in a number of fibres. A moth-eaten appearance is the most common finding (Fig. 8.5B). The areas of moth-eaten structure show focally degenerated myofibrils with loss of cross-striation on electron microscopy.

The presence of numerous fibres with 'sarcoplasmic masses' is a striking and diagnostic finding for myotonic dystrophy (Fig. 8.5A). Sarcoplasmic masses are regions in a muscle fibre in which myofibrils have been disorganized, reduced in numbers and partly replaced by PAS-positive and high oxidative enzyme material (Fig. 8.5B). The mass is therefore not a completely degenerated region like a necrotic segment invaded by macrophages, but an area of focal myofibrillar degeneration. They are mostly located in the subsarcolemmal zones and rarely in the deep sarcoplasm (Fig. 8.5A). The mass sometimes occupies the entire subsarcolemmal zone so that the concentric band of homogeneous cytoplasm surrounds a core of normal-looking myofibrils on cross section. In longitudinal section, the masses may extend along the whole length of the fibre (Åström & Adams 1982).

Sarcoplasmic masses can also be seen in various other neuromuscular disorders but are not as prominent and extensive as in myotonic dystrophy. In a biopsy described by Schröder and Adams (1968), 98% of the fibres had sarcoplasmic masses. Although sarcoplasmic masses are predominantly seen in the advanced stages, this tends to differ from muscle to muscle. They were present in all muscles examined postmortem in one reported patient, with a frequency ranging from 0.2% in the vastus lateralis to 53% in the extensor digitorum longus muscle (Adams & Rebeiz 1966).

Since the fibres with sarcoplasmic masses are

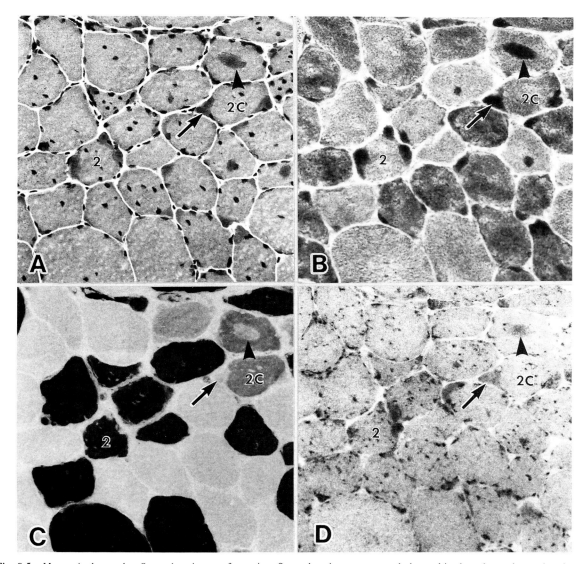

Fig. 8.5 Myotonic dystrophy. Sarcoplasmic mass formation. Sarcoplasmic masses, mostly located in the subsarcolemmal region (arrows), and rarely in the deep sarcoplasm (arrowheads), are stained basophilic on H&E (A), and darkly with NADH–TR (B); they are seen predominantly in type 1 fibres (C). In this picture, type 2 (2) fibres also have the masses. Type 2C (2C) fibres are increased in number. Thirty-one-year-old male. A, H&E; B, NADH–TR; C, routine ATPase; D, acid phosphatase. A–D (serial sections) ×250

usually atrophic type 1 fibres (Fig. 8.5C), the mass formation is closely related to muscle fibre atrophy in this disorder. In addition, the masses have an increased acid phosphatase activity (Fig. 8.5D) suggesting an active autophagic phenomenon scavenging degenerate myofibrils in these areas.

On electron microscopy, the masses contain sparse disoriented myofibrils, aggregates of mitochondria, glycogen particles, occasional lipofuscin granules, ribosomes, lysosomal vacuoles and myelin bodies (Fig. 8.6A, B).

Abnormalities in sarcotubular and sarcolemmal membranes are described by several authors

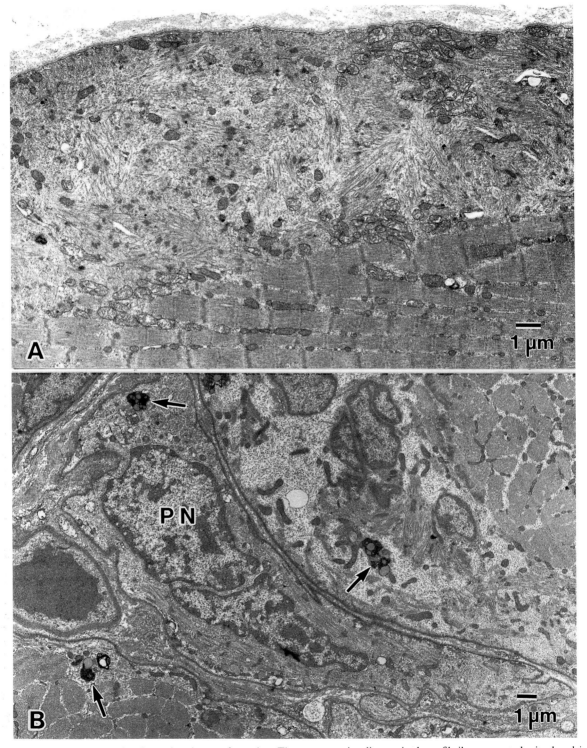

Fig. 8.6 Myotonic dystrophy. Sarcoplasmic mass formation. The mass contains disorganized myofibrils, aggregated mitochondria (A), and increased amounts of glycogen and lipofuscin granules (arrow) (B). Lipofuscin granules are also increased in an atrophic fibre with a pyknotic nuclear clump (PN), and a normal-appearing fibre below (B). Seventeen-year-old male. A, B, electron micrographs

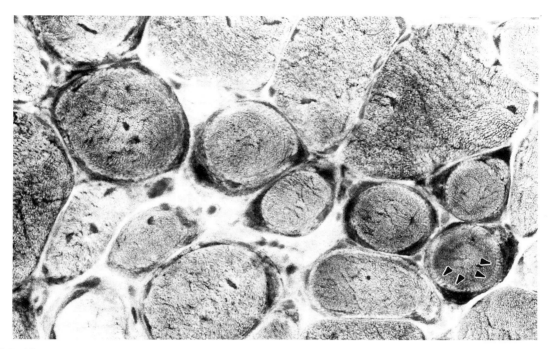

Fig. 8.7 Myotonic dystrophy. Ring fibres. The ring fibres are recognizable at higher frequency in the field where numerous sarcoplasmic masses are present. Note circumferential ring myofibrils (arrowheads) oriented at right angles to the long axis of the muscle fibre. Fifty-year-old male. PAS, ×450

(Samaha et al 1967, Schröder & Adams 1968, Schröder & Becker 1972). Even in fibres with a normal myofibrillar structure, the sarcoplasmic reticulum may be swollen and proliferated (Mussini et al 1970, Schotland 1970), forming peculiar geometric arrangements of terminal cisternae (Schröder & Adams 1968, Schröder & Becker 1972). The transverse tubules are also markedly proliferated forming honeycomb structures which range from 0.2 × 0.2 μm to 1.5 × 4.9 μm in size (Schotland 1970, Casanova & Jerusalem 1979). Morphometric analysis of the sarcotubular system revealed a significant increase of these membrane profiles (Casanova & Jerusalem 1979). The above ultrastructural abnormalities are not specific for myotonic dystrophy but are also seen in various other neuromuscular diseases. Although their significance remains to be determined, abnormalities of the sarcotubular system may be related to the altered contractile properties (myotonia) of the muscles (Schröder & Becker 1972). In an experimentally induced myotonia

after clofibrate administration in rats, the earliest change was a dilatation of the transverse tubules suggesting that the sarcotubular abnormalities preceded the more extensive morphological abnormalities in muscle fibres (Ontell et al 1979).

Ring fibres (ringbinden) characterized by aberrant cross-striated myofibrils spirally or radially oriented around the long axis of the muscle fibre (spiral annulet) are present in greater numbers in myotonic dystrophy than in other neuromuscular diseases (Fig. 8.7) (Heidenhain 1918, Wohlfart 1951, Engel 1962, Bethlem & Wijngaarden 1963, Schotland et al 1966). These structures probably result from focal disorganization of myofibrils because they are frequently associated with sarcoplasmic masses and lobulated fibres (Bethlem & Wijngaarden 1963, Schotland et al 1966).

Fingerprint inclusions (Tomé & Fardeau 1973), nemaline and cytoplasmic bodies are recognizable in atrophic fibres and are probably non-specific findings resulting from focal myofibrillar degeneration (Fig. 8.4D).

Mitochondrial abnormalities

Although occasional abnormalities including an increased number of enlarged mitochondria with abnormal cristae have been described by many authors (Aleu & Afifi 1964, Klinkerfuss 1967, Schröder & Adams 1968, Korényi-Both et al 1975, Casanova & Jerusalem 1979), these have been thought to be a secondary non-specific finding. An ultrastructural morphometric study failed to demonstrate significant differences in mito-chondrial percentage of fibre volume and mean mitochondrial size between normal and diseased muscles (Casanova & Jerusalem 1979). Recent histochemical studies have indicated that ragged red fibres (RRF) are present with higher frequency than in other neuromuscular diseases (Fig. 8.8A) (Carpenter & Karpati 1984, Ono et al 1986, Naka-gawa et al 1989, Yamamoto et al 1989). They are predominantly seen in the biceps brachii muscle and very rarely in leg muscles. Although Ono et al (1986) found no relationship between the incidence of RRF, age and duration of illness, RRF were found mostly in patients over 40 years of age and in severely damaged muscles (Fig. 8.8). The mitochondrial abnormalities therefore appear to become apparent as the disease progresses.

With cytochrome c oxidase stain, RRF and some scattered otherwise normal fibres show focal lack of enzyme activity (Fig. 8.8B). The number of such fibres is usually greater than those of RRF (Yamamoto et al 1989).

Scattered RRF and fibres with focal cytochrome c oxidase deficiency are also constant and diagnostic morphological features in chronic progressive external ophthalmoplegia including the Kearns–Sayre syndrome (Johnson et al 1983, Müller–Höcker et al 1983, Yamamoto & Nonaka 1988). Four of five myotonic dystrophy patients with RRF had limited ocular muscle movement and three had ptosis (Nakagawa et al 1989). In addition to myofibrillar degeneration (Kuwabara & Lessell 1976), the mitochondrial abnormality may therefore be responsible at least in part for ocular muscle weakness in this disorder. Patients with RRF had a mild decrease in the activities of the electron transfer chain enzymes succinate coenzyme Q reductase and cytochrome c oxidase in biopsied muscles (Nakagawa et al 1989).

On electron microscopy, the RRF are filled with numerous enlarged mitochondria of various sizes with markedly proliferated cristae (Fig. 8.8C, D) and rare crystalline inclusions (Ono et al 1986). Lipid droplets are increased in number. Further study is necessary to understand the re-lationship between these mitochondrial abnormal-ities and the pathogenesis of myotonic dystrophy.

Muscle spindles

One of the unique morphological features of myotonic dystrophy is an abnormality of muscle spindles which may contain a large number of very thin intrafusal fibres with abnormal inner-vation patterns (Daniel & Strich 1964, Swash 1972, Heene 1973, Swash & Fox 1975a, b, Maynard et al 1977, Stranock & Davis 1978a, b). Since only one spindle in our 25 biopsies from biceps brachii muscles contained an increased number of intrafusal fibres, proximal muscles seem to be less involved than distal muscles in which most spindles are abnormal (Swash 1972, Swash & Fox 1975a). The numerous small muscle fibres in muscle spindles are thought to result from a process of longitudinal splitting of the parent intrafusal fibres due to mechanical stresses, perhaps associated with the myotonia or myotonic after-discharges in the muscles (Swash 1972, Swash & Fox 1975a, b, Heene 1973, Stranock & Davis 1978a). Since the dividing intrafusal fibres are commonly seen in mid-polar sections, the fibre fragmentation probably starts in the equatorial zone of the spindle, spreading outward towards the poles (Swash & Fox 1975a, Stranock & Davis 1978a). Rows and clumps of pyknotic nuclei similar to those seen in extrafusal fibres may also be seen in some intrafusal fibres (Daniel & Strich 1964).

Abnormal patterns of innervation, including proliferation of sensory and motor terminals and degenerated endings, are thought to result from degenerating and re-innervating nerve terminals following muscle fibre fragmentation.

Peripheral nerve involvement

Although morphological abnormalities in peri-

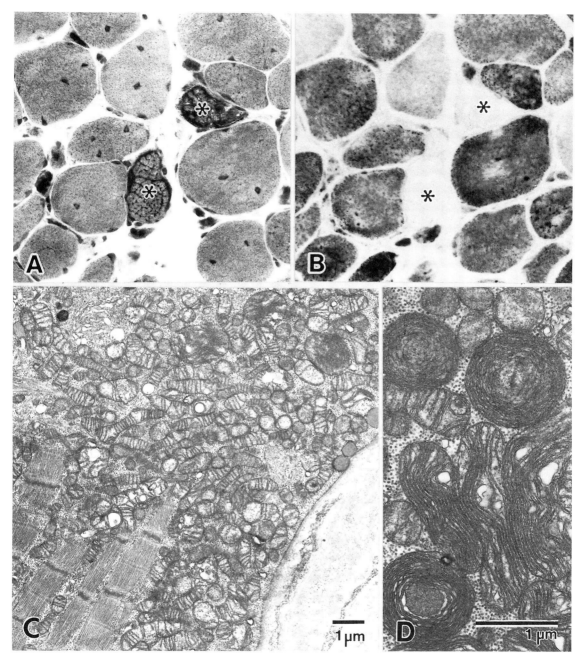

Fig. 8.8 Myotonic dystrophy. Abnormal mitochondria. Ragged-red fibres (asterisk) are commonly seen in aged patients with advanced muscle pathology (A). In addition, cytochrome c oxidase activity is absent in the ragged-red fibres (B). On electron microscopy, the mitochondria are increased in number and size (C), and contain markedly proliferated cristae (D). Fifty-five-year-old female. A, modified Gomori trichrome; B, cytochrome c oxidase. A, B (serial sections) ×280, C, D, electron micrographs

pheral nerve have been described in a number of previous reports (MacDermot 1961, Allen et al 1969, Coërs et al 1973, Kito et al 1973, Cros et al 1988), their significance is still controversial (Pollock & Dyck 1976, Harper 1986). Although we did not carry out morphometric or ultrastructural studies, none of the intramuscular nerves in biopsies from our patients showed a reduced number of myelinated fibres on routine histochemical staining. However, an abnormal neural factor affecting muscle fibres should be considered (Panayiotopoulos & Scarpalezos 1976, 1977) because of the common finding of an abnormal fibre type distribution including fibre type grouping (Fig. 8.2E), type 2B fibre deficiency and type 1 fibre predominance (Fig. 8.2F).

CONGENITAL (NEONATAL, INFANTILE) MYOTONIC DYSTROPHY

Since the first description by Vanier (1960), congenital myotonic dystrophy has come to be recognized as a distinctive clinical entity manifesting with severe muscle weakness and hypotonia from early infancy. The incidence of this disorder ranges from 1.5 per 100 000 population in the San-in district in Japan (Takeshita et al 1981) to 6 per 100 000 live births in South Wales (O'Brien & Harper 1984) and approximately one per 3500 live births in a district in Sweden (Wesström et al 1986).

In almost all patients the condition is maternally transmitted; only in one of 70 patients from 54 sibships was it reported to be transmitted paternally (Harper 1975). Two-thirds of the affected mothers have minimal or no objective symptoms but have myotonia on clinical and electrophysiological examination. Since the symptoms in the affected mothers and in other relatives are not more severe than usual, it is difficult to explain the severity of the congenital myotonic dystrophy on the basis of genetic heterogeneity. An intrauterine factor, as yet unidentified, is believed to affect fetal development in patients with congenital myotonic dystrophy (Harper & Dyken 1972, Sarnat et al 1976, Tanaka et al 1981, Young et al 1981, Farkas-Bargeton et al 1988).

Many affected infants have generalized muscular hypotonia and weakness (floppy infant), respira-

tory insufficiency, feeding difficulty and decreased deep tendon reflexes from early life. Occasionally, severe respiratory failure at birth requires mechanical ventilation and results in a high early mortality. The facial muscles are involved, resulting in a characteristic and virtually diagnostic facial expression: an open mouth with a tent-shaped or inverted V-shaped upper lip. All patients are mentally retarded to some degree.

The muscular hypotonia, weakness, and respiratory insufficiency improve with further development. Although there is often a marked delay in developmental milestones, most patients learn to walk alone. Myotonia usually becomes manifest after 6 years of age. When these patients reach adulthood, the more typical clinical characteristics of myotonic dystrophy including myotonia, muscle weakness, cardiopulmonary involvement, cataract and abnormalities of the endocrine system become manifest.

Muscle pathology

Infantile stage

The most significant and common histological abnormality in the skeletal muscle is muscle fibre immaturity (Karpati et al 1973, Aicardi et al 1974, Bossen et al 1974, Farkas et al 1974, Sarnat & Silbert 1976, Argov et al 1980, Sahgal et al 1983a, Silver et al 1984, Iannaccone et al 1986, Neuen-Jacob et al 1987, Tanabe & Nonaka 1987, Farkas-Bargeton et al 1988). All muscle fibres are of small calibre with variation in fibre size. The fibres are round in contour and embedded in an oedematous interstitium. They have basophilic cytoplasm and occasional internally-placed vesicular nuclei, showing the histological characteristics of myotubes. Unlike the multiple internal nuclei seen in the late-onset form of the disease, in the congenital form only single central nuclei are seen in fibres in cross-section. The central nuclei decrease in number with development, reflecting muscle fibre immaturity. Fibre necrosis, sarcoplasmic masses and ring fibres are not recognizable.

While the muscle fibre type distribution may vary from fascicle to fascicle, it always shows significant abnormalities. Type 1 fibres are hypotrophic as compared with type 2 fibres in most of the

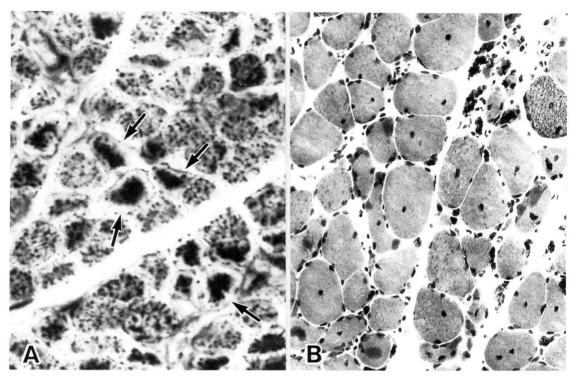

Fig. 8.9 Congenital myotonic dystrophy. In the early infantile stage (A), all muscle fibres are small and show histochemical characteristics of immaturity, with a peripheral halo (arrows) on oxidative enzyme staining. The overall muscle histology is similar to that seen in the late-onset disease when patients are in adulthood (B). There is marked variation in fibre size with nuclear changes, sarcoplasmic mass formation and interstitial fibrosis. Eleven-day-old male (A), and 39-year-old male (B). A, NADH-TR, ×900; B, H&E, ×180

patients (Karpati et al 1973, Farkas et al 1974, Argov et al 1980, Tanabe & Nonaka 1987). Undifferentiated type 2C fibres are markedly increased in number, especially in patients under one year of age (Farkas-Bargeton et al 1977, Sahgal et al 1983a, Neuen-Jacob et al 1987, Tanabe & Nonaka 1987). An increase in number of the type 2C fibres suggests a marked delay in muscle fibre differentiation into mature type 1, 2A or 2B fibres. Type 1 fibre predominance is the additional common finding. The overall histochemical findings are similar to those seen in congenital fibre type disproportion in which type 1 fibres are hypotrophic and predominant with occasional findings of muscle fibre immaturity. A reduced oxidative enzyme activity at the periphery (peripheral halo) (Fig. 8.9A), which is a characteristic finding in myotubes, is recognized in a number of muscle fibres in severely affected infants (Aicardi et al

1974, Farkas et al 1974, Neuen-Jacob et al 1987, Tanabe & Nonaka 1987, Farkas-Bargeton et al 1988). The peripheral halo is known to be present in normal fetal muscle up to the 33rd week of gestation (Farkas-Bargeton et al 1977).

On electron microscopy, many muscle fibres also have the morphological characteristics of immature fibres in the myotubular stage of development. The satellite cells, which are present with high frequency in early developing muscles, are also increased in numbers, again confirming the concept of muscle fibre immaturity (Tanabe & Nonaka 1987).

An early infantile death may occur from respiratory muscle involvement. In reported autopsied cases the diaphragm contained small fibres with fetal characteristics (Bossen et al 1974, Sarnat & Silbert 1976, Silver et al 1984), and scattered necrotic fibres (Sarnat & Silbert 1976).

Muscle spindles were thick-walled and contained a large number of small intrafusal fibres in preterm infants (Sahgal et al 1983a, b). On electron microscopy, the intrafusal fibres had similar morphology to that seen in the developing muscle spindle, leading these authors to the conclusion that the abnormal muscle spindles in the congenital form are also due to impaired maturation (Sahgal et al 1983b). Since an increased number of intrafusal fibres are recognized in some infants who have no myotonia clinically or electrophysiologically, they may not result from splitting or fragmentation of intrafusal fibres from mechanical stress as has been proposed in late-onset myotonic dystrophy.

Child to adulthood

The overall muscle pathology is similar to that seen in late-onset myotonic dystrophy (Dodge et al 1965, Watters & Williams 1967, Tanabe & Nonaka 1987, Wakai et al 1988). Muscle fibres no longer show evidence of immaturity; type 2C fibres are less frequent and fibres with a peripheral halo are absent. Myonuclei are increased in number, and fibres with multiple centrally-placed nuclei become evident. Necrotic and regenerating fibres may be seen in some patients. Type 1 fibre atrophy and predominance progress, and sarcoplasmic masses and fibrosis also appear (Fig. 8.9B) (Tanabe & Nonaka 1987, Wakai et al 1988).

MYOTONIA CONGENITA

Patients with myotonia congenita, first described by Thomsen (1876), have two different modes of inheritance, an autosomal dominant (Thomsen's disease) and an autosomal recessive pattern (Becker 1977, 1979, Kuhn et al 1979). Although the concept of a continuum of myotonic dystrophy and Thomsen's disease had been discussed, the two disorders have been proven to be distinct by clinical and genetic studies (Höweler et al 1980) and linkage analysis using chromosome 19 markers (Koch et al 1989).

The onset of myotonia in Thomsen's disease is usually in infancy. The myotonia is the most troublesome symptom which involves the eyelids, hands and legs. The symptom is aggravated by cold and is diminished by repetitive muscle activity. Muscle weakness is absent except in adult patients with a long history of myotonia. Muscle hypertrophy is frequent and thought to be the result of continuous muscle over-activity.

In the more common form with autosomal recessive inheritance, the myotonia is similar to that seen in the autosomal dominant form but appears slightly later, usually after 3 years of age. Myotonic symptoms sometimes progress rapidly during childhood. Muscle hypertrophy is more marked than in Thomsen's disease. The contention proposed by Becker that an enzymatic defect is the cause of the disease in the recessive form and a structural abnormality in the dominant form has yet to be proven.

Muscle pathology

Although no apparent degenerative changes are recognized on conventional histological examination (Engel & Brooke 1966), there may be excessive variation in fibre size, involving both type 1 and type 2 fibres from the early stage of the disease. In the younger patients under 6 years of age, type 1, 2A and 2B fibres are distributed in a normal mosaic pattern with type 2B fibre atrophy both in patients with Thomsen's disease (Fig. 8.10A) and in the autosomal recessive form. Undifferentiated type 2C fibres are slightly increased in number. No hypertrophic or degenerative fibres are recognized in the early stage of the disease except for a 6-year-old patient described by Hofmann et al (1966) who had necrotic fibres with phagocytosis, central chains of sarcolemmal nuclei and occasional true hypertrophy in the intercostal muscle.

From young adulthood, although mild non-specific abnormalities are recognized in routine histopathological preparations, an almost constant histochemical finding is type 2B fibre deficiency (Crews et al 1976, Heene 1986, Heene et al 1986) (Fig. 8.10B). Since the type 2B fibre deficiency is seen in later childhood and adult life, the phenomenon may be induced by continuous myotonic discharges (Heene 1986), as seen in myotonic dystrophy and paramyotonia congenita (Heene et al 1986). Type 1 and type 2A fibres are hypertrophic in almost a half of all biopsies. Muscle fibre hypertrophy becomes prominent as the

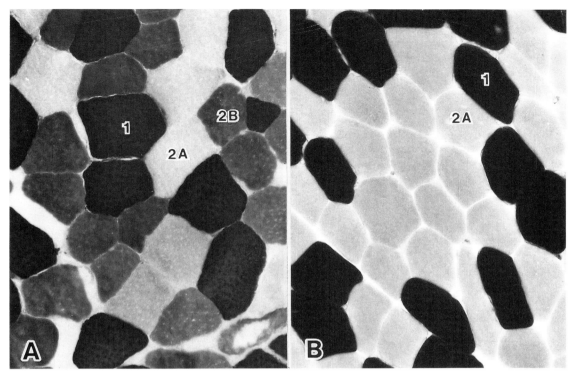

Fig. 8.10 Myotonia congenita. Except for a mild variation in sizes of type 1 (1), 2A (2A), and 2B (2B) fibres, no morphological abnormalities are seen in this biopsy from a 6-year-old male with Thomsen's disease (A). In addition to a moderate variation in type 1 (1) and 2A (2A) fibre size, with mild type 2A fibre atrophy, type 2B fibres are completely absent in a 13-year-old female with the autosomal recessive form (B). A, B, ATPase with pre-incubation at pH 4.6. A ×300, B, ×200

disease progresses (Wohlfart 1951), predominantly in patients with the autosomal recessive form (Schröder & Becker 1972).

Most biopsies show normal to mild non-specific structural abnormalities in muscle fibres (Norris 1962, Samaha et al 1967, Engel & Brooke 1966, Fisher et al 1975). In the advanced stage, especially in aged patients, certain structural changes may be recognizable such as marked variation in fibre size, hypertrophic fibres, centrally placed nuclei, and fibre necrosis (Schröder & Becker 1972, Kuhn et al 1979, Sun & Streib 1983). If there are severe dystrophic changes, one should suspect either an error in diagnosis (for instance myotonic dystrophy instead of myotonia congenita) or the superimposition of another disease (Åström & Adams 1982).

On electron microscopy, the sarcoplasmic reticulum and the transverse tubules are normal (Samaha et al 1967, Korényi–Both et al 1975, Schröder & Becker 1972, Fisher et al 1975) in muscles from patients with autosomal recessive inheritance.

Intracytoplasmic tubular aggregates, proliferated derivatives of the sarcoplasmic reticulum, were identified in three of five patients with autosomal dominant inheritance (Schröder & Becker 1972). The tubular aggregates were similar to those seen in periodic paralysis (see Ch. 9). The significance of these structures remains unknown. An increased number of enlarged mitochondria at electron microscopic level was described by Kuhn et al (1979).

In a biopsy from a 17-year-old patient, two muscle spindles were morphologically normal (Swash & Schwartz 1983).

PARAMYOTONIA CONGENITA

Since the first description of paramyotonia congenita by Eulenburg (1886), there has been considerable controversy as to its nosological status. It has been thought to be a variant of myotonia congenita, a variant of myotonic dystrophy, or a disorder similar to hyperkalemic periodic paralysis. However, since there is no genetic linkage between myotonic dystrophy, myotonia congenita and paramyotonia congenita (Bender et al 1989), the latter is considered to be a distinct entity, but one which is possibly related to primary hyperkalaemic periodic paralysis (adynamia episodica hereditaria) (Gamstorp 1956).

Paramyotonia congenita has been defined by the following criteria: (i) single autosomal dominant gene inheritance with complete or nearly complete penetrance; (ii) myotonia which becomes manifest in childhood, which is frequently paradoxical, and which is much increased by cold and relieved by warming; (iii) episodes of flaccid muscle weakness which may be precipitated with or without cold; (iv) the condition is not progressive; (v) muscle wasting, as seen in myotonic dystrophy, is not present.

Muscle pathology

There is no specific diagnostic morphological feature to identify paramyotonia congenita. Most biopsies have shown only mild pathological changes such as variation in fibre size with hypertrophic and atrophic fibres, and increased numbers of centrally placed nuclei (Drager et al 1958, Hudson 1963, Garcin et al 1966, Thrush et al 1972, Schiffer et al 1976). Almost complete lack of differentiation into type 1 and 2 fibres on oxidative enzyme and ATPase stains was described in two patients (Thrush et al 1972), while others showed normal muscle fibre type differentiation (Schiffer et al 1976, Friis et al 1985).

Disorganized intermyofibrillar networks with a moth-eaten appearance, target fibres (Engel & Brooke 1966), and focally disarrayed myofibrils are commonly seen on electron microscopy (Isch et al 1968, Julien et al 1971).

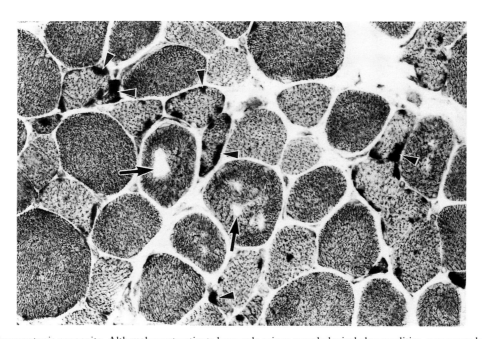

Fig. 8.11 Paramyotonia congenita. Although most patients have only minor morphological abnormalities, some may have a marked variation in fibre size, occasional tubular aggregates (arrowheads) and intracytoplasmic vacuoles (arrows). Twenty-two-year-old female who had mild muscle weakness. NADH–TR, ×350

Intracytoplasmic inclusions of 'tubular aggregates' are the additional common finding in the muscle fibres in this disorder (Fig. 8.11) (Julien et al 1971, Schiffer et al 1976, Schröder & Becker 1972). The presence of the tubular aggregates is not a disease-specific finding but is seen most commonly in hypokalaemic periodic paralysis. They are mostly present in type 2B fibres, and are basophilic in staining with haematoxylin and eosin, and brilliant red with the modified Gomori trichrome technique (Dubowitz 1973, 1987). They are stained darkly on NADH–TR, non-specific esterase and AMP deaminase, but lack the mitochondrial enzymes succinate dehydrogenase and cytochrome c oxidase (Meijer 1988). On electron microscopy the tubules are uniform in size and shape, and possess double membranes with an outer diameter of 50–70 nm and an inner diameter of about 35 nm. They are laid parallel in tightly packed bundles.

Intracytoplasmic vacuoles, occasionally seen in the chronic form of periodic paralysis, are also recognizable in some patients with paramyotonia congenita (Norris 1962, Thrush et al 1972, Schiffer et al 1976, Friis et al 1985).

SCHWARTZ–JAMPEL SYNDROME (CHONDRODYSTROPHIC MYOTONIA, OSTEOCHONDRO-MUSCULAR DYSTROPHY)

Schwartz and Jampel (1962) first described two sibs who had congenital blepharophimosis (narrowing of the palpebral aperture throughout life) in association with generalized muscle weakness and contracture of multiple joints. Thereafter, a number of similar patients have been described in the literature (Aberfeld et al 1965, Huttenlocher et al 1969, Mereu et al 1969, Aberfeld et al 1970, Saadat et al 1972, Beighton 1973, Fowler et al 1974, van Huffelen et al 1974, Brown et al 1975, Cao et al 1978, Fariello et al 1978, Pavone et al 1978, Scribaum & Ionasescu 1981, Ferrannini et al 1982, Milachowski et al 1982, Kuriyama et al 1985).

Although the disease has been thought to be inherited as an autosomal recessive trait (Schwartz & Jampel 1962, Huttenlocher et al 1969, Aberfeld et al 1970, Brown et al 1975, Fariello et al 1978),

an autosomal dominant inheritance was suggested in one family (Ferrannini et al 1982). This unique neuromuscular disorder is characterized clinically by an unusual pinched and immobile facial expression with blepharophimosis (blepharospasm), dwarfism, chondrodystrophic bone abnormalities with multiple joint contractures, muscle weakness, myotonia and an EMG pattern of continuous muscle fibre activity, even at rest. Some severely affected patients may have muscle weakness, stiffness, myotonia and skeletal abnormalities dating from birth (Fowler et al 1974, Cao et al 1978). Most patients show normal or slightly delayed motor milestones during infancy. Joint stiffness and contractures are recognizable usually before one year of age. Cold liquids may produce paroxysms of 'choking'. Narrowed palpebral fissures and an immobile facial expression become manifest from one to two years of age with a slow progression thereafter. Skeletal muscles appear hypertrophic in approximately half of all patients, though there is slowly progressive muscle weakness.

Slightly to moderately elevated serum creatine kinase levels are described in almost all patients.

Muscle pathology

Except for some patients who showed normal muscle histology (Aberfeld et al 1970) or only fat infiltration (Mereu et al 1969) on light microscopy, muscle biopsies show myopathic changes of various degrees. There is variation in fibre size with hypertrophic and atrophic fibres (Fig. 8.12) (Schwartz & Jampel 1962, Aberfeld et al 1965, Huttenlocher et al 1969, Fowler et al 1974, Cao et al 1978, Fariello et al 1978, Ferrannini et al 1982).

There are no disease-specific abnormalities in fibre type distribution: described in the literature are type 2 fibre hypertrophy (Fowler et al 1974), type 2 fibre predominance (Cao et al 1978, Ferrannini et al 1982), mild type 1 fibre predominance and type 2 fibre atrophy (Ferrannini et al 1982). A biopsy from a 30-month-old boy had some neuropathic features in addition to myopathic changes, namely, mild grouping of type 1 or 2 fibres and small groups of atrophic fibres. Muscle fibre necrosis and regeneration were described in two patients (Fowler et al 1974, Fariello et al

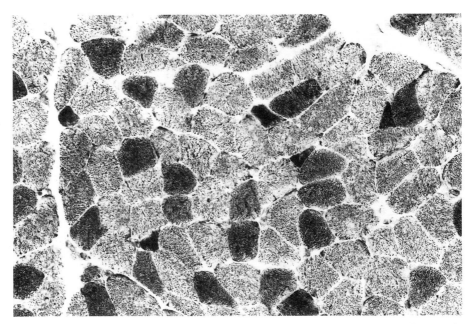

Fig. 8.12   Schwartz-Jampel syndrome. Except for a mild variation in fibre size and mildly disorganized intermyofibrillar networks, no pathognomonic abnormalities are recognizable. Eighteen-month-old male with severe symptoms from the neonatal period. NADH–TR, ×290

1978). Fibres with centrally-placed nuclei are increased in number, and interstitial fibrosis and fat tissue replacement become prominent as the disease progresses.

The ultrastructural findings are non-specific, comprising focal myofibrillar degeneration (Huttenlocher et al 1969, Fariello 1978) with autophagocytosis (Mereu et al 1969), dilatation of sarcotubular systems (Huttenlocher et al 1969, Aberfeld et al 1970, Fowler et al 1974, Pavone et al 1978), and mild mitochondrial abnormalities (Huttenlocher et al 1969, Pavone et al 1978).

REFERENCES

Aberfeld D C, Hinterbuchner L P, Schneider 1965 Myotonia, dwarfism, diffuse bone disease and unusual ocular and facial abnormalities (a new syndrome). Brain 88: 313

Aberfeld D C, Namba T, Vya M V, Grob D 1970 Chondrodystrophic myotonia: report of two cases. Archives of Neurology 22: 455

Adams R D, Rebeiz J J 1966 Histopathologie der myotonischen Erkrankungen. In: Kuhn E (ed) Progressive Muskeldystrophie, Myotonie, Myasthenie. Springer-Verlag, Berlin, p 191

Adie W J, Greenfield J G 1923 Dystrophia myotonica (myotonia atrophica). Brain 46: 73

Aicardi J, Conti D, Goutières F 1974 Les formes néo-natales de la dystrophie myotonique de Steinert. Journal of the Neurological Sciences 22: 149

Aleu F P, Afifi A K 1964 Ultrastructure of muscle in myotonic dystrophy. Preliminary observations. American Journal of Pathology 45: 221

Allen D E, Johnson A G, Woolf A L 1969 The intramuscular nerve endings in dystrophia myotonica — a biopsy study by vital staining and electron microscopy. Journal of Anatomy 105: 1

Argov V, Gardner-Medwin D, Johnson M A, Mastaglia F L 1980 Congenital myotonic dystrophy. Fiber type abnormalities in two cases. Archives of Neurology 37: 693

Åström K E, Adams R D 1979 The pathological reactions of the skeletal muscle fiber. In: Vinken P J, Bruyn G W, Ringel S P (eds) Handbook of clinical neurology, vol 40, Diseases of muscle. North-Holland, Amsterdam, p 197

Åström K E, Adams R D 1982 Myotonic disorders. In: Mastaglia F L, Walton J N (eds) Skeletal muscle pathology. Churchill Livingstone, Edinburgh, p 266

Batten F E, Gibb H P 1909 Myotonia atrophica. Brain 32: 187

Becker P E 1977 Syndromes associated with myotonia: Clinical-genetic classification. In: Rowland L P (ed) Pathogenesis of human muscular dystrophies. Excerpta Medica, Amsterdam, p 699

Becker P E 1979 Heterozygote manifestation in recessive

generalized myotonia. Human Genetics 46: 325

Beighton P 1973 The Schwartz syndrome in southern Africa. Clinical Genetics 4: 548

Bender K, Senff H, Steiert A, Lagodny H, Wienker T F, Koch M 1989 Linkage studies of myotonia congenita and paramyotonia congenita. Clinical Genetics 36: 92

Bethlem J A A P, van Wijngaarden G K 1963 The incidence of ringed fibres and sarcoplasmic masses in normal and diseased muscle. Journal of Neurology, Neurosurgery and Psychiatry 26: 326

Borg J, Edström L, Butler-Browne G S, Thornell L-E 1987 Muscle fibre type composition, motoneuron firing properties, axonal conduction velocity and refractory period for foot extensor motor units in dystrophia myotonica. Journal of Neurology, Neurosurgery and Psychiatry 50: 1036

Bossen E H, Shelburne J D, Verkauf B S 1974 Respiratory muscle involvement in infantile myotonic dystrophy. Archives of Pathology 97: 250

Brooke M H, Engel W K 1969 The histographic analysis of human muscle biopsies with regard to fiber types. 3. Myotonias, myasthenia gravis, and hypokalemic periodic paralysis. Neurology (Minneapolis) 19: 469

Brooke M H, Williamson E, Kaiser K K 1971 The behaviour of four fiber types in developing and reinnervated muscle. Archives of Neurology 25: 360

Brown S B, Garcia-Mullin R, Murai Y 1975 The Schwartz–Jampel syndrome (myotonic chondrodystrophy) in the adult. Neurology (Minneapolis) 25: 365

Brunner H G, Smeets H, Lambermon M M, Coerwinkel-Driessen M, van Oost B A, Wieringa B, Ropers H H 1989 A multipoint linkage map around the locus for myotonic dystrophy on chromosome 19. Genomics 5: 589

Cao A, Cinachetti C, Calisti L, De Virgiliis S, Ferreli A, Tangheroni W 1978 Schwartz–Jampel syndrome. Clinical, electrophysiological and histopathological study of a severe variant. Journal of the Neurological Sciences, 35: 175

Carpenter S, Karpati G 1984 Pathology of skeletal muscle. Churchill Livingstone, New York

Casanova G, Jerusalem F 1979 Myopathology of myotonic dystrophy. A morphometric study. Acta Neuropathologica (Berlin) 45: 231

Cöers C, Telerman-Toppet N, Gerard J-M 1973 Terminal innervation ratio in neuromuscular disease. II. Disorders of lower motor neuron, peripheral nerve and muscle. Archives of Neurology 29: 215

Crews J, Kaiser K K, Brooke M H 1976 Muscle pathology of myotonia congenita. Journal of the Neurological Sciences 28: 449

Cros D, Harnden P, Pouget J, Pellissier J F, Gastaut J L, Serratrice G 1988 Peripheral neuropathy in myotonic dystrophy: a nerve biopsy study. Annals of Neurology 23: 470

Cullen M J, Fulthorpe J J 1975 Stages in fibre breakdown in Duchenne muscular dystrophy: an electron microscopic study. Journal of the Neurological Sciences 24: 179

Daniel P M, Strich S J 1964 Abnormalities in the muscle spindles in dystrophia myotonica. Neurology (Minneapolis) 14: 310

Dodge P R, Gamstorp I, Byers R K, Russell P 1965 Myotonic dystrophy in infancy and childhood. Pediatrics 35: 3

Drager G A, Hammill J F, Shy G M 1958 Paramyotonia congenita. Archives of Neurology and Psychiatry 30: 1

Dubowitz V 1973 Muscle biopsy: a modern approach. Saunders, Philadelphia

Dubowitz V 1987 Muscle biopsy: a practical approach.

Baillière Tindall, London

Eiberg H, Mohr J, Nielsen L, Simonsen N 1983 Genetics and linkage relationships of the C3 polymorphism: discovery of C3-Se linkage and assignment of LES-C3-DM-Se-PEPD-Lu synteny to chromosome 19. Clinical Genetics 24: 159

Engel W K 1962 Chemocytology of striated annulets and sarcoplasmic masses in myotonic dystrophy. Journal of Histochemistry and Cytochemistry 19: 229

Engel W K, Brooke M H 1966 Histochemistry of the myotonic disorders. In: Kuhn E (ed) Progressive Muskeldystrophie, Myotonie, Myasthenie. Springer-Verlag, Berlin, p 203

von Eulenburg A 1886 Uber eine familiäre, durch 6 Generationen verfolgbare Form congenitaler Paramyotonie. Neurologisches Zentralblatt 5: 265

Fariello R, Meloff K, Murphy E G, Reilly B J, Armstrong D 1978 A case of Schwartz-Jampel syndrome with unusual muscle biopsy findings. Annals of Neurology 3: 93

Farkas E, Tomé F M S, Fardeau M, Arséno-Nunes M L, Dreyfus P, Diebler M F 1974 Histochemical and ultrastructural study of muscle biopsies in 3 cases of dystrophia myotonica in the newborn child. Journal of the Neurological Sciences 21: 273

Farkas-Bargeton E, Diebler M F, Arséno-Nunes M L, Wehrlé R, Rosenberg B 1977 Etude de la maturation histochimique, quantitative et ultrastructurale du muscle foetal humain. Journal of the Neurological Sciences 31: 245

Farkas-Bargeton E, Barbet J P, Dancea S, Wehrle R, Checouri A Dulac O 1988 Immaturity of muscle fibers in the congenital form of myotonic dystrophy: its consequences and its origin. Journal of the Neurological Sciences 83: 145

Ferrannini E, Perniola T, Krajewska G, Serlenga L, Trizio M 1982 Schwartz–Jampel syndrome with autosomal-dominant inheritance. European Neurology 21: 137

Fisher E R, Danowski T S, Ahmad U, Breslau P, Nolan S, Stephan T 1975 Electron microscopical study of a family with myotonia congenita. Archives of Pathology 99: 607

Fowler W M, Layzer R B, Taylor R G, Eberle E D, Sims G E, Munsat T L, Philippart M, Wilson P W 1974 The Schwartz–Jampel syndrome. Its clinical, physiological and histological expressions. Journal of the Neurological Sciences 22: 127

Friis M L, Johnsen T, Saltin B, Paulson O B 1985 Skeletal muscle in paramyotonia congenita: biochemistry, histochemistry and morphology. Acta Neurologica Scandinavica 71: 62

Fukuhara N, Kumamoto T, Tsubaki T 1980 Rimmed vacuoles. Acta Neuropathologica (Berlin) 51: 229

Gamstorp I 1956 Adynamia episodica hereditaria. Acta Paediatrica Scandinavica. Supplement 108: 1

Garcin R, Legrain M, Rondot P, Fardeau M 1996 Étude clinique et métabolique d'une observation de paramyotonie congénitale d'Eulenburg. Documents ultrastructuraux concernant la biopsie musculaire. Revue Neurologique (Paris) 115: 295

Grimby G, Hedberg M, Henriksson K-G, Johansson G, Wigerstad-Lossing I, Seleden U, Orndahl G 1988 Muscle function and morphology in myotonic dystrophy. Acta Medica Scandinaviaca 224: 349

Harper P S 1975 Congenital myotonic dystrophy in Britain. II. Genetic basis. Archives of Disease in Childhood 50: 514

Harper P S 1986 Myotonic disorders. In: Engel A G, Banker B Q (eds) Myology vol 2. McGraw-Hill, New York, p 1267

Harper P S, Dyken R R 1972 Early-onset dystrophia myotonica. Evidence supporting a maternal environmental factor. Lancet ii: 53

Heene R 1973 Histological and histochemical findings in

muscle spindles in dystrophia myotonica. Journal of the Neurological Sciences 18: 369

Heene R 1986 Evidence of myotonic origin of type 2B muscle fibre deficiency in myotonia and paramyotonia congenita. Journal of the Neurological Sciences 76: 357

Heene R, Gabriel R-R, Manz F, Schimrigk K 1986 Type 2B muscle fibre deficiency in myotonia and paramyotonia congenita. A genetically determined histochemical fibre type pattern? Journal of the Neurological Sciences 73: 23

Heidenhain M 1918 Über progressive Veränderungen der Muskulatur bei Myotonia atrophica. Beiträge zur Pathologischen Anatomie und zur Allgemeinen Pathologie 64: 198

Hofmann W W, Alston W, Rowe G 1966 A study of individual neuromuscular junctions in myotonia. Electroencephalography and Clinical Neurophysiology 21: 521

Höweler C J, Busch H F M, Bernini L F, van Loghem E, Khan P M, Nijenhuis L E 1980 Dystrophia myotonica and myotonia congenita concurring in one family. A clinical and genetic study. Brain 103: 497

Hudson A J 1963 Progressive neurological disorder and myotonia congenita associated with paramyotonia. Brain 86: 811

Hulsebos T, Wieringa B, Hochstenbach R et al 1986 Toward early diagnosis of myotonic dystrophy: construction and characterization of a somatic cell hybrid with a single human der(19) chromosome. Cytogenetics and Cell Genetics 43: 47

Huttenlocher P R, Landwirth J, Hanson V, Gallagher B B, Bensch K 1969 Osteo-chondro-muscular dystrophy. A disorder manifested by multiple skeletal deformities, myotonia, and dystrophic changes in muscle. Pediatrics 44: 945

Iannaccone S T, Bove K E, Vogler C, Azzarelli B, Muller J 1986 Muscle maturation delay in infantile myotonic dystrophy. Archives of Pathology and Laboratory Medicine 110: 405

Isch F, Stoebner P, Warter J M 1968 Paramyotonie congénitale de von Eulenburg: étude des observations d'une enfant et de sa mère. Revue Neurologique (Paris) 118: 214

Johnson M A, Turnbull D M, Dick P J, Sherratt H S A 1983 A partial deficiency of cytochrome c oxidase in chronic progressive external ophthalmoplegia. Journal of the Neurological Sciences 60: 31

Julien J, Vital C, Vallat J M, Martin M F 1971 Paramyotonie d'Eulenburg. Journal of the Neurological Sciences 13: 447

Karpati G, Carpenter S, Watters G V, Eisen A A, Andermann F 1973 Infantile myotonic dystrophy. Histochemical and electron microscopic features in skeletal muscle. Neurology (Minneapolis) 23: 1066

Kito S, Yamamoto M, Fujimori N, Itoga K, Kosaka K 1973 Studies on myotonic dystrophy: 1. Ultrastructural lesions of the muscle and the nerve in myotonic dystrophy. 2. Insulin and HGH responses in myotonic dystrophy. In: Kakulas B A (ed) Basic research in myology. Excerpta Medica, Amsterdam, p 651

Klinkerfuss G H 1967 An electron microscopic study of myotonic dystrophy. Archives of Neurology 16: 181

Koch M, Harley H, Sarfarazi M, Bender K, Wienker T, Zoll B, Harper P S 1989 Myotonia congenita (Thomsen's disease) excluded from the region of the myotonic dystrophy locus on chromosome 19. Human Genetics 82: 163

Korényi-Both A, Lapis K, Gallai M, Szobor A 1975 Fine structural alterations of muscle fibers in diseases accompanied by myotonia. Beiträge zur Pathologie 156: 241

Korneluk P G, MacKenzie A E, Nakamura Y, Dubé I, Jacob P, Hunter A G W 1989 A reordering of human chromosome 19 long-arm DNA markers and identification of markers flanking the myotonic dystrophy locus. Genomics 5: 596

Kuhn E, Fiehn W, Seiler D, Schröder J-M 1979 The autosomal recessive (Becker) form of myotonia congenita. Muscle and Nerve 2: 109

Kuriyama M, Shinmyozu K, Osame M, Kawahira M, Igata A 1985 Schwartz–Jampel syndrome associated with von Willebrand's disease. Journal of Neurology 232: 49

Kuwabara T, Lessell S 1976 Electron microscopic study of extraocular muscles in myotonic dystrophy. American Journal of Ophthalmology 82: 303

MacDermot V 1961 The histology of the neuromuscular junction in dystrophia myotonica. Brain 84: 75

Maynard J A, Cooper R R, Ionasescu V V 1977 An ultrastructure investigation of intrafusal muscle fibers in myotonic dystrophy. Virchows Archiv. A. Pathological Anatomy and Histology 373: 1

Meijer A E F H 1988 Histochemical features of tubular aggregates in diseased human skeletal muscle fibres. Journal of the Neurological Sciences 86: 73

Mereu T R, Porter I H, Hug G 1969 Myotonia, shortness of stature, and hip dysplasia. Schwartz–Jampel syndrome. American Journal of Diseases of Children 117: 470

Milachowski K, Keyl W, Witt T N 1982 Das Schwartz–Jampel Syndrom. Orthopädische und neurologische Probleme der chondrodystrophien Myotonie. Zeitschrift für Orthopädie und ihre Grenzgebiete 120: 657

Müller-Höcker J, Pongratz D, Hübner G 1983 Focal deficiency of cytochrome-c-oxidase in skeletal muscle of patients with progressive external ophthalmoplegia. Virchows Archiv A, Pathological Anatomy and Histopathology 402: 61

Mussini I, DiMauro S, Angelini C 1970 Early ultrastructural and biochemical changes in muscle in dystrophia myotonica. Journal of the Neurological Sciences 10: 585

Nakagawa M, Higuchi I, Yamano T, Fukunaga H, Osame M 1989 A study of mitochondrial electron transfer chain in myotonic dystrophy. Clinical Neurology (Tokyo) 29: 1110

Neuen-Jacob E, Voit Th, Turski J, Lenard H G, Wechsler W 1987 Neonatal myotonic dystrophy in a premature infant: clinical and morphological findings. Clinical Neuropathology 6: 236

Nonaka I, Takagi A, Sugita H 1981a The significance of type 2C muscle fibres in Duchenne muscular dystrophy. Muscle and Nerve 4: 326

Nonaka I, Sunohara N, Ishiura S, Satoyoshi E 1981b Familial distal myopathy with rimmed vacuole and lamellar (myeloid) body formation. Journal of the Neurological Sciences 51: 141

Norris F H 1962 Unstable membrane potential in human myotonic muscle. Electroencephalography and Clinical Neurophysiology 26: 98

O'Brien T A, Harper P S 1984 Course, prognosis and complications of childhood-onset myotonic dystrophy. Developmental Medicine and Child Neurology 26: 62

Ono S, Kurisaki H, Inouye K, Mannen T 1968 'Ragged-red' fibres in myotonic dystrophy. Journal of the Neurological Sciences 74: 247

Ontell M, Paul H S, Adibi S A, Martin J L 1979 Involvement of transverse tubules in induced myotonia. Journal of Neuropathology and Experimental Neurology 38: 596

Panayiotopoulos C P, Scarpalezos S 1976 Dystrophia myotonica. Peripheral nerve involvement and pathogenetic implications. Journal of the Neurological Sciences 27: 1

Panayiotopoulos C P, Scarpalezos S 1977 Dystrophia

myotonica. A model of combined neural and myopathic muscle atrophy. Journal of the Neurological Sciences 31: 261

Pavone L, Mollica F, Grasso A, Cao A, Gullotta F 1978 Schwartz–Jampel syndrome in two daughters of first cousin. Journal of Neurology, Neurosurgery and Psychiatry 41: 161

Pollock M, Dyck P J 1976 Peripheral nerve morphometry in myotonic dystrophy. Archives of Neurology 33: 33

Pongratz D, Schultz D, Koppenwallner Ch, Hübner G 1979 Wertigkeit der Muskelbiopsie in der Diagnostik der Dystrophia myotonica (Curschmann-Steinert). Klinische Wochenschrift 57: 215

Roses A D, Harper P S, Bossen E H 1979 Myotonic muscular dystrophy. In: Vinken P J, Bruyn G W, Ringel S P (eds) Handbook of clinical neurology, vol 40: Diseases of muscle. North-Holland, Amsterdam, p 485

Saadat M, Mokfi H, Vakil H, Ziai M 1972 Schwartz syndrome: myotonia with blepharophimosis and limitations of joints. Journal of Pediatrics 81: 348

Sahgal V, Bernes S, Sahgal S, Lischwey C, Subramani V 1983a Skeletal muscle in preterm infants with congenital myotonic dystrophy. Morphologic and histochemical study. Journal of the Neurological Sciences 59: 47

Sahgal V, Sahgal S, Bernes S, Subramani V 1983b Ultrastructure of muscle spindle in congenital myotonic dystrophy. A study of preterm infant muscle muscle spindles. Acta Neuropathologica (Berlin) 61: 207

Salviati S, Biasia E, Betto R, Betto D D 1986 Fast to slow transition induced by experimental myotonia in rat FDL muscle. Pflügers Archiv. European Journal of Physiology 406: 266

Samaha F J, Schroeder J M, Rebeiz J, Adams R D 1967 Studies on myotonia. Biochemical and electron microscopic studies on myotonia congenita and myotonia dystrophica. Archives of Neurology 17: 22

Sarnat H B, Silbert S W 1976 Maturational arrest of fetal muscle in neonatal myotonic dystrophy. A pathologic study of four cases. Archives of Neurology 33: 466

Sarnat H B, O'Conner T, Byrne P A 1976 Clinical effects of myotonic dystrophy on pregnancy and the neonate. Archives of Neurology 33: 459

Schiffer D, Giordana M T, Monga G, Mollo F 1976 Histochemistry and electron microscopy of muscle fibres in a case of congenital paramyotonia. Journal of Neurology 211: 125

Schimmelpfeng J, Jockusch H, Heimann P 1987 Increased density of satellite cells in the absence of fibre degeneration in muscle of myotonic mice. Cell and Tissue Research 249: 351

Schmalbruch H 1975 Segmental fiber breakdown and defects of the plasmalemma in diseased human muscles. Acta Neuropathologica (Berlin) 33: 129

Schotland D L 1970 An electron microscopic investigation of myotonic dystrophy. Journal of Neuropathology and Experimental Neurology 29: 241

Schotland D L, Spiro D, Carmel P 1966 Ultrastructural studies of ring fibers in human muscle disease. Journal of Neuropathology and Experimental Neurology 25: 431

Schröder J M, Adams R D 1968 The ultrastructural morphology of the muscle fiber in myotonic dystrophy. Acta Neuropathologica (Berlin) 10: 218

Schröder J M, Becker P E 1972 Anomalien des T-Systems und des sarkoplasmatischen Reticulums bei der Myotonie, Paramyotonie und Adynamie. Virchows Archiv. Abteilung A. Pathologische Anatomie 357: 319

Schwartz O, Jampel R S 1962 Congenital blepharophimosis associated with a unique generalized myopathy. Archives of Ophthalmology 68: 82

Scribaum N, Ionassescu V 1981 Schwartz–Jampel syndrome: a case report. Stimulatory effect of calcium and A23187 calcium ionophore for protein synthesis in muscle cell cultures. European Neurology 20: 46

Shaw D J, Meredith A L, Sarfarazi M, Huson S M, Brook J D, Myklebost O, Harper P S 1985 The apolipoprotein CII gene: subchromosomal localisation and linkage to the myotonic dystrophy locus. Human Genetics 70: 271

Silver M M, Banerjee D, Hudson A J 1983 Segmental myofiber necrosis in myotonic dystrophy. An immunoperoxidase study of immunoglobulins in skeletal muscle. American Journal of Pathology 112: 294

Silver M M, Vilos G A, Silver M D, Shaheed W S, Turner K L 1984 Morphologic and morphometric analyses of muscle in the neonatal myotonic dystrophy syndrome. Human Pathology 15: 1171

Steinert H 1909 Myopathologische Beiträge. I. Über das klinische und anatomische Bild des Muskelschwunds der Myotoniker. Deutsche Zeitschrift für Nervenheilkunde 37: 58

Stranock S D, Davis J N 1978a Ultrastructure of the muscle spindle in dystrophia myotonica. I. The intrafusal muscle fibres. Neuropathology and Applied Neurobiology 4: 393

Stranock S D, Davis J N 1978b Ultrastructure of the muscle spindle in dystrophia myotonica. II. The sensory and motor nerve terminals. Neuropathology and Applied Neurobiology 4: 407

Sun S F, Streib E W 1983 Autosomal recessive generalized myotonia. Muscle and Nerve 6: 143

Swash M 1972 The morphology and innervation of the muscle spindle in dystrophia myotonica. Brain 95: 357

Swash M, Fox K P 1975a Abnormal intrafusal muscle fibres in myotonic dystrophy: a study using serial sections. Journal of Neurology, Neurosurgery and Psychiatry 38: 91

Swash M, Fox K P 1975b The fine structure of the spindle abnormality in myotonic dystrophy. Neuropathology and Applied Neurobiology 1: 171

Swash M, Schwartz M S 1983 Normal muscle spindle morphology in myotonia congenita: the spindle abnormality in myotonic dystrophy is not due to myotonia alone. Clinical Neuropathology 2: 75

Takeshita K, Tanaka K, Nakashima T, Kasagi S 1981 Survey of patients with early onset myotonic dystrophy in San-in district Japan. Japanese Journal of Human Genetics 26: 295

Tanabe Y, Nonaka I 1987 Congenital myotonic dystrophy. Changes in muscle pathology with ageing. Journal of the Neurological Sciences 77: 59

Tanaka K, Takeshita K, Takita M 1981 Deoxycholic acid, a candidate for the maternal intrauterine factor in early onset myotonic dystrophy. Lancet i: 1046

Thomsen J 1876 Tonische Krämpfe in willkürlich beweglichen Muskeln infolge von ererbter psychischer Disposition (Ataxia muscularis ?). Archiv fur Psychiatrie und Nervenkrankheiten 6: 702

Thrush D C, Morris C J, Salmon M V 1972 Paramyotonia congenita: a clinical, histochemical and pathological study. Brain 95: 537

Tomé F M S, Fardeau M 1973 'Fingerprint inclusions' in muscle fibers in dystrophia myotonica. Acta Neuropathologica (Berlin) 24: 62

van Huffelen A C, Gabreëls F J M, van Lypen-vd Horst J S, Slooff J L, Stadhouders A M, Korten J J 1974

Chondrodystrophic myotonia. A report of two unrelated Dutch patients. Neuropädiatrie 5: 71

Vanier T M 1960 Dystrophia myotonica in childhood. British Medical Journal 2: 1284

Vassilopoulos D, Lumb E M 1980 Muscle nuclear changes in myotonic dystrophy. European Neurology 19: 237

Wakai S, Kameda K, Okabe M, Nagaoka M, Minami R, Tachi N 1988 Histopathological study of the biopsied muscles from juvenile patients with congenital myotonic dystrophy. Acta Paediatrica Japonica 30: 7

Watters G V, Williams T W 1967 Early onset myotonic dystrophy. Clinical and laboratory findings in five families and a review of the literature. Archives of Neurology 17: 137

Wechsler W, Hager H 1961 Elektronenmikroskopische Untersuchungen bei myotonischer Muskeldystrophie. Archiv für Psychiatrie und Nervenkrankheiten 201: 668

Wesström G, Bensch J, Schollin J 1986 Congenital myotonic dystrophy. Incidence, clinical aspects and early prognosis. Acta Paediatrica Scandinavica 75: 849

Wohlfart G 1951 Dystrophia myotonica and myotonia congenita. Histopathologic studies with special reference to changes in the muscle. Journal of the Neuropathology and Experimental Neurology 10: 109

Yamamoto M, Nonaka I 1988 Skeletal muscle pathology in chronic progressive external ophthalmoplegia. Acta Neuropathologica (Berlin) 76: 558

Yamamoto M, Koga Y, Ohtaki E, Nonaka I 1989 Focal cytochrome c oxidase deficiency in various neuromuscular diseases. Journal of the Neurological Sciences 91: 207

Young R S K, Gang D L, Zalneraitis E L, Krishnamoorthy K S 1981 Dysmaturation in infants of mothers with myotonic dystrophy. Archives of Neurology 38: 716

9. Periodic paralysis and electrolyte disorders

Fernando M. S. Tomé   Kristian Borg

INTRODUCTION

The periodic paralyses are characterized by intermittent attacks of flaccid muscle weakness or paralysis, without sensory loss or psychic disturbances, and are usually associated with changes in serum potassium levels.

These conditions are usually inherited and are referred to as familial periodic paralyses: the first familial cases were reported in 1887 by Cousot. According to the clinical picture and serum potassium levels during the attacks, two main types are recognized — hypokalaemic and hyperkalaemic — of which the first is more frequent than the second. However, although fewer families are affected by the hyperkalaemic type, in each affected family many more of its members suffer from the disease than in the hypokalaemic type. A familial normokalaemic type of periodic paralysis has also been reported, but this is rare and its existence has been contested. Sporadic cases of hypokalaemic periodic paralysis also occur and may be primary or secondary; the latter are, in general, caused by severe potassium depletion or are associated with thyrotoxicosis, particularly in Oriental subjects.

Detailed descriptions of periodic paralysis were published in the last century (see Talbott 1941, Sagild 1959, Buruma & Schipperheyn 1979) but it is not possible to know exactly which type many of those cases represented. In fact, the decrease in plasma potassium levels during attacks was first reported in 1934 by Biemond & Daniels. Its importance was later stressed in 1937 by Aitken et al who demonstrated that attacks could be provoked by giving glucose and insulin, and were accompanied by a fall in serum potassium levels.

They expressed the view that the fall in serum potassium was accompanied by the passage of sugar from the blood into the tissues. Gammon (1938) confirmed the lowering of serum potassium during the attacks and thought that is was due to diffusion of potassium from the serum into the muscles to correct the muscular inexcitability and weakness.

The occurrence of attacks of periodic paralysis associated with an increase in serum potassium was well documented by Gamstorp (1956) in an extensive study of two families of Swedish origin. She named the condition adynamia episodica hereditaria but it is more commonly called hyperkalaemic periodic paralysis.

Paralytic attacks not correlated with changes in serum potassium were reported by Tyler et al (1951) in a family with 33 affected members. Some authors have regarded these cases as belonging to a normokalaemic form of periodic paralysis (Bradley 1969a,b, Buruma & Schipperheyn 1979) while others have included them in the hyperkalaemic type (McArdle 1963). Brooke (1977) examined four new members of this kinship and concluded that the disease was of the hyperkalaemic type.

The report generally quoted in reference to the normokalaemic variety is that of Poskanzer & Kerr (1961), based on the study of a family with 21 affected members. These authors stated that the plasma potassium remained normal throughout attacks. Another family, in whom three members were thought to have normokalaemic periodic paralysis, was reported by Meyers et al (1972). During the episodes of paralysis experienced by the propositus, no alteration was found in serum potassium levels. This patient was later reinvestigated (Chesson et al 1979) after an increase in the frequency and duration of the attacks and the development of persistent weakness, and it was then observed that some attacks were associated with hypokalaemia and others with hyperkalaemia. Hence the condition was referred to as biphasic periodic paralysis.

In paramyotonia congenita of Eulenburg (1886), in which myotonia is precipitated by cold, attacks of flaccid paralysis may be provoked by giving potassium (French & Kilpatrick 1957). Several authors have suggested that paramyotonia congenita cannot be clearly distinguished from hyperkalaemic periodic paralysis (Layzer et al 1967).

The various types of periodic paralysis can be differentiated clinically and biochemically, but all may present similar morphological changes in the muscle fibres. Using classical histological methods, the most striking change seen is vacuolation of fibres, as first illustrated by Goldflam (1895). Electron microscopy has demonstrated that the vacuoles arise from the sarcoplasmic reticulum and the T system (see A. G. Engel 1970) and has shown the presence of a particular type of tubular aggregates originating from the sarcoplasmic reticulum (Gruner 1966): these aggregates correspond to the regions of the muscle fibres giving a strong reaction with some histochemical techniques (see W. K. Engel et al 1970).

Many theories have been advanced with regard to the physiopathology of periodic paralysis. A dysfunction of the muscle fibre membrane was first demonstrated in the hypokalaemic type (see Engel & Lambert 1969) but also exists in the hyperkalaemic type as was shown by electrophysiological and biochemical studies. On the basis of results from in vitro studies it has been suggested that the paralysis, in both the hypokalaemic and hyperkalaemic types, results from an inexcitability of the muscle fibres because of a membrane depolarization caused by an abnormality in sodium channel function (see Rüdel and Ricker 1985). For further information the reader is referred to the following articles: Gordon & Kao (1977), Johnsen & Beck-Nielsen (1979), Samaha (1979), Clausen et al (1980), Hofmann et al (1983).

In this chapter the main clinical features of the various types of periodic paralysis will be mentioned and the morphological changes in muscle fibres described. The changes in secondary hypokalaemia and hyperkalaemia, in osteomalacia, and in certain other electrolyte disorders, will be referred to briefly.

HYPOKALAEMIC PERIODIC PARALYSIS

Clinical aspects

Hypokalaemic periodic paralysis is usually primary. In 80 to 90% of cases it is inherited as an autosomal dominant trait with almost 100% penetrance in males and very low penetrance in females. The disease is manifest about twice as often in males as in females (Sagild 1959). It occurs all over the world but has rarely been reported in black races (Corbett & Nuttall 1975). According to Helweg-Larsen et al (1955) its incidence in Denmark is 0.8 per 100 000 inhabitants. In general the attacks appear in the second decade of life and tend to decline in the thirties. They vary greatly in degree, the most severe usually occurring at night, following a day of vigorous muscular exercise. The patient may awake in the early hours of the morning with weakness or flaccid paralysis of all four limbs. In most cases the weakness begins in the shoulders (or trunk) and thighs, then spreads gradually to the legs, arms and neck. It is usually symmetrical but proximal segments are more affected than distal. The reflexes are reduced or abolished and the affected muscles do not respond to mechanical or electrical stimulation. Disturbances of sensation, coordination or consciousness do not occur and the patient is able to speak.

In very severe attacks there may be diplopia, dysarthria and some difficulty in breathing. Death, probably due to paralysis of the respiratory muscles, has been recorded (e.g. six patients of the family studied by Holtzapple (1905) died in an attack) but nowadays is exceptional (Ionasescu et al 1974). Cardiac involvement, and even death due to disturbance of atrioventricular conduction, have been reported (Levitt et al 1972). However, Schipperheyn et al (1978) did not find any evidence of cardiac involvement by echocardiographic and electrocardiographic examination performed between attacks in nine patients. The smooth muscles are not affected.

Most patients, in addition to severe attacks, also have mild attacks in which only the lower limbs may be involved. Sometimes patients are able to 'walk off' an attack by briefly exercising the affected muscles. Premonitory symptoms of varying nature may be experienced by some patients a few hours before the attacks. The duration of the attacks varies from a few hours to 3 days; recovery is fairly rapid and movements reappear first in the muscles more recently and less severely involved. Minor disturbances such as stiffness or tiredness of the legs may last for several days after the attacks. Between attacks the patients are usually asymptomatic. However, with time, some may develop permanent weakness and atrophy of the most affected limb muscles (see Dyken et al 1969, Buruma et al 1985). It is believed that the permanent weakness results from muscle damage induced by the attacks (Bekény 1961, Pearson 1964, A. G. Engel 1970). Myotonic 'lid lag' can be elicited between attacks in some patients (Resnick & Engel 1967).

The frequency of attacks is variable; they may occur at intervals of a few days or several years. They may be precipitated by various factors including rest after exertion, cold and damp, carbohydrate-rich meals, alcohol ingestion and emotional stress. For diagnostic purposes it may be possible to elicit an attack by the administration of glucose and insulin. Attacks can be relieved by giving potassium chloride. Occasional patients require intravenous potassium administration. The potassium should be given in a mannitol solution since glucose- and saline-containing solutions further decrease the serum potassium level (Griggs et al 1983). During an attack the serum potassium level is generally low (below 3.4 mmol/l) and there is no increase in the urinary potassium excretion. During recovery from an attack the serum potassium rises to levels higher than normal. Of the various treatments that have been proposed, the most effective is, paradoxically, acetazolamide (Griggs et al 1970) which was first used to treat the hyperkalaemic form of the disorder (McArdle 1962). Acetazolamide may also improve inter-attack muscle weakness (Links et al 1988). Patients who become unresponsive or deteriorate with this drug may benefit by administration of dichlorophenamide, a more potent carbonic anhydrase inhibitor (Dalakas and Engel 1983).

Histopathology

The first microscopic study of muscle in periodic paralysis was reported by Oppenheim (1891) who described waxy degeneration of the fibres in a biopsy of the patient described by Westphal (1885). This patient suffered from attacks which were probably of the hypokalaemic type, and developed permanent muscle weakness. It was Goldflam (1895, 1897) who, in a study of biopsies from five patients, described and illustrated in expressive drawings the presence of *vacuoles* within the muscle fibres. He considered the vacuoles to be the result of myofibrillary rarefaction and regarded them as specific for the disease. Vacuolation of fibres was subsequently reported in America by Crafts (1900) and in Britain by Singer & Goodbody (1901) in a biopsy examined by Collier. The British authors thought that the vacuoles ('fissuring') were 'artefact in nature' and this view was shared by others, including Biemond & Daniels (1934). However, also in 1901, Buzzard (who reported a case, probably of the hyperkalaemic form) wrote that Singer might be wrong in regarding the vacuoles as artefacts. Numerous studies have since shown that vacuolation of the fibres is a real change, characteristic of periodic paralysis, and is particularly abundant in biopsies taken at the height of an attack or in patients who have had frequent attacks or have developed permanent muscular weakness (Pearson 1964, Olivarius & Christensen 1965, Engel et al 1965). Shy et al (1961) suggested that vacuolation is reversible because the vacuoles were smaller and more dispersed through the muscle fibres in a biopsy taken 10 hours after an attack than in one taken from the contralateral muscle during the same attack. In certain biopsies the vacuoles are present in as many as 90% of the fibres (Griggs et al 1970). The vacuolation may be generalized but its degree varies from muscle to muscle, as reported by Ionasescu et al (1974) in a necropsy examination. In this case the vacuolation was severe in the temporalis and gastrocnemius muscles, and mild in the rectus abdominis.

The vacuoles (Fig. 9.1) are round or oval, and

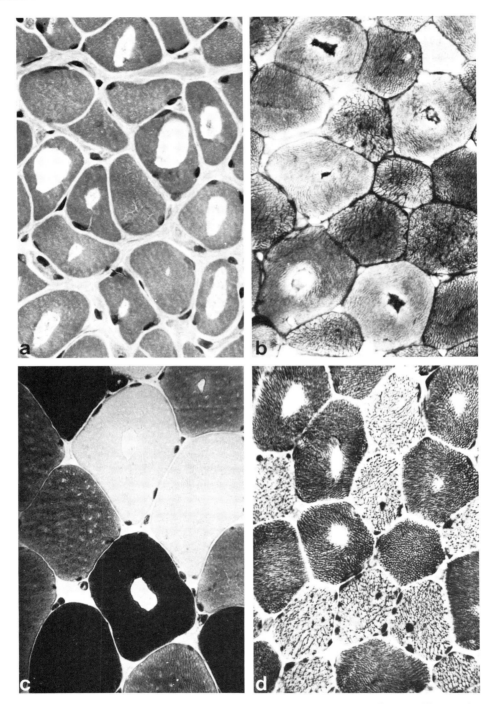

Fig. 9.1 Hypokalaemic periodic paralysis. Vacuolation of muscle fibres in frozen cryostat sections. (a) The vacuoles vary in size and may look empty or contain a tenuous matrix. H&E. (b) They may be intensely stained with PAS. (c) They may be found in type 1 (dark), 2A (light) and 2B (intermediate) muscle fibres. ATPase pH 4.65. (d) They may predominate in type 1 fibres and coexist in the same biopsy with strongly reactive zones in type 2 fibres, corresponding to tubular aggregates. NADH–TR; all ×400

vary in size, measuring up to 100 μm in diameter and 400 μm in length. They may be single or multiple and usually lie near the centre of the fibre. Large vacuoles may be formed by the coalescence of small vacuoles. They may be empty or may contain granular or hyaline material. Several authors have shown that the contents of some vacuoles are often PAS-positive, as seen in Figure 9.1b. However, this does not necessarily indicate that the vacuoles contain glycogen. Calcium has also been found within vacuoles (A. G. Engel 1970). The vacuoles occur in all types of muscle fibres (Fig. 9.1c). In a case reported by Ionasescu et al (1971) they predominated in type 1 fibres and this was also observed in one of our cases (Fig. 9.1d).

Electron-microscopic studies of the vacuoles in hypokalaemic periodic paralysis have been reported by many authors including Shy et al (1961), Howes et al (1966), Biczyskowa et al (1969), MacDonald et al (1969), Gordon et al (1970), Ionasescu et al (1971), Ionasescu et al (1974), Buruma & Bots (1978), Pellissier et al (1980), Martin et al (1984) and particularly A. G. Engel (1966, 1970, 1973). Engel discribed four steps in the formation and evolution of these vacuoles: evolving vacuole, intermediate-stage vacuole, mature vacuole, and remodelling.

The *evolving vacuole* is a large, poorly delimited region of the fibre, made up of numerous vesicles originating from the sarcoplasmic reticulum. Some contain electron-dense material that may be arranged in concentric rings and probably contains calcium. Somewhat similar appearances were described by Weller & McArdle (1971) who called this change basophilic granular degeneration due to deposits of calcium resembling hydroxyapatite crystals. They found them in two cases of primary, one case of secondary hypokalaemic (associated with thyrotoxicosis) and three cases of hyperkalaemic periodic paralysis. In the evolving vacuole the vesicles are sometimes associated with T tubules of bizarre shape, osmiophilic membranes and various products of cytoplasmic degeneration. This type of vacuole can be identified in semi-thin sections (as illustrated in a case of hyperkalaemic periodic paralysis in Fig. 9.5a) particularly by phase-contrast microscopy.

The *intermediate-stage vacuole* is a well-demarcated space, of varying size, with a curvilinear or irregular outline, which is limited by a distinct membrane and contains remnants of cytoplasmic structures which merge within an amorphous matrix of low electron-density. According to A. G. Engel (1970, 1973), in the process of the formation of this vacuole the T system proliferates and acts as a source of membranes to entrap the components of the envolving vacuole.

The *mature vacuole* (Fig. 9.2) is formed when most of the contents of the intermediate-stage vacuole disappear by means of various degrading mechanisms, but the matrix persists in its interior. This is the commonest type of vacuole. Tubules and honeycomb structures of T-system origin surround and communicate with the intermediate-stage or mature vacuoles. Engel (1973) showed that horseradish peroxidase used as an extracellular marker penetrates the intermediate-stage and mature vacuole via the tubules of the T system indicating continuity with the extracellular space.

Remodelling of intermediate-stage and mature vacuoles results from rupture of the limiting membrane that surrounds the sarcoplasmic invaginations which project into the vacuoles. The rupture of the vacuolar membrane permits the entry of sarcoplasm and glycogen into the vacuoles and also the release of extracellular fluid, contained in them, into the surrounding myofilamentary space.

A. G. Engel (1970) observed acid-phosphatase-positive regions in many fibres, particularly within the vacuoles or adjacent to them. This suggests that an autophagic mechanism is involved in the degradation of vacuolar contents. The degradation may be effected by macrophages which may occassionally be found within the vacuoles, and also by other mechanisms.

The vacuoles are not specific for the hypokalaemic type. They also occur in other forms of periodic paralysis and in other muscle disorders (see Ch. 3). However, in the hypokalaemic variety vacuolation of muscle fibres is frequent and widespread.

Among the other changes that may be found in periodic paralysis, the most characteristic are the collections of structures referred to as *tubular aggregates* (Figs 9.3 and 9.4). These consist of collections of long, straight tubules, 40–80 nm (average 55 nm) in diameter, disposed in hexagonal

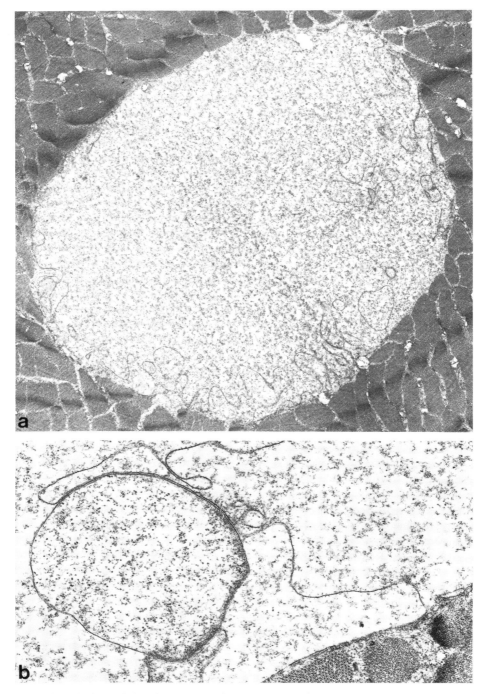

Fig. 9.2 Hypokalaemic periodic paralysis. Ultrastructure of the vacuoles. (a) A large membrane-bound central vacuole contains a finely granular matrix; the membrane has ruptured in places and projects into the vacuole. ×5500. (b) Details of the ruptured membrane and the contents of a vacuole. ×20 000

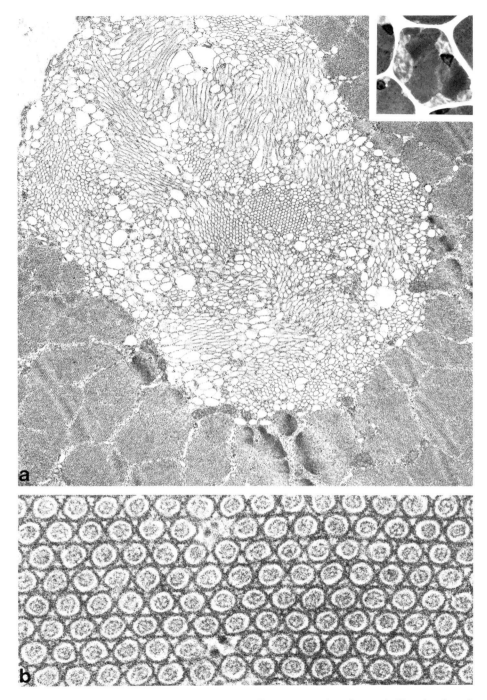

Fig. 9.3 Hypokalaemic periodic paralysis. Tubular aggregates. (a) Transverse section of a muscle fibre showing a large collection of tubules cut transversely and obliquely. ×10 000. *Inset*: The tubular aggregates lie around the edge of the fibres. Semithin section. Toluidine blue; ×400. (b) The tubules are in hexagonal array and contain a moderately electron-dense core. ×100 000

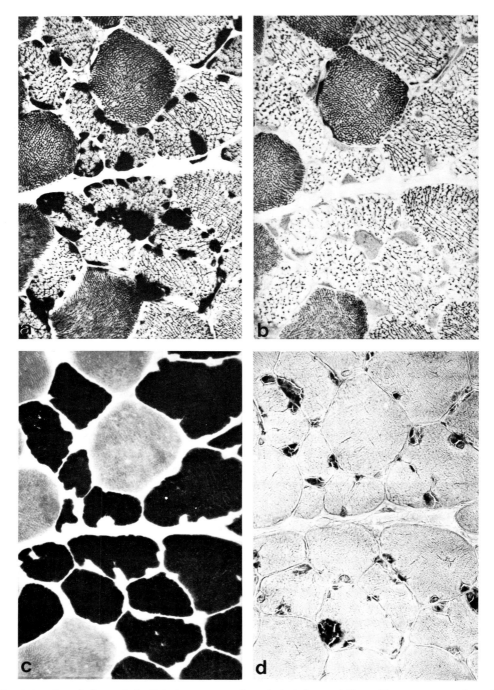

Fig. 9.4   Hypokalaemic periodic paralysis. Tubular aggregates lie exclusively in type 2 fibres. They appear as regions of intense staining with NADH–TR (a), are unstained with succinic dehydrogenase (b) and ATPase at pH 9.4 (c), and stain bright red with Gomori's trichrome (d). Serial frozen cryostat sections; ×400

arrays. Their origin from the sarcoplasmic reticulum is generally accepted (see W. K. Engel et al 1970). They often show a finely granular core, about 35 nm in diameter, separated by a clear space of about 10 nm from the wall of the tubule which is about 8 nm thick. The periphery of this central core is sometimes more dense than the inner part and may appear to form the wall of an 'inner tubule'. This appearance may be exaggerated under certain fixation conditions. In transverse sections one or a few inner tubules sometimes lie within a large tubule, as has been reported by Gruner (1966) and by others.

The tubular aggregates may be large and are usually situated at the periphery of the fibres. Sometimes, however, they seem to be confined to more central regions but serial sections usually show that they are in continuity with subsarcolemmal tubular aggregates. Their existence can be suspected in semi-thin sections of epoxy-embedded material (Fig. 9.3a inset) and is clearly recognized in frozen cryostat sections treated with appropriate histochemical techniques (Fig. 9.4), as first reported by W. K. Engel (1964). He initially regarded them as mitochondrial aggregates because of the intense reaction which they had with regard to staining some enzymes that were considered to be located in mitochondria, particularly NADH–tetrazolium reductase (Fig. 9.4a). However, he also observed that with succinate dehydrogenase (Fig. 9.4b) and α-glycerophosphate dehydrogenase (menadione-linked) the aggregates are unstained. They lack myofibrillar material, as is seen with the myosin ATPase reaction (Fig. 9.4c). This technique shows that the tubular aggregates lie exclusively in type 2 fibres, as reported by W. K. Engel. In some cases they appear to involve nearly all the type 2 fibres but predominate in type 2B. The zones containing tubular aggregates are basophilic with haematoxylin–eosin and reddish-purple with the modified Gomori trichrome stain (Fig. 9.4d). With PAS and phosphorylase reactions these areas are not always clearly seen. In paraffin sections the tubular aggregates appear to be located in irregular spaces which cannot often be distinguished with certainty from artefacts.

The tubular aggregates are seen also in the hyperkalaemic form in which they were first identified by Gruner (1966). In the hypokalaemic form they were first reported by Odor et al (1967). Tubular aggregates may also be seen in various other disorders (Pearse & Johnson 1970, Morgan-Hughes et al 1970, Lewis et al 1971, Mair & Tomé 1972, etc.) and in 'otherwise normal individuals' receiving drugs for a long time (W. K. Engel et al 1970). They have also been observed in experimental animals, after the injection of botulinum (Duchen 1971) or tetanus (Duchen 1973) toxin into muscle fibres, and in perhexiline maleate intoxication (Fardeau et al 1979). Schiaffino et al (1977) induced their formation by anoxia in isolated skeletal muscles of the rat.

Besides the vacuoles and tubular aggregates which can occur in the same biopsy (Fig. 9.1d) and occasionally in the same fibre, other non-specific changes may sometimes also be seen in hypokalaemic periodic paralysis. These include: variation in the size of the muscle fibres; atrophic fibres (preferentially type 2 — Brooke & Engel 1969); hypertrophic and split fibres; increase in nuclei with frequent internal nuclei; whorling of the intramyofibrillar network; increased glycogen and proliferation of the interstitial collagenous tissue. In some fibres, streaming of Z lines, filamentous or cytoplasmic bodies, mitochondrial inclusions and pyknotic nuclei may occasionally be seen. The split fibres may have deep indentations of their surface, which enlarge towards the centre of the fibre to form rounded pockets which sometimes enclose collagen fibres, fibroblasts and blood capillaries. In any given section the communication of these pockets with the extracellular space may not be apparent and therefore they may be taken for vacuoles. However, these pockets can be easily identified by electron microscopy, which reveals the extracellular nature of their contents, as well as the presence of the plasma membrane and basal lamina of the indented muscle fibre surrounding the pockets (see A. G. Engel 1970, Gérard et al 1978). In a few cases of hypokalaemic periodic paralysis, degenerating or necrotic fibres are found. Regenerating zones may also occur in some fibres.

HYPERKALAEMIC PERIODIC PARALYSIS

Clinical aspects

This form of periodic paralysis was named adynamia episodica hereditaria by Gamstorp (1956) who reported 138 cases in two families. It is inherited as an autosomal dominant trait with complete, or almost complete, penetrance but sporadic cases have occasionally been reported (Dyken and Timmons 1963, Riggs et al 1981). Recent linkage studies have suggested that the gene of the sodium charnee α-subunit (chromosome 17q) is the gene of hyperkalaemic periodic paralysis (Fontaine et al 1990). Both sexes are affected equally. The attacks appear at an early age (often in infancy and generally before 10 years). They always occur after exercise followed by a short rest. Cold, missing a meal or emotional upsets may also provoke attacks. Before the attacks the patients may have pain, numbness or tingling in the legs (Bradley 1969a). The weakness usually starts in the legs and very rapidly progresses to the arms. The tendon reflexes are diminished or lost in the affected muscle groups. Myotonia, particularly of the eye muscles, is very frequent but may be detected only on electromyographic examination. In the family reported by Samaha (1965), myotonia was constantly observed at the beginning of the attacks and declined with the progression of the weakness. Chvostek's sign can often be elicited. The severity of the attacks varies but in general is mild; only exceptionally is there complete paralysis of the limbs. The respiratory muscles are very rarely involved and death during an attack has not been recorded. The attacks may appear at any time, during the day or night, but most often they occur during the day and the patient is often able to abort them by mild active movements of the involved muscles. However, the weakness may return with rest. Furthermore, if the patients insist on postponing the attack by repetitive movements they may experience pain in the calves associated with hardening and tenderness of calf muscles (McArdle 1962). The attack may be deferred by taking a light meal or sugar. The duration of the attacks is usually brief: they reach their peak within 30 to 60 minutes, fade rapidly and disappear in 2 or 3 hours. As in the hypo-

kalaemic form, the muscles to recover first are those last and least involved. Some motor disability accompanied by dull pain in the affected muscles may persist for several days after the attacks (Sagild 1959). In long-standing cases, permanent weakness or wasting may occur; it has been reported by many authors, including McArdle (1962), Pearson (1964), Saunders et al (1968) and Thomas et al (1978). Hypertrophy of calf muscles has been described (Gamstorp 1963, Bradley 1969a, Thomas et al 1978). Cardiac arrhythmia was reported by Klein et al (1963) in two cases and by Lisak et al (1972) in one case.

The frequency of the attacks is variable. Usually they are more frequent but much less severe than in hypokalaemic periodic paralysis. They may occur several times a day or several days a week (about three-quarters of the patients reported by Gamstorp in 1956 had an attack at least once a week). Sometimes they are interspersed by intervals of months or even years. Often they become less frequent with increasing age. Pregnancy may be an aggravating factor (McArdle 1962, Gamstorp 1963).

The attacks may be provoked by exercise, or by ingesting potassium chloride or sodium bicarbonate and as a rule develop within 30 minutes. Injection of glucose and insulin during an induced attack improves the power of the weak muscles. The administration of glucocorticoids can also induce an attack (Streeten et al 1971). During attacks the serum potassium levels are usually raised (6–7 mmol/l) but may be normal or even reduced (Pearson 1964). Bradley (1969a) demonstrated that venous blood drained from muscles that are not involved in an attack does not show an increase in its serum potassium concentration. Hyperkalaemia during the interictal period was observed by Lewis et al (1979) in two patients in whom the serum potassium was studied in venous blood taken every hour during a 36-hour period. These authors suggested that the increased potassium during the attacks may reflect a continuous alteration of potassium regulation. After provoked attacks, the serum potassium decreases rapidly and often falls to a level below that observed during the attack. Electrocardiographic changes accompany variation in the serum potassium levels. The total muscle potassium content is reduced between attacks (Gamstorp 1962) and is even lower during them (Carlson & Pearson 1964). Increased serum creatine kinase activity has been found during and between attacks, particularly in patients with permanent weakness. The drugs most useful in the prevention of attacks are acetazolamide (McArdle 1962) and chlorothiazide (Samaha 1965). β-Adrenergic treatment with salbutamol has also proved effective (Wang and Clausen 1976).

Histopathology

The first histological studies of muscle in hyperkalaemic periodic paralysis were reported by Tyler at al (1951) in three members of a large family which was considered by several authors to have the normokalaemic form. As previously mentioned, the hyperkalaemic nature of the attacks in other members of the same family was identified by Brooke (1977). The most important histological change described by Tyler et al was the presence of vacuoles in scattered muscle fibres. Brooke studied the histochemistry of muscle biopsies from four members of the family reported by Tyler et al and found vacuoles and tubular aggregates in two cases. The other changes commonly seen in this family were variation of fibre size, internal nuclei, increased number and pyknosis of nuclei, fibre splitting and fibrosis. In one case there were also marked changes of the inner architecture of the fibres, with moth-eaten and whorled fibres. Muscle biopsy studies have been reported by many other authors. In a few cases no pathological change was noted with classic histological methods (Gamstorp 1956, Sagild 1959, Klein et al 1960, Samaha 1965). However, in most reports the changes described were similar to those reported by Tyler et al (1951) and Brooke (1977).

The most characteristic changes in hyperkalaemic periodic paralysis are the *vacuoles* and *tubular aggregates*, which have features identical to those observed in hypokalaemic periodic paralysis. The only differences are quantitative: in the hyperkalaemic form both the vacuoles and the tubular aggregates are found in fewer biopsies and in fewer fibres than in the hypokalaemic form. According to Pearson (1973), the less extensive vacuolation of the muscle fibres in the hyperkalaemic form corresponds to the much less common permanent clinical weakness. The vacuolation also appears to be more prominent during the attacks than in the intervals. In the formation and evolution of the vacuoles, the same steps described by A. G. Engel (1970) in hypokalaemic periodic paralysis may be observed. As already mentioned in the description of the histopathological changes in the hypokalaemic form, Weller & McArdle (1971) found basophilic granular degeneration of sarcoplasm with calcium deposits in three cases. This change (Fig. 9.5a) had already been illustrated in the hyperkalaemic type by Gruner & Porte (1959) and referred to by Bradley (1969a) and corresponds to that observed by A. G. Engel (1970) in some evolving vacuoles.

Vacuolation of muscle fibres has been reported by many authors including Gruner & Porte (1959), Bekény et al (1961), Pearson (1964), Gruner (1966), Thomas et al (1966), van Bogaert et al (1967), MacDonald et al (1968), Bradley (1969a,b), Weller & McArdle (1971), Ionasescu et al (1971), Schröder & Becker (1972), Ionasescu et al (1973), Thomas et al (1978) and Pellissier et al (1980). Tubular aggregates have been reported less frequently (Gruner 1966, Engel et al 1970, Schröder & Becker 1972, Ionasescu et al 1973, Thomas et al 1978, Pellissier et al 1980). However, in six cases studied in our laboratory, the tubular aggregates appeared to be as frequent as vacuoles. The tubular aggregates are found exclusively in type 2 fibres and predominantly in type 2B.

Among the other changes described commonly in the literature is dilatation of the sarcoplasmic reticulum, first reported by Gruner & Porte (1959). It was also found by Danowski et al (1975) in the biopsies of two clinically normal children of an affected mother, who had four other (affected) children. These authors suggested that dilatation of the sarcoplasmic reticulum is the initial lesion. Serpiginous and convoluted tubules (Fig. 9.5b), membranes of sarcoplasmic reticulum origin and honeycomb structures arising from the T system may be observed in degenerating fibres, as reported by MacDonald et al (1968). In a case of hyperkalaemic periodic paralysis, Schröder and Becker (1972) described small electron-dense precipitates ('incrustations') situated on the sarco-

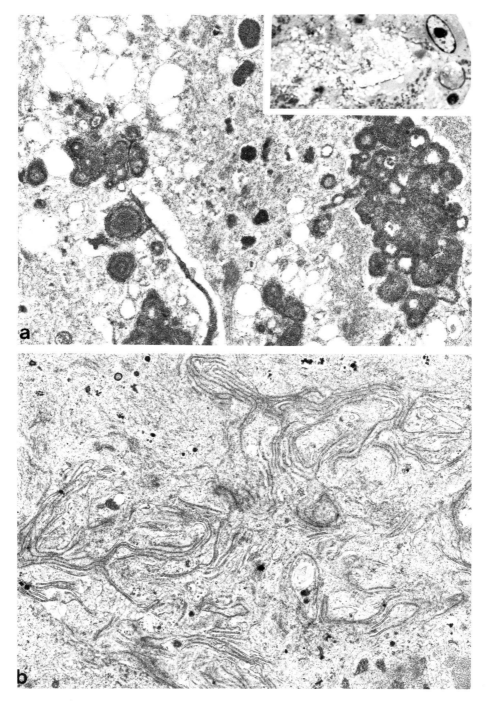

Fig. 9.5   Hyperkalaemic periodic paralysis. (a) A degenerating muscle fibre contains electron-dense concentric structures and many vacuoles. ×21 000. *Inset*: Semi-thin section of the same fibre showing multiple vacuoles. ×1000. (b) Serpiginous tubules arising from the sarcoplasmic reticulum and small dense particles in a degenerating muscle fibre. ×10 000

plasmic side of the T system, on the outer surface of the plasma membrane and on pinocytotic vesicles. Their significance is unknown. In some cases of hyperkalaemic periodic paralysis, particularly in those with permanent muscular weakness, various degenerative changes of the muscle fibres may be observed in addition to the vacuoles and tubular aggregates. These include disorganization of the myofibrillar pattern, sarcoplasmic masses, target fibres, membranous and myelin bodies, and occasionally necrotic fibres with autophagic vacuoles. An increase in muscle fibre nuclei and the presence of centrally located nuclei are often observed. Groups of atrophied fibres may also be found. In one of the cases reported by Thomas et al (1978), who did not have any permanent weakness, there was scattered atrophy of type 2 fibres.

The morphological changes in hyperkalaemic periodic paralysis do not enable one to distinguish it from the hypokalaemic form. However, the changes in the hyperkalaemic form are generally less marked than in the hypokalaemic.

NORMOKALAEMIC PERIODIC PARALYSIS

Clinical aspects

This form is not clearly defined. It resembles the hyperkalaemic form, and whether or not it should be distinguished as a separate form has been a matter of controversy. As previously mentioned and as reported by Gamstorp (1956), the attacks in hyperkalaemic periodic paralysis are sometimes not accompanied by an increase in serum potassium. Four new members of the family reported by Tyler et al (1951) as normokalaemic were subsequently shown to be suffering from hyperkalaemic attacks (Brooke 1977).

Only the family reported by Poskanzer & Kerr (1961) is cited by most authors as a true example of normokalaemic periodic paralysis. In this family the disease affected 21 members and was inherited as an autosomal dominant trait. The attacks started in childhood, occurred at intervals of 1–3 months and lasted for 2 days to 3 weeks. They were often severe, with quadriplegia and involvement of the masticatory muscles. The attacks were not accompanied by a rise in a serum potassium but could be provoked or aggravated by

potassium and relieved by administration of sodium chloride.

Histopathology

In a muscle biopsy from one of the patients reported by Poskanzer & Kerr, taken during an attack and studied by classic histological methods, scattered muscle fibres contained vacuoles and showed degenerative changes. In another biopsy from the same patient, taken six years later and examined by electron microscopy, tubular aggregates were found within a muscle fibre (Bradley 1969b). In a biopsy from another patient from the same family, dilatation of the sarcoplasmic reticulum and occasional vacuoles were observed (Bradley 1969b).

BIPHASIC PERIODIC PARALYSIS

Meyers et al (1972) reported a mother and son who had suffered from attacks of paralysis since the age of 12 and 17 years, respectively. A brother of the mother was also affected. The attacks usually lasted for hours and were not accompanied by changes in the serum potassium levels.

Muscle biopsies taken from the son during an attack and during an asymptomatic period showed similar changes: vacuoles in type 2 muscle fibres, small fibres and tubular aggregates which were identified by electron microscopy. Light microscopy of the mother's biopsy showed some vacuoles, internal nuclei, a ring fibre and occasional small fibres. Electron microscopy revealed dilated vesicles originating in the sarcoplasmic reticulum, but no tubular aggregates.

The son was studied again, seven years later (Chesson et al 1979). He had noted an increased frequency and duration of attacks and had developed mild persistent weakness. Some attacks were associated with hypokalaemia and others with hyperkalaemia. The disorder was therefore referred to as biphasic periodic paralysis. Two muscle biopsies were performed, one between attacks and the other immediately after an attack associated with hyperkalaemia. Both biopsies showed the presence of tubular aggregates, but vacuolation of the fibres was observed only in the biopsy taken shortly after the attack.

PARAMYOTONIA CONGENITA

Clinical aspects

The relationship of this disease to hyperkalaemic periodic paralysis is controversial. The paramyotonia congenita first described by Eulenburg (1886), is inherited as an autosomal dominant trait and characterized clinically by myotonic episodes which are provoked or aggravated by cold. Repetitive muscular activity may aggravate the myotonia (paradoxical myotonia) rather than improve it. In a few cases there are attacks of weakness similar to those observed in hyperkalaemic periodic paralysis. They are sometimes associated with a slightly raised serum potassium level or may eventually be provoked by potassium ingestion (French & Kilpatrick 1957). However, the attacks of weakness may also be associated with low (Delwaide et al 1971, Streib 1989) or normal potassium levels (Streib 1987). Becker (1970) described patients who, besides paramyotonia, had longer periods of weakness independent of cold and named this disorder paralysis periodica paramyotonia. In addition to these symptoms, abnormal fatiguability was reported in two patients (Lundberg et al 1974). These two patients had a normal serum potassium level. Furthermore, in the four families studied by Layzer et al (1967) there were individuals with myotonia only and others with both myotonia and attacks of weakness. These authors regarded the paramyotonia congenita as identical to hyperkalaemic periodic paralysis. de Silva et al (1990) found three members of a single family, each having clinical and electro-physiological features of either hyperkalaemic periodic paralysis or of paramyotonia congenita, and suggested that the two disorders represent two extremes of the spectrum of a single genetic entity. Several other authors believe that these conditions are distinct entities, but 'pure' cases of paramyotonia congenita are rare. The paramyotonic symptoms respond to treatment with tocainide, a lidocaine derivative (Ricker et al 1980, Ricker et al 1983, Streib 1987).

Histopathology

The cases published under the heading of paramyotonia congenita in which muscle biopsies have been performed include those of Drager et al (1958), Garcin et al (1966), Isch et al (1968), Castaigne et al (1971), Julien et al (1971), Sigwald et al (1971), Schröder & Becker (1972), Thrush et al (1972), Schiffer et al (1976), Wegmüller et al (1979), Friis et al (1985) and Heene et al (1986). In most cases the changes in muscle fibres are unremarkable or uncharacteristic. The fibres may show variation in size, with some atrophy and some hypertrophy. Internal nuclei, focal areas of degeneration or regeneration of some fibres, and filamentous bodies have been reported. In one case, Isch et al (1968) found a collection of convoluted tubules with a 'truffle-like' appearance. Vacuolation of the fibres has been reported in a few cases but was not prominent (Castaigne et al 1971, Julien et al 1971, Schröder & Becker 1972, Thrush et al 1972, Schiffer et al 1976, Friis et al 1985). Tubular aggregates have rarely been described (Castaigne et al 1971, Schröder & Becker 1972, Schiffer et al 1976). However, many of these cases cannot be considered to be 'pure' cases of paramyotonia congenita. A type 2B myofibre deficiency has been reported in patients with paramyotonia congenita (Heene 1986, Heene et al 1986). This finding was thought to be related to chronic myotonia. However, a normal proportion of type 2B fibres was reported in another study (Friis et al 1985).

THYROTOXIC PERIODIC PARALYSIS

Clinical aspects

The association of periodic paralysis and thyrotoxicosis occurs mainly in Asiatics but has been observed incidentally in Caucasians. Bernhard et al (1972) reported six Californian cases, five of whom were of Mexican or Filipino ancestry. Two per cent of the Japanese and 1.8% of southern Chinese patients with thyrotoxicosis have attacks of periodic paralysis (MacFadzean & Yeung 1967). A genetic explanation for this predominance in Orientals was provided by Yeo et al (1978), who found that Chinese patients with thyrotoxic periodic paralysis had HLA antigens BW46 or BW46/B40 (common to patients with Graves' disease) and A2 BW22 and AW19 B17 (not present in patients without thyrotoxic periodic paralysis). Thus, the occurrence of Graves' disease in patients who have both these haplotypes would permit the development of periodic paralysis. This HLA antigenic association in the same individual appears to be much more frequent among Orientals than Caucasians.

Thyrotoxic periodic paralysis is usually sporadic and occurs in the third or fourth decades (see Engel 1961). Males are affected much more frequently than females. The first attack of paralysis generally occurs after the thyrotoxicosis has been diagnosed but occasionally the attack may disclose the Graves' disease (Singer et al 1977, Shulkin et al 1989). The paralytic attacks are similar in many respects to those of primary hypokalaemic periodic paralysis. They are also accompanied by low serum potassium levels and may be relieved or prevented by giving potassium chloride. According to Engel (1972), the distinction between primary and thyrotoxic hypokalaemic periodic paralysis can be made by the following pharmacological test: in primary hypokalaemic periodic paralysis the intra-arterial injection of minute doses of epinephrine causes prompt paralysis of small hand muscles on the side of the injection, even in the absence of a generalized attack, while in thyrotoxic periodic paralysis the test is negative.

The treatment of thyrotoxicosis abolishes the periodic paralysis. However, the attacks may recur with relapse of the thyrotoxicosis. β-blockade with propranolol also prevents the paralytic attacks (Conway et al 1974).

Histopathology

The study of muscle biopsies in thyrotoxic periodic paralysis has been reported by many including Satoyoshi et al (1963), Jackman & Jones (1964), Engel (1966), Mussini et al (1968), Norris et al (1968, 1971), Schutta & Armitage (1969), Brody & Dudley (1969), Resnick et al (1969), Bergman et al (1970a,b), Dunkle et al (1970), Weller & McArdle (1971), Takagi et al (1973), Cheah et al (1975), and Pellissier et al (1980). In various cases, changes were not observed or were mild. In other cases they were similar to those in primary hypokalaemic periodic paralysis. However, vacuolation of muscle fibres is much less frequent and usually not very marked. Tubular

aggregates have been observed in very few cases (Mussini et al 1968, Bergman et al 1970b, Dunkle et al 1970). As in hypokalaemic periodic paralysis, the changes are usually more marked during than between attacks (Norris et al 1971), but even during attacks the biopsies may be normal (Cheah et al 1975). The latter authors in a light-microscopic study of 17 biopsies could not establish a relationship between the histological changes and the duration of the thyrotoxicosis, the duration of the periodic paralysis or the number of attacks. In an electron-microscopic study of 10 of these biopsies they did not find any relationship between the degree of ultrastructural change and the severity of the muscle weakness or the hypokalaemia during attacks.

The ultrastructural change that has been most frequently reported is dilatation of the sarcoplasmic reticulum. Such dilatation, as well as honeycomb structures in communication with T tubules, were clearly illustrated by Schutta & Armitage (1969) in a biopsy taken 12 hours after an induced paralysis. In this case mitochondrial inclusions and concentric laminated bodies were also seen.

It is possible that some of the morphological changes that have been described in thyrotoxic periodic paralysis may be due to an asymptomatic myopathy which is frequent in hyperthyroidism not complicated by periodic paralysis. (see Engel 1972).

HYPOKALAEMIC PARALYSIS OF OTHER ORIGINS

Clinical aspects

Muscle weakness may occur in many conditions in which serum potassium levels are decreased, and is often referred to as *hypokalaemic myopathy*. Hypokalaemia may have various causes, particularly inadequate intake, excessive loss by sweating and in gastrointestinal or renal loss of potassium (see Lindeman 1976, Nardone et al 1978). Acute episodes of weakness, resembling attacks of hypokalaemic periodic paralysis, are common in aldosteronism (see Conn et al 1964) and may also occur after chronic ingestion of liquorice (see Garcin et al 1961). In aldosteronism there is metabolic alkalosis and increased urinary loss of potassium. Liquorice contains ammonium glycyrrhizate which is a potent mineralocorticoid and experimentally can produce pseudoaldosteronism (see Conn et al 1968). In other causes of renal depletion of potassium (e.g. carbenoxolone administration—Mohamed et al 1966, the use of diuretics—Oh et al 1971, Jensen et al 1977), as well as in increased gastrointestinal loss of potassium (e.g. the use of laxatives—Van Horn et al 1970, chronic diarrhoea—Coërs et al 1972) the weakness is generally progressive over a few days and not periodic. The serum levels of muscle enzymes are usually markedly raised. In severe cases there may be myoglobinuria. The treatment of the weakness usually requires large doses of potassium over a period. The muscle disturbances do not recur after removal of the aetiological factors (e.g. withdrawal of drugs; ablation of an adrenal tumour in aldosteronism).

Hypokalaemia in alcoholic myopathy has been reported by Martin et al (1971), Khurana & Kalyanaraman (1977) and Rubenstein & Wainapel (1977). In three of the four cases reported by these authors, the onset of the weakness was preceded by a period of diarrhoea. In the 4th case (case 1 of Rubenstein & Wainapel) there was abundant sweating. Thus it has been suggested that the alcoholic myopathy might be due to potassium deficiency resulting from excessive loss of this ion. However, other pathogenetic mechanisms have also been proposed (see Knochel et al 1975).

Histopathology

The change most often reported in the various conditions in which muscle weakness is associated with hypokalaemia is vacuolation of muscle fibres (Heitzman et al 1962, Gross et al 1966, Oh et al 1971, Coërs et al 1972, Gallai 1977, Khurana & Kalyanaraman 1977, Atsumi et al 1979, Bautista et al 1979, Ruff 1979, Okamoto et al 1983). The vacuoles are neither as marked nor as frequent as those seen in primary hypokalaemic periodic paralysis. Necrotic and regenerating fibres are common, particularly in cases with myoglobinuria. In a few cases, atrophied fibres have been noted, occasionally in small groups (Hashimoto et al 1980). Atrophy of type 2A fibres was seen in one

case (Bautista et al 1979) but histochemical studies have been undertaken only rarely. Inflammatory infiltrates have occasionally been reported (Becker et al 1987, Severance et al 1989). Electron-microscopic findings were reported by Gross et al (1966), Gallai (1977), Jensen et al (1977), Atsumi et al (1979), Bautista et al (1979), Hashimoto et al (1980) and Okamoto et al (1983). The changes described include dilatation of the sarcoplasmic reticulum, vacuolation of some fibres and a few minor abnormalities. Tubular aggregates were observed in one patient with paretic attacks and slight permanent weakness associated with hyperaldosteronism (Gallai 1977). Intranuclear inclusions, consisting of fibrillary bundles, were reported in one case of hypokalaemia due to medication with diuretics (Okamoto et al 1983). Some ultrastructural changes in motor end-plates were described, in one case, by Hashimoto et al (1980). According to several authors there is regression of the changes after recovery. In a second biopsy taken from patients when the muscle disturbances have disappeared, abnormalities were minimal or absent (Sambrook et al 1972, Jensen et al 1977, Atsumi et al 1979).

EXPERIMENTAL HYPOKALAEMIA

The morphological changes in muscle due to potassium deficiency have been studied in dogs and rats (see De Coster 1979, Corbett & Pollock 1981). In most experiments the animals were fed with a potassium-deficient diet which, in the study of Corbett & Pollock (1981), was associated with an ion-exchange resin. In those of De Coster (1979) a diuretic (chlorothiazide) was used, together with normal food. In all the experiments, marked hypokalaemia was observed within a few weeks. Severe muscular weakness was seen in the dogs (Smith et al 1950, Tate et al 1978) but not in rats (Smith et al 1950, De Coster 1979). In both species there was retardation of growth, and death occurred if the potassium-deficient diet was continued. Smith et al (1950) observed morphological changes in the heart and kidney of the rat but not the dog. However, other authors have found some changes in the heart and kidney of dogs (see Tate et al 1978). Morphological changes have been found in skeletal muscles in both species, but the changes appear to be more marked in the dog than in the rat. Smith et al (1950) did not find any change in the rat. Gustafson et al (1973) have shown that, in rats fed on a potassium-restricted diet, the content of potassium decreased more markedly in skeletal muscle than in the heart.

The changes in skeletal muscle include vacuolation of some fibres, necrotic and regenerating fibres, and infiltration with mononuclear cells around degenerating fibres. Electron-microscopic studies showed membrane-bound vacuoles, dilatation of the sarcoplasmic reticulum and T tubules, membranous bodies and disruption of mitochondria (Kao & Gordon 1977, De Coster 1979, Corbett & Pollock 1981). Tubular aggregates have not been reported so far. Some changes in motor end-plates were described in the gastrocnemius muscle of the rat by De Coster (1979).

The muscle changes in experimental animals resemble somewhat those changes observed in human hypokalaemic myopathy. However, in the experimental model, vacuoles in the muscle fibres are less frequent and the necrosis and phagocytosis of the fibres are more marked than in the human myopathy.

SECONDARY HYPERKALAEMIA

Hyperkalaemia may arise in numerous clinical conditions including metabolic acidosis, renal failure, Addison's disease and hypoaldosteronism, and as a result of intravenous potassium administration and the use of potassium-retaining diuretics (see Whang 1976, DeFronzo 1980).

Muscle twitching, fatiguability and even episodes of weakness leading to flaccid quadriplegia may be observed in secondary hyperkalaemia. However, cardiac symptoms (hypotension and arrhythmias) precede and prevail over the skeletal muscle disturbances. The electrocardiographic changes reflect the changes in the serum potassium levels. Death may be caused by cardiac arrest.

Detailed studies of muscle biopsies in cases of secondary hyperkalaemia have not been reported.

MUSCLE CHANGES IN OSTEOMALACIA

Muscle weakness is common in osteomalacia but it is difficult to know whether it is due to a direct muscle effect or is secondary to limitation of movement due to skeletal pain. Many authors have attributed the weakness to an 'osteomalacic myopathy' (see Smith & Stern 1969, Dastur et al 1975, Schott & Willis 1976, Serratrice et al 1978). The main clinical features of this muscle disorder are easy fatiguability, progressive weakness predominating in the proximal limb muscles, hypotonia and a slow waddling gait. The tendon reflexes are usually brisk. The changes in the serum levels of calcium, inorganic phosphorus and alkaline phosphatase depend on the condition causing the osteomalacia. For example, in cases of severe vitamin D deficiency, there are hypocalcaemia, hypophosphataemia and raised serum levels of alkaline phosphatase. In these cases the muscle disturbances regress with vitamin D administration. In cases of different origin the treatment of the underlying condition is essential.

Muscle biopsy studies have been reported by various authors (see Mallette et al 1975, Schott & Willis 1975, Skaria et al 1975, Serratrice et al 1978). The changes are, as a rule, mild and consist mainly of scattered atrophic fibres with occasional clumping of the sarcolemmal nuclei. Necrosis and phagocytosis of fibres have not been reported. Histochemical studies have shown preferential atrophy of type 2 fibres (Mallette et al 1975, Schott & Willis 1975, Serratrice et al 1978) and occasional ragged-red fibres (Mallette et al 1975, Serratrice et al 1978). These changes can be observed in many muscle disorders. Ultrastructural changes revealed only slight and non-specific myofibrillary changes in some fibres (Dastur et al 1975, Schott & Willis 1975, Boudouresques et al 1977, Serratrice et al 1978).

Most authors regard the origin of the muscle disturbances in osteomalacia as myopathic and relate them to a disturbance of vitamin D metabolism (see Smith & Stern 1969, Schott & Willis 1975). Muscle changes (particularly type 2 fibre atrophy) have been induced in rats fed on a vitamin-D-deficient diet (Swash et al 1979). Mallette et al (1975) considered that the changes were neuropathic in nature and resembled those found in primary hyperparathyroidism. It is possible that, in many patients, the muscle changes are related to associated nutritional deficiencies (Dastur et al 1975, Skaria et al 1975). Ageing and disuse atrophy may be other factors.

MUSCLE CHANGES IN OTHER ELECTROLYTE DISTURBANCES

Muscle weakness, although rarely the predominant clinical symptom, may arise as result of changes in the serum concentration of phosphorus, calcium, sodium, magnesium and other electrolytes. In most cases, several ions may be involved simultaneously. Little has been reported concerning the pathology of the muscle in these conditions. Some pathological conditions will be mentioned briefly here.

Hypophosphataemia may occur in many clinical conditions and is sometimes accompanied by muscle dysfunction (see Knochel 1977). Hypophosphataemia may have a role in precipitating the myopathy of chronic alcoholism (Knochel et al 1975). In hypophosphataemia following hyperalimentation, muscle weakness is common. The central nervous system may be involved and death may ensue (see Silvis & Paragas 1972).

The muscle changes seen in osteomalacia associated with hypophosphataemia have already been mentioned. In other conditions associated with hypophosphataemia there are only a few reports on the muscle changes, and these provide little information. They include that of Furlan et al (1975), concerning a patient with hypophosphataemia related to hyperalimentation, whose biopsy was said to show evidence of denervation atrophy. Another report (Moser & Fessel 1974) concerning a patient with hypophosphataemia caused by excessive use of antacids stated that there were no histological abnormalities in the muscle.

Hyperphosphataemia does not apparently cause any muscular symptoms.

Hypocalcaemia may be attributable to many causes: its clinical manifestations vary in different individuals (see Juan 1979), the most significant being tetany. Muscle biopsies have been studied in hypocalcaemia associated with hypothyroidism, the findings being briefly described. In one case the muscle was said to be normal (Shane et al

1980) and in another to show myopathic changes (Snowdon et al 1976).

Hypercalcaemia associated with muscular lesions has been observed particularly in renal failure subsequent to rhabdomyolysis (see Cadnapaphornchai et al 1980). The rise in serum calcium results probably from the inability of the kidney to excrete calcium which has been released from muscle fibres undergoing necrosis. The necrosis is manifest in the histological examination, as is also some evidence of regeneration.

In severe *hyponatraemia* or *hypernatraemia*, associated with hypo-osmolarity or hyperosmolarity respectively, the principal symptoms are related to involvement of the central nervous system and muscle disturbances are usually not prominent. However, rhabdomyolysis has been described in connection with hyponatraemia (Alamartine et al 1987). Hyponatraemia may have many origins (see Moses & Miller 1974) and in many cases the most important symptoms are those of the underlying disease. Hypernatraemia may be due to hypothalamic lesions. In these cases muscle paralysis may occur and is probably due to both hypernatraemia and reduction of total body potassium (see Alford et al 1973). There are few reports on muscle biopsy findings in hyponatraemia and hypernatraemia and these give little information.

Hypomagnesaemia may induce hypocalcaemia (see Juan 1979) and patients with this condition may experience muscle disturbances (see Weigmann & Kaye 1977, Juan 1982). Pall et al (1987) described scattered atrophic muscle fibres in an alcoholic patient with hypomagnesaemia and hypocalcaemia. The myopathy responded well to magnesium supplementation. In magnesium deficiency in rats a few minor changes in the muscle fibres have been noted (see Robeson et al 1980).

Hypermagnesaemia may be attributable to oral or rectal administration of magnesium-containing cathartics and may be accompanied by severe muscular weakness due to neuromuscular block (Swift 1979, Castelbaum et al 1989). As far as we know, histological studies of muscle in this condition have not been reported.

In conclusion, this brief survey of the changes

in muscle associated with disorders of electrolytes other than potassium shows that there is scanty evidence of structural changes. Those described are mild and non-specific. The lack of information on this topic may be due to lack of interest and inadequate methods of investigation.

ACKNOWLEDGEMENTS
We are indebted to Drs M. Fardeau and W. G. P. Mair for their suggestions regarding the manuscript, to Mmes J. Godet-Guillain, M. Chevallay and H. Collin, and Miss J. Reix for their assistance in the study of the muscle biopsies on which this work is based, and to Miss A. Rouche for her help and skill in preparing the photographs.

REFERENCES

Aitken R S, Allott E N, Castleden L I M 1937 Observations in a case of familial periodic paralysis. Clinical Science 3: 34

Alamartine E, Gerard M, Boyer F, Robert D 1987 Rhabdomyolyse itérative par hyponatrémie. La Presse Médicale 16: 490

Alford F P, Scoggins B A, Wharton C 1973 Symptomatic normovolemic essential hypernatraemia: a clinical and physiologic study. American Journal of Medicine 54: 359

Atsumi T, Ishikawa S, Miyatake T, Yoshida M 1979 Myopathy and primary aldosteronism: electronmicroscopic study. Neurology (Minneapolis) 29: 1348

Bautista J, Gli-Neciga E, Gil-Peralta A 1979 Hypokalemic periodic paralysis in primary hyperaldosteronism. European Neurology 18: 415

Becker N J, Hinman M, Giles M N, Kepes J J, Abdou N I 1987 Polymyositis with hypokalemia: Correction with potassium replacement in the absent of steroids. Journal of Rheumatology 14: 1042

Becker P E 1970 Paramyotonia congenita (Eulenberg) In: P E Becker, W Lenz, F Vogel, G G Wendt (eds) Advances in human genetics, vol 3. Thieme, Stuttgart, p 1

Bekény G 1961 Über irreversible Muskelveränderungen bei der paroxysmalen Lahmung auf Grund bioptischer Muskeluntersuchungen. Deutsche Zeitschrift für Nervenheilkunde 182: 119

Bekény G, Hasznos T, Solti, F 1961 Über die hyperkalämische Form der paroxysmalen Lahmung. Zur Frage der Adynamia episodica hereditaria. Deutsche Zeitschrift für Nervenheilkunde 182: 92

Bergman R A, Afifi A K, Dunkle L M, Johns R J 1970a Muscle pathology in hypokalemic periodic paralysis with hyperthyroidism: high resolution light microscopic study of a case. Johns Hopkins Medical Journal 126: 88

Bergman R A, Afifi A K, Dunkel L M, Johns R J 1970b Muscle pathology in hypokalemic periodic paralysis with hyperthyroidism: a light and electron microscopic study. Johns Hopkins Medical Journal 126: 100

Bernhard J D, Larson M A, Norris F H 1972 Thyrotoxic periodic paralysis in Californians of Mexican and Filipino ancestry. California Medicine 116: 70

Biczyskowa W, Fidziánska A, Jedrzejowska H 1969 Light and electron microscopic study of the muscles in hypokalemic periodic paralysis. Acta neuropathologica (Berlin) 12: 329

Biemond A, Daniels A P 1934 Familial periodic paralysis and its transition into spinal muscular atrophy. Brain 57: 91

Boudouresques J, Khalil R, Vigouroux R A, Pellissier J F, Maestraci D, Cros D 1977 Myopathie ostéomalacique. A propos d'une observation. Revue Neurologique 133: 709

Bradley W G 1969a Adynamia episodica hereditaria. Clinical pathological and electrophysiological studies in an affected family. Brain 92: 345

Bradley W G 1969b Ultrastructural changes in adynamia episodica hereditaria and normokalemic familial periodic paralysis. Brain 92: 379

Brody I A, Dudley A W 1969 Thyrotoxic hypokalemic periodic paralysis. Archives of Neurology (Chicago) 21: 1

Brooke M H 1977 A clinician's view of neuromuscular diseases. Williams & Wilkins, Baltimore

Brooke M H, Engel W K 1969 The histographic analysis of human muscle biopsies with regard to fiber types. 3. Myotonias, myasthenia gravis and hypokalemic periodic paralysis. Neurology (Minneapolis) 19: 469

Buruma O J S, Schipperheyn J J 1979 Periodic paralysis. In: Vinken P J, Bruyn G W, Ringel S P (eds) Diseases of muscle. Part II, volume 41, Handbook of clinical neurology. North-Holland Publishing Company, Amsterdam, p 147

Buruma O J S, Bots G T A M, Went L N 1985 Familial hypokalemic periodic paralysis. 50-year follow-up of a large family. Archives of Neurology 42: 28

Buruma O J S, Bots G T A M 1978 Myopathy in familial hypokalaemic periodic paralysis independent of paralytic attacks. Acta Neurologica Scandinavica 57: 171

Buzzard E F 1901 Three cases of family periodic paralysis, with a consideration of the pathology of the disease. Lancet 2: 1564

Cadnapaphornchai P, Taher S, McDonald F D 1980 Acute drug-associated rhabdomyolysis: an examination of its diverse renal manifestations and complications. American Journal of the Medical Sciences 280: 66

Carlson M J, Pearson C M 1964 Familial hyperkalemic periodic paralysis with myotonic features. Journal of Pediatrics 64: 853

Castaigne P, Laplane D, Escourolle R, Fardeau M, Poirier J, Turpin J C 1971 Etude clinique, histologique et ultrastructurale d'une variété de paramyotonie d'Eulenburg. In: Serratrice. G, Roux H (eds) Actualités de pathologie neuro-musculaire. Expansion Scientifique Française, Paris, p 333

Castelbaum A R, Donofrio P D, Walker F O, Troost B T 1989 Laxative abuse causing hypermagnesemia, quadriparesis, and neuromuscular junction defect. Neurology 39: 746

Cheah J S, Tock E P C, Kan S P 1975 The light and electron microscopic changes in the skeletal muscles during paralysis in thyrotoxic periodic paralysis. American Journal of the Medical Sciences 269: 365

Chesson A L, Schochet S S, Peters B H 1979 Biphasic periodic paralysis. Archives of Neurology (Chicago) 36: 700

Clausen T, Wang P, Orskov H, Kristensen O 1980

Hyperkalemic periodic paralysis. Relationships between changes in plasma water, electrolytes, insulin and catecholamines during attacks. Scandinavian Journal of Clinical & Laboratory Investigation 40: 211

Coërs C, Telerman-Toppet N, Cremer M 1972 Acute quadriparesis with muscle spasms related to electrolyte disturbances in steatorrhea. American Journal of Medicine 52: 849

Conn J W, Knopf R F, Nesbit R M 1964 Clinical characteristics of primary aldosteronism from an analysis of 145 cases. American Journal of Surgery 107: 159

Conn J W, Rovner D R, Cohen E L 1968 Licorice-induced pseudo-aldosteronism: hypertension, hypokalemia, aldosteronopenia and suppressed plasma renin activity. Journal of the American Medical Association 205: 492

Conway M J, Seibel J A, Eaton P 1974 Thyrotoxicosis and periodic paralysis: improvement with beta blockade. Annals of Internal Medicine 81: 332

Corbett V A, Nuttall F Q 1975 Familial hypokalemic periodic paralysis in blacks. Annals of Internal Medicine 83: 63

Corbett A J, Pollock M 1981 Experimental potassium depletion myopathy. Journal of the Neurological Sciences 49: 193

Cousot G 1887 Paralysie périodique. Revue de Médicine 7: 190

Crafts L M 1900 A fifth case of family periodic paralysis. American Journal of the Medical Sciences 119: 651

Dalakas M C, Engel W K 1983 Treatment of 'permanent' muscle weakness in familial hypokalemic periodic paralysis. Muscle and Nerve 6: 82

Danowski T S, Fisher E R, Vidalon C, Vester J W, Thompson R, Nolan S et al 1975 Clinical and ultrastructural observations in a kindred with normo-kalemic periodic paralysis. Journal of Medical Genetics 12: 20

Dastur D K, Gagrat B M, Wadia N H, Desai M M, Bharucha E P 1975 Nature of muscular changes in osteomalacia: light- and electron-microscope obervations. Journal of Pathology 117: 211

De Coster W J P 1979 Experimental hypokalemia: ultrastructural changes in rat gastrocnemius muscle. Acta neuropathologica (Berlin) 45: 79

DeFronzo R A 1980 Hyperkalemia and hyporeninemic hypoaldosteronism. Kidney International 17: 118

Delwaide P-J, Penders C-A, Daubresse J C, Dodinval P, Reznik M 1971 Paramyotonie familiale et crises parétiques avec hypokaliémie. Revue Neurologique 125: 287

de Silva S M, Kuncl R W, Griffin J W, Cornblatt D R, Chavonstie S 1990 Paramyotonia congenita or hyperkalemic periodic paralysis? Clinical and electrophysiological features of each entity in one family. Muscle and Nerve 13: 21

Drager G A, Hammill J F, Shy G M 1958 Paramyotonia congenita. Archives of Neurology and Psychiatry 80: 1

Duchen L W 1971 Changes in the electron microscopic structure of slow and fast skeletal muscle fibres of the mouse after the local injection of botulinum toxin. Journal of the Neurological Sciences 14: 61

Duchen L W 1973 The local effects of tetanus toxin on the electron microscopic structure of skeletal muscle fibres of the mouse. Journal of the Neurological Sciences 19: 169

Dunkle L M, Diggs, C H, Bergman R A, Johns R J 1970 A light and electron microscopic study of a second case of hypokalemic periodic paralysis with hyperthyroidism. Johns Hopkins Medical Journal 126: 225

Dyken M L, Timmons G D 1963 Hyperkalemic periodic paralysis with hyocalcemic episode. Absence of an autosomal dominant pedigree pattern. Archives of Neurology 9: 508

Dyken M, Zeman W, Rusche T 1969 Hypokalemic periodic

paralysis. Children with permanent myopathic weakness. Neurology (Minneapolis) 19: 691

Engel A G 1961 Thyroid function and periodic paralysis. American Journal of Medicine 30: 327

Engel W K 1964 Mitchondrial aggregates in muscle disease. Journal of Histochemistry and Cytochemistry 12: 46

Engel A G 1966 Electron microscopic observations in primary hypokalaemic and thyrotoxic periodic paralyses. Mayo Clinic Proceedings 41: 797

Engel A G 1970 Evolution and content of vacuoles in primary hypokalaemic periodic paralysis. Mayo Clinic Proceedings 45: 774

Engel A G 1972 Neuromuscular manifestations of Graves' disease. Mayo Clinic Proceedings 47: 919

Engel A G 1973 Vacuolar myopathies: multiple etiologies and sequential structural studies. In: Pearson C M, Mostofi F K (eds) The striated muscle. Williams and Wilkins, Baltimore, p 301

Engel A G, Lambert E H 1969 Calcium activation of electrically inexcitable muscle fibres in primary hypokalemic periodic paralysis. Neurology (Minneapolis) 19: 851

Engel A G, Lambert E H, Rosevear J W, Tauxe W N 1965 Clinical and electromyographic studies in a patient with primary hypokalemic periodic paralysis. American Journal of Medicine 38: 626

Engel W K, Bishop D W, Cunningham G G 1970 Tubular aggregates in type 2 muscle fibers, ultrastructural and histochemical correlation. Journal of Ultrastructural Research 31: 507

Eulenburg A 1886 Ueber eine familiäre, durch 6 Generationen verfolgbare Form congenitaler Paramyotonic. Neurologisches Centralblatt 5: 265

Fardeau M, Tomé F M S, Simon P 1979 Muscle and nerve changes induced by perhexiline maleate in man and mice. Muscle and Nerve 2: 24

Fontaine B, Khurana T S, Hoffman E P, Bruns G A P, Haines, J L et al 1990 Hyperkalaemic periodic paralysis and the adult muscle sodium α-subunit gene. Science 250: 1000

French E B, Kilpatrick R 1957 A variety of paramyotonia congenita. Journal of Neurology, Neurosurgery and Psychiatry 20: 40

Friis M L, Johnsen T, Saltin B, Paulson O B 1985 Skeletal muscle in paramyotonia congenita: biochemistry, histochemistry and morphology. Acta Neurologica Scandinavica 71: 62

Furlan A J, Hanson M, Cooperman A, Farmer R G 1975 Acute areflexic paralysis: association with hyperalimentation and hypophosphatemia. Archives of Neurology (Chicago) 32: 706

Gallai M 1977 Myopathy with hyperaldosteronism: an electron-microscopic study. Journal of the Neurological Sciences 32: 337

Gammon G D 1938 Relation of potassium to family periodic paralysis. Proceedings of the Society for Experimental Biology and Medicine 38: 922

Gamstorp I 1956 Adynamia episodica hereditaria. Acta paediatrica (Uppsala) 45 suppl 108: 1

Gamstorp I 1962 A study of transient muscular weakness. Clinical, biochemical and electromyographic findings during attacks of periodic paralysis and adynamia episodica hereditaria. Acta neurologica scandinavica 38: 3

Gamstorp I 1963 Adynamia episodica hereditaria and myotonia. Acta neurologica scandinavica 39: 41

Garcin R, Goulon M, Tournilhac M, Amor B 1961 Nouvelle observation de paralysies avec hypokaliémie et alcalose métabolique secondaires à l'ingestion excessive et prolongée d'extrait de réglisse après cure de desintoxication éthylique.

Revue Neurologique 104: 461

Garcin R, Legrain M, Rondot P, Fardeau M 1966 Etude clinique et métabolique d'une observation de paramyotonie congénitale d'Eulenburg. Documents ultrastucturaux concernant la biopsie musculaire. Revue Neurologique 115: 295

Gérard J M, Khoubesserian K, Telerman-Toppet N, Barsy Th de, Coërs C 1978 Paralysie périodique familiale avec hypokaliémie, hyperaldostéronisme et vacuolisation extra-cellulaire. Revue Neurologique 134: 761

Goldflam S 1895 Weitere Mittheilung über die paroxysmale, familiäre Lähmung. Deutsche Zeitschrift für Nervenheilkunde 7: 1

Goldflam S 1897 Dritte Mittheilung über die paroxysmale, familiäre Lähmung. Deutsche Zeitschrift für Nervenheilkunde 11: 242

Gordon A M, Kao I 1977 Membranes, electrolytes, periodic paralysis. In: Rowland L P (ed) Pathogenesis of human muscular dystrophies. Proceedings of the Fifth International Scientific Conference of the Muscular Dystrophy Association, International Congress Series no. 404, Excerpta Medica, Amsterdam, p 762

Gordon A M, Green J R, Lagunoff D 1970 Studies on a patient with hypokalemic familial periodic paralysis. American Journal of Medicine 48: 185

Griggs R C, Engel W K, Resnick J S 1970 Acetazolamide treatment of hypokalemic periodic paralysis: prevention of attacks and improvement of persistent weakness. Annals of Internal Medicine 73: 39

Griggs R C, Resnick J, Engel W K 1983 Intravenous treatment of hypokalemic periodic paralysis. Archives of Neurology 40: 539

Gross E G, Dexter J D, Roth R G 1966 Hypokalemic myopathy with myoglobinuria associated with licorice ingestion. New England Journal of Medicine 274: 602

Gruner J E 1966 Anomalies du réticulum sarcoplasmique et prolifération de tubules dans le muscle d'une paralysie périodique familiale. Comptes Rendus des Séances de la Société de Biologie et de ses Filiales (Paris) 160: 193

Gruner J E, Porte A 1959 Les lésions musculaires dans la paralysie périodique familiale. Revue Neurologique 101: 501

Gustafson A B, Shear L, Gabuzda G J 1973 Protein metabolism in vivo in kidney, liver, muscle and heart of potassium-deficient rats. Journal of Laboratory and Clinical Medicine 82: 287

Hashimoto S, Akai F, Semba E, Sakatani K, Hiruma S, Nagaoka M et al 1980 Neuronal changes of hypokalemic myopathy. A light- and electron-microscopic study on muscle biopsy. Journal of the Neurological Sciences 44: 169

Heene R 1986 Evidence of myotonic origin of type 2B muscle fibre deficiency in myotonia and paramyotonia congenita. Journal of the Neurological Sciences 76: 357

Heene R, Gabriel R-R, Manz F, Schimrigk K 1986 Type 2B Muscle fibre deficiency in myotonia and paramyotonia congenita. A genetically determined histochemical fibre type pattern? Journal of the Neurological Sciences 73: 23

Heitzman E J, Patterson J E, Stanley M M 1962 Myoglobinuria and hypokalemia in regional enteritis. Archives of Internal Medicine 110: 117

Helweg-Larsen H F, Hauge M, Sagild U 1955 Hereditary transient muscular paralysis in Denmark. Genetic aspects of family periodic paralysis and family periodic adynamia. Acta genetica et statistica medica 5: 263

Hofmann W W, Adornato B T, Reich H 1983 The relationship of insulin receptor to hypokalemic periodic paralysis. Muscle and Nerve 6: 48

Holtzapple G E 1905 Periodic paralysis. Journal of the American Medical Association 45: 1224

Howes E L, Price H M, Pearson C M, Blumberg J M 1966 Hypokalemic periodic paralysis: electronmicroscopic changes in the sarcoplasm. Neurology (Minneapolis) 16: 242

Ionasescu V, Radu H, Nicolescu P 1971 Ultrastructural changes in hypokalaemic periodic paralysis. Revue Roumaine de Neurologie 8: 419

Ionasescu V, Zellweger H S, Schochet S S, Conway T W 1973 Biochemical abnormalities of muscle ribosomes during attacks of hyperkalaemic periodic paralysis. Journal of the Neurological Sciences 19: 389

Ionasescu V, Schochet S S, Powers J W, Koob K, Conway T W 1974 Hypokalaemic periodic paralysis. Journal of the Neurological Sciences 21: 419

Isch F, Stoebner P, Warter J M 1968 Paramyotonie congénitale de von Eulenburg: étude des observations d'une enfant et de sa mère. Revue Neurologique 118: 214

Jackman R L, Jones R E 1964 Hyperthyroidism and periodic paralysis. Archives of Internal Medicine 113: 657

Jensen O B, Mosdal C, Reske-Nielsen E 1977 Hypokalemic myopathy during treatment with diuretics. Acta neurologica scandinavica 55: 465

Johnsen T, Beck-Nielsen H 1979 Insulin receptors, insulin secretion and glucose disappearance rate in patients with periodic hypokalaemic paralysis. Acta endocrinologica 90: 272

Juan D 1979 Hypocalcemia. Differential diagnosis and mechanisms. Archives of Internal Medicine 139: 1166

Juan D 1982 Clinical review: the clinical importance of hypomagnesemia. Surgery 91: 510

Julien J, Vital C, Vallat J M, Marin F 1971 Paramyotonie d'Eulenburg. Journal of the Neurological Sciences 13: 447

Kao I, Gordon A M 1977 Alteration of skeletal muscle cellular structures by potassium depletion. Neurology (Minneapolis) 27: 855

Khurana R, Kalyanaraman K 1977 Hypokalemic vacuolar myopathy of chronic alcoholism: a histological and histochemical study. Diseases of the Nervous System 38: 287

Klein R, Egan T, Usher P 1960 Changes in sodium, potassium and water in hyperkalemic familial periodic paralysis. Metabolism 9: 1005

Klein R, Ganelin R, Marks J F, Usher P, Richards C 1963 Periodic paralysis with cardiac arrhythmia. Journal of Pediatrics 62: 371

Knochel J P 1977 The pathophysiology and clinical characteristics of severe hypophosphatemia. Archives of Internal Medicine 137: 203

Knochel J P, Bilbrey G L, Fuller T J, Carter N W 1975 The muscle cell in chronic alcoholism: the possible role of phosphate depletion in alcoholic myopathy. Annals of the New York Academy of Sciences 252: 274

Layzer R B, Lovelace R E, Rowland L P 1967 Hyperkalemic periodic paralysis. Archives of Neurology (Chicago) 16: 455

Levitt L P, Rose L I, Dawson D M 1972 Hypokalemic periodic paralysis with arrhythmia. New England Journal of Medicine 286: 253

Lewis D D, Pallis C, Pearse A G E 1971 Myopathy with tubular aggregates. Journal of the Neurological Sciences 13: 381

Lewis E D, Griggs R C, Moxley R T 1979 Regulation of plasma potassium in hyperkalemic periodic paralysis. Neurology (Minneapolis) 29: 1131

Lindeman R D 1976 Hypokalemia: causes, consequences and correction. American Journal of the Medical Sciences 272: 5

Links T J, Zwarts M J, Oosterhuis H J G H 1988 Improvement

of muscle strength in familial hypokalaemic periodic paralysis with acetazolamide. Journal of Neurology, Neurosurgery and Psychiatry 51: 1142

Lisak R P, Lebeau J, Tucker S H, Rowland L P 1972 Hyperkalemic periodic paralysis and cardiac arrhythmia. Neurology (Minneapolis) 22: 810

Lundberg P O, Stalberg E, Thiele D 1974 Paralysis periodica paramyotonia: A clinical and neurophysiological study. Journal of the Neurological Sciences 21: 309

McArdle B 1962 Adynamia episodica hereditaria and its treatment. Brain 85: 121

McArdle B 1963 Metabolic myopathies. The glycogenosis affecting muscle and hypo- and hyperkalemic periodic paralysis. American Journal of Medicine 35: 661

MacDonald R D, Rewcastle N B, Humphrey J G 1968 The myopathy of hyperkalemic periodic paralysis: an electron microscopic study. Archives of Neurology (Chicago) 19: 274

MacDonald R D, Rewcastle N D, Humphrey J G 1969 Myopathy of hypokalaemic periodic paralysis. Archives of Neurology (Chicago) 20: 565

MacFadzean A J S, Yeung R 1967 Periodic paralysis complicating thyrotoxicosis in Chinese. British Medical Journal 1: 451

Mair W G P, Tomé F M S 1972 Atlas of the ultrastructure of diseased human muscle. Churchill Livingstone, Edinburgh and London

Mallette L E, Pattern B M, Engel W K 1975 Muscular disease in secondary hyperparathyroidism. Annals of Internal Medicine 82: 474

Martin J B, Craig J W, Eckel R E 1971 Hypokalemic myopathy in chronic alcoholism. Neurology (Minneapolis) 21: 1160

Martin J J, Ceuterick C, Mercelis R, Amrom D 1984 Familial periodic paralysis with hypokalaemia. Study of a muscle biopsy in the myopathic stage of the disorder. Acta Neurologica Belgica 84: 233

Meyers K R, Gilden D H, Rinaldi C F, Hansen J L 1972 Periodic muscle weakness, normokalemia and tubular aggregates. Neurology (Minneapolis) 22: 269

Mohamed S D, Chapman R S, Crooks J 1966 Hypokalaemia, flaccid quadriparesis and myoglobinuria with carbenoxolone (Biogastrone). British Medical Journal 1: 1581

Morgan-Hughes J A, Mair W G P, Lascelles P T 1970 A disorder of skeletal muscle associated with tubular aggregates. Brain 93: 873

Moser C R, Fessel W J 1974 Rheumatic manifestation of hypophosphatemia. Archives of Internal Medicine 134: 674

Moses A M, Miller M 1974 Drug-induced dilutional hyponatremia. New England Journal of Medicine 291: 1234

Mussini I, DiMauro S, Margreth A 1968 Hypertrophy and proliferative changes of the SR in periodic paralysis. Abstracts of the 4th European Regional Conference on Electron Microscopy. Tipographia Poliglotta Vaticana, Rome, p 309

Nardone D A, MacDonald W J, Girard D E 1978 Mechanisms in hypokalemia: clinical correlation. Medicine (Baltimore) 57: 435

Norris F H, Panner B J, Stormont J M 1968 Thyrotoxic periodic paralysis. Metabolic and ultrastructural studies. Archives of Neurology (Chicago) 19: 88

Norris F H Jr, Clarck E C, Biglieri E G 1971 Studies in thyrotoxic periodic paralysis. Journal of the Neurological Sciences 13: 431

Odor D L, Patel A N, Pearce L A 1967 Familial hypokalaemic periodic paralysis with permanent myopathy. Journal of Neuropathology and Experimental Neurology 26: 98

Oh S J, Douglas J E, Brown R A 1971 Hypokalemic vacuolar myopathy associated with chlorthalidone treatment. Journal of the American Medical Association 216: 1858

Okamoto K, Uchiyama T, Sato S, Harigaya Y, Hirai S 1983 A case of hypokalemic myopathy with two types of filamentous intranuclear inclusions. Clinical Neurology 24: 379 (in Japanese)

Olivarius B F, Christensen E 1965 Histopathological muscular changes in familial periodic paralysis. Acta neurologica scandinavica 41: 1

Oppenheim H 1891 Neue Mittheilungen über den von Professor Westphal beschriebene Fall von periodischer Lähmung aller vier Extremitäten. Charité-Annalen 16: 350

Pall H S, Williams A C, Heath D A, Sheppard M, Wilson R 1987 Hypomagnesaemia causing myopathy and hypocalcaemia in an alcoholic. Postgraduate Medical Journal 63: 665

Pearse A G E, Johnson M 1970 Histochemistry in the study of normal and diseased muscle with special reference to myopathy with tubular aggregates. In: Walton J N, Canal N, Scarlato G (eds) Proceedings of the International Congress on Muscle Diseases. International Congress Series no. 199, Excerpta Medica, Amsterdam, p 25

Pearson C M 1964 The periodic paralysis: differential features and pathological observations in permanent myopathic weakness. Brain 87: 341

Pearson C M 1973 Pathological features of the periodic paralyses. In: Pearson C M, Mostofi F K (eds) The striated muscle. Williams and Wilkins, Baltimore, p 427

Pellissier J F, Faugere M C, Gambarelli D, Toga M 1980 Les paralysies périodiques. Etude histologique, histochimique et ultrastructurale du muscle, à propos de cinq observations. Archives d'Anatomie et de Cytologie Pathologiques 28: 5

Poskanzer D C, Kerr D N S 1961 A third type of periodic paralysis with normokalemia and favourable response to sodium chloride. American Journal of Medicine 31: 328

Pearson C M, Engel W K 1967 Myotonic lid lag in hypokalaemic periodic paralysis. Journal of Neurology, Neurosurgery and Psychiatry 30: 47

Resnick J S, Dorman J D, Engel W K 1969 Thyrotoxic periodic paralysis. American Journal of Medicine 47: 831

Ricker K, Haas A, Rüdel R, Böhlen R, Mertens H G 1980 Successful treatment of paramyotonia congenita (Eulenberg): muscle stiffness and weakness prevented by tocainide. Journal of Neurology, Neurosurgery and Psychiatry 43: 268

Ricker K, Böhlen R, Rohkamm R 1983 Different effectiveness of tocainide and hydrochlorothiazide in paramyotonia congenita with hyperkalemic episodic paralysis. Neurology 33: 1615

Riggs J E, Moxley R T, Griggs R C, Horner F A 1981 Hyperkalemic periodic paralysis: an apparent sporadic case. Neurology 31: 1157

Robeson B L, Martin W G, Friedman M H 1980 A biochemical and ultrastructural study of skeletal muscle from rats fed a magnesium-deficient diet. Journal of Nutrition 110: 2078

Rubenstein A E, Wainapel S F 1977 Acute hypokalemic myopathy in alcoholism. A clinical entity. Archives of Neurology (Chicago) 34: 553

Rüdel R, Ricker K 1985 The primary periodic paralyses. Trends in Neurosciences 8: 467

Ruff R L 1979 Insulin-induced weakness in hypokalemic myopathy. Annals of Neurology 6: 139

Sagild U 1959 Hereditary transient paralysis with special reference to the metabolism of potassium: familial periodic paralysis. Familial episodic adynamia. Munksgaard, Copenhagen

Samaha F J 1965 Hyperkalemic periodic paralysis. Archives of Neurology (Chicago) 12: 145

Samaha F J 1979 Molecular aspects of muscle disease. In: Baum H, Gergely J (eds) Molecular Aspects of Medicine. Pergamon Press, Oxford vol 2, no. 5, p 293

Sambrook M A, Heron J R, Aber G M 1972 Myopathy in association with primary aldosteronism. Journal of Neurology, Neurosurgery and Psychiatry 35: 202

Satoyoshi E, Murakami K, Kowa H, Kinoshita M, Nishiyama Y 1963 Periodic paralysis in hyperthyroidism. Neurology (Minneapolis) 13: 746

Saunders M, Ashworth B, Emery A E H, Benedikz J E G 1968 Familial myotonic periodic paralysis with muscle wasting. Brain 91: 295

Schiaffino S, Severin E, Cantini M, Sartore S 1977 Tubular aggregates induced by anoxia in isolated rat skeletal muscle. Laboratory Investigation 37: 223

Schiffer D, Giordana M T, Monga G, Mollo F 1976 Histochemistry and electron microscopy of muscle fibres in a case of congenital paramyotonia. Journal of Neurology 211: 125

Schipperheyn J J, Buruma O J S, Voogd P J 1978 Hypokalaemic periodic paralysis and cardiomyopathy. Acta neurologica scandinavica 58: 374

Schott G D, Willis M R 1975 Myopathy in hypophosphataemic osteomalacia presenting in adult life. Journal of Neurology, Neurosurgery and Psychiatry 38: 297

Schott G D, Willis M R 1976 Muscle weakness in osteomalacia. Lancet i: 626

Schröder J M, Becker P E 1972 Anomalien des T-Systems und des Sarkoplasmatischen Reticulums bei der Myotonie, Paramyotonie und Adynamie. Virchows Archiv A: Pathological Anatomy and Histology 357: 319

Schutta H S, Armitage J L 1969 Thyrotoxic hypokalemic periodic paralysis. Journal of Neuropathology and Experimental Neurology 28: 321

Serratrice G, Pellissier J F, Cross D 1978 Les atteintes musculaires des ostéomalacies: étude clinique, histoenzymologique et ultrastructurale de 10 cas. Revue du Rhumatisme 45: 621

Severance H W, Holt T, Patrone N A, Chapman L 1989 Profound muscle weakness and hypokalemia due to clay ingestion. Southern Medical Journal 81: 272

Shane E, McClane K A, Olarte M R, Bilezikian J P 1980 Hypoparathyroidism and elevated muscle enzymes. Neurology (Minneapolis) 30: 192

Shulkin D, Olson B R, Levey G S 1989 Case report: thyrotoxic periodic paralysis in a Latin-American taking acetazolamide. American Journal of the Medical Sciences 297: 337

Shy G M, Wanko T, Rowley P T, Engel A G 1961 Studies in familial periodic paralysis. Experimental Neurology 3: 53

Sigwald J, Rondot P, Fardeau M, Godet-Guillan J 1971 Paramyotonie congénitale d'Eulenburg. Etude clinique, biologique, histologique et ultrastructurale d'une nouvelle observation familiale. Revue Neurologique 124: 439

Silvis S E, Paragas P D, 1972 Paresthesias, weakness, seizures and hypophosphatemia in patients receiving hyperalimentation. Gastroenterology 62: 513

Singer H D, Goodbody F W 1901 A case of family periodic paralysis with a critical digest of the literature. Brain 24: 257

Singer B, Thomas M, Rozensztajn L 1977 Paralysie périodique sporadique chez un français de 41 ans révélatrice d'une maladie de Basedow. Annales de Médecine Interne 128: 533

Skaria J, Katiyar B C, Srivastava T P, Dube B 1975 Myopathy and neuropathy associated with osteomalacia. Acta Neurologica Scandinavica 51: 37

Smith R, Stern G 1969 Muscular weakness in osteomalacia and hyperparathyroidism. Journal of the Neurological Sciences 8: 511

Smith S G, Black-Schaffer B, Lasater T E 1950 Potassium deficiency syndrome in the rat and the dog: a description of the muscle changes in the potassium-depleted dog. Archives of Pathology 49: 185

Snowdon J A, Macfie A C, Pearce J B 1976 Hypocalcaemic myopathy with paranoid psychosis. Journal of Neurology, Neurosurgery and Psychiatry 39: 48

Streeten D H P, Dalakos T G, Fellerman H 1971 Studies on hyperkalemic periodic paralysis. Evidence of changes in plasma Na and Cl and induction of paralysis by adrenal glucocorticoids. Journal of Clinical Investigation 50: 142

Streib E W 1987 Paramyotonia congenita: successful treatment with tocainide. Clinical and electrophysiological findings in seven patients. Muscle and Nerve 10: 155

Streib E W 1989 Hypokalemic paralysis in two patients with paramyotonia congenita (PC) and known hyperkalemic/exercise-induced weakness. Muscle and Nerve 12: 936

Swash M, Schwartz M S, Sargeant M K 1979 Osteomalacic myopathy: an experimental approach. Neuropathology and Applied Neurobiology 5: 295

Swift T R 1979 Weakness from magnesium-containing cathartics: electrophysiologic studies. Muscle and Nerve 2: 295

Takagi A, Schotland D L, DiMauro S, Rowland L P 1973 Thyrotoxic periodic paralysis. Function of sarcoplasmic reticulum and muscle glycogen. Neurology (Minneapolis) 23: 1008

Talbott J H 1941 Periodic paralysis, a clinical syndrome. Medicine (Baltimore) 20: 85

Tate C L, Bagdon W J, Bokelman D L 1978 Morphologic abnormalities in potassium-deficient dogs. American Journal of Pathology 93: 103

Thomas C, Babin E, Isch F 1966 De l'unité de la paralysie périodique. Revue Neurologique 115: 262

Thomas C, Schweitzer R, Isch F, Collin H, Fardeau M 1978 Données nouvelles sur la généalogie, la clinique et l'histologie d'une famille atteinte de paralysie pérodique hyperkaliémique. Revue Neurologique 134: 45

Thrush D C, Morris C J, Salmon M V 1972 Paramyotonia congenita: a clinical, histochemical and pathological study. Brain 95: 537

Tyler F H, Stephens F E, Gunn F D, Perkoff G T 1951 Studies in disorders of muscle. VII. Clinical manifestations and inheritance of a type of periodic paralysis without hypopotassemia. Journal of Clinical Investigation 30: 492

van Bogaert L, Kissel P, Schmitt J, Martin J J, Claes C, Duc M et al 1967 Syndrome myopathique au cours d'une maladie de Gamstorp. Etude anatomique. Acta Neurologica Belgica 67: 133

van Horn G, Drori J B, Schwartz F D 1970 Hypokalemic myopathy and elevation of serum enzymes. Archives of Neurology (Chicago) 22: 335

Wang P, Clausen T 1976 Treatment of attacks in hyperkalaemic familial periodic paralysis by inhalation of salbutamol. Lancet i: 221

Wegmüller E, Ludin H P, Mumenthaler M 1979 Paramyotonia congenita. A clinical, electrophysiological and histological study of 12 patients. Journal of Neurology 250: 251

Weller R O, McArdle B 1971 Calcification within muscle fibres in periodic paralysis. Brain 94: 263

Westphal C 1885 Ueber einen merkwürdigen Fall von periodischer Lähmung aller vier Extremitäten mit gleichzeitigen Erlöschen der elektrischen Erregbarkeit während der Lähmung. Berliner klinische Wochenschrift 22: 489

Whang R 1976 Hyperkalemia: diagnosis and treatment. American Journal of the Medical Sciences 272: 19

Wiegmann T, Kaye M 1977 Hypomagnesemic hypocalcemia: early serum calcium and late parathyroid hormone increase with magnesium therapy. Archives of Internal Medicine 137: 953

Yeo P P B, Chan S H, Lui K F, Wee G B, Lim P, Cheah J S 1978 HLA and thyrotoxic periodic paralysis. British Medical Journal 2: 930

10. Mitochondrial diseases

J. A. Morgan-Hughes

INTRODUCTION

Mitochondrial diseases due to known biochemical abnormalities can be separated into those with specific defects which primarily disrupt the pathways of oxidative metabolism and energy transfer and those which affect other mitochondrial functions not directly associated with the synthesis of adenosine triphosphate (ATP). The former disorders, which are expressed in skeletal muscle and include the lipid storage myopathies as well as the mitochondrial myopathies and encephalomyopathies, comprise the largest group and will be the subject of this review. The latter disorders, which include defects of the urea cycle, ketone body production and the catabolism of branched chain amino acids, take place mainly in the liver and will not be considered further.

Since the pioneer studies of Luft and colleagues over 30 years ago (Luft et al 1962) a growing number of defects of oxidative metabolism have been identified and recent strategies are rapidly providing new insights into the underlying molecular and genetic mechanisms. Since 1988, no fewer than nine different disease-related abnormalities of the mitochondrial genome have been described and a genetic classification based on these advances is already beginning to emerge (Shoffner & Wallace 1990). In this chapter, these advances will be considered against the background of a more traditional biochemical classification based on the site of the metabolic block as shown in Table 10.1.

BIOCHEMISTRY

Mitochondria are elongated and often branched structures which measure about 0.1 μm in diameter. In normal human muscle they occupy up to 4% of the total fibre volume (Jerusalem et al 1975) and are located beneath the plasma membrane and between the myofibrils on each side of the Z disc. They consist of two membranes separated by the intermembrane space. The smooth outer membrane is permeable to most small molecules. The inner membrane which encloses the matrix space is invaginated into folds or cristae and is impermeable to most hydrophilic and ionized metabolites. The rapid transport of these molecules into and out of the mitochondrial matrix is mediated by specific carriers located within the inner membrane itself (LaNoue & Schoolwerth, 1979).

The primary function of mitochondria is the provision of ATP. The matrix space, bounded by the inner membrane, is the exclusive site of the Krebs cycle and the enzymes involved in the oxidation of pyruvate and fatty acids. Reducing equivalents generated by these and other oxidations are transferred to molecular oxygen by the enzyme complexes and mobile carriers of the respiratory chain assembled in the lipid bilayer of the mitochondrial inner membrane. The two main substrates oxidized by muscle mitochondria are pyruvate and non-esterified free fatty acids.

Pyruvate, the product of glycolysis, is derived partly from blood-borne glucose but mainly from endogenous glycogen which is synthesized and stored in the muscle fibres under resting conditions. Muscle pyruvate production is maximal at high work intensities and during the initial phase of submaximal exercise when glycogen is the obligate or preferred fuel (Bergstrom & Hultman 1967). Once formed in the cell cytosol, pyruvate

Table 10.1 Biochemical classification of mitochondrial diseases

Site of defect	References
1. Mitochondrial substrate transport	
Primary muscle carnitine deficiency	Engel & Angelini (1973), Rebouche & Engel (1984)
Primary systemic carnitine deficiency	Treem et al (1988), Tein et al (1990), Stanley et al (1990a)
Secondary carnitine deficiency	Engel (1986), Stanley (1987)
Carnitine palmitoyltransferase deficiencies (CPT 1 & 2)	
Muscular form (?CPT2 deficiency)	DiMauro & Papadimitriou (1986), Zierz & Engel (1985, 1987)
Hepatic form (?CPT1 deficiency)	Tein et al (1989), Bonnefont et al (1990), Demaugre et al (1990)
2. Mitochondrial substrate utilization	
Fatty acid oxidation	
Long-chain acyl-CoA dehydrogenase (LCAD) deficiency	Vianey-Liaud et al (1987), Hale et al (1990a)
Medium-chain acyl-CoA dehydrogenase (MCAD) deficiency	Vianey-Liaud et al (1987), Stanley et al (1990b)
Short-chain acyl-CoA dehydrogenase (SCAD) deficiency	Turnbull et al (1990), Naito et al (1990)
Long-chain 3-hydroxyacyl-CoA dehydrogenase deficiency	Wanders et al (1989), Hale et al (1990b)
Multiple acyl-CoA dehydrogenation (MAD) deficiency	Vianey-Liaud et al (1987)
Electron transfer flavoprotein (ETF) deficiency	Frerman & Goodman (1985, 1989)
Severe variant (glutaric aciduria type II)	Amendt & Rhead (1986), Goodman et al (1990)
Mild variant (ethylmalonic-adipic aciduria)	Ikeda et al (1986b)
ETF-dehydrogenase deficiency (glutaric aciduria type II)	Frerman & Goodman (1985), Goodman et al (1990)
Riboflavin responsive multiple acyl-CoA dehydrogenation (RR-MAD) deficiency	Gregersen (1985), Rhead & Roettger (1986), DiDonato et al (1989) Gregersen et al (1990)
Pyruvate oxidation	
Pyruvate dehydrogenase (E_1) deficiency	Robinson et al (1987a, 1989), Old & DeVivo (1989)
Dihydrolipoamide acetyltransferase (E_2) deficiency	Brown et al (1989)
Protein X deficiency	Robinson et al (1990)
Dihydrolipoamide dehydrogenase (E_3) deficiency	Matuda et al (1984), Robinson et al (1989)
Phospho-E_1 phosphatase deficiency	Robinson et al (1987a, 1989)
3. Krebs cycle enzymes	
Fumarase deficiency	Zinn et al (1986), Gellera et al (1990)
Dihydrolipoamide dehydrogenase (E_3) deficiency	Naito et al (1988)
4. The mitochondrial respiratory chain	
NADH-CoQ reductase (Complex I) deficiency	Morgan-Hughes et al (1987, 1988, 1990a and b, Koga et al (1988)
Succinate-CoQ reductase (Complex II) deficiency	Rivner et al (1989), Haller et al (1990)
Coenzyme Q_{10} deficiency	Ogasahara et al (1989)
CoQ-cytochrome c reductase (Complex III) deficiency	Kennaway (1988), Morgan-Hughes et al (1990b)
Cytochrome c oxidase (Complex IV) deficiency	DiMauro et al (1988), Lombes et al (1989)
Multiple respiratory enzyme deficiencies	Mizusawa et al (1988), Yoneda et al (1989a), Zheng et al (1989) Morgan-Hughes et al (1990a and b)
5. The energy transducing system	
H^+-ATPase (Complex V) deficiency	Schotland et al (1976), Clark et al (1984)
Luft's disease	Luft et al (1962), DiMauro et al (1976)

may be reduced to lactate, transaminated to alanine, or oxidized by mitochondria. The proportion oxidized will depend on the availability of oxygen and the reduced state of the mitochondrial and cytosolic compartments. Pyruvate is transported across the mitochondrial inner membrane in exchange for hydroxyl ions by the monocarboxylate translocase (Denton & Halestrapp 1980) where it undergoes oxidative decarboxylation to acetyl CoA (Fig. 10.1). This is mediated by the pyruvate dehydrogenase complex (PDC).

Mammalian PDC is composed of multiple copies of three catalytic enzymes, pyruvate dehydrogenase (E_1), dihydrolipoamide acetyltransferase (E_2), and dihydrolipoamide dehydrogenase (E_3), two regulatory enzymes, E_1-specific kinase and phospho-E_1 phosphatase, and a recently identified lipoyl-containing protein of uncertain

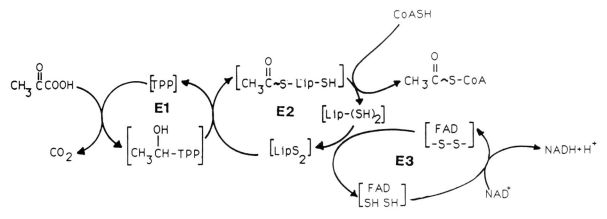

Fig 10.1 Scheme to show the reaction sequence of pyruvate oxidation. E_1 = pyruvate dehydrogenase; E_2 = dihydrolipoamide acetyltransferase; E_3 = dihydrolipamide dehydrogenase; FAD = flavin adenine dinucleotide; NAD^+ = nicotinamide adenine dinucleotide and its reduced form NADH; TPP = thiamin diphosphate; $LipsS_2$ and $Lips(SH)_2$ = oxidized and reduced lipoyl moiety

function called protein X (Reed & Yeaman 1987, De Marcucci et al 1986, Roche et al 1989). The lipoyl-bearing E_2 monomers form the structural core to which multiple copies of the other components are attached. E_1 is a tetramer composed of two non-identical subunits ($\alpha_2\beta_2$), and E_3 is a homodimer containing one molecule of flavin adenine dinucleotide (FAD) per monomer. E_3 is also a component of the α-ketoglutarate dehydrogenase and branched-chain α-keto acid dehydrogenase complexes and is involved in the glycine cleavage system.

The activity of the PDC is regulated by product inhibition (NADH, acetyl CoA) and by phosphorylation (inactivation) and dephosphorylation (activation) of serine residues on the $E_1\alpha$ mediated by the E_1-specific kinase and phospho-E_1phosphatase respectively (Yeaman et al 1978, Reed 1981). $E_1\alpha$ has been assigned to the human X-chromosome (Brown et al 1989a) and E_3 to chromosome 7 (Otulakowski et al 1988). In common with other nuclear-encoded mitochondrial proteins, PDC subunits are synthesized as precursors with amino-terminal signal peptides that guide them to their correct mitochondrial location (Lindsay 1989).

Free fatty acids (FFAs) are the major substrates oxidized by muscle at rest, particularly in the post-absorptive state and during prolonged periods of endurance exercise when glycogen stores are depleted (Newsholme 1981). They are derived

from: (i) endogenous triglycerides which are stored as fine neutral lipid droplets, especially in the type 1 muscle fibres, (ii) circulating FFAs complexed with plasma albumin, and (iii) triglycerides of circulating lipoproteins which are hydrolysed to FFAs by lipoprotein lipase on the endothelial surface of intramuscular capillaries (Schulz 1990). It is uncertain whether the uptake of FFAs by skeletal muscle occurs by simple diffusion or requires an active carrier mechanism. An energy-dependent uptake mechanism which involves a specific 40 kD fatty-acid binding protein has been identified in rat hepatocytes (Stemmel et al 1986).

Having entered the muscle fibres, FFAs may be esterified and stored as neutral lipid droplets, incorporated into membrane phospholipids, or undergo β-oxidation in the mitochondrial matrix. Long-chain FFAs are transported across the mitochondrial inner membrane by the carnitine-acylcarnitine translocase (Pande & Parvin 1976). They are first activated to their CoA thioesters by long-chain acyl-CoA synthetase located in the mitochondrial outer membrane (Fig. 10.2). Activation requires ATP and CoASH. Long-chain acyl-CoA thioesters are converted to acylcarnitines by carnitine palmitoyltransferase 1, recently relocated to the mitochondrial outer membrane (Murthy & Pande 1987). The transfer of long-chain acylcarnitine esters across the inner membrane occurs in exchange for free carnitine

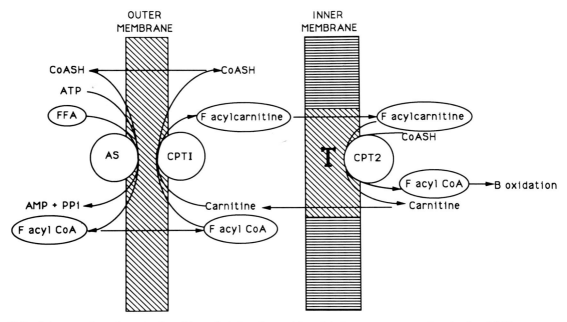

Fig. 10.2 Scheme to show the activation of long-chain free fatty acids and their transport across the mitochondrial inner membrane. AS = long-chain acyl-CoA synthetase; CPT1, CPT2 = carnitine palmitoyl transferases; T = carnitine-acylcarnitine translocase

and is catalysed by the translocase (Fig. 10.2). Carnitine palmitoyltransferase 2, which is bound to the inner face of the mitochondrial inner membrane, reverses the reaction to form long-chain acyl-CoA thioesters, the primary substrates of β-oxidation. Medium and short-chain FFAs diffuse directly across the inner membrane and are activated to their CoA thioesters by acyl-CoA synthetases in the matrix space before entering the β-oxidation pathway.

In addition to dietary sources, L-carnitine (β-hydroxy-γ-trimethylaminobutyric acid), a quaternary amine, is synthesized mainly in the liver and kidney and transported to muscle and other tissues via the blood (Bremer 1983, Bieber 1988). Carnitine levels in most tissues are 20 to 50 times higher than in plasma due to the presence of a high-affinity Na^+-dependent carrier-mediated uptake mechanism (Bremer 1983) which is now thought to be the site of the defect in primary systemic carnitine deficiency (Eriksson et al 1988, Treem et al 1988).

It is uncertain whether the two mitochondrial CPT activities represent two distinct enzymes or one enzyme in two different locations (Hoppel & Brady 1985). Recent studies suggest, however, that CPT1 and CPT2 differ in their physical properties, molecular size and immunological characteristics (Murthy & Pande 1987, Zammit et al 1988, McGarry et al 1990).

Fatty acyl-CoA thioesters are oxidized to acetyl-CoA in the mitochondrial matrix by the repeat action of a four-enzyme sequence which consists of acyl-CoA dehydrogenase, enoyl-CoA hydratase, 3-hydroxyacyl-CoA dehydrogenase, and 3-oxoacyl-CoA thiolase, as depicted in Fig. 10.3 (Schulz 1990). Fatty acyl-CoA is shortened by two carbon units with each round of β-oxidation. Each enzyme exists in two or three molecular forms with different chain-length specificities. Mammalian acyl-CoA dehydrogenases are homotetrameric mitochondrial flavoproteins, containing one molecule of FAD per monomer (Naito et al 1989a). They are synthesized in the cytosol as precursors with leader peptides and imported into mitochondria by an energy-dependent mechanism (Ikeda et al 1987). In common with other acyl-CoA dehydrogenases, they donate electrons to the

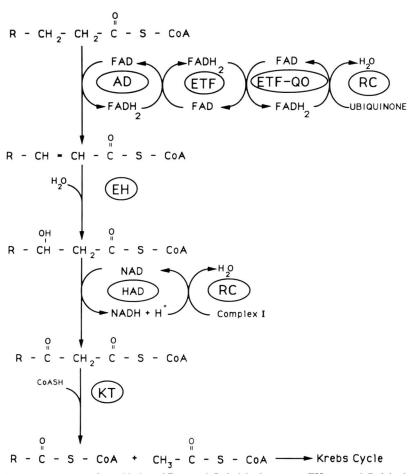

Fig. 10.3   Scheme to show one sequence of β-oxidation. AD = acyl-CoA dehydrogenase; EH = enoyl-CoA hydratase; HAD = 3-hydroxyacyl-CoA dehydrogenase; KT = 3-oxoacyl-CoA thiolase; ETF = electron transfer flavoprotein; ETF-QO = ETF dehydrogenase; RC = respiratory chain

respiratory chain via the electron transfer flavoprotein (ETF) and ETF-dehydrogenase (Fig. 10.3). Human ETF is a heterodimer composed of one α and one β subunit and contains one molecule of FAD per dimer. Both subunits are nuclear encoded and imported into mitochondria by an energy-dependent mechanism. The α subunit has a 3 kDa signal peptide but the β subunit does not appear to have a cleavable presequence (Finocchiano et al 1990). ETF dehydrogenase is a 68 kDa protein containing FAD which interacts with ETF and a tetranuclear iron–sulphur cluster which donates electrons directly to Coenzyme Q (Fig. 10.3).

The mitochondrial respiratory chain and oxidative phosphorylation system is the major site of energy transfer in mammalian cells (Hatefi 1985). The components of the system are depicted schematically in Fig. 10.4. The respiratory chain is composed of four oligomeric complexes linked by the mobile carriers Coenzyme Q_{10} and cytochrome c. It transfers reducing equivalents (H or e^-) generated in the matrix space to molecular oxygen to form water. According to the chemiosmotic hypothesis, originally proposed by Mitchell, redox energy generated by electron transfer is coupled at three sites (Complex I, III and IV) to vectorial transmembrane proton translocation (Mitchell 1976). Because the inner membrane is impermeable to protons this generates an electrical

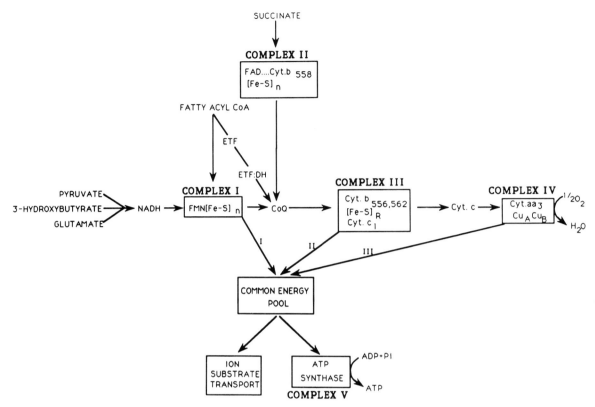

Fig. 10.4 Scheme to show the mitochondrial respiratory chain Complexes (I–V) and energy coupling sites. FMN = flavin mononucleotide; FAD = flavin adenine dinucleotide; FeS = iron–sulphur protein; ETF = electron transfer flavoprotein; ETF: QO = ETF dehydrogenase; CoQ = coenzyme Q_{10}; b, c_1, c, aa_3 = mitochondrial cytochromes, I, II and III = energy coupling sites

potential ($\Delta\psi$) and pH difference (ΔpH), which together comprise the protonic energy or proton-motive force Δp. Δp is used to drive ATP synthesis and the translocation of ions and other metabolites across the inner membrane. When ADP is available (state 3 respiration) the inward movement of protons is channelled through the proton-translocating ATPase (Complex V) which spans the inner membrane. ATP formed in the matrix space is transported out of the mito-chondrion in exchange for ADP by the adenine nucleotide translocase during state 3 respiration. When Δp is used to drive cation transport, stimulated respiration is not associated with ATP synthesis. The electrical potential ($\Delta\psi$) is also essential for the import of most nuclear-encoded mitochondrial proteins (Pfanner & Neupert 1990b).

Mitochondrial biogenesis depends on the co-ordinated function of two distinct genetic systems, one in the nucleus and the other in the mito-chondrion (Attardi & Schatz 1988). Human mitochondrial DNA is a closed, circular, double-stranded molecule, 16 569 base pairs in length (Anderson et al 1981); it codes for the small and large ribosomal RNAs, a complete set of 22 transfer RNAs and 13 of the 67 or so proteins of the oxidative phosphorylation system (Tables 10.2 and 10.3). They include seven subunits of Complex I, apocytochrome b of Complex III, the three larger subunits of Complex IV and subunits 6 and 8 of Complex V (Anderson et al 1981, Chomyn et al 1985, 1986). The two rRNAs, 14 tRNAs and 12 of the 13 open reading frames are transcribed from the G-rich heavy (H) strand and only eight tRNAs and ND6 are encoded on the C-rich light (L) strand. Except for a short non-coding segment in the displacement loop (D-loop) region, the H

Table 10.2 Mitochondrial genes

12S ribosomal RNA gene
16S ribosomal RNA gene
22 transfer RNA genes
13 protein coding genes
    Subunits ND1, 2, 3, 4L, 4, 5 and 6 of Complex I
    Apocytochrome b of Complex III
    Subunits I, II and III of Complex IV
    Subunits 6 and 8 of Complex V

Table 10.3 Respiratory chain polypeptides

	No. of subunits	No. encoded by mtDNA
Complex I	25–28	7 (ND1, 2, 3, 4, L4, 5 and 6)
Complex II	5	0
Complex III	11	1 (apocytochrome b)
Complex IV	13	3 (COX I, II, III)
Complex V	13	2 (subunits 6 and 8)

strand is saturated with flush-ended genes, all of which lack introns (Attardi & Schatz 1988). The genes are so tightly packed that there are few intervening non-coding stretches and some of the open reading frames even overlap (Anderson et al 1981).

Both strands of human mtDNA are transcribed as polycistronic RNA molecules from independent promoters in the D-loop region close to the origin of H-strand replication (Clayton 1984). The primary transcripts, which contain all the information encoded on each DNA strand are then catalytically cleaved to form tRNAs, rRNAs and mRNAs by RNA processing enzymes (Attardi et al 1985, Attardi & Schatz 1988). The smaller transcripts are matured post-transcriptionally by base modification of the transfer and ribosomal RNAs and polyadenylation of the mRNA precursors. For most structural genes post-transcriptional polyadenylation provides the terminal codon (Clayton, 1984). Because mitochondrial messages lack 5' end leaders, mitochondrial ribosomes probably recognize single codons such as AUG or AUA as start signals. The code itself also differs from the universal genetic code in that mitochondria read AUA as methionine rather than isoleucine and UGA as tryptophan rather than as 'stop'. Because all mitochondria in the zygote are derived from the ovum, mammalian mitochondrial genes are exclusively maternally inherited (Giles et al 1980). Each organelle contains up to 10 genomic DNA molecules and most human cells contain several hundred mitochondria (Robin & Wong 1988).

The remaining polypetides of the oxidative phosphorylation system (and all other mitochondrial proteins) are encoded by nuclear genes and synthesized on free cytoplasmic polysomes, mostly as precursors with amino-terminal amphiphilic targeting presequences which guide them to their correct locations in the mitochondria (Schatz 1987, Pfanner & Neupert 1990a,b). In order to be successfully imported into mitochondria, the newly synthesized cytosolic precursors must be kept in a loosely folded configuration (Razzow et al 1989). This is achieved by interaction with cytosolic heat-shock proteins and requires the hydrolysis of ATP (Mirakami et al 1988). Membrane translocation occurs via receptors on the mitochondrial surface at sites of close membrane contact and for most proteins depends on an electrical potential ($\Delta\psi$) across the inner membrane (Pfanner & Neupert 1990a,b). Imported subunits have their presequences cleaved by the combined action of a matrix peptidase and processing-enhancing protein before being assembled with their mtDNA encoded subunits into supramolecular complexes in the mitochondrial inner membrane (Hawlitschek et al 1988). Little is known about the assembly mechanism in mammalian cells but studies of yeast mutants suggest that it may be an ordered and sequential process (Grivell 1989). It depends on the addition of prosthetic groups and the presence of one or more matrix heat-shock proteins (hsp60) which are thought to catalyse the gradual refolding of imported proteins in an ATP-mediated reaction (Ostermann et al 1989). Nuclear genes specify all components of the machinery for import, processing and assembly and also control the replication and expression of mtDNA.

MYOPATHOLOGY

Except for the rare hepatic form of CPT deficiency, all disorders listed in Table 10.1 are expressed and can be identified in skeletal muscle, despite the fact that myopathy may be undetectable

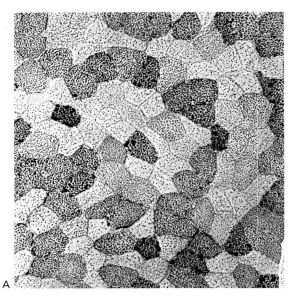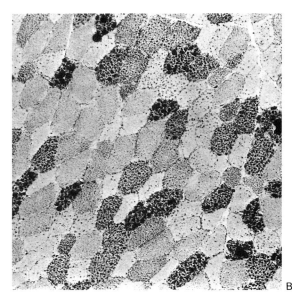

A

B

Fig. 10.5 Transverse sections of the vastus lateralis muscle stained with Sudan black B: **A**, from a patient with a defect of Complex I and secondary carnitine deficiency. ×120; **B**, from a patient with a riboflavin-responsive lipid storage myopathy. ×120. Note the excess lipid in a high proportion of the fibres in both cases

clinically, or may be only a minor feature of the disease. The muscle biopsy appearances, although non-specific, often provide the initial diagnostic clue and in many instances have prompted investigations which have led to the discovery of the defect.

As might be predicted, defects of mitochondrial fatty acid oxidation cause abnormal lipid storage, especially in the type 1 and type 2a fibres which normally have a high oxidative capacity (Fig. 10.5). Such changes typically occur in primary muscle carnitine deficiency in which there is impaired uptake of carnitine by muscle (Engel & Angelini 1973), and in primary systemic carnitine deficiency caused by a genetic defect of the high-affinity carnitine uptake mechanism in kidney and muscle (Eriksson et al 1988, 1989, Treem et al 1988, Tein et al 1990, Stanley et al 1990a). Lipid storage in muscle also occurs in a variety of other inborn metabolic errors which cause secondary carnitine deficiency (Engel 1986, Stanley 1987). They include long-chain acyl-CoA dehydrogenase deficiency (Fig. 10.6), medium-chain acyl-CoA dehydrogenase deficiency (Zierz et al 1988) and short-chain acyl-CoA dehydrogenase deficiency (Turnbull et al 1984, Coates et al 1988), riboflavin-

responsive multiple acyl-CoA dehydrogenation deficiency (DiDonato et al 1986, 1989, 1990, Turnbull et al 1988), and defects of the mitochondrial respiratory chain (Morgan-Hughes et al 1984, Scholte et al 1983, Clark et al 1984). It is uncertain whether the lipid storage seen in these conditions is due to deficiency of carnitine or to the primary biochemical error. In patients with respiratory chain disorders or riboflavin-responsive multiple acyl-CoA dehydrogenation defects, however, the changes usually resolve either partially or completely with carnitine supplementation. In CPT deficiency, a muscle biopsy taken between attacks of myoglobinuria is usually normal but modest triglyceride storage has been reported (Hostetler et al 1978).

At an ultrastructural level, the lipid bodies appear as rounded empty spaces which lack a limiting membrane and are characteristically situated in rows between the myofibrils and beneath the plasma membrane (Fig. 10.7). Muscle mitochondria may be increased and often tend to cluster at the edges of the lipid bodies (Fig. 10.7). Mitochondria may also show structural abnormalities including concentrically arranged cristae and paracrystalline inclusions. In patients with respira-

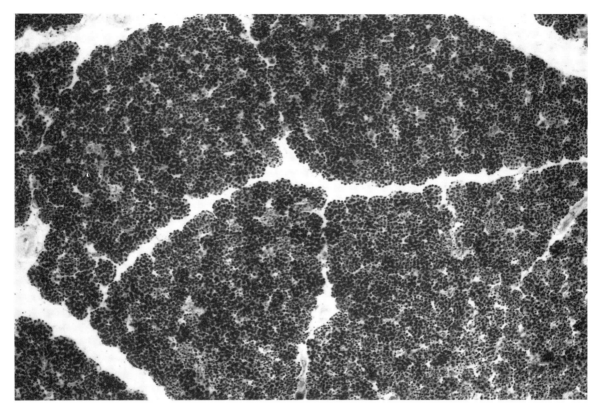

Fig. 10.6 Transverse section of the quadriceps femoris muscle from an infant with long-chain fatty acyl CoA dehydrogenase deficiency. Stained with Sudan black B. Note that all fibres are packed with excess lipid. ×160

tory chain dysfunction, the muscle biopsy may show ragged red changes as well as lipid storage.

The morphological hallmark of a mitochondrial myopathy is the *ragged red fibre* (Olson et al 1972) which contains large peripheral and intermyofibrillar collections of mitochondria. Mitochondrial aggregates are readily seen in fresh frozen sections where they appear as red-staining granular deposits with the modified Gomori trichrome stain (Engel & Cunningham 1963), and show an intense reaction for the exclusively intramitochondrial enzyme succinate dehydrogenase (Figs 10.8a and 10.9a). In some cases the fibres are rimmed with red-staining material but do not have a ragged appearance (Fig. 10.8b). Affected fibres also contain an excess of glycogen granules and increased numbers of fine neutral lipid droplets (Fig. 10.9b). The ragged red changes are usually segmental and when viewed in longitudinal sections

they do not extend continuously throughout the length of the fibres. An interesting feature of ragged red fibres in some, but not all cases, is their failure to stain histochemically for cytochrome c oxidase (COX) activity (Johnson et al 1983, 1988, Morgan-Hughes & Landon 1983). COX-negative fibres are invariably present in patients with progressive external ophthalmoplegia (PEO) and the Kearns–Sayre syndrome (Fig. 10.10) but they also occur in other mitochondrial encephalomyopathies and in patients with myopathy alone. In several of these disorders, particularly those associated with PEO, COX-negative fibres may considerably out-number ragged red fibres and sometimes represent the only detectable histochemical abnormality (Turnbull et al 1985). The number of COX-negative fibres also increases as the disease progresses (Bresolin et al 1987, Koga et al 1988a).

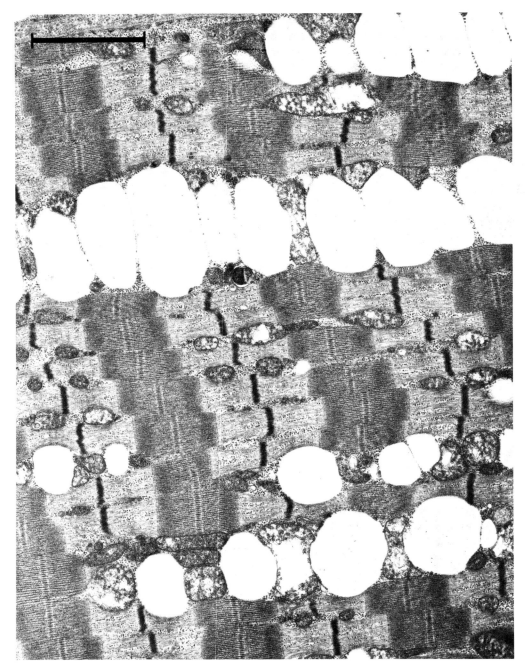

Fig. 10.7   Systemic carnitine deficiency. Electron micrograph of a fibre rich in lipid droplets, illustrating their tendency to accumulate in rows between the myofibrils. Bar represents 2 μm

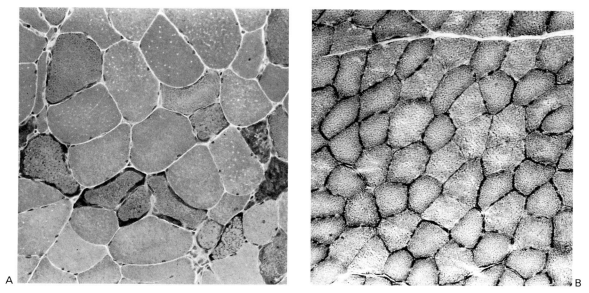

Fig. 10.8 Transverse sections of the vastus lateralis muscles from two patients with a mitochondrial myopathy associated with weakness and exercise intolerance and a deficiency of Complex I: **A**, modified Gomori trichrome stain to show typical ragged red fibres. ×250; **B**, succinate dehydrogenase stain to show rimmed fibres. ×200

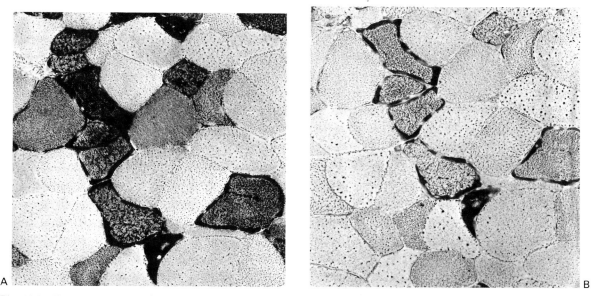

Fig. 10.9 Transverse sections of the vastus lateralis muscle from the patient shown in Fig. 10.8, **A**, succinate dehydrogenase stain to show intense activity in ragged red fibre. ×250; **B**, Sudan black B to show excess lipid droplets in the ragged red and non-ragged red fibres. ×250

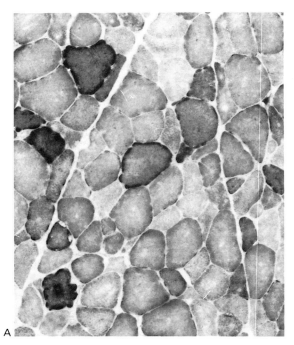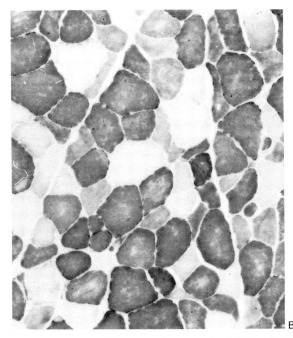

A   B

Fig. 10.10 Consecutive transverse sections of the vastus lateralis muscle from a patient with progressive external ophthalmoplegia, a deficiency of Complex I and a partially deleted population of mtDNA in muscle, to show absence of cytochrome c oxidase activity in the ragged red fibres: **A**, succinate dehydrogenase. ×220; **B**, cytochrome c oxidase. ×220

Loss of COX activity, like the ragged red changes, is segmental and does not extend throughout the length of the fibre.

Recent in situ hybridization studies of patients with PEO who harbour large heteroplasmic deletions of mtDNA suggest that focal loss of COX activity may be caused by failure to translate the transcripts of partially deleted genomes (Mita et al 1989, Shoubridge et al 1990). In these studies, fibre segments lacking COX activity were packed with mutant mtDNA whereas those with normal COX activity contained only wild type genomes. The abundant mtDNA transcripts in the COX negative segments containing mainly deleted mtDNA were not translated into proteins (Mita et al 1989). A similar mechanism may explain the presence of COX-negative fibres in other mitochondrial myopathies with mutations of the mitochondrial genome, particularly those affecting mitochondrial tRNA genes (Shoffner et al 1990, Goto et al 1990). Focal loss of muscle COX activity, however, is not confined to mitochondrial myopathies. It also occurs in cardiac and skeletal

muscle as an age-related phenomenon (Müller-Hocker 1988, 1990) and in various neuromuscular diseases including myotonic dystrophy, nemaline myopathy and limb–girdle dystrophy (Yamamoto et al 1989). It is not yet known whether the COX-negative fibres in these conditions are caused by age-related mutations of the mitochondrial genome.

At an ultrastructural level, muscle mitochondria are typically embedded in a glycogen-rich sarcoplasm and display a variety of changes in their fine structure (Figs. 10.11–10.17). Individual organelles are usually enlarged, sometimes grossly so, and may possess over-abundant distorted cristae which are unduly branched (Fig. 10.16a), flattened peripherally or concentrically arranged (Figs. 10.12 and 10.13). Elongated mitochondria with straight transverse cristae also occur (Fig. 10.14). Various intramitochondrial inclusions have been described, the most common being paracrystalline structures which are located either within the cristae or in the intermembrane space (Figs. 10.11–10.16). Both types of crystal may occur in the same fibre

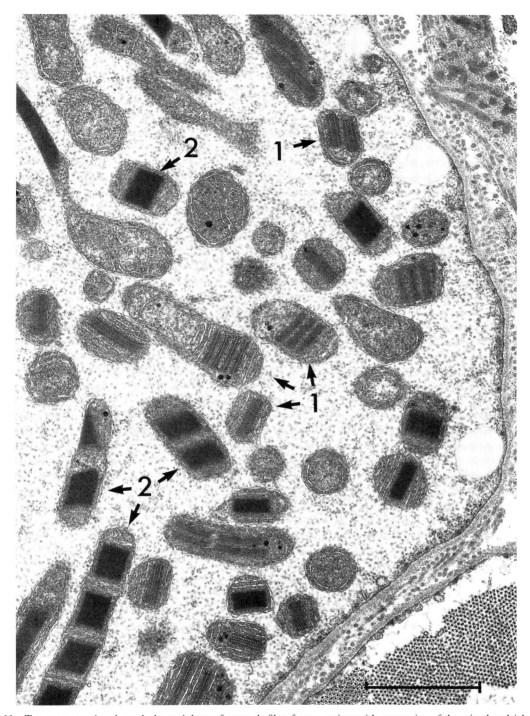

Fig. 10.11 Transverse section through the periphery of a muscle fibre from a patient with a mutation of the mitochondrial tRNA$^{\text{Leu (UUR)}}$ gene at position 3243, who presented with ataxia, dementia, sensorineural deafness and peripheral neuropathy. Note the numerous enlarged mitochondria embedded in a glycogen-rich sarcoplasm. Some of the mitochondria contain type I inclusions whereas others contain type 2 inclusions. Bar = 1 μm

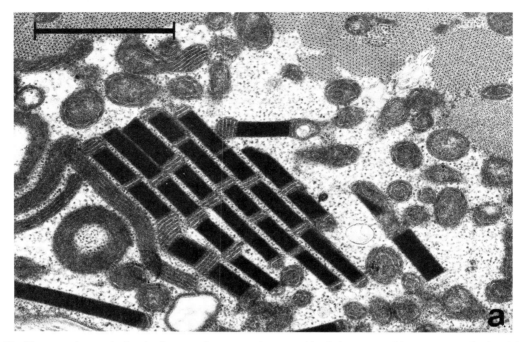

Fig. 10.12 Electron micrograph showing intermembrane crystals arranged in chains separated by transverse mitochondrial cristae. Bar represents 2 μm

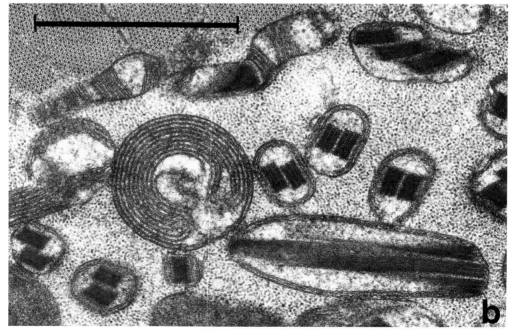

Fig. 10.13 Electron micrograph showing mitochondria containing 'parking lot' inclusions or multiple concentric cristae embedded in glycogen. Bar represents 2 μm

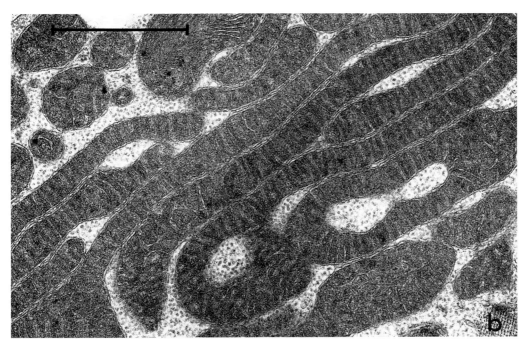

Fig. 10.14 Electron micrograph of the vastus lateralis muscle to show elongated mitochondria with regular transverse cristae from a patient with PEO, an isolated transient stroke and a mutation at position 3243 in the mitochondrial tRNA$^{\text{Leu (UUR)}}$ gene. Bar = 1 μm

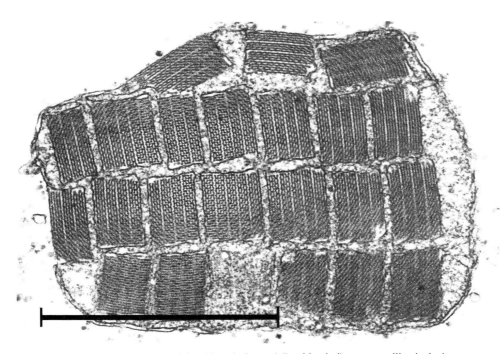

Fig. 10.15 An enlarged mitochondrion containing 22 typical type 1 ('parking lot') paracrystalline inclusions

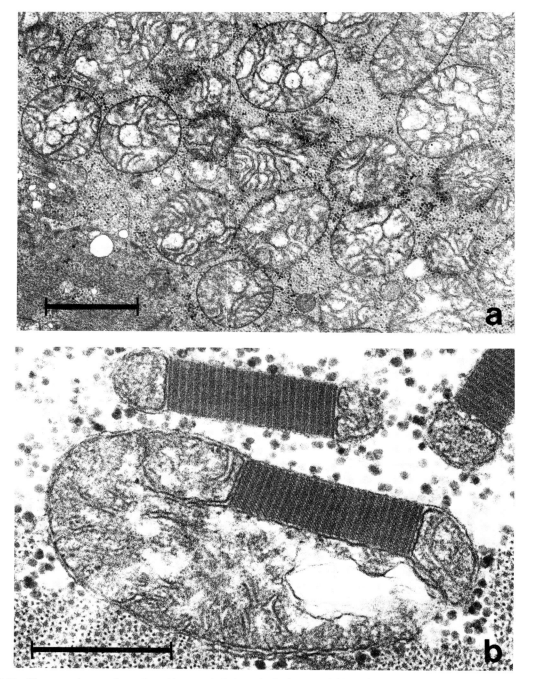

Fig. 10.16   Electron micrographs to show (a) excessively branched cristae, and (b) typical examples of an intermembranal type 2 paracrystalline inclusion

(Fig. 10.11) and occasionally in the same mitochondrion. The mitochondrial matrix may appear empty or vacuolated or contain osmiophilic or other electron dense bodies (Fig. 10.17). There is no correlation between the ultrastructural features and the site of the biochemical defect, or the type of mtDNA mutation. The electron micrographs shown in Figs. 10.11 and 10.14 were obtained

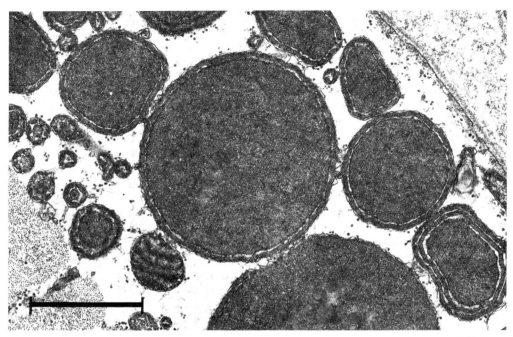

Fig. 10.17   Left vastus medialis muscle from a patient with a mitochondrial myopathy due to a defect in the NADH CoQ-reductase complex. Note the grossly enlarged peripherally located mitochondria with concentric cristae and dense matrix cores. Bar represents 1 μm

from two patients who both harboured a transitional mutation at nucleotide position 3243 in the mitochondrial tRNA$^{\text{Leu(UUR)}}$ gene. One patient (Fig. 10.11) had typical crystalloids of both types, whereas the other had elongated mitochondria without paracrystalline inclusions (Fig. 10.14).

The nature of the paracrystalline inclusions remains unknown. Previous studies had shown that they are composed of protein but are enzymatically inert (Bonilla et al 1975). In a recent immunoelectronmicroscopic study, however, they were shown to be immunoreactive for mitochondrial creatine kinase (Stadhouders et al 1990).

DISORDERS OF SUBSTRATE TRANSPORT

Defects of mitochondrial substrate transport block the entry of long-chain fatty acids into mitochondria where they are further metabolized by the β-oxidation pathway.

Carnitine deficiency

This deficiency has been identified as a secondary phenomenon in a large number of inborn metabolic errors and is particularly common in the organic acidurias, disorders of β-oxidation and defects of the respiratory chain (see Engel 1986, Stanley 1987, Angelini et al 1987). The mechanism of secondary carnitine deficiency in these disorders is thought to relate to its detoxifying role in converting acyl-CoA compounds which accumulate as a consequence of the metabolic block, into innocuous acylcarnitines, thereby releasing CoA for other metabolic reactions (Bremer 1983, Stumpf et al 1985). The acylcarnitine esters formed in the matrix space are transported out of mitochondria and excreted virtually unchanged in the urine. In the presence of an inadequate carnitine intake, the increased urinary excretion of acylcarnitines imposes a considerable drain on carnitine stores and may eventually lead to carnitine depletion.

In some patients, however, carnitine deficiency appears to be due to a primary defect of carrier-mediated carnitine transport across the plasma membrane (Bremer 1983). The myopathic form was identified by Engel and Angelini in a 24-year-old woman with a lipid storage myopathy who had life-long muscle weakness which became progressively worse in her late teens (Engel & Angelini

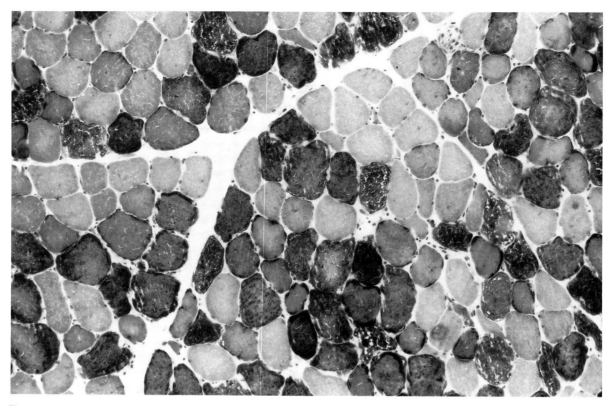

Fig. 10.18a

1973). Carnitine levels were normal in liver and plasma but were severely reduced in muscle. Renal reabsorption of carnitine was normal, but the uptake of labelled carnitine by the patient's muscle was impaired (Rebouche & Engel 1984).

In 1988 Eriksson and colleagues identified a more widespread genetic defect of carnitine transport in a 4-year-old girl with hypertrophic cardiomyopathy and lipid storage myopathy, whose brother had died of a similar disorder at the age of 18 months (Eriksson et al 1988). Carnitine levels were severely reduced in plasma, heart, muscle and cultured skin fibroblasts and the renal reabsorption of carnitine was markedly impaired. In a subsequent study these authors showed that the low concentration of carnitine in the patient's fibroblasts was due to a severe defect of the carrier-mediated carnitine uptake mechanism (Eriksson et al 1989).

Since these observations a further 14 patients with 'primary systemic carnitine deficiency' have been reported (Treem et al 1988, Tein et al 1990, Stanley et al 1990a). Some of these cases have presented in early infancy with hypoketotic hypoglycaemic coma induced by fasting, whereas others have developed hypertrophic or dilated cardiomyopathy and lipid storage myopathy in early childhood. Psychomotor retardation, seizures, normochromic or hypochromic anaemia, disturbances of bowel function, and failure to thrive have been additional features in some cases. Several patients have had affected siblings suggesting autosomal recessive transmission. All 14 patients have had a severe renal carnitine leak associated with very low levels of carnitine in various tissues including plasma, liver, muscle and heart. In contrast to defects of β-oxidation, urinary dicarboxylic acids are not increased, even during an acute metabolic crisis. Carnitine uptake in cultured skin fibroblasts has been negligible in all cases, indicating a primary defect of the high affinity carrier-mediated uptake mechanism.

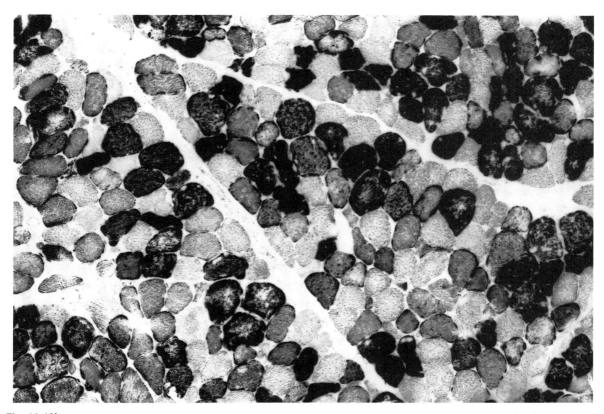

Fig. 10.18b

Fig. 10.18 Transverse sections of the vastus lateralis muscle from a patient with a severe defect of Complex I who presented with lifelong weakness and exercise intolerance. Note the high proportion of ragged red fibres. a: Gomori trichrome stain. ×165; b: succinate dehydrogenase stain. ×165

Intermediate rates of carnitine uptake in the parents of affected children are consistent with autosomal recessive inheritance. Treatment with oral carnitine results in dramatic improvement in cardiac function and muscle strength, but does not correct the renal carnitine leak or restore the muscle carnitine concentration. This would suggest that the carnitine transport defect demonstrated in fibroblast cultures is also present in kidney and muscle.

Carnitine palmitoyltransferase (CPT) deficiency

This causes two distinct syndromes. The more common myopathic form identified in 1973 (DiMauro & DiMauro 1973) presents with episodes of muscle pain, weakness and myoglobinuria in childhood or adult life (DiMauro & Papadimitriou

1986). Attacks are usually brought on by prolonged vigorous exercise especially in the cold or after fasting, or a high fat, low carbohydrate intake. They are also induced by intercurrent infection or emotional stress, but in some cases occur without any apparent precipitating cause. Renal failure is relatively uncommon. In a severe attack the weakness may be profound and may lead to respiratory distress but the bulbar muscles are usually spared. EMG, serum CK and muscle biopsy are usually normal between attacks. During an attack, however, the serum CK is markedly raised and a muscle biopsy may show modest lipid storage. Ketogenesis on fasting may be decreased or delayed. The defect has been demonstrated in liver, leukocytes and platelets, as well as in skeletal muscle, but may or may not be present in cultured fibroblasts (DiMauro and Papadimitriou 1986).

Although CPT deficiency is the most common of the known genetic causes of myoglobinuria (Tonin et al 1990) the precise nature of the defect remains unclear. Depending upon the type of assay used, the deficiency has involved CPT1 in some cases and CPT2 in others. More recent studies, however, have discounted evidence for two distinct forms of muscle CPT and suggest that the myopathic phenotype may be caused by altered regulatory properties of the mutant enzyme rather than by loss of catalytic activity (Zierz & Engel 1985, 1987).

The rare hepatic form of CPT deficiency presents in early infancy with episodes of hypoketotic, hypoglycaemic coma induced by fasting or by intercurrent infection (Bougneres et al 1981, Demaugre et al 1988, 1990, Tein et al 1989, Bonnefont et al 1990). Recent studies of cultured fibroblasts and muscle from three patients with the hepatic form and four with the myopathic form suggest that the two syndromes of CPT deficiency are caused by different mutations (Bonnefont et al 1990). Fibroblasts from patients with the hepatic form showed selective deficiency of CPT1, whereas those from patients with the myopathic form showed selective deficiency of CPT2. The activities of both CPT1 and CPT2 were normal in muscle from hepatic patients, but muscle from one myopathic case confirmed selective deficiency of CPT2 (Tein et al 1989, Bonnefont et al 1990). These results were confirmed by immunological studies using antibodies which probably recognized CPT2 (Demaugre et al 1990, Bonnefont et al 1990). These studies also suggest that there may be at least two distinct isoforms of CPT1, one expressed in fibroblasts and the other in skeletal muscle.

DISORDERS OF SUBSTRATE UTILIZATION: DEFECTS OF FATTY ACID OXIDATION

Long-chain acyl-CoA dehydrogenase (LCAD) deficiency

This is an autosomal recessive disorder which typically presents with hypoketotic hypoglycaemic coma in infancy or early childhood (Hale et al 1983, 1985, 1990a, Coates et al 1986, Amendt et al 1988). The metabolic crises which are precipitated by fasting or by intercurrent infection are characterized by generalized hypotonic weakness and increasing lethargy which may lead to coma and death, usually from cardiorespiratory arrest (Hale et al 1983, 1985, Vianey-Liaud et al 1987). Hepatomegaly and hypertrophic cardiomyopathy have been reported in half the cases and seizures may also occur (Hale et al 1983, 1985). Hypotonic weakness may persist between attacks. Onset in early infancy heralds a poor prognosis. Five out of eight patients who presented within the first six months of life died of the disease, compared with one out of six who presented after this age (Hale et al 1990a). Two patients, one with and one without previous attacks of hypoglycaemic coma, subsequently developed episodes of exercise-related myalgia and myoglobinuria in early childhood (Hale et al 1990a).

The urinary organic acid profile is normal between attacks, but samples taken during fasting or in an acute crisis show increased levels of medium-chain dicarboxylic acids (Hale et al 1985, 1990a, Vianey-Liaud et al 1987). The increased urinary excretion of acetylcarnitine during attacks has been attributed to peroxisomal β-oxidation (Corkey et al 1988). Total and free plasma carnitine concentrations are significantly reduced and the esterified fraction is increased. Liver biopsy shows excess fat in hepatocytes and ultrastructural abnormalities of mitochondria (Treem et al 1986). The enzyme defect has been identified in fibroblasts and leukocytes. LCAD activity in fibroblasts from the parents of affected children is half that of controls, confirming autosomal recessive inheritance.

Treatment is aimed at correcting the hypoglycaemia and maintaining a high carbohydrate intake especially during intercurrent illnesses. Supplementation of the diet with medium-chain triglyceride oil which effectively bypasses the metabolic block has also been advocated (Hale et al 1990a). Oral carnitine lowers the serum free fatty acid level during fasting but has little effect on the clinical course of the disorder.

Medium-chain acyl-Co-A dehydrogenase (MCAD) deficiency

MCAD deficiency, identified biochemically in 1983 (Stanley et al 1983, Divry et al 1983, Rhead et al 1983) appears to be the most common of the known inborn errors of mitochondrial fatty acid oxidation (Vianey-Liaud et al 1987, Stanley et al 1990b). The disorder, which typically presents in infancy, may cause: (i) sudden infant death (Howat et al 1985, Roe et al 1986, Allison et al 1988); (ii) episodes of hypoketotic hypoglycaemia and metabolic encephalopathy resembling the Reye syndrome (Coates et al 1985, Bougneres et al 1985, Roe et al 1986, Stanley et al 1990b); or (iii) a carnitine-deficient lipid storage myopathy with, or without, recurrent Reye-like attacks (Coates et al 1985, Engel 1986, Zierz et al 1988). Biochemical screening of the siblings of MCAD-deficient probands indicates that the enzyme defect may remain completely asymptomatic (Roe et al 1986, Duran et al 1986, Stanley et al 1990b).

The attacks of metabolic encephalopathy are precipitated by fasting or by intercurrent infection and are characterized by nausea, vomiting, hypotonic weakness and increasing lethargy which may lead to seizures, coma, and death from cardiorespiratory failure, or from cerebral oedema with uncal herniation (Stanley et al 1983, 1990b, Roe et al 1985). In a recent review of 64 patients with MCAD deficiency, death occurred during the first attack in 25% (Stanley et al 1990b). The median age of presentation was 15 months with a range of 2–47 months. Hepatomegaly is an inconstant feature but liver biopsy invariably shows excess fat in hepatocytes (Treem et al 1986). Most patients are well between attacks, but some have persistent proximal weakness and exercise intolerance associated with systemic carnitine deficiency and lipid storage on muscle biopsy (Coates et al 1985, Zierz et al 1988). They included several patients who were previously reported to have primary systemic carnitine deficiency (Engel et al 1981, Rebouche & Engel 1984, Cruse et al 1984).

In patients with MCAD deficiency total carnitine levels are significantly reduced in plasma, liver and muscle, and the esterified fraction of serum carnitine may be increased, particularly after fasting or during an acute metabolic crisis. The mechanism of secondary carnitine deficiency in this disorder remains unknown but may be related to excessive excretion of acylcarnitines, particularly octanoylcarnitine or to impaired renal carnitine conservation (Stanley et al 1990b).

In addition to hypoglycaemia, which may be profound, and inappropriately low levels of ketones in plasma and urine, the acute metabolic crises are associated with a rapid rise in plasma medium-chain fatty acids and their metabolites (Duran et al 1988). The plasma ammonia and serum transaminase levels may be elevated and there is a moderate but usually well-compensated metabolic acidosis. During an acute crisis or on fasting there is a massive dicarboxylic aciduria consisting mainly of adipic, suberic, and sebacic acids, and increased urinary excretion of 5-hydroxyhexanoic acid, octanoylcarnitine and the glycine conjugates n-hexanoylglycine, 3-phenylpropionylglycine and suberylglycine (Roe et al 1986, 1990, Rinaldo et al 1988, 1990). Dicarboxylic acids arise from microsomal omega-oxidation of monocarboxylic acids and may be chain-shortened by peroxisomal β-oxidation (Gregersen 1985, Gregersen et al 1990). The urinary organic acid profile is characteristic of MCAD deficiency. Octanoylcarnitine and the glycine conjugates are excreted even between attacks and serve as important diagnostic markers of the disease.

Recent studies indicate that MCAD deficiency is genetically heterogeneous. Biosynthesis and processing of MCAD protein in MCAD-deficient cultured fibroblasts from a number of patients with the disorder has been normal (Ikeda et al 1986a, Strauss et al 1990). This would suggest mutations in parts of the molecule which are essential for catalytic activity or for substrate or co-factor binding. In one patient, however, the mutation involved the signal peptide of the MCAD precursor protein and prevented its import into mitochondria (Strauss et al 1990).

In common with other defects of β-oxidation, treatment is aimed at correcting the hypoglycaemia and maintaining a high carbohydrate intake. Treatment with carnitine supplements has been recommended by some authors (Roe et al 1990) but not by others (Stanley et al 1990b).

Short-chain acyl-CoA dehydrogenase (SCAD) deficiency

Four female patients have been described with widely differing clinical features (Turnbull et al 1984, Amendt et al 1987, Coates et al 1988). The first reported case was a 46-year-old woman with a 6-year history of proximal muscle weakness and exertional myalgia, secondary carnitine deficiency and a lipid storage myopathy (Turnbull et al 1984). The urinary metabolites consisted mainly of ethylmalonic and methylsuccinic acids. The patient was unresponsive to steroids or DL-carnitine, but improved slightly with riboflavin (Turnbull et al 1990). SCAD activity was markedly reduced in skeletal muscle but was normal in cultured fibroblasts (Coates et al 1988).

In three patients with SCAD deficiency, the defect was present in cultured fibroblasts. Two presented in the neonatal period with feeding difficulties, lethargy, metabolic acidosis, aminoaciduria and increased levels of lactate and ethylmalonate in the urine (Amendt et al 1987). One patient improved following treatment with intravenous fluids, but the other died on the sixth postnatal day. Autopsy showed cerebral oedema and fatty infiltration of the liver. The fourth patient presented with feeding difficulties and vomiting in the neonatal period and went on to develop progressive muscular weakness, ptosis, hypotonia, hepatomegaly, psychomotor retardation and microcephaly (Coates et al 1988). There was a mild generalized aminoaciduria with increased levels of dicarboxylic acids and β-hydroxybutyrate. Muscle biopsy at 8 months showed lipid storage in the type 1 fibres. Total carnitine levels were reduced in plasma and muscle and the esterified fractions were increased. The patient improved with regular feeding via a gastrostomy tube.

Further studies in the three patients with SCAD deficiency in cultured fibroblasts (Amendt et al 1987, Coates et al 1988) indicated genetic heterogeneity (Naito et al 1989a,b, 1990). Cultured cells from two cases synthesized a normal sized variant SCAD protein with normal stability, but cells from the third case synthesized a labile SCAD variant. This patient was later shown to be a compound heterozygote with two unique mutant alleles (Naito et al 1990).

Long-chain 3-hydroxyacyl-CoA dehydrogenase deficiency

This enzyme occupies the third step in the β-oxidation pathway. It catalyses the reversible dehydrogenation of 3-hydroxyacyl-CoA to 3-ketoacyl-CoA and donates electrons to NAD (Fig. 10.3).

Three infants with a deficiency of this enzyme have been reported (Wanders et al 1989, Hale et al 1990b). The clinical features resemble those of LCAD deficiency and consist of episodes of hypoketotic hypoglycaemia, hepatomegaly, muscular weakness and hypertrophic cardiomyopathy. The attacks are precipitated by fasting or by intercurrent infection and are associated with a predominantly long-chain 3-hydroxydicarboxylic aciduria. Secondary carnitine deficiency and increased levels of long-chain acylcarnitines in muscle and liver have been described (Hale et al 1990b). The defect has been identified in cultured fibroblasts. As in LCAD deficiency treatment is aimed at correcting the hypoglycaemia and maintaining a high carbohydrate intake particularly during intercurrent illness. Medium chain triglyceride oil was beneficial in one case (Wanders et al 1989).

Multiple acyl-CoA dehydrogenation (MAD) deficiency

At least three variants have been described (Vianey-Liaud et al 1987).

Glutaric aciduria type II

The severe variants are caused by a deficiency of the electron-transfer flavoprotein (ETF) or ETF-dehydrogenase (ETF-DH) (Frerman & Goodman 1985). Patients present at, or soon after, birth with severe metabolic acidosis, hypoketotic hypoglycaemia and a characteristic odour of 'sweaty feet'. Some cases have renal cystic dysplasia and congenital anomalies of the face, abdominal wall and external genitalia (Vianey-Liaud et al 1987). These patients usually but not invariably have a deficiency of ETF-DH and always succumb within the first few weeks. In patients lacking renal cysts and other congenital anomalies, the disease may run a slightly more benign clinical course, but early onset heralds a poor prognosis. The deficiency in these cases usually involves ETF.

Deficiencies of ETF and ETF-DH affect all enzymes which feed reducing equivalents into the respiratory chain via this pathway. They include

LCAD, MCAD and SCAD, isovaleryl-CoA dehydrogenase, 2-methyl-branched chain acylCoA dehydrogenase, glutaryl-CoA dehydrogenase and sarcosine and dimethylglycine dehydrogenases. This is reflected in the urinary organic acid profile (Vianey-Liaud et al 1987). Immunoblots in patients with ETF deficiency have usually shown absence of both subunits (Frerman & Goodman 1985), but in one case only the β subunit was lacking (Goodman et al 1990). Studies of the biosynthesis and processing of the α and β subunits of ETF in cultured fibroblasts from three patients with glutaric aciduria type II showed defective synthesis of the α subunit (Ikeda et al 1986a,b).

Ethylmalonic adipic aciduria

The mild variant is due to a deficiency of ETF. It typically presents in infancy or childhood with episodes of vomiting, hypoglycaemia and metabolic acidosis and may be associated with hepatomegaly. Some cases, however, have presented rather later with a lipid storage myopathy and secondary carnitine deficiency (DiDonato et al 1986). Patients with the milder variant may show a response to riboflavin, suggesting that the defect may involve FAD (Gregerson 1985, Gregerson et al 1986, 1990). Several patients with riboflavin-responsive MAD deficiency have presented with a lipid storage myopathy and secondary carnitine deficiency (Turnbull et al 1988, DiDonato et al 1989, 1990). In these cases the reduced activities of SCAD and MCAD are associated with loss of the enzyme proteins on Western blot analysis. These changes appear to be reversed by riboflavin supplementation (DiDonato et al 1989).

DEFECTS OF PYRUVATE OXIDATION

Defects of the PDC have been identified as important causes of lactic acidosis and cerebral dysfunction in infancy and childhood (Stansbie et al 1986, Robinson et al 1987a, 1989, Brown et al 1988, 1989b, Old & DeVivo 1989). In the majority of patients the defect has involved the E_1 component of the complex but a few cases have been reported with specific deficiencies of E_2 (Ho et al 1989, Robinson et al 1990), E_3 (Munnich et al 1982, Matuda et al 1984, Robinson et al 1989),

phospho-E_1 phosphatase (Naito et al 1988) or protein X (Robinson et al 1990). The defect appears to be generalized but the amount of residual enzyme activity may vary widely between tissues even from the same patient. In a few cases the defect has been present in liver, muscle, kidney, brain or lymphocytes but not in cultured fibroblasts (Willems et al 1974, Kerr et al 1988, Ho et al 1989) and in one patient it appeared to be restricted to the brain (Prick et al 1981a).

In its most severe form PDC deficiency presents with a rapidly fatal metabolic acidosis in the neonatal period (Robinson et al 1987a, 1989). The acidosis is usually refractory to treatment but correction of the acid–base balance and the administration of large doses of thiamine and dichloroacetate, which are thought to activate any residual E_1, may sustain life for several weeks. Neurological abnormalities include profound generalized hypotonic weakness, areflexia, seizures, psychomotor retardation, and respiratory difficulties with episodes of apnoea indicative of brain stem dysfunction. Dysmorphic features and microcephaly are common (Robinson et al 1987a, 1989, Robinson 1988, Brown et al 1989b, Old & DeVivo 1989). Most patients with the severe form die within the first few weeks or months of life, but a few survive infancy although they are left with severe neurological disability (Old & DeVivo 1989).

Patients with a less severe or episodic lactic acidaemia without major changes in acid-base balance typically present in late infancy or early childhood with a progressive encephalopathy exhibiting many of the clinical and morphological features of Leigh's syndrome (Miyabayashi et al 1985, Kretzschmar et al 1987, Robinson 1988, Robinson et al 1987a, 1989, Brown et al 1988, 1989b, Old & DeVivo 1989). In many cases the encephalopathy leads to a severe vegetative state with death before the age of 3. In a few cases, however, it runs a more protracted clinical course with survival into late childhood or adolescence (Brown et al 1988). Clinical features include severe mental retardation, myoclonic or generalized seizures, hypotonia, spasticity, dystonic rigidity, cerebellar ataxia, cortical blindness, optic atrophy, ocular motor and bulbar abnormalities, Cheyne-Stokes respiration, dysmorphic features and microcephaly. Lactate and pyruvate levels may be normal in the blood but are usually elevated in the CSF (Brown et al 1988, 1989b).

Less severe deficiencies of the PDC are compatible with survival and typically present with intermittent ataxia in childhood (Robinson et al 1987a, 1989). The attacks are often precipitated by intercurrent infection, emotional stress or a high carbohydrate intake. Blass and co-workers first drew attention to this type of disorder and a few additional cases have been reported (Blass et al 1970, 1971, Robinson et al 1987a, 1989).

Immunoblotting of fibroblast extracts has been used to further characterize the defect, particularly in patients with a deficiency of the E_1 component (Wicking et al 1986, Ho et al 1986, 1989, Brown et al 1987, Kerr et al 1987, 1988, Old & DiVivo 1989, Robinson et al 1989). Analysis of the data from one of these studies illustrates the different patterns of abnormality which have been observed (Old & DeVivo 1989). The four girls and two out of the seven boys included in the study had normal patterns for the E_1, E_2 and E_3 components. The remaining five boys had alterations of the E_1 α subunit and normal patterns for E_2 and E_3. Four of these boys, however, also showed a reduction of the E_1 β subunit. The simultaneous reduction of both E_1 subunits would suggest that in the absence of one component, the other is unable to form a stable tetramer and is rapidly degraded. This was supported by Northern analysis in four male patients lacking the $E_1\alpha$ and $E_1\beta$ subunits (Ho et al 1989). Fibroblast RNA from all four cases had apparently normal amounts and sizes of specific $E_1\beta$ mRNAs. In two of these cases, however, both species of specific $E_1\alpha$ mRNAs were decreased (Ho et al 1989). Another study also suggested that a mutant $E_1\alpha$ subunit may disturb normal assembly of the E_1tetramer (Endo et al 1989). These authors identified a 4-bp frame shift deletion in the $E_1\alpha$ gene from a male patient with exercise intolerance and markedly reduced E_1 activity in cultured fibroblasts (Miyabayashi et al 1985). The deduced sequence of the deleted gene suggested that the $E_1\alpha$ subunit would be larger than normal. Studies of complex formation in pulse-labelled transformed lymphocytes, followed by immunoprecipitation with anti-E_2 antibody showed that the $E_1\alpha$ and $E_1\beta$ subunits co-

precipitated with E_2 in control mitochondria but that both subunits were missing in mitochondria isolated from the patient's cells (Endo et al 1989). The preponderance of boys with $E_1\alpha$ deficiency is consistent with the recent assignment of $E_1\alpha$ to Xp22.13–22.1 (Brown et al 1989a).

Patients with the severe clinical phenotypes usually show extensive cerebral pathology with cystic lesions and areas of spongiform change, vascular proliferation and loss of myelin in the brain stem, basal ganglia and cerebral hemispheres. Developmental anomalies, including microcephaly and agenesis of the corpus callosum are not uncommon. Although deficiencies of the PDC are expressed in skeletal muscle, muscle biopsies have been relatively normal and have not shown any major alterations in the mitochondrial structure.

DISORDERS OF THE KREBS CYCLE

Specific deficiencies of only two Krebs cycle enzymes have been described.

Fumarase deficiency has been identified in three patients who presented with a progressive encephalopathy in early infancy (Zinn et al 1986, Petrova-Benedict et al 1987, Gellera et al 1990). Clinical features included feeding difficulties, lethargy, severe psychomotor retardation, hypotonia and microcephaly. Seizures occurred in one case (Gellera et al 1990) and another had epileptiform discharges on EEG (Zinn et al 1986). CT brain scan in two cases showed cerebral atrophy (Zinn et al 1986, Gellera et al 1990). Urinary organic acid analysis showed increased levels of fumarate and succinate in all three cases. Two patients died in the 7th and 8th months respectively but the third was still alive at 6 months. The enzyme defect was demonstrated in various tissues, including brain, liver, kidney, heart and cultured fibroblasts. Both cytosolic and mitochondrial forms of fumarase were barely detected in two cases (Zinn et al 1986, Gellera et al 1990) but the third patient showed some residual mitochondrial enzyme activity (Petrova-Benedict et al 1987).

Fumarase is a tetrameric enzyme which catalyzes the reversible hydration of fumarate to L-malate. It is a component of the Krebs cycle, but it is also present in the cytosol. The mitochondrial and cytosolic forms are encoded by a single gene on the long arm of human chromosome 1 (van Someren et al 1974). In common with many other enzymes present in both the mitochondrial and cytosolic compartments, the two forms of fumarase are generated from different transcriptional starts.

Dihydrolipoamide dehydrogenase deficiency has been described in six patients who presented with a severe lactic acidosis and progressive encephalopathy in early infancy (Munnich et al 1982, Matuda et al 1984, Robinson et al 1989). Autopsy studies have shown loss of myelin with cystic lesions in the basal ganglia, thalamus and brain stem, consistent with Leigh's syndrome. All cases showed a combined deficiency in the activities of PDC, α-ketoglutarate dehydrogenase and branched-chain keto-acid dehydrogenase complexes with elevated levels of lactate, pyruvate, α-ketoglutarate and branched-chain aminoacids in the blood. These cases are further discussed under defects of pyruvate oxidation.

DISORDERS OF THE RESPIRATORY CHAIN

Because of the complexities of biogenesis and the dual genetic control of the component proteins, defects of the respiratory chain have a considerable potential for molecular and genetic heterogeneity. Nuclear mutations may alter the sequence, transcription or translation of respiratory chain polypeptides, components of the import or processing machinery, or products required for the replication or expression of the mitochondrial genome. Mutations of mtDNA may similarly affect respiratory chain subunits and may also alter the expression of functionally related nuclear genes (Parikh et al 1987). Bigenomic mismatch mutations leading to incompatibility between closely associated respiratory chain subunits represent another theoretical possibility. In the last few years considerable progress has been made in unravelling the molecular genetic basis of some of these disorders (see later section).

Defects of Complex I (NADH–ubiquinone oxidoreductase)

Complex I catalyses the transfer of reducing equivalents from NADH to coenzyme Q (Hatefi

1985). The reaction is coupled to vectorial proton translocation and generates a protonic electrochemical potential (Δp) across the inner membrane (Senior 1988). Complex I is the largest of the respiratory chain enzymes and contains 25 to 28 different polypeptides, 7 of which are encoded by mitochondrial genes (Chomyn et al 1985, Chomyn & Lai 1990, Capaldi et al 1988, Attardi & Schatz 1988). The remaining subunits are nuclear encoded and are synthesized on cytoplasmic polysomes as precursors with N-terminal amphiphilic signal sequences which direct them into the correct mitochondrial compartment (Hartl et al 1989, Pfanner & Neupert 1990a,b). The redox groups include FMN and at least eight iron-sulphur centres (Hatefi 1985, Capaldi et al 1988). The function of the other Complex I polypeptides is not known but some mtDNA-encoded subunits are thought to contribute to the hydrophobic shell which surrounds the catalytic core (Chomyn et al 1985). The product of the mitochondrial gene ND1, however, may be involved in the reduction of coenzyme Q.

Defects predominantly or exclusively affecting Complex I have been identified in over 80 cases (Table 10.4). They can be separated into four broad clinical categories but within each subgroup there is considerable clinical, biochemical and genetic heterogeneity.

The fatal infantile form

This presents with severe lactic acidosis at, or soon after, birth and leads to death from cardiorespiratory insufficiency in early infancy (Moreadith et al 1984, 1987, Robinson et al 1986, 1987b, Hoppel et al 1987, Zheng et al 1989). Clinical features include breathing and feeding difficulties, failure to thrive and profound generalized hypotonic weakness. Mental regression, seizures, hypertrophic cardiomyopathy and hepatocellular dysfunction may also occur. The biochemical defect appears to be systemic and has been demonstrated in liver, kidney, heart and cultured fibroblasts, as well as in skeletal muscle. Autopsy studies in four cases have confirmed multisystem involvement. The brain was microscopically and biochemically normal in one case (Zheng et al 1989). In two other cases, however,

Table 10.4 Defects of Complex I: clinical phenotypes in 82 cases

Syndrome	No. of cases	References
Fatal infantile form	5	Moreadith et al (1984, 1987) Robinson et al (1986) Hoppel et al (1987) Zheng et al (1989)
Myopathy with limb weakness and exercise intolerance: pigmentary retinopathy (3 cases), cardiomyopathy (1 case)	18	Morgan–Hughes et al (1979, 1985, 1987, 1990a) Land et al (1981) Scholte et al (1983, 1987) Arts et al (1987) Clark et al (1984) Roodhooft et al (1986) Schapira et al (1988) Koga et al (1988a) Watmough et al (1989, 1990)
Syndromes with PEO±pigmentary retinopathy, deafness, cardiomyopathy, CNS disease	17	Morgan–Hughes et al (1987, 1990a,b) Sherratt et al (1984, 1986) Scholte et al (1987, 1990) Schapira et al, (1988) Johnson et al (1988) Holt et al (1989a)

Progressive encephalomyopathy
    Dementia (37 cases)
    Seizures (29 cases)
    Strokes (29 cases)
    Short stature (20 cases)
    Deafness (17 cases)
    Ataxia (14 cases)
    Cardiomyopathy (9 cases)
    Pigmentary retinopathy (5 cases)
    Involuntary movements (4 cases)
    Sensory neuropathy (3 cases)
	42	Senior & Jungas (1974)
		Prick et al (1981b)
		Morgan–Hughes et al (1982, 1984, 1985, 1987, 1990a)
		Hayes et al (1985)
		Nishizawa et al (1987)
		Kobayashi et al (1987)
		van Erwen et al (1987)
		Ichiki et al (1988)
		Koga et al (1988a)
		Byrne et al (1988)
		Yoneda et al (1989a)
		Schapira et al (1988, 1990a)
		Sakuta & Nonaka (1989)

there were extensive spongiform changes (Robinson et al 1986, Hoppel et al 1987), and a third patient showed ventricular enlargement and low-density areas in the subcortical white matter on CT brain scan (Moreadith et al 1984). Muscle biopsy performed in three cases showed the typical changes of a mitochondrial myopathy (Moreadith et al 1984, Hoppel et al 1987, Zheng et al 1989). Liver and heart mitochondria were structurally abnormal in two out of the three patients in which these tissues was examined (Moreadith et al 1984, Zheng et al 1989). The defect was confined to Complex I in four cases, but in a fifth patient Complex IV activity and cytochrome aa$_3$ were also significantly reduced in heart, liver and muscle (Zheng et al 1989).

Two patients had one or more affected siblings,

and the parents of a third case were first cousins (Robinson et al 1986, Hoppel et al 1987). The remaining two cases were sporadic. Specific activities of respiratory chain enzymes in muscle mitochondria from the parents of one sporadic case were normal (Zheng et al 1989).

Immunoblots of Complex I from liver and heart of one patient showed virtual absence of the 75 kDa and 13 kDa iron–sulphur proteins and reduced amounts of the 49 kDa and 30 kDa subunits (Moreadith et al 1987).

Myopathy with limb weakness and exercise intolerance, often associated with exercise-related muscle pain but without pigmenturia, have been the main presenting features in 18 cases (Table 10.4). In most patients symptoms began in childhood or adolescence, but one was weak at birth

(Roodhooft et al 1986) and another remained asymptomatic until the fifth decade (Morgan-Hughes et al 1985). Five patients had isolated or infrequent attacks of increased weakness or paralysis which, when severe, were accompanied by headache, nausea and vomiting (Morgan-Hughes et al 1987, 1990a). In two cases the attacks were shown to be due to a severe metabolic acidosis (Morgan-Hughes et al 1979, Schapira et al 1988). Precipitating factors included intercurrent infection, unaccustomed exercise and the intake of modest amounts of alcohol. Identical twin brothers had pigmentary retinopathy, which was asymptomatic (Morgan-Hughes et al 1987) and a 21-year-old girl developed unexplained congestive heart failure at the age of 11 years which resolved spontaneously after several months (Morgan-Hughes et al 1985, Wiles et al 1986). All patients in this group showed a variable lactic acidaemia which was made worse by exercise. Muscle biopsy in all cases showed the typical changes of a mitochondrial myopathy (Fig. 10.18). Carnitine deficiency with, or without, lipid storage on muscle biopsy occurred in some cases (Morgan-Hughes et al 1985, 1987, Scholte et al 1983, Roodhooft et al 1986).

The 18 cases included cousins whose mothers were said to be affected (Koga et al 1988a,b), identical twin brothers (Morgan-Hughes et al 1987), an affected mother and son (Scholte et al 1987) and an affected mother and daughter (Morgan-Hughes et al 1987, 1990a). Of the remaining 10 cases 4 had affected siblings (Morgan-Hughes et al 1987, Watmough et al 1990), one had an affected maternal uncle (Roodhoft et al 1986) and five were sporadic.

Phosphorus nuclear magnetic resonance spectroscopy (^{31}P NMR) of muscle typically shows a low PCr/Pi ratio at rest, an abnormally rapid fall during exercise and delayed recovery of PCr after exercise (Radda et al 1982, Arnold et al 1985, Argov et al 1987). Despite the high blood lactate levels observed during exercise, the changes in intracellular pH as determined by ^{31}P NMR are relatively small. The rapid recovery of intracellular pH after exercise suggests that muscle has developed a more efficient adaptive mechanism for handling increased lactate loads. These patterns of abnormality appeared to be specific for respiratory chain dysfunction and have been observed in

defects of Complex III and Complex IV as well as Complex I (Eleff et al 1984, Arnold et al 1985, Argov 1989). They differ from the changes recorded in other metabolic myopathies in which muscle energy production is impaired (Argov 1989).

In addition to the rate-limiting defect in Complex I, about half the patients in this group have had a partial deficiency of Complex IV with reduced levels of cytochrome aa$_3$ and/or cytochrome oxidase activity in isolated muscle mitochondria (Roodhooft et al 1986, Schapira et al 1988, Koga et al 1988a, Morgan-Hughes et al 1990a, Watmough et al 1990). In one case cytochrome b was also abnormally low (Watmough et al 1990). Immunoblots of muscle Complex I performed in seven patients showed a generalized and proportional reduction of all cross-reacting bands in four (Morgan-Hughes et al 1988, Watmough et al 1989, 1990). In the remaining three cases, there was selective loss of the 24 kDa iron–sulphur protein in two (Morgan-Hughes et al 1988, Schapira et al 1988) and 24 kDa and 13 kDa iron–sulphur proteins in one (Morgan-Hughes et al 1988, Cooper et al 1990). All three of these patients also showed selective loss of subunit II in Complex IV (Morgan-Hughes et al 1988, Cooper et al 1990). One of these cases was subsequently shown to have an A to G transitional mutation at nucleotide position 3243 in the dihydrouridine loop of the mitochondrial tRNA$^{Leu(UUR)}$ gene (Hammans et al 1991).

Progressive external ophthalmoplegia (PEO) with, or without, limb weakness was the major presenting feature in 17 cases (Table 10.4). Pigmentary retinopathy was documented in seven cases, short stature in two, and sensorineural deafness in two (Morgan-Hughes et al 1987, Sherratt et al 1984, Holt et al 1989a,b; Morgan-Hughes et al 1990a). Two cases had cardiac conduction defects and/or CNS disease consistent with the Kearns–Sayre syndrome (Holt et al 1989a,b). As in cases with isolated limb weakness, cytochrome aa$_3$ and/or the activity of cytochrome c oxidase were below the control range in over half the cases (Sherratt et al 1984, 1986, Johnson et al 1988, Holt et al 1989a,b, Morgan-Hughes et al 1990a). All cases in which the family history was documented were sporadic. A high proportion of patients in this group have heteroplasmic deletions of mitochondrial DNA described in a later section (Holt et al 1989a,b, Morgan-Hughes et al 1990a).

Immunoblots of Complex I in three cases showed a mild generalized reduction of all cross-reacting bands in one and a normal profile in two (Morgan-Hughes et al 1988, Schapira et al 1988).

Encephalomyopathy

This is the commonest clinical presentation in patients with Complex I deficiency and accounts for over half the cases (Table 10.4). Symptoms have usually appeared in childhood or early adult life, but one patient developed progressive ataxia, dementia and muscle weakness in the seventh decade (Morgan-Hughes et al 1987, Truong et al 1990), and two presented in early infancy (Prick et al 1981b, Koga et al 1988a & b). Patients in this group have presented with a variable combination of clinical features which include muscle weakness, headache, vomiting, mental regression, cerebellar ataxia, myoclonic or generalized seizures, visual failure, sensorineural deafness or recurrent stroke-like episodes (Morgan-Hughes et al 1982, 1987, 1988, 1990a, Petty et al 1986, Koga et al 1988a, Ichiki et al 1988, Sakuta & Nonaka 1989). Stroke-like episodes usually associated with seizures and intellectual decline were the major clinical features in 29 out of the 42 cases (69%). The remaining cases usually presented with a combination of dementia, cerebellar ataxia, sensorineural deafness and muscle weakness. Dystonic and choreoathetoid movements have been noted in some cases (Petty et al 1986, Truong et al 1990) and Parkinsonian features were particularly prominent in one (van Erwen et al 1987). Short stature was documented in 20 cases, deafness in 17, cerebellar ataxia in 14, and pigmentary retinopathy in 5, including 4 patients with recurrent strokes (Morgan-Hughes et al 1987, Koga et al 1988a). Cardiomyopathy occurred in nine (Morgan-Hughes et al 1987, Nishizawa et al 1987, Kobayashi et al 1987, Ichiki et al 1988, Koga et al 1988a, Yoneda et al 1989a) and sensory neuropathy in three (Morgan-Hughes et al 1987). Most patients with encephalopathy showed clinical and electromyographic evidence of myopathy, but the weakness was often slight, and in some cases was clinically undetectable.

The family history was positive in six cases (14%) and one patient was the product of a first cousin marriage (Yoneda et al 1989a). Four patients had similarly affected siblings (Morgan-Hughes et al 1987, 1988, Byrne et al 1988, Koga et al 1988a). One had an affected maternal uncle (Nishizawa et al 1987), and one female had an affected son (Morgan-Hughes et al 1987, Schapira et al 1988).

Laboratory investigations have confirmed the widespread nature of the disease process and have shown prominent EEG changes, raised lactate levels with an increased lactate:pyruvate ratio in the blood and in the CSF and various abnormalities on CT brain scan. These include cerebral and cerebellar atrophy, low-density areas in the sub-cortical white matter and calcification in the basal ganglia (Morgan-Hughes et al 1982, Ichiki et al 1988, Koga et al, 1988a, Yoneda et al 1989a). Phosphorus nuclear magnetic resonance spectro-scopy (^{31}P NMR) has demonstrated a reduced phosphorylation potential in the brain of one case (Hayes et al 1985) and three other patients were shown to have a significant reduction in cerebral oxygen utilization, as determined by positron emission tomography (Frackowiak et al 1988).

Autopsy studies have shown multiple necrotic foci with haemorrhage and spongiform change in the cerebral cortex, subcortical white matter, basal ganglia, and brain stem. Some cases have shown diffuse fatty infiltration of the liver, hypertrophic cardiomyopathy, and a proliferative glomerular nephritis (Ohama et al 1987). Marked proliferation of mitochondria in smooth muscle and in endo-thelial cells of cerebral blood vessels suggests that the recurrent stroke-like episodes may be due to a mitochondrial angiopathy (Ohama et al 1987). Similar mitochondrial proliferation has been demonstrated in the smooth muscle and, to a lesser extent, in the endothelial cells, of intra-muscular arterioles (Sakuta & Nonaka 1989).

In common with other Complex I deficiency phenotypes, the rate-limiting defect in Complex I is often associated with a partial deficiency of cytochrome c oxidase activity and/or a reduced level of cytochrome aa_3 in muscle mitochondria (Ichiki et al 1988, Koga et al 1988a, Byrne et al 1988, Yoneda et al 1989a, Schapira et al 1988, 1990a, Morgan-Hughes et al 1988, 1990a). Immunoblots of Complex I have usually shown a generalized reduction of all cross-reacting bands (Nishizawa et al 1987, Morgan-Hughes et al 1988, Schapira et al 1988, Yoneda et al 1989a). In a few cases, however, there has been a disproportionate and severe deficiency of one or more Complex I polypeptides encoded by nuclear genes (Morgan-Hughes et al 1988, Ichiki et al 1988, Schapira et al 1990a). Five out of the nine patients with the encephalopathic form of Complex I deficiency studied in our laboratory have subsequently been shown to have the A to G transitional mutation at position 3243 in the mitochondrial tRNa$^{Leu(UUR)}$ gene (Hammans et al 1991). They included two patients with specific deficiencies of nuclear encoded Complex I polypeptides, one of whom has been reported in detail previously (Schapira et al 1990a).

Defects of Complex II (succinate–ubiquinone oxidoreductase)

Complex II catalyses the transfer of electrons from succinate to ubiquinone (Hatefi 1985). It consists of four or five polypeptides all encoded by nuclear genes. The largest subunit contains covalently bound flavin and the second largest subunit contains the iron–sulphur clusters. The smaller subunits which contain haem b are essential for succinate–ubiquinone oxidoreductase activity and probably anchor the larger subunits to the mitochondrial inner membrane. Nine patients with defects probably involving Complex II have been reported (Table 10.5).

Severe myopathy in infancy, with lactic acidosis, carnitine deficiency and ragged red fibres in biopsied muscle occurred in two cases (Sengers et al 1983, Behbehani et al 1984). CT brain scan in one case showed cerebral and cerebellar atrophy but there were no clinical signs of CNS disease (Sengers et al 1983). In both cases the diagnosis of Complex II deficiency was inferred on the basis of low or undetectable levels of succinate cytochrome c reductase activity in skeletal muscle.

Limb weakness and exercise intolerance were the presenting features in a 22-year-old man (Haller et al 1990) and a 14-year-old girl (Garavaglia et al 1990). Succinate oxidation was severely impaired in muscle mitochondria from both cases and, in the man succinate dehydrogenase activity was virtually undetectable biochemically and on histochemical staining of biopsied muscle (Haller et al 1990).

The activities of succinate dehydrogenase, succinate-CoQ reductase and succinate cytochrome c reductase were markedly reduced in muscle mitochondria in one patient with the Kearns–Sayre syndrome (Rivner et al 1989). An immunoblot of Complex II was normal. Mitochondrial DNA was not examined.

Encephalomyopathy occurred in four cases. They included two siblings aged 7 and 9 years, with short stature, dementia, cerebellar ataxia, myoclonic jerks and occasional generalized seizures (Riggs et al 1984). Myopathy was not evident clinically but a muscle biopsy in each case showed ragged red fibres with prominent lipid storage. In both patients there was a partial deficiency of succinate–cytochrome c reductase in muscle homogenates, but the activities of succinate dehydrogenase, NADH–cytochrome c reductase, and cytochrome c oxidase were normal. A three-

Table 10.5 Defects of Complex II: clinical presentations in 9 cases

Syndrome	No. of cases	References
Severe myopathy in infancy with lactic acidosis	2	Sengers et al (1983) Behbehani et al (1984)
Myopathy with weakness and exercise intolerance	2	Haller et al (1990) Garavaglia et al (1990)
Kearns–Sayre syndrome	1	Rivner et al (1989)
Encephalomyopathy	4	Riggs et al (1984) Martin et al (1988) Sperl et al (1988)

year-old boy who presented with severe psycho-motor retardation had symmetrical hypodense areas in the basal ganglia on CT brain scan, resembling Leigh's syndrome (Martin et al 1988). The activities of succinate dehydrogenase and succinate cytochrome c reductase were normal in muscle homogenates, but succinate oxidation by isolated muscle mitochondria was significantly reduced, as was pyruvate oxidation. It was suggested that these paradoxical results may have been due to an abnormality of one of the Co-Q binding proteins (Martin et al 1988). A fourth patient reported by Sperl et al, (1988) was a 3-month-old girl with lactic acidosis, severe developmental delay, renal tubular dysfunction and signs of liver involvement. There were no ragged red fibres on muscle biopsy. Succinate cytochrome c reductase activity was greatly reduced in muscle, and low in liver, but the activities of succinate dehydrogenase and cytochrome c oxidase were normal.

Defects of Complex III (ubiquinone–cytochrome c oxidoreductase)

Complex III catalyses the transfer of electrons from dihydroubiquinone to cytochrome c (Hatefi 1985). The reaction is coupled to transmembrane proton translocation. The complex contains 11 subunits and 3 redox centres. These consist of two b haems thought to be associated with a single hydrophobic polypeptide encoded by mitochondrial DNA, a c_1 haem which appears to be associated with two unlike polypetides and a dinuclear iron–sulphur cluster carried by the Rieske protein. The complex also contains core proteins I and II, subunit VI and subunit VIII, but the functions of these components are unknown. With the exception of apocytochrome b all subunits are encoded by nuclear genes. Sixteen patients with defects of Complex III have been described (Table 10.6). Fourteen of these cases have recently been reviewed (Kennaway 1988).

Limb weakness and exercise intolerance dominated the clinical picture in five patients. Symptoms began in childhood or adolescence except in one patient who was hypotonic and weak at birth and did not walk until the age of 2 years (Schapira et al 1990b). All five patients had a variable lactic acidaemia, induced or made worse by exercise, and all except one case (Schapira et al 1990b) had ragged red fibres on muscle biopsy. The concentration of reducible cytochrome b as determined by spectral analysis was significantly reduced in three cases, and in one of these cytochrome c_1 was undetectable (Morgan-Hughes et al 1977, Darley-Usmar et al 1983, Kennaway et al 1984, Hayes et al 1984). The mitochondrial cytochromes were normal in two cases, suggesting that the defects may have involved the Rieske iron–sulphur protein. The family history was negative in all cases.

Progressive external ophthalmoplegia occurred in six patients (Morgan-Hughes et al 1987, Holt et al 1989a). Pigmentary retinopathy was present in one and another patient had a combination of cerebellar

Table 10.6 Defects of Complex III: clinical presentations in 16 cases

Syndrome	No. of cases	References
Limb weakness and exercise intolerance	5	Hayes et al (1984) Morgan–Hughes et al (1977, 1987, 1990a) Darley-Usmar et al (1983) Kennaway et al (1984) Reichmann et al (1986) Schapira et al (1990b)
Syndromes with PEO±pigmentary retinopathy, deafness, cardiomyopathy, CNS disease	6	Morgan-Hughes et al (1987, 1990a) Holt et al (1989a)
Early or late onset encephalomyopathy	4	Spiro et al (1970) Morgan-Hughes et al (1982, 1987 and 1990a) Scholte et al (1987)
Histiocytoid cardiomyopathy	1	Papadimitriou et al (1984)

ataxia, myoclonic jerks and a peripheral sensory neuropathy. The mitochondrial cytochromes were normal in four cases, but cytochrome aa_3 was reduced in two and in one of these cytochrome b was also low. Four cases in this group were subsequently shown to have large deletions of muscle mtDNA and a fifth patient, who suffered a transient hemiparesis in middle age, had an A to G transitional mutation at nucleotide position 3243 in the mitochondrial $tRNA^{Leu(UUR)}$ gene, (Hammans et al 1991). Two patients both with large mtDNA deletions had affected relatives. One female patient had an affected daughter and a male patient had an affected niece, the daughter of his unaffected sister (Holt et al 1989a, Morgan-Hughes et al 1990a).

Encephalopathy occurred in four patients. One presented in early infancy with severe mental retardation, hypotonia and failure to thrive (Scholte et al 1987). Muscle mitochondria isolated from the patient at 7 months oxidized pyruvate, succinate and duroquinol at a reduced rate, but ascorbate oxidation was normal. Succinate cytochrome c oxidase activity was low in muscle and liver, but succinate dehydrogenase activity was normal. Spectral analysis of the mitochondrial cytochromes showed a slow rate of reduction of cytochrome aa_3 by succinate, and a marked deficiency of cytochromes $c_1 + c$. In the second biopsy taken at 2.8 years the changes were more severe. Three patients presented with an encephalomyopathy in childhood or adult life (Spiro et al 1970, Morgan-Hughes et al 1982). A father and son had a complex hereditary disorder, characterized by dementia, cerebellar ataxia and muscle weakness. Additional features in the son included choreoretinitis, myoclonus, ptosis and partial external ophthalmoplegia. Spectral analysis of the mitochondrial cytochromes in each case showed low levels of reducible cytochrome b and a partial deficiency of cytochrome a. The third patient presented with myoclonic jerks in her early 30s and later went on to develop progressive muscle weakness, cerebellar ataxia and dementia (Morgan-Hughes et al 1982). Lactate levels were increased in blood and CSF, an EEG showed atypical spike and slow wave activity and a CT brain scan showed cerebral and cerebellar atrophy, with calcification of the basal ganglia. Difference spectra (reduced minus oxidized) of the mitochondrial cytochromes at 77 Kelvin showed a deficiency of reducible cytochrome b and a shift in its absorbance peak (Morgan-Hughes et al 1982).

Isolated histiocytoid cardiomyopathy has been described in association with a severe deficiency of reducible cytochrome b in heart muscle from a 4-week-old girl with cardiomegaly who died of cardiac arrest (Papadimitriou et al 1984). Succinate cytochrome c reductase and rotenone sensitive NADH cytochrome c reductase activity were markedly reduced. Morphological studies of the heart showed enlarged muscle fibres with accumulations of abnormal mitochondria.

Immunoblots of muscle Complex III in two patients with muscle weakness and exercise intolerance, have shown different patterns of abnormality. In one patient there was a severe deficiency of cytochrome b, core proteins I and II, the Rieske iron–sulphur protein and subunit VI (Darley-Usmar et al 1983). This patient had a dramatic and lasting clinical response to treatment with menadione (vitamin K_3) and ascorbate which was confirmed by ^{31}P NMR (Eleff et al 1984, Kennaway 1988). The findings in the second patient pointed to defective translocation of the Rieske precursor protein from the cytosol into the mitochondria (Schapira et al 1990b). There were no ragged red fibres on muscle biopsy (Fig. 10.19), but with histochemical stains there was virtual absence of succinate dehydrogenase in the muscle fibres, with normal activity in the intramuscular blood vessels (Fig. 10.20). At an ultrastructural level there were large collections of abnormal mitochondria containing dense granular matrix inclusions (Fig. 10.21) which, on energy dispersive X-ray microanalysis contained substantial quantities of iron (Schapira et al 1990b). Biochemical studies showed a defect of Complexes I–III and confirmed the severe deficiency of succinate dehydrogenase activity. Immunoblots of mitochondrial protein showed virtual absence of the Rieske iron–sulphur protein of Complex III and the 27.2 kDa iron–sulphur protein of Complex II. Homogenate and cytosolic blots using subunit specific antiserum, showed that the Rieske precursor protein was present in an amount similar to that seen in controls. Unlike the Rieske protein, however, the 27.2 kDa subunit of Complex II was

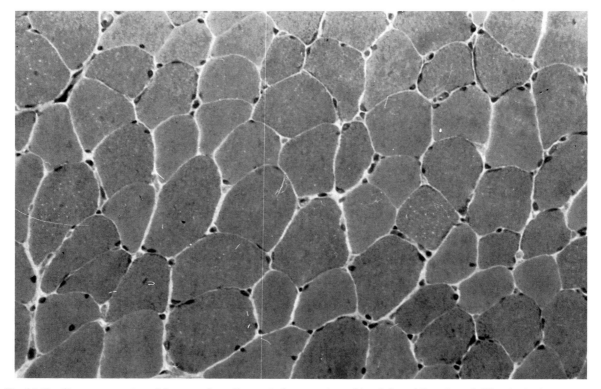

Fig. 10.19 Transverse section of the vastus lateralis muscle from a patient with a defect of Complexes I–III and selective deficiencies of the Rieske protein and the 27.2 kDa protein of Complex II (see text). Note the absence of ragged red fibres. Gomori trichrome stain. ×350

also markedly deficient in homogenate and cytosolic blots, suggesting either reduced synthesis or increased degradation of this protein.

The combined molecular abnormality encountered in this patient is difficult to explain on the basis of a single gene defect, unless the two proteins are isoforms which seems unlikely. It is possible, however, that certain iron–sulphur proteins may be encoded by a cluster of genes on nuclear DNA. If this were the case, a mutation affecting a single coding sequence could lead to reduced synthesis of the 27.2 kDa polypeptide of Complex II and alter the Rieske presequence, thereby preventing its receptor-mediated import into mitochondria. A limited base change resulting in a small alteration in molecular mass would not be detected by gel electrophoresis. Mutations which alter or eliminate targeting sequences have been identified for the mitochondrial matrix enzymes methylmalonyl-CoA mutase (Ledley et al 1990) and MCAD (Strauss et

al 1990) and for the peroxisomal enzyme alanine/glyoxylate aminotransferase (Purdue et al 1990). The presence of large deposits of sequestrated iron in the matrix of a high proportion of the muscle mitochondria from this case would be consistent with the hypothesis that the iron–sulphur clusters are assembled into iron–sulphur proteins within the mitochondria after translocation of the apoproteins.

A severe deficiency of co-enzyme Q_{10} in muscle from two sisters aged 14 and 12 has recently been described (Ogasahara et al 1989). They both had weakness and exercise intolerance, associated with episodes of myoglobinuria. The younger sister developed generalized seizures at the age of 7 and the older sister had a progressive cerebellar syndrome from the age of 12. Both patients had lactic acidaemia and mitochondrial abnormalities with lipid storage on muscle biopsy. The activities of Complex I, III and IV were normal and that of

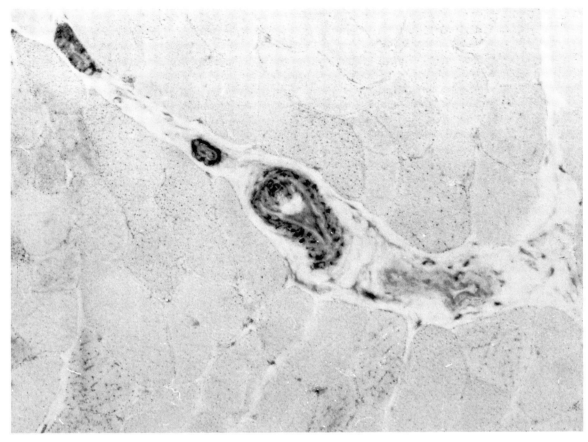

Fig. 10.20 Transverse section of the vastus lateralis muscle from the same patient shown in Fig. 10.19. Stained for succinate dehydrogenase activity. Note the virtual absence of enzyme activity in the muscle fibres, but normal activity in the intramuscular blood vessels. ×350

Complex II was increased. The coenzyme Q_{10} content of muscle mitochondria was reduced to about 5% of the mean control value in each case. Coenzyme Q_{10} levels in the serum and in cultured fibroblasts were normal. These results pointed to a defect of a tissue-specific isoenzyme involved in the biosynthesis of coenzyme Q_{10} in muscle and brain mitochondria (Ogasahara et al 1989).

Defects of Complex IV (cytochrome c oxidase)

Cytochrome c oxidase (COX), the terminal component of the respiratory chain, catalyses the irreversible transfer of four electrons from the single electron donor cytochrome c to molecular oxygen (Hatefi 1985; Capaldi 1990). The reaction con-

sumes four protons to form water and is also coupled to transmembrane proton translocation. The mammalian enzyme is composed of 13 different polypeptides (Kadenbach et al 1987). It carries four redox centres consisting of two haems (a and a_3) each associated with an atom of copper (Cu_A, Cu_B). The redox centres and transmembrane proton translocation, are associated with the three larger subunits (I, II and III) which form the catalytic core of the enzyme. These subunits are encoded by mitochondrial genes (Anderson et al 1981). The remaining subunits are encoded by nuclear genes and synthesized on free cytoplasmic polysomes mostly as precursor proteins with N-terminal amphiphilic targeting presequences which direct them into the correct mito-

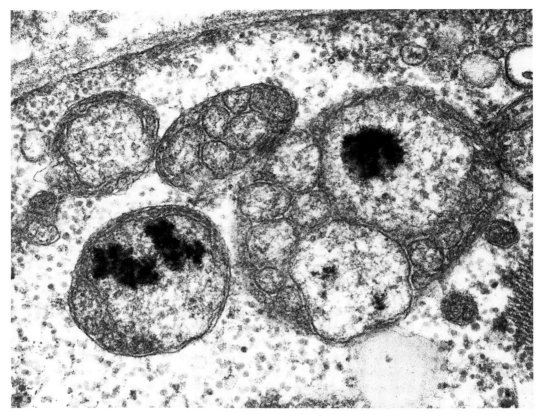

Fig. 10.21 Electron micrograph of the periphery of a muscle fibre from the same patient as shown in Figs 10.19 and 10.20. Note the presence of enlarged mitochondria with distorted cristae containing dense granular matrix inclusions which contained substantial quantities of iron (see text). Bar = 0.5 μm

chondrial compartment (Hartl et al 1989). The function of the nuclear-encoded subunits is largely unknown but a regulatory role has been proposed (Kadenbach 1986, Kadenbach et al 1989, Capaldi 1990). Isoforms of some of these subunits have been identified (Kuhn-Nentwig & Kadenbach 1985, Schlerf et al 1988, Capaldi 1990).

In common with defects of other respiratory complexes, COX deficiency has been identified in a clinically heterogeneous group of disorders which may affect the brain, heart or kidney, as well as skeletal muscle. The main clinical presentations are summarized in Table 10.7.

The fatal infantile myopathy begins soon after birth and usually leads to death from respiratory insufficiency during the first year. It is characterized by severe lactic acidosis, profound generalized hypotonic weakness, breathing and feeding difficulties and failure to thrive (DiMauro et al 1988). The myopathy may occur in isolation (Bresolin et al 1985) or may be associated with cardiomyopathy (Rimoldi et al 1982, Sengers et al 1984, Zeviani et al 1986) or more commonly with the De-Toni–Fanconi–Debré syndrome (van Biervliet et al 1977, DiMauro et al 1980, Zeviani et al 1985, Nonaka et al 1988).

Muscle biopsy in most cases has shown ragged red fibres with abundant glycogen and increased numbers of neutral lipid droplets (Bresolin et al 1985, Nonaka et al 1988). In a few cases, however, ragged red fibres were not seen (Rimoldi et al 1982, Nonaka et al 1988). In sections stained histochemically COX activity is virtually undetectable in the extrafusal fibres, but is present in the intrafusal fibres of the muscle spindles and in the smooth muscle of intramuscular blood vessels

Table 10.7 Defects of Complex IV (cytochrome c oxidase): clinical presentation in 69 cases

Phenotype	No. of cases	Reference
1. Fatal infantile myopathy ± Fanconi syndrome or cardiomyopathy	20	DiMauro et al (1988) Nonaka et al (1988) Tritschler et al (1991)
2. Benign infantile myopathy	6	DiMauro et al (1983) Zeviani et al (1987) Nonaka et al (1988) Tritschler et al (1991)
3. Limb weakness and exercise intolerance	1	Haller et al (1989)
4. Leigh's syndrome	24	Willems et al (1977) Miyabayashi et al (1985, 1987) Robinson et al (1987b) DiMauro et al (1987) Arts et al (1987) Ogier et al (1988) Nonaka et al (1988) Shepherd et al (1988) Miranda et al (1989) Koga et al (1990)
5. Alpers' syndrome	2	Prick et al (1983)
6. Childhood or adult encephalopathy	8	Angelini et al (1986) Servidie et al (1987) Nonaka et al (1987)
7. Progressive external ophthalmoplegia and KSS	6	Byrne et al (1985) Johnson et al (1983, 1988) Bresolin et al (1987)
8. Myoclonic epilepsy and RRF (MERRF)	2	Berkovic et al (1989) Lombes et al (1989)

(Zeviani et al 1985, Nonaka et al 1988). Biochemical studies of skeletal muscle have shown virtual absence of COX activity in all cases. Difference (reduced–minus–oxidized) spectra of the mitochondrial cytochromes have confirmed lack of an aa_3 peak and in some cases have shown a partial deficiency of cytochrome b (van Biervliet et al 1977, DiMauro et al 1980, Minchom et al 1983, Sengers et al 1984, Bresolin et al 1985). Cases with renal involvement had a partial deficiency of COX activity and cytochrome aa_3 in kidney (van Biervliet et al 1977, DiMauro et al 1980). In two patients with cardiomyopathy, enzyme activity in the heart was normal in one (Rimoldi et al 1982) but markedly reduced in the other (Zeviani et al 1986). In all cases studied, COX activity has been normal in clinically unaffected tissues including brain, liver, kidney, heart and cultured fibroblasts (van Biervliet et al 1977, DiMauro et al 1980, Stansbie et al 1982, Minchom et al 1983, Bresolin

et al 1985). Secondary carnitine deficiency has also been described (Müller-Hocker et al 1983). Immunotitration by ELISA has shown that the amount of immunologically detectable enzyme protein is markedly reduced in skeletal muscle but the subunit composition of the mutant enzyme, as determined by immunoprecipitation and SDS-PAGE, is normal (Bresolin et al 1985, Zeviani et al 1985). In a recent immunohistochemical study of muscle from four cases, however, there was absence of the nuclear-encoded COX subunits VIIa VIIb (Tritschler et al 1991).

Five cases have had one or more affected siblings suggesting autosomal recessive inheritance (van Biervliet et al 1977, Stansbie et al 1982, Minchom et al 1983, Müller-Hocker et al 1983, Nonaka et al 1988).

Mutations of mtDNA have not, so far, been reported in the fatal infantile form of COX deficiency. Recently, however, a severe depletion of mtDNA has been identified in four patients with this condition (Moraes et al 1991). In two cases the myopathy was associated with the De-Toni–Fanconi–Debré syndrome. The other two were second cousins previously described by Boustany et al (1983) and by Aprille (1985). One of these patients had an isolated myopathy with PEO and died of respiratory failure at 12 weeks. Her cousin died of hepatic failure at the age of 9 months. In all four cases there was severe depletion of mtDNA in affected tissues and severe deficiency of COX activity (Moraes et al 1991). These findings suggested a disturbance of mtDNA replication but sequence analysis of mtDNA replication origins failed to reveal any abnormality that could account for the low copy number (Moraes et al 1991).

The benign infantile myopathy has been described in six cases (Table 10.7). The disorder presents soon after birth with generalized hypotonic weakness, feeding and breathing difficulties and severe lactic acidosis but tissues other than skeletal muscle are not affected. Infants with this disorder improve spontaneously during the first year and are virtually normal by the age of 3 years. Muscle COX activity, as determined histochemically or by enzyme assay, is virtually undetectable in samples taken at or soon after birth, but gradually increases as the child's clinical condition improves. The ragged red changes observed in early muscle biopsies similarly disappear. Immunotitration by ELISA has shown normal amounts of immunologically detectable enzyme protein, even in muscle taken early in the course of the disease, a finding which distinguishes this disorder from the fatal infantile form (Zeviani et al 1987). In a recent study of four patients using immunohistochemical techniques, however, muscle taken early in the course of the disease lacked the nuclear encoded COX subunits VIIa and b, and also subunit II which is encoded by mitochondrial DNA (Tritschler et al 1991). Immunostaining for all three subunits returned to normal as the patients improved.

Five cases were sporadic but one had an affected sibling (Tritschler et al 1991). The gradual appearance of COX activity in skeletal muscle during the first few months after birth would suggest a nuclear mutation, possibly affecting a tissue-specific fetal COX isoform (Zeviani et al 1987).

Limb weakness, exercise intolerance, and lactic acidosis were the major clinical features in a 27-year-old woman with a marked deficiency of COX and low levels of cytochrome aa$_3$ and b in skeletal muscle (Haller et al 1989). She walked late and was never able to run or play games at school. A muscle biopsy showed excess lipid predominantly in the type 1 fibres, abundant glycogen granules and increased numbers of normal looking mitochondria but there were no definite ragged red changes with the Gomori trichrome stain. COX activity was absent in virtually all the muscle fibres histochemically and was severely reduced when assayed enzymatically. Cytochromes aa$_3$ and b were also markedly reduced but succinate–cytochrome c reductase activity was normal. Total and free muscle carnitine levels were less than half control values.

Leigh's syndrome appears to be the most common clinical presentation of COX deficiency, and has been reported in over 20 cases (Table 10.7). Most patients have presented in infancy or early childhood with a variable combination of clinical features, including developmental delay, mental regression, seizures, anorexia, vomiting, breathing difficulties, dysphagia, cerebellar ataxia, intention tremor, nystagmus, optic atrophy, deafness, ptosis, ophthalmoplegia, hypotonic weakness, spasticity, failure to thrive and peripheral neuropathy. Hypertrophic cardiomyopathy (DiMauro et al 1987) and renal dysfunction with aminoaciduria, hypercalcuria and hyperphosphaturia, features consistent with the Fanconi syndrome, have been described (Ogier et al 1988). Lactic acidosis and elevated lactate levels with an increased lactate:pyruvate ratio in the CSF are common findings. CT brain scan may show low-density areas in the subcortical white matter, basal ganglia, mid brain or pons, associated with cortical, brain stem or cerebellar atrophy.

On histochemical analysis, COX activity is barely detectable in the extrafusal muscle fibres, but unlike the fatal infantile myopathy, enzyme activity is also lacking in muscle spindles and in the smooth muscle of intramuscular blood vessels (Nonaka et al 1988, Koga et al 1990). Ragged red fibres have only been reported in one case (Arts et al 1987). Autopsy studies have shown that COX activity is reduced to a variable extent in all tissues including brain, heart, liver, kidney, skeletal muscle and cultured fibroblasts (Miyabayashi et al 1987, DiMauro et al 1987, Arts et al 1987, Koga et al 1990). However, COX activity was normal in the liver of one patient (Willems et al 1977) and in the liver and cultured fibroblasts of another (DiMauro et al 1987). A less marked deficiency of Complex I has been reported in some cases (Nonaka et al 1988, Koga et al 1990). Spectral analysis of the mitochondrial cytochromes in one patient showed that cytochromes aa_3 and b were decreased in heart, skeletal muscle, liver, kidney and brain, and cytochromes $c+c_1$ were also decreased in heart and liver (Koga et al 1990). In the two patients studied by DiMauro and colleagues (1987), cytochrome aa_3 was decreased in muscle from one case, but was probably normal in brain and muscle from the other. The amount of immunologically detectable enzyme protein has been variable. In some cases it has been decreased (DiMauro et al 1987, Miyabayashi et al 1987, Koga et al 1990) whereas in others it has been normal (DiMauro et al 1987, Miranda et al 1989). Specific subunit deficiencies have also been reported in one patient (Koga et al 1990).

Several patients have had affected siblings (Miyabayashi et al 1987, Arts et al 1987, Miranda et al 1989) and two sporadic cases were the products of first cousin marriages (Arts et al 1987, Koga et al 1990). These findings would suggest autosomal recessive inheritance. Further evidence for a nuclear gene mutation has been obtained by studying somatic cell hybrids produced by fusing COX-positive Helacot cells with transformed COX-deficient fibroblasts from an infant with Leigh's syndrome whose brother had died from the disease (Miranda et al 1989). The resulting hybrid cells which contained mtDNA almost exclusively derived from the COX-deficient Leigh fibroblasts showed normal or elevated COX activity. These findings would suggest that a Helacot nuclear gene was responsible for correcting the enzyme defect in hybrid cells (Miranda et al 1989).

Leigh's syndrome has also been described in association with deficiencies of the pyruvate dehydrogenase complex (Robinson et al 1987a, 1989) and defects of Complex I (Robinson et al 1986, 1987a,b, Hoppel et al 1987). In the overwhelming majority of patients with Leigh's syndrome, however, the biochemical defect remains unknown (Miyabayashi et al 1985).

Alpers' syndrome is thought to be distinct from Leigh's syndrome (Egger et al 1987) although the clinical features and course of the disease are somewhat similar. A partial deficiency of COX activity in muscle has been described in two unrelated patients with this condition (Prick et al 1983). The older of the two cases had ragged red fibres in biopsied muscle.

Childhood and adult encephalomyopathies have also been described in association with partial COX deficiency in skeletal muscle (Angelini et al 1986, Servidei et al 1987, Nonaka et al 1988). The clinical features have been variable but have included mental impairment, cerebellar ataxia, myoclonus, seizures, intention tremor, ptosis, ophthalmoplegia, nystagmus, hearing loss, recurrent stroke-like episodes and progressive muscle weakness. Laboratory studies have shown elevated lactate levels in the blood and in the CSF, EEG abnormalities and cerebral atrophy or low density areas in the cerebral white matter on CT brain scan. Muscle biopsy in most cases has shown ragged red fibres and only faint or patchy staining for COX activity. Complex I activity has been significantly reduced in some cases (Nonaka et al 1988). The amount of immunologically detectable enzyme protein was reduced in muscle from a 52-year-old man with seizures, hearing loss and muscle weakness, who showed cerebral atrophy on CT brain scan (Servidie et al 1987).

The Kearns–Sayre syndrome and myoclonic epilepsy with ragged red fibres have also been associated with partial COX deficiency in some cases (Johnson et al 1983, 1988, Byrne et al 1985, Bresolin et al 1987, Berkovic et al 1989, Lombes et al 1989b). The patient with myoclonic epilepsy described by Lombes and colleagues (1989b) was the last affected member of the family originally reported by Tsairis et al (1973) who first drew attention to this distinctive disorder. The patient died of cardiorespiratory arrest at the age of 36. COX activity was reduced in heart, brain, liver and kidney, as well as in skeletal muscle, but the activities of other respiratory chain enzymes were essentially normal (Lombes et al 1989b). Immunoblot analysis and immunohistological studies indicated a selective deficiency of subunit II which, is encoded by mtDNA (Lombes et al 1989b).

Multiple respiratory enzyme deficiencies

Combined deficiencies of the respiratory chain enzymes appear to be the rule rather than the exception, particularly in patients with mutations of the mitochondrial genome or depletion of mtDNA (Wallace et al 1988a,b, Shoffner et al 1989, Holt et al 1989a,b, Moraes et al 1989a,b, 1991). Combined deficiencies of Complexes I and IV, III and IV, and I, III and IV, have also been identified in a number of patients without detectable mutations of the mitochondrial genome (Zheng et al 1989, Morgan-Hughes et al 1990a, Bindoff et al 1991). Whether the changes in such cases occur at the level of transcription, translation or assembly, or result from accelerated degradation remains to be determined.

Defects of Complex V (H$^+$-ATPase)

Complex V utilizes the proton electrochemical gradient (Δp) generated by electron transport to catalyse the phosphorylation of ADP to form ATP (Hatefi 1985). It occupies the final step in the oxidative phosphorylation pathway. The complex comprises a catalytic component (F$_1$) and a membrane component (F$_0$) which contains the proton channel. Mammalian H$^+$-ATPase is composed of at least 13 different polypeptides, two of which (subunits 6 and 8) are encoded by mitochondrial genes (Anderson et al 1981, Chomyn et al 1985). The functions of subunits 6 and 8 are obscure.

Only two patients with deficiency of H$^+$-ATPase have been described (Schotland et al 1976, Clark et al 1984). The first was a 37-year-old woman who presented with a life-long history of mild non-progressive weakness. A muscle biopsy showed prominent mitochondrial changes with abundant paracrystalline inclusions (Schotland et al 1976). Studies of freshly isolated muscle mitochondria showed very low oxygen uptake rates with both NAD-linked and FAD-linked substrates which were restored to normal by the addition of the uncoupling agent 2,4-dinitrophenol. P/O ratios and the rate and extent of mitochondrial Ca^{2+} uptake were normal. These results suggested a defect of phosphorylation which involved all three coupling sites and was distal to the common energy pool. Further study showed that the limitation of electron transport was associated with a deficiency of basal, Mg^{2+}-stimulated and 2,4-dinitrophenol-stimulated mitochondrial ATPase activity.

The second patient, a 17-year-old boy, originally presented in childhood with weakness and abnormal fatigue on exertion, growth retardation, sensorineural deafness and recurrent episodes of unexplained vomiting. Investigations at this time showed calcification of the basal ganglia and a lipid storage myopathy with muscle carnitine deficiency (Smythe et al 1975). On treatment with oral carnitine the vomiting stopped and there was gradual improvement in muscle strength (Hoskins et al 1977), but he subsequently went on to develop progressive dementia, cerebellar ataxia, pigmentary retinopathy, myoclonic jerks and a peripheral sensory neuropathy. A repeat muscle biopsy at the age of 17 showed peripheral accumulations of mitochondria in many of the fibres with virtual disappearance of lipid storage. The total muscle carnitine concentration was now within the normal range. Studies of isolated muscle mitochondria showed low respiratory rates with both NAD-linked and FAD-linked substrates which were enhanced almost 2-fold by the addition of Ca^{2+} or the uncoupling agent FCCP (Clark et al 1984). Basal and uncoupler-stimulated mitochondrial ATPase activity was less than 10% of control values in the patient's mitochondrial preparation.

Luft's disease

Only two patients with a mitochondrial myopathy and severe euthyroid-hypermetabolism have been described (Luft et al 1962, DiMauro et al 1976). Both patients were women who had suffered from severe heat intolerance, hyperhidrosis, polyphagia, polydypsia without polyuria and mild muscle weakness and fatigue since childhood or early adolescence. A muscle biopsy in each case showed peripheral accumulations of structurally abnormal mitochondria, many of which contained electron-dense osmiophilic bodies or paracrystalline inclusions. Freshly isolated muscle mitochondria had retained a capacity to synthesize ATP from added ADP and Pi but they continued to respire at an almost maximal rate even in the absence of ADP. Endogenous mitochondrial ATPase activity was greatly increased and showed negligible enhancement following the addition of uncoupler. The spectrum and content of the mitochondrial cytochromes were normal in the second case (DiMauro et al 1976). Studies of mitochondrial calcium transport suggested that the stimulated rate of mitochondrial respiration in the absence of ADP was associated with an inability of the mitochondria to retain Ca^{2+}. Calcium uptake by mitochondria is energy-linked and can be supported by electron transport or by ATP hydrolysis. In Luft's disease continuous recycling of Ca^{2+} between the cytosol and the mitochondrial matrix could account for the high and sustained respiratory rates in the absence of ADP. The presence of a retained phosphorylative capacity would suggest, however, that when ADP was available, phosphorylation took precedence over calcium transport.

Loss of the normal respiratory control adequately accounted for the patient's clinical condition as it suggested that the redox energy generated by the high basal or State 4 ($-$ADP) respiratory activity, which approached that recorded under State 3 ($+$ADP) conditions, was being dissipated as heat and thereby inducing the hypermetabolic state.

DISEASE-ASSOCIATED ABNORMALITIES OF THE MITOCHONDRIAL GENOME

Since 1988 (Holt et al 1988a), no fewer than nine different disease-related abnormalities of the mitochondrial genome have been identified. These are listed together with their associated phenotypes in Table 10.8. Seven of these abnormalities which either eliminate or alter mitochondrial tRNA genes or severely reduce mtDNA copy number are associated with abnormal mitochondrial proliferation (ragged red fibres) in skeletal muscle (types 1–7, Table 10.8). The two transitional mutations, which alter structural genes, are not associated with significant mitochondrial proliferation (types 8 and 9, Table 10.8).

Heteroplasmic deletions of mtDNA

Two populations of mtDNA, one normal (wild type) and the other with large uniform deletions up to 8 kb in size, have been identified in: (i) oculoskeletal myopathy with or without pigmentary retinopathy and/or sensorineural deafness; (ii) the Kearns–Sayre syndrome (KSS) as defined by Berenberg et al (1977); and (iii) Pearson's bone marrow/pancreas syndrome. This disorder presents with sideroblastic anaemia in early infancy and is associated with vacuolization of bone marrow precursors, hepatomegaly and pancreatic exocrine dysfunction (Pearson et al 1979).

Combined data from two recent publications (Moraes et al 1989a, Holt et al 1989a) showed that 62 out of 168 patients (40%) with mitochondrial myopathies, defined morphologically, had a variable proportion of deleted mtDNAs in muscle, detectable by Southern blot analysis. Deletions were present in 28 of 57 patients with oculoskeletal myopathy (49%), 15 of 16 with PEO plus retinopathy and/or deafness (94%) and 19 of 24 with KSS (79%). Deletions of mtDNA were not detected in 35 other patients with PEO, including 5 with KSS, or in patients with limb weakness alone, various encephalomyopathies, Leigh's syndrome, Luft's disease, the fatal or benign forms of COX deficiency, congenital lactic acidosis, or mitochondrial ATPase deficiency (Moraes et al 1989a). Similar results have been reported by others (Shoffner et al 1989, Gerbitz et al 1990, Johns et al 1989). In all cases the deletions have eliminated two or more open reading frames, together with the intervening tRNA genes, but they do not appear to have extended to the origins of transcription or translation of the H or L strands of mtDNA (Fig 10.22). Although the deleted regions differ in size and location between cases, in any one individual the deleted molecules are identical. The relative proportions of deleted mtDNAs in muscle have ranged from 20 to 80% in different cases (Moraes et al 1989a, Holt et al 1989a). Post mortem studies of KSS have confirmed that the same deletion identified in muscle is present in variable proportions in other tissues, including extraocular muscles, cerebrum, cerebellum, liver, kidney and heart (Shanske et al 1990, Zeviani et al 1990a). Deleted molecules have also been identi-

Table 10.8 Diseases associated with abnormalities of the mitochondrial genome

Genotype	Phenotype	References
A. With ragged red fibres		
1. Large single deletions (heteroplasmic)	PEO±limb weakness	Holt et al (1988a,b, 1989a)
	PEO±retinopathy and/or deafness	Zeviani et al (1988)
	Kearns–Sayre syndrome	Moraes et al (1989a)
		Mita et al (1989)
		Schoffner et al (1989)
		Gerbitz et al (1990)
	Pearson's bone marrow/pancreas syndrome	Rotig et al (1989)
		van Oost et al (1990)
		Larsson et al (1990)
		McShane et al (1991)
	(Parkinson's disease)	Ikebe et al (1990)
2. Tandem duplications (heteroplasmic)	Kearns–Sayre syndrome	Poulton et al (1989)
3. Large multiple deletions (pleioplasmic)	Autosomal dominant PEO	Zeviani et al (1989, 1990b)
	Autosomal dominant encephalomyopathy	Cormier et al (1990)
	Ptosis, optic atrophy, peripheral neuropathy	Yuzaki et al (1989)
	Kearns–Sayre syndrome ?aut. dominant	Otsuka et al (1990)
	Recurrent myoglobinuria	Ozawa et al (1990)
	(Idiopathic cardiomyopathy)	Ohno et al (1991)
4. A→G transition at np 8344 in the Tψc loop of tRNA^{Lys} (heteroplasmic)	Myoclonic epilepsy and ragged red fibres (MERRF)	Shoffner et al (1990)
		Yoneda et al (1990)
		Zeviani et al (1991)
		Hammans et al (1991)
5. A→G transition at np 3243 in the dihydrouridine loop of tRNA$^{\text{Leu(UUR)}}$ (heteroplasmic)	Encephalopathy with strokes (MELAS)	Goto et al (1990)
	PEO±stroke	Kobayashi et al (1990)
	Ataxia, dementia, deafness	Hammans et al (1991)
	Myopathy only	
6. A→G transition at np 4317 in Tψc loop of tRNA^{Ile} (heteroplasmic)	Encephalopathy with strokes and fatal cardiomyopathy	Tanaka et al (1990)
7. mtDNA depletion	COX-deficient fatal infantile myopathy ± De-Toni–Franconi–Debré syndrome. COX-deficient fatal infantile hepatopathy	Moraes et al (1991)
B. Without ragged red fibres		
8. G→A transition at np 11788 in ND4 (homoplasmic or heteroplasmic)	Leber's hereditary optic neuropathy	Wallace et al (1988)
		Singh et al (1989)
		Holt et al (1989c)
		Vilkki et al (1989, 1991)
		Yoneda et al (1989b)
9. T→G transition at np 8993 in H$^+$-ATPase (heteroplasmic)	Maternally inherited multisystem disease with dementia, ataxia, retinopathy, and neuropathy	Holt et al (1990)

fied in cloned myoblast and fibroblast cultures, derived from patients with KSS (Moraes et al 1989b). Because of their low concentration in blood, mutant molecules are difficult to detect by Southern analysis, but they can usually be identified by selective polymerase chain reaction amplification across the break-point regions (Johns et al 1989, Zeviani et al 1990a). This is in contrast to Pearson's syndrome, where deleted mtDNAs are present in higher concentration in the blood and are readily detectable by Southern analysis (Rotig et al 1989) even long after the child has recovered from sideroblastic anaemia (McShane et al 1991). Patients who survive Pearson's syndrome in infancy subsequently develop KSS in childhood (Larsson et al 1990, McShane et al 1991). The change in phenotype seen in this and in other disorders associated with mtDNA mutations (Fukuhara 1985, Byrne et al 1988, Zupanc et al 1989) illustrates the difficulties of clinical classification.

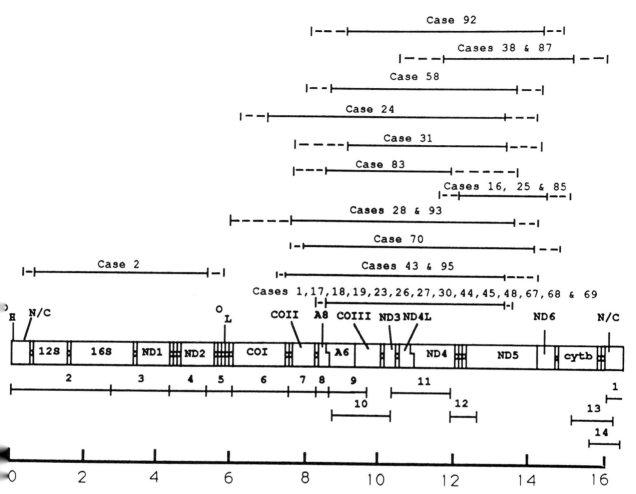

Fig. 10.22 Linearized map of the mitochondrial genome showing extent of the mtDNA deletions in 30 patients with mitochondrial myopathies. ND-Complex I subunits, cyt b = cytochrome b; CO = cytochrome oxidase subunits; A6 and A8 = ATP⁺-ase subunits; 12S and 16S = ribosomal RNAs; ǂ = transfer RNAs; O_H and O_L = origins of heavy and light strand replication; N/C = non-coding regions. The interrupted lines at either end of deletions represent their upper and lower limits, defined by the presence or absence of restriction sites

Seventeen different mtDNA deletions from 28 patients have been characterized by sequencing the break-point regions after polymerase chain reaction (PCR) amplification (Mita et al 1990). In 20 cases (71%), each harbouring one of nine different deletions, the break-point regions contained short nucleotide sequences 5–13 bp in size, which occur in the normal genome as perfect direct repeats immediately flanking the 5' and 3' ends of the deleted region (Class I deletions) (Fig. 10.23). The commonest of these which occurred in 12 cases was a 4977 bp deletion flanked by the

largest of the direct repeats, 13 bp in length. The deletion which extends from nucleotide position 8483 in the ATPase 8 gene to position 13460 in ND5 results in a frame-shift within the fusion gene and a premature stop codon 12 nucleotides down from the break-point (Schon et al 1989, Holt et al 1989b, Mita et al 1990). In the remaining 8 cases (29%), each harbouring a different deletion (Class II deletions) the break-points were not flanked by perfect direct repeats (Mita et al 1990). The presence of perfect direct repeats in about 50% of mtDNA deletions suggests that they may

DELETED mtDNA

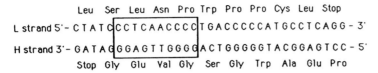

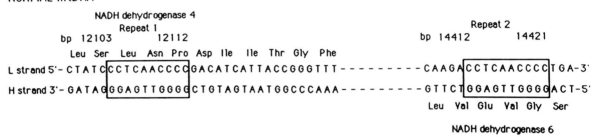

Fig. 10.23 The deletion junction in mutant mtDNA (top) to show a 10 bp bridging sequence which is present in normal mtDNA (bottom) as perfect direct repeats flanking the deleted region

arise from homologous recombination, or from slippage and mispairing of short homologous sequences during replication (Schon et al 1989, Johns et al 1989, Shoffner et al 1989, Mita et al 1990).

None of the deletions identified so far is specific for any one clinical phenotype. For example, the common deletion which accounts for one-third of all cases occurs in Pearson's syndrome (Rotig et al 1989, McShane et al 1991), KSS and patients with mild oculoskeletal weakness beginning much later in life (Moraes et al 1989a, Holt et al 1989a, Mita el al 1990). This would suggest that clinical phenotype is determined as much by the distribution and dose of deleted mtDNAs in different tissues as by the size or the position of the deletion itself. Most deletions eliminate several tRNA genes as well as open reading frames, so that protein coding sequences not encompassed by the deletion would not be translated unless complementation occurred. This would require the presence of normal mtDNAs alongside deleted mtDNAs within

the same organelle. Heteroplasmic mitochondria containing only one or two deleted copies might function quite well, whereas organelles homoplasmic for the deletion would be non-functional. Little is known about the distribution of wild type and mutant mtDNAs within individual organelles.

Almost all patients with single mtDNA deletions are sporadic and only two have been reported with similarly affected relatives (Holt et al 1989a). Deleted molecules have not been detected by Southern blot analysis in blood or muscle from three unaffected mothers of patients with KSS (Moraes et al 1989a), or by PCR amplication of muscle mtDNA from two sisters of another case (Shoffner et al 1989). These results suggest that large deletions are not maternally transmitted, but arise as fresh mutations either during oogenesis or embryonic development. Why this should occur is obscure. The mitochondrial genome, however, is known to have a much higher mutation rate than nuclear DNA (Wallace 1987), and it is conceivable that certain nucleotide substitutions might render the molecule more prone to deletion, particularly at a stage of rapid replication. Such an hypothesis could explain the presence of different mtDNA deletions in a mother and daughter with PEO and short stature described by Ozawa et al (1988). The timing of the deletional event may also be important in determining clinical phenotype. If it occurred at the blastocyst stage and the replication of deleted molecules outstripped that of the wild type genomes (being smaller, deleted mtDNAs may have a replicational advantage), the mutation may be expressed as Pearson's syndrome or KSS. If it occurred after the cells had differentiated, the mutation may be expressed as an oculoskeletal myopathy starting later in life (Shoffner & Wallace 1990).

The precise role of deleted mtDNAs in the pathogenesis of these diseases remains unclear. In situ hybridization experiments on muscle from patients with deletions have shown that the mutant molecules are concentrated in segments of the fibres which lack COX activity and usually, but not invariably, show ragged red changes with other stains (Mita et al 1989, Shoubridge et al 1990). These studies have also shown that deleted mtDNAs are transcriptionally active but the abundant mtRNAs are not translated into proteins (Mita et al 1989) despite the presence of apparently normal levels of wild type mtDNA in the same fibre segment (Shoubridge et al 1990). Translational failure in these fibre segments has been attributed either to lack of indispensable mt tRNA genes, eliminated by the deletion (Mita et al 1989) or to interference with expression of wild type mtDNAs by the overabundant mutant molecules (Shoubridge et al 1990). Similar results have been obtained by examining mtDNA transcription and translation directly in cloned fibroblast cultures containing 60% deleted genomes (Nakase et al 1990). Failure to translate the transcripts of deleted mtDNAs would imply that mutant and wild type molecules are segregated in different organelles. This would mean that all deletions would share a common biochemical phenotype, as mitochondria homoplasmic for the deletion would lack all four complexes containing mtDNA encoded subunits, irrespective of the size or location of the deletion. That this may not be the case for all deletions, however, is suggested by recent biochemical

studies which have shown that there is some correlation between the size and position of the deletion and the site of respiratory chain blockade (Holt et al 1989a, Morgan-Hughes et al 1990b, 1991). In five out of six patients with Complex I defects, the deletion was confined to genes encoding Complex I subunits together with the intervening tRNAs. Moreover, in one of these cases COX-negative fibres were not observed (Holt et al 1989a).

Heteroplasmic tandem duplications of mtDNA have been identified in two patients with the Kearns–Sayre syndrome (Poulton et al 1989). These duplicated molecules may represent dimers composed of one deleted and one wild type genome.

Deletions of mtDNA in other conditions

The common mtDNA deletion of 4977 bp has been detected by PCR amplication using the primer shift method in the striatum from five patients with idiopathic Parkinson's disease, and from two out of six age-matched controls (Ikebe et al 1990). Although the proportion of deleted mtDNAs was low, it appeared to be higher in Parkinsonian patients than in controls. This is an interesting observation, particularly as it has been shown that Complex I activity is significantly reduced in substantia nigra (Schapira et al 1990c) and in blood platelets (Parker et al 1989a) from patients with idiopathic Parkinson's disease, and that 1-methyl-4-phenylpyridium (MPP^+) a known powerful inducer of Parkinsonism (Langston et al 1983) also inhibits Complex I (Ramsay et al 1989).

Multiple deletions of mtDNA

Zeviani and colleagues (1989) identified multiple deletions of muscle mtDNA in four members of a large pedigree with an autosomal dominant mitochondrial myopathy, characterised by PEO, limb weakness, cataract and premature death (Zeviani et al 1989). Sequence analysis of mutant mtDNAs showed that the deletions all originated in a 12-nucleotide stretch of the D-loop template and ranged from 8 to 12.5 kb in length. The deletion break-points were different in the four cases suggesting that they were not transmitted from one generation to the next but arose de novo by some common mechanism. These results pointed to a mutation of a nuclear gene involved in mtDNA replication (Zeviani et al 1989). A second family with dominantly inherited PEO and multiple deletions of muscle mtDNA has subsequently been reported by the same group (Zeviani et al 1990b).

At least 12 different deletions of muscle mtDNA were identified in two brothers with a mitochondrial myopathy, characterized by PEO, optic atrophy and peripheral axonal neuropathy whose parents were first cousins (Yuzaki et al 1989). These patients were originally reported by Mizusawa et al (1988) and were shown to have partial deficiencies of Complex I and Complex IV in isolated muscle mitochondria. In contrast to the dominantly inherited disorders described by Zeviani et al (1989, 1990b), most of the deletions in the two brothers did not arise in the D-loop region and were flanked by direct repeats (Yuzaki et al 1989). Multiple deletions of muscle mtDNA have also been identified by Southern blot analysis in another patient with KSS whose brother and son were also affected (Otsuka et al 1990). In this patient the amount of muscle mtDNA was markedly decreased.

Multiple mtDNA deletions have been identified by Southern blot hybridization in two brothers with recurrent myoglobinuria (Ohno et al 1991) and by PCR amplification using the primer shift method in idiopathic cardiomyopathy (Ozawa et al 1990).

TRANSITIONAL MUTATIONS OF MITOCHONDRIAL tRNA GENES

Myoclonic epilepsy with ragged red fibres (MERRF)

This maternally inherited mitochondrial disease was originally described by Tsairis et al (1973). The clinical features vary widely, even amongst affected members of the same pedigree (Fukuhara et al 1980, Fukuhara 1983, Rosing et al 1985). Mild muscle weakness or neurosensory hearing loss may be the sole clinical manifestations. In its fully developed form, however, the syndrome is characterized by progressive myoclonus, cerebellar ataxia, sensorineural deafness, dementia and muscle weakness (Fukuhara 1983, Rosing et al 1985). Less common features include generalized seizures, hemicranial headache, optic atrophy, foot deformity, pyramidal signs and peripheral sensory loss. Stroke-like episodes are rare but have been described (Kuriyama et al 1984, Fukuhara 1985, Byrne et al 1988). Pigmentary retinopathy has only occurred in one case (Morgan-Hughes et al 1982) and cardiomyopathy has not, so far, been reported. Even the most mildly affected cases gradually become worse with age (Rosing et al 1985). COX-negative fibres and structural abnormalities of muscle mitochondria are consistent findings.

An A to G transition at nucleotide position 8344 in the pseudouridine loop ($T\psi C$) of the mitochondrial tRNA^{Lys} gene (see Fig. 10.24) has been identified in 16 out of 20 independent MERRF pedigrees (Shoffner et al 1990, Yoneda et al 1990, Zeviani et al 1991, Hammans et al 1991). In the original study (Shoffner et al 1990) the tRNA^{Lys} mutation was present in muscle from eight maternal lineage relatives of a large Georgia MERRF family (Rosing et al 1985) and from two unrelated MERRF cases but was absent in 75 controls. The mutation was heteroplasmic in all three pedigrees and comprised between 78% and 98% of the total muscle mtDNA (Schoffner et al 1990). In the large MERRF pedigree there appeared to be some correlation between the percentage of mutant mtDNA in muscle and disease severity when age was taken into account. The differences were marginal, however, even between cases of comparable age. One patient with 6% wild type mtDNA had the full MERRF syndrome, whereas her male cousin (of similar age) with 4% wild type mtDNA had only mild muscle weakness (Shoffner et al 1990). Previous studies of the proband had shown a combined deficiency of Complexes I, IV and V and reduced synthesis of the larger mtDNA encoded proteins in lymphoblastoid cells. (Wallace et al 1988a).

Zeviani and co-workers (1991) identified the same tRNA^{Lys} mutation in muscle of 11 patients from 5 out of 7 Italian MERRF families. Three cases in one pedigree were asymptomatic. The mutation was absent in muscle from 14 controls, a large number of patients with mitochondrial and

Normal tRNA^{Lys}

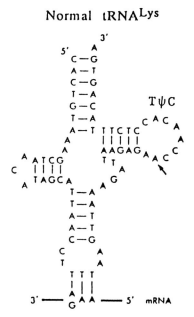

Mutant tRNA^{Lys}

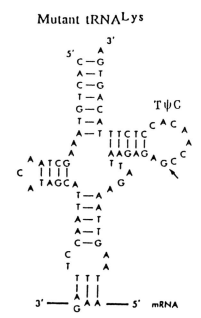

Fig. 10.24 Comparison of wild type and mutant tRNA^{Lys}

non-mitochondrial neurological diseases and two unrelated patients with the full MERRF syndrome (Zeviani et al 1991). These authors also identified the tRNA^{Lys} mutation in autopsy samples of brain, cerebellum, heart, liver and kidney from one case (Zeviani et al, 1991). Similar results were reported by Hammans and colleagues (1991) who found the mutation at position 8344 in muscle and blood from six MERRF families. The mutation was absent in controls and in other mitochondrial diseases and also in two patients displaying the full MERRF phenotype. One case lacking the tRNA^{Lys} mutation had pigmentary retinopathy and severe deficiency of reducible cytochrome b in muscle mitochondria (Morgan-Hughes et al 1982). The other, without pigmentary retinopathy, had generalized loss of respiratory chain activity with absence of the aa₃ peak, and a reduced amount of cytochrome b on spectral analysis (Morgan-Hughes et al 1990a).

The TψC loop of tRNA^{Lys} is thought to interact with the ribosomal surface (Rich & RagBhandary 1976), so that a mutation in this region is likely to affect incorporation of lysine residues into mitochondrial proteins. The biochemical findings in the proband of the large

Georgia MERRF pedigree would be consistent with this hypothesis (Wallace et al 1988a).

The effect of the tRNA^{Lys} mutation on respiratory chain function and mitochondrial protein synthesis has been studied directly by transferring myoblast mitochondria harbouring the mutation into two genetically distinct human cell lines which had been rendered completely devoid of mtDNA by prolonged exposure to low concentrations of ethidium bromide (King & Attardi 1989, Chomyn et al 1991). Transformants which became homoplasmic for the tRNA^{Lys} mutation showed a severe defect of mitochondrial protein synthesis and a marked reduction in oxygen consumption and COX activity (Chomyn et al 1991).

Mitochondrial myopathy, encephalopathy, lactic acidosis and stroke-like episodes

The acronym MELAS was introduced by Pavlakis and colleagues to identify a distinctive clinical syndrome associated with ragged red fibres, characterized by normal early development, stunted growth, focal or generalized seizures and recurrent cerebral insults resembling strokes (Pavlakis et al 1984). Absence of ophthalmoplegia, pigmentary retinopathy and heart block, and lack of myoclonus, optic atrophy and sensory neuropathy, distinguished MELAS from two other distinctive syndromes, KSS and MERRF.

Recently an A to G transition at position 3243 in the dihydrouridine loop of the mitochondrial tRNA$^{Leu(UUR)}$ gene has been identified in several patients with this syndrome (see Fig. 10.25). In the original study (Goto et al 1990) the mutation was present in muscle from 26 of 31 patients with mitochondrial encephalomyopathies and stroke-like episodes (MELAS) and one patient with PEO, but was absent in 50 controls. A further six patients with MELAS and the tRNA$^{Leu(UUR)}$ mutation were reported by Kobayashi and co-workers (Kobayashi et al 1990). In a more recent study Hammans and colleagues have identified the same mutation in muscle and/or blood from 15 cases with variable clinical phenotypes (Hammans et al 1991). Seven patients had neurological syndromes with multiple stroke-like episodes, including two cases who had been reported in detail previously (Schapira et al 1988, 1990a). Of the remaining eight cases three had PEO, two of whom had suffered a single stroke in middle life, four had a syndrome of ataxia, dementia and deafness without

strokes, and one had a pure myopathy with exercise intolerance (Hammans et al 1991). This patient had a combined defect of Complexes I and IV, with specific deficiencies of the 24 kDa and 13 kDa iron–sulphur protein of Complex I and subunit II of complex IV (case YD, Cooper et al 1990).

The mechanism of the tRNA$^{Leu(UUR)}$ gene mutation in disease pathogenesis remains unknown, but in addition to affecting the function of tRNA^{Leu} it may interfere with H strand transcription termination (see Attardi et al 1990). Transcription of the H strand may terminate at the 16SrRNA-tRNA$^{Leu(UUR)}$ boundary by a mechanism which provides for the higher rate of synthesis of rRNA species when compared with mRNAs transcribed from the same strand (Attardi et al 1990). A protein which binds to this region of mtDNA and may be involved in H strand transcription termination has been identified (Kruse et al 1989). A mutation of the dihydrouridine loop of the tRNA$^{Leu(UUR)}$ gene may affect the binding of this protein.

An A to G transition at position 4317 in the mitochondrial tRNA isoleucine gene (tRNA^{Ile}) has recently been demonstrated in heart muscle from a

Normal tRNA$^{Leu(UUR)}$

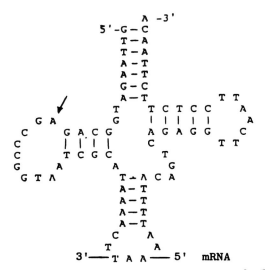

Mutant tRNA$^{Leu(UUR)}$

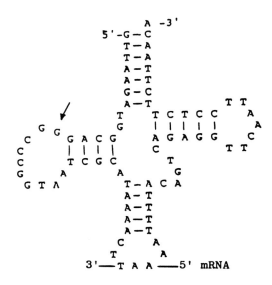

Fig. 10.25 Comparison of wild type and mutant tRNA$^{Leu\ (UUR)}$

boy with a MELAS type syndrome who died of congestive heart failure at the age of 1 year (Tanaka et al 1990).

Depletion of mtDNA

Severe depletion of mtDNA, identified in four patients with the fatal infantile form of COX deficiency (Moraes et al 1991), has been discussed in a previous section (see COX deficiency). An acquired depletion of muscle mtDNA with ragged red fibres on muscle biopsy has recently been described in association with long-term use of the anti-AIDS drug Zidovudine (Arnaudo et al 1991). All nine patients receiving Zidovudine for nine months or longer developed a myopathy with ragged red fibres and variable depletion of muscle mtDNA. These changes were reversible as the muscle mtDNA content returned to normal after treatment was discontinued. Zidovudine is a thymidine analogue which serves as a substrate for DNA polymerase gamma and may affect the function of this enzyme which is essential for mtDNA replication (Arnaudo et al 1991).

TRANSITIONAL MUTATIONS IN MITOCHONDRIAL PROTEIN CODING GENES

Although Leber's hereditary optic neuropathy (LHON) and the maternally inherited multisystem disease described by Holt and colleagues (1990) must now be regarded as mitochondrial diseases, they are not associated with significant proliferation (ragged red fibres) of muscle mitochondria. The G to A transition at nucleotide position 11788 in the mitochondrial ND4 gene identified in 9 out of 11 LHON pedigrees by Wallace and coworkers (1988b), converts the 340th amino acid of subunit 4 from a highly conserved arginine to histidine, and results in loss of an SfaM1 restriction site (Wallace et al 1988b, Singh et al 1989). The mutation which may be homoplasmic (Wallace et al 1988b) or heteroplasmic (Holt et al 1989c, Vilkki et al 1989) occurs in about 50% of all LHON pedigrees world-wide. Although Complex I activity was decreased in platelet mitochondria from members of a large Australian LHON family (Parker et al 1989b), previously studied by Wallace

(1970), this pedigree was subsequently shown not to harbour the ND4 mutation (Howell & McCullough 1990). The above findings indicate that LHON, like other distinctive mitochondrial disease syndromes, is genetically heterogeneous.

The maternally inherited mitochondrial disease described by Holt and co-workers (1990) presented with a variable combination of clinical features including developmental delay, retinitis pigmentosa of the bone corpuscle type, seizures, ataxia and peripheral neuropathy. The mtDNA mutation in this family, which was heteroplasmic, involved a T to G transition at position 8993 in the mitochondrial ATPase subunit 6 gene. This base substitution converts a highly conserved hydrophobic leucine to a hydrophilic arginine at position 156 in ATPase subunit 6. Mitochondrial metabolism was not studied.

CONCLUSIONS

Mitochondria have inhabited eukaryocytes and their ancestors for nearly 2 billion years, but it is only in the last three decades that they have been implicated in the pathogenesis of human disease. Since 1988, the study of mitochondrial DNA in mitochondrial diseases has clearly established that role, but it has also brought with it a number of unexpected surprises which are difficult to reconcile with clinical observation. How is it, for example, that apparently identical deletion mutations of the mitochondrial genome can cause a fatal blood dyscrasia in infancy, a devastating brain disease in adolescence or non-progressive ptosis in late adult life? Is it merely a question of the dose and the way in which deleted and wild type genomes are segregated during mitotic cell division or are there other factors involved? Having arisen, presumably de novo, from a single clonal event, why are deleted mtDNAs, unlike their single base change counterparts, not handed down to the next generation, and if they are what eliminates them? How is it that mitochondria, which are translationally incompetent and presumably non-functional survive, let alone become the dominant species?

These and other questions relating to the mechanisms of expression of mutant mtDNAs remain to be determined, but the pleiotropic effects of these genetic abnormalities suggest that the nuclear background may be important in determining the biochemical and clinical phenotypes at least in some of these disorders. That this may be the case is suggested in a recent study of Leber's hereditary optic neuropathy, a disease known to be associated with mutant mitochondrial genes which is predominantly expressed in the male (Vilkki et al 1991). These authors have shown that the liability to develop optic atrophy in LHON families with or without the ND4 gene mutation is linked to the DXS7 locus on the proximal short arm of the X chromosome (Vilkki et al, 1991).

ACKNOWLEDGEMENTS

I would like to thank Dr David Landon for kindly providing the electron micrographs shown in this chapter. I am also grateful to Professors John Clark, Tony Schapira and Anita Harding for their helpful discussion, and Drs Mary Sweeney and Simon Hammans for allowing me to quote their unpublished results. The work quoted in this chapter was supported by the Muscular Dystrophy Group of Great Britain and Northern Ireland, the Medical Research Council, the Wellcome Trust, the Brain Research Trust, and the Research Trust for Metabolic Diseases of Childhood. I would also like to thank the physicians at the National Hospital and elsewhere for referring patients, Miss Marjorie Ellison for technical assistance and Mrs Pat Stafford for preparing the manuscript.

REFERENCES

Allison F, Bennett M J, Variend S, Engel P C 1988 Acylcoenzyme A dehydrogenase deficiency in heart tissue from infants who died unexpectedly with fatty change in the liver. Br Med J 296: 11–12

Amendt B A, Rhead W J 1986 The multiple acyl-coenzyme A dehydrogenase disorders, glutaric aciduria Type II and ethylmalonic-adipic aciduria. J Clin Invest 78: 205–213

Amendt B A, Greene C, Sweetman L et al 1987 Short-chain acyl-Coenzyme A dehydrogenase deficiency. Clinical and biochemical studies in two patients. J Clin Invest 79: 1303–1309

Amendt B A, Moon A, Teel L, Rhead W J 1988 Long-chain acyl-Coenzyme deficiency: biochemical studies in fibroblasts from three patients. Pediatr Res 23: 603–605

Anderson S, Bankie A T, Barrell B G, et al 1981 Sequence and organisation of the human mitochondrial genome. Nature 290: 457–465

Angelini C, Bresolin N, Pegolo G, Bet L, Rinaldo P, Trevisan C, Vergani L 1986 Childhood encephalomyopathy with cytochrome c oxidase deficiency, ataxia, muscle wasting, and mental impairment. Neurology 36: 1048–1052

Angelini C, Trevisan C, Isaya G, Pegolo G, Vergani L 1987 Clinical varieties of carnitine and carnitine palmytoyl transferase deficiency. Clin Biochem 20: 1–7

Aprille J R 1985 Tissue specific cytochrome deficiency in human infants. In: Quagliariello E (ed) Achievement and perspectives of mitochondrial research. Elsevier Science, Amsterdam, pp 465–476

Argov Z 1989 Phosphorous magnetic resonance spectroscopy (^{31}P NMR) as a tool for in vivo monitoring of mitochondrial muscle disorders. In: Azzi A, Drahota Z, Papa S (eds) Molecular basis of membrane-associated diseases. Springer-Verlag, Berlin, pp 183–199

Argov Z, Bank W J, Maris J, Peterson P, Chance B 1987 Bioenergetic heterogeneity of human mitochondrial myopathies: phosphorus magnetic resonance spectroscopy study. Neurology 37: 257–262

Arnaudo E, Dalakas M, Shanske S, Moraes C T, DiMauro S, Schon E A 1991 Depletion of muscle mitochondrial DNA in AIDS patients with AZT-induced myopathy. Lancet i: 508–510

Arnold D L, Taylor D J, Radda G K 1985 Investigation of human mitochondrial myopathies by phosphorous magnetic resonance spectroscopy. Ann Neurol 18: 189–196

Arts W F M, Scholte H R, Loonen M C B, Przyrembel H, Fernandes J, Trijbels J M F, Luyt-Houwen I E M 1987 Cytochrome c oxidase deficiency in subacute necrotising encephalomyelopathy. J Neurol Sci 77: 108–115

Attardi G, Schatz G 1988 Biogenesis of mitochondria. Ann Rev Cell Biol 4: 290–333

Attardi G, Doersen C, Gaines G, King M, Montoya J, Guerrier-Takuda C, Altman S 1985 New insights into the mechanisms of RNA synthesis and processing in human mitochondria. In: Quagliariello E, Slater E L, Palmieri F, Saccone C, Kroon A M (eds) Achievements and perspectives of mitochondrial research vol II. Elsevier Science, New York pp 145–163

Attardi G, Chomyn A, King M P, Kruse B, Polosa P L, Murdter N N 1990 Biogenesis and assembly of the mitochondrial respiratory chain. Structural, genetic and pathological aspects. Biochem Soc Trans 18: 509–513

Behbehani A W, Goebel H, Osse G et al 1984 Mitochondrial myopathy with lactic acidosis and deficient activity of muscle succinate cytochrome-c-oxidoreductase. Eur J Pediatr 143: 67–71.

Berenberg R A, Pellock J M, Di Mauro S et al 1977 Lumping or splitting? 'Ophthalmoplegia-plus' or Kearns–Sayre syndrome? Ann Neurol 1: 37–54

Bergstrom J, Hultman E 1967 A study of glycogen metabolism during exercise in man. Scand J Clin Lab Invest 19: 218–228

Berkovic S F, Carpenter S, Evans A et al 1989 Myoclonus epilepsy and ragged red fibres (MERRF). 1. A clinical, pathological, biochemical, magnetic resonance spectrographic and positron emission tomographic study. Brain 112: 1231–1260

Bieber L L 1988 Carnitine. Ann Rev Biochem 57: 261–283

Bindoff L A, Desnuelle C, Birth-Machin M A et al 1991 Multiple defects of the mitochondrial respiratory chain in a mitochondrial encephalopathy (MERRF): a clinical, biochemical and molecular study. J Neurol Sci 102: 17–24

Blass J P, Avignan J, Unlendorf B W 1970 A defect in pyruvate decarboxylase in a child with intermittent movement disorder. J Clin Invest 49: 423–432

Blass J P, Kark A P, Engel W K 1971 Clinical studies of a patient with pyruvate decarboxylase deficiency. Arch Neurol 25: 449–460

Bonilla E, Schotland D L, DiMauro S, Aldover B 1975 Electron cytochemistry of cristaline inclusions in human skeletal muscle mitochondria. J Ultrastruc Res 51: 404–408

Bonnefont J-P, Tein I, Saudubray J-M, Demaugre F 1990 Hepatic and muscular forms of palmytoyl carnitine transferase deficiency. In: Tanaka K, Coates P M (eds) Fatty acid oxidation: clinical, biochemical and molecular aspects. Alan R Liss Inc, New York pp 451–456

Bougneres P F, Saudubray J M, Marsac C, Bernard O, Odievre M, Girard J 1981 Fasting hypoglycaemia resulting from hepatic carnitine palmytoyl transferase deficiency. J Pediatr 98: 742–746

Bougneres P F, Rocchiccioli F, Kolvraa S et al 1985 Medium-chain acyl-CoA dehydrogenase deficiency in two siblings with a Reye-like syndrome. J Pediatr 106: 918–921

Boustany R N, Aprille J R, Halperin J, Levy H, DeLong G R 1983 Mitochondrial cytochrome deficiency presenting as a myopathy with hypotonia, external ophthalmoplegia, and lactic acidosis in an infant and as fatal hepatopathy in a second cousin. Ann Neurol 14: 462–470

Bremer J (1983) Carnitine — metabolism and functions. Physiol Rev 63: 1420–1480

Bresolin N, Zeviani M, Bonilla E et al 1985 Fatal infantile cytochrome c oxidase deficiency: decrease of immunologically detectable enzyme in muscle. Neurology 35: 802–812

Bresolin N, Moggio M, Bet L et al 1987 Progressive cytochrome c oxidase deficiency in a case of Kearns-Sayre syndrome: morphological, immunological and biochemical studies in muscle biopsies and autopsy tissue. Ann Neurol 21: 564–572

Brown G K, Scholen R D, Hunt S M, Harrison J R, Pollard A C 1987 Hyperammonaemia and lactic acidosis in a patient with pyruvate dehydrogenase deficiency. J Inher Metab Dis 10: 359–366

Brown G K, Haan E A, Kirby D M, Scholen R D, Wraith J E, Rogers J G, Danks D M 1988 'Cerebral' lactic acidosis: defects in pyruvate metabolism with profound brain damage and minimal systemic acidosis. Eur J Pediatr 147: 10–14

Brown R M, Dahl H-H, M, Brown G K 1989a X-chromosome localisation of the functional gene for the E₁ α subunit of the human pyruvate dehydrogenase complex. Genomics 4: 174–181

Brown R M, Scholem R D, Kirby D M, Dahl H-H M 1989b The clinical and biochemical spectrum of human pyruvate dehydrogenase complex deficiency. Ann NY Acad Sci 537: 360–368

Byrne E, Dennett X, Trounce I, Henderson R 1985 Partial cytochrome oxidase (aa₃) deficiency in chronic progress external ophthalmoplegia. Histochemical and biochemical studies. J Neurol Sci 71: 257–271

Byrne E, Trounce I, Dennett X, Gilligan B, Morley J B, Marzuki S 1988 Progression from MERRF to MELAS phenotype in a patient with combined respiratory Complex I and IV deficiencies. J Neurol Sci 88: 327–337

Capaldi R A 1990 Structure and function of cytochrome c oxidase. Ann Rev Biochem 59: 569–596

Capaldi R A, Halphen D G, Zhang Y-Z, Yamamura W 1988

Complexity and tissue specificity of the mitochondrial respiratory chain. J Bioenerg Biomembr 20: 291–311

Chomyn A, Lai S T 1990 Regulation of expression of nuclear and mitochondrial genes for mammalian NADH dehydrogenase, In: Quagliariello E, Papa S, Palmieri S, Saccone C (eds) Structure, function and biogenesis of energy transfer systems. Elsevier, Amsterdam, pp 179–185

Chomyn A, Mariottini P, Cleeter M W J et al 1985 Six unidentified reading frames of human mitochondrial DNA encode components of the respiratory chain NADH dehydrogenase. Nature 314: 592–597

Chomyn A, Cleeter M W J, Ragan C I, Riley M, Doolittle R F, Attardi G 1986 URF6, the last unidentified reading frame of human mitochondrial DNA codes for an NADH dehydrogenase subunit. Science 234: 614–618

Chomyn A, Meola G, Bresolin N, Lia S T, Scarlato G, Attardi G 1991 In vitro genetic transfer of protein synthesis and respiration defects to mitochondrial DNA-less cells with myopathy patient mitochondria. Mol Cell Biol (in press)

Clark J B, Hayes D J, Morgan-Hughes J A, Byrne E 1984 Mitochondrial myopathies: disorders of the respiratory chain and oxidative phosphorylation system. J Inher Metab Dis 7: 62–68

Clayton D A 1984 Transcription of the mammalian mitochondrial genome. Ann Rev Biochem 53: 573–594

Coates P M, Hale D E, Stanley C A, Corkey B E, Cortner J A 1985 Genetic deficiency of medium-chain acyl Coenzyme A dehydrogenase: studies in cultured skin fibroblasts and peripheral mononuclear leukocytes. Pediatr Res 19: 672–676

Coates P M, Hale D E, Stanley C A, Kelley R I, Corkey B E 1986 Diagnosis of acyl-CoA dehydrogenase deficiencies. SSIEM Symposium 24, Amersfort, pp 9–12

Coates P M, Hale D E, Finocchiaro G, Tanaka K, Winter S C 1988 Genetic deficiency of short-chain Acyl-Coenzyme A dehydrogenase in cultured fibroblasts from a patient with muscle carnitine deficiency and severe skeletal muscle weakness. J Clin Invest 81: 171–175

Cooper J M, Schapira A H V, Holt I J, Toscano A, Harding A E, Morgan-Hughes J A, Clark J B 1990 Biochemical and molecular aspects of human mitochondrial respiratory chain disorders. Biochem Soc Trans 18: 517–519

Corkey B E, Hale D E, Glennon M C, Kelley R I, Coates P M, Stanley C A 1988 Unusual hepatic acyl CoA profiles in patients with Reye's syndrome. J Clin Invest 82: 782–788

Cormier V, Rotig A, Tardieu M, Saudubray J M, Munnich A 1990 Autosomal dominant deletions of the mitochondrial genome in a case of progressive encephalomyopathy. J Neurol Sci (suppl to vol 98, pp 217, abst 1.18.10)

Cruse R P, Di Mauro S, Towfighi J, Trevisan C 1984 Familial systemic carnitine deficiency. Arch Neurol 41: 301–305

Darley-Usmar V M, Kennaway N G, Buist N R M, Capaldi R A 1983 Deficiency in ubiquine cytochrome c reductase in a patient with mitochondrial myopathy and lactic acidosis. Proc Natl Acad Sci 80: 5103–5106

De Marcucci O G L, Hodgson J A, Lindsay J G 1986 The Mr-50 000 polypeptide of mammalian pyruvate dehydrogenase complex participates in acetylation reactions. Eur J Biochem 158: 587–594

Demaugre F, Bonnefont J P, Mitchell G et al 1988 Hepatic and muscular presentations of carnitine palmytoyltransferase deficiency. Two distinct entities. Pediatr Res 24: 308–311

Demaugre F, Bonnefont J P, Cepanec C, Scholte J, Saudubray J M, Le Roux J P 1990 Immune quantitative analysis of human carnitine palmytoyl transferase I and II defects. Pediatr Res 27: 497–500

Denton R M, Halestrapp A P 1980 Pathways and regulation of pyruvate metabolism. In: Burman D, Holton J B, Pennock C A (eds) Inherited disorders of carbohydrate metabolism. MTP Press, Lancaster, pp 209–238

DiDonato S, Frerman F E, Rimoldi M S, Rinaldo P, Taroni F, Wiesmann U M 1986 Systemic carnitine deficiency due to lack of electron transfer flavoprotein: ubiquinone oxido reductase. Neurology 36: 957–963

DiDonato S, Gellera C, Peluchetti D, Uziel G, Antonelli A, Lus G, Rimoldi M 1989 Normalization of short-chain acylcoenzyme A dehydrogenase after riboflavin treatment in a girl with multiple acylcoenzyme A dehydrogenase-deficient myopathy. Ann Neurol 25: 479–484

DiDonato S, Gellera C 1990 Short-chain and medium-chain acyl Co-A dehydrogenases are lowered in riboflavine-responsive lipid myopathies with multiple acylCoA dehydrogenase deficiency. In: Tanaka K, Coates P M (eds) Fatty acid oxidation: clinical, biochemical and molecular aspects. Alan R Liss Inc, New York pp 325–332

DiMauro S, DiMauro P M M 1973 Muscle carnitine palmytoyltransferase deficiency and myoglobinuria. Science 182: 929–931

DiMauro S, Papadimitriou A 1986 Carnitine palmytoyltransferase deficiency. In: Engel A G, Banker B Q (eds) Myology. McGraw-Hill, New York pp 1697–1708

DiMauro S, Bonilla E, Lee C P, Schotland D, Scarpa A, Conn H, Chance B 1976 Luft's disease; further biochemical and ultrastructural studies of skeletal muscle in the second case. J Neurol Sci 27: 217–232

DiMauro S, Mendell J R, Sahenk Z, Bachman D, Scarpa A, Scofield R M, Reiner C 1980 Fatal infantile mitochondrial myopathy and renal dysfunction due to cytochrome-c-oxidase deficiency. Neurology 30: 795–804

DiMauro S, Nicholson J F, Hays A P, Eastwood A B, Papadimitriou A, Koenigsberger R, DeVivo D C 1983 Benign infantile mitochondrial myopathy due to reversible cytochrome c oxidase deficiency. Ann Neurol 14: 226–234

DiMauro S, Servidei S, Zeviani M et al 1987 Cytochrome c oxidase deficiency in Leigh syndrome. Ann Neurol 22: 498–506

DiMauro S, Zeviani M, Rizzuto R et al 1988 Molecular defects in cytochrome oxidase in mitochondrial diseases. J Bioenerg Biomembr 20: 353–365

Divri P, David M, Gregsen N et al 1983 Dicarboxylic aciduria due to medium chain acyl CoA dehydrogenase defect. A cause of hypoglycaemia in childhood. Acta Paediatr Scand 72: 943–949

Duran M, Hofkamp M, Rhead W J, Saudubray J M, Wadman S K 1986 Sudden child death and 'healthy' affected members with medium-chain acyl-Coenzyme A dehydrogenase deficiency. Pedriatr 78: 1052–1057

Duran M, Bruinvis L, Ketting D, de Klerk J B C, Wadman S K 1988 Cis-4 decanoic acid in plasma: a characteristic metabolite in medium-chain acyl-CoA dehydrogenase deficiency. Clin Chem 34: 548–551

Egger J, Harding B N, Boyd S G, Wilson J, Erdohazi M 1987 Progressive neuronal degeneration of childhood (PNDC) with liver disease. Clin Pediatr 26: 167–173

Eleff S, Kennaway N G, Buist N R M, Darley-Usmar V M, Kapaldi R A, Bank W J, Chance B 1984 ^{31}P NMR study of improvement in oxidative phosphorylation by vitamins K_3 and C in a patient with a defect in electron transport at Complex III in skeletal muscle. Proc Natl Acad Sci 81: 3529–3533

Endo H, Hasegawa K, Narisawa K, Tada K, Kagawa Y, Ohta

S 1989 Identification of a gene for the pyruvate dehydrogenase $E_1\alpha$ subunit with a deletion of four nucleotides from a patient with pyruvate dehydrogenase complex deficiency. Ann NY Acad Sci 573: 458–460

Engel A G 1986 Carnitine deficiency syndromes and lipid storage myopathies. In: Engel A G, Banker B Q (eds) Myology. McGraw Hill, New York pp 1663–1696

Engel A G, Angelini C 1973 Carnitine deficiency of human skeletal muscle with associated lipid storage myopathy: a new syndrome. Science 179: 899–902

Engel W K, Cunningham G G 1963 Rapid examination of muscle tissue: an improved trichrome stain method for fresh-frozen biopsy sections. Neurology (Minneap) 13: 919–923

Engel A G, Rebouche C J, Wilson D M, Glasgow A M, Romshe C A, Cruse R P 1981 Primary systemic carnitine deficiency II. Renal handling of carnitine. Neurology 31: 819–825

Eriksson B O, Lindsedt S, Nordin I 1988 Hereditary defect in carnitine membrane transport is expressed in skin fibroblasts. Eur J Pediatr 147: 662–663

Eriksson B O, Gustafson B, Lindstedt S, Nordin I 1989 Transport of carnitine into cells in hereditary carnitine deficiency. J Inher Met Dis 12: 108–111

Finocchiano G, Ikeda Y, Ito M, Tanaka K 1990 Biosynthesis, molecular cloning and sequencing of electron transfer flavoprotein. In: Tanaka K, Coates P M (eds) Fatty acid oxidation: clinical, biochemical and molecular aspects. Alan R Liss Inc, New York, pp 637–652

Frackowiak R S J, Herold S, Petty R K H, Morgan-Hughes J A 1988 The cerebral metabolism of glucose and oxygen measured with positron tomography in patients with mitochondrial diseases. Brain 111: 1009–1024

Frerman F E, Goodman S I 1985 Deficiency of electron transfer flavoprotein or electron transfer flavoprotein ubiquinone oxidoreductase in glutaric acidemia Type II fibroblasts. Proc Natl Acad Sci 82: 4517–4520

Frerman F E, Goodman S I 1989 Glutaric acidemia Type II defects of the mitochondrial respiratory chain. In: Scriver C R, Beaudet A L, Sly W S Valle D (eds) The metabolic basis of inherited disease, McGraw-Hill, New York, pp 915–931

Fukuhara N 1983 Myoclonus epilepsy and mitochondrial myopathy. In: Scarlato G, Cerri C (eds) Mitochondrial pathology and muscle diseases. Piccin Medical Books, Padua, pp 89–110

Fukuhara N 1985 Stroke-like episodes in MERRF. Ann Neurol 18: 368

Fukuhara N, Tokiguchi S, Shirakawa K, Tsubaki T 1980 Myoclonus epilepsy associated with ragged red fibres (mitochondrial abnormalities): disease entity or a syndrome? J Neurol Sci 47: 117–133

Garavaglia B, Antozzi C, Girotti F, Peluchetti D, Rimoldi M, Zeviani M, DiDonato S 1990 A mitochondrial myopathy with Complex II deficiency. Neurology 40 (suppl 1): 294

Gellera C, Uziel D, Rimoldi M, Zeviani M, Laverda A, Carrara F, DiDonato S 1990 Fumarase deficiency is an autosomal recessive encephalopathy affecting both the mitochondrial and the cytosolic enzymes. Neurology 40: 495–499

Gerbitz K D, Obermaier-Kusser B, Zierz S, Pongratz D, Muller-Höcker, Lestienne P 1990 Mitochondrial myopathies: divergences of genetic deletions, biochemical defect and the clinical syndromes. J Neurol 237: 5–10

Giles R E, Blanc H, Cann H M, Wallace D C 1980 Maternal inheritance of human mitochondrial DNA. Proc Natl Acad Sci 77: 6715–6719

Goodman S I, Loehr J P, Frerman F E, 1990 Clinical and
biochemical aspects of glutaric acidemia Type II. In: Tanaka
K, Coates P M (eds) Fatty acid oxidation: clinical,
biochemical and molecular aspects. Alan R Liss Inc,
pp 465–476

Goto Y, Nonaka I, Horai S 1990 A mutation in the tRNA^Leu
(UUR) gene, associated with the MELAS subgroup of
mitochondrial encephalomyopathies. Nature 348: 651–653

Gregersen N 1985 The acyl-CoA dehydrogenation deficiencies.
Scand J Clin Lab Invest 45 (suppl 174): 1–60

Gregersen N, Fjord Christensen M, Christensen E, Kolvraa S
1986 Riboflavin responsive multiple acyl-CoA
dehydrogenation deficiency: assessment of three years of
Riboflavine treatment. Acta Paediatr Scand 75: 676–681

Gregersen N, Rhead W, Christensen E 1990 Riboflavine
responsive glutaric aciduria Type II. In: Tanaka K, Coates
P M (eds) Fatty acid oxidation: clinical, biochemical and
molecular aspects. Alan R Liss Inc, New York pp 477–494

Grivell L A 1989 Nucleo-mitochondrial interactions in yeast
mitochondrial biogenesis. Eur J Biochem 182: 477–493

Hale D E, Coates P M, Stanley C A, Lortner J A, Hall C L 1983
Long-chain acyl-CoA dehydrogenase deficiency. Pediatr Res
17: 390 (abstr)

Hale D E, Batshaw M L, Coates P M, Frerman F E, Goodman
S I, Singh I, Stanley C A 1985 Long-chain acyl Coenzyme A
dehydrogenase deficiency; an inherited cause of non-ketotic
hypoglycaemia. Pediatr Res 19: 666–671

Hale D E, Stanley C A, Coates P M 1990a The long-chain acyl-
CoA dehydrogenase deficiency. In: Tanaka K, Coates P M
(eds) Fatty acid oxidation: clinical, biochemical and
molecular aspects. Alan R Liss Inc, New York pp 303–311

Hale D E, Thorp C, Braat K, Wright J H, Roe C R, Coates
P M, Hashimoto T, Glasgow A M 1990b The
L-3-Hydroxyacyl-CoA dehydrogenase deficiency. In: Tanaka
K, Coates P M (eds) Fatty acid oxidation: clinical,
biochemical and molecular aspects. Alan R Liss Inc, New
York pp 503–510

Haller R G, Lewis S F, Estabrook R W, DiMauro S, Servidei
S, Foster D W 1989 Exercise intolerance, lactic acidosis and
abnormal cardiopulmonary regulation in exercise associated
with adult skeletal muscle, cytochrome c oxidase deficiency.
J Clin Invest 84: 155–161

Haller R G, Henriksson K G, Jorfeldt L, Areskog N-H, Lewis
S F 1990 Muscle succinate dehydrogenase deficiency:
exercise pathophysiology of a novel mitochondrial myopathy.
Neurology 40 (suppl 1): 413

Hammans S R, Sweeney M, Brockington M, Morgan-Hughes
J A, Harding A E 1991 Non-invasive molecular genetic
diagnosis of mitochondrial encephalopathies. (in press)

Hartl F U, Pfanner N, Nicholson D, Neupert W 1989
Mitochondrial protein import. Biochem Biophys Acta
988: 1–45

Hatefi Y 1985. The mitochondrial electron transport and
oxidativephosphorylation system. Ann Rev Biochem
54: 1015–1069

Hawlitschek G, Schneider H, Schmidt B, Tropschug M, Hartl
S U, Neupert W 1988 Mitochondrial protein import:
identification of processing peptidase and of the PEP, a
processing enhancing protein. Cell 53: 795–806

Hayes D J, Lecky B R F, Landon D N, Morgan-Hughes J A,
Clark J B 1984 A new mitochondrial myopathy: biochemical
studies revealing a deficiency in the cytochrome b-c_1
complex (Complex III) of the respiratory chain. Brain 107:
1165–1177

Hayes D J, Hilton-Jones D, Arnold D L, Galloway G, Styles P,

Duncan J, Radda G K 1985 A mitochondrial
encephalomyopathy. A combined 31P magnetic resonance
and biochemical investigation. J Neurol Sci 71: 105–118

Ho L, Hu C-W C, Packman S, Patel M S 1986 Deficiency of
the pyruvate dehydrogenase component in pyruvate
dehydrogenase complex-deficient human fibroblasts. J Clin
Invest 78: 844–847

Ho L, Wexler I D, Kerr D S, Patel M S 1989 Genetic defects in
human pyruvate dehydrogenase. Ann NY Acad Sci
573: 347–359

Holt I J, Harding A E, Morgan-Hughes J A 1988a Deletions of
mitochondrial DNA in patients with mitochondrial
myopathies. Nature 331: 717–719

Holt I J, Cooper J M, Morgan-Hughes J A, Harding A E 1988b
Deletions of muscle mitochondrial DNA. Lancet i: 1462

Holt I J, Harding A E, Cooper J M, Schapira A H V, Toscano
A, Clark J B, Morgan-Hughes J A, 1989a Mitochondrial
myopathies: clinical and biochemical features of 30 patients
with major deletions of muscle mitochondrial DNA. Ann
Neurol 26: 699–708

Holt I J, Harding A E, Morgan-Hughes J A 1989b Deletions of
muscle mitochondrial DNA in mitochondrial myopathies:
sequence analysis and possible mechanisms. Nuc Acid Res
17: 4465–4469

Holt I J, Miller D H, Harding A E 1989c Genetic heterogeneity
and mitochondrial DNA heteroplasmy in Leber's hereditary
optic neuropathy. J Med Genet 26: 739–743

Holt I J, Harding A E, Petty R K H, Morgan-Hughes J A 1990
A new mitochondrial disease associated with mitochondrial
DNA heteroplasmy. Am J Hum Genet 46: 428–433

Hoppel C L, Brady L 1985 Carnitine palmytoyl transferase and
transport of fatty acids. In Martonosi A N (ed) The enzymes
of biological membranes, vol 2. Plenum, New York,
pp 139–175

Hoppel C L, Kerr D S, Dahms B, Roessmann U 1987
Deficiency of reduced nicotinamide adenine dinucleotide
dehydrogenase component of Complex I of mitochondrial
electron transport. J Clin Invest 80: 71–77

Hoskins G P, Cavanagh N P C, Smythe D P L, Wilson J 1977
Oral treatment of carnitine myopathy. Lancet i: 853

Hostetler K Y, Hoppel C L, Romine J S, Sipe J C, Gross S R,
Higginbottom P H 1978 Partial deficiency of muscle
carnitine palmytoyltransferase with normal ketone
production. New Engl J Med 298: 553–557

Howat A J, Bennett M J, Variend S, Shaw L, Engel P C 1985
Defects in the metabolism of fatty acids in the sudden infant
death syndrome. Br Med J 290: 1771–1773.

Howell N, McGullough D 1990 An example of Leber
hereditary optic neuropathy not involving a mutation in the
mitochondrial ND4 gene. Am J Hum Genet 47: 629–634

Ichiki T, Tanaka M, Nishikimi M, Suziki H, Ozawa T,
Kobayashi M, Wada Y 1988 Deficiency of subunits of
Complex I and mitochondrial encephalomyopathy. Ann
Neurol 23: 287–294

Ikebe S, Tanaka M, Ohno K et al 1990 Increase of deleted
mitochondrial DNA in the striatum in Parkinson's disease
and senescence. Biochem Biophys Res Comm
170: 1044–1048

Ikeda Y, Hale D E, Keese S M, Coates P M, Tanaka K 1986a
Biosynthesis of variant MCAD in cultured fibroblasts from
patients with MCAD deficiency. Pediatr Res 20: 843–847

Ikeda Y, Keese S M, Tanaka K 1986b Biosynthesis and
mitochondrial processing of electron transfer flavoprotein: a
defect in the α-subunit synthesis is a primary lesion in
glutaric aciduria Type II. J Clin Invest 78: 997–1002

Ikeda Y, Keese S M, Fenton W A, Tanaka K 1987
    Biosynthesis of four rat liver mitochondrial acylCoA
    dehydrogenases in vitro synthesis: import into mitochondrial
    and processing of their precursors in a cell free system and in
    cultured cells. Arch Biochem Biophys 252: 662–674
Jerusalem F, Engel A G, Peterson H A 1975 Human muscle
    fibre fine structure: morphometric data on controls.
    Neurology (Minneap) 25: 127–134
Johns D R, Rutledge S L, Stine O C, Hurko O 1989 Directly
    repeated sequences associated with pathogenic mitochondrial
    DNA deletions. Proc Natl Acad Sci 86: 8059–8062
Johnson M A, Turnbull D M, Dick D J, Sherratt H S A 1983 A
    partial deficiency of cytochrome c oxidase in chronic
    progressive external ophthalmoplegia. J Neurol
    Sci 60: 31–35
Johnson M A, Kadenbach B, Droste N, Old S L, Turnbull
    D M 1988 Immunocytochemical studies of cytochrome
    oxidase subunits in skeletal muscle of patients with partial
    cytochrome oxidase deficiencies. J Neurol Sci 87: 75–90
Kadenbach B 1986 Regulation of respiration and ATP
    synthesis in higher organisms; hypothesis. J Bioenerg
    Biomembr 18: 39–54
Kadenbach B, Kuhn-Nentwig L, Buge U 1987 Evolution of a
    regulatory enzyme. Cytochrome c oxidase (Complex IV).
    Curr Top Bioenerg 15: 113–161
Kadenbach B, Huther F-J, Buge U, Schlerf A, Johnson M A,
    1989 Regulatory complexity of cytochrome c oxidase and its
    defective manifestation in mitochondrial diseases. In: Azzi
    A, Drahota Z, Papa S (eds) Molecular basis of membrane-
    associated diseases. Springer-Verlag, Berlin, pp 216–227
Kennaway N G 1988 Defects in the cytochrome bc₁ complex in
    mitochondrial diseases. J Bioenerg Biomembr 20: 325–352
Kennaway N G, Buist M R M, Darley-Usmar V M et al 1984
    Lactic acidosis and mitochondrial myopathy associated with
    deficiency of several components of Complex III of the
    respiratory chain. Pediatr Res 18: 991–999
Kerr D S, Ho L, Berlin C M et al 1987 Systemic deficiency of
    the first component of the pyruvate dehydrogenase complex.
    Pediatr Res 22: 312–318
Kerr D S, Berry S A, Lusk M M, Ho L, Patel M S 1988 A
    deficiency of both subunits of pyruvate dehydrogenase which
    is not expressed in fibroblasts. Pediatr Res 24: 95–100
King M P, Attardi G 1989 Human cells lacking mtDNA:
    repopulation with exogenous mitochondria by
    complementation. Science 246: 500–503
Kobayashi Y, Morishita H, Sugiyama N et al 1987 Two cases
    of NADH-Coenzyme Q reductase deficiency: relationship to
    MELAS syndrome. J Pediatr 110: 223–227
Kobayashi Y, Momoi M Y, Tominaga K et al 1990 A point
    mutation in the mitochondrial tRNA^Leu(UUR) gene in
    MELAS (mitochondrial myopathy, encephalopathy, lactic
    acidosis and strokelike episodes). Biochem Biophys Res
    Commun 173: 816–822
Koga Y, Nonaka I, Sunohara N, Yamanaka R, Kumagae K
    1988a Variability in the activity of respiratory chain enzymes
    in mitochondrial myopathies. Acta Neuropathol (Berlin)
    76: 135–141
Koga Y, Nonaka I, Kobayashi M, Tojyo M, Nihei K 1988b
    Findings in muscle in Complex I (NADH) CoenzymeQ
    reductase deficiency. Ann Neurol 24: 749–756
Koga Y, Nonaka I, Nakoa M et al 1990 Progressive
    cytochrome c oxidase deficiency in a case of Leigh's
    encephalomyelopathy. J Neurol Sci 95: 63–76
Kretzschmar H A, DeArmond S J, Coch T K, Patel M S,
    Newth C J L, Schmidt K A, Packman S 1987 Pyruvate

dehydrogenase complex deficiency as a cause of subacute
    necrotizing encephalopathy (Leigh's disease). Pediatr
    79: 370–373
Kruse B, Narasimham N, Attardi G 1989 Termination of
    transcription in human mitochondria: identification and
    purification of a DNA binding protein factor that promotes
    termination. Cell 58: 391–397
Kuhn-Nentwig L, Kadenbach B 1985 Isolation and properties
    of cytochrome c oxidase from rat liver and quantification of
    immunological differences between isoenzymes from various
    rat tissues with subunit-specific antisera. Eur J Biochem
    149: 147–158
Kuriyama M, Umezaki H, Fukuda Y, Osame M, Koike K,
    Tateishi J, Igata A 1984 Mitochondrial encephalomyopathy
    with lactate–pyruvate elevation and brain infarctions.
    Neurology 34: 72–77
Land J M, Morgan-Hughes J A, Clark J B 1981 Mitochondrial
    myopathy. Biochemical studies revealing a deficiency of
    NADH–cytochrome b reductase activity. J Neurol Sci
    50: 1–13
Langston J W, Ballard P, Terud J W, Irwin I 1983 Chronic
    Parkinsonism in humans due to a product of meperidine-
    analog synthesis. Science 219: 979–980
LaNoue K F, Schoolwerth A C 1979 Metabolite transport in
    mitochondria. Ann Rev Biochem 48: 871–922
Larsson N G, Holme E, Kristiansson B, Oldfors A, Tulinius M
    1990 Progressive increase of the mutated mitochondrial
    DNA fraction in Kearns–Sayre syndrome. J Neurol Sci
    98: 214 (abst)
Ledley F D, Jansen R, Nham S-U, Fenton W A, Rosenberg
    L E 1990 Mutation eliminating mitochondrial leader
    sequence of methylmalonyl-CoA mutase causes mut⁰
    methylmalonic acidemia. Proc Natl Acad Sci 87: 3147–3150
Lindsay J G 1989 Targeting of 2-oxo acid dehydrogenase
    complexes to the mitochondrion. Ann NY Acad Sci
    573: 254–266
Lombes A, Bonilla E, DiMauro S 1989a Mitochondrial
    encephalomyopathies. Rev Neurol (Paris) 145: 671–689
Lombes A, Mendell J R, Nakase H et al 1989b Myoclonic
    epilepsy and ragged-red fibres with cytochrome oxidase
    deficiency: neuropathology, biochemistry and molecular
    genetics. Ann Neurol 26: 20–33
Luft R, Ikkos D, Palmieri G, Ernster L, Afzelius B 1962 A
    case of severe hypermetabolism of nonthyroid origin with a
    defect in the maintenance of mitochondrial respiratory
    control: a correlated clinical, biochemical and morphological
    study. J Clin Invest 41: 1776–1804
McGarry J D, Woeltje K F, Schroder J G, Cox W F, Foster
    D W 1990 Carnitine palmytoyltransferase — structure/
    function/regulatory relationships. In: Tanaka K, Coates P M
    (eds) Fatty acid oxidation: clinical biochemical and
    molecular aspects. Alan R Liss Inc, New York pp 193–208
McShane M A, Hammans S R, Sweeney M, Holt I J, Beattie
    H J, Brett E M, Harding A E 1991 Pearson syndrome and
    mitochondrial encephalomyopathy in a patient with a
    deletion of mtDNA. Am J Hum Genet 48: 39–42
Martin J J, Van de Vyver F L, Scholte H R, Roodhooft A M,
    Ceuterick L, Martin L, Luyt-Houwen I E M 1988 Defect in
    succinate oxidation by isolated muscle mitochondria in a
    patient with symmetrical lesions in the basal ganglia.
    J Neurol Sci 84: 189–200
Matuda S, Kitano A, Sakaguchi Y, Yoshino M, Saheki T 1984
    Pyruvate dehydrogenase subcomplex with lipoamide
    dehydrogenase deficiency in a patient with lactic acidosis and
    branched chain ketoaciduria. Clin Chim Acta 140: 59–64

Minchom P E, Dormer R L, Hughes I A et al 1983 Fatal infantile mitochondrial myopathy due to cytochrome c oxidase deficiency. J Neurol Sci 60: 453–463

Mirakami H, Pain D, Blobel G 1988 70-kD heat shock-related protein is one of at least two distinct cytosolic factors stimulating protein import into mitochondria. J Cell Biol 107: 2051–2057

Miranda A F, Ishii S, DiMauro S, Shay J W 1989 Cytochrome c oxidase deficiency in Leigh's syndrome. Genetic evidence for a nuclear DNA-encoded mutation. Neurology 39: 697–702

Mita S, Schmidt B, Schon E A, DiMauro S, Bonilla E 1989 Detection of 'deleted' mitochondrial genomes in cytochrome-c oxidase-deficient muscle fibers of a patient with Kearns–Sayre syndrome. Proc Natl Acad Sci 86: 9509–9513

Mita S, Rizzuto R, Moraes C T et al 1990 Recombination via flanking direct repeats is a major cause of large-scale deletions of human mitochondrial DNA. Nuc Acid Res 18: 561–567

Mitchell P 1976 Possible molecular mechanisms of the proton motive function of cytochrome systems. J Theot Biol 62: 327–367

Miyabayashi S, Ito T, Narisawa K, Tada K 1985 Biochemical study in 28 children with lactic acidosis, in relation to Leigh's encephalomyopathy. Eur J Pediatr 143: 278–283

Miyabayashi S, Ito T, Abukawa D et al 1987 Immunochemical study in three patients with cytochrome c oxidase deficiency presenting Leigh's encephalomyelopathy. J Inher Metab Dis 10: 289–292

Mizusawa H, Watanabe M, Kanazawa I et al 1988 Familial mitochondrial myopathy associated with peripheral neuropathy; partial deficiencies of Complex I and Complex IV. J Neurol Sci 86: 171–184

Moraes C T, DiMauro S, Zeviani M et al 1989a Mitochondrial DNA deletions in progressive external ophthalmoplegia and Kearns–Sayre syndrome. New Eng J Med 320: 1293–1299

Moraes C T, Schon E A, DiMauro S, Miranda A F 1989b Heteroplasmy of mitochondrial genomes in clonal cultures from patients with Kearn's–Sayre syndrome. Biochem Biophys Res Comm 160: 765–771

Moraes C T, Shanske S, Tritschler H-J et al 1991 mtDNA depletion with variable tissue expression: a novel genetic abnormality in mitochondrial diseases. Am J Hum Genet 48: 492–501

Moreadith R W, Bapshaw M L, Ohnishi T et al 1984 Deficiency of the iron–sulfur clusters of mitochondrial reduced nicotinamide–adamine dye nucleotide–ubiquinone oxidoreductase (Complex I) in an infant congenital lactic acidosis. J Clin Invest 74: 685–697

Moreadith R W, Pleeter M W J, Ragan C R, Batshaw M L, Lehninger A L 1987 Congenital deficiency of two polypeptide subunits of the iron–protein fragment of mitochondrial Complex I. J Clin Invest 79: 463–467

Morgan–Hughes J A, Landon D N 1983 Mitochondrial respiratory chain deficiencies in man. Some histochemical and fine-structural observations. In: Scarlato G, Cerri C (eds) Mitochondrial pathology in muscle diseases. Piccin Medical Books, Padua, pp 21–37

Morgan–Hughes J A, Darveniza P, Kahn S N, Landon D N, Sherratt R M, Land J M, Clark J B 1977 A mitochondrial myopathy characterised by a deficiency in reducible cytochrome b. Brain 100: 617–640

Morgan–Hughes J A, Darveniza P, Landon D N, Land J M, Clark J B 1979 A mitochondrial myopathy with a deficiency

of respiratory chain NADH–CoQ reductase activity. J Neurol Sci 43: 27–46

Morgan–Hughes J A, Hayes D J, Clark J B, Landon D N, Swash M, Stark R J, Rudge P 1982 Mitochondrial encephalomyopathies. Biochemical studies in two cases revealing defects in respiratory chain. Brain 105: 553–582

Morgan–Hughes J A, Hayes D J, Clark J B 1984 Mitochondrial myopathies. In: Serratrice G et al (eds) Neuromuscular diseases. Raven Press, New York, pp 79–87

Morgan–Hughes J A, Hayes D J, Cooper J M, Clark J B 1985 Mitochondrial myopathies: deficiencies localised to Complex I and Complex III of the mitochondrial respiratory chain. Biochem Soc Trans 13: 648–650

Morgan–Hughes J A, Cooper J M, Schapira A H V, Hayes D J, Clark J B 1987 The mitochondrial myopathies. Defects of the mitochondrial respiratory chain and oxidative phosphorylation system. In: Ellingson R J, Murray N M F, Halliday A M (eds) The London symposia. Elsevier, Amsterdam, pp 103–114

Morgan–Hughes J A, Schapira A H V, Cooper J M, Clark J B 1988 Molecular defects of NADH–Ubiquinone oxidoreductase (Complex I) in mitochondrial diseases. J Bioenerg Biomemb 20: 365–383

Morgan–Hughes J A, Cooper J M, Holt I J, Harding A E, Schapira A H V, Clark J B 1990a Mitochondrial myopathies: clinical defects. Biochem Soc Trans 18: 523–525

Morgan–Hughes J A, Schapira A H V, Cooper J M, Holt I J, Harding A E, Clark J B 1990b The molecular pathology of respiratory-chain dysfunction in human mitochondrial myopathies. Biochim Biophys Acta 1018: 217–222

Morgan–Hughes J A, Cooper J M, Schapira A H V, Sweeney M, Holt I J, Harding A H V, Clark J B 1991 The molecular pathology of human respiratory chain defects. Rev Neurol (Paris) 147: 450–454

Müller–Hocker J 1988 Cytochrome c oxidase deficient cardiomyocytes in the human heart. An age-related phenomenon. Amer J Pathol 134: 1167–1171

Müller–Hocker J 1990 Cytochrome c oxidase deficient fibres in the limb muscle and diaphragm of man without muscular disease: an age-related alteration. J Neurol Sci 100: 14–21

Müller–Hocker J, Pongratz D, Deusel T, Trijbels J M F, Endres W, Hubner G 1983 Fatal lipid storage myopathy with deficiency of cytochrome c oxidase and carnitine. Virchows Arch (Pathol Anat) 399: 11–23

Munnich A, Saudubray J M, Taylor J et al 1982 Congenital lactic acidosis, α-ketoglutaric aciduria and variant form of maple syrup urine disease due to a single enzyme defect. Dihydrolipoyl dehydrogenase deficiency. Acta Paediatr Scand 71: 167–171

Murthy M S R, Pande S V 1987 Some differences in the properties of carnitine palmytoyltransferase activities of the mitochondrial outer and inner membranes. Biochem J 248: 727–733

Naito E, Kuroda Y, Takeda E, Yokota J, Kobashi H, Miyao M 1988 Detection of pyruvate metabolism disorders by culture of skin fibroblasts with dichloroacetate. Pediatr Res 23: 561–564

Naito E, Ozasa H, Ikeda Y, Tanaka K 1989a Molecular cloning and nucleotide sequence of complimentary DNAs encoding human short chain acyl-Coenzyme A dehydrogenase and the study of the molecular basis of human short chain acyl-Coenzyme A dehydrogenase deficiency. J Clin Invest 83: 1605–1613

Naito E, Indo Y, Tanaka K 1989b Short chain acyl-Coenzyme A dehydrogenase (SCAD) deficiency: immunochemical demonstration of molecular heterogeneity due to variant SCAD with differing stability. J Clin Invest 84: 1671–1674

Naito E, Indo Y, Tanaka K 1990 Identification of two variant short chain acyl-Coenzyme A dehydrogenase alleles, each containing a different point mutation in a patient with short chain acyl-Coenzyme A dehydrogenase deficiency. J Clin Invest 85: 1575–1582

Nakase H, Moraes C T, Rizzuto R, Lombes A, DiMauro S, Schon E A 1990 Transcription and translation of deleted mitochondrial genomes in Kearns–Sayre syndrome: implications for pathogenesis. Am J Hum Genet 46: 418–427

Newshome E A 1981 The glucose/fatty acid cycle and physical exhaustion. In: Human muscle fatigue: physiological mechanisms. Ciba Foundation Symposium 82. London, Pitman Medical, pp 89–96

Nishizawa M, Tanaka K, Shinozawa K, Kuwabara T, Atsumi T, Miyatake T, Ohama E 1987 A mitochondrial encephalomyopathy with cardiomyopathy. A case revealing a defect of Complex I in the respiratory chain. J Neurol Sci 78: 189–201

Nonaka I, Koga Y, Shikura K et al 1988 Muscle pathology in cytochrome c oxidase deficiency. Acta Neuropathol 77: 152–160

Ogasahara S, Engel A G, Frens D, Mack D 1989 Muscle coenzyme Q deficiency in familial mitochondrial encephalomyopathy. Proc Natl Acad Sci 86: 2379–2382

Ogier H, Lombes A, Scholte H R et al 1988 deToni–Fanconi–Debré syndrome with Leigh syndrome revealing severe muscle cytochrome c oxidase deficiency. J Pediatr 112: 734–739

Ohama E, Ohara S, Ikuta F, Tanaka K, Nishizawa M, Miyatake T 1987 Mitochondrial angiopathy in cerebral blood vessels of mitochondrial encephalomyopathy. Acta Neuropathol (Berlin) 74: 226–233

Ohno K, Tanaka M, Sahashi K, Ibi T, Sato W, Takahashi A, Ozawa T 1991 Mitochondrial DNA deletions in inherited recurrent myoglobinuria. Ann Neurol 29: 364–369

Old S E, DeVivo D C 1989 Pyruvate dehydrogenase complex deficiency; biochemical and immunoblot analysis of cultured skin fibroblasts. Ann Neurol 26: 746–751

Olson W, Engel W K, Walsh G O, Einaugler R 1972 Oculo-craniosomatic neuromuscular disease with 'ragged-red' fibers: histochemical and ultrastructural changes in limb muscles of a group of patients with idiopathic progressive external ophthalmoplegia. Arch Neurol 26: 193–211

Ostermann J, Horwich A L, Neupert W, Hartl F U 1989 Protein folding in mitochondria requires complex formation with hsp60 and ATP hydrolysis. Nature 341: 125–130

Otsuka M, Niijima K, Mizuno Y, Yoshida M, Kagawa Y, Ohta S 1990 Marked decrease of mitochondrial DNA with multiple deletions in a patients with familial mitochondrial myopathy. Biochem Biophys Res Commun 167: 680–685

Otulakowski G B H, Robinson B H, Willard F 1988 Gene for lipoamide dehydrogenase maps to human chromosome 7. Somatic Cell Mol Genet 14: 411–414

Ozawa T, Yoneda M, Tanaka M et al 1988 Maternal inheritance of deleted mitochondrial DNA in a family with mitochondrial myopathy. Biochem Biophys Res Comm 154: 1240–1247

Ozawa T, Tanaka M, Sugiyama S et al 1990 Multiple mitochondrial DNA deletions exist in cardiomyocytes of patients with hypertrophic or dilated cardiomyopathy. Biochem Biophys Res Commun 170: 830–836

Pande S V, Parvin R 1976 Characterisation of carnitine acylcarnitine translocase system of heart mitochondria. J Biol Chem 251: 6683–6691

Papadimitriou A, Neustein H B, DiMauro S, Stanton R, Bresolin N 1984 Histiocytoid cardiomyopathy of infancy deficiency of reducible cytochrome b in heart mitochondria. Pediatr Res 18: 1023–1028

Parikh V S, Morgan M M, Scott R, Clements L S, Butow R A 1987 The mitochondrial genotype can influence nuclear gene expression in yeast. Science 235: 576–580

Parker W D, Boyson F J, Parks J K 1989a Abnormalities of the electron transport chain in idiopathic Parkinson's disease. Ann Neurol 26: 719–723

Parker W D, Oley C A, Parks J K 1989b A defect in mitochondrial electron transport activity (NADH-coenzyme Q reductase) in Leber's hereditary optic neuropathy. N Engl J Med 320: 1331–1333

Pavlakis S G, Phillips P C, Di Mauro S, DeVivo D C, Rowlands L P, 1984 Mitochondrial myopathy, encephalopathy, lactic acidosis and strokelike episodes: a distinctive clinical syndrome. Ann Neurol 16: 481–488

Pearson H A, Lobel J S, Kocoshis S A et al 1979 A new syndrome of refractory sideroblastic anaemia with vacuolisation of marrow precursors and exocrine pancreatic dysfunction. J Pediatr 95: 976–984

Petrova–Benedict R, Robinson B H, Stacey T E, Mistry J, Chalmers R A 1987 Deficient fumarase activity in an infant with fumaricacidemia and its distribution between the different forms of the enzyme seen in isoelectric focusing. Am J Hum Genet 40: 257–266

Petty R K H, Harding A E, Morgan–Hughes J A, 1986 The clinical features of mitochondrial myopathy. Brain 109: 915–938

Pfanner N, Neupert W 1990a The mitochondrial protein import apparatus. Ann Rev Biochem 59: 331–353

Pfanner N, Neupert W 1990b A mitochondrial machinery for membrane translocation of precursor proteins. Biochem Soc Trans 18: 513–515

Poulton J, Deadman M E, Gardiner R M 1989 Duplication of mitochondrial DNA in mitochondrial myopathy. Lancet i: 236–240

Prick M, Gabreels F, Renier W, Trijbels F, Jaspar H, Lamers K, Kok J, 1981a Pyruvate dehydrogenase deficiency restricted to brain. Neurology 31: 398–404

Prick M J J, Gabreels F J M, Renier W O, Trijbels J M F, Sengers R C A, Sloof J L 1981b Progressive infantile poliodystrophy; association with disturbed pyruvate oxidation in muscle and liver. Arch Neurol 38: 767–772

Prick M J J, Gabreels F J M, Trijbels J M F et al 1983 Progressive poliodystrophy (Alper's disease) with a defect in cytochrome aa₃; a report of two unrelated patients. Clin Neurol Neurosurg 85: 57–70

Purdue P E, Takada Y, Danpure C J 1990 Identification of mutations associated with peroxisome-to-mitochondrion mistargeting of alanine/glyoxylate aminotransferase in primary hyperoxaluria Type 1. J Cell Biol 111: 2341–2351

Radda G K, Bore P J, Gadian D G, Ross B D, Styles P, Taylor D J, Morgan–Hughes J A 1982 ^{31}P NMR examination of two patients with NADH CoQ reductase deficiency. Nature 295: 608–609

Ramsay R R, Youngster S K, Nicklas W J, McKeown K A, Jin Y-Z, Heikkila R E, Singer T P 1989 Structural dependence of the inhibition of mitochondrial respiration and of NADH oxidase by 1-methyl-4-phenylpyridinium (MPP⁺) analogs and their energized accumulation by mitochondria. Proc Natl Acad Sci 86: 9168–9172

Razzow J, Guiard B, Wienhues U, Herzog V, Hartl F U, Neupert W 1989 Translocation arrest by reversible folding of a precursor protein imported into mitochondria. A means to quantitate translocation contact sites. Cell 109: 1421–1428

Rebouche C J, Engel A G, 1984 Kinetic compartmental analysis of carnitine metabolism in the human carnitine deficiency syndrome: evidence for alterations in tissue carnitine transport. J Clin Invest 73: 857–867

Reed L J 1981 Regulation of mammalian pyruvate dehydrogenase complex by a phosphorylation-dephosphorylation cycle. Curr Top Cell Regul 18: 95–106

Reed L J, Yeaman S J 1987 Pyruvate dehydrogenase. The Enzymes. 18: 77–95

Reichmann H, Rokhamm R, Zeriani M, Servidei S, Richer K, Di Mauro S 1986 Mitochondrial myopathy due to complex III deficiency with normal reducible cytochrome b concentration. Arch Neurol 43: 957–961

Rhead W J, Roettger V 1986 Defective mitochondrial FAD uptake in riboflavin responsive (RR) multiple acyl-CoA dehydrogenation deficiency (MAD). SSIEM 24th Annual Symposium, Amersfoort

Rhead W J, Amendt B A, Fritchman K S, Felts S J 1983 Dicarboxylic aciduria: deficient (1-^{14}C) octanoate oxidation and medium-chain acyl-CoA dehydrogenase in fibroblasts. Science 221: 73–75

Rhead W J, Wolff J A, Lipson M et al 1987 Clinical and biochemical variation and family studies in multiple acyl-CoA dehydrogenation disorders. Pediatr Res 21: 371–376

Rich A, RagBhandary U L 1976 Transfer RNA: molecular structure, sequence and properties. Annu Rev Biochem 45: 805–806

Riggs J E, Schochet S S, Fakadeg A V et al 1984 Mitochondrial encephalomyopathy with decreased succinate-cytochrome-c reductase activity. Neurology 34: 48–53

Rimoldi M, Bottacchi E, Rossi L, Cornelio F, Uziel G, DiDonato S 1982 Cytochrome-c-oxidase deficiency in muscle of a floppy infant without mitochondrial myopathy. J Neurol 227: 201–207

Rinaldo P, O'Shea J J, Coates P M, Hale D E, Stanley C A, Tanaka K 1988 Medium chain acyl-CoA dehydrogenase deficiency; diagnosis by stable isotope dilution measurement of urinary n-hexanoylglycine and 3-phenylpropionylglycine. New Engl J Med 319: 1308–1313

Rinaldo P, O'Shea J J, Welch R D, Tanaka K 1990 Diagnosis of medium chain acyl-CoA dehydrogenase deficiency by stable isotope dilution analysis of urinary acylglycines; retrospective and prospective studies and comparison of its accuracy to acylcarnitine identification by FAB/MASS spectrometry. In: Tanaka K, Coates P M (eds) Fatty acid oxidation: clinical, biochemical and molecular aspects. Alan R. Liss Inc, New York, pp 411–418

Rivner M H, Shamsnia M, Swift T R et al 1989 Kearns–Sayre syndrome and Complex II deficiency. Neurology 39: 693–696

Robin E D, Wong R 1988 Mitochondrial DNA molecules and virtual number of mitochondria per cell in mammalian cells. J Cell Physiol 136: 507–513

Robinson B H 1988 Cell culture studies on patients with mitochondrial diseases: molecular defects in pyruvate dehydrogenase. J Bioenerg Biomembr 20: 313–323

Robinson B H, Ward J, Goodyer P, Baudet A 1986 Respiratory chain defects in the mitochondria of cultured skin fibroblasts from three patients with lacticacidemia. J Clin Invest 77: 1422–1427

Robinson B H, MacMillan H, Petrova–Benedict R, Sherwood W G 1987a Variable clinical presentation in patients with defective E_1 component of the pyruvate dehydrogenase complex. J Pediatr 111: 525–533

Robinson B H, DeMeirleir L, Glarun M, Sherwood G, Becker L 1987b Clinical presentation of patients with mitochondrial respiratory chain defects in NADH-Coenzyme q reductase and cytochrome oxidase: clues to the pathogenesis of Leigh disease. J Pediatr 110: 216–222

Robinson B H, Chun K, Mackay N, Otulakowski G, Petrova–Benedict R, Willard H 1989 Isolated and combined deficiencies of the α-keto acid dehydrogenase complexes. Ann NY Acad Sci 573: 337–346

Robinson B H, Mackay N, Petrova–Benedict R, Ozalp I, Coskun T, Stacpoole P W 1990 Defects in the E_2 lipoyl transacetylase and the X-lipoyl containing component of the pyruvate dehydrogenase complex in patients with lactic acidemia. J Clin Invest 85: 1821–1824

Roche T E, Rahmatullah M, Powers–Greenwood S L, Radke G A, Gopalkrishnan S, Chang C L 1989 The lipoayl-containing components of the mammalian pyruvate dehydrogenase complex: structural comparison and subdomain roles. Ann NY Acad Sci 573: 66–75

Roe C R, Millington D S, Maltby D A, Bohan T P, Kahler S G, Chalmers R A 1985 Diagnostic and therapeutic implications of medium-chain acylcarnitines in medium-chain acyl-CoA dehydrogenase deficiency. Pediatr Res 19: 459–466

Roe C R, Millington D S, Maltby D A, Kinnebrew P 1986 Recognition of medium-chain acyl-coA dehydrogenase deficiency in asymptomatic siblings of children dying of sudden infant death or Reye-like syndromes. J Pediatr 108: 13–18

Roe C R, Millington D S, Kahler S G, Kodo N, Norwood D L 1990 Carnitine homeostatis in the organic acidurias. In: Tanaka K, Coates P M (eds) Fatty acid oxidation: clinical biochemical and molecular aspects. Alan R Liss Inc, New York, pp 383–402

Roodhooft A M, Van Acker K J, Martin J J, Ceuterick C, Scholte H R, Luyt-Houwen E M 1986 Benign mitochondrial myopathy with deficiency of NADH-CoQ reductase and cytochrome c oxidase. Neuropediatrics 17: 221–226

Rosing H S, Hopkins L C, Wallace D C, Epstein C M, Weidenheim K 1985 Maternally inherited mitochondrial myopathy and myoclonic epilepsy. Ann Neurol 17: 228–235

Rotig A, Colonna M, Bonnefont J P, Blanche S, Fischer A, Saudubray J M, Munnich A 1989 Mitochondrial DNA deletion in Pearson's marrow/pancreas syndrome. Lancet i: 902–903

Sakuta R, Nonaka I 1989 Vascular involvement in mitochondrial myopathy. Ann Neurol 25: 594–601

Schapira A H V, Cooper J M, Morgan–Hughes J A, Patel S D, Cleeter M J W, Ragan C I, Clark J B 1988 Molecular basis of mitochondrial myopathies: polypeptide analysis in Complex I deficiency. Lancet i: 500–503

Schapira A H V, Cooper J M, Manneschi L, Vital C, Morgan–Hughes J A, Clark J B 1990a A mitochondrial encephalomyopathy with specific deficiencies of two respiratory chain polypeptides and a circulating autoantibody to a mitochondrial matrix protein. Brain 113: 419–432

Schapira A H V, Cooper J M, Morgan–Hughes J A, Landon D N, Clark J B 1990b Mitochondrial myopathy with a defect of mitochondrial protein transport. New Eng J Med 323: 37–42

Schapira A H V, Cooper J M, Dexter D, Clark J B, Jenner P,

Marsden C D 1990c Mitochondrial Complex 1 deficiency in Parkinson's disease. J Neuro Chem 54: 823–827

Schatz G 1987 Signals guiding proteins to their correct locations in mitochondria. Eur J Biochem 165: 1–6

Schlerf A, Droste M, Winter M, Kadenbach B 1988 Characterisation of two different genes (CDNA) for cytochrome c oxidase subunit VIa from heart and liver of the rate. EMBO J 7: 2387–2391

Scholte H R, Busch H F M, Barth P G et al 1983 Carnitine deficiency and mitochondrial respiratory chain blockage. In: Scarlatto G, Serri C, (eds) Mitochondrial pathology in muscle diseases. Piccin Medical Books, Padua, pp 215–228

Scholte H R, Busch H F M, Luyt-Houwen I E M, Vaandrager–Verduin M H M, Przyrembel H, Arts W F M 1987 Defects in oxidative phosphorylation. Biochemical investigations in skeletal muscle and expression of the lesion in other cells. J Inher Metab Dis 10(suppl 1): 81–97

Scholte H R, Agsteribbe E, Busch H F M et al 1990 Oxidative phosphorylation in human muscle in patients with ocular myopathy and after general anaesthesia. Biochim Biophys Acta 1018: 211–216

Schon E A, Rizzuto R, Moraes C T, Nakase H, Zeviani M, DiMauro S 1989 A direct repeat is a hot spot for large-scale deletion of human mitochondrial DNA. Science 244: 346–348

Schotland D L, Di Mauro S, Bonilla E, Scarpa A, Lee C P 1976 Neuromuscular disorder associated with a defect in mitochondrial energy supply. Arch Neurol 33: 475–479

Schulz H 1990 Mitochondrial β-oxidation. In: Tanaka K, Coates P M (eds) Fatty acids oxidation: clinical, biochemical and molecular aspects. Alan R Liss Inc, New York, pp 23–36

Sengers R C A, Fischer J C, Trijbels J M F, Ruitenbeek W, Stadhouders A M, Ter Laak H J, Jaspar H H 1983 A mitochondrial myopathy with a defective respiratory chain and carnitine deficiency. Eur J Pediatr 140: 332–337

Sengers R C A, Trijbels J M F, Bakkeren J A J M et al 1984 Deficiency of cytochrome b and aa₃ in muscle from a floppy infant with cytochrome oxidase deficiency. Eur J Pediatr 141: 178–180

Senior A E 1988 ATP synthesis by oxidative phosphorylation. Phys Rev 68: 177–220

Senior B, Jungas R L 1974 A disorder resulting from an enzymatic defect of the respiratory chain. Pediatr Res 8: 438a

Servidei S, Lazaro R P, Bonilla E, Barron K D, Zeviani M, DiMauro S 1987 Mitochondrial encephalomyopathy and partial cytochrome c oxidase deficiency. Neurology 37: 58–63

Shanske S, Moraes C T, Lombes A et al 1990 Widespread tissue distribution of mitochondrial DNA deletions in Kearns–Sayre syndrome. Neurology 40: 24–28

Shepherd I M, Birch–Machin M A, Johnson M A et al 1988 Cytochrome oxidase deficiency: immunological studies of skeletal muscle mitochondrial fractions. J Neurol Sci 87: 265–274

Sherratt H S A, Cartlidge N E F, Johnson M A, Turnbull D M 1984 Mitochondrial myopathy with partial cytochrome oxidase deficiency and impaired oxidation of NADH-linked substrates. J Inher Metab Dis 7(suppl 2): 107–108

Sherratt H S A, Johnson M A, Turnbull D M 1986 Defects of Complex I and Complex III in chronic progressive external ophthalmoplegia. Ann NY Acad Sci 488: 508–510

Shoffner J M, Wallace D C 1990 Oxidative phosphorylation

diseases. Disorders of two genomes. Adv Hum Genet 19: 267–330

Shoffner J M, Lott M T, Voljavec A S, Soueidan S A, Costigan D A, Wallace D C 1989 Spontaneous Kearns–Sayre/chronic external ophthalmoplegia plus syndrome, associated with a mitochondrial DNA deletion: a slip-replication model and metabolic therapy. Proc Natl Acad Sci 86: 7952–7956

Shoffner J M, Lott M T, Lezza A M S, Seibel P, Ballinger S W, Wallace D C 1990 Myoclonic epilepsy and ragged-red fiber diseases (MERRF) is associated with a mitochondrial DNA tRNA^{Lys} mutation. Cell 61: 931–937

Shoubridge E A, Carpati G, Hastings K E M 1990 Deletion mutants are functionally dominant over wild-type mitochondrial genomes in skeletal muscle fiber segments in mitochondrial disease. Cell 62: 43–49

Singh G, Lott M T, Wallace D C 1989 A mitochondrial DNA mutation as a cause of Leber's hereditary optic neuropathy. N Engl J Med 320: 1300–1305

Smythe D P L, Lake B D, MacDermot J, Wilson J 1975 Inborn error of carnitine metabolism ('carnitine deficiency') in man. Lancet i: 1198–1199

Sperl W, Ruitenbeek W, Trijbels J M F, Sengers R C A, Stadhouders A N, Guggenbichler J P 1988 Mitochondrial myopathy with lactic acidaemia, Fanconi-De Toni-Debré syndrome and a disturbed succinate: cytochrome (c) oxido reductase activity. Eur J Pediatr, pp 418–421

Spiro A J, Moore C L, Prineas J W, Strasberg P M, Rapin I 1970 A cytochrome-related inherited disorder of the nervous system and muscle. Arch Neurol 23: 103–112

Stadhouders A, Jap P, Wallimann Th 1990 Biochemical nature of mitochondrial crystals. J Neurol Sci 98: 304 (abst)

Stanley C A 1987 New genetic defects in mitochondrial fatty acid oxidation and carnitine deficiency. Adv Pediatr 34: 59–88

Stanley C A, Hale D E, Coates P M et al 1983 Medium-chain acyl-CoA dehydrogenase deficiency in children with non-ketotic hypoglycaemia and low carnitine levels Pediatr Res 17: 877–884

Stanley C A, Treem W R, Hale D E, Coates P M 1990a A genetic defect in carnitine transport causing primary carnitine deficiency. In: Tanaka K, Coates P M (eds) Fatty acid oxidation: clinical, biochemical and molecular aspects. Alan R Liss Inc, New York, pp 457–464

Stanley C A, Hale D E, Coates P M 1990b Medium-chain acyl-CoA dehydrogenase deficiency. In: Tanaka K, Coates P M (eds) Fatty acid oxidation: clinical, biochemical and molecular aspects. Alan R Liss Inc, New York, pp 291–302

Stansbie D, Dormer R L, Hughes J A, Minchom P E 1982 Mitochondrial myopathy with skeletal muscle cytochrome oxidase deficiency. J Inhert Metab Dis 5(suppl 1): 27–28

Stansbie D, Wallace S J, Marsac C 1986 Disorders of the pyruvate dehydrogenase complex. J Inher Metab Dis 9: 105–119

Stemmel W, Strohmeyer G, Berk P D 1986 Hepatocellular uptake of oleate is energy dependent, sodium linked, and inhibited by an antibody to a hepatocyte plasma membrane fatty acid binding protein. Proc Natl Acad Sci 83: 3584–3588

Strauss A W, Duran M, Zhang Z, Alpers R, Kelly D P 1990 Molecular analysis of medium chain acyl-CoA dehydrogenase deficiency. In: Tanaka K, Coates P M (eds) Fatty acid oxidation: clinical, biochemical and molecular aspects. Alan R Liss Inc, New York, pp 609–623

Stumpf D A, Parker W D, Angelini C 1985 Carnitine

deficiency, organic acidemias and Reye's syndrome. Neurology 35: 1041–1045

Tanaka M, Ino H, Ohno K et al 1990 Mitochondrial mutation in fatal infantile cardiomyopathy. Lancet ii: 1452

Tein I, Demaugre F, Bonnefont J P, Saudabray J M 1989 Normal muscle CPT_1 and CPT_2 activities in hepatic presentation patients with CPT_1 deficiency in fibroblasts, J Neurol Sci 92: 229–245

Tein I, DeVivo D C, Bierman F et al 1990 Impaired skin fibroblast carnitine uptake in primary systemic carnitine deficiency manifested by childhood carnitine-responsive cardiomyopathy. Pediatr Res 28: 247–255

Tonin P, Lewis P, Servidei S, Di Mauro S 1990 Metabolic causes of myoglobinuria. Ann Neurol 27: 181–185

Treem W R, Witzleben C A, Piccoli D A, Stanley C A, Hale D E, Coates P M, Watkins J B 1986 Medium-chain and long-chain acyl-CoA dehydrogenase deficiency. Clinical, pathological and ultra-structural differentiation from Reye's syndrome. Hepatology 6: 1270–1278

Treem W R, Stanley C A, Finegold D N, Hale D E, Coates P M 1988 Primary carnitine deficiency due to a failure of carnitine transport in kidney, muscle and fibroblasts. New Engl J Med 319: 1331–1336

Tritschler H J, Bonilla E, Lombes A et al 1991 Differential diagnosis of fatal and benign cytochrome c oxidase-deficient myopathies of infancy: an immunohistochemical approach. Neurology 41: 300–305

Truong D D, Harding A E, Scaravelli S, Smith S J M, Morgan–Hughes J A, Marsden C D 1990 Movement disorders in mitochondrial myopathy: a study of 9 cases with 2 autopsy studies. Mov Dis 5: 109–117

Tsairis P, Engel W K, Kark P 1973 Familial myoclonic epilepsy syndrome associated with skeletal muscle mitochondrial abnormalities. Neurol 23: 408

Turnbull D M, Bartlett K, Stevens D L et al 1984 Short-chain Acyl-CoA dehydrogenase deficiency associated with a lipid storage myopathy and secondary carnitine deficiency. N Eng J Med 311: 1232–1236

Turnbull D M, Johnson M A, Dick D J, Cartlidge N E F, Sherratt H S A 1985 Partial cytochrome oxidase deficiency without subsarcolemmal accumulations of mitochondria in chronic progressive external ophthalmoplegia. J Neurol Sci 70: 93–100

Turnbull D M, Shepherd M, Ashworth B et al 1988 Lipid storage myopathy associated with low acyl-CoA dehydrogenase activities. Brain 111: 815–828

Turnbull D M, Shepherd I M, Bartlett K, Sherratt H S A 1990 Short-chain acyl-CoA dehydrogenase deficiency. In: Tanaka K, Coates P M (eds) Fatty acid oxidation: clinical, biochemical and molecular aspects. Alan R Liss Inc, New York, pp 313–324

van Biervliet J P G M, Bruinvis I, Ketting D, DeBree P K, van der Heiden C, Wadman K 1977 Hereditary mitochondrial myopathy with lactic acidaemia, a De-Toni–Fanconi–Debré syndrome, and a defective respiratory chain in voluntary striated muscle. Pediatr Res 11: 1088–1092

van Erwen P M M, Gabreels F J M, Ruitenbeek W, Renler W O, Fischer J C 1987 Mitochondrial encephalomyopathy. Association with an NADH dehydrogenase deficiency. Arch Neurol 44: 775–778

van Oost B A, Weusten M, Ruitenbeck W, Sperl W, Sengers R 1990 Detection of deleted mitochondrial DNA in blood and muscle of a patient with Pearson's syndrome. J Neurol Sci 98 (suppl): 215 (abstr 1.118.5)

van Someren H, van Henegouven H B, Westerveld A, Bootsma

D 1974 Synteny of the human loci for fumarate hydratase and UDPG pyrophosphorylase with chromosome 1 markers in somatic cell hybrids. Cytogenet Cell Genet 13: 551–557

Vianey–Liaud C, Divry P, Gregersen N, Mathieu M 1987 The inborn errors of mitochondrial fatty acid oxidation. J Inher Metab Dis 10(suppl 1): 159–198

Vilkki J, Savontaus M-L, Nikoskelainen E K 1989 Genetic heterogeneity in Leber heredetary optic neuroretinopathy revealed by mitochondrial DNA polymorphism. Am J Hum Genet 45: 206–211

Vilkki J, Ott J, Savontaus M-L, Aula P, Nikoskelainen E K 1991 Optic atrophy in Leber hereditary optic neuroretinopathy is probably determined by an X-chromosomal gene closely linked to DXS7. Am J Hum Genet 48: 486–491

Wallace D C 1970 A new manifestation of Leber's disease and a new explanation for the agency responsible for its unusual pattern of inheritance. Brain 93: 131–132

Wallace D C 1987 Maternal genes: mitochondrial diseases. In: Birth defects; original article series, vol 23, pp 137–190. March of Dimes Birth Defects Foundation, Alan R Liss, New York.

Wallace D C, Zheng X, Lott M T et al 1988a Familial mitochondrial encephalomyopathy (MERRF): genetic, pathophysiological and biochemical characterisation of a mitochondrial DNA disease. Cell 55: 601–610

Wallace D C, Singh G, Lott M T et al 1988b Mitochondrial DNA mutation associated with Leber's hereditary optic neuropathy. Science 242: 1427–1430

Wanders R J A, Duran M, Ijlst L et al 1989 Sudden infant death and long-chain 3-hydroxyacyl-CoA dehydrogenase. Lancet ii: 52–53

Watmough M J, Birch–Machin M A, Bindoff L A et al 1989 Tissue specific defect of Complex I of the mitochondrial respiratory chain. Biochem Biophys Res Comm 160: 623–627

Watmough M J, Bindoff L A, Birch–Machin M A et al 1990 Impaired mitochondrial β-oxidation in a patient with an abnormality of the respiratory chain. J Clin Invest 85: 177–184

Wicking C A, Scholem R D, Hunt S M, Brown G K 1986 Immunochemical analysis of normal and mutant forms of human pyruvate dehydrogenase. Biochem J 239: 89–96

Wiles C M, Morgan–Hughes J A, Rose P E, Weston M J 1986 Breathlessness and weakness in a 22 year old woman. Hospital Update 12: 31–42

Willems J L, Monnens L A H, Trijbels J M F, Sengers R A C, Veerkamp J H 1974 Pyruvate decarboxylase deficiency in liver. New Engl J Med 290: 406–407

Willems J L, Monnens L A H, Trijbels J M F, Veerkamp J H, Meyer A E, van Dam K, van Haelst U 1977 Leigh's encephalomyelopathy in a patient with cytochrome c oxidase deficiency in muscle tissue. Pediatr 60: 850–857

Yamamoto M, Koga Y, Ohtaki E, Nonaka I 1989 Focal cytochrome c oxidase deficiency in various neuromuscular diseases. J Neurol Sci 91: 207–213

Yeaman S J, Hutcheson E T, Roche T E et al 1978 Sites of phosphorylation on pyruvate dehydrogenase from bovine kidney and heart. Biochemistry 17: 2364–2370

Yoneda M, Tanaka M, Nishikimi M et al 1989a Pleiotropic molecular defects in energy-transducing complexes in mitochondrial encephalomyopathy (MELAS). J Neurol Sci 92: 143–158

Yoneda M, Tsuji S, Yamaguchi T, Inuzuka T, Miyatake T, Horai S, Ozawa T 1989b Mitochondrial DNA mutation in family with Leber's hereditary optic neuropathy. Lancet i: 1076–1077

Yoneda M, Tanno Y, Horai S, Ozawa T, Miyatake T, Tsuji S 1990 A common mitochondrial DNA mutation in the tRNA^{Lys} of patients with myoclonus epilepsy associated with ragged-red fibres. Biochem Int 21: 789–796

Yuzaki M, Ohkoshi N, Kanazawa I, Kagawa Y, Ohta S 1989 Multiple deletions in mitochondrial DNA at direct repeats of the non-D-loop regions in cases of familial mitochondrial myopathy. Biochem Biophys Res Commun 164: 1352–1357

Zammit V A, Corstorphine C G, Kelliher M G 1988 Evidence for distinct functional molecular sizes of carnitine palmytoyl transferases I and II in rat liver mitochondria. Biochem J 250: 415–420

Zeviani M, Nonaka I, Bonilla E, Okino E, Moggio M, Jones S, Di Mauro S 1985 Fatal infantile mitochondrial myopathy and renal dysfunction caused by cytochrome c oxidase deficiency: immunological studies in a new patient. Ann Neurol 17: 414–417

Zeviani M, van Dyke D H, Servidei S 1986 Myopathy and fatal cardiopathy due to cytochrome c oxidase deficiency. Arch Neurol 43: 1198–1202

Zeviani M, Peterson P, Servidei S, Bonilla E, DiMauro S 1987 Benign reversible muscle cytochrome c oxidase deficiency: a second case. Neurology 37: 64–67

Zeviani M, Moraes C T, DiMauro S, Nakase H, Bonilla E, Schon E A, Rowland L P 1988 Deletions of mitochondrial DNA in Kearns–Sayre syndrome. Neurology 38: 1339–1346

Zeviani M, Servidei S, Gellera C, Bertini E, DiMauro S, DiDonato S 1989 An autosomal dominant disorder with multiple deletions of mitochondrial DNA starting at the D-loop region. Nature 339: 309–311

Zeviani M, Gellera C, Pannacci M, Uziel G, Prell A, Servidei S, Didonato S 1990a Tissue distribution and transmission of mitochondrial DNA deletions in mitochondrial myopathies. Ann Neurol 28: 94–97

Zeviani M, Bresolin N, Moggio M et al 1990b Familial mitochondrial myopathy with autosomic dominant inheritance. J Neurol Sci 98(suppl): 205 (abstr 1.15.7)

Zeviani M, Amati P, Bresolin N, Antozzi C, Piccolo G, Toscano A, DiDonato S 1991 Rapid detection of the A→G$^{(8344)}$ mutation of mtDNA in Italian families with myoclonus, epilepsy and ragged-red fibers (MERRF). Am J Hum Genet 48: 203–211

Zheng X, Shoffner J M, Lott M T, Voljavec A S, Krawiecki M S, Winn K, Wallace D C 1989 Evidence in a lethal infantile mitochondrial disease for a nuclear mutation affecting respiratory Complexes I and IV. Neurology 39: 1203–1209

Zierz S, Engel A G 1985 Regulatory properties of a mutant carnitine palmytoyltransferase in human skeletal muscle. Eur J Biochem 149: 207–214

Zierz S, Engel A G 1987 Are there two forms of carnitine palmytoyltransferase in muscle? Neurol 37: 1785–1790

Zierz S, Engel A G, Romshe C A 1988 Assay of acyl-CoA dehydrogenases in muscle and liver and identification of four new cases of medium-chain acyl-CoA dehydrogenase deficiency associated with systemic carnitine deficiency. In: DiDonato S (ed) Advances in neurology, vol 48. Molecular genetics of neurological and neuromuscular diseases. Alan R Liss, New York

Zinn A B, Kerr D W, Hoppel C L 1986 Fumarase deficiency: a new cause of mitochondrial encephalomyopathy. New Engl J Med 315: 469–475

Zupanc M L, Moraes C T, Shanske S, DiMauro S 1989 Deletion of mitochondrial DNA in a patient with features of the Kearns–Sayre and MELAS syndrome. Ann Neurol 26: 436

11. Skeletal muscle storage diseases: myopathies resulting from errors in carbohydrate and fatty acid metabolism

S. DiMauro   E. Bonilla   A. P. Hays   E. Ricci

INTRODUCTION

Disorders of glycogen or lipid metabolism cause two main syndromes, one dominated by progressive weakness, the other by exercise-induced cramps with or without acute muscle necrosis and myoglobinuria (Fig. 11.1).

Myopathy can be the only clinical expression or it can be part of a multisystem disorder: this usually depends on whether the defective enzyme exists as a muscle-specific isoform or, instead, is a 'house-keeping' protein common to all tissues. Most muscle-specific isozymes are also developmentally regulated: an immature or 'fetal' isoform is expressed early in myogenesis, and a mature or 'adult' isozyme, under separate genetic control, is expressed by mature muscle (Miranda et al 1982).

From the pathological point of view, vacuolation of muscle fibres is the light microscopic hallmark of these disorders. The vacuoles are periodic acid–Schiff- (PAS)-positive in glycogenoses and oil red O- (ORO)-positive in lipid storage myopathies. However, the severity of the vacuolar changes varies greatly in different diseases and in different patients with the same disease. Therefore, while glycogen or lipid storage, when present, are important clues, their absence does not exclude a biochemical defect of glycogen or lipid metabolism. Histochemical enzyme stains, when available, are excellent diagnostic tools, but there are pitfalls. For instance regenerating fibres, such as are seen after an episode of myoglobinuria, may express the 'fetal' form of a muscle-specific enzyme whose adult form is missing, thus giving a false-positive reaction. Ultrastructural studies are rarely needed for diagnosis, but may provide useful additional clues, such as the intralysosomal accumulation of glycogen in acid maltase deficiency or the

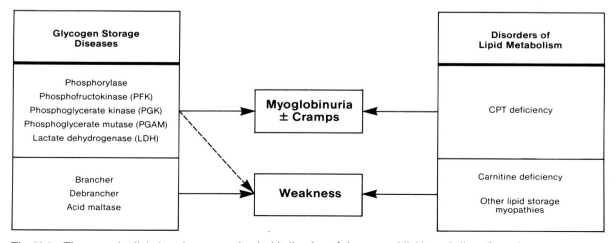

Fig. 11.1 The two main clinical syndromes associated with disorders of glycogen and lipid metabolism of muscle

abnormal granulo-filamentous structure of the polysaccharide in branching enzyme deficiency.

Even when glycogen or lipid storage are present, they do not necessarily reflect primary biochemical defects of glycogen or lipid metabolism. For example, mitochondrial myopathies affecting the respiratory chain may impair intermediate metabolism globally and cause accumulation of glycogen and triglycerides in addition to mitochondrial proliferation. One such condition, initially labelled 'mitochondria-lipid-glycogen' (MLG) disease (Jerusalem et al 1973), was later found to be associated with a benign form of cytochrome c oxidase deficiency (DiMauro et al 1983a).

The pathogenesis of symptoms and signs in glycogenoses and lipid metabolism disorders remains uncertain, despite extensive work in this area. Exercise intolerance and recurrent myoglobinuria have been attributed to acute shortage of energy due to the metabolic block. In agreement with this general concept are the circumstances that precipitate symptoms and signs. In blocks of glycogen metabolism, the crucial source of energy for intense exercise, cramps are invariably associated with exertion, and especially strenuous activities. In blocks of long-chain fatty acid oxidation, the principal muscle 'fuel' during prolonged exercise and during fasting, attacks of myoglobinuria are precipitated by protracted exercise, especially when associated with fasting. Although an 'energy crisis' appears compelling, experimental evidence is lacking: no depletion of ATP could be demonstrated biochemically or by ^{32}P-NMR spectroscopy. The pathogenesis of weakness is equally obscure: energy shortage, mechanical damage to the fibres, and fibre loss have been considered, but none of these mechanisms is completely satisfactory (Rowland et al 1986a).

MUSCLE GLYCOGENOSES

There are nine well-documented enzyme defects affecting glycogen metabolism or glycolysis in muscle (Fig. 11.2). For each disease we will review briefly the typical clinical presentation and clinical variants, muscle pathology, biochemistry, and molecular genetic data.

Acid maltase deficiency

Acid maltase deficiency (AMD, glycogenosis type II) causes two major clinical syndromes, a severe, generalized and invariably fatal disease of infancy, or a myopathy starting in childhood or adult life.

Infantile AMD (Pompe's disease) manifests in the first weeks or months of life with generalized hypotonia and weakness (floppy baby syndrome), although muscle bulk may be increased, and macroglossia is not infrequent. There is massive cardiomegaly and less pronounced hepatomegaly. Death due to cardiac or respiratory failure invariably occurs before 2 years of age and usually before the end of the first year.

In *childhood AMD* the onset of weakness is also very early in life, but there is no cardiopathy, and the clinical picture is characterized by myopathy involving mostly axial and proximal limb muscles. Because calf enlargement is common, in boys the disorder may mimic Duchenne muscular dystrophy. There is early involvement of the respiratory muscles, and death usually occurs during the second or third decade because of ventilatory failure.

Adult AMD is also confined clinically to the skeletal muscles and manifests as a slowly progressive myopathy similar to limb–girdle dystrophy or polymyositis. Early involvement of the respiratory muscles (acute respiratory insufficiency may be the presenting problem) and the 'irritative' features in the electromyograph (EMG) (see below) are clues to the correct diagnosis.

The serum CK activity is variably but consistently increased in all three forms. The EMG shows myopathic features together with fibrillation potentials, positive waves, bizarre high frequency discharges and myotonic discharges. Pulmonary function studies show more or less severe restrictive lung disease.

Muscle biopsy shows vacuolar myopathy. In the infantile form, all fibres contain numerous, sometimes confluent, vacuoles giving a 'lacework' appearance (Fig. 11.3A). In the childhood and adult variants, vacuoles are less numerous and in some adult patients the biopsy may appear virtually normal even with the PAS stain (Fig. 11.3B). In these cases, the correct diagnosis may be indicated by the acid phosphatase stain showing foci of

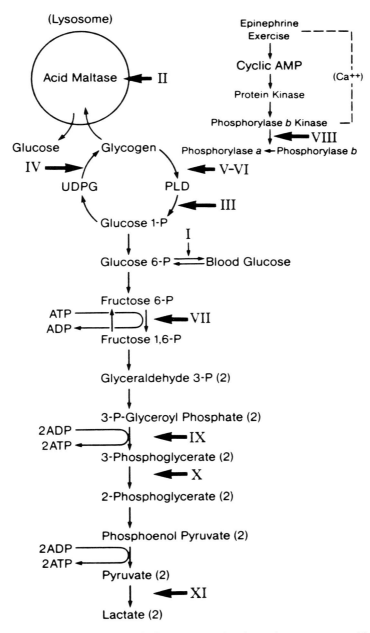

Fig. 11.2 Scheme of glycogen metabolism and glycolysis. Roman numerals refer to glycogenoses caused by deficiencies of the following enzymes: I = glucose-6-phosphatase; II = acid maltase; III = debrancher; IV = brancher; V = muscle phosphorylase; VI = liver phosphorylase; VII = phosphofructokinase; IX = phosphoglycerate kinase (PGK); X = phosphoglycerate mutase (PGAM); XI = lactate dehydrogenase (LDH). (From DiMauro et al 1986, with permission)

reactivity in non-vacuolated fibres (Fig. 11.3C). Electron microscopy shows glycogen storage in two locations, within lysosomal sacs and free in the cytoplasm, where it may form very large pools

compressing and distorting the myofibrils (Figs. 11.4 and 11.5).

Acid maltase (acid alpha-1,4- and alpha-1, 6-glucosidase) is a lysosomal enzyme capable of

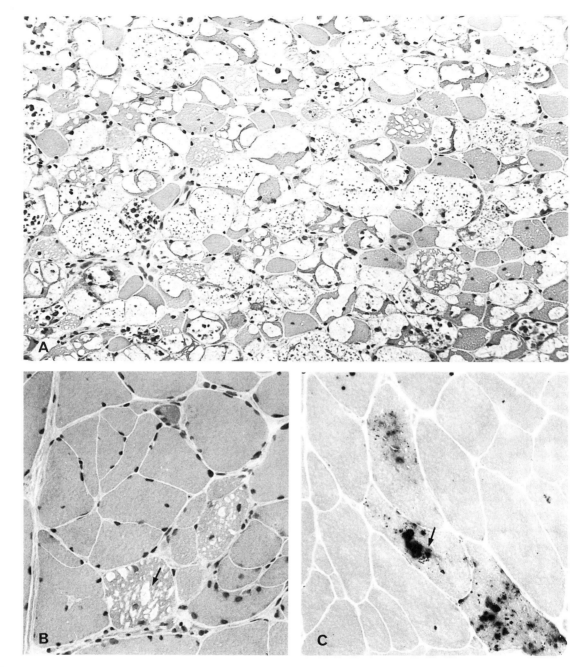

Fig. 11.3 Acid maltase deficiency (AMD). (A) frozen section from the muscle biopsy of an infant with infantile AMD (Pompe's disease) stained with haematoxylin–eosin (H&E) shows vacuoles in almost all fibres. ×200. (B) Frozen section from the muscle biopsy of a patient with adult-onset AMD stained with H&E shows vacuoles (arrow) in scattered fibres. ×250. (C) Frozen section from the muscle biopsy of a patient with late-onset AMD shows increased acid phosphatase activity (arrow) in a few fibres. ×220

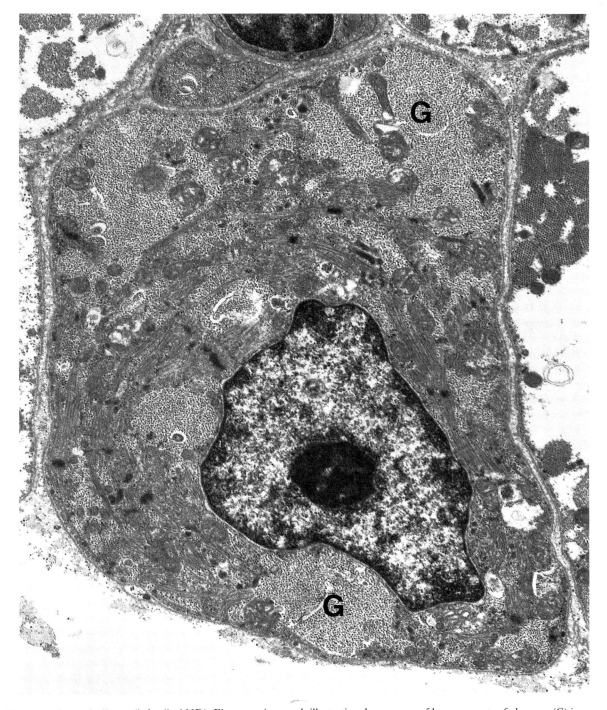

Fig. 11.4 Pompe's disease (infantile AMD). Electron micrograph illustrating the presence of large amounts of glycogen (G) in a muscle fibre. There is also disruption and faulty arrangement of contractile elements. ×20 000

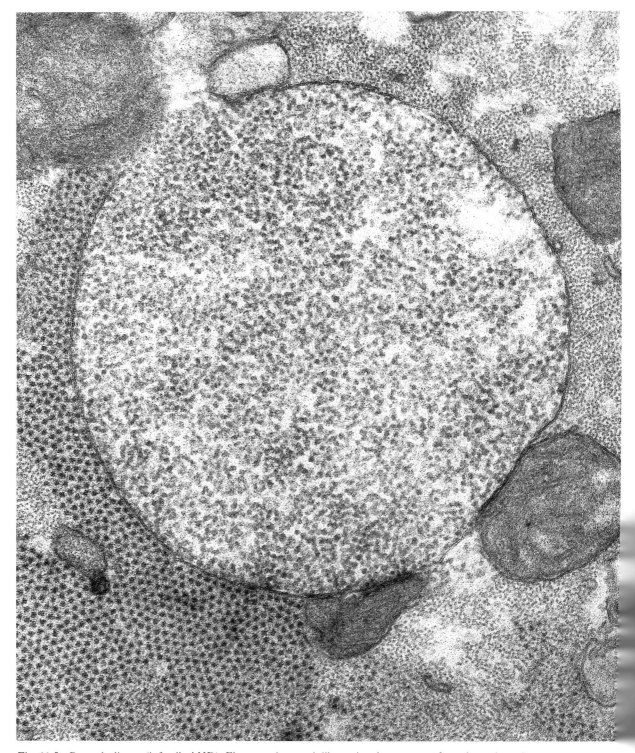

Fig. 11.5 Pompe's disease (infantile AMD). Electron micrograph illustrating the presence of membrane-bound glycogen. ×100 000

digesting glycogen completely to glucose. A defect of this enzyme should result in progressive accumulation of glycogen within lysosomes. While intralysosomal glycogen is in fact seen, the origin of the abundant free glycogen seen in skeletal and cardiac muscle in Pompe's disease is difficult to explain. Assuming that glycogen is discharged from overloaded lysosomes, it is not clear why it should not be degraded by the normal glycogenolytic enzymes present in the cytoplasm.

In infantile AMD, glycogen concentration is markedly increased in all tissues, especially cardiac and skeletal muscle. In childhood and adult AMD, glycogen storage is limited to skeletal muscle, and the concentration varies considerably from case to case and from muscle to muscle.

Because there are no tissue-specific isozymes and acid maltase deficiency is expressed in all tissues in all three clinical variants, it is difficult to explain the striking clinical heterogeneity that characterizes this disease. Initial biochemical studies had shown some residual enzyme activity in tissues from patients with childhood and adult AMD but virtually none in patients with infantile AMD (Mehler & DiMauro 1977). The importance of the relative amount of residual activity in determining the severity of the clinical phenotype has been confirmed in recent elegant studies of fibroblasts from 30 patients (Reuser et al 1987). Acid maltase, like other lysosomal enzymes, is normally synthesized as a large precursor, which is then glycosylated, phosphorylated and finally trimmed down to form enzymatically active polypeptides (Hasilik & Neufeld 1980a,b). In cultured fibroblasts from two patients with Pompe's disease, radiolabelling experiments showed that neither the precursor nor the smaller polypeptides were formed (Hasilik & Neufeld 1980a,b). Reuser et al (1987) studied both biosynthesis and in situ localization of AM and its precursors in cultured fibroblasts from 30 patients, 11 with infantile AMD, 3 with childhood AMD, and 16 with adult AMD. They found that the precursor was detectable in all but one of the mutant cell lines, while the intermediate and the mature forms of the enzyme were partially or totally lacking. Thus, by combining clinical features and definition of the nature of the residual AM polypeptides, they distinguished at least 10 different mutant phenotypes.

That the situation is even more complex, however, was documented by the same group of investigators when they conducted similar studies in South African patients of different ethnic origin (van der Ploeg et al 1989). An AM precursor of reduced size was found in two sisters with infantile AMD: the precursor appeared to be glycosylated and phosphorylated normally, but was not processed to the mature enzyme. Complete lack of the precursor was found in two other unrelated patients with infantile AMD.

This remarkable biochemical heterogeneity is now being explored at the molecular level, using a partial-length cDNA clone for AM (Martiniuk et al 1990). Taking into account residual enzyme activity and the results of immunochemistry and Northern analysis in cultured fibroblasts from 14 patients, Martiniuk et al (1990) distinguished at least six different types of mutations, three for the infantile form and three for the adult-onset form. Lack of AM mRNA was found by van der Ploeg et al (1989) in the two infants lacking the precursor protein.

The locus for AM has been assigned to chromosome 17 (D'Ancona et al 1979, Solomon et al 1979, Weil et al 1979), and all three forms of AMD are transmitted as autosomal recessive traits. Heterozygotes can be identified because they express a partial enzyme defect in various tissues, and prenatal diagnosis can be reliably established by measuring AM activity in cultured amniotic fluid cells or in biopsies of chorionic villi.

Debrancher deficiency

Debrancher deficiency (glycogenosis type III; Cori–Forbes disease) is typically a benign disease of childhood characterized by hepatomegaly, growth retardation, fasting hypoglycaemia, and hypoglycaemia-related seizures. These symptoms usually remit spontaneously with age (Smit et al 1990). Although hypotonia or mild weakness are reported in affected children, clinical myopathy is not common. However, a group of patients develop a neuromuscular disease later in life, in the third or fourth decade, long after the liver symptoms have disappeared (DiMauro et al 1979, Cornelio et al 1984, Smit et al 1990). There is often wasting of the legs and of intrinsic hand muscles, which may suggest Charcot–Marie–Tooth disease or motor neurone disease, and the course is slowly progressive. In a few cases, the myopathy starts in childhood and is accompanied by stunted growth and delayed motor milestones. Only two patients had exercise intolerance, cramps and premature fatigue (Ozand et al 1967, Murase et al 1973), and myoglobinuria has been reported in one patient (Brown 1986). Although clinical cardiopathy is unusual, laboratory data suggest that the heart is often involved (Moses et al 1989, Smit et al 1990).

Serum CK is markedly increased in patients with myopathy. There is no rise of blood glucose after glucagon or epinephrine administration indicating that the liver is also affected. Forearm ischaemic exercise causes no rise or an abnormally small rise of venous lactate. Electromyography shows myopathic features together with fibrillation, positive sharp waves, and myotonic discharges. Nerve conduction velocities can be decreased.

Muscle biopsy shows severe vacuolar myopathy, the vacuoles containing PAS-positive material which is digested by diastase (Fig. 11.6). By electron microscopy, the vacuoles correspond to large pools of free and apparently normal glycogen. Glycogen storage is also seen in intramuscular nerves and in endothelial cells (Powell et al 1985); studies of sural nerve biopsies showed glycogen accumulation both in Schwann cells and in axons (Ugawa et al 1986, Moses et al 1986). Excessive glycogen was also seen in skin biopsies (Sancho et al 1990) and in cultured muscle fibres (Miranda et al 1981).

The debranching enzyme removes the peripheral branches of glycogen after they have been maximally shortened by phosphorylase. This is a two-step reaction catalyzed by two distinct activities of the same enzyme protein: oligo-1,4-1, 4-glucantransferase and alpha-1,6-glycosidase. Genetic heterogeneity of debrancher deficiency is suggested by the observation that patients may

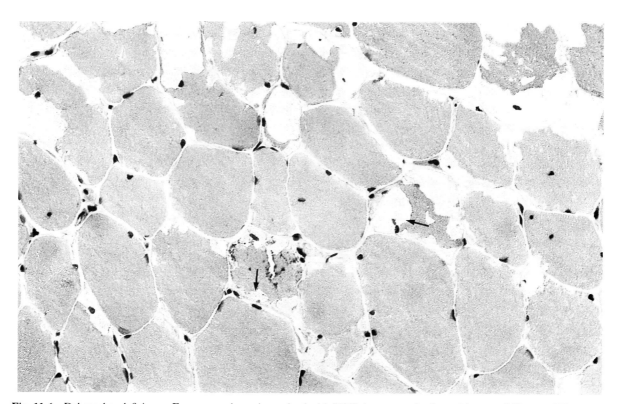

Fig. 11.6 Debrancher deficiency. Frozen muscle section stained with H&E shows vacuoles (arrow) in several fibres. ×228

lack only one of the two activities or, more often, both (van Hoof & Hers 1967, DiMauro et al 1979).

Glycogen concentration in muscle is markedly increased and, as expected, the polysaccharide has the structure of phosphorylase-limit dextrin (PLD) with abnormally short peripheral branches. Anaerobic glycolysis in vitro shows no lactate production by muscle extracts with endogenous substrate, while some lactate is formed from exogenous glycogen because the peripheral branches of the normal polysaccharide can be degraded by phosphorylase (Servidei & DiMauro 1989). As expected, lactate is produced normally with the addition of hexose-phosphate glycolytic intermediates.

Using antibodies against debranching enzyme purified from porcine skeletal muscle, Chen et al (1987) showed lack of cross-reacting material in liver and muscle from five of five patients with debrancher deficiency. Although this must be the most common situation, represented enzymatically by the loss of both transferase and alpha-1, 6-glucosidase activities, it is to be expected that patients with selective loss of one but not the other enzymatic function should have cross-reacting material corresponding to a mutant protein. Northern analysis of mRNA isolated from lymphoid cells in four cases provided evidence of genetic heterogeneity: two patients had decreased amount of message, one had a truncated mRNA, and the fourth had normal mRNA (Ding et al 1989).

As indicated above, the pathogenesis of weakness is puzzling. It cannot be simply due to the mechanical disruption of the fibres by glycogen accumulation because similar changes are seen in muscle of patients without weakness. On the other hand, it is not easily explained by energy shortage secondary to the metabolic block because deficiency of phosphorylase, which is only one step removed from debrancher, typically causes exercise intolerance, cramps and myoglobinuria rather than weakness.

Branching enzyme deficiency

Branching enzyme deficiency (glycogenosis type IV; Andersen's disease) is characterized by liver disease, with failure to thrive and progressive cirr-

hosis; death from hepatic failure or gastrointestinal bleeding usually occurs before 4 years of age (Brown 1986, Servidei & DiMauro 1989). Cardiomyopathy dominated the clinical picture in three older children and may be less rare than previously thought (Farrans et al 1966, Servidei et al 1987a, Tonin et al unpublished): the presence of PAS-positive, diastase-resistant storage material in endomyocardial or skeletal muscle biopsies suggests the diagnosis. Myopathy is rarely the predominant clinical feature, but severe hypotonia, muscle wasting, and contractures were described in three children (Fernandes & Huijing 1968, Zellweger et al 1972).

Branching enzyme attaches short glucosyl chains with alpha-1,6-glucosyl bonds to naked peripheral chains of glycogen, thus starting new chains that will be elongated by glycogen synthetase. A defect of branching enzyme, therefore, results in the production of an abnormal polysaccharide similar to amylopectin, with longer peripheral chains and fewer branching points than normal glycogen.

Muscle biopsy shows deposits of a basophilic, intensely PAS-positive material, which is partially resistent to diastase digestion. Ultrastructurally, the abnormal polysaccharide consists of filamentous and finely granular material often associated with normal-looking glycogen particles. Although the abnormal polysaccharide has been demonstrated in skin, liver, muscle, heart and central nervous system, the amount varies markedly in different tissues from the same patient. Despite the uneven distribution of the storage material, there is no evidence of tissue-specific brancher isozymes, and the defect appeared to be generalized in a postmortem study (Servidei et al 1987a).

Branching enzyme deficiency seems to be transmitted as an autosomal recessive trait.

Myophosphorylase deficiency

The first patient was described in 1951 by McArdle who elegantly demonstrated that the disorder was due to a block of glycogen breakdown (McArdle 1951). The enzyme defect, however, was identified 8 years later (Mommaerts et al 1959, Schmidt & Mahler 1959). Myophosphorylase deficiency (glycogenosis type V, McArdle disease) causes exercise intolerance with myalgia, premature fatigue, and cramps of exercising muscles, relieved by rest. Two types of activity are more likely to cause symptoms: (i) brief exercise of great intensity, such as sprinting or lifting heavy loads; and (ii) less intense but sustained activity, such as climbing stairs or walking uphill.

Many patients experience a 'second wind' phenomenon: if they slow down or pause briefly at the first appearance of myalgia, they can then resume exercising without problems. Three main adaptive processes seem to precede the second wind: (i) increased cardiac output and blood flow to exercising muscles; (ii) increased utilization of glucose and premature mobilization of free fatty acids; and (iii) increased EMG activity, probably due to recruitment of additional motor units to compensate for the failure of force generation in muscle fibres (Braakhekke et al 1986).

However, the adaptive processes are not always sufficient: acute muscle necrosis and myoglobinuria after strenuous exercise occur in about 50% of patients and are often complicated by renal failure. Fixed weakness is seen in about one-third of cases and tends to be more common in older patients (DiMauro & Bresolin 1986a).

Clinical variants of myophosphorylase deficiency are not frequent and fall into four groups: (i) a very mild syndrome of 'tiredness' or 'poor stamina' which is often considered 'functional'; (ii) progressive weakness, often in the sixth or seventh decade, without prior history of cramps or myoglobinuria; (iii) mild congenital weakness (Cornelio et al 1983); and (iv) fatal infantile myopathy with onset soon after birth and death in infancy from respiratory failure (DiMauro & Hartlage 1978). Biochemical studies have failed to provide an explanation for the clinical heterogeneity. The resting serum CK activity is variably but consistently increased. The resting EMG is

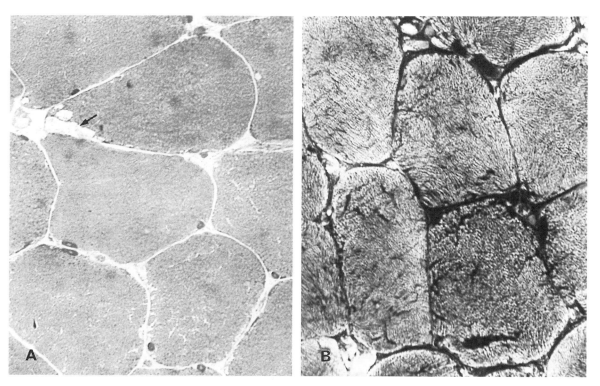

Fig. 11.7 Myophosphorylase deficiency (McArdle's disease). (A) Frozen muscle section stained with H&E shows subsarcolemmal (arrow) vacuoles. ×320. (B) Frozen section stained with PAS shows subsarcolemmal and intermyofibrillar accumulation of glycogen. ×291

normal, but no electrical activity is recorded from muscle during cramps, which are, therefore, real contractures. Forearm ischaemic exercise testing causes no increase of venous lactate.

The muscle biopsy shows subsarcolemmal and intermyofibrillar vacuoles filled with glycogen (Fig. 11.7A, B). However, glycogen accumulation can be so mild that no vacuoles are seen in the light microscope. Ultrastructurally, there are deposits of normal looking free glycogen and occasional alterations of mitochondria or sarcoplasmic reticulum (Fig. 11.8). The histochemical reaction for phosphorylase shows no staining of muscle fibres while smooth muscle of intramuscular vessels stains normally. However, 'false positive' staining of regenerating muscle fibres (which express the fetal isozyme) is often present, especially if the biopsy is obtained soon after an episode of myoglobinuria (Mitsumoto 1979).

Phosphorylase activity is undetectable in muscle in most cases. Glycogen concentration is increased two or three times above normal, but it can be normal in mild cases. The structure of glycogen is normal. Anaerobic glycolysis in vitro shows lack of lactate production with both endogenous and exogenous glycogen, but normal lactate formation after addition of glucose-l-phosphate or other hexose-phosphate glycolytic intermediates (Servidei & DiMauro 1989).

Most patients with McArdle's disease lack immunologically reactive protein in muscle: virtually no protein was found in 41 of 48 cases by SDS-PAGE and ELISA (Servidei et al 1988). These results suggest that phosphorylase deficiency is usually due to synthetic failure of the enzyme protein. However, Northern analysis of muscle mRNA has shown evidence of genetic heterogeneity: some patients lack mRNA, others have

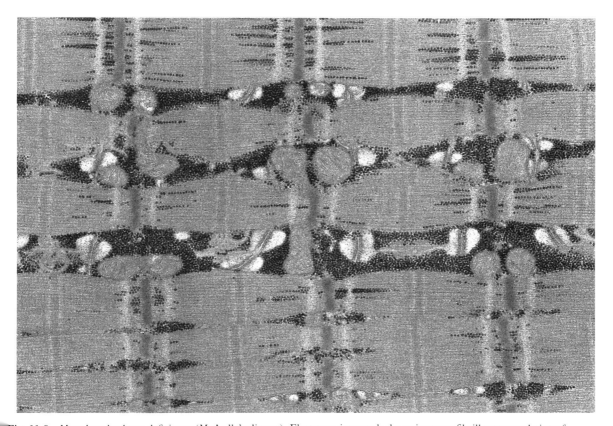

Fig. 11.8   Myophosphorlyase deficiency (McArdle's disease). Electron micrograph shows intermyofibrillar accumulation of glycogen. ×23 250

decreased amounts of normal message, still others have abnormal mRNA (Gautron et al 1987, Servidei et al 1988).

McArdle's disease is inherited as an autosomal recessive trait and the gene encoding the mature muscle isozyme of phosphorylase has been assigned to the long arm of chromosome 11 (Lebo et al 1984). Reports of autosomal dominant transmission (Schimrigk et al 1967, Chui & Munsat 1976) are probably explained by the presence in a family of manifesting heterozygotes in whom the residual phosphorylase activity in muscle has fallen below a critical threshold (Schmidt et al 1987).

Muscle phosphofructokinase (PFK) deficiency

Muscle PFK deficiency (glycogenosis type VII; Tarui disease) resembles McArdle's disease in its clinical presentation: intolerance to intense exercise, with premature fatigue, cramps (contractures), and, less frequently, myoglobinuria (Rowland et al 1986b). Differential diagnosis from McArdle's disease may be suggested by some laboratory tests (see below), but ultimately requires biochemical studies of muscle. Clinical heterogeneity is illustrated by two main variants: (i) late-onset, slowly progressive proximal weakness without cramps or myoglobinuria (Serratrice et al 1969, Hays et al 1981, Danon et al 1988); and (ii) fatal infantile myopathy (Guibaud et al 1979, Danon et al 1981a, Servidei et al 1986). All typical cases had a mild compensated haemolytic trait, and a few patients had jaundice or gout.

Serum CK activity is variably increased. Forearm ischaemic exercise test gives a flat lactate response. Most typical cases have moderate reticulocytosis, increased serum bilirubin, and increased uric acid. The pathogenesis of hyperuricaemia and gout is directly related to exercise ('myogenic hyperuricaemia') and due to excessive release of uric acid precursors, such as inosine and hypoxanthine, by exercising muscles (Mineo et al 1987). Electromyography shows myopathic changes in patients with weakness.

Muscle biopsy shows glycogen storage under the sarcolemma and between myofibrils. Besides normal-looking glycogen particles, an abnormal polysaccharide resembling that seen in branching enzyme deficiency is found in biopsies from patients with late-onset myopathy (Fig. 11.9A, B;

Agamanolis et al 1980, Hays et al 1981, Danon et al 1988). This polysaccharide is intensely PAS-positive, but resistant to diastase digestion. Ultrastructurally, the abnormal storage material is indistinguishable from the amylopectin-like glycogen that accumulates in branching enzyme deficiency or from the polyglucosan of Lafora disease and polyglucosan body disease, and consists of granular and filamentous structures. We have suggested that the amylopectin-like polysaccharide may originate from an imbalance between the activities of glycogen synthetase and brancher due to the abnormal accumulation of glucose-6-phosphate, a physiological activator of the synthetase (Hays et al 1981).

PFK activity in muscle of patients is usually negligible, but biochemical data have to be interpreted with caution due to the extreme lability of the enzyme. Glycogen concentration in muscle is usually two to three times higher than normal. Anaerobic glycolysis in vitro shows that no lactate is formed with glycogen or any of the hexose-phosphates except fructose-1,6-diphosphate, which is below the level of the enzymatic block (Servidei & DiMauro 1989).

PFK is a tetrameric protein under the control of three structural genes which encode three different subunits, called M for muscle, L for liver, and P for platelet (Vora et al 1983b). The subunits are variably expressed in different tissues. Mature muscle contains the homotetramer M4. Erythrocytes express both M and L subunits and random tetramerization produces five isozymes, the homotetramers M4 and L4 and three hybrid forms. In PFK deficiency, genetic defects of the M subunit cause total lack of activity in muscle and a partial enzyme defect in erythrocytes. An unstable M subunit has been described in one patient with late-onset myopathy (Vora et al 1987, Danon et al 1988) and in two with haemolysis but without muscle symptoms (Waterbury & Frenkel 1972, Etiemble et al 1976). Tissues that do not express the M subunit, such as liver and kidney, are predictably spared in Tarui's disease. The lack of clinical involvement of heart and brain, which do express the M subunit, must be due to the protective effect of the non-muscle isozymes.

Immunological studies in muscle or erythrocytes from patients had shown either the presence or absence of cross-reacting material, suggesting

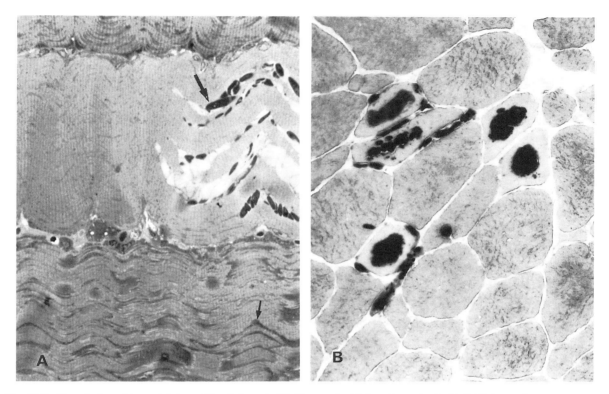

Fig. 11.9 Phosphofructokinase deficiency (Tarui disease). (A) Epon-embedded section stained with PAS shows glycogen accumulation (small arrow) in one fibre, and storage of abnormal polysaccharide (large arrow) in another fibre. ×900. (B) Frozen section stained with lugol shows dark material in several fibers. ×230

biochemical heterogeneity. Recently, the first molecular genetic error underlying PFK deficiency was documented by Tarui and coworkers in a member of the original family described by the same group (Nakajima et al 1990). A point mutation in the genomic DNA caused a splicing error resulting in a 75-base in-frame deletion in the cDNA. The mutant protein would miss 25 amino acids in an area of crucial importance for catalytic activity, thus explaining the enzyme defect.

The disease is transmitted by autosomal recessive inheritance. The genes encoding subunits M, P, and L have been localized on chromosomes 1, 10 and 21 (Vora et al 1982, Vora et al 1983a, van Keuren et al 1986).

Phosphorylase b kinase deficiency

Based on the mode of transmission and tissue involvement, four main clinical variants of phosphorylase b kinase deficiency can be recognized (van der Berg & Berger 1990): (i) an X-linked recessive disorder dominated by benign infantile hepatomegaly sometimes accompanied by mild hypoglycaemia and remitting spontaneously around puberty, the enzyme defect being expressed in liver and erythrocytes; (ii) an autosomal recessive form manifesting in childhood with hepatomegaly and weakness, in which the enzyme defect was documented in liver, muscle, and erythrocytes; (iii) an autosomal recessive form manifesting in adolescents or young adults and characterized by myopathy alone (Ohtani et al 1982, Iwamasa et al 1983, Abarbanel et al 1986, Servidei et al 1987b, Clemens et al 1990), with exercise intolerance, myalgia, and cramps; one patient had distal myopathy (Clemens et al 1990) and another myoglobinuria (Abarbanel et al 1986); and (iv) a probable autosomal recessive variant described in two infants with isolated cardiomyopathy; the heart showed severe glycogen storage and was the only tissue affected (Servidei et al 1987b).

In patients with myopathy, glycogen concentration in muscle is increased two or three times. Phosphorylase kinase activity is markedly decreased or absent. A clue to the diagnosis may come from measurement of phosphorylase activity in muscle: total phosphorylase is normal, but the active form of the enzyme (phosphorylase a) is reduced or absent. Forearm ischaemic exercise may be normal in these patients, either because of the presence of phosphorylase b or because other mechanisms of phosphorylase activation are triggered by exercise.

The clinical heterogeneity of phosphorylase b kinase deficiency is not too surprising considering the complexity of the enzyme, which is composed of four subunits, alpha, beta, gamma, and delta, each present as a tetramer (Kilimann 1990). The gamma subunits are catalytic, the alpha and beta subunits play a regulatory role through phosphorylation, and the delta subunits are identical to calmodulin and confer calcium sensitivity upon the enzyme. An alpha' isozyme has been identified in heart and slow-twitch muscle fibres, but other tissue-specific isoforms may exist. The gene for the alpha subunit has been assigned to the X chromosome (Francke et al 1989), that for the beta subunit to chromosome 16 (Francke et al 1989), and that for the gamma subunit to chromosome 7 (Chamberlain et al 1987).

Defects of terminal glycolysis

Within a short time interval in 1980–1981 three new enzyme defects were recognized — PGAM, PGK, and LDH deficiencies — all three affecting terminal glycolysis (Fig. 11.2) and all three causing recurrent myoglobinuria (DiMauro & Bresolin 1986b). Laboratory tests give similar results in the three disorders. Forearm ischaemic exercise causes some increase of lactate, but less than normal. Muscle biopsy may be normal or may show moderate glycogen storage and, accordingly, glycogen concentration is normal or mildly increased. Anaerobic glycolysis in vitro shows an incomplete block below the PFK reaction because

lactate production is decreased (but not absent) with all hexose-phosphate glycolytic intermediates. Outside episodes of myoglobinuria, electromyography is normal.

Phosphoglycerate kinase (PGK) deficiency

PGK deficiency can be clinically silent or can cause two main syndromes: (i) haemolytic anaemia, seizures, and mental retardation in infancy or childhood; and (ii) exercise intolerance and recurrent myoglobinuria in children or young adults. Because PGK is a single polypeptide encoded by a gene on the X chromosome and there is no evidence of tissue-specific isozymes (except in spermatogenic cells), the enzyme defect should be generalized. Despite this, and for reasons that are not clear, muscle alone was involved in three patients with intolerance to vigorous exercise, cramps, and recurrent myoglobinuria (Rosa et al 1982, DiMauro et al 1983b, Tonin et al 1989). Recently, however, an 11-year-old boy was reported who had a combination of the two syndromes, mental retardation, seizures, and myoglobinuria (Sugie et al 1989). Studies of physical and kinetic characteristics of PGK in different patients have shown different alterations, such that no two mutations appear to be identical.

Phosphoglycerate mutase (PGAM) deficiency

PGAM deficiency has been reported in four patients, two men and two women (DiMauro et al 1981, 1982, Bresolin et al 1983, Kissel et al 1985, Vita et al 1990), and we have studied a fifth patient in collaboration with Dr Gerald Fenichel (Vanderbilt University, Nashville, Tennessee). All patients had intolerance to intense exercise, with myalgia, cramps, and myoglobinuria.

Human PGAM is a dimeric enzyme containing, in different tissues, different proportions of a muscle homodimer (MM), a brain homodimer (BB), and a hybrid isozyme (MB). Electrophoresis of normal adult muscle PGAM shows marked predominance of the MM band, accounting for about 95% of the total activity, and very faint MB and BB bands. In muscle from patients, only the BB band could be seen, suggesting a genetic defect of the M subunit (DiMauro et al 1981).

Full-length cDNAs have been obtained and

sequenced for both PGAM-M (Shanske et al 1987) and PGAM-B (Sakoda et al 1988), and the gene encoding PGAM-M has been assigned to chromosome 7 (Edwards et al 1990). All patients were sporadic cases, but a partial enzyme defect was found in one set of parents, consistent with autosomal recessive inheritance (Bresolin et al 1983).

Lactate dehydrogenase deficiency

LDH deficiency was reported in two young men with recurrent myoglobinuria after intense exercise (Kanno et al 1980, Bryan et al 1990). The enzyme defect in the first patient was suspected because, during an attack of myoglobinuria, the predictably very high serum concentration of CK was not accompanied by an increase of LDH.

LDH is a tetrameric enzyme composed of two subunits, one (M) predominant in skeletal muscle, the other (H) predominant in cardiac muscle. There are five isozymes, the two homotetramers M4 and H4 and three heterotetramers. Electrophoretic studies of muscle extracts in the two patients showed that only the H4 isozyme was present and suggested a genetic defect of the M subunit. Bicycle ergometer studies in the second patient showed that maximal exercise raised blood pyruvate but not lactate, with a paradoxical fall of the lactate/pyruvate ratio (Bryan et al 1990).

Biochemical studies in family members of one patient showed that the defect was inherited as an autosomal recessive trait (Kanno et al 1980). The gene encoding LDH-M has been localized to chromosome 11 (Boone et al 1972).

Cardiomyopathy, mental retardation and autophagic vacuolar myopathy

Seven male patients have been reported with a familial disorder characterized by non-obstructive hypertrophic cardiomyopathy, proximal myopathy, and variably severe mental retardation, with age of onset between $2\frac{1}{2}$ and 19 years (Danon et al 1981b, Riggs et al 1983, Bergia et al 1986, Byrne et al 1986, Hart et al 1987). Cardiomyopathy dominated the clinical picture and caused death in the second or third decade. Muscle biopsy showed autophagic vacuoles and accumulation of intralysosomal and free glycogen. This picture suggested

acid maltase deficiency but acid maltase activity was normal in all cases, and glycogen concentration was increased in muscle of some but not all patients. Because women were less severely affected than men, X-linked dominant transmission was suggested (Hart et al 1987).

While there is little doubt that this is a lysosomal disease, it is not certain that glycogen metabolism is specifically impaired in this condition, and the aetiology remains unknown.

Other glycogenoses

A polysaccharide ultrastructurally and biochemically similar to the amylopectin-like material seen in branching enzyme deficiency and, less commonly, in PFK deficiency accumulates in two other conditions, Lafora disease and polyglucosan body storage disease (DiMauro 1989).

Lafora disease

This is characterized by the triad of epilepsy, myoclonus, and dementia. Typically, onset is in adolescence and progression is rapid, with death occurring in most cases between 17 and 24 years of age. Transmission is autosomal recessive. The pathological hallmark of the disease is the presence in the central nervous system of the bodies first described by Lafora in 1911: round, basophilic, strongly PAS-positive intracellular structures varying in size from 3 to 30 μm in diameter. Lafora bodies are seen only in neuronal perikarya and processes, especially in cerebral cortex, substantia nigra, thalamus, globus pallidus and dentate nucleus. Ultrastructurally, they are not membrane-bound and consist of two components, amorphous electron-dense granules and irregular filaments. Irregular deposits of a similar material are found in liver, skeletal and cardiac muscle, retina and skin. Despite the similarities of the storage material in Lafora disease and branching enzyme deficiency, brancher activity is normal in Lafora disease (Gambetti et al 1971), and the biochemical cause remains obscure.

Polyglucosan body disease

This has been described in about 15 patients and

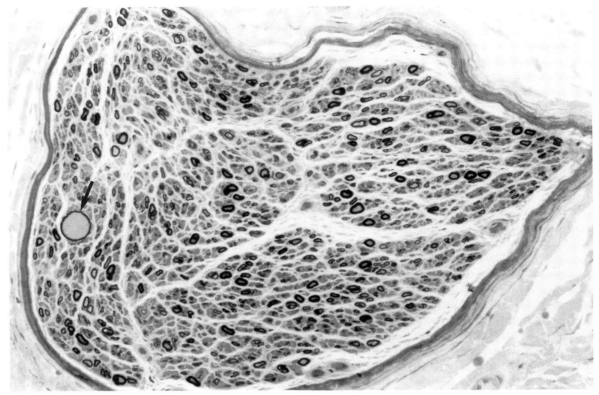

Fig. 11.10 Polyglucosan body disease. Epon-embedded section of a sural nerve biopsy shows a body (arrow) in a myelinated axon. ×855

is characterized by upper motor neuron involvement, peripheral neuropathy, sphincter problems and, in many but not all cases, dementia. Onset is in the fifth or sixth decade (Gray et al 1988). Sural nerve biopsy shows the characteristic bodies located mostly in the axoplasm of myelinated fibres, but also in unmyelinated fibres and in Schwann cells (Fig. 11.10). Post mortem studies have shown that the bodies are widespread, suggesting a generalized metabolic abnormality. However, the cause of the disease is not known.

Therapy

Therapeutic trials in patients with glycogenoses have been largely unsuccessful. In AMD, several strategies of enzyme replacement were attempted in the infantile form: while some exogenous AM could be found in liver, delivery of the enzyme to muscle, heart and brain proved an insurmountable task. Van der Ploeg et al (1988) recently succeeded in delivering a precursor of AM isolated from human urine and rich in mannose-phosphate into muscle cells in culture.

Various dietary regimens have been suggested. Infants and young children with debrancher deficiency should be protected from fasting hypoglycaemia with frequent feedings and nocturnal gastric infusions of glucose and uncooked corn starches (Moses 1990). A high-protein diet has been advocated in AMD (Slonim et al 1983, Isaacs et al 1986, Umpleby et al 1989), debrancher deficiency (Slonim et al 1984) and phosphorylase deficiency, especially in cases with muscle wasting (Slonim & Goans 1985). The goal was to correct excessive muscle protein catabolism, to provide alternative sources of energy to muscle in the form of branched-chain aminoacids, and to favour liver gluconeogenesis. Although the results are not striking, the benign nature of these interventions and the lack of more effective measures make a high-protein diet worth trying.

Patients with childhood or adult-onset AMD are likely to develop respiratory insufficiency early in the course of the disease and should be provided with respiratory muscle training initially (Martin et al 1983), and with respiratory assistance when the vital capacity falls below 25%.

DISORDERS OF LIPID METABOLISM

This generic heading is more appropriate than 'lipid storage myopathies' or 'triglyceride storage myopathies' because, while accumulation of lipid droplets within muscle fibres may be quite impressive in some conditions, it is absent or only transient in others. Under the light microscope, lipid storage is usually revealed with the oil red O (ORO) stain, which is specific for triglycerides. However, more information can be obtained with the Nile red stain, which not only reveals triglyceride droplets but also highlights membranes as red-orange fluorescent structures (Bonilla & Prelle 1987). This is particularly useful in mitochondrial myopathies where mitochondrial proliferation may be overshadowed by the accompanying lipid storage.

Long-chain fatty acids (LCFA) are a crucial source of energy for muscle, especially in two circumstances: (i) prolonged exercise, which cannot be sustained indefinitely by the limited muscle glycogen stores or by blood glucose (largely derived from liver glycogen); and (ii) during fasting, when both muscle and liver glycogen are depleted. The relative roles of carbohydrate and lipid 'fuels' at rest and during exercise have been the subject of several excellent reviews to which the reader is referred for details (Havel 1972, Felig & Wahren 1975, Lewis & Haller 1989).

The major steps of lipid metabolism in muscle are illustrated in Fig. 11.11. LCFA, the 'currency' of lipid metabolism, can derive from exogenous or endogenous sources. Exogenous, blood-borne sources are represented by plasma LCFA bound to albumin, plasma triglycerides in the form of very low density lipoproteins (VLDL), and chylomicrons. Fatty acids are released from VLDL by a

triglyceride lipase (lipoprotein lipase) which is located on the endothelial surface of capillaries. Endogenous sources of LCFA are triglycerides stored in the lipid droplets that are normally present in muscle in close proximity to mitochondria. Fatty acids are liberated from these triglycerides through the action of a poorly studied intracellular triglyceride lipase.

Irrespective of their origin, once within the muscle cell, LCFA are activated to acyl-CoA at the expense of ATP by a thiokinase bound to the outer mitochondrial membrane. Because the inner mitochondrial membrane is impermeable to LCFAcyl-CoA, the acyl residues are transferred to carnitine by carnitine palmitoyltransferase I (CPT I), which is bound to the inner face of the outer mitochondrial membrane (Murthy & Pande 1987). As carnitine esters, LCFA can cross the inner membrane by a process of exchange diffusion catalyzed by a carnitine–acylcarnitine translocase located in the inner membrane. Once inside the mitochondrial matrix, a second transferase (CPT II), bound to the inner face of the inner membrane, catalyzes the formation of LCFAcyl-CoA from LCFAcylcarnitine and intramitochondrial CoA. The LCFAcylCoA is now ready to undergo beta-oxidation.

The first step in beta-oxidation requires three flavin adenine dinucleotide (FAD)-dependent dehydrogenases with different specificities for carbon chain length: short-chain acylCoA dehydrogenase (SCAD), medium-chain acylCoA dehydrogenase (MCAD), and long-chain acylCoA dehydrogenase (LCAD). The second step of beta-oxidation is catalyzed by an enoylCoA hydratase. The third step requires two NAD-dependent 3-hydroxyacylCoA dehydrogenases, one with optimal activity for short-chain substrates, the other reacting preferentially with long-chain substrates. The final step of beta-oxidation is catalyzed by two 3-ketoacylCoA thiolases, acetoacetylCoA thiolase and general ketothiolase. At every 'turn' of this cyclic process one molecule of acetylCoA is formed (and enters the Krebs cycle) and the LCFAcylCoA, now two carbon atoms shorter, undergoes a new series of beta-oxidation reactions. The electron equivalents generated by the FAD-dependent dehydrogenases are carried to coenzyme Q by an electron-transferring flavoprotein (ETF)

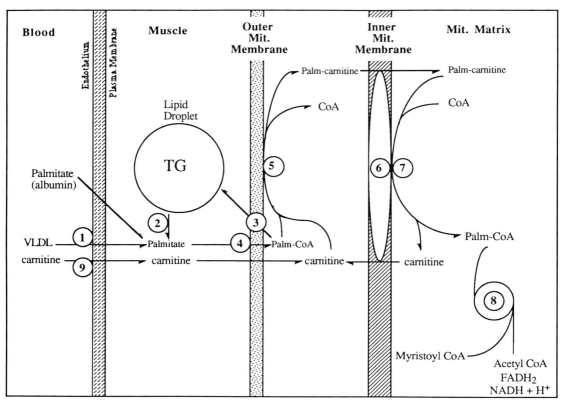

Fig. 11.11 Schematic representation of long-chain fatty acid metabolism in muscle. Blood-borne substrates are represented by fatty acids bound to albumin and by triglycerides in the form of very-low-density lipoproteins (VLDL). Endogenous lipid stores are triglycerides (TG) in lipid droplets. Enzymes or enzyme complexes are indicated by circled numbers adjacent to or within the membrane to which they are bound. Mit. = mitochondrial; 1 = lipoprotein lipase; 2 = intracellular, neutral tri-, di- and mono-glyceride lipase; 3 = triglyceride synthetic pathway; 4 = palmitoylCoA synthetase; 5 = CPT I; 6 = carnitine–acylcarnitine translocase; 7 = CPT II; 8 = beta-oxidation pathway; 9 = active transport system of carnitine. (Modified from DiMauro and Papadimitriou 1986, with permission)

through the action of an iron–sulphur flavoprotein ETF-dehydrogenase (ETF-DH).

A rational biochemical classification of the disorders of lipid metabolism affecting muscle has been proposed by DiDonato et al (1989a).

Carnitine deficiencies

Myopathic carnitine deficiency

First reported by Engel and Angelini in 1973, this is characterized clinically by slowly progressive and fluctuating axial and proximal limb weakness and, pathologically, by severe lipid storage myopathy (Figs 11.12 and 11.13). The fact that non-muscle tissues appear clinically spared and

that carnitine concentration is normal in serum distinguishes this form from systemic carnitine deficiency and suggests a primary defect of the active transport of carnitine from blood into muscle, a hypothesis supported by kinetic compartmental analysis in one patient (Rebouche & Engel 1984). However, primary forms of purely myopathic carnitine deficiency may not exist and previously reported cases might have been due to unrecognized systemic deficiencies or to defects of beta-oxidation (DiDonato et al 1989a).

Systemic carnitine deficiency

This deficiency was first described by Karpati et al (1975) in an 11-year-old boy with recurrent

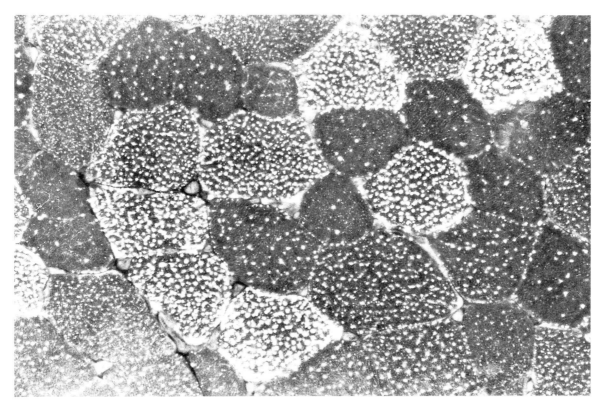

Fig. 11.12   Carnitine deficiency. Frozen muscle section stained with Nile red shows lipid accumulation in several fibres. ×276

episodes of hepatic encephalopathy since the age of 3 and progressive weakness since the age of 10. Numerous other patients were reported with similar Reye-like episodes, lipid storage myopathy, and low levels of carnitine in muscle, blood and other tissues (hence the label 'systemic'). Because carnitine is synthesized in liver and kidney but not in most other tissues, a block in the synthetic pathway could explain the generalized nature of the defect. However, no such block could be identified, and it soon became apparent that most cases of systemic carnitine deficiency are, in fact, secondary to other inborn errors of metabolism, most commonly MCAT, but also other defects of beta-oxidation, various organic acidaemias, defects of branched-chain aminoacid metabolism and defects of the respiratory chain (Engel 1986). In these disorders, there is a tendency for acylCoAs to accumulate. These potentially toxic compounds are esterified to acylcarnitines which are excreted in the urine, leading to a net carnitine loss. Carnitine supplementation has been successful in many of these patients, particularly during the acute attacks.

A special form of systemic carnitine deficiency is associated with *childhood cardiomyopathy*, which is often familial and fatal if untreated. There is also weakness (with or without hypoketotic hypoglycaemic encephalopathy), low serum and tissue carnitine levels, and severe renal carnitine leak. There is good evidence that this disorder is a primary carnitine deficiency due to a defect in the specific high-affinity, low-concentration, carrier-mediated uptake mechanism (Treem et al 1988, Eriksson et al 1988, Tein et al 1990a). Although the defect has been documented in cultured fibroblasts, the same uptake system is probably shared by skeletal and cardiac muscle, thus explaining the lipid storage myopathy and the cardiopathy. Oral L-carnitine supplementation causes dramatic

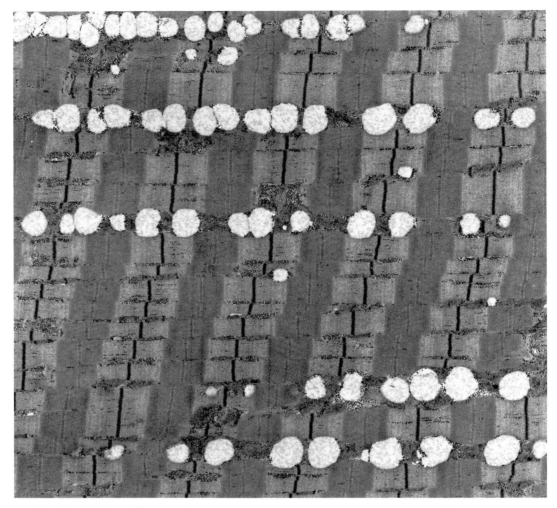

Fig. 11.13 Carnitine deficiency. Electron micrograph illustrating the presence of several lipid droplets in a segment of a muscle fibre. ×12 000

clinical improvement in cardiac function, strength, and growth. Given the frequent history of unexplained sibling death in these families and the beneficial effect of carnitine, early identification of presymptomatic siblings is of the greatest importance.

Carnitine palmitoyltransferase (CPT) deficiency

Myopathic CPT deficiency

This was first described by DiMauro and Melis DiMauro in 1973, and numerous reports have

followed (DiMauro & Papadimitriou 1986). In a recent review of 77 consecutive adult patients with myoglobinuria (Tonin et al 1990), CPT deficiency accounted for the highest number of biochemically documented enzymopathies (17 of 36), followed by phosphorylase deficiency (10 of 36).

The clinical picture is rather stereotyped: these patients are normal and usually vigorous individuals, predominantly young men, who, after prolonged though not necessarily strenuous exercise, develop myalgia, 'tightness', and weakness of exercising muscles followed by myoglobinuria, with the attending risk of renal insufficiency. The other major precipitating factor is prolonged fasting, either alone or in association with exercise, while minor causative factors include cold exposure, lack of sleep and intercurrent infection. Unlike patients with McArdle's disease or other glycogenoses, who are 'warned' of impending myoglobinuria by painful cramps, patients with CPT deficiency have no such warning signs and, therefore, tend to have multiple episodes. Also, while only exercising muscles are damaged in the glycogenoses, all muscles may be affected in CPT deficiency, especially after prolonged fasting, thus explaining the occurrence of respiratory insufficiency in some patients (DiMauro & Papadimitriou 1986).

Forearm ischaemic exercise results in a normal rise of venous lactate. Prolonged fasting, which should be carried out only under close medical supervision because of the risk of myoglobinuria, causes a sharp rise of serum CK and decreased or delayed production of ketone bodies in some patients (DiMauro and Papadimitriou 1986).

The muscle biopsy can be completely normal or show some degree of lipid storage, which is usually much less marked than in patients with carnitine deficiency.

The enzyme defect has been documented in tissues other than muscle, including liver, leukocytes, and cultured fibroblasts, suggesting that there are no tissue-specific isozymes, but raising the question of why only muscle should be clinically affected. Another related question is whether both CPT I and CPT II are affected by the genetic defect (as would be expected if they were the same protein) or one enzyme is specifically involved (if, in fact, the two proteins are different). Recent work, in animals and in humans, has convincingly demonstrated that CPT I and II are different proteins, and immunological studies (Singh et al 1988, Demaugre et al 1990) have confirmed previous, more controversial, biochemical evidence that CPT II is specifically affected in myopathic CPT deficiency.

Hepatic CPT deficiency

This was initially documented in an infant with severe hypoglycemic hypoketotic encephalopathy (Bougneres et al 1981), and a second patient with similar clinical features has been reported recently (Tein et al 1989). Biochemical studies in cultured fibroblasts from these patients suggested that CPT I was specifically affected in the hepatic form of CPT deficiency. The observation that both CPT I and II were normal in muscle from patients with the hepatic form further suggested that there may be at least two isoforms of CPT I, one expressed in muscle, the other expressed in liver and fibroblasts (Tein et al 1989).

Defects of β-oxidation

Defects of β-oxidation have been described largely in the paediatric population and liver dysfunction with hepatic encephalopathy usually overshadows muscle involvement. However, this area of metabolism has not been systematically explored in patients with biochemically undefined myopathies. For example, Tein et al (1990b) reviewed 93 cases of childhood myoglobinuria and divided them into two main groups: 'exertional' myoglobinuria which is precipitated by exercise; 'toxic' myoglobinuria which follows intercurrent infections. A specific enzymopathy could be identified in 34% of the exertional cases but in only 11% of the toxic cases. Defects of β-oxidation may explain some of these often fatal disorders.

Defects of LCAD

These are dominated by liver and heart involvement, but chronic myopathy has been described in patients surviving past infancy (Treem et al 1986), and one of two sisters who had presented with episodes of non-ketotic hypoglycaemia in childhood developed, at about the age of 20, recurrent myoglobinuria (Stanley 1987). A 47-year-old man with weakness, wasting and lipid storage myopathy also had LCAD deficiency in muscle; the observation that he produced ketones normally with fasting suggested that the liver was not affected (DiDonato et al 1988a).

MCAD deficiency

This is the most common disorder of β-oxidation, and, probably, the most common cause of systemic carnitine deficiency. As mentioned above, weakness and lipid storage myopathy are typical features, but the clinical syndrome is dominated by recurrent episodes of hepatic encephalopathy similar to Reye's syndrome. The gene encoding MCAD has been assigned to chromosome 1 (Matsubara et al 1986).

SCAD deficiency

This has been described in a few infants with variably severe syndromes including failure to thrive, developmental delay, hypotonia, and metabolic acidosis, but also in a 46-year-old woman with a pure myopathy, characterized by proximal weakness and myalgia (Turnbull et al 1984). Because she produced ketone bodies normally in response to fasting and SCAD activity was normal in fibroblasts, the biochemical defect seemed to be confined to skeletal muscle.

Multiple acylCoA dehydrogenation (MAD) deficiencies

These are characterized by excretion of numerous organic acids in the urine, and are usually explained biochemically by defects in the common final pathway linking FAD-dependent dehydrogenases to the respiratory chain, that is ETF or ETF-DH. As expected and as reflected by the patterns of organic acid excretion, defects of ETF or ETF-DH impair not only beta-oxidation but also the oxidation of branched-chain amino acids, ethyl-malonic and dicarboxylic acids, and sarcosine. Because the predominant organic acid excreted in the urine is glutaric acid, these biochemical defects are also collectively known as *glutaric aciduria type II* (glutaric aciduria type I is due to a specific defect of glutarylCoA dehydrogenase).

These disorders are clinically heterogeneous, ranging from fatal neonatal acidosis to late-infantile forms with hypotonia, hypoglycaemia and acidosis. Progressive weakness and wasting were important clinical features in two patients, a 19-year-old girl and an 8-year-old boy, with lipid storage myopathy and systemic carnitine deficiency (Dusheiko et al 1979, DiDonato et al 1986). Both also had recurrent crises reminiscent of Reye's syndrome.

Riboflavine-responsive MAD deficiency (RR-MAD)

This typically causes episodic nausea, vomiting, lethargy with hypoglycaemia and metabolic acidosis, but myopathy dominated the clinical picture in two patients, who did not improve with carnitine administration but responded dramatically to riboflavine supplementation (DeVisser et al 1986; DiDonato et al 1989b). In one of these patients, a 12-year-old girl, SCAD was immunologically absent in muscle but 'reappeared' after treatment with riboflavine. It has been suggested that RR-MAD may be due to an abnormality of riboflavine metabolism decreasing the availability of FAD in mitochondria. Low intramitochondrial FAD concentration could somehow either down-regulate the synthesis or accelerate the breakdown of flavoprotein enzymes (DiDonato et al 1989b).

Other defects of β-oxidation

Two new defects of β-oxidation, one involving the short-chain 3-hydroxyacylCoA dehydrogenase (SCHAD) and the other involving the long-chain 3-hydroxyacylCoA dehydrogenase (LCHAD), have been described in children with hypoketotic hypoglycaemic encephalopathies (Hale and Thorpe 1989, Wanders et al 1989). Two more patients with blocks at this level of the respiratory chain have been identified. One was a girl with LCHAD who suffered from hypoketotic hypoglycaemia, hepatomegaly, cardiomyopathy, hypotonia, pigmentary retinopathy, and peripheral neuropathy, and died at 1 year of cardiorespiratory arrest (Garavaglia et al 1990). The other was a girl with SCHAD who, between the ages of 13 and 16 suffered three episodes of myoglobinuria and hypoglycaemic encephalopathy and died at the age of 16 of hypertrophic cardiomyopathy (Tein et al 1990).

Finally, partial defects of β-oxidation may be secondary to defects of the respiratory chain, as documented by Watmough et al (1990) in muscle from a patient with complex I deficiency.

Triglyceride storage disease

Five patients have been reported with what

appears to be a distinct disorder, characterized by congenital ichthyosis, myopathy, and lipid storage in many tissues, including fibroblast and muscle cultures (Chanarin et al 1975, Miranda et al 1979, Angelini et al 1980, DiDonato et al 1988b, Radom et al 1987). The stored lipid was identified as triglyceride by thin-layer chromatography and blood and muscle carnitine concentrations, and the activities of CPT and acid lipase were normal (Miranda et al 1979). Impaired oxidation of fatty acids was reported in one case (Angelini et al 1980), but studies of cultured fibroblasts from two other patients showed normal oxidation of fatty acids and revealed a specific impairment in the degradation of endogenously synthesized triglycerides (DiDonato et al 1988b). The enzyme defect may involve the intracellular neutral triglyceride lipase, but this remains to be documented.

ACKNOWLEDGEMENTS

Part of the work described here was supported by Centre Grant NS 11766 from the National Institute of Neurological and Communicative Disorders and Stroke and by a Grant from the Muscular Dystrophy Association, and by a generous donation from Libero and Graziella Danesi, Milano, Italy. Dr Enzo Ricci is supported by a fellowship from the Unione Italiana Lotta contro la Distrofia Muscolare (UILDM), Sezione Laziale 'Giulia Testore'.

REFERENCES

Abarbanel J M, Bashan N, Potashnik R, Moses R, Herishanu Y 1986 Adult muscle phosphorylase b kinase deficiency. Neurology 36: 560

Agamanolis D P, Askari A D, DiMauro S, Hays A P, Kumar K, Lipton M, Raynor A 1980 Muscle phosphofructokinase deficiency: two cases with unusual polysaccharide accumulation and immunologically active enzyme protein. Muscle and Nerve 3: 456

Angelini C, Philippart M, Borrone C, Bresolin N, Cantini M, Lucke S 1980 Multisystem triglyceride storage disorder with impaired long-chain fatty acid oxidation. Annals of Neurology 7: 5

Bergia B, Sybers H D, Butler J 1986 Familial lethal cardiomyopathy with mental retardation and scapuloperoneal muscular dystrophy. Journal of Neurology, Neurosurgery and Psychiatry 49: 1423

Bonilla E, Prelle A 1987 Application of Nile blue and Nile red, two fluorescent probes, for detection of lipid droplets in human skeletal muscle. Journal of Histochemistry and Cytochemistry 35: 619

Boone C M, Chen T R, Ruddle F H 1972 Assignment of LDH-A locus in man to chromosome c-11 using somatic cell hybrids. Proceedings of the National Academy of Sciences of the USA 69: 510

Bougneres P F, Saudubray J M, Marsac C, Bernard O, Odievre M, Girard J 1981 Fasting hypoglycemia resulting from hepatic carnitine palmitoyltransferase deficiency. Journal of Pediatrics 98: 742

Braakhekke J P, deBruin M I, Stegeman D F, Wevers R A, Binkhorst R A, Joosten E M G 1986 The second wind phenomenon in McArdle's disease. Brain 109: 1087

Bresolin N, Ro Y I, Reyes M, Miranda A F, DiMauro S 1983 Muscle phosphoglycerate mutase (PGAM) deficiency: a second case. Neurology 33: 1049

Brown B I 1986 Debranching and branching enzyme deficiencies. In: Engel A G, Banker B Q (eds) Myology, vol 2. McGraw-Hill, New York, p 1635

Bryan W, Lewis S F, Bertocci L, Gunder M, Ayyad K, Gustafson P, Haller R G 1990 Muscle lactate dehydrogenase deficiency: a disorder of anaerobic glycolysis associated with exertional myoglobinuria. Neurology 40 (supplement 1): 203

Byrne E, Bennet X, Crotty B et al 1986 Dominantly inherited cardioskeletal myopathy with lysosomal glycogen storage and normal acid maltase levels. Brain 109: 523

Chamberlain J S, Van Tuinen P, Reeves A A, Philip B A, Caskey C T 1987 Isolation of cDNA clones for the catalytic gamma subunit of mouse muscle phosphorylase kinase: expression of mRNA in normal and mutant Phk mice. Proceedings of the National Academy of Sciences of the USA 84: 2886

Chanarin I, Patel A, Slavin G, Wills E J, Andrews T M, Stewart G 1975 Neutral lipid storage disease: a new disorder of lipid metabolism. British Medical Journal 1: 203

Chen Y T, He J K, Ding J H, Brown B I 1987 Glycogen debranching enzyme: purification, antibody characterization, and immunoblot analyses of type III glycogen storage disease. American Journal of Human Genetics 41: 1002

Chui L A, Munsat T L 1976 Dominant inheritance of McArdle syndrome. Archives of Neurology 33: 636

Clemens P R, Yamamoto M, Engel A G 1990 Adult phosphorylase b kinase deficiency. Annals of Neurology 28: 529

Cornelio F, Bresolin N, DiMauro S, Mora M, Balestrini M R 1983 Congenital myopathy due to phosphorylase deficiency. Neurology 33: 1383

Cornelio F, Bresolin N, Singer P A, DiMauro S, Rowland L P 1984 The clinical varieties of neuromuscular disease in debrancher deficiency. Archives of Neurology 41: 1027

D'Ancona G C, Wurm J, Croce C M 1979 Genetics of type II glycogenosis: assignment of the human gene for alpha-glucosidase to chromosome 17. Proceedings of the National Academy of Sciences of the USA 76: 4526

Danon M J, Carpenter S, Manaligod J R, Schliselfeld L H 1981a Fatal infantile glycogen storage disease: deficiency of phosphofructokinase and phosphorylase b kinase. Neurology 31: 1303

Danon M J, Oh S J, DiMauro S, Manaligod J R, Eastwood A, Naidu S, Schliselfeld L H 1981b Lysosomal glycogen storage disease with normal acid maltase. Neurology 31: 51

Danon M J, Servidei S, DiMauro S, Vora S 1988 Late-onset muscle phosphofructokinase deficiency. Neurology 38: 956

Demaugre F, Bonnefont J P, Cepanec C, Scholte J, Saudubray J M, Leroux J P 1990 Immunoquantitative analysis of human carnitine palmitoyltransferase I and II defects. Pediatric Research 27: 497

DeVisser M, Scholte J, Schutgens R B H et al 1986 Riboflavin-responsive lipid storage myopathy and glutaric aciduria type II of early adult onset. Neurology 36: 367

DiDonato S, Frerman F E, Rimoldi M, Rinaldo P, Taroni F, Wiesmann U N 1986 Systemic carnitine deficiency due to lack of electron transfer flavoprotein:ubiquinone oxidoreductase. Neurology 36: 957

DiDonato S, Gellera C, Rimoldi M, Peluchetti D, Antozzi C 1988a Long-chain acylCoA dehydrogenase deficiency in muscle of an adult with lipid myopathy. Neurology 38 (supplement 1): 269

DiDonato S, Garavaglia B, Strisciuglio P, Borrone C, Andria G 1988b Multisystem triglyceride storage disease is due to a specific defect in the degradation of endocellularly synthesized triglycerides. Neurology 38: 1107

DiDonato S, Garavaglia B, Bloisi W, Colombo I, Finocchiaro G 1989a Biochemical and molecular aspects of beta-oxidation defects in skeletal muscle. In: Benzi G (ed) Advances in myochemistry, vol 2. John Libbey, London, p 151

DiDonato S, Gellera C, Peluchetti D, Uziel G, Antonelli A, Lus G, Rimoldi M 1989b Normalization of short-chain acylcoenzyme A dehydrogenase after riboflavin treatment in a girl with multiple acylcoenzyme A dehydrogenase-deficient myopathy. Annals of Neurology 25: 479

DiMauro S 1989 Disorders of carbohydrate metabolism. In: Rowland L P (ed) Merritt's textbook of neurology, 8th edn Lea and Febiger, Philadelphia, p 530

DiMauro S, Bresolin N 1986a Phosphorylase deficiency. In: Engel A G, Banker B Q (eds) Myology, vol 2. McGraw-Hill, New York, p 1585

DiMauro S, Bresolin N 1986b Newly recognized defects of distal glycolysis. In: Engel A G, Banker B Q (eds) Myology, vol 2. McGraw-Hill, New York, p 1619

DiMauro S, Hartlage P L 1978 Fatal infantile form of muscle phosphorylase deficiency. Neurology 28: 1124

DiMauro S, Papadimitriou A 1986 Carnitine palmitoyltransferase (CPT) deficiency. In: Engel A G, Banker B Q (eds) Myology, vol 2. McGraw-Hill, New York p 1697

DiMauro S, Melis DiMauro P 1973 Muscle carnitine palmitoyltransferase deficiency and myoglobinuria. Science 182: 929

DiMauro S, Hartwig G B, Hays A P et al 1979 Debrancher deficiency: neuromuscular disorder in five adults. Annals of Neurology 5: 422

DiMauro S, Miranda A F, Khan S, Gitlin K, Friedman R 1981 Human muscle phosphoglycerate mutase deficiency: a newly discovered metabolic myopathy. Science 212: 1277

DiMauro S, Miranda A F, Olarte M, Friedman R, Hays A P 1982 Muscle phosphoglycerate mutase deficiency. Neurology 32: 898

DiMauro S, Nicholson J F, Hays A P, Eastwood A B, Papadimitriou A, Koenigsberger R, DeVivo D C 1983a

Benign infantile mitochondrial myopathy due to reversible cytochrome c oxidase deficiency. Annals of Neurology 13: 679

DiMauro S, Dalakas M, Miranda A F 1983b Phosphoglycerate kinase (PGK) deficiency: Another cause of recurrent myoglobinuria. Annals of Neurology 13: 11

DiMauro S, Miranda A F, Sakoda S et al 1986 Metabolic myopathies. American Journal of Medical Genetics 25: 635

Ding J H, Harris D A, Bing-Zi Y, Chen Y T 1989 Cloning of the cDNA for human muscle glycogen debrancher, the enzyme deficient in type III glycogen storage disease. Pediatric Research 25: 140A

Dusheiko G, Kew M C, Joffe B I, Lewin J R, Mantagos S, Tanaka K 1979 Recurrent hypoglycemia associated with glutaric aciduria type II in an adult. New England Journal of Medicine 301: 1405

Edwards Y H, Sakoda S, Schon E A, Povey S 1990 The gene for human muscle-specific phosphoglycerate mutase, PGAMM, mapped to chromosome 7 by polymerase chain reaction. Genomics 5: 948

Engel A G 1986 Carnitine deficiency syndromes and lipid storage myopathies. In: Engel A G, Banker B Q (eds) Myology, vol 2. McGraw-Hill, New York, p 1663

Engel A G, Angelini C 1973 Carnitine deficiency of human skeletal muscle with associated lipid storage myopathy. A new syndrome. Science 179: 899

Eriksson B O, Lindstedt S, Nordin I 1988 Hereditary defect in carnitine membrane transport is expressed in skin fibroblast. European Journal of Pediatrics 221: 662

Etiemble J, Kahn A, Boivin P 1976 Hereditary hemolytic anemia with erythrocyte phosphofructokinase deficiency. Human Genetics 31: 193

Farrans V J, Hibbs R G, Wash J J, Burch G E 1966 Cardiomyopathy, cirrhosis of the liver and deposits of a fibrillar polysaccharide. American Journal of Cardiology 17: 457

Felig P, Wahren J 1975 Fuel homeostasis in exercise. New England Journal of Medicine 293: 1978

Fernandes J, Huijing F 1968 Branching enzyme deficiency glycogenosis: studies in therapy. Archive Diseases of Childhood 43: 347

Francke U, Darras B T, Zander N F, Kilimann M W 1989 Assignment of human genes for phosphorylase kinase subunits alpha (PHKA) to Xq12–q13 and beta to 16q12–q13 (PHKB). American Journal of Human Genetics 45: 276

Gambetti P L, DiMauro S, Hirt L, Blume R P 1971 Myoclonic epilepsy with Lafora bodies. Archives of Neurology 25: 483

Garavaglia B, Dionisi Vici C et al 1990 Peripheral neuropathy and pigmentary retinal degeneration in a cardiomyopathic infant with long-chain 3-hydroxyacylCoA dehydrogenase deficiency. Abstracts of the 5th International Congress of Inborn Errors of Metabolism, Asilomar, abstract W17.5

Gautron S, Daegelen D, Mennecier F, Dubocq D, Kahn A, Dreyfus J C 1987 Molecular mechanisms of McArdle's disease (muscle glycogen phosphorylase deficiency). Journal of Clinical Investigation 79: 275

Gray F, Gherardi R, Marshall A, Janota I, Poirier J 1988 Adult polyglucosan body disease (APBD). Journal of Neuropathology and Experimental Neurology 47: 459

Guibaud P, Carrier H, Mathieu M, Dorche C, Parehoux B, Bethenod M, Larbre F 1979 Observation familiale de dystrophie musculaire congenitale par deficit en phosphofructokinase. Archives Francais de Pediatrie 35: 1105

Hale D E, Thorpe C 1989 Short-chain 3-OH-acylCoA

dehydrogenase deficiency. Pediatric Research 25: 199A

Hart Z H, Servidei S, Peterson P L, Chang C H, DiMauro S 1987 Cardiomyopathy, mental retardation, and autophagic vacuolar myopathy. Neurology 37: 1065

Hasilik A, Neufeld E F 1980a Biosynthesis of lysosomal enzymes in fibroblasts: synthesis as precursors of higher molecular weight. Journal of Biological Chemistry 255: 4937

Hasilik A, Neufeld E F 1980b Biosynthesis of lysosomal enzymes in fibroblasts: Phosphorylation of mannose residues. Journal of Biological Chemistry 255: 4946

Havel R J 1972 Caloric homeostasis and disorders of fuel transport. New England Journal of Medicine 287: 1186

Hays A P, Hallett M, Delfs J, Morris J, Sotrel A, Shevchuk M M, DiMauro S 1981 Muscle phosphofructokinase deficiency: abnormal polysaccharide in a case of late-onset myopathy. Neurology 31: 1077

Isaacs H, Savage N, Badenhorst M, Whistler T 1986 Acid maltase deficiency: a case study and review of the pathophysiological changes and proposed therapeutic measures. Journal of Neurology, Neurosurgery and Psychiatry 49: 1011

Iwamasa T, Fukuda S, Tokumitsu S, Ninomiya N, Mtsuda J, Osame M 1983 Myopathy due to glycogen storage disease. Experimental and Molecular Pathology 38: 405

Jerusalem F, Angelini C, Engel A G, Groover R V 1973 Mitochondria–Lipid–Glycogen (MLG) disease of muscle. Archives of Neurology 29: 162

Kanno T, Sudo K, Takeuchi I, Kanda S, Honda N, Nishimura Y, Oyama K 1980 Hereditary deficiency of lactate dehydrogenase M-subunit. Clinica Chimica Acta 108: 267

Karpati G, Carpenter S, Engel A G, Watters G, Allen J, Rothman S, Klassen G, Mamer O 1975 The syndrome of systemic carnitine deficiency. Neurology 25: 16

Kilimann M W 1990 Molecular genetics of phosphorylase kinase: cDNA cloning, chromosomal mapping and isoform structure. Journal of Inherited Metabolic Diseases 13: 435

Kissel J T, Beam W, Bresolin N, Gibbons G, DiMauro S, Mendell J R 1985 The physiologic assessment of a newly described myopathy, phosphoglycerate mutase deficiency, through incremental exercise testing. Neurology 35: 828

Lebo R V, Gorin F, Fletterick R J, Kao F-T, Cheung M-C, Bruce B D, Kan Y W 1984 High-resolution chromosome sorting and DNA spot-blot analysis assign McArdle syndrome to chromosome 11. Science 225: 57

Lewis S F, Haller R G 1989 Skeletal muscle disorders and associated factors that limit exercise performance In: Pandolf K (ed) Exercise and sport sciences reviews, vol 17. Williams and Wilkins, Baltimore, p 67

Martin R J, Sufit R L, Ringel S P, Hudgel D W, Hill P L 1983 Respiratory improvement by muscle training in adult onset acid maltase deficiency. Muscle and Nerve 6: 201

Martiniuk F, Mehler M, Tzall S, Meredith G, Hirschhorn R 1990 Extensive genetic heterogeneity in patients with acid alpha glucosidase deficiency as detected by abnormalities of DNA and mRNA. American Journal of Human Genetics 47: 73

Matsubara Y, Kraus J P, Yang-Feng T L, Francke U, Rosenberg L E, Tanaka K 1986 Molecular cloning of cDNAs encoding rat and human medium chain acyl-CoA dehydrogenase and assignment of the gene to human chromosome 1. Proceedings of the National Academy of Sciences of the USA 83: 6543

McArdle B 1951 Myopathy due to a defect in muscle glycogen breakdown. Clinical Science 10: 13

Mehler M, DiMauro S 1977 Residual acid maltase activity in late-onset acid maltase deficiency. Neurology 27: 178

Mineo I, Kono N, Hara N et al 1987 Myogenic hyperuricemia: a common pathophysiologic feature of glycogenosis types III, V, and III. New England Journal of Medicine 317: 75

Miranda A F, DiMauro S, Eastwood A B et al 1979 Lipid storage myopathy, ichthyosis, and stheatorrhea. Muscle and Nerve 2: 1

Miranda A F, DiMauro S, Antler A, Stern L Z, Rowland L P 1981 Glycogen debrancher deficiency is reproduced in muscle culture. Annals of Neurology 9: 283

Miranda A F, Shanske S, DiMauro S 1982 Developmentally regulated isozyme transitions in normal and diseased muscle. In: Pearson M L, Epstein H F (eds) Muscle development: molecular and cellular control. Cold Spring Harbor Laboratory, New York, p 515

Mitsumoto H 1979 McArdle disease: phosphorylase activity in regenerating muscle fibers. Neurology 29: 258

Mommaerts W F H M, Illingworth B, Pearson C M, Guillory R J, Seraydarian K 1959 A functional disorder of muscle associated with the absence of phosphorylase. Proceedings of the National Academy of Sciences of the USA 45: 791

Moses S W 1990 Muscle glycogenosis. Journal of Inherited Metabolic Diseases 13: 452

Moses S W, Gadoth N, Bashan N, Ben-David E, Slonim A, Wanderman K L 1986 Neuromuscular involvement in glycogen storage disease type III. Acta Paediatrica Scandinavica 75: 289

Moses S W, Wanderman K L, Myroz A, Friedman M 1989 Cardiac involvement in glycogen storage disease type III. European Journal of Pediatrics 431: 1

Murase T, Ikeda H, Muro T, Nakao K, Sugita H 1973 Myopathy associated with type III glycogenosis. Journal of the Neurological Sciences 20: 287

Murthy M S R, Pande S V 1987 Malonyl-CoA building site and the overt carnitine palmitoyltransferase activity reside on the opposite sides of the outer mitochondrial membrane Proceedings of the National Academy of Sciences of the USA 84: 378

Nakajima H, Kono N, Yamasaki T et al 1990 Genetic defect in muscle phosphofructokinase deficiency. Journal of Biological Chemistry 265: 9392

Ohtani I, Matsuda I, Iwasama T, Tamari H, Origuchi Y, Miike T 1982 Infantile glycogen storage myopathy in a girl with phosphorylase kinase deficiency. Neurology 32: 833

Ozand P, Tokatli M, Amiri S 1967 Biochemical investigation of an unusual case of glycogenosis. Journal of Pediatrics 71: 225

Powell H C, Haas R, Hall C L, Wolff J A, Nyhan W, Brown B I 1985 Peripheral nerve in type III glycogenosis: selective involvement of unmyelinated fiber Schwann cells. Muscle and Nerve 8: 667

Radom J, Salvayre R, Negre' A, Maret A, Douste-Blazy L 1987 Metabolism of neutral lipids in cultured fibroblasts from multisystemic (or type 3) lipid storage myopathy. European Journal of Biochemistry 164: 703

Rebouche C J, Engel A G 1984 Kinetic compartmental analysis of carnitine metabolism in the human carnitine deficiency syndromes: evidence for alterations in tissue carnitine transport. Journal of Clinical Investigation 73: 857

Reuser A J J, Kroos M, Willemsen R, Swallow D, Tager J M, Galjaard H 1987 Clinical diversity in glycogenosis type II. Biosynthesis and in situ localization of acid alpha-glucosidase in mutant fibroblasts. Journal of Clinical Investigation 79: 1689

Riggs J E, Schochet S S, Gutmann L, Shanske S, Neal W A, DiMauro S 1983 Lysosomal glycogen storage disease without acid maltase deficiency. Neurology 33: 873

Rosa R, Claude G, Fardeau M, Calvin M C, Rapin M, Rosa J 1982 A new case of phosphoglycerate kinase deficiency: P G K Creteil associated with rhabdomyolysis and lacking hemolytic anemia. Blood 60: 84

Rowland L P, Layzer R B, DiMauro S 1986a Pathophysiology of metabolic disorders. In: Asbury A K, McKhann G M, McDonald W I (eds) Diseases of the nervous system, vol 1. W B Saunders, Philadelphia, p 197

Rowland L P, Layzer R B, DiMauro S 1986b Phosphofructokinase deficiency. In: Engel A G, Banker B Q (eds) Myology. McGraw-Hill, vol 2. New York, p 1603

Sakoda S, Shanske S, DiMauro S, Schon E A 1988 Isolation of a cDNA encoding the B isozyme of human phosphoglycerate mutase (PGAM) and characterization of the PGAM gene family. Journal of Biological Chemistry 263: 16899

Sancho S, Navarro C, Fernandez J M, Dominguez C, Ortega A, Roig M, Cervera C 1990 Skin biopsy findings in glycogenosis type III: Clinical, biochemical, and electrophysiological correlations. Annals of Neurology 27: 480

Schimrigk K, Mertens H G, Ricker K, Fuhr J, Eyer P, Pette D 1967 McArdle syndrome (Myopathie bei fehlender Muskelphosphorylase). Klinische Wochenschrifte 45: 1

Schmidt R, Mahler R 1959 Chronic progressive myopathy with myoglobinuria: demonstration of a glycogenolytic defect in the muscle. Journal of Clinical Investigation 38: 2044

Schmidt B, Servidei S, Gabbai A A, Silva A C, Sousa Boulle de Oliveira A, DiMauro S 1987 McArdle disease in two generations: autosomal recessive transmission with manifesting heterozygote. Neurology 37: 1558

Serratrice G, Monges A, Roux H, Aquaron R, Gambarelli D 1969 Forme myopatique du deficit en phosphofructokinase. Revue Neurologique 120: 271

Servidei S, DiMauro S 1989 Disorders of glycogen metabolism of muscle. Neurologic Clinics 7: 159

Servidei S, Bonilla E, Diedrich R G et al 1986 Fatal infantile form of phosphofructokinase deficiency. Neurology 36: 1465

Servidei S, Riepe R E, Langston C et al 1987a Severe cardiopathy in branching enzyme deficiency. Journal of Pediatrics 111: 51

Servidei S, Metlay L A, Chodosh J, DiMauro S 1987b Fatal infantile cardiopathy due to phosphorylase b kinase deficiency. Journal of Pediatrics 113: 82

Servidei S, Shanske S, Zeviani M, Lebo R, Fletterick R, DiMauro S 1988 McArdle disease: biochemical and molecular genetic studies. Annals of Neurology 24: 774

Shanske S, Sakoda S, Hermodson M A, DiMauro S, Schon E A 1987 Isolation of cDNA encoding the muscle-specific subunit of human phosphoglycerate mutase. Journal of Biological Chemistry 262: 14 612

Singh R, Shepherd I M, Derrick J P, Ramsay R R, Sherratt H S A, Turnbull D M 1988 A case of carnitine palmitoyltransferase II deficiency in human skeletal muscle. FEBS Letters 241: 126

Slonim A E, Goans P J 1985 Myopathy in McArdle syndrome: improvement with a high-protein diet. New England Journal of Medicine 312: 355

Slonim A E, Coleman R A, McElligot M A et al 1983 Improvement in muscle function in acid maltase deficiency by high-protein therapy. Neurology 33: 34

Slonim A E, Coleman R A, Moses S W 1984 Myopathy and growth failure in debrancher enzyme deficiency:

improvement with high-protein nocturnal enteral therapy. Journal of Pediatrics 105: 906

Smit G P A, Fernandes J, Leonard J V, Matthews E E, Moses S W, Odievre M, Ullrich K 1990 The long-term outcome of patients with glycogen storage diseases. Journal of Inherited Metabolic Diseases 13: 411

Solomon E, Swallow D, Burgess S, Evans L 1979 Assignment of the human acid alpha-glucosidase gene to chromosome 17 using somatic cell hybrids. Annals of Human Genetics 42: 273

Stanley C A 1987 New genetic defects in mitochondrial fatty acid oxidation and carnitine deficiency. Advances in Pediatrics 34: 59

Sugie H, Sugie Y, Nishida M, Masataka I, Tsurui S, Suzuki M, Miyamoto R, Igarashi Y 1989 Recurrent myoglobinuria in a child with mental retardation: phosphoglycerate kinase deficiency. Journal of Child Neurology 4: 95

Tein I, Demaugre F, Bonnefont J P, Saudubray J M 1989 Normal muscle CPT1 and CPT2 activities in hepatic presentation patients with CPT1 deficiency in fibroblasts. Tissue specific isoforms of CPT1? Journal of the Neurological Sciences 92: 229

Tein I, DeVivo D C, Bierman F et al 1990a Impaired skin fibroblast carnitine uptake in primary systemic carnitine deficiency manifested by childhood carnitine-responsive cardiomyopathy. Pediatric Research 28: 247

Tein I, DiMauro S, DeVivo D C 1990b Recurrent childhood myoglobinuria. Advances in Pediatrics 37: 77

Tein I, DeVivo D C, Clarke J T R, Zinman H, Laxer R, DiMauro S 1990c Short-chain L-3-hydroxyacyl-CoA dehydrogenase deficiency: a new cause for recurrent myoglobinuria and encephalopathy. Annals of Neurology (in press)

Tonin P, Shanske S, Brownell A K, Wyse J P, DiMauro S 1989 Phosphoglycerate kinase (PGK) deficiency: a third case with recurrent myoglobinuria. Neurology 39 (suppl 1): 359

Tonin P, Lewis P, Servidei S, DiMauro S 1990 Metabolic causes of myoglobinuria. Annals of Neurology 27: 181

Treem W R, Witzleben C A, Piccoli D A, Stanley C A, Hale D E, Coates P M, Watkins J B 1986 Medium-chain and long-chain acylCoA dehydrogenase deficiency: clinical, pathologic and ultrastructural differentiation from Reye's syndrome. Hepatology 6: 1270

Treem W R, Stanley C A, Finegold D N, Hale D E, Coates P M 1988 Primary carnitine deficiency due to a failure of carnitine transport in kidney, muscle and fibroblasts. New England Journal of Medicine 319: 1331

Turnbull D M, Bartlett K, Stevens D L et al 1984 Short-chain acylCoA dehydrogenase deficiency associated with a lipid storage myopathy and secondary carnitine deficiency. New England Journal of Medicine 311: 1232

Ugawa Y, Inoue K, Takemura T, Iwamasa T 1986 Accumulation of glycogen in sural nerve axons in adult-onset type III glycogenosis. Annals of Neurology 19: 294

Umpleby A M, Trend P St J, Chubb D et al 1989 The effect of a high protein diet on leucine and alanine turnover in acid maltase deficiency. Journal of Neurology, Neurosurgery and Psychiatry 52: 954

van der Berg I E T, Berger R 1990 Phosphorylase b kinase deficiency in man: a review. Journal of Inherited Metabolic Diseases 13: 442

van der Ploeg A T, Loonen M C B, Bolhuis P A, Busch H M F, Reuser A J J, Galjaard H 1988 Receptor mediated uptake of acid alpha-glucosidase corrects lysosomal storage in cultured skeletal muscle. Pediatric Research 24: 90

van der Ploeg A T, Hoefsloot L J, Hoogeveen-Westerveld M, Petersen E, Reuser A J J 1989 Glycogenosis type II: protein and DNA analysis in five South African families from various ethnic origins. American Journal of Human Genetics 44: 787

van Hoof F, Hers H G 1967 The subgroups of type III glycogenosis. European Journal of Biochemistry 2: 265

van Keuren M, Drabkin H, Hart I, Harker D, Patterson D, Vora S 1986 Regional assignment of human liver-type 6-phosphofructokinase to chromosome 21q22.3 by using somatic cell hybrids and a monoclonal anti-L antibody. Human Genetics 74: 34

Vita G, Toscano A, Bresolin N, Meola G, Barbiroli B, Baradello A, Messina C 1990 Muscle phosphoglycerate mutase (PGAM) deficiency in the first Caucasian patient. Neurology 40 (suppl 1): 296

Vora S, Durham S, de Martinville B, George D L, Francke U 1982 Assignment of the human gene for muscle-type phosphofructokinase (PFKM) to chromosome 1 (region cen-q32) using somatic cell hybrids and monoclonal anti-M antibody. Somatic Cell Genetics 8: 95

Vora S, Miranda A F, Hernandez E, Francke U 1983a Regional assignment of the human gene for platelet-type phosphofructokinase (PFKP) to chromosome 10p: novel use of polyspecific rodent antisera to localize human enzyme genes. Human Genetics 63: 374

Vora S, Davidson M, Seaman C et al 1983b Heterogeneity of the molecular lesions in inherited phosphofructokinase deficiency. Journal of Clinical Investigation 72: 1995

Vora S, DiMauro S, Spear D, Harker D, Danon M J 1987 Characterization of the enzymatic defect in late-onset muscle phosphofructokinase deficiency; a new sub-type of glycogen storage disease type VII. Journal of Clinical Investigation 80: 1479

Wanders R J A, Duran M, Ijlst L et al 1989 Sudden infant death and long-chain 3-hydroxyacyl-CoA dehydrogenase. Lancet ii: 52

Waterbury L, Frenkel E P 1972 Hereditary non-spherocytic hemolysis with erythrocytes phosphofructokinase deficiency. Blood 39: 415

Watmough N J, Bindoff L A, Birch-Machin M A et al 1990 Impaired mitochondrial beta-oxidation in a patient with an abnormality of the respiratory chain. Journal of Clinical Investigation 85: 177

Weil D, Cong N V, Gross M S, Frezal J 1979 Localization du gene de l'alpha-glucosidase acide sur le segment 21 qter du chromosome 17 par l'hybridation cellulaire interspecifique. Human Genetics 52: 249

Zellweger H, Mueller S, Ionasescu V, Schochet S S, McCormick W F 1972 Glycogenosis IV: a new cause of infantile hypotonia. Journal of Pediatrics 80: 842

12. Inflammatory myopathies

F. L. Mastaglia   J. N. Walton

INTRODUCTION

The inflammatory myopathies are the largest group of acquired myopathies of adult life and may also occur during infancy and childhood. They represent a heterogeneous group of conditions having in common the presence of inflammatory infiltrates in the skeletal muscles, usually in association with muscle fibre destruction. For practical purposes they can be subdivided into those which are due to a known viral, bacterial, protozoal or other microbial agent, and those in which no such agent can be identified and in which immunological mechanisms are involved or have been implicated. The latter group includes the various forms of polymyositis and dermatomyositis, which in non-tropical regions are the commonest of the inflammatory myopathies, and which are collectively referred to as the *idiopathic inflammatory myopathies*. A classification of the inflammatory myopathies is given in Table 12.1.

While the hallmark of these conditions is the presence of an inflammatory infiltrate, the mere presence of inflammatory cells in a muscle biopsy does not, in itself, necessarily indicate that the basic process is an inflammatory one. Thus mononuclear phagocytic cells within or in the immediate vicinity of necrotic muscle fibres may be observed in focal traumatic lesions (e.g. 'needle myopathy') or in necrotizing myopathies such as Duchenne dystrophy. Focal interstitial or perivascular accumulations of mononuclear inflammatory cells may also be found in denervated (Mastaglia & Walton 1971, Jennekens et al 1975) or dystrophic muscle, as in certain cases of facioscapulohumeral muscular dystrophy (Munsat et al 1972, Bacq et al 1985), and are considered to be 'reactive' or

Table 12.1 Classification of the inflammatory myopathies

A. Due to an infective agent
Viral
Bacterial
Fungal
Protozoal
Helminthic

B. Idiopathic
Generalized
  Polymyositis
  Dermatomyositis
  Inclusion-body myositis
  Granulomatous myositis
  Eosinophilic myositis

Focal
  Focal interstitial myositis
  Focal eosinophilic myositis
  Localized nodular myositis
  Monomelic myositis
  Orbital myositis
  Inflammatory pseudotumour
  Proliferative myositis

secondary in nature. This chapter is concerned with those conditions in which muscle inflammation is part of an infective process or is thought to be of importance in the pathogenesis of the muscle damage.

INFLAMMATORY MYOPATHIES DUE TO MICROBIAL AGENTS AND PARASITES

Viral infections

A variety of DNA and RNA viruses can cause an acute myopathy (Table 12.2). The resulting clinical syndromes range from a localized self-limited form of myositis to a more generalized necrotizing myopathy associated with myoglobinuria (*acute*

Table 12.2 Syndromes of acute viral myositis and causative agents

Benign acute myositis
Influenza A & B
Parainfluenza
Adenovirus 2

Acute myoglobinuric myositis
Influenza A & B
Parainfluenza 3
Coxsackie A9, B2, B3, B5
Echovirus 9
Adenovirus 21
Herpes simplex 2
Epstein–Barr virus

Epidemic pleurodynia
Coxsackie B1, B3, B4, B5

rhabdomyolysis). Certain viruses have also been implicated in the pathogenesis of some cases of chronic myositis and certain congenital muscle disorders.

Post-influenzal myositis

In addition to the diffuse myalgia which occurs during an attack of influenza, a post-influenzal form of myositis may occur and is well-documented in the literature (Lundberg 1957, Middleton et al 1970, Chou 1988). This distinctive syndrome usually occurs during the first week after an attack of influenza. It is characterized by severe pain, tenderness, and sometimes swelling of the calf muscles, but sometimes also of the thigh and upper limb muscles, and usually resolves completely over the course of about one week. Serum creatine kinase (CK) levels are usually elevated.

Muscle biopsy shows scattered segmental muscle fibre necrosis and in some cases, regenerative activity, even in some clinically unaffected muscles, but these changes are not always present (Farrell et al 1980). The inflammatory infiltrate, which consists of polymorphonuclear and mononuclear cells, particularly in a perivascular distribution, is usually sparse and may be absent in some biopsies. Electron microscopy does not show viral particles in muscle fibres but distinctive intracytoplasmic vacuoles with internal 'filopodial' microvilli have been described in some cases (Bore et al 1983, Chou 1988).

The syndrome has been reported particularly in children during outbreaks of influenza A or B infection (Middleton et al 1970, Mejlszenkier et al 1973, Dietzman et al 1976) but sporadic cases may also occur in adults (Congy et al 1980). The pathogenesis of this form of myositis is uncertain. Direct invasion of muscle by the virus has been postulated, and the susceptibility of human muscle to the virus has been demonstrated in tissue culture (Armstrong et al 1978). However, attempts to isolate the virus from muscle biopsy specimens have usually been unsuccessful.

Acute myoglobinuric viral myositis

A number of different viruses may rarely cause a more widespread form of acute myositis and rhabdomyolysis with associated myoglobinaemia and myoglobinuria leading, in some cases, to acute oliguric renal failure (Mastaglia & Ojeda 1985, Chou 1988). The influenza A virus has been most frequently implicated and, less often, influenza B, parainfluenza 3, Coxsackievirus B2, B3, B5, A9, Echovirus 9, adenovirus 21, herpes simplex type 2, and Epstein–Barr virus as well as *Mycoplasma pneumoniae*.

The condition develops during the febrile phase of the viral illness and is characterized by diffuse myalgia, muscle tenderness, weakness and at times swelling, especially of proximal muscle groups; myoglobinuria leading to discoloration of the urine is usually an early feature. Serum CK levels are markedly elevated. Although most patients recover, the condition may have a fatal outcome, particularly in elderly patients who develop renal failure or other complications. The biopsy findings in reported cases were of scattered muscle fibre necrosis and, in some cases associated regenerative activity and a mild inflammatory cellular infiltrate which may, however, be absent (Chou 1988). The condition is presumed to result from direct viral invasion leading to cytolysis of muscle fibres. However, a viral agent has only rarely been isolated from muscle in such cases (Gamboa et al 1979).

Epidemic pleurodynia

Epidemic pleurodynia, or Bornholm disease, is a

localized form of myositis of the muscles of the chest or abdominal wall and, less frequently, the back or shoulder muscles, which can result from infection by a number of different strains of Coxsackie B virus (B1, 3, 4, 5). Children are more often affected than adults and the condition is characterized by the acute onset of severe localized myalgia and muscle tenderness which is aggravated by breathing, coughing or movement, and which is usually accompanied by fever, headache and symptoms of an upper respiratory tract infection. There are few reports of muscle biopsy findings in the literature. An acute inflammatory reaction has been found in some cases (Lepine et al 1952) while others have had normal biopsy findings.

Reye's syndrome

The finding in some cases of Reye's syndrome of muscle changes similar to those occurring in the liver, namely accumulation of fatty droplets and mitochondrial swelling, led to the suggestion that there may also be a viral myositis in this condition (Hanson & Urizar 1977, Alvira & Mendoza 1985). An influenza A virus was isolated from muscle in a case of Reye's syndrome in which virions were also identified in muscle fibres by electron microscopy (Partin et al 1976). However, other reports of picornavirus–like paracrystalline arrays in post mortem specimens of muscle are now considered to represent artefacts due to ribosomal crystallization or to the formation of glycogen complexes (Chou 1988).

Chronic viral infections

Although a number of viruses have been implicated in cases of chronic inflammatory myopathy, virus isolation from muscle has been only rarely reported. Several different strains of Echovirus have been isolated from cerebrospinal fluid or, rarely, from muscle in patients with an X-linked recessive agammaglobulinaemia with associated meningoencephalitis and a dermatomyositis–like syndrome (Mease et al 1981, Crennan et al 1986).

Coxsackie group A viruses, which are strongly myotropic in suckling mice, were isolated in two rather atypical cases of chronic myositis in an infant and an 11-year-old girl (see Tang et al

1975). Serological evidence of Coxsackie B virus infection has been found in some cases of dermatomyositis or polymyositis and the presence of enterovirus RNA has been demonstrated in muscle biopsy specimens from some cases of dermatomyositis and polymyositis using in situ hybridization techniques (Bowles et al 1987, Rosenberg et al 1989). An experimental model with clinical and histological similarities to human polymyositis has been induced by inoculation of mice with certain strains of Coxsackie B1 virus (Strongwater et al 1984, Ytterberg 1987).

Intrauterine viral infections

Experimental studies have shown that prenatal infection with Coxsackie A2 virus in chick embryos (Drachman et al 1976) or Akabane virus (an Arbovirus) in calves and hamsters causes severe myositis with arthrogrypotic deformities (Sato et al 1980). These observations have led to the suggestion that an intrauterine viral infection may be responsible for certain cases of arthrogryposis or infantile polymyositis in humans (Kinoshita et al 1980).

Post-viral fatigue-myalgia syndrome

This debilitating syndrome is a not uncommon sequel to infection with various viruses, in particular influenza, Epstein–Barr, herpes and enteroviruses (e.g. Coxsackie B virus). Routine histological and histochemical examination of muscle tissue in this condition is usually normal although mild non-specific changes in muscle fibre ultrastructure have been reported (Aström et al 1982). In one study it was found that about 30% of patients with this condition had Coxsackie B virus-specific IgM antibodies in the serum, while in another series approximately 20% of cases were found to have enterovirus-specific RNA in muscle biopsy specimens (Archard et al 1988, Yousef et al 1988).

Acquired immunodeficiency syndrome (AIDS)

Up to 80% of patients with HIV infection develop a clinical or subclinical neuromuscular disorder (Dalakas & Pezeshkpour 1988, Dalakas et al 1989).

Table 12.3 Neuromuscular disorders associated with HIV infection

Myopathies
Polymyositis
Giant cell myositis
Rod body myopathy
Necrotizing myopathy with microvesicular change
Proximal weakness with type II fibre atrophy
Zidovudine myopathy

Neuropathies
Guillain–Barré syndrome
Chronic inflammatory demyelinating
Mononeuritis multiplex
Small fibre axonal sensory neuropathy
Large fibre ataxic neuropathy
Cauda equina syndrome
Myeloradiculoneuropathy

The disorders that have been reported in patients with AIDS are listed in Table 12.3

Of the myopathies, the most frequently encountered is an inflammatory myopathy which resembles polymyositis both clinically and histopathologically (Dalakas & Pezeshkpour 1988, Lange et al 1988, Simpson & Bender 1988, Dalakas et al 1990). This may occur in patients with AIDS or the AIDS-related complex, as well as in individuals who are HIV-negative at the time of presentation (Simpson & Bender 1988). The severity of the histological changes in muscle biopsies has varied in reported cases, some having florid necrosis and inflammatory cellular infiltration while in other cases these changes have been inconspicuous (Fig. 12.1). It has been shown that the majority of the perivascular and endomysial infiltrating cells are CD8$^+$ (suppressor-cytotoxic) lymphocytes or macrophages suggesting that the myopathy is T-cell-mediated (Dalakas et al 1990). As in polymyositis and inclusion body myositis (see below) invasion of muscle fibres by these cells can be demonstrated (Fig. 12.2). In some cases the presence of HIV in some of the interstitial inflammatory cells has been demonstrated using immunocytochemical techniques. However, attempts to demonstrate the virus with in situ hybridization techniques have so far been unsuccessful (Dalakas & Pezeshkpour 1988, Simpson & Bender 1988). While it therefore seems likely that the inflammatory myopathy associated with AIDS is immunologically-mediated, it remains unclear whether direct invasion of muscle by the virus plays any part in initiating the autoimmune attack.

In one reported case in which multinucleated giant cells were a prominent feature in the muscle lesions a direct HIV infection of muscle was postulated (Bailey et al 1987). In another patient with HIV infection and polymyositis, HIV could not be demonstrated in muscle but evidence of muscle infection with HTLV-1 was found (Wiley et al 1989), as has also been found in other patients with associated polymyositis and HTLV-1-associated myelopathy (Evans et al 1989, Masson et al 1989, Salazar–Grueso et al 1990). A necrotizing inflammatory myopathy has also been found to occur in about 50% of primates with simian AIDS due to infection with the SRV-1 retrovirus (Dalakas et al 1986). The virus was isolated from affected muscles in these animals, and was shown to infect muscle cultures.

In other AIDS patients with a proximal myopathic syndrome the myopathy has been non-inflammatory with granular fibre degeneration, fibre atrophy, rod-body formation and prominent cytoplasmic bodies in some cases (Dalakas & Pezeshkpour 1988, Simpson & Bender 1988, Simpson et al 1990, Panegyres et al 1990). Panegyres et al (1990) have also described a necrotizing myopathy with an unusual segmental microvesicular change due to dilatation of the sarcoplasmic reticulum in some AIDS patients (Fig. 12.1). Muscle biopsies from AIDS patients with a myopathy may also show neurogenic changes if there is an associated peripheral neuropathy or myeloradiculoneuropathy (Bailey et al 1987, Lange et al 1988, Dalakas & Pezeshkpour 1988, Verma et al 1990).

Bacterial myositis

Acute suppurative myositis

Suppurative myositis is uncommon but may complicate penetrating or crush injuries, decubitus skin lesions, osteomyelitis, infectious arthritis or septicaemia, or may develop spontaneously. It is more frequent in tropical and sub-tropical regions where it is referred to as *pyomyositis*. This is more frequent in men than in women, and usually develops without any antecedent illness although

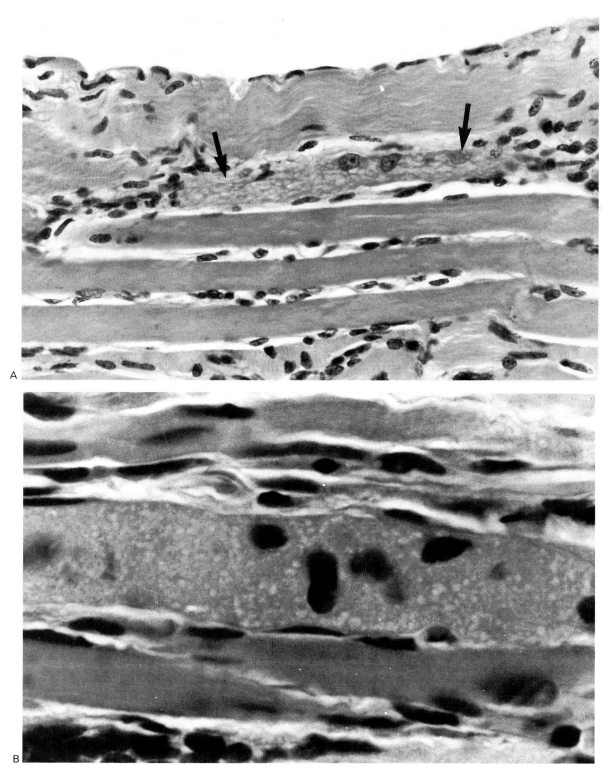

Fig. 12.1   AIDS myopathy. (A) Interstitial infiltration with mononuclear cells; muscle fibre showing vesicular degeneration (arrows). H&E, ×595. (B) Muscle fibre showing segmental vesicular degeneration and nuclear pyknosis. H&E, ×1510. (B reproduced with permission from Panegyres et al 1990)

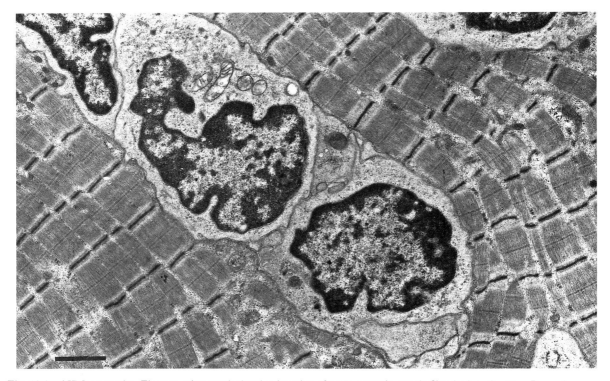

Fig. 12.2 AIDS myopathy. Electron micrograph showing invasion of a non-necrotic muscle fibre by lymphocytes. Bar = 2 μm. (Courtesy of Professor J. M. Papadimitriou)

in some cases there is a history of minor trauma or an upper respiratory tract infection (Chiedozi 1979, Ojeda & Mastaglia 1988a). The organism most frequently involved is *Staphylococcus aureus*. Organisms less frequently involved include group A β-haemolytic streptococci, *Escherichia coli*, *Yersinia* and anaerobes. Single or multiple muscle abscesses may develop. The muscles most frequently affected are the glutei, quadriceps, hamstrings, iliopsoas and shoulder muscles. There is usually a peripheral polymorphonuclear leukocytosis with elevation of the erythrocyte sedimentation rate and, in tropical cases, an eosinophilia. Serum creatine kinase activity may be elevated if there is extensive muscle destruction. Deep-seated lesions may be localized by computerized tomography, ultrasonography or gallium scanning.

Pathologically, in the early stages there is interstitial oedema with a mixed polymorphonuclear and mononuclear cellular infiltrate. Muscle fibres in the centre of the lesions undergo hyaline necrosis and phagocytosis and regeneration may subsequently occur. In the later stages the abscess cavity is surrounded by granulation tissue and there may be irreversible loss of muscle tissue with permanent scarring.

Clostridial myositis (gas gangrene)

Gas gangrene is rare in civilian life but may still occur when there is contamination of open wounds or compound limb fractures by organisms belonging to the clostridial group of anaerobic bacteria (Adams et al 1965, Willis & Willis 1972, Kissane 1985). Less frequently, it may follow clostridial infection of an ulcerated ischaemic limb, intramuscular injections, or intestinal or biliary tract surgery (Ojeda & Mastaglia 1988a). The three major organisms which cause gas gangrene are *Cl. perfringens* (*welchii*), *Cl. novyi* (*oedematiens*) and *Cl. septicum*. The organisms flourish in anaerobic conditions and in the presence of foreign material and necrotic debris and produce multiple exotoxins and enzymes (e.g. haemolysins, lecithinases, collagenase and hyaluronidase). These cause rapidly spreading necrosis of muscle fibres and interstitial tissues, vascular congestion, fibrin exudation, intense polymorphonuclear infiltration and haemorrhage. The inflammatory response is variable and may be minimal or absent in some cases. Muscle regeneration occurs if the infection is controlled and necrotic tissue is removed but is usually ineffective and there is often marked muscular atrophy and fibrosis in survivors.

Other forms

Tuberculous and syphilitic infections of muscle are now rare. Tuberculous infection may occur as a result of spread from a neighbouring site of infection in the spine or chest ('cold abscess') or of haematogenous spread (*miliary tuberculosis*). The latter results in multiple small miliary foci (*tuberculous polymyositis*) and occasionally larger lesions which may produce localized painful muscle swellings. Muscle biopsy may be of diagnostic value in miliary tuberculosis and may demonstrate caseating or non-caseating granulomas containing acid-fast bacilli. Granulomatous lesions, which are usually asymptomatic, may also occur in muscle and in peripheral nerves in some cases of leprosy. The finding of granulomatous inflammation with denervation atrophy in a muscle biopsy should therefore suggest the possibility of Hansen's disease.

A necrotizing inflammatory myopathy with widespread muscle pain and weakness has been described in patients with septicaemia (Hamilton et al 1987). Extensive myonecrosis leading to myoglobinuric acute renal failure has also been reported to occur in some patients with septicaemia (Kalish et al 1982) or pneumococcal pneumonia (Hroncich & Rudinger 1989).

Fungal infections

A number of fungal agents may cause focal or diffuse muscle involvement (Grove 1988). *Candida myositis* may develop as part of disseminated candidiasis and has been reported in patients with acute leukaemia (Jarowski et al 1978). The resulting clinical syndrome is characterized by fever, a papular or erythematous skin rash and diffuse muscle pain and tenderness. A muscle biopsy and staining of sections with methanamine–silver will allow identification of the organism and the institution of appropriate therapy (Kressel et al 1978). The fungus induces necrosis of muscle fibres with surrounding haemorrhage and inflammation, but inflammatory changes may be inconspicuous particularly in immunosuppressed patients.

Localized muscle involvement with abscess and sinus formation may occur in actinomycosis and coccidioidomycosis (Adams et al 1965). Muscle nodules or masses may occur in patients with localized or generalized sporotrichosis.

Protozoal infections

Toxoplasmosis

Myalgia may be a prominent symptom in acute acquired toxoplasmosis in children or adults. However, actual *Toxoplasma* infection of muscle is rare. A multifocal myositis may occur as part of disseminated toxoplasmosis in immunocompromized individuals but meningoencephalitis, myocarditis and pneumonitis are usually more prominent features (Grove 1988). A muscle biopsy may disclose the organism in such cases. Cysts, which are 20 to 60 μm in diameter, and which contain multiple bradyzoites, may be found in healthy muscle fibres in Giemsa–stained sections in patients with latent or chronic infection, and free tachyzoites may also be found interstitially between muscle fibres and may be demonstrated using fluorescein-labelled anti-*Toxoplasma* antibodies (Hendrickx et al 1979). Within the foci of myositis necrotic muscle fibres are surrounded and infiltrated by polymorphonuclear leukocytes, lymphocytes and plasma cells. However, otherwise normal muscle fibres may contain cysts without surrounding inflammation and, conversely, in some areas of intense inflammation parasites may be absent.

A possible link between toxoplasmosis and polymyositis/dermatomyositis has been suggested because of the finding of active *Toxoplasma* infection or, more often, of serological evidence of toxoplasmosis in some cases of polymyositis or dermatomyositis. Magid & Kagen (1983) found raised *Toxoplasma* antibody titres in 50% of 58 patients with polymyositis or dermatomyositis and evidence of recent infection in 24% of cases as shown by the presence of IgM antibodies. The

Table 12.4 Parasitic and fungal infections of muscle*

Fungal
Candidiasis
Actinomycosis
Coccidioidomycosis
Sporotrichosis

Protozoal
Toxoplasmosis
Sarcosporidiosis
Trypanosomiasis
Microsporidiosis
Amoebiasis

Helminthic
Trichinosis
Cysticercosis
Echinococcosis

---

* For further information on clinical aspects of these
  conditions the reader is referred to the reviews by Grove
  (1988) and by Pallis & Lewis (1988).

explanation of this finding remains uncertain. In some cases of dermatomyositis with elevated *Toxoplasma* antibody titres it has been postulated that *Toxoplasma* infection may cause an inflammatory myopathy as a result of the deposition of non-specific immune complexes in the walls of intramuscular blood vessels (Quilis & Damjanov 1982, Schröter et al 1987).

Sarcosporidiosis (Sarcocystosis)

Sarcosporidiosis is the only protozoal infection in which skeletal muscle is the primary site of infection (Grove 1988). Invasion of skeletal muscles by *Sarcocystis* in man is uncommon and is usually asymptomatic, the organism being found in muscle quite accidentally (Adams et al 1965). In some cases, however, there has been muscle aching, tenderness, weakness and loss of tendon reflexes. The parasitic cysts, which are filled with many sporozoites, are initially found within individual muscle fibres (Fig. 12.3) and may enlarge to lengths of 1–5 mm. Inflammatory changes may be inconspicuous.

American trypanosomiasis (Chagas' disease)

In this condition, which is indigenous to South America, there is typically a disseminated focal polymyositis, myocarditis and encephalomyelitis, but more widespread visceral involvement may

also occur (Adams et al 1965). In the muscle, parasites are localized within individual muscle fibres and form small thin-walled cysts which are loaded with trypanosomes and which may be difficult to distinguish from *Toxoplasma* pseudocysts. There is interstitial infiltration with lymphocytes, plasma cells and large mononuclear cells, usually with destruction of muscle fibres and fibrosis (Grove 1988).

Other protozoal infections

Microsporidial myositis has been described in a patient with the acquired immunodeficiency syndrome (Ledford et al 1985). There has also been a report of a patient with an amoebic suppurative necrotizing myositis (Mastaglia & Ojeda 1985). Other organisms such as *Plasmodium falciparum*, which are carried in the blood stream, may sometimes be seen incidentally in muscle sections.

Helminth infections

Trichinosis

This is the most frequent and best-known form of parasitic infection of muscle. The causative agent, *Trichinella spiralis*, is a nematode which is acquired by man as a result of ingesting raw or inadequately processed pork or other types of meat or meat products (Grove 1988). After penetration through the mucosa of the small intestine, the larvae enter the lymphatic system and the bloodstream and are disseminated throughout the body. The stage of muscular invasion begins towards the end of the first week and lasts for several weeks, during which there is myalgia, muscle tenderness and sometimes weakness. This may be generalized or limited to certain muscle groups such as the ocular muscles. Periorbital and conjunctival oedema, chemosis and subconjunctival haemorrhage and in some cases a macular, petechial or urticarial rash, may also occur. In some cases the clinical picture closely resembles that of dermatomyositis (Herrera et al 1985). An eosinophil leukocytosis is present in over 90% of cases and aids diagnosis. Serum CK activity may be elevated.

The diagnosis may be confirmed by muscle biopsy, which will usually demonstrate the para-

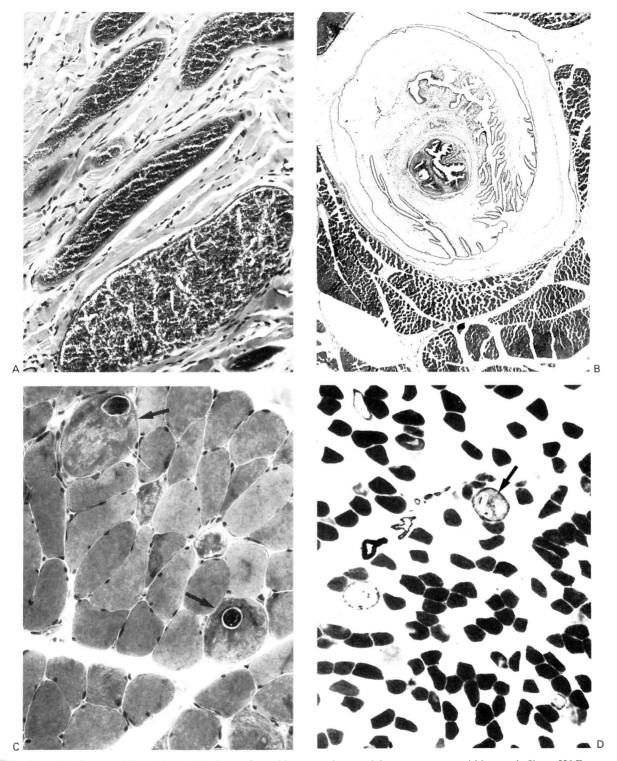

Fig. 12.3   (A) Sarcosporidiosis of muscle in the rat. Several large parasite-containing cysts are seen within muscle fibres. H&E, ×1520. (B) *Cysticercus cellulosae* cyst in pig muscle. H&E, ×38. (C, D) Muscle trichinosis in a 35-year-old woman. Parasites at different stages of development are seen in a number of muscle fibres (arrows). (C) Gomori trichrome, ×304. (D) Myosin ATPase, pH 4.2 ×95

sites at various stages of development and encystment (Fig. 12.3). Individual muscle fibres may undergo segmental necrosis. An interstitial inflammatory infiltrate, mainly of eosinophils and neutrophils with some lymphocytes, plasma cells and other mononuclear cells, is usually prominent around muscle fibres containing the parasites, and also more diffusely in the interstitium and surrounding small blood vessels (Gross & Ochoa 1979). The capsules of the cysts may calcify and the parasites may remain viable for prolonged periods within these capsules, although the greater proportion are thought to die.

Cysticercosis

This condition is common in India and Eastern Europe, being encountered less frequently in other parts of the world, and results from infestation with the encysted larval stage of the tapeworm *Taenia solium* as a result of ingesting raw or inadequately cooked pork (Grove 1988). The larval parasites (*Cystericercus cellulosae*) invade the intestine and undergo haematogenous dissemination to all parts of the body, muscle and brain being common sites of invasion. As in trichinosis, the invasion stage may be associated with muscular tenderness, fever and eosinophilia, although commonly no history of this stage is obtained and evidence of muscular or central nervous system lesions may only be found many years later when the patient presents with a myopathy or with epilepsy or other neurological problems.

In addition to the myalgic form of myopathy, which occurs during the early stages of muscle invasion, pseudohypertrophic and nodular forms of myopathy have also been described (Sawhney et al 1976). In the latter form, nodules may be palpated in the tongue and in other muscles, while in the pseudohypertrophic form (which is probably the rarest) gross hypertrophy of multiple limb muscles may occur, producing a picture which may superficially resemble pseudohypertrophic muscular dystrophy (Sawhney et al 1976).

The cysts, which may be found in a biopsy from an affected muscle, are situated in the interstitial connective tissue septa and may be associated with a mild interstitial infiltrate of neutrophil and eosinophill polymorphonuclear leukocytes and lymphocytes (Adams et al 1965) although this is not always so (Fig. 12.3). The parasites ultimately become calcified after a period of 1–5 years and calcified cysts may be found in muscle radiographs many years after the stage of acute infestation.

Echinococcosis

Muscular echinococcosis is extremely rare and much less frequent than hepatic or pulmonary involvement, even in countries in which hydatid disease is common such as South America, New Zealand, Australia and Iceland. Of 1802 hydatid cysts reported to the Australasian Hydatid Registry, only 5% were in muscle (Grove 1988). In the case of *Echinococcus granulosus*, the embryo parasites lodge in small capillaries in the muscle and subsequently form small cysts which enlarge to reach a diameter of up to one centimetre. The cysts are usually solitary and are surrounded by a zone of granulomatous inflammation and eosinophil infiltration, the surrounding muscle fibres being compressed and atrophic. Rupture of individual cysts may lead to the formation of a large number of daughter cysts. Cysts may continue to enlarge and present as a painless slowly enlarging tumour in the muscle. The muscles most commonly affected are those of the posterior trunk, the inner thigh, the neck and the upper arm.

Muscular involvement due to *Echinococcus alveolaris* is even less frequent, but has been reported from Germany in five members of a family with myotonia congenita (Schimrigk & Emser 1978).

IDIOPATHIC INFLAMMATORY MYOPATHIES

In those parts of the world in which bacterial and parasitic forms of myositis are rare, most cases of myositis encountered in clinical practice fall into the category of 'idiopathic inflammatory myopathy'. This heterogeneous group of conditions includes the various syndromes of polymyositis and dermatomyositis occurring in childhood and adult life, as well as the other forms of inflammatory myopathy listed in Table 12.5.

Table 12.5 Classification of polymyositis (PM) and dermatomyositis (DM)

Childhood
Infantile myositis
Juvenile DM

Adult life
Isolated PM
Isolated DM
PM or DM associated with malignancy
PM or DM associated with connective tissue diseases
PM or DM associated with immune deficiency states
PM or DM associated with other systemic disorders
Drug-induced PM or DM
Inclusion body myositis

Polymyositis and dermatomyositis

Classification

These conditions have been classified in various ways on the basis of the age at presentation, clinical and histopathological features, associated conditions and proposed pathogenetic mechanisms (Walton & Adams 1958, Barwick & Walton 1963, World Federation of Neurology 1968, Bohan & Peter 1975, Carpenter & Karpati 1981, Mastaglia & Ojeda 1985). The ultimate classification awaits further clarification of the aetiopathogenesis. The classification in Table 12.5 separates conditions that have distinctive clinical or pathological features or that are thought to have different underlying mechanisms or initiating factors.

Clinical features

These conditions may occur at any age from infancy and throughout adult life, but particularly in the fifth and sixth decades. The overall incidence is of the order of 4–5 per million population (Rose & Walton 1966, Medsger et al 1970). Women are more frequently affected than men (DeVere & Bradley 1975, Pearson & Bohan 1977). The conditions vary in their mode of onset, rate of progression, and in the presence and extent of dermal, particular and other manifestations.

In the most *acute cases*, profound generalized muscle weakness, pain and tenderness develop over a period of days with markedly elevated serum enzyme levels and myoglobinuria which may lead to acute oliguric renal failure (Walton 1964, Pirovino et al 1979). These patients are acutely ill, often with high fever, dysphagia and joint pains, and in some cases these is oedema of the limbs and face (Walton 1965). In some cases there is an associated malignancy (e.g. of the breast or lung). The condition must be distinguished from other forms of acute rhabdomyolysis due to drugs, toxins, metabolic disturbances, or viral infections (see above).

In *subacute cases* of polymyositis and dermatomyositis, which may occur in isolation or in association with a malignancy or a collagen–vascular disease the condition evolves over a period of weeks or months and there is non-selective weakness, particularly of the pelvic and shoulder-girdle muscles, which is out of proportion to the degree of muscular atrophy. The neck muscles are frequently weak, while the facial and ocular muscles are rarely involved (Arnett & Michels 1973). The tendon reflexes are preserved and often surprisingly brisk (Walton 1965).

The skin changes in typical cases of dermatomyositis include an erythematous rash in a 'butterfly' distribution on the face, a lilac (heliotrope) discoloration of the upper eyelids and periorbital areas, an erythematous rash with dermal scaling and atrophy over the dorsal aspects of the metacarpophalangeal and interphalangeal joints (*Gottron's papules*), and periungual erythema and telangiectasis. A similar rash may be present over the knees, elbows and malleoli. In chronic cases, particularly in childhood, subcutaneous calcification (*calcinosis cutis*) may occur over the heels, elbows and knuckles and sometimes more diffusely over the limbs.

Dysphagia, Raynaud's phenomenon and articular symptoms are common in patients with subacute polymyositis and dermatomyositis, especially in cases with an associated collagen–vascular disease (Walton 1965). Cardiac involvement leading to arrhythmias, heart block or cardiac failure may occur in some cases, as may pulmonary and other systemic manifestations (Mastaglia & Ojeda 1985, Plotz et al 1989). In juvenile dermatomyositis there may be an associated systemic vasculitis leading to ischaemic lesions in other organs such as the gastrointestinal tract (Banker & Victor 1966).

In the *chronic form* of polymyositis the onset is

insidious and the clinical course may extend over many years, with slowly progressive weakness and atrophy often involving the distal as well as the proximal limb and girdle muscles. Such cases usually respond poorly to treatment with corticosteroids and other immunosuppressive agents. It is likely that many such patients have *inclusion-body myositis* (p. 475).

Occasional cases of polymyositis are atypical clinically. These include cases in which the facial muscles are affected as part of a *facioscapulohumeral* syndrome (Rothstein et al 1971, Bates et al 1973). Such cases are to be distinguished from familial cases of facioscapulohumeral muscular dystrophy with a prominent inflammatory reaction in the muscles (Munsat et al 1972). Other unusual presentations include patients in whom the muscular involvement is confined to a single muscle (Ruff & Seattle 1983), to one limb (*monomelic myositis*) (Stark 1978), or to the lower limbs for prolonged periods and others with focal myositis presenting with localized painful swellings in one or more limb muscles (*localized nodular myositis*) (Cumming et al 1977, Heffner & Barron 1981). Most cases of this type go on to develop a more diffuse form of polymyositis (Cumming et al 1977).

Diagnosis

Confirmation of the diagnosis of polymyositis depends upon the finding of increased serum levels of CK (Vignos & Goldwyn 1972) and of myoglobin (Kagen 1977, Nishikai & Reichlin 1977), which are indices of muscle fibre destruction; the finding of typical electromyographic changes in limb and paraspinal muscles (Walton & Adams 1958, Barwick & Walton 1963, DeVere & Bradley 1975); and ultimately on the demonstration of a necrotizing inflammatory myopathy by muscle biopsy. A proximal upper or lower limb muscle which has not previously been examined electromyographically is most suitable for biopsy. It has been suggested that ^{99m}Tc polyphosphate muscle scanning may help in choosing the biopsy site (Brown et al 1976) but this technique is not widely used. An open or conchotome biopsy is preferable to a needle biopsy because a larger tissue sample can be taken (see Ch. 2), thereby

making it less likely that the biopsy may miss a muscle lesion. However, even with an open biopsy and careful selection of the biopsy site, in a small proportion of cases the biopsy is normal, reflecting the focal nature of the muscle lesions.

Histopathology

The histological hallmark of these conditions is the finding of muscle fibre necrosis and regeneration (occurring pari passu), and the presence of interstitial and perivascular infiltrates of mononuclear inflammatory cells. In cases of active polymyositis or dermatomyositis before treatment all of these changes are usually found; however in early, mild or partially treated cases not all of the changes may be present.

The patterns and severity of the histological changes vary in the different clinical subgroups. In the most acute cases of polymyositis or dermatomyositis there may be extensive necrosis and breakdown of a large proportion of muscle fibres (*acute rhabdomyolysis*) (Fig. 12.4A). In such cases there is usually also evidence of profuse regenerative activity, with active myoblast and myotube formation within the sarcolemmal tubes of muscle fibres which have undergone necrosis and phagocytosis. Inflammatory changes may be absent or inconspicuous in such cases, although a careful search of serial sections from different tissue blocks will usually disclose an infiltrate of lymphocytes, plasma cells, histiocytes and sometimes polymorphonuclear leukocytes in the endomysium and perimysium as well as mononuclear phagocytic cells within necrotic muscle fibres.

In the more common subacute and chronic cases of polymyositis or dermatomyositis the histopathological changes are of variable severity and certain basic differences in the patterns of muscle fibre necrosis and inflammatory infiltration can be recognized between cases of polymyositis and dermatomyositis (Table 12.6) although there is some overlap between the two groups (Carpenter & Karpati 1981, Ringel et al 1986, Comola et al 1987, Rosenberg & Ringel 1988).

In *polymyositis* there is usually scattered necrosis of single muscle fibres, which appear hyalinized or show loss of staining in the early stages and are subsequently invaded by mononuclear phagocytic

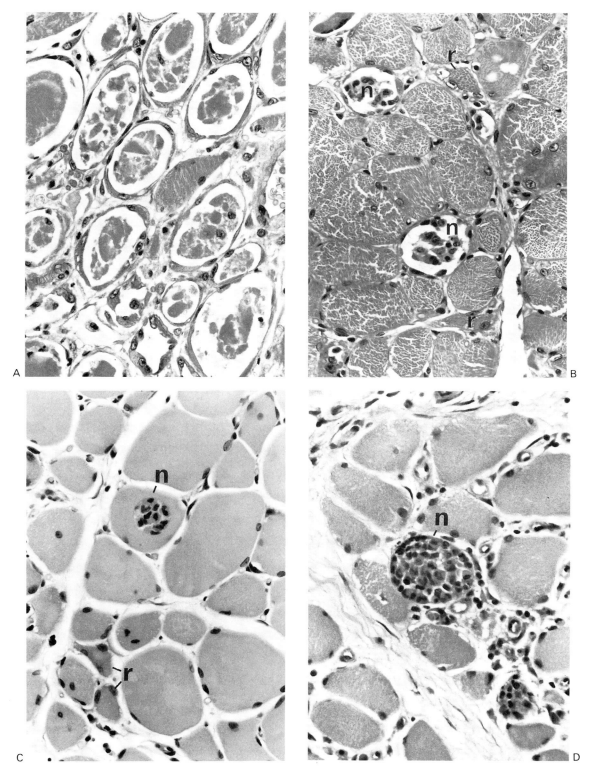

Fig. 12.4   (A) Extensive muscle fibre necrosis and early regeneration in a 61-year-old man with acute myositis associated with bronchogenic carcinoma. H&E, ×348. (B, C, D) Single fibre necrosis (n) and phagocytosis in cases of adult polymyositis. r = regenerating fibres. H&E, ×348

Table 12.6   Major histopathological features of polymyositis, dermatomyositis and inclusion-body myositis

	Polymyositis	Adult dermatomyositis	Juvenile dermatomyositis	Inclusion-body myositis
Myofibre necrosis	Single fibres	Single fibres or groups	Single fibres or groups; microinfarcts	Single fibres (sparse)
Perifascicular atrophy	—	Yes	Common	—
Rimmed vacuoles	—	—	—	Common
Filamentous inclusions	—	—	—	Common
Capillary numbers	Normal	Reduced	Reduced	Normal or increased
Microvascular changes	—	Yes	Common	—
Inflammatory infiltrates	EM>PM/PV	PM/PV>EM	PM/PV>EM	EM>PV/PM
Autoinvasive CD8$^+$ cells	Common	Rare	Rare	Common

EM = endomysial; PM = perimysial; PV = perivascular.

cells (Figs 12.4, 12.5). Basophilic fibres at various stages of regeneration are also seen singly or in small groups distributed focally and randomly throughout the muscle. Muscle fibre breakdown and regeneration may be occurring pari passu in the same or in adjoining muscle fibres. The inflammatory cell infiltrate is predominantly intra-fascicular (endomysial), surrounding muscle fibres, rather than in the interfascicular septa although perivascular infiltrates may also be found. The inflammatory cells consist mainly of lymphocytes, plasma cells and macrophages. Lymphocytes and macrophages may be seen at the periphery of non-necrotic muscle fibres and focal invasion of muscle fibres by these cells is a characteristic finding. Electron microscopy shows that the processes of these cells may extend into the muscle fibre without loss of cell membrane integrity (Fig. 12.5) (Mastaglia & Currie 1971).

Immunocytochemical studies using monoclonal antibody markers have shown that most of the lymphocytes in the cellular infiltrates are activated T cells with a mixture of CD8$^+$ (suppressor/cytotoxic) and CD4$^+$ (helper–inducer) cells, as well as macrophages (Rowe et al 1981, Giorno et al 1984, Engel & Arahata 1984, Arahata & Engel 1984, Olsson et al 1985, Arahata & Engel 1986). The immunoelectron-microscopic studies of Arahata & Engel (1986) have shown that most of the mononuclear cells invading non-necrotic muscle fibres are CD8$^+$ cytotoxic lymphocytes which are at times associated with macrophages. In these studies it was found that the CD8$^+$ cells were closely apposed to muscle fibres and that spike-like processes of these cells invaginated the plasma membrane of non-necrotic muscle fibres and induced the formation of honeycomb arrays

(Fig. 12.5C). These observations support the previous evidence that cell-mediated cytotoxicity is responsible for the muscle fibre injury in poly-myositis and are similar to those described previously in muscle homografts undergoing rejection and following the addition of cytotoxic lymphocytes to muscle cultures (Mastaglia et al 1974, 1975). The demonstration of class I MHC antigen expression on the surface of non-necrotic muscle fibres being invaded by lymphocytes (Karpati et al 1988, Emslie-Smith et al 1989) is also in accord with the view that the muscle fibre damage in polymyositis is caused by cytotoxic T lymphocytes as these cells require the presence of class I MHC molecules on target cells to exert their action.

In *dermatomyositis*, particularly in juvenile patients, isolated muscle fibre necrosis is a rare finding. More often, portions of a muscle fascicle, or even entire fascicles of muscle fibres as well as interstitial tissues may be necrotic and the lesions resemble microinfarcts (Figs 12.6, 12.7). Other characteristic findings include *perifascicular atrophy* (Fig. 12.8) in which there is non-selective atrophy of type I and II fibres at the periphery of muscle fascicles, and central areas of myofibrillar loss resembling cores or core-targetoids in muscle fibres (Fig. 12.6). However, these changes are not necessarily found in all cases. More consistent is the finding of microvascular changes including capillary loss, particularly at the periphery of muscle fascicles (Carpenter & Karpati 1981, De Visser et al 1989, Emslie-Smith & Engel 1990), which is thought to be responsible for the peri-fascicular atrophy, and necrosis and thrombosis of capillaries, arterioles and venules which account for the occurrence of microinfarction. Capillary endothelial cells often show ultrastructural changes such as swelling and the presence of tubuloreticular inclusions (Fig. 12.9). The frequent finding of immunoglobulins and complement components, including the C5b–9 membrane attack complex, in blood vessel walls suggests that the basic process leading to muscle injury in dermatomyositis is an immune complex vasculopathy (Crowe et al 1982, Whitaker & Engel 1972, Kissel et al 1986, De Visser et al 1989, Emslie-Smith & Engel 1990).

In contrast to polymyositis in which the inflammatory cell infiltrate is predominantly intrafascicular, in dermatomyositis the infiltrates are principally perimysial and perivascular although in some cases there may also be mild intrafascicular inflammation. Analysis of mononuclear cell subsets in dermatomyositis has shown a high percentage of B cells and a high $CD4^+/CD8^+$ ratio at perivascular and perimysial sites with close proximity of $CD4^+$ cells (helper cells) to B cells at all sites of cell accumulation suggesting a helper T-cell-dependent stimulation of B cells to secrete immunoglobulins (Engel & Arahata 1986). Invasion of non-necrotic muscle fibres by cytotoxic T cells is rare in dermatomyositis (Engel & Arahata 1986).

Other non-specific changes in damaged muscle fibres, which can be demonstrated by using histochemical or immunocytochemical techniques, include the accumulation of calcium (Oberc & Engel 1977, Bodensteiner & Engel 1978), of immunoglobulins and other serum proteins (Whitaker & Engel 1972, Oxenhandler et al 1977a, Sufit et al 1981), of complement components including the C5b–9 membrane lysis complex (Whitaker & Engel 1972, Engel & Biesecker 1982, Morgan et al 1984), and of lysosomal proteases such as cathepsin D (Whitaker et al 1981). Immunoglobulin deposition may also be found in the sarcolemma of undamaged muscle fibres and in interstitial connective tissues but is non-specific (Whitaker & Engel 1972, Isenberg 1983).

Changes in muscle fibre size and architecture are common in subacute and chronic cases of polymyositis and dermatomyositis. Muscle fibre atrophy is usually seen in some part of the biopsy, the most typical appearance being that of perifascicular atrophy which occurs in dermatomyositis (see above). A similar non-selective atrophy of both fibre types may also be seen more randomly or focally within fascicles in some cases. In some cases there is more diffuse selective atrophy of type 2 fibres and, less frequently, of type 1 fibres (Dubowitz & Brooke 1973, Jerusalem et al 1980, Comola et al 1987). Small angulated fibres may also be seen in some biopsies and, when numerous or grouped may be a clue to the presence of an associated neurogenic process. Muscle fibre hypertrophy is rare in polymyositis but does occur in some chronic cases. Architectural changes in muscle fibres are common and may take various forms. These include 'moth-eaten' and 'whorled' fibres, fibres with darkly staining central zones in oxidative enzyme preparations, cytoplasmic bodies, and fibres showing target or targetoid change with central loss of ATPase staining (Fig. 12.6) (Dubowitz & Brooke 1973, Jerusalem et al 1980).

Increased histochemical staining of the endomysial and perimysial connective tissue for 5'-nucleotidase (El-Shammaa et al 1984) and increased alkaline phosphatase staining in endomysial capillaries and perimysial connective tissues (Armbrustmacher & Griffin 1981, Cros et al 1980) are commonly found in cases of inflammatory myopathy. The use of these techniques, and of histochemical staining for acid phosphatase and esterases, can be of help in the interpretation of muscle biopsies from such cases particularly when the inflammatory changes are inconspicuous (see Ch. 3).

Associated conditions

As already indicated, polymyositis and dermatomyositis may occur in isolation as organ-specific autoimmune disorders involving the skeletal muscles alone or with additional skin involvement. In another group of patients, who may have either polymyositis or dermatomyositis, this occurs as part of a systemic collagen vascular disorder such as systemic lupus erythematosus, progressive systemic sclerosis (scleroderma), rheumatoid arthritis, mixed connective tissue disease or Sjögren's syndrome. The inflammatory myopathy in such cases is presumed to be another manifestation of the systemic disease and associated derangements of immune function, but the

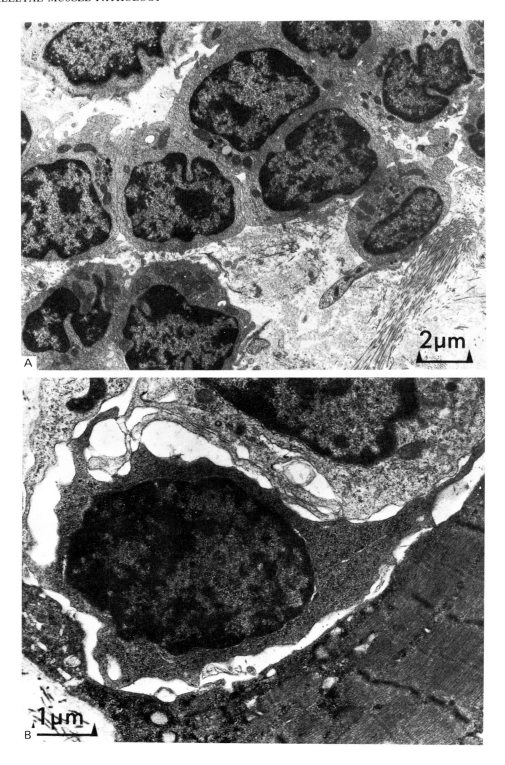

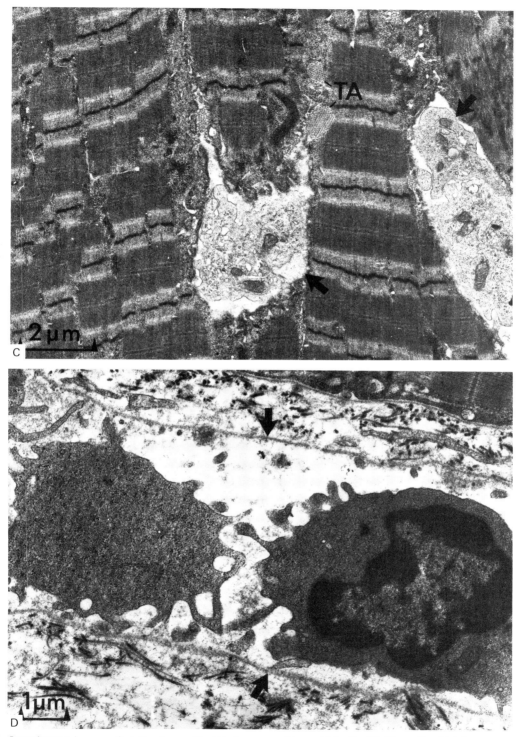

Fig. 12.5 Lymphocytes in cases of adult polymyositis. (A) Aggregate of interstitial cells. (B) Two cells which have penetrated the basal lamina of a muscle fibre to lie in close proximity to its plasma membrane. (C) Processes of cells (arrows) which have invaginated the plasma membrane of a muscle fibre. Honeycomb tubular arrays (TA) (of probable T-system origin) are present close to one area of invagination. (D) Two cells within the empty 'sarcolemmal tube' of a muscle fibre which has undergone necrosis and phagocytosis. The arrows indicate the basal lamina of the muscle fibre. (A and B reproduced, with permission, from Walton 1981)

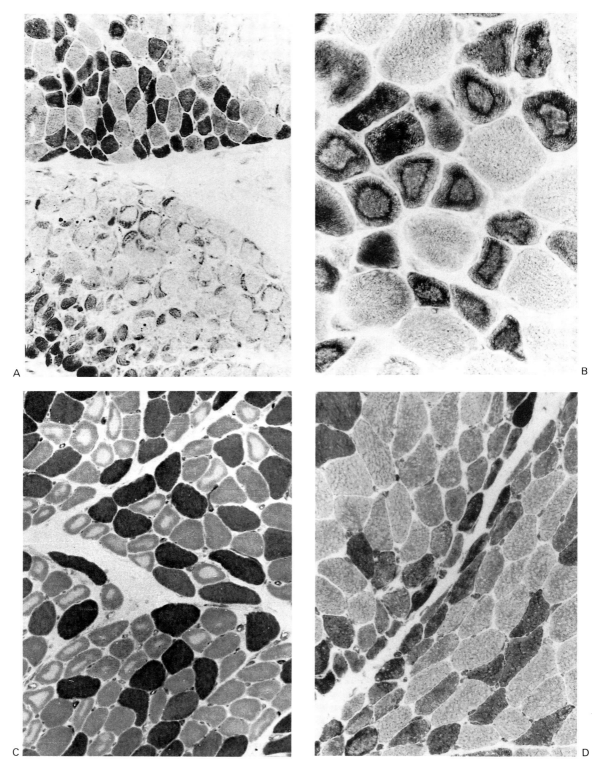

Fig. 12.6 Adult dermatomyositis. (A) Large group muscle fibre necrosis. Almost all the muscle fibres in the lower fascicle have undergone necrosis and are regenerating. (B) Target fibres. (C) Central loss of enzyme activity in type 1 fibres. (D) Perifascicular atrophy. (A, B, D) NAD–tetrazolium reductase. (C) Myosin ATPase (pH 9.4). A ×88, B ×282, C ×128, D ×140

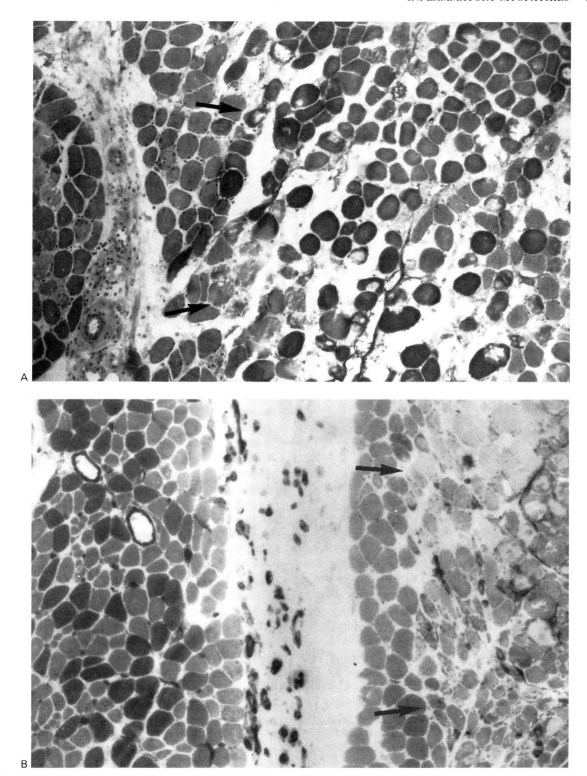

Fig. 12.7   Muscle microinfarcts in two cases of adult dermatomyositis. The arrows indicate the edges of the lesions while muscle fibres at the periphery of the affected fascicle and in the adjoining fascicle are spared. (A) H&E, ×134 (B) Myosin ATPase (pH 9.4), ×134

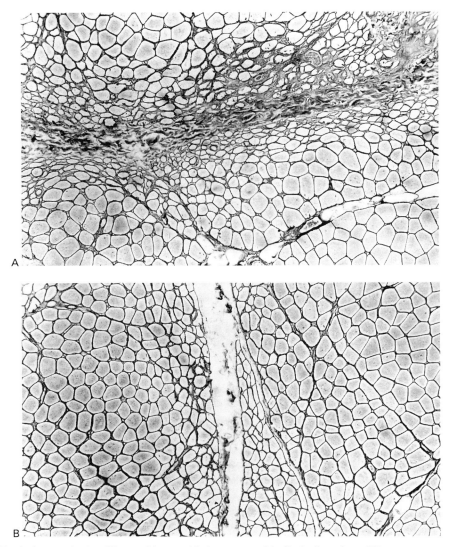

Fig. 12.8 Perifascicular atrophy in a 37-year-old man with dermatomyositis. Reticulin stain, ×100

mechanisms involved have not been clearly defined and may well be different in the different diseases.

Polymyositis or dermatomyositis may also be associated with other autoimmune disorders including myasthenia gravis (Behan et al 1982), pernicious anaemia (Mastaglia & Kakulas 1967), Hashimoto's thyroiditis (Dahan et al 1984), fibrosing alveolitis, coeliac disease (Henriksson et al 1982), and scleromyxoedema (Harvey et al 1986); with paraproteinaemias such as Waldenstrom's macroglobulinaemia (Ringel et al 1979) or benign monoclonal gammopathy (Telerman-Toppet et al 1982); with immune deficiency states such as hypocomplementaemia (Leddy et al 1975), agammaglobulinaemia (Gotoff et al 1972) and the acquired immunodeficiency syndrome (see above); and in graft-versus-host disease after bone marrow transplantation (Anderson et al 1982, Reyes et al 1983, Urbano-Marquez et al 1986).

The association with malignancy is well known and has been confirmed in some recent case-control studies (Manchul et al 1985) but not in

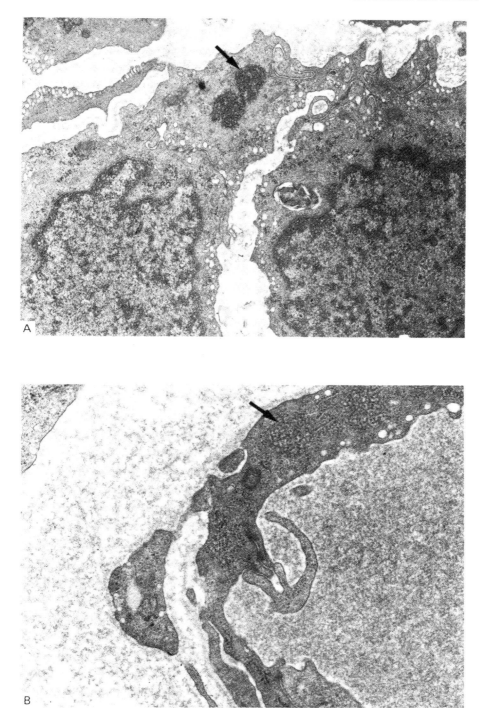

Fig. 12.9   Tubuloreticular inclusions (arrows) in capillary endothelial cells in juvenile dermatomyositis. A ×18 340, B ×23 760. (Courtesy of Dr B Q Banker)

others (Lakhanpal et al 1986). The overall incidence of malignancy among patients with polymyositis or dermatomyositis in different series has varied from 7–24% (Rowland et al 1977, Bohan & Peter 1975, Sela & Shoenfeld 1988). The risk of an underlying malignancy at the time of presentation is usually regarded as being higher in adult patients with dermatomyositis while patients with juvenile dermatomyositis or with an associated collagen vascular disease have a low risk of having a malignancy. Some series have found no difference in the risk of malignancy in adult patients with polymyositis or dermatomyositis (Manchul et al 1985). The range of associated malignancies is very extensive, but the most frequent association is with carcinoma of the breast or ovary in females and of the lung and gastrointestinal tract in males (Barnes 1976, Callen 1984). It remains uncertain whether or not there is any direct pathogenetic link between the tumour and the myositis or dermatomyositis in such cases. It is possible that both are related to derangements of immunoregulatory function.

Pathogenesis

As discussed earlier in this chapter, and in Ch. 4, as well as in other reviews (Mastaglia & Ojeda 1985, Targoff & Reichlin 1988, Lisak 1988) there is now considerable evidence that the muscle damage in polymyositis is mediated by cytotoxic T lymphocytes whose action is class I MHC restricted, while in dermatomyositis an immune complex vasculopathy appears to be the primary process. However, the possibility that more than one immunopathological mechanism is involved in both polymyositis and dermatomyositis and that different mechanisms may predominate in different subtypes of these disorders cannot be excluded at the present time. For example, it remains to be determined whether the various autoantibodies to nuclear and cytoplasmic antigens that have been described in patients with polymyositis and other subgroups of patients with inflammatory myopathies have a pathogenetic role or merely represent epiphenomena.

The nature of the target antigens in muscle in these conditions, and the factors responsible for the loss of tolerance also remain unclear. There is

some evidence that immunoregulatory mechanisms may be impaired in patients with polymyositis or dermatomyositis (see Ch. 4) (Walker et al 1982) and it has been postulated that a disturbance of immunoregulation during viral infections (e.g. HIV infection), following vaccination or during treatment with certain drugs such as D-penicillamine, or in patients with an associated malignancy, results in loss of tolerance and initiates an autoimmune reaction directed against muscle antigens in certain individuals who may be genetically predisposed (Mastaglia & Walton 1982, Mastaglia & Ojeda 1985).

The recent demonstration of enterovirus RNA in muscle in some cases of polymyositis and dermatomyositis (Yousef et al 1990) suggests that direct viral infections of muscle may also play a more direct pathogenetic role in these conditions by initiating an immune response which also damages muscle tissue (Chou 1988). It has been postulated that this may result from a homology in amino acid sequences between certain antigenic components of the viral agent and muscle antigens ('molecular mimicry') (Walker & Jeffrey 1986).

Infantile myositis

There have been a number of reports of an inflammatory myopathy presenting in the first year of life, and sometimes in the neonatal period, with widespread muscle weakness, atrophy and hypotonia and elevated serum CK levels. Histological changes include scattered muscle fibre necrosis, regeneration and atrophy, an endomysial and perivascular mononuclear cell infiltrate and increased interstitial connective and adipose tissue (Carpenter & Karpati 1981). Misshapen myonuclei containing microtubular and actin-like filamentous inclusions were a feature in one case (Carpenter & Karpati 1981) while in another there was perifascicular muscle fibre atrophy and vascular deposition of immunoglobulins and complement (Roddy et al 1986). The aetiology of these cases and their relationship to juvenile and adult cases of dermatomyositis and polymyositis is uncertain. In some congenital cases with arthrogryposis the possibility of an intrauterine infection has been suggested (Kinoshita et al 1980).

Inclusion-body myositis

This is a distinct variety of inflammatory myopathy with characteristic clinical and pathological features (Chou 1967, 1988, Yunis & Samaha 1971, Mastaglia & Ojeda 1985, Lotz et al 1989). The condition is not usually associated with skin changes or with malignancy or collagen vascular diseases. However there have been recent reports of an association with Sjögren's syndrome (Chad et al 1982, Gutmann et al 1985), SLE (Yood & Smith 1985), scleroderma (Tomé et al 1981, Somer et al 1986), immune thrombocytopoenia (Riggs et al 1984), coeliac disease (Hughes & Esiri 1975), sarcoidosis (Danon et al 1986) and malignancy (Lotz et al 1989) in a small number of cases. There is slowly progressive, usually painless, weakness, often involving distal as well as proximal limb muscles and some cases have dysphagia. The rate of progression varies, some patients being severely handicapped even after two years (Carpenter & Karpati 1981), although in the majority the disease is very slowly progressive over a period of 10–20 years. Serum CK levels may be normal or mildly to moderately elevated. Some cases have an associated peripheral neuropathy and both neuropathic and myopathic changes are commonly found on electromyography (Eisen et al 1983, Sawchuk et al 1983, Ringel et al 1987). Corticosteroids and immunosuppressive treatment are usually ineffective, although occasional cases do respond.

Histopathology

Although the diagnosis can be suspected on clinical grounds, muscle biopsy is necessary for confirmation, distinctive changes being seen both with light and electron microscopy. Bluish granular inclusions distributed around the edges of slit-like vacuoles (*rimmed vacuoles*) are seen in muscle fibres in cryostat sections stained with haematoxylin and eosin (Fig. 12.10). The granules are removed by lipid solvents and are not seen in paraffin-embedded sections. They often, but not always, show acid phosphatase activity and on electron microscopy are found to be composed of polymorphic lamellated membranous structures (*myeloid bodies*) (Fig. 12.11). In addition, eosino-philic hyaline cytoplasmic inclusions are present in some muscle fibres in most cases (Fig. 12.10D). Occasional necrotic or regenerating muscle fibres may be seen and groups of atrophic fibres are often present. Cytoplasmic bodies and 'ragged red' fibres may also be present in some cases.

The inflammatory infiltrates, which comprise mainly lymphocytes and macrophages, are predominantly endomysial and less frequently perimysial and perivascular in location (Fig. 12.10). Immunohistochemical analysis has shown a predominance of $CD8^+$ cytotoxic lymphocytes which surround and invade non-necrotic muscle fibres (Arahata & Engel 1984, 1986). Capillary numbers are often increased, when assessed in semi-thin epoxy resin sections, in contrast to the reduction in capillary numbers at the periphery of muscle fascicles in cases of dermatomyositis (Carpenter et al 1976).

The other distinctive feature, which is not found in other types of inflammatory myopathy, and which is considered to be essential for the diagnosis of inclusion body myositis is the finding on electron microscopy of intranuclear and cytoplasmic masses of filamentous microtubules (Fig. 12.12). The cytoplasmic filaments measure 17–21 nm in diameter and the nuclear filaments 10–14 nm (Lotz et al 1989). It was thought that these structures were viral in nature because of their resemblance to the nucleocapsids of myxoviruses and paramyxoviruses (Chou 1968). However, with the exception of one case in which an adenovirus (type 2) was isolated from muscle tissue (Mikol et al 1982), viral serological studies and attempts at viral isolation from muscle have been negative. The nature of the filamentous inclusions therefore remains uncertain. Chou (1986) reported immunostaining for mumps virus antigens in the nuclear and cytoplasmic inclusions in eight cases of inclusion-body myositis and postulated that the condition is due to a chronic persistent mumps virus infection. However, Nishino et al (1989) failed to confirm these findings and found no evidence of mumps virus nucleocapsid gene using an in-situ hybridization technique. Other ultrastructural changes in muscle fibres include abnormal mitochondria containing paracrystalline inclusions, which have been particularly prominent in some cases (Chou 1969).

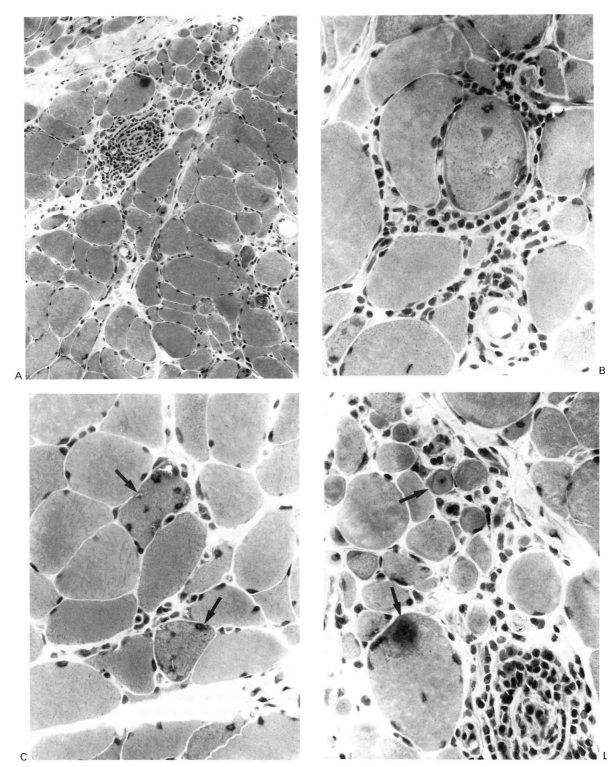

Fig. 12.10 Inclusion body myositis in a 66-year-old male: (A) Perivascular and endomysial mononuclear cell infiltrate; rounded and angulated atrophic fibres singly and in groups. (B) Endomysial infiltrate of mononuclear cells between muscle fibres. (C) Two fibres with 'rimmed' vacuoles (arrows). (D) Cytoplasmic inclusions in two muscle fibres (arrows). H&E; A ×147, B–D ×368

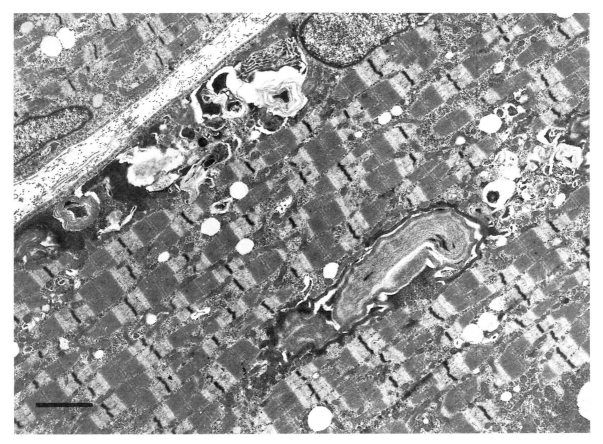

Fig. 12.11 Inclusion-body myositis in a 53-year-old man. Electron micrograph of a muscle fibre with 'rimmed' vacuoles showing focal accumulations of multilamellated membranes ('myeloid' bodies) and electron-dense material. Bar = 2 μm

Lotz et al (1989) have defined the following essential pathological features for the diagnosis of inclusion body myositis: (i) at least one rimmed vacuole per high power field; (ii) at least one group of atrophic fibres per high power field; (iii) an endomysial inflammatory infiltrate with lymphocytes invading non-necrotic muscle fibres; (iv) electron-microscopic demonstration of the typical filamentous inclusions; a minimum of three vacuolated muscle fibres should be examined.

Granulomatous myositis

Sarcoidosis

Several different forms of muscle involvement may occur in sarcoidosis (Table 12.7). Asympto-matic granulomas are commonly present in muscle in the acute stages of the disease (Silverstein & Siltzbach 1969), being found in 50–60% of patients who have a muscle biopsy. Their presence provides a useful means of confirming the diagnosis (Phillips & Phillips 1956, Wallace et al 1958). A clinically evident myopathy is unusual, being found in only 3 of 800 patients in one series (Silverstein & Siltzbach 1969) and in 2 of 500 patients in another series (Douglas et al 1973). In some cases palpable nodules may be present in some muscles, while others may develop a proximal myopathy with muscle pain, weakness and atrophy. Marked swelling or pseudohypertrophy of the muscles of the calves and thighs has also been reported (Douglas et al 1973). Such sympto-matic myopathies usually develop in the chronic

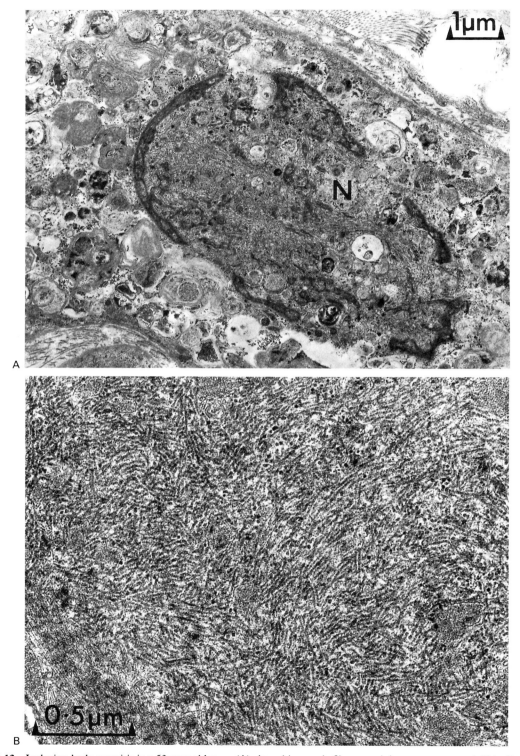

Fig. 12.12 Inclusion-body myositis in a 53-year-old man. (A) Atrophic muscle fibre containing numerous myeloid bodies and a degenerate nucleus in which bundles of filaments are present. (B) Accumulation of 16–18 nm filamentous microtubules in the cytoplasm of a muscle fibre. Bar = 1 μm A, 0.5 μm B

stages of the disease and there is usually evidence of involvement of other organs by the disease process. There have also been a number of reports of patients with sarcoidosis presenting with the clinical picture of dermatomyositis (Itoh et al 1980, Lipton et al 1988). It remains uncertain whether sarcoidosis can be confined solely to the skeletal muscles.

Table 12.7 Causes of granulomatous inflammation in skeletal muscle

---

Sarcoidosis
Asymptomatic granulomas
Proximal myopathy (with clinical features of polymyositis or
    dermatomyositis)
Nodular form
Pseudohypertrophic form

Other causes
Parasitic infections
Tuberculosis
Leprosy
AIDS
Collagen–vascular disease
Wegener's granulomatosis
Crohn's disease
Giant-cell myositis with thymoma
Intramuscular injections

The characteristic lesions in sarcoidosis are found within muscle fibre fascicles or in interstitial connective tissue septa (Fig. 12.13) and have the appearance of sharply circumscribed granulomatous nodules which are composed of histiocytes, epithelioid cells and Langhans giant cells, with a light lymphocytic infiltrate sometimes associated with a few plasma cells, mast cells and neutrophil polymorphonuclear leukocytes. The lesions tend to replace or displace the muscle fibres, which may become atrophic; active necrosis and regeneration are uncommon (Hewlett & Brownell 1975). Histochemical examination may show type 2 fibre atrophy in some cases, while in others perifascicular atrophy or fibre type grouping may be found (Hewlett & Brownell 1975, Lipton et al 1988). The latter finding and the finding of grouped neurogenic atrophy in such cases would point to an associated peripheral neuropathy (Adams et al 1965).

A form of giant-cell polymyositis leading to widespread muscle weakness with increased serum CK activity may also occur in association with giant-cell myocarditis in patients with a thymoma;

it may become manifest either before the thymoma or after its removal (Namba et al 1974). The 'giant cells' in the muscle lesions in such cases are, in fact, abnormal multinucleated muscle fibres ('myogenic giant cells') rather than the Langhans-type giant cells which are characteristic of granulomatous inflammation.

Other causes

Granulomatous muscle lesions similar to those of sarcoidosis may occur in leprosy, Crohn's disease (Menard et al 1976), parasitic infections and after intramuscular injections of diphtheria and tetanus toxoid, pertussis vaccine (Mrak 1982) and of drugs such as chlorpromazine (Brumback and Staton 1983). They may also occur in miliary or generalized tuberculosis, in which case there is usually evidence of caseous necrosis within the granulomas.

Eosinophilic myositis

A number of different forms of eosinophilic myositis have been described.

Eosinophilic polymyositis

This rare form of inflammatory myopathy occurs as part of the systemic *hypereosinophilic syndrome* which is characterized by eosinophilia, anaemia, hypergammaglobulinaemia, cardiac and pulmonary involvement, skin changes, peripheral neuropathy and encephalopathy (Layzer et al 1977). The typical presentation of the myositis is with a localized tender swelling of one of the calf or thigh muscles with elevated serum CK activity, leading subsequently to the development of a more extensive proximal myopathy (Layzer et al 1977, Stark 1979). The myopathy may be the dominant or presenting feature of the illness and it is important to be aware that it may be the initial manifestation of a systemic disorder. The condition must be distinguished from trichinosis, and other forms of parasitic muscle infestation and from localized nodular myositis (see below). The response to treatment with corticosteroids has been good in most reported cases (Layzer et al 1977, Stark 1979). The histological changes consist of scattered muscle fibre necrosis and an endomysial and peri-

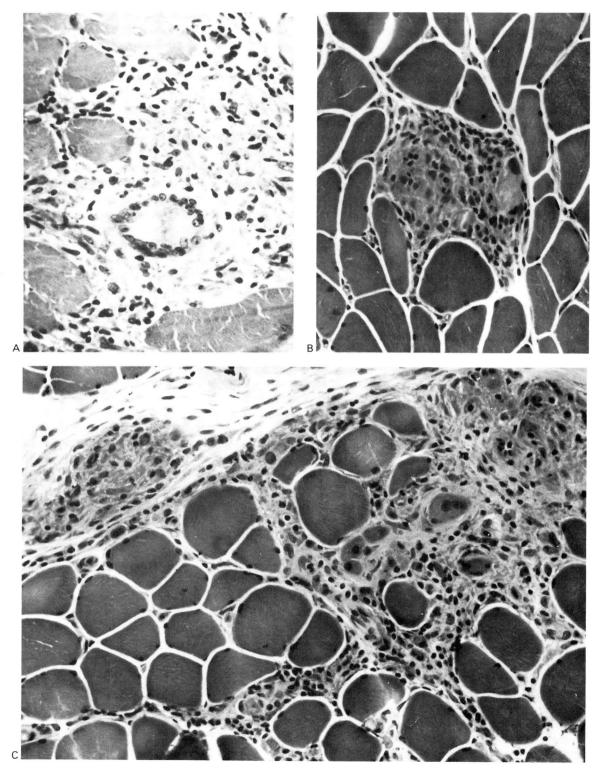

Fig. 12.13 Granulomatous myositis in a 42-year-old woman. Non-caseating granulomas are present within muscle fascicles as well as in the perimysium in C. H&E, ×500

vascular inflammatory infiltrate comprising large numbers of eosinophils together with lymphocytes and plasma cells. In some cases, interstitial areas of granulomatous inflammation have been noted (Layzer et al 1977).

Eosinophilic perimyositis

This condition usually presents with muscle pain and tenderness and sometimes as a relapsing myalgic syndrome, usually without other systemic manifestations or elevation of the serum CK level or erythrocyte sedimentation rate but with a peripheral blood eosinophilia (Serratrice et al 1980, Fang et al 1988, Lakhanpal et al 1988). The inflammatory infiltrate, which comprises mixed mononuclear cells and some eosinophils, is concentrated in the perimysial connective tissue and perivascular spaces with infiltration of the walls of perimysial blood vessels in some cases. Perifascicular muscle fibre necrosis suggestive of ischaemic microinfarction was found in one reported case (Fang et al 1988) while in another case larger areas of intrafascicular ischaemic damage were present (Serratrice et al 1980). The nosological position of such cases and their relationship to cases of dermatomyositis, eosinophilic polymyositis, scleromyxoedema and eosinophilic fasciitis (Shulman's syndrome, see below), in which eosinophilic perimysial inflammation may also occur, remains uncertain.

An interstitial form of eosinophilic myositis may also occur in patients treated with L-tryptophan (Hertzman et al 1990, Silver et al 1990, Flannery et al 1990).

Focal eosinophilic myositis

This form is confined to a single muscle or group of muscles, such as those of the calf, and is not associated with systemic manifestations, although the serum CK activity and erythrocyte sedimentation rate may be elevated and there is a peripheral blood eosinophilia (Lakhanpal et al 1988). A relapsing form, which sometimes occurs in alcoholics, has also been described (Symmans et al 1986, Kamm et al 1987).

Angiopathic myositis

This term could aptly be applied to the muscle lesions found in cases of juvenile dermatomyositis and certain forms of systemic arteritis, such as polyarteritis nodosa (Fig. 12.14), Churg–Strauss vasculitis and Wegener's granulomatosis, in which the muscle lesions basically consist of microinfarcts but in which there may also be some inflammatory cellular infiltration in the nearby muscle tissue (see Ch. 20). Within such focal lesions there is pan-necrosis involving not only muscle fibres but also the interstitial tissues. While frank arteritic lesions and perivascular infiltrates may be found, endomysial and perimysial inflammatory infiltrates are uncommon. Lesions of this type have also been described in *localized nodular myositis* (Allen et al 1980) (see below).

Neuromyositis

The term neuromyositis is used to refer to cases of polymyositis or dermatomyositis with associated clinical features suggestive of peripheral nerve involvement, such as subjective or objective sensory changes, or depression of deep tendon reflexes (Walton & Adams 1958). Such a combination of an inflammatory myopathy and a peripheral neuropathy may occur in patients with collagen–vascular disease, with a malignancy or with AIDS (see above). From a histopathological point of view, the coincident finding of a necrotizing inflammatory myopathy and evidence of neurogenic atrophy in the biopsy could aptly also be referred to as neuromyositis. A form of neuromyopathy characterized by proximal muscle wasting and weakness, depression of tendon reflexes and electromyographic features of both denervation and myopathy is relatively common in patients with various forms of malignancy (Croft & Wilkinson 1965, Campbell & Paty 1974), but the pathological changes in the proximal limb and girdle muscles in such cases are poorly documented.

CONNECTIVE TISSUE DISORDERS

Although there is a high incidence of histological abnormalities in muscle in patients with systemic lupus erythematosus (SLE), rheumatoid arthritis, scleroderma, Sjögren's syndrome and mixed connective tissue disease (MCTD), the occurrence of classical polymyositis or dermatomyositis is

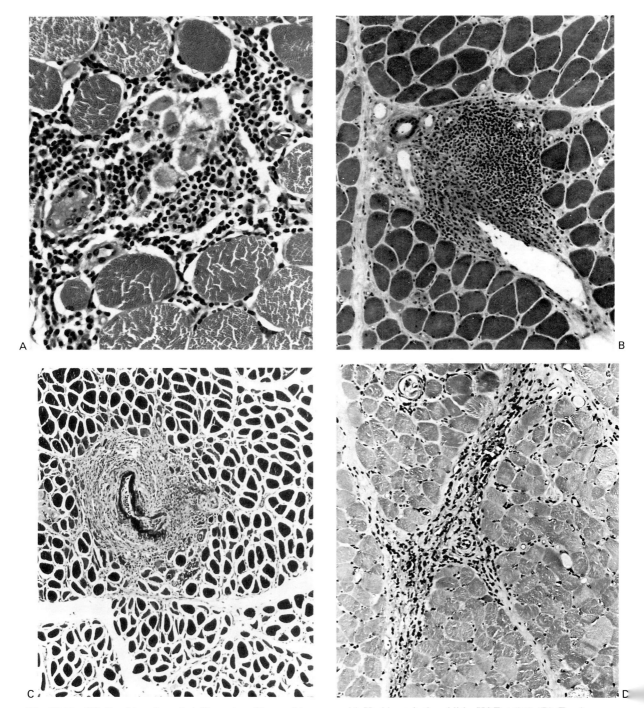

Fig. 12.14 (A) Focal lymphocytic infiltrate in a 43-year-old woman with Hashimoto's thyroiditis. H&E, ×360. (B) Focal perivascular infiltrate of mononuclear cells in a patient with a mixed connective tissue disease. H&E, ×360. (C) Necrotizing panarteritis in a case of polyarteritis nodosa. H&E, ×105. (D) Perimysial fibrosis and lymphocytic infiltrate in a case of scleromyxoedema. H&E, ×154

uncommon in patients with these conditions (Mastaglia & Ojeda 1985, Zilko 1988).

Systemic lupus erythematosus

In SLE, 5–11% of patients have been found to have a necrotizing myopathy in different series (Foote et al 1982). The myopathy is usually present at the time of presentation or develops during an acute flare-up of the disease and the prognosis for recovery is good, in contrast to patients with rheumatoid arthritis or scleroderma who develop polymyositis (DeVere & Bradley 1975, Zilko 1988). Immunofluorescence studies frequently show evidence of immunoglobulin and complement deposition in blood vessel walls and in muscle fibre basement membranes, even in patients without a clinical myopathy (Oxenhandler et al 1982).

Scleroderma

Only 5–10% of patients with scleroderma develop an overt inflammatory myopathy although a higher proportion are found to have a mild non-specific myopathy on muscle biopsy with type 2 fibre atrophy, focal perivascular and perimysial mononuclear cell infiltrates and increased interstitial connective tissue (Zilko 1988). The cellular infiltrates consist mainly of T-cells and macrophages, some of which are activated, but invasion of muscle fibres is rare and it appears that there is a cell-mediated immune response against a connective tissue or vascular element (Engel & Arahata 1986).

In some patients with linear scleroderma (*morphoea*) a localized form of inflammatory myopathy occurs with lymphocytic infiltration and perifascicular muscle fibre atrophy and fibrosis in the underlying muscles (Miike et al 1983, Medsger 1985).

Rheumatoid arthritis

Classical polymyositis may occur in patients with rheumatoid arthritis but is rare, and in some patients appears to be precipitated by treatment with D-penicillamine (Carroll et al 1987). In addition, it has been claimed that there is a distinct form of rheumatoid myositis in which there is local synthesis of IgM and rheumatoid factor and deposition of immunoglobulins and complement, particularly in patients with systemic disease and a very high erythrocyte sedimentation rate (Halla et al 1984). More frequently, perivascular and perimysial mononuclear cell infiltrates, vasculitis, type 2 fibre atrophy and other non-specific myopathic changes are found even when there is no clinical evidence of a myopathy (Magyar et al 1977).

Sjögren's syndrome

Polymyositis, dermatomyositis and inclusion body myositis may occur in patients with Sjögren's syndrome but are uncommon. Ringel et al (1982) who reported three patients with Sjögren's syndrome and polymyositis and one with dermatomyositis, found prominent microvascular changes with a mononuclear cell infiltrate consisting predominantly of plasma cells around small vessels and capillaries as well as immune complex deposition. These authors suggested that the myositis in Sjögren's disease is due to small vessel injury by autoantibodies or circulating immune complexes.

Mixed connective tissue disease (MCTD)

An inflammatory myopathy characterized by focal muscle fibre necrosis, perifascicular atrophy and perivascular and interstitial lymphocytic infiltration is common in patients with this condition in which features of scleroderma, SLE and arthritis coexist and high titres of speckled antinuclear antibody and antibodies to ribonucleoprotein are present in the serum (Sharp et al 1972, Zilko 1988). In addition immunoglobulin deposition is common on muscle fibres, in blood vessel walls and in perimysial connective tissue (Oxenhandler et al 1977b). Such patients usually respond well to corticosteroid therapy.

FOCAL FORMS OF MYOSITIS

Focal interstitial myositis

Focal aggregates of lymphocytes or mixed mononuclear cells in the perimysium, perivascular spaces or at times even within muscle fascicles are a non-specific finding in patients with a variety of conditions. First described by Aschoff (1904) in patients with rheumatic fever, they may also occur in myasthenia gravis ('lymphorrhages', see Ch. 17), in collagen vascular diseases such as rheumatoid arthritis, systemic lupus erythematosus including drug-induced cases (Mastaglia & Argov 1981), scleroderma, Sjögren's syndrome and in other autoimmune diseases such as Hashimoto's thyroiditis and Graves' disease (Fig. 12.14). In most instances, focal interstitial myositis is an incidental finding which is not associated with clinical evidence of a myopathy. However, it may be symptomatic in some cases of polymyalgia associated with a collagen–vascular disease or with autoimmune thyroid disease (Mastaglia et al 1988). Moreover, it may be the only histological finding in biopsies from some patients with polymyositis or dermatomyositis (Adams & Kakulas 1985).

Adams et al (1965) suggested that simple lymphocytic infiltration of muscle should be regarded as a form of 'lymphocytosis of muscle' and that the term 'interstitial myositis' should be used only for cases in which there are mixed inflammatory cellular infiltrates including not only lymphocytes but also plasma cells and histiocytes and some associated degenerative changes in muscle fibres. Pure lymphocytosis is a very non-specific finding which may be encountered even in random muscle sections taken at autopsy from patients dying of the effects of trauma, malignancy, vascular or a variety of other diseases (Kakulas & Mastaglia 1966).

Localized nodular myositis

This term was introduced by Cumming et al (1977) for a group of patients with a focal form of necrotizing inflammatory myopathy presenting as a localized painful mass in the thigh or calf and less frequently in the upper limb muscles and subsequently going on to develop similar lesions in other sites. In fact, many of these cases proceed to develop a widespread inflammatory myopathy which is difficult to distinguish from polymyositis (Cumming et al 1977, Heffner & Barron 1980). Histological examination shows myofibre necrosis,

which may be very extensive and resemble a microinfarct, as well as regeneration and endomysial and perimysial accumulation of lymphocytes, macrophages and other cell types. In some cases there has been an associated vasculitis (Allen et al 1980). The differential diagnosis of localized nodular myositis includes focal forms of arteritis involving the calf muscles, myositis ossificans, eosinophilic myositis, proliferative myositis, pseudosarcomatous fasciitis, pyomyositis, granulomatous and parasitic muscle lesions (Wilson & Hawkins 1989).

Orbital myositis

This is a rare condition of adolescents or young adults which presents clinically with a painful ophthalmoplegia which responds to corticosteroids. In most cases only one of the extraocular muscles is affected and can be shown to be enlarged by computed tomography or ultrasonography (Hankey et al 1987). Biopsy of the affected muscle shows diffuse infiltration with lymphocytes and other mononuclear cells as well as invasion of muscle fibres (Bullen & Young 1982). An inflammatory ocular myopathy may also occur rarely in systemic lupus erythematosus, systemic sclerosis or other connective tissue disorders, and in sarcoidosis. Lymphocytic infiltrates may also be found in the extraocular muscles in thyroid eye disease (see Ch. 13).

Inflammatory pseudotumour

This benign condition, which can occur in children or adults, manifests as a localized painful swelling in the thigh, calf, forearm, trunk or back muscles, which increases in size over a period of a few weeks to two years (Heffner et al 1977). On macroscopic examination the lesion is usually pale and of a rubbery consistency. Histological examination shows irregularity of fibre size with fibre hypertrophy and splitting as well as scattered necrotic and regenerating fibres, endomysial and perimysial lymphocytic infiltrates and interstitial fibrosis. In some cases there is a prominent eosinophil cellular infiltrate (see Serratrice et al 1985, Ojeda and Mastaglia 1988b) while in others there are changes of denervation and re-innervation (Heffner & Barron 1980).

Proliferative myositis is another type of inflammatory pseudotumour in which there is aberrant muscle regeneration and marked interstitial connective tissue proliferation producing a pseudosarcomatous appearance (Enzinger & Dulcey 1967). The condition usually occurs in areas subjected to repeated trauma (see Ch. 22) but similar lesions may at times also occur in other areas.

Other conditions

Focal areas of myositis may also occur in certain parasitic infections, granulomatous disorders such sarcoidosis, and in muscles underlying plaques of localized scleroderma (Miike et al 1983) and foci of panniculitis (Palliyath & Garcia 1982).

POLYMYALGIA RHEUMATICA

This well-defined syndrome, which typically occurs in individuals over the age of 50 years, is characterized by pain and stiffness in proximal muscle groups, particularly around the neck and shoulders, which responds dramatically to treatment with corticosteroids. The erythrocyte sedimentation rate is usually markedly elevated (over 80 mm/h) but may be normal in some cases. In some cases the condition is associated with symptomatic or subclinical cranial (giant cell) arteritis (Dixon et al 1966, Fauchald et al 1972). Other reported associations are with rheumatoid arthritis, other collagen vascular diseases, malignancy and primary biliary cirrhosis (Huskisson et al 1977, Robertson & Batstone 1978, Bird et al 1979). In the majority of cases of polymyalgia rheumatica the muscle biopsy is normal or shows non-specific changes such as type 2 fibre atrophy and, in some cases, architectural changes in muscle fibres such as cytoplasmic bodies, moth-eaten and whorled fibres (Brooke & Kaplan 1972). Focal interstitial myositis may be found in some cases with an associated collagen vascular disease or other autoimmune disorder. In some patients a biopsy shows inflammatory changes in the fascia overlying painful areas in the extremities (Simon & Sufit 1982).

FASCIITIS

Inflammation of the fascia which invests the skeletal muscles occurs in a number of different conditions and may be responsible for a clinical picture of diffuse muscular pain, aching and tenderness in the extremities. Fascial inflammation may occur in some patients with dermatomyositis or inflammatory myopathy associated with connective tissue diseases. Simon & Sufit (1982) have emphasized the value of performing an open muscle biopsy and including the overlying fascia in patients who are suspected of having an inflammatory myopathy particularly when there is prominent myalgia. Fascial inflammation may also be found in some patients with fibrositis but is the exception rather than the rule (Simon & Sufit 1982).

In the condition of eosinophilic fasciitis (Shulman's syndrome) there is painful swelling and induration of the skin and soft tissues of the extremities and trunk leading to the development of weakness and contractures in the limbs and there is usually a marked eosinophilia in the peripheral blood and hypergammaglobulinaemia (Shulman 1974). Biopsy of the fascia shows collagenous hypertrophy and infiltration with lymphocytes, plasma cells and, in about 50% of cases, eosinophils. A number of cases have been reported in which there has been extension of the fascial inflammation into the epimysial and perimysial connective tissue of the underlying muscle while in some cases perifascicular atrophy, myofibre necrosis and phagocytosis and eosinophilic infiltration of the muscle have been found (Faugere et al 1981, Simon & Sufit 1982). A form of eosinophilic fasciitis presenting as a scleroderma-like syndrome has also been reported in some patients treated with L-tryptophan (Varga et al 1990, Silver et al 1990).

Two other forms of fasciitis have been described. These are nodular fasciitis ('pseudosarcomatous fasciitis') which typically presents as a rapidly growing mass on the upper extremity or the trunk, and necrotizing fasciitis which is a potentially serious streptococcal or staphylococcal infection of the fascia which usually develops after minor trauma (see Simon & Sufit 1982).

REFERENCES

Adams R D, Kakulas B A 1985 Disease of muscle: pathological foundation of clinical myology, 4th edn. Harper-Row, New York, p 514

Adams R D, Denny–Brown D, Pearson C M 1965 Diseases of muscle. A study in pathology. Hoeber, New York

Allen I, Mullally B, Mawhinney H, Sawhney B, McKee P 1980 The nodular form of polymyositis — a possible manifestation of vasculitis. Journal of Pathology 131: 183

Alvira M M, Mendoza M 1985 Reye's syndrome: a viral myopathy? New England Journal of Medicine 292: 1297

Anderson B A, Young V, Kean W F et al 1982 Polymyositis in chronic graft vs host disease. Archives of Neurology 39: 188

Arahata K, Engel A G 1984 Monoclonal antibody analysis of mononuclear cells in myopathies. I: Quantitation of subsets according to diagnosis and sites of accumulation and demonstrations and counts of muscle fibers invaded by T-cells. Annals of Neurology 16: 198

Arahata K, Engel A G 1986 Monoclonal antibody analysis of mononuclear cells in myopathies. III: Immunoelectron microscopy aspects of cell-mediated muscle fiber injury. Annals of Neurology 19: 112

Archard L C, Bowles N E, Behan P O, Bell E J, Doyle D 1988 Postviral fatigue syndrome: persistence of enterovirus RNA in muscle and elevated creatine kinase. Journal of the Royal Society of Medicine 81: 326

Armbrustmacher V W, Griffin J L 1981 Pathology of inflammatory and metabolic myopathies. Pathology Annual 16: 15

Armstrong C L, Miranda A F, Hsu K C, Gamboa E T 1978 Susceptibility of human skeletal muscle culture to influenza virus infection. Journal of Neurological Sciences 35: 43

Arnett F C, Michels R G 1973 Inflammatory ocular myopathy in systemic sclerosis (scleroderma). A case report and review of the literature. Archives of Internal Medicine 132: 740

Aschoff L 1904 Zur Myocarditisfrage. Verhandlungen Deutsche Gesellschaft Pathologie 8: 46

Aström E, Friman G, Pilström L 1982 Human skeletal muscle in viral and mycoplasma infections. Ultrastructural morphometry and its correlations to enzyme activities. Uppsala Journal of Medical Science 82: 191

Bacq M, Telerman-Toppet N, Coërs C 1985 Familial myopathies with restricted distribution, facial weakness and inflammatory changes in affected muscles. Journal of Neurology 231: 295

Bailey R O, Turok D I, Jautmann B P Singh J K 1987 Myositis and acquired immunodeficiency syndrome. Human Pathology 18: 749

Banker B Q, Victor M 1966 Dermatomyositis (systemic angiopathy) of childhood. Medicine 45: 261

Barnes B E 1976 Dermatomyositis and malignancy. A review of the literature. Annals of Internal Medicine 84: 68

Barwick D D, Walton J N 1963 Polymyositis. American Journal of Medicine 35: 646

Bates D, Stevens J C, Hudgson P 1973 'Polymyositis' with involvement of facial and distal musculature. One form of the facioscapulohumeral syndrome? Journal of the Neurological Sciences 19: 105

Behan W M H, Barkas T, Behan P O 1982 Detection of immune-complexes in polymyositis. Acta Neurologica Scandinavica 65: 320

Bird H A, Esselinck W, Dixon A St J, Mowat A G, Wood P H N 1979 An evaluation of criteria for polymyalgia rheumatica. Annals of the Rheumatic Diseases 38: 434

Bodensteiner J B, Engel A G 1978 Intracellular calcium accumulation in Duchenne dystrophy and other myopathies: a study of 567 000 muscle fibers in 114 biopsies. Neurology 28: 439

Bohan A, Peter J B 1975 Polymyositis and dermatomyositis. New England Journal of Medicine 292: 344

Bore K E, Hilton P K, Partin J et al 1983 Morphology of acute myopathy associated with influenza B infection. Pediatric Pathology 1: 51

Bowles N E, Dubowitz V, Sewry C A, Archard L C 1987 Dermatomyositis, polymyositis and Coxsackie-B-virus infection. Lancet i: 1004

Brooke M H, Kaplan H 1972 Muscle pathology in rheumatoid arthritis, polymyalgia rheumatica, and polymyositis. A histochemical study. Archives of Pathology 94: 101

Brown M, Swift T R, Spies S M 1976 Radioisotope scanning in inflammatory muscle disease. Neurology (Minneapolis) 26: 517

Brumback R A, Staton R D 1983 Muscle granulomas after injection (letter). Muscle and Nerve 6: 387

Bullen C L, Young B R 1982 Chronic orbital myositis. Archives of Ophthalmology 100: 1749

Callen J P 1984 Myositis and malignancy. Clinics in Rheumatic Diseases 19: 117

Campbell M H, Paty D W 1974 Carcinomatous neuromyopathy. 1. Electrophysiological studies. Journal of Neurology, Neurosurgery and Psychiatry 37: 131

Carpenter S, Karpati G 1981 The major inflammatory myopathies of unknown cause. Pathology Annual 16: 205

Carpenter S, Karpati G, Rothman S, Watters G 1976 The childhood type of dermatomyositis. Neurology (Minneapolis) 26: 952

Carroll G J, Will R K, Peter J B, Garlepp M J, Dawkins R L 1987 Penicillamine induced polymyositis and dermatomyositis. Journal of Rheumatology 14: 995

Chad D, Good P, Adelman L, Bradley W G, Mills J 1982. Inclusion body myositis associated with Sjögren's syndrome. Archives of Neurology 39: 186

Chiedozi L 1979 Pyomyositis. Review of 205 cases in 112 patients. American Journal of Surgery 137: 255

Chou S M 1967 Myxovirus-like structures in a case of human chronic polymyositis. Science 158: 1453

Chou S M 1968 Myxovirus-like structures and accompanying nuclear changes in chronic polymyositis. Archives of Pathology 86: 649

Chou S M 1969 'Megaconial' mitochondria observed in a case of chronic polymyositis. Acta Neuropathologica (Berlin) 12: 68

Chou S M 1986 Inclusion body myositis: a chronic persistent mumps myositis? Human Pathology 17: 765

Chou S M 1988 Viral myositis. In: F L Mastaglia (ed) Inflammatory diseases of muscle. Blackwell Scientific Publications, Oxford, ch 7, p 125

Comola M, Johnson M A, Howel D, Brunsdon C 1987 Spatial distribution of muscle necrosis in biopsies from patients with inflammatory muscle disorders. Journal of the Neurological Sciences 82: 229

Congy F, Hauw J J, Wang A, Moulias R 1980 Influenzal acute myositis in the elderly. Neurology (Minneapolis) 30: 877

Crennan J M, van Scoy R E, McKenna C H, Smith T F 1986 Echovirus polymyositis in patients with hypogammaglobulinemia. Failure of high-dose intravenous gammaglobulin therapy and review of the literature. American Journal of Medicine 81: 35

Croft P B, Wilkinson M 1965 The incidence of carcinomatous neuromyopathy in patients with various types of carcinoma. Brain 88: 427

Cros D, Pearson C, Verity M A 1980 Polymyositis–dermatomyositis. Diagnostic and prognostic significance of muscle alkaline phosphatase. American Journal of Pathology 101: 159

Crowe W E, Bove K E, Levinson J E, Hilton P K 1982 Clinical and pathogenetic implications of histopathology in childhood poly-dermatomyositis. Arthritis and Rheumatism 25: 126

Cumming W J K, Weiser R, Teoh R, Hudgson P, Walton J N 1977 Localised nodular myositis: a clinical and pathological variant of polymyositis. Quarterly Journal of Medicine 184: 531

Dahan V, Geny M, Frey G 1984 Polymyositis associated with autoimmune thyroiditis. Presse Medicale 13: 563

Dalakas M C, Pezeshkpour G H 1988 Neuromuscular diseases associated with human immunodeficiency virus infection. Annals of Neurology 23(suppl): S38

Dalakas M C, London W T, Gravell M, Sever J L 1986 Polymyositis in an immunodeficiency disease in monkeys induced by a tape D retrovirus. Neurology 36: 569

Dalakas M C, Wichman A, Sever J 1989 AIDS and the nervous system. Journal of the American Medical Association 261: 2396

Dalakas M C, Illa I, Pezeshkpour G H, Laukaitis J P, Cohen B, Griffin J L 1990 Mitochondrial myopathy caused by long-term zidovudine therapy. New England Journal of Medicine 322: 1098

Danon M J, Perurena O H, Ronan S, Manaligod J R 1986 Inclusion body myositis associated with systemic sarcoidosis. Canadian Journal Neurological Science 13: 334

DeVere R, Bradley W G 1975 Polymyositis: its presentation, morbidity and mortality. Brain 98: 637

De Visser M, Emslie-Smith A M, Engel A G 1989 Early ultrastructural alterations in adult dermatomyositis. Capillary abnormalities precede other structural changes in muscle. Journal of the Neurological Sciences 94: 181

Dietzman D E, Schaller J G, Ray C G, Reed M E 1976 Acute myositis associated with influenza B infection. Archives of Disease in Childhood 51: 135

Dixon A St J, Beardwell C, Kay A, Wanka J, Wong Y T 1966 Polymyalgia rheumatic and temporal arteritis. Annals of the Rheumatic Diseases 25: 203

Douglas A C, Macleod J G, Matthews J D 1973 Symptomatic sarcoidosis of skeletal muscle. Journal of Neurology, Neurosurgery and Psychiatry 36: 1034

Drachman D B, Weiner L P, Price D L, Chase J 1976 Experimental arthrogryposis caused by viral myopathy. Archives of Neurology (Chicago) 33: 362

Dubowitz V, Brooke M H 1973 Muscle biopsy: a modern approach. Saunders, Philadelphia

Eisen A, Berry K, Gibson G 1983 Inclusion body myositis (IBM): myopathy or neuropathy? Neurology, Cleveland 33: 1109

El-Shammaa N A, Fishbein W N, Armbrustmacher V W 1984 Interstitial 5'-nucleotidase stain for frozen biopsy specimens of skeletal muscle. Archives of Pathology Laboratory Medicine 108: 251

Emslie-Smith A M, Engel A G 1990 Microvascular changes in early and advanced dermatomyositis: a quantitative study. Annals of Neurology 27: 343

Emslie-Smith A M, Arahata K, Engel A G 1989 Major histocompatibility complex class I antigen expression, immunolocalization of interferon subtypes, and T cell-mediated cytotoxicity in myopathies. Human Pathology 20: 224

Engel A G, Arahata K 1984 Monoclonal antibody analysis of mononuclear cells in myopathies. II. Phenotypes of autoinvasive cells in polymyositis and inclusion body myositis. Annals of Neurology 16: 209

Engel A G, Arahata K 1986 Mononuclear cells in myopathies: quantitation of functionally distinct subsets, recognition of antigen-specific cell-mediated cytotoxicity in some diseases, and implications for the pathogenesis of the different inflammatory myopathies. Human Pathology 17: 704

Engel A G, Biesecker G 1982 Complement activation in muscle fiber necrosis: demonstration of the membrane attack complex in necrotic fibers. Annals of Neurology 12: 289

Enzinger F M, Dulcey F 1967 Proliferative myositis. Report of thirty-three cases. Cancer 20: 2213

Evans B K, Gore I, Harrell L E, Arnold T, Oh S J 1989 HTLV-I-associated myelopathy and polymyositis in a US native. Neurology 39: 1572

Fang M A, Verity A, Paulus H E 1988 Subacute perimyositis. Journal of Rheumatology 15: 1291

Farrell M K, Partin J C, Bova K E, Jacobs R, Hilton P K 1980 Epidemic influenza myopathy in Cincinnati in 1977. Journal of Pediatrics 96: 545

Fauchald P, Rygvold O, Oystese B 1972 Temporal arteritis and polymyalgia rheumatica. Clinical and biopsy findings. Annals of Internal Medicine 77: 845

Faugere M C, Mussini J M, Pellisier J F, Henin D, Gray F, Brousse N 1981 Eosinophilic myositis and Shulman syndrome. Semaine Hôpital 57(3–4): 158

Flannery M T, Wallach P M, Espinoza L R, Dohrenwend M P, Moscinski L C 1990 A case of the eosinophilia–myalgia syndrome associated with use of an L-tryptophan product. Annals of Internal Medicine 112: 300

Foote R A, Kimbrough S M, Stevens J C 1982 Lupus myositis. Muscle and Nerve 5: 65

Gamboa E T, Eastwood A B, Hays A P, Maxwell J, Penn A S 1979 Isolation of influenza virus from muscle in myoglobinuric polymyositis. Neurology (Minneapolis) 29: 1323

Giorno R, Barden M T, Kohler P F, Ringel S P 1984 Immunohistochemical characterization of the mononuclear cells infiltrating muscle of patients with inflammatory and noninflammatory myopathies. Immunology and Immunopathology 30: 405

Gotoff S P, Smith R D, Sugar D 1972 Dermatomyositis with cerebral vasculitis in a patient with agammaglobulinemia. American Journal of Diseases of Children 123: 53

Gross B, Ochoa J 1979 Trichinosis: clinical report and histochemistry of muscle. Muscle and Nerve 2: 394

Grove D I 1988 Parasitic and fungal infections of muscle. In: Mastaglia F L (ed) Inflammatory diseases of muscle. Blackwell Scientific Publications, Oxford, ch 9 p 164

Gutmann L, Govindan S, Riggs J E, Schochet S S 1985 Inclusion body myositis and Sjögren's syndrome. Archives of Neurology, Chicago 42: 1021

Halla J T, Koopman W J, Fallahi S, Oh S J, Gay R E, Schrohenloher R E 1984 Rheumatoid myositis: clinical and histological features and possible pathogenesis. Arthritis and Rheumatism 27: 737

Hamilton I, Sharp R A, Anderson J M, Kerr M R 1987 Polymyositis complicating staphylococcal septicaemia. Scottish Medical Journal 32: 149

Hankey G J, Silberg P L, Edis R H, Nicholl A M 1987 Orbital myositis: a study of six cases. Australian and New Zealand Journal of Medicine 17: 585

Hanson P A, Urizar R E 1977 Ultrastructural lesions of muscle and immunofluorescent deposits in vessels in Reye's syndrome: a preliminary report of serial muscle biopsies. Annals of Neurology 1: 431

Harvey J M, Mastaglia F L, Zilko P J, Ojeda V J, Cheah P S 1986 Scleromyxoedema and inflammatory myopathy: a clinicopathologic study of three patients. Australian and New Zealand Journal of Medicine 16: 329

Heffner R R, Barron S A 1980 Denervating changes in focal myositis, a benign inflammatory pseudotumour. Archives of Pathology and Laboratory Medicine 104: 261

Heffner R R, Barron S A 1981 Polymyositis beginning as a focal process. Archives of Neurology 38: 439

Heffner R R, Armbrustmacher V W, Earle K M 1977 Focal myositis. Cancer 40: 301

Hendrickx G F M, Verhage J, Jennekens F G I, van Knapen D V M 1979 Dermatomyositis and toxoplasmosis. Annals of Neurology 5: 393

Henriksson K G, Hallert C, Norrby K, Walan A 1982 Polymyositis and adult coeliac disease. Acta Neurologica Scandinavica 65: 301

Herrera R, Varela E, Morales G, Del Rio A, Gallardo J M 1985 Dermatomyositis-like syndrome caused by trichinae. Report of two cases. Journal of Rheumatology 12: 782

Hertzman P A, Blevins W L, Mayer J, Greenfield B, Ting M, Gleich G J 1990 Association of the eosinophilia–myalgia syndrome with the ingestion of tryptophan. New England Journal of Medicine 322: 869

Hewlett R H, Brownell B 1975 Granulomatous myopathy: its relationship to sarcoidosis and polymyositis. Journal of Neurology, Neurosurgery and Psychiatry 38: 1090

Hroncich M E, Rudinger A N 1989 Rhabdomyolysis with pneumococcal pneumonia: a report of two cases. American Journal of Medicine 86: 467

Hughes J T, Esiri M M 1975 Ultrastructural studies in human polymyositis. Journal of the Neurological Sciences 25: 347

Huskisson E C, Dieppe P A, Balme H W 1977 Complicated polymyalgia. British Medical Journal 4: 1459

Isenberg D A 1983 Immunoglobulin deposition in skeletal muscle in primary muscle disease. Quarterly Journal of Medicine 52: 297

Itoh J, Akiguchi I, Midorikawa R, Kameyama M 1980 Sarcoid myopathy with typical rash of dermatomyositis. Neurology 30: 1118

Jarowski C I, Fialk M A, Murray H W et al 1978 Fever, rash and muscle tenderness: a distinctive clinical presentation of disseminated candidiasis. Archives of Internal Medicine 138: 544

Jennekens F G I, Busch H F M, van Hemel N M, Hoogland R A 1975 Inflammatory myopathy in scapulo-ilio-peroneal atrophy with cardiopathy. A study of two families. Brain 98: 709

Jerusalem F, Simona F, Fontana A 1980 Myopathological and immunological findings in the diagnosis and pathogenesis of polymyositis and dermatomyositis. Nervenartz 51: 255

Kagen L J 1977 Myoglobinemia in inflammatory myopathies. Journal of the American Medical Association 237: 1448

Kakulus B A, Mastaglia F L 1966 Type and incidence of lesions found in a human necropsy survey of skeletal muscle. Proceedings of the Australian Association of Neurologists 4: 35

Kalish S B, Tallman M S, Cook F V Blumen E A 1982

Polymicrobial septicemia associated with rhabdomyolysis, myoglobinuria and acute renal failure. Archives of Internal Medicine 142: 133

Kamm M A, Dennett X, Byrne E 1987 Relapsing eosinophilic myositis — a cause of pseudothrombophlebitis in an alcoholic. Journal of Rheumatology 14: 831

Karpati G, Pouliot Y, Carpenter S 1988 Expression of immunoreactive major histocompatibility complex products in human skeletal muscles. Annals of Neurology 23: 64

Kinoshita M, Iwasaki Y, Wada E, Segawa M 1980 A case of congenital polymyositis — a possible pathogenesis of 'Fukuyama type congenital muscular dystrophy'. Clinical Neurology 20: 911

Kissane J 1985 Bacterial diseases. In: Kissane J (ed) Anderson's pathology, 8th edn. Mosby, St Louis, p 284

Kissel J T, Mendell J R, Rammohan K W 1986 Microvascular deposition of complement membrane attack complex in dermatomyositis. New England Journal of Medicine 314: 329

Kressel B, Szewczyk C, Tuazon C U 1978 Early clinical recognition of disseminated candidiasis by muscle and skin biopsy. Archives of Internal Medicine 138: 429

Lakhanpal S, Bunch T W, Ilstrup D M, Melton L J 1986 Polymyositis–dermatomyositis and malignant lesions: does an association exist? Mayo Clinic Proceedings 61: 645

Lakhanpal S, Duffy J, Engel A G 1988 Eosinophilia associated with perimyositis and pneumonitis. Mayo Clinic Proceedings 63: 37

Lange D J, Britton C B, Younger D S, Hays A P 1988 The neuromuscular manifestations of human immunodeficiency virus infections. Archives of Neurology 45: 1084

Layzer R B, Shearn M A, Satya-Murti S 1977 Eosinophilic polymyositis. Annals of Neurology 1: 65

Leddy T P, Griggs R C, Klemperer M H, Frank M M 1975 Hereditary complement (C2) deficiency with dermatomyositis. American Journal of Medicine 58: 83

Ledford D K, Overman M D, Gonzalvo A, Cali A, Mester S M, Lockey R F 1985 Microsporidiosis myositis in a patient with the acquired immunodeficiency syndrome. Annals Internal Medicine 102: 628

Lepine P, Pesse G, Sautter V 1952 Biopsies musculaires avec examen histologique et isolement du virus Coxsackie chez l'homme attein de myalgie epidemique (Maladie de Bornholm). Bulletin de l'Academie Nationale de Médecine (Paris) 136: 66

Lipton J H, McLeod B D, Brownell K W 1988 Dermatomyositis and granulomatous myopathy associated with sarcoidosis. Canadian Journal of Neurological Science 15: 426

Lisak R P 1988 The immunology of neuromuscular disease. In: J N Walton (ed) Disorders of voluntary muscle, p 345. Churchill Livingstone, Edinburgh

Lotz B P, Engel A G, Nishino H, Stevens J C, Litchy W J 1989 Inclusion body myositis. Brain 112: 727

Lundberg A 1957 Myalgia cruris epidemica. Acta Paediatrica Scandinavica 46: 18

Magid S K, Kagen I J 1983 Serologic evidence for acute toxoplasmosis in polymyositis–dermatomyositis. American Journal of Medicine 75: 313

Magyar E, Talerman A, Mohacsy J, Wouters H W, de Bruijn W C 1977 Muscle changes in rheumatoid arthritis. Virchows Archiv A Pathology, Anatomy and Histology 373: 267

Manchul L A, Jin A, Pritchard K I et al 1985 The frequency of malignant neoplasms in patients with polymyositis–dermatomyositis. Archives of Internal Medicine 145: 1835

Masson C, Chaunu M P, Henin D et al 1989 HTLV-1-associated myelopathy with polymyositis and systemic abnormalities. Revue Neurologique 145: 839

Mastaglia F L, Argov Z 1981 Immunologically mediated drug-induced neuromuscular disorders. In: Schlumberger (ed) Pseudo-allergic reactions. S Karger, Basel

Mastaglia F L, Currie S 1971 Immunological and ultrastructural observations on the role of lymphoid cells in the pathogenesis of polymyositis. Acta Neuropathologica (Berlin) 18: 1

Mastaglia F L, Kakulas B A 1967 Rheumatoid arthritis, polyarteritis, polymyositis, gastritis and Hashimoto's thyroiditis. Medical Journal of Australia 1: 1135

Mastaglia F L, Ojeda V J 1985 Inflammatory myopathies: Part 1. Annals of Neurology 17: 215

Mastaglia F L, Walton J N 1971 Histological and histochemical changes in skeletal muscle from cases of chronic juvenile and early adult spinal muscular atrophy (the Kugelberg–Welander syndrome). Journal of the Neurological Sciences 12: 15

Mastaglia F L, Walton J N 1982 Inflammatory myopathies. In: Mastaglia F L and Walton J N (eds) Skeletal muscle pathology. Churchill Livingstone p 360

Mastaglia F L, Dawkins R L, Papadimitriou J M 1974 Lymphocyte–muscle cell interactions in vivo and in vitro. Journal of the Neurological Sciences 22: 261

Mastaglia F L, Dawkins R L, Papadimitriou J M 1975 Mechanisms of cell-mediated myotoxicity: morphological observations in muscle grafts and in muscle exposed to sensitized spleen cells in vivo. Journal of the Neurological Sciences 25: 269

Mastaglia F L, Sarnat H B, Ojeda V J, Kakulas B A 1988 Myopathies associated with hypothyroidism: a review based upon 13 cases. Australian and New Zealand Journal of Medicine 18: 799

Mease P J, Ochs H D, Wedgwood R J 1981 Successful treatment of echovirus meningoencephalitis and myositis–fasciitis with intravenous immune globulin therapy in a patient with X-linked agammaglobulinemia. New England Journal of Medicine 304: 1278

Medsger T A 1985 Systemic sclerosis (scleroderma), eosinophilic fasciitis and calcinosis. In: McCarty D J (ed) Arthritis and allied conditions. Lea and Febiger, Philadelphia, p 994

Medsger T A, Dawson W N, Masi A T 1970 The epidemiology of polymyositis. American Journal of Medicine 48: 715

Mejlszenkier J D, Safran A P, Healy J J, Embree L, Quellette E M 1973 The myositis of influenza. Archives of Neurology (Chicago) 29: 441

Menard D B, Haddard H, Blain J G, Beaudry R, Devroede G, Masse S 1976 Granulomatous myositis and myopathy associated with Crohn's colitis. New England Journal of Medicine 295: 818

Middleton P J, Alexander R M, Szymanski M T 1970 Severe myositis during recovery from influenza. Lancet ii: 533

Miike T, Ohtani Y, Hattori S, Ono T, Kageshita T, Matsuda I 1983 Childhood-type myositis and linear scleroderma. Neurology (Cleveland) 33: 928

Mikol J, Felton–Papaiconomou A, Ferchal F, Perol Y, Gautier B, Haguenau M, Pepin B 1982 Inclusion-body myositis: clinicopathological studies and isolation of an adenovirus type 2 from muscle biopsy specimen. Annals of Neurology 11: 576

Morgan B P, Sewry C A, Siddle K, Luzio J P, Campbell A K 1984 Immunolocalization of complement component C9 on

necrotic and non-necrotic muscle fibers in myositis using monoclonal antibodies: a primary role of complement in autoimmune cell damage. Immunology 52: 181

Mrak R E 1982 Muscle granulomas following intramuscular injection. Muscle and Nerve 5: 637

Munsat T L, Piper D, Cancilla P, Mednick J 1972 Inflammatory myopathy with facioscapulohumeral distribution. Neurology (Minneapolis) 22: 335

Namba T, Brunner N G, Grob D 1974 Idiopathic giant cell polymyositis. Archives of Neurology (Chicago) 31: 27

Nishikai M, Reichlin M 1977 Radioimmunoassay of serum myoglobin in polymyositis and other conditions. Arthritis and Rheumatism 20: 1514

Nishino H, Engel A G, Rima B K 1989 Inclusion body myositis: the mumps virus hypothesis. Annals of Neurology 25: 260

Oberc M A, Engel W K 1977 Ultrastructural localization of calcium in normal and abnormal skeletal muscle. Laboratory Investigation 36: 566

Ojeda V J, Mastaglia F L 1988a Bacterial myositis In: Mastaglia F L (ed) Inflammatory diseases of muscle. Blackwell Scientific Publications, ch 8, p 154.

Ojeda V J, Mastaglia F L 1988b Miscellaneous conditions In: Mastaglia F L (ed) Inflammatory diseases of muscle. Blackwell Scientific Publications, ch 10, p 185

Olsson T, Henriksson K G, Klareskog L, Forsum U 1985 HLA-DR expression, T lymphocyte phenotypes, OKM1 and OKT9 reactive cells in inflammatory myopathy. Muscle and Nerve 8: 419

Oxenhandler R, Adelstein E H, Hart M N 1977a Immunopathology of skeletal muscle. Human Pathology 8: 321

Oxenhandler R, Hart M, Corman C, Sharp G C, Adelstein E 1977b Pathology of skeletal muscle in mixed connective tissue disease. Arthritis and Rheumatism 20: 985

Oxenhandler R, Hart M N, Bickel J, Scearce D, Durham J, Irvin W 1982 Pathologic features of muscle in systemic lupus erythematosus: a biopsy series with comparative clinical and immunopathologic observations. Human Pathology 13: 745

Pallis C A, Lewis P D 1988 Involvement of human muscle by parasites. In: Walton J N (ed), Disorders of voluntary muscle, 5th edn. Churchill Livingstone, Edinburgh, p 611

Palliyath S, Garcia C A 1982 Multifocal interstitial myositis associated with localized lipoatrophy. Archives of Neurology 39: 722

Panegyres P K, Papadimitriou J M, Hollingsworth P N, Armstrong J A, Kakulas B A 1990 Vesicular changes in the myopathies of AIDS. Ultrastructural observations and their relationship to zidovudine treatment. Journal of Neurology, Neurosurgery and Psychiatry. 53: 649

Partin J C, Schubert W K, Partin J S et al 1976 Isolation of influenza virus from liver and muscle biopsy specimens from a surviving case of Reye's syndrome. Lancet ii: 599

Pearson C M, Bohan A 1977 The spectrum of polymyositis and dermatomyositis. Medical Clinics of North America 61: 439

Phillips R W, Phillips A M 1956 The diagnosis of Boeck's sarcoid by skeletal muscle biopsy. Archives of Internal Medicine 98: 732

Pirovino M, Neff M S, Sharon E 1979 Myoglobinuria and acute renal failure with acute polymyositis. New York State Journal of Medicine 79: 764

Plotz P H, Dalakas M, Leff R L, Love L A, Miller F W, Cronin M E 1989 Current concepts in the idiopathic inflammatory myopathies: polymyositis, dermatomyositis, and related disorders. Annals of Internal Medicine 111: 143

Quilis M R, Damjanov I 1982 Dermatomyositis as an immunologic complication of toxoplasmosis. Acta Neuropathologica 58: 183

Reyes M G, Noronha P, Thomas W, Hereda R 1983 Myositis of graft versus host disease. Neurology 33: 1222

Riggs J E, Schochet S S, Gutmann L et al 1984 Inclusion body myositis and chronic immune thrombocytopenia. Archives of Neurology 41: 93

Ringel S P, Thorne E G, Phanuphak P, Lava N S, Kohler P S 1979 Immune complex vasculitis, polymyositis and hyperglobulinemic purpura. Neurology (Minneapolis) 29: 682

Ringel S P, Forstot J Z, Tan E M, Wehling C, Griggs R C, Butcher D 1982 Sjögren's syndrome and polymyositis or dermatomyositis. Archives of Neurology 39: 157

Ringel S P, Carry M R, Aguilera A J, Starcevich J M 1986 Quantitative histopathology of the inflammatory myopathies. Archives of Neurology 43: 1004

Ringel S P, Kenny C E, Neville H E, Giorno R, Carry M R 1987 Spectrum of inclusion body myositis. Archives of Neurology 44: 1154

Robertson J C, Batstone G F 1978 Polymyalgia rheumatica and primary biliary cirrhosis. British Medical Journal 4: 1128

Roddy S M, Ashwal S, Peckham N, Mortensen S 1986 Infantile myositis: a case diagnosed in the neonatal period. Paediatric Neurology 2: 241

Rose A L, Walton J N 1966 Polymyositis: a survey of 89 cases with particular reference to treatment and prognosis. Brain 89: 747

Rosenberg N L, Ringel S P 1988 Adult polymyositis and dermatomyositis. In: Mastaglia F L (ed) Inflammatory diseases of muscle. Blackwell Scientific Publications, Oxford, ch 5, p 87

Rosenberg N L, Rotbart H A, Abzug M J et al 1989 Evidence for a novel picornavirus in human dermatomysitis. Annals of Neurology 26(2): 204

Rothstein T L, Carlson C B, Sumi S M 1971 Polymyositis with facioscapulohumeral distribution. Archives of Neurology (Chicago) 25: 313

Rowe D J, Isenberg D A, McDougall J, Beverley P C L 1981 Characterization of polymyositis using monoclonal antibodies to human leukocyte antigen. Clinical and Experimental Immunology 45: 290

Rowland L P, Clark C, Olarte M 1977 Therapy for dermatomyositis and polymyositis. Advances in Neurology 17: 64

Ruff F L, Seattle W A 1983 Inflammatory myopathy restricted to a single muscle. Neurology 33 (suppl 2): 236

Salazar–Grueso E F, Holzer T J, Gutierrez R A et al 1990 Familial spastic paraparesis syndrome associated with HTLV-I infection. New England Journal of Medicine 323: 732

Sato T, Arahata K, Mori H 1980 Virus induced arthrogryposis multipex congenita in animals. In: Ebashi S (ed) Muscular dystrophy. Japan Medical Research Foundation, Tokyo p 493

Sawchuk J A, Kula R W, Sher J H, Shafiq S A, Clark L M 1983 Clinicopathologic investigations in patients with inclusion body myositis (IBM). Neurology 33: 237

Sawhney B B, Chopra J S, Banerji A K, Wahi P L 1976 Pseudohypertrophic myopathy in cysticercosis. Neurology (Minneapolis) 26: 270

Schimrigk K, Emser W 1978 Parasitic myositis by Echinococcus alveolaris. Report of a family with myotonia congenita. European Neurology 17: 1

Schröter H M, Sarnat H B, Matheson D S, Seland T P 1987 Juvenile dermatomyositis induced by toxoplasmosis. Journal of Child Neurology 2: 101

Sela O, Shoenfeld Y 1988 Cancer in autoimmune diseases. Seminars in Arthritis and Rheumatism 18: 77

Serratrice G, Pellissier J F, Cros D, Gastaut J L, Brindisi G 1980 Relapsing eosinophilic perimyositis. Journal of Rheumatology 7: 199

Serratrice G, Pellissier J F, Lachard A, Pouget J, Lachard J 1985 Myosite localisée avec eosinophilie. Presse Médicale 14: 533

Sharp G C, Irvin W S, Tan E M, Gould R G, Holman H R 1972 Mixed connective tissue disease — apparently distinct rheumatic disease syndrome associated with a specific antibody to an extractable nuclear antigen (ENA). American Journal of Medicine 52: 148

Shulman L E 1974 Diffuse fasciitis with hypergammaglobulinaemia and eosinophilia: a new syndrome? Journal of Rhematology 1: 46

Silver R M, Heyes M P, Maize J C, Quearry B, Vionnet–Fuasset M, Sternberg E M 1990 Scleroderma, fasciitis and eosinophilia associated with the ingestion of tryptophan. New England Journal of Medicine 322: 874

Silverstein A, Siltzbach L E 1969 Muscle involvement in sarcoidosis. Archives of Neurology (Chicago) 21: 235

Simon D B, Sufit R L 1982 Clinical spectrum of fascial inflammation. Muscle and Nerve 5: 525

Simpson D M, Bender A N 1988 Human immunodeficiency virus-associated myopathy: analysis of 11 patients. Annals of Neurology 24: 79

Simpson D M, Bender A N, Farraye J, Mendelson S G, Wolfe D E 1990 Human immunodeficiency virus wasting syndrome may represent a treatable myopathy. Neurology 40: 535

Somer H, Haltia M, Somer T 1986 'Inclusion body myositis': in scleroderma: improvement with steroids. Muscle and Nerve 9: 220

Stark R J 1978 Polymyositis presenting with severe weakness involving only one arm. Australian and New Zealand Journal of Medicine 8: 544

Stark R J 1979 Eosinophilic polymyositis. Archives of Neurology (Chicago) 36: 721

Strongwater S L, Dorovini–zis K, Ball R D, Schintzer T J 1984 A murine model of polymyositis induced by Coxsackievirus B1 (Tucson strain). Arthritis and Rheumatism 27: 433

Sufit R L, Barden M T, Ringel S P, Tan E N 1981 Antibodies in inflammatory myopathies. Annals of Neurology 10: 83

Symmans W A, Beresford C H, Bruton D et al 1986 Cyclic eosinophilic myositis and hyperimmunoglobulin-E. Annals of Internal Medicine 104: 26

Tang T T, Sedmak G V, Siegesmund K A, McCreadie S R 1975 Chronic myopathy associated with Coxsackie virus type A9. A combined electron microscopical and virus isolation study. New England Journal of Medicine 292: 608

Targoff I N, Reichlin M 1988 Immunological aspects. In: Mastaglia F L (ed) Inflammatory diseases of muscle. Blackwell Scientific Publications, Oxford ch 3, p 37

Telerman–Toppet N, Wittek M, Bacq M, Dajez P, Coërs C, Fassotte A 1982 Benign monoclonal gammopathy and relapsing polymyositis. Muscle and Nerve 5: 490

Tomé F M S, Fardeau M, Lebon P et al 1981 Inclusion body myositis. Acta Neuropathologica suppl VII, p 287

Urbano–Marquez A, Estruch R, Grau J M, Granena A, Martin–Ortega E, Palou J, Rozman C 1986 Inflammatory myopathy associated with chronic graft-versus-host disease. Neurology 36: 1091

Varga J, Peltonen J, Uitto J, Jimenez S 1990 Development of diffuse fasciitis with eosinophilia during L-trytophan treatment: demonstration of elevated type I collagen gene expression in affected tissues. Annals of Internal Medicine 112: 344

Verma R K, Ziegler D W, Kepes J J 1990 HIV-related neuromuscular syndrome simulating motor neuron disease. Neurology 40: 544

Vignos P J, Goldwyn J 1972 Evaluation of laboratory tests in diagnosis and management of polymyositis. American Journal of the Medical Sciences 263: 291

Walker E J, Jeffrey P D 1986 Polymyositis and molecular mimicry, a mechanism of autoimmunity. Lancet ii: 605

Walker G L, Mastaglia F L, Roberts D F 1982 Search for genetic influence in idiopathic inflammatory myopathy. Acta Neurologica Scandinavica 66: 432

Wallace S G, Latte R, Malia J P, Ragan C 1958 Muscle involvement in Boeck's sarcoid. Annals of Internal Medicine 48: 497

Walton J N 1964 Some diseases of muscle. Lancet i: 447

Walton J N 1965 Neuromuscular diseases. Proceedings of the 8th International Congress of Neurology, Vienna, p 127

Walton J N 1981 Disorders of voluntary muscle, 4th edn. Churchill Livingstone, Edinburgh

Walton J N, Adams R D 1958 Polymyositis. Livingstone, Edinburgh

Whitaker J N, Engel W K 1972 Vascular deposits of immunoglobulin and complement in idiopathic inflammatory myopathy. New England Journal of Medicine 286: 333

Whitaker J N, Bertorinin T E, Mendell J R 1981 Immunocytochemical studies of cathepsin D in human skeletal muscle. Annals of Neurology 10: 91

Wiley C A, Nerenberg M, Cros D, Soto–Aguilar M C 1989 HTLV-1 polymyositis in a patient also infected with the human immunodeficiency virus. New England Journal of Medicine 320: 992

Willis R A, Willis A T 1972 Principles of Pathology and Bacteriology, 3rd edn. Butterworths, London, p 158

Wilson D C, Hawkins S A 1989 Recurrent localised myositis. Journal of Neurology, Neurosurgery and Psychiatry 52: 411

World Federation of Neurology, Research Group on Neuromuscular Diseases 1968 Classification of the neuromuscular disorders. Journal of the Neurological Sciences 6: 165

Yood R A, Smith T W 1985 Inclusion body myositis and systemic lupus erythematosus. Journal of Rheumatology 12: 568

Yousef G E, Bell E J, Mann G F, Murugesan V, Smith D G, McCartney R A, Mowbray J F 1988 Chronic enterovirus infection in patients with postviral fatigue syndrome. Lancet i: 146

Yousef G E, Isenberg D A, Mowbray J F 1990 Detection of enterovirus specific RNA sequences in muscle biopsy specimens from patients with adult onset myositis. Annals of the Rheumatic Diseases 49: 310

Ytterberg S R 1987 Coxsackievirus B1 induced murine polymyositis: acute infection with active virus is required for myositis. Journal of Rheumatology 14: 12

Yunis E J, Samaha F J 1971 Inclusion body myositis. Laboratory Investigation 25: 240

Zilko P J 1988 Myopathy in connective tissue diseases other than polymyositis. In: F L Mastaglia (ed) Inflammatory diseases of muscle. Blackwell Scientific Publications, ch 6, p 107

13. Endocrine myopathies

Peter Hudgson   Pat Kendall-Taylor

INTRODUCTION

Muscle weakness is a well-recognized component of the clinical presentation of many disorders of endocrine function, and may predominate or even be the presenting feature in some. The accessibility of muscle tissue has provided a convenient means of studying the generalized disturbances of metabolism accompanying endocrine disorders but, in spite of this, our knowledge of the breakdown of normal muscle structure and function in these situations is imprecise, to say the least. Indeed, in all but a few of the conditions we will be considering in this chapter, pathological changes in muscle are absent or inconspicuous. Stark evidence for this can be found in recent authoritative reviews of the subject (Ruff 1986, Engel 1988) which devote many pages to endocrine myopathies as a whole with only two illustrations altogether! Further to this, Ruff's (1986) encyclopaedic review, which contained 316 references in all, had only one reference to his own work, which was non-clinical, dated 1985, with none other more recent than 1982, the date of publication of the first edition of this book. Many others dated back to the 19th century! None the less, striking morphological abnormalities do arise in certain situations, as we hope to show, particularly in the dysthyroid myopathies, and these may provide useful guides to the mode of action of the relevant hormones upon muscle tissue.

DYSTHYROID MYOPATHIES

Whether or not skeletal muscle disease develops in association with autoimmune thyroiditis (AIT) appears to have no clear relationship to the extent of thyroid dysfunction. This is well recognized in patients with ophthalmic Graves' disease but has recently become obvious also in young and middle-aged women with AIT and polymyositis (Emslie–Smith 1987). Nevertheless, certain clinicopathological correlates can be established with reasonable confidence and these are discussed below.

Thyrotoxicosis

General weakness and atrophy of muscles, localized paresis of the extra-ocular muscles and the syndromes of myasthenia gravis and of periodic paralysis may all be seen in hyperthyroidism. Clinical evidence of proximal muscle weakness is evident in most patients with thyroid overactivity and may even be the presenting manifestation. An element of fatiguability may raise a suspicion of associated myasthenia, although this is relatively rare. Appropriate physiological studies show that the small distal muscles are also affected. Very occasionally, involvement of the respiratory and bulbar musculature may occur (Gaan 1967). Muscular atrophy may also be seen but it is seldom a prominent feature. In contrast to hypothyroidism, the tendon reflexes are brisk and the relaxation phase shortened.

Serum enzymes of muscle origin are surprisingly little changed, even in patients with symptomatic muscle weakness. Creatine kinase (CK) levels may be normal or slightly lowered in hyperthyroidism, in comparison with the raised levels often found in hypothyroidism. Electromyography may demonstrate the presence of 'myopathic' motor unit action potentials in up to 90% of all cases, irrespective of their clinical state (Havard et al 1963,

Ramsay 1966). In view of this, the paucity of pathological data in hyperthyroidism is disappointing, although it is perhaps not surprising because the instinct of most physicians is to avoid invasive investigations when a clear-cut diagnosis can be made on clinical and non-invasive laboratory grounds. Certainly, our own experience in this area is limited, and a recent review of the literature on ultrastructural studies (Cullen et al 1988) failed to reveal more than a few case reports with no comprehensive and systematic studies, especially those involving electron microscopy. In fact, the first suggestion of any 'specific' histopathological abnormalities in the dysthyroid myopathies generally was made by Asbøe–Hansen et al (1952) in limb muscle from 10 out of 10 cases of malignant exophthalmos, 9 out of 10 cases of thyrotoxicosis without eye involvement, and one out of seven cases of myxoedema. These workers claimed to have found small PAS-positive crescents (containing mucopolysaccharide) immediately beneath the sarcolemma in material from some of the patients, although this observation has not been confirmed, as far as we are aware. Certainly we have never seen these structures in biopsy muscle from patients with thyrotoxicosis, although they have been reported subsequently in hypothyroidism (see below).

In the majority of cases, routine histopathological studies show little or nothing (Havard et al 1963, Engel 1966a, Ramsay 1966, Gruener et al 1975), Ramsay reporting non-specific changes in only 25% of the biopsies from his patients and Gruener and his colleagues finding only nonselective fibre atrophy in their material at the light-microscopic level. In fact, the only reported change which would be accepted as genuinely abnormal nowadays would be the 'focal perivascular lymphorrhages' which may well have been due to associated inflammatory muscle disease. Engel (1966a) described the light- and electron-microscopic findings in two cases of thyrotoxic myopathy, reporting only 'small clear spaces' in a few fibres seen with phase-contrast microscopy (see his Fig. 3A, B). With the benefit of hindsight, these 'small clear spaces' seem likely to have been artefacts. However, he found a number of abnormalities at the ultrastructural level, including numerous papillary projections

from the normally smooth sarcolemma of the muscle fibres, large subsarcolemmal deposits of glycogen (Engel related these to the PAS-positive crescents described by Asbøe–Hansen et al 1952), focal dilatation of the T tubules, and mitochondrial degeneration. Engel considered that the last two changes were likely to be relevant to the pathogenesis of thyrotoxic myopathy, and it seems only reasonable to suggest that the mitochondrial changes in particular may have been induced by excessive circulating thyroxine. Gustaffson et al (1965) described proliferation of mitochondria in muscle from hypothyroid rats, and the mitochondrial volume in rat liver can be increased by a single injection of T4. Repeated injections cause mitochondrial swelling with the formation of intramitochondrial myelin whorls and structureless deposits (O'Brien & Klitgaard 1965). More recently, Peter et al (1970b) related the hypermetabolism of thyrotoxic myopathy to an actual increase in the population of mitochondria, which has a close parallel in so-called 'non-thyroidal hypermetabolism' (Luft's disease, see Ch. 10). Ultrastructural abnormalities similar to those described by Engel (1966a) have been recorded by Gruener et al (1975).

In an experimental study, Johnson et al (1980a) found a decrease in the percentage of type 1 fibres in fast- and slow-twitch muscles and an increase in the percentage of type 2a (slow-twitch) and type 2c (intermediate) fibres in hyperthyroid rats. In addition, both the contraction and relaxation phases of the isometric twitch of soleus (slow-twitch) were accelerated and the rate of development of maximum tetanic tension was increased. Johnson and her colleagues speculated that these changes may have been induced by a neural mechanism (see below).

Personal experience with human material is limited, although the histochemical findings in a Cantonese subject with severe thyrotoxic myopathy closely resembled those seen in the experimental situation.

Ophthalmic Graves' disease

The ocular manifestations of Graves' disease consist of exophthalmos, lid retraction, periorbital swelling and sometimes ophthalmoplegia, together with varying degrees of conjunctival irritation and chemosis. These may be associated with hyperthyroidism or may occur in the syndrome of ophthalmic Graves' disease, where the patient is not clinically hyperthyroid and gives no past history of hyperthyroidism. Increase in muscle bulk in the orbit can contribute to the exophthalmos. Ophthalmoplegia is associated with autoimmune thyroiditis (AIT) and is not seen in patients with hyperthyroidism resulting from other causes. In some instances the limitation of upward and/or lateral gaze may be due to tethering, adhesions and fibrosis of the inferior rectus and medial rectus respectively.

The orbital muscles may be greatly swollen (Fig. 13.1) and there is an increase in the orbital connective tissue. Mucopolysaccharides (glycos-

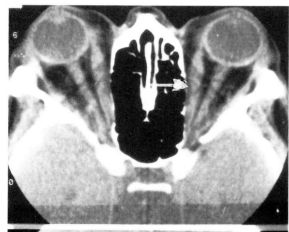
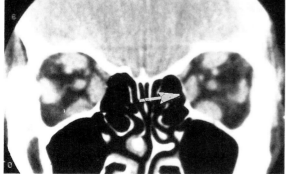

Fig. 13.1 Computerised axial tomographic scan of the orbits from an adult male with ophthalmic Graves' disease and left proptosis. Marked enlargement of the left superior rectus muscle is shown (arrows)

aminoglycans) accumulate in the ground substance, especially hyaluronic acid and chondroitin sulphates which bind water and increase the orbital swelling. Cellular infiltration with lymphocytes, plasma cells and mast cells (Riley 1972, Spoor et al 1980) reflects the underlying autoimmune nature of the disorder. The fat content of the orbit may be increased but this is not a usual feature. Cellular and water accumulation, less often fat, contribute to the swelling of the orbital muscles and retrobulbar connective tissue.

Electron microscopy of fibrotic muscles reveals myofibrillar disorganization, loss of cross-striations and eventually fibroblastic multiplication and replacement (Kroll & Kuwabara 1966, Spoor et al 1980, Hufnagel et al 1984).

The lid retraction of Graves' disease results from spasm of the striated muscle of levator palpebrae superioris, accentuated in some cases by sympathetic overactivity of its smooth muscle component. Little is known of the biochemical and ultrastructural abnormalities which must accompany this functional change. The histochemical changes have been reviewed by Ringel et al (1978).

The pathogenesis of the ocular changes of Graves' disease remains uncertain, although there is general agreement that the increased levels of circulating thyroid hormones contribute little other than lid retraction. One of many theories is that which postulates that damage to the orbital tissues may result from binding of thyroglobulin–antithyroglobulin immune complexes to cell membranes, particularly of muscle (Kriss et al 1975) but recent studies have not supported this view. However, the most attractive hypothesis to emerge in the recent past is that the target organ, i.e. extra-ocular muscle, is attacked selectively by specific auto-antibodies (polyclonal IgG?) to their surface antigens (Perros & Kendall–Taylor 1989). This proposition has yet to be confirmed independently but seems hardly surprising in context. In the light of this, it is perhaps surprising that patients with thyroid-associated ophthalmopathy do not usually have concomitant inflammatory muscle disease (see above, p 493). However, eye muscle has some characteristics not found in skeletal muscle, and it is possible that the autoimmune response is directed to autoantigens occurring predominantly in eye muscle. The curious predilection for the inferior and medial recti remains to be explained.

Thyrotoxic periodic paralysis (TPP)

TPP is defined as the occurrence of an episode, or episodes, of muscular weakness in a thyrotoxic patient. It occurs particularly in males of Asian origin although it is seen occasionally in females and in Caucasians as well. In Singapore it is more often associated with the HLA type BW46 (SIN 2), and the presence of types BW22 and BW17 appears to increase the risk of paralysis (Cheah 1978). Au & Yeung (1972), using the erythrocyte membrane system as a model, suggest that the underlying defect rests in an inherited abnormality of the ATPase activity of the sarcolemma, which is unmasked by high extracellular glucose and thyrotoxicosis.

Engel (1966b) reported that biopsies obtained from weak muscles from a patient with thyrotoxic periodic paralysis appeared to be normal under the light microscope. At the ultrastructural level, variable numbers of muscle fibres contained numerous small vacuoles ranging from 0.1 to 0.7 μm in diameter, lined by a unit membrane, some containing small amounts of low-density amorphous material. Engel considered that these vacuoles were dilated terminal cisternae of the SR and he described these as the earliest abnormality seen in 'primary' hypokalaemic periodic paralysis. In addition, he reported occasional subsarcolemmal glycogen accumulations but no other morphological abnormalities. Similar abnormalities have been described during and between attacks (Bergman et al 1970, Takagi et al 1973). Mitochondrial changes, for example swelling, pleomorphism, matrical pallor and reduction of cristae, are likely to be attributable to concomitant hyperthyroidism. Large masses of interfibrillar glycogen and subsarcolemmal deposits have been reported (Takagi et al 1973).

Hypothyroid myopathy

Disordered muscle function may be a dominant feature of hypothyroidism and is present in virtually all patients with overt thyroid failure. Commonly, patients complain of generalized aches and pains, with muscle stiffness and sometimes cramps which may simulate rheumatic disorders (Golding 1970). Hoffmann's syndrome of increased muscle volume and slowness of contraction without weakness is a rare but striking association of hypothyroidism. Prolongation of the relaxation phase of the tendon reflexes is characteristic of hypothyroidism and may be of diagnostic value.

Increased activity of serum enzymes of muscle origin is common in hypothyroidism, although of little diagnostic value because of the lack of specificity of the finding. It has been claimed that serum CK levels are significantly increased in the majority of patients with overt hypothyroidism (Fleisher et al 1965). Males tend to have higher values and the increased activity is confined to the muscle isoenzyme (Goto 1974). Serum lactate dehydrogenase levels are often raised in hypothyroidism, the isoenzyme pattern resembling that seen after myocardial infarction. In some patients, levels of serum aspartate aminotransferase (SAsT) are also increased (Fleisher et al 1965).

Despite the frequency of hypothyroidism in the general population, the literature on its myopathology is relatively sparse. There seems to be a consensus that the brunt of disruption inflicted by thyroid hormone deficiency upon the muscle cell is borne by the structure of the mitochondrion on the one hand and by carbohydrate metabolism on the other. Certainly, there are several references to the presence of PAS-positive crescents within the muscle cell in hypothyroidism and related disorders (Asbøe–Hansen et al 1952, Kirchheiner 1962, Scarlato & Spinnler 1967), this material being resistant to predigestion with amylase in the case described by Scarlato & Spinnler (1967). Godet–Guillain & Fardeau (1970) suggested that these phenomena may simply have been produced by unorthodox fixation. In addition, excessive amounts, or focal accumulations, of glycogen have been reported in material examined electron-microscopically from children with hypertrophic myopathy (Kocher–Debré–Sémélaigne syndrome) (Spiro et al 1970, Afifi et al 1974) and adult hypothyroidism (Norris & Panner 1966). In this context, the observation that muscle acid maltase activity may be reduced in adult hypothyroidism (Hurwitz et al 1970, McDaniel et al 1977) may be relevant.

In addition, Spiro et al (1970) demonstrated type 1 fibre atrophy, major alterations in oxidative enzyme activity, peripheral crescents, and distension of the sarcoplasmic reticulum, in a child with hypothyroidism and increased muscle bulk. These changes resolved fully after treatment with thyroid hormone.

As mentioned previously with reference to thyrotoxicosis, it seems only reasonable to suggest that the mitochondria would be the prime target for thyroid dysfunction, and the first description of the ultrastructural pathology of hypothyroidism (Norris & Panner 1966) emphasized the frequency and severity of degenerative changes in these organelles. Norris & Panner described widespread focal non-specific degenerative changes in muscle mitochondria with scattered inclusions, some of which were paracrystalline and others simple dense bodies. Subsequently, Godet–Guillain & Fardeau (1970) described frequent paracrystalline inclusions in material from a patient with an atrophic form of hypothyroid myopathy.

A number of other less specific abnormalities have been recorded in some of the accounts mentioned above. In particular, Godet–Guillain & Fardeau reported focal myofibrillar degeneration accompanied by evidence of local lysosomal enzyme activity (autophagic vacuole formation), proliferation of the SR with dilatation of its terminal cisternae, peripheral and internal sarcoplasmic masses and striated annulets or ring fibres, and commented upon the similarity of these changes to those seen in myotonic dystrophy, in which there is also an increase in muscle tone.

These observations have been supported by the findings of Cullen et al (1988) who found areas of degeneration and myeloid bodies in the mitochondria both of muscle fibres and of endothelial cells as the commonest abnormality in a study of hypothyroid myopathy. They also found paracrystalline inclusions and calcific granules in mitochondria and, in two cases, 'core-like' areas without enzyme activity which contained fine granular material (Fig. 13.2).

Turning to experimental hypothyroidism,

emphasis has been placed on disordered oxidative metabolism once again. Gustaffson et al (1965) and Meijer (1972) described an increase both in the volume and in the number of mitochondria in liver and muscle from thyroidectomized rats. Johnson et al (1980b) found significant increases in the percentage of type 1 fibres in both fast- and slow-twitch muscles of hypothyroid rats, particularly the latter (Fig. 13.3). They also showed that this phenomenon could be prevented by denervation. Reasoning from this, they suggested that functional conversion of type 2 to type 1 fibres (and vice versa) can be induced by altered discharge patterns of anterior horn cells in the presence of thyroid hormone deficiency (or excess). No evidence of structural damage to anterior horn cells or of denervation/re-innervation in the affected muscles was found. These observations have been reflected in the reports of higher-than-normal percentages of type 1 fibres in muscle from hypothyroid humans (McKeran et al 1975, Wiles et al 1979) which decrease only very slowly with replacement therapy (McKeran et al 1975). Wiles et al (1979) found a corresponding reduction in percentages of type 1 fibres in only one of their patients with hyperthyroidism. The striking muscular hypertrophy, which is so often a feature of Hoffmann's syndrome (Walton 1990), is still unexplained as muscle biopsy in such cases often fails to reveal any morphological abnormality.

It is quite clear that no sweeping generalizations can be made about the pathogenetic significance of the morphological and histochemical abnormalities described above. It seems equally clear, however, that they underline the importance of the intimate relationship between thyroid function and both glycolytic and oxidative metabolism. In addition, they re-emphasize the value of muscles as an accessible target tissue for study of the pathophysiology of intermediary metabolism and of the role of neural control both in the clinical and in the experimental situation.

Medullary carcinoma of the thyroid

It would be inappropriate to conclude this section without a brief mention of the congenital myopathy which is but one of the myriad of dysplastic

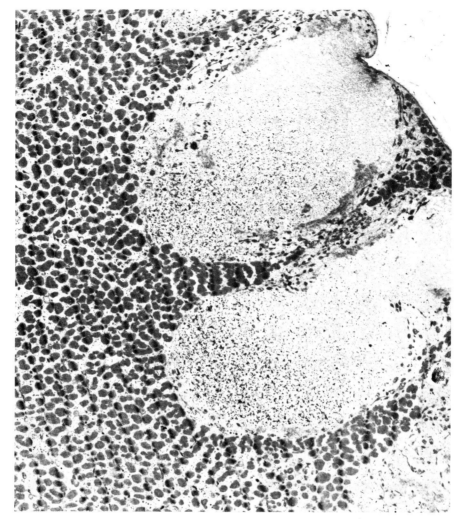

Fig. 13.2 Hypothyroid myopathy in a 20-year-old female. Electron micrograph showing peripheral areas devoid of myofibrils and containing granular material; ×27 500

associations of medullary carcinoma of the thyroid, formerly called Sipple's syndrome and now termed multiple endocrine neoplasia (MEN) type III (or IIb). Medullary carcinoma of the thyroid, which arises from the parafollicular or C cells, produces calcitonin, but the high circulating level apparently does not have any deleterious effects on the affected subject. Skin pigmentation often accompanies the myopathy, as first described by Cunliffe et al (1970). The latter has some features in common with what McKusick (1972) calls 'marfanoid myopathy', a condition associated with a variety of dysplastic states (and which is almost certainly *neurogenic* in some cases). This myopathy is characterized pathologically by an overwhelming predominance of type 1 fibres, similar to that seen in central core disease (Cunliffe et al 1970 — see their Fig. 4a,b), with a variety of non-specific changes at the ultrastructural level.

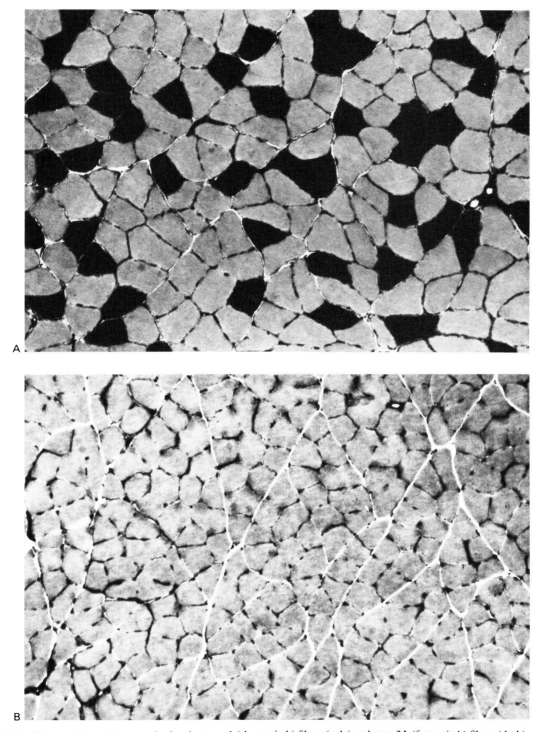

Fig. 13.3 (A) normal rat soleus muscle showing type 1 (slow-twitch) fibres (pale) and type 2A (fast-twitch) fibres (dark). (B) Hypothyroid rat soleus showing loss of type 2A fibres due to conversion into type 1 (slow-twitch). Myofibrillar ATPase pH 9.5; ×120

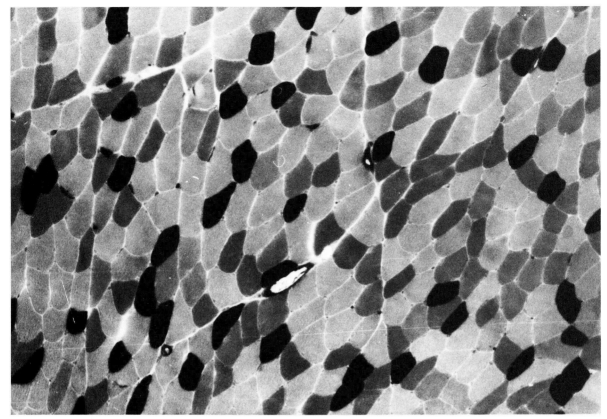

Fig. 13.4 Quadriceps muscle biopsy from a hyperthyroid patient showing an abnormally low percentage of type 1 fibres. 'Reversal' ATPase after pH 4.6 preincubation. Type 1 fibres dark, type 2A pale, type 2B intermediate; ×140

MYOPATHIES ASSOCIATED WITH DISORDERS OF ADRENAL CORTICOSTEROID METABOLISM

Muscle dysfunction in Addison's disease and/or in disorders of sodium concentration

Muscular weakness and fatiguability are common features of hypoadrenalism, whatever its cause, and remit rapidly with appropriate corticosteroid replacement. Hyperkalaemia and/or hypernatraemia in primary adrenal failure may contribute to the muscle dysfunction. There are no reliable reports of the morphological changes in muscle responsible for these symptoms.

The possibility that changes in intracellular sodium concentration may cause a myopathy was raised by a single case, seen by one of us (PH), in which fluctuating muscle weakness was associated with alterations in serum sodium concentration produced by a presumed bronchogenic metastasis in the floor of the third ventricle. This lesion must have involved the hypothalamic thirst centres, because the patient periodically 'forgot' to drink, at which time his serum sodium concentration rose rapidly and he developed profound proximal muscle weakness with a myopathic electromyogram (EMG). Both his weakness and the EMG abnormalities resolved when he was rehydrated. A biopsy taken during a myopathic attack appeared to be normal under the light microscope, although examination of ultrathin sections showed dilatation of the terminal cisternae of the SR (Hudgson & Pearce 1969).

The myopathy of naturally occurring Cushing's syndrome

Proximal muscle weakness is a common clinical finding in Cushing's syndrome (as clearly described by Cushing (1932) in cases of basophil adenomas of the pituitary body) and is thought to be due to a direct effect of cortisol on muscle cell metabolism. It remits with successful treatment of the underlying condition (Müller & Kugelberg 1959), in a similar manner to thyrotoxic myopathy, which it resembles clinically. Perhaps the most interesting observation made with the light microscope is the apparently consistent increase in the number of lipid droplets in type 1 fibres (Harriman & Reed 1972). This may be a reflection of the known capacity of cortisol to liberate free fatty acids from neutral fat stored in adipose tissue, although why it should accumulate preferentially in skeletal muscle is not clear. Type 2 fibre atrophy has also been reported in Cushing's syndrome (Pleasure et al 1970).

The mechanism of production of muscle weakness in this situation is also obscure, but it may be an 'overload' block of utilization by mitochondria (muscle fibres do not function normally when they contain too much fat, for example in carnitine or CPT deficiency — see Ch. 11). Certainly there is some experimental evidence to suggest that mitochondrial structure and oxidative metabolism may be impaired by the administration of synthetic corticosteroids (Bullock et al 1971, Vignos & Greene 1973) although Peter et al (1970a) found that muscle mitochondria from rats treated with triamcinolone respired normally. Further to this, Shoji & Pennington (1977) and Rannels et al (1978) reported inhibition of protein synthesis, caused by impairment of mRNA synthesis, in experimental corticosteroid myopathy. As far as we are aware, there have not been any comparable studies on muscle from patients with Cushing's syndrome.

There do not appear to be any other gross histological or histochemical abnormalities in this disorder, apart from a characteristic type 2 fibre atrophy also seen in steroid myopathy; the rather meagre ultrastructural data available do not shed any further light on the problem.

When cortisol overproduction is severe, particularly in the ectopic ACTH syndrome, hypokalaemia any contribute to the muscle weakness, although hypokalaemia per se is unlikely to be a major factor in the aetiology of the myopathy in most patients with Cushing's syndrome.

Iatrogenic steroid myopathy

The propensity of most of the naturally occurring and synthetic corticosteroid agents used therapeutically to produce side-effects exactly similar to the clinical features of Cushing's disease, has been well recognized for many years. Prominent among these side-effects is muscle weakness, first described by Perkoff et al (1959). This may be severe and permanent, although its development is usually related closely to dose and duration of therapy and possibly to the type of synthetic steroid employed, the 9,α-fluorinated group allegedly being the worst offender (Golding et al 1961). Once again, our understanding of the pathology and pathogenesis of this form of steroid myopathy is imprecise, probably because only a very small minority of such cases are subjected to biopsy. However, we have had the opportunity to study patients occasionally in whom a repeat biopsy was carried out to clarify diagnostic uncertainty, for example, in a patient with chronic polymyositis receiving long-term corticosteroid therapy, who deteriorated after initial improvement and who then proved to have a steroid myopathy (Lane et al 1989). In almost all such cases, histochemical studies have demonstrated a type 2 fibre atrophy (Fig. 13.5) with little or no evidence of any necrobiotic changes within the muscle fibres. This experience was adumbrated by the experimental study of Livingstone et al (1981) who administered dexamethasone to rats for 14 days, producing a moderately severe type 2b fibre atrophy.

Unfortunately, ultrastructural data on the steroid myopathies are sparse, and the abnormalities described to date have been entirely non-specific, contributing little or nothing to our understanding of pathogenetic mechanisms. Thickening of the basement membrane of muscle fibres was reported by Afifi et al (1968) and by Mastaglia et al (1970b), and focal aggregations of mitochondria with 'degenerative' changes, for example vacuolation in some, were described by

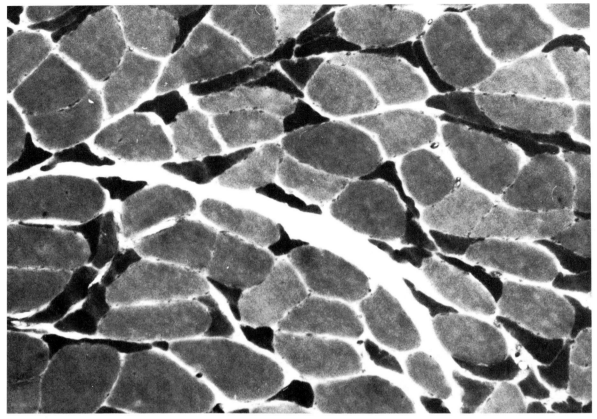

Fig. 13.5 Muscle biopsy (deltoid) showing severe type 2 fibre atrophy in a patient with polymyositis after prolonged treatment with steroids. Myofibrillar ATPase pH 9.5; ×165

Pearce (1964) and Engel (1966a). Some of these changes at least may have been artefactual, possibly attributable to suboptimal fixation, although similar abnormalities have been reported in experimental steroid myopathy in the rat and rabbit (D'Agostino & Chiga 1966, Ritter 1967, Afifi & Bergman 1969, Freund–Mölbert et al 1973). Other reported abnormalities include an increase in intermyofibrillar sarcoplasm and an apparent increase in glycogen (Pearce 1964, D'Agostino & Chiga 1966, Ritter 1967), the latter observation being consistent with the increase in glycogen synthetase activity in muscle in experimental steroid myopathy, demonstrated by Shoji et al (1974). In addition, D'Agostino & Chiga (1966), Harriman & Reed (1972) and Freund–Mölbert et al (1973) reported an increase in the number of lipid droplets in muscle fibres in iatrogenic steroid myopathy as well as Cushing's disease, although

this is not seen with the light microscope in our experience. Afifi & Bergman (1969) and Freund–Mölbert et al (1973) described both necrosis and calcification of muscle fibres in acute, high-dose animal experiments, an experience paralleled by the reports of an acute necrobiotic myopathy developing in patients with status asthmaticus treated with large intravenous doses of hydrocortisone (MacFarlane & Rosenthal 1977, van Marle & Woods 1980, Knox et al 1986).

Nelson's syndrome

A proportion of patients who were subjected to bilateral adrenalectomy for Cushing's syndrome developed generalized skin pigmentation and, later, proximal muscle weakness which may be fatiguable (Prineas et al 1968). The presence of a myopathy can be confirmed by electromyography in these patients, and biopsy shows an increase in the number of lipid droplets in the type 1 fibres, assessed histochemically or electron-microscopically. The clinicopathological features of this condition are thought to be caused by an extra-adrenal action of the very high serum ACTH levels which develop after adrenalectomy.

Conn's syndrome

Some patients with aldosterone-secreting cortical adenomas develop either paralytic attacks (Conn 1955) or progressive proximal muscle weakness, and can be shown to have a vacuolar myopathy associated with their potassium loss.

Acromegalic myopathy

In acromegaly, muscular enlargement is common but muscle strength is inappropriately less than would be expected from the increased bulk. Mastaglia et al (1970a) described a myopathy associated with untreated acromegaly in nine patients, and Mastaglia (1973) later analysed the pathological data from this group. He described a variety of non-specific histological, histochemical and

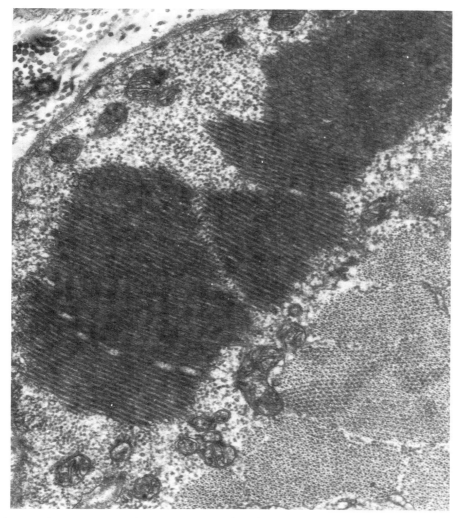

Fig. 13.6 An electron-microscope section of a muscle biopsy obtained from a patient with acromegaly. Densely staining tubular aggregates are seen at the periphery of a muscle fibre; ×28 000. (From Hudgson & Mastaglia 1974 In: Walton J N (ed) Disorders of voluntary muscle, 3rd edn. Churchill Livingstone, Edinburgh, ch 10, p 397)

ultrastructural abnormalities in this material, and the most interesting finding was the presence of coiled membranous inclusions and tubular aggregates (Fig. 13.6) in one case. The biological significance of the tubular aggregates is uncertain but their histochemical reactions for oxidative enzyme activity suggest that their behaviour is similar to that of the outer lamina of the mitochondrial membrane. Their most consistent clinical association is with patients presenting with cramping muscle pains on exertion.

Mastaglia et al (1970a) observed type 1 fibre hypertrophy and type 2 atrophy as did Nagulesparen et al (1976), who found atrophy particularly affecting type 2A fibres. The atrophy was not that of simple disuse, which affects largely type 1 fibres, while the hypertrophy was not that seen after exercise, which is most often present in type 2 fibres. It seems most unlikely that the hypertrophy is a result of the excess growth-hormone secretion, acting directly on muscle and increasing circulatory levels of insulin-like growth factor (KF-1).

Acromegalic cardiomyopathy is a well-recognized although rare complication of the disease and is not fully explained by the hypertension which often accompanies acromegaly. It may present as heart failure, and cardiac enlargement is present. Asymmetrical hypertrophy of the interventricular septum is observed on echocardiography (Hearne et al 1975). The relationship of the cardiomyopathy to the myopathy of acromegaly remains uncertain.

MUSCLE DYSFUNCTION IN DISORDERS OF CALCIUM METABOLISM (see also Ch. 9)

As appears to be the case with many of the other endocrine 'myopathies', profound muscle weakness and/or pain due to gross disturbances of calcium metabolism may be accompanied by little, if any, evidence of morphological change within the muscle cell. In fact, the most consistent finding with the light microscope is a simple type 2 fibre atrophy irrespective of the nature of the underlying metabolic error. We have seen this in hypercalcaemia caused by a parathyroid adenoma (in a patient presenting with intense muscle pain) and in hypocalcemia and osteomalacia attributable to a variety of causes. These include adult coeliac

disease (Schott & Wills 1976), chronic renal failure (Floyd et al 1974) (both conditions may actually *present* with a slowly progressive limb–girdle myopathy) and primary hypoparathyroidism (Snowdon et al 1976). Floyd et al (1974) described a variety of non-specific ultrastructural abnormalities in biopsy material from their patients with 'uraemic' myopathy, including a 'finger-print' body in one, but these gave no help as far as pathogenetic mechanisms were concerned. They invoked a number of possible factors, including a direct effect of as yet undefined products of end-stage renal failure, intracellular acidosis, deficiency of, or resistance to, vitamin D (or more likely lack of 1,25-dihydroxycholecalciferol) and/or hypocalcaemia. In those patients with severe bone disease, the latter two factors were considered to be causes as likely as any of the others. In addition, muscle ischaemia has been involved as a possible pathogenetic mechanism in patients with 'uraemic' hyperparathyroidism who develop muscle weakness associated with focal calcium deposits and medial calcification in muscle arterioles (Richardson et al 1969, Goodhue et al 1972). Cholod et al (1970) also found arteriolar thickening and expansion of the capillary basement membranes in material from two cases of familial hyperparathyroidism and inferred that these changes may have induced muscle ischaemia and thence weakness in these patients.

More recently, Pleasure et al (1979), in an experimental study of vitamin D deficiency in chicks, found that in vitro transport of $^{45}Ca^{2+}$ by the sarcoplasmic reticulum (SR) was reduced and that the calcium content of muscle was much lower than in normal controls. These abnormalities were unrelated to changes in plasma calcium and phosphate concentrations and were reflected physiologically by delayed relaxation of tension after tetanic stimulation.

HYPOGONADISM

Patients who are hypogonadal from any cause usually suffer from lack of muscle strength, and examination may reveal reduction in muscle bulk. These features resolve with appropriate hormone replacement. It has been common practice in some athletic communities to use anabolic steroids and occasionally testosterone itself, to increase performance. There have been no reported studies of the pathology of muscle in hypogonadal patients or in athletes self-treated with androgens.

MUSCLE DYSFUNCTION IN DIABETES MELLITUS

It is clear from a review of the recent literature that skeletal muscle dysfunction in diabetes mellitus is due principally to ischaemia and/or denervation atrophy. The latter is, of course, produced by the various peripheral neuropathies associated with diabetes, including so-called diabetic amyotrophy (see below). The commonest cause of muscle ischaemia in diabetes is obliterative disease of arteries of all sizes because of accelerated atherosclerosis and this has led to actual infarction of muscle in rare instances (Banker & Chester 1973). In gross muscle infarction, the patients present with excruciatingly painful localized swellings which develop suddenly in the large muscles of the lower limbs. According to Banker & Chester (1973), regeneration of these lesions is ineffective for three reasons: the patients often have repeated haemorrhages into the infarcts when they persist with ambulation; collateral circulation is poor because of diffuse arterial obliteration; and effective regeneration depends upon integrity of the peripheral nervous system, which is often abnormal.

In addition, in a series of ultrastructural studies, diabetic microangiopathy has been shown to affect the microvasculature of skeletal muscle. Siperstein et al (1968) measured the mean internal and external radii of muscle capillaries in a group of normal subjects and pre-diabetic and diabetic patients. By this means they were able to demonstrate thickening of the capillary basement membranes (up to a maximum of twice the normal width) in 50% of both the diabetic and pre-diabetic groups. The authors considered that these changes were unrelated to the age or weight of the patients or to the severity or duration of their disease, and they did not believe that they were induced by hyperglycaemia per se. Reske–Nielsen et al (1977) studied the capillaries in 32 muscle biopsies from patients with juvenile-onset diabetes and found increased pinocytotic activity in the endothelial

cells, irrespective of the duration of the disease. However, they found that capillary basement membrane thickening was restricted to material from patients with long-standing diabetes. In this context, it is of interest that Barbosa et al (1980) were unable to demonstrate basement membrane thickening in either HLA-identical or non-identical sibs of patients with insulin-dependent diabetes, in a search for markers for pre-diabetes. However, the HLA-identical sibs had significantly more intense immunofluorescent staining for albumin in the extracellular membranes of skeletal muscle than either the HLA-non-identical sibs or the controls. In addition, both sib groups had significantly more intense immunofluorescent staining for IgG in these membranes, than the normal controls. These workers suggested that such abnormal staining for protein in the extracellular membranes was an expression of pre-diabetes and that it might be associated with mild or intermittent glucose intolerance.

Direct associations between diabetes mellitus and primary muscle disease are uncommon except in the case of dystrophia myotonica, where approximately 30% of all affected subjects have an abnormal insulin response to a carbohydrate load. In addition, a close association between early-onset diabetes, mitochondrial myopathy and cerebellar ataxia has been defined in six generations of a family with a facioscapulohumeral syndrome, studied in the Newcastle laboratories (Hudgson et al 1972, Worsfold et al 1973, Mechler et al 1981). This disorder appears to be determined by an autosomal dominant mode of inheritance, with incomplete penetrance and variable expression, probably consistent with mitochondrial inheritance. It is characterized pathologically in muscle by the presence of large numbers of morphologically abnormal mitochondria, many of which contain pleomorphic inclusions (Cullen et al 1988 — see their Figs. 8.14 and 8.15). Biochemical studies (Worsfold et al 1973) have shown that oxidative phosphorylation is only loosely coupled in muscle from these patients, but the fundamental metabolic defect has yet to be unmasked. The diabetes in members of this family tends to be rather brittle, and one patient is also subject to frequent and severe lactic acidaemic attacks.

The only other possible association of which we

are aware is the late-onset proximal myopathy developing in four diabetic sisters, who also had 'senile' cataracts and Dupuytren's contractures (Swash et al 1970). Biopsies from these patients showed mild and rather patchy necrobiotic changes, with no histochemical abnormalities and no inclusions of any kind. Swash and his colleagues emphasized that none of these patients had either clinical or electromyographic evidence of myotonia, but were unable to suggest a suitable nosological category for this condition. Follow-up information on this sibship and on two of their children who had diabetes but no evidence of muscle disease at the time of writing, would be of considerable interest.

Diabetic amyotrophy

This entity is firmly associated with the name of Garland who, in 1955, studied 12 patients with poorly controlled diabetes associated with asymmetrical weakness, pain and wasting of the quadriceps in particular (and sometimes of other muscle groups), with loss of the knee reflexes but no sensory loss. Biopsies revealed a pattern of single muscle fibre atrophy which differed from the usual pattern of neurogenic atrophy, according to Locke et al (1963). Muscle enzymes remain within the normal range, and histochemical studies are inconclusive in differentiating a neuropathy from a myopathy, although appropriate electrophysiological studies will often demonstrate delayed femoral nerve conduction. This condition, which should probably be regarded as a manifestation of diabetic femoral mononeuritis, may be the presenting manifestation of the disease in the elderly. It may be either unilateral or bilateral and it usually improves with the passage of time and with improved control of diabetes.

Pathologically, one would expect to see denervation atrophy in biopsy specimens of muscle from these patients and, certainly, this was so in the patients studied by Shafiq et al (1968). In addition, they found scattered subsarcolemmal collections of diamond-shaped crystals in semi-thin (1–1.5 μm) araldite sections stained with methylene blue. Ultrastructurally, these crystals contained either parallel rows of electron-dense material with a periodicity of approximately 1200 nm, or a much finer rectangular lattice. Their significance remains obscure.

MISCELLANEOUS DISORDERS

Patients with gastrin-secreting adenomas of the islets of Langerhans may develop severe, generalized muscle weakness with a vacuolar myopathy, caused by loss of potassium from the gut. An ischaemic myopathy has been described in patients with carcinoid tumours.

CONCLUSION

In view of the complexity and variety of the metabolic derangements underlying the disorders discussed above, it is not surprising, although disappointing, to find so little 'specific' myopathology underlying the often severe accompanying muscle weakness. However, this underlines the old pathological truism, that tissues which are highly specialized from the functional standpoint are limited in the ways in which they can react to stresses of various kinds. It also emphasizes our ignorance of the pathophysiological basis for disordered muscle function at the molecular level in these conditions.

ACKNOWLEDGEMENTS

The authors wish to thank Miss Sarah Barwick for typing the manuscript.

REFERENCES

Afifi A K, Bergman R A 1969 Steroid myopathy. A study of the evolution of the muscle lesion in rabbits. Johns Hopkins Medical Journal 124: 66

Afifi A K, Bergman R A, Harvey J C 1968 Steroid myopathy. Clinical, histologic and cytologic observations. Johns Hopkins Medical Journal 123: 158

Afifi A K, Najjar S S, Mire-Salman J, Bergman R A 1974 The myopathology of the Kocher-Debré Sémélaigne syndrome. Journal of the Neurological Sciences 22: 445

Asbøe-Hansen G, Iversen K, Wickman B 1952 Malignant exophthalmos: muscular changes and thyrotropin content in serum. Acta endocrinologica (Copenhagen) 11: 376

Au K S, Yeung R 1972 Thyrotoxic periodic paralysis. Periodic variation in the muscle calcium pump activity. Archives of Neurology (Chicago) 26: 543

Banker B Q, Chester C S 1973 Infarction of thigh muscle in the diabetic patient. Neurology (Minneapolis) 23: 667

Barbosa J, Chavers B, Steffes M et al 1980 Muscle extracellular membrane immunofluorescence and HLA as possible markers in prediabetes. Lancet ii: 330

Bergman R A, Afifi A K, Dunkle L M, Johns R G 1970 Muscle pathology in hypokalemic periodic paralysis with myasthenia gravis and Eaton–Lambert syndrome. Annals of the New York Academy of Sciences 183: 88

Bullock G R, Christian R A, Peters R F, White A M 1971 Rapid mitochondrial enlargement in muscle in response to triamcinolone acetonide and its relation to the ribosomal defect. Biochemical Pharmacology 20: 943

Cheah J S 1978 Thyrotoxic periodic paralysis in Singapore. In: Proceedings of the 6th Asian and Oceanian Congress of Endocrinology, Singapore, vol 1, p 282

Cholod E J, Haust M D, Hudson A J, Lewis F N 1970 Myopathy in primary familial hyperparathyroidism. Clinical and morphologic studies. American Journal of Medicine 48: 700

Conn J W 1955 Primary aldosteronism, a new clinical syndrome. Journal of Laboratory and Clinical Medicine 45: 661

Cullen M J, Hudgson P, Mastaglia F L 1988 Ultrastructural studies of diseased muscle. In: Walton J N (ed) Disorders of voluntary muscle, 5th edn. Churchill Livingstone, Edinburgh, p 284

Cunliffe W J, Hudgson P, Fulthorpe J J et al 1970 A calcitonin-secreting medullary thyroid carcinoma with mucosal neuromas, marfanoid features, myopathy and pigmentation. American Journal of Medicine 48: 120

Cushing H 1932 Basophic adenomas of pituitary body and their clinical manifestations (pituitary basophilism). Bulletin of the Johns Hopkins Hosp 50: 137

D'Agostino A N, Chiga M 1966 Corticosteroid myopathy in the rabbit. A light and electronmicroscopic study. Neurology (Minneapolis) 16: 247

Emslie-Smith A M 1987 Personal Communication to P Hudgson

Engel A G 1966a Thyrotoxic and corticosteroid-induced myopathies. Mayo Clinic Proceedings 41: 785

Engel A G 1966b Primary hypokalemic and thyrotoxic periodic paralyses. Mayo Clinic Proceedings 41: 797

Engel A G 1988 Metabolic and endocrine myopathies. In: Walton J N (ed) Disorders of voluntary muscle, 5th edn. Churchill Livingstone, Edinburgh, p 811

Fleisher G A, McConahey W M, Panko W M 1965 Serum creatine kinase, lactic dehydrogenase and glutamic-oxaloacetic transaminase in thyroid disease and pregnancy. Mayo Clinic Proceedings 40: 300

Floyd M F, Ayyar D R, Barwick D D, Hudgson P, Weightman D 1974 Myopathy in chronic renal failure. Quarterly Journal of Medicine (New Series) 43: 109

Freund–Mölbert E, Ketelsen U-P, Beckmann R 1973 Ultrastructural study of experimental steroid myopathy. In: Kakulas B A (ed) Basic research in myology. Excerpta Medica, Amsterdam, p 593

Gaan D 1967 Chronic thyrotoxic myopathy with involvement of respiratory and bulbar muscles. British Medical Journal 3: 415

Garland H G 1955 Diabetic amyotrophy. British Medical Journal 2: 1287

Godet–Guillain J, Fardeau M 1970 Hypothyroid myopathy.

Histological and ultrastructural study of an atrophic form. In: Walton J N, Canal N, Scarlato G (eds) Muscle diseases. Excerpta Medica, Amsterdam, p 512

Golding D N 1970 Hypothyroidism as a cause of rheumatic pain. Annals of Rheumatic Diseases 29: 10

Golding D N, Murray S M, Pearce G W, Thompson M 1961 Corticosteroid myopathy. Annals of Physical Medicine 6: 171

Goodhue W W, Davis J N, Porro R S 1972 Ischemic myopathy in uremic hyperparathyroidism. Journal of the American Medical Association 221: 911

Goto I 1974 Serum creatine phosphokinase isoenzymes in hypothyroidism, convulsions, myocardial infarction and other diseases. Clinica Chimica Acta 52: 27

Gruener R P, Stern L Z, Payne C, Hannapel L 1975 Hyperthyroid myopathy. Intracellular electrophysiological correlates of biopsied human intercostal muscle. Journal of the Neurological Sciences 24: 339

Gustaffson R, Tata J R, Lindberg O, Ernster L 1965 The relationship between the structure and activity of rat skeletal muscle mitochondria after thyroidectomy and thyroid hormone treatment. Journal of Cell Biology 26: 555

Harriman D G F, Reed L 1972 The incidence of lipid droplets in human muscle in neuromuscular disorders. Journal of Pathology 106: 1

Havard C W H, Campbell E D R, Ross H B, Spence A W 1963 Electromyographical and histological findings in patients with thyrotoxicosis. Quarterly Journal of Medicine (New Series) 32: 145

Hearne M J, Sherber H S, De Leon A C 1975 Asymmetrical septal hypertrophy in acromegaly — an endocardiographical study. Circulation (suppl II) 52: 130

Hudgson P, Pearce G W 1969 Ultramicroscopic studies of diseased muscle. In: Walton J N (ed) Disorders of voluntary muscle, 2nd edn. Churchill, London, Ch 9

Hudgson P, Bradley W G, Jenkison M 1972 Familial 'mitochondrial' myopathy. I. Clinical, electrophysiological and pathological findings. Journal of the Neurological Sciences 16: 343

Hufnagel T J, Hickey W F, Cobbs W H, Jakoriec F A, Iwamoto T, Eagle R C 1984 Immunohistochemical and ultrastructural studies on the exenterated orbital tissues of a patient with Graves' disease. Ophthalmology 91: 1411

Hurwitz L, McCormick D, Allen I V 1970 Reduced muscle α-glucosidase (acid maltase) activity in hypothyroid myopathy. Lancet i: 67

Johnson M A, Mastaglia F L, Montgomery A 1980a The histochemical and contractile properties of hyperthyroid myopathy. Lancet i: 67

Johnson M A, Mastaglia F L, Montgomery A, Pope B, Weeds A G 1980b A neurally mediated effect of thyroid hormone deficiency on slow-twitch skeletal muscle. In: Pette D (ed) Plasticity of muscle. De Gruyter, Berlin, p 607

Kirchheiner B 1962 Specific muscle lesions in pituitary–thyroid disorders. Acta Medica Scandinavica 172: 559

Knox A J, Mascie-Taylor B H, Muers M F 1986 Acute hydrocortisone myopathy in acute severe asthma. Thorax 41: 411

Kriss J P, Konishi J, Herman M 1975 Studies on the pathogenesis of Graves' ophthalmopathy (with some related observations regarding therapy). Recent Progress in Hormone Research 31: 533

Kroll A J, Kuwabara T 1966 Dysthyroid ocular myopathy: anatomy, histology and electron microscopy. Archives of Ophthalmology 76: 244

Lane R J M, Emslie-Smith A M, Mosquera I A, Hudgson P

1989 Clinical and biochemical responses to treatment in polymyositis: a prospective study. Journal of the Royal Society of Medicine 82: 333

Livingstone I R, Johnson M A, Mastaglia F L 1981 Effects of dexamethasone on fibre subtypes in rat muscle. Neuropathology and Applied Neurobiology 7: 381

Locke S, Lawrence D G, Legg M A 1963 Diabetic amylotrophy. American Journal of Medicine 34: 775

McDaniel H G, Pittman C S, Oh S J, DiMauro S 1977 Carbohydrate metabolism in hypothyroid myopathy. Metabolism 26: 867

MacFarlane I A, Rosenthal F D 1977 Severe myopathy after status asthmaticus. Lancet ii: 615

McKeran R O, Slavin G, Andrews T M, Ward P, Mair W G P 1975 Muscle fibre type changes in hypothyroid myopathy. Journal of Clinical Pathology 28: 659

McKusick V A 1972 Heritable disorders of connective tissue, 4th edn. Churchill Livingstone, Edinburgh, ch 4

Mastaglia F L 1973 Pathological changes in skeletal muscle in acromegaly. Acta Neuropathologica (Berlin) 24: 273

Mastaglia F L, Barwick D D, Hall R 1970a Myopathy in acromegaly. Lancet ii: 907

Mastaglia F L, McCollum J P K, Larson P F, Hudgson P 1970b Steroid myopathy complicating McArdle's disease. Journal of Neurology, Neurosurgery and Psychiatry 33: 111

Mechler F, Fawcett P R W, Mastaglia F L, Hudgson P 1981 Mitochondrial myopathy. A study of clinically affected and asymptomatic members of a six-generation family. Journal of the Neurological Sciences 50: 191

Meijer A E F H 1972 Mitochondria with defective respiratory control of oxidative phosphorylation isolated from muscle tissues of thyroidectomised rabbits. Journal of the Neurological Sciences 26: 305

Müller R, Kugelberg E 1959 Myopathy in Cushing's syndrome. Journal of Neurology, Neurosurgery and Psychiatry 22: 314

Nagulesparen M, Trickey R, Davies M J, Jenkins J S 1976 Muscle changes in acromegaly. British Medical Journal 4: 914

Norris F H Jr, Panner B J 1966 Hypothyroid myopathy. Archives of Neurology (Chicago) 14: 574

O'Brien T W, Klitgaard H M 1965 Electron microscopic study of in vivo effects of thyroxine on rat liver metabolism. Journal of Cell Biology 27: 74A (abstract)

Pearce G W 1964 Tissue culture and electron microscopy in muscle disease. In: Walton J N (ed) Disorders of voluntary muscle, 1st edn. Churchill, London, ch 9

Perkoff G T, Silber R, Tyler F H, Cartwright G E, Wintrobe M M 1959 Studies in disorders of muscle. XII. Myopathy due to the administration of therapeutic amount of 17-hydroxycorticosteroids. American Journal of Medicine 26: 891

Perros P, Kendall-Taylor P 1989 The pathogenesis of thyroid-associated ophthalmopathy. Journal of Endocrinology 122: 201

Peter J B, Verhaag D A, Worsfield M 1970a Studies of steroid myopathy. Examination of the possible effects of triamcinolone on mitochondria and sarcotubular vesicles of rat skeletal muscle. Biochemical Pharmacology 19: 1627

Peter J B, Worsfield M, Stempel K 1970b Mechanism of hypermetabolism and of rapid contraction and relaxation of muscle in hyperthyroidism. In: Walton J N Canal N, Scarlato G (eds) Muscle diseases. Excerpta Medica, Amsterdam, p 506

Pleasure D E, Walsh G O, Engel W K 1970 Atrophy of skeletal muscle in patients with Cushing's syndrome. Archives of Neurology (Chicago) 22: 118

Pleasure D E, Wyszynski B, Sumner A et al 1979 Skeletal muscle calcium metabolism and contractile force in vitamin D-deficient chicks. Journal of Clinical Investigation 64: 1157

Prineas J W, Hall R, Barwick D D, Watson A G 1968 Myopathy associated with pigmentation following adrenalectomy for Cushing's syndrome. Quarterly Journal of Medicine (New Series) 37: 63

Ramsay I D 1966 Muscle dysfunction in hyperthyroidism. Lancet ii: 931

Rannels S R, Rannels D E, Pegg A E, Jefferson L S 1978 Glucocorticoid effects on peptide side-chain initiation in skeletal muscle and heart. American Journal of Physiology 235: E134

Reske–Nielsen E, Harmsen A, Vorre P 1977 Ultrastructure of muscle biopsies in recent, short-term and long-term juvenile diabetes. Acta Neurologica Scandinavica 55: 345

Richardson J A, Herron G, Reitz R, Layzer R 1969 Ischemic ulcerations of the skin and necrosis of muscle in azotemic hyperparathyroidism. Annals of Internal Medicine 71: 129

Riley F C 1972 Orbital pathology in Graves' disease. Mayo Clinic Proceedings 47: 975

Ringel S P, Wilson W B, Barden M T, Kaiser K K 1978 Histochemistry of human extraocular muscle. Archives of Ophthalmology 96: 1067

Ritter R A 1967 The effect of cortisone on the structure and function of skeletal muscle. Archives of Neurology (Chicago) 17: 493

Ruff 1986 Endocrine myopathies (hyper- and hypofunction of adrenal, thyroid, pituitary, and parathyroid glands and iatrogenic steroid myopathy). In: Engel A G, Banker B Q (eds) Myology. McGraw-Hill, New York, ch 65

Scarlato G, Spinnler H 1967 La miopatica ipotiroidea. Revisione clinica e istopatologica con illustrazione d'un caso. Sistema Nervoso 19: 96

Schott G D, Wills M R 1976 Muscle weakness in osteomalacia. Lancet i: 626

Shafiq S A, Milhorat A T, Gorycki M A 1968 Crystals in muscle fibres in patients with diabetic amyotrophy and neuropathy. Neurology (Minneapolis) 18: 8785

Shoji S, Pennington R J T 1977 The effect of cortisone on protein breakdown and synthesis in rat skeletal muscle. Molecular and Cellular Endocrinology 6: 159

Shoji S, Takagi A, Sugita H, Toyokura Y 1974 Muscle glycogen metabolism in steroid-induced myopathy in rabbits. Experimental Neurology 45: 1

Siperstein M D, Unger R H, Madison L L 1968 Studies of muscle capillary basement membranes in normal subjects, diabetic and prediabetic patients. Journal of Clinical Investigation 47: 1973

Snowdon J A, Macfie A C, Pearce J B 1976 Hypocalcaemic myopathy with paranoid psychosis. Journal of Neurology, Neurosurgery and Psychiatry 39: 48

Spiro A J, Hirano A, Beilin R L, Finkelstein J W 1970 Cretinism with muscular hypertrophy (Kocher–Debre–Sémélaigne syndrome). Archives of Neurology (Chicago) 23: 340

Spoor T C, Martinez A J, Kennerdell J S, Mark L E 1980 Dysthyroid and myasthenic myopathy of the medical rectus: a clinical pathologic report. Neurology (Minneapolis) 30: 939

Swash M, van den Noort S, Craig J W 1970 Late-onset proximal myopathy with diabetic mellitus in four sisters. Neurology (Minneapolis) 20: 693

Takagi A, Schotland D L, DiMauro S, Rowland L P 1973

Thyrotoxic periodic paralysis. Function of sarcoplasmic reticulum and muscle glycogen. Neurology (Minneapolis) 23: 1008

van Marle W, Woods K L 1980 Acute hydrocortisone myopathy. British Medical Journal 3: 271

Vignos P J Jr, Greene R 1973 Oxidative respiration of skeletal muscle in experimental corticosteroid myopathy. Journal of Laboratory and Clinical Medicine 81: 365

Walton of Detchant, Lord (J N Walton) 1990 Method in medicine. The Harveian Oration, Royal College of Physicians, London

Wiles C M, Young A, Jones D A, Edwards R H T 1979 Muscle relaxation rate, fibre-type composition and energy turnover in hyper- and hypo-thyroid patients. Clinical Science 57: 375

Worsfold M, Park D C, Pennington R J T 1973 Familial 'mitochondrial' myopathy. 2. Biochemical findings. Journal of the Neurological Sciences 19: 261

14. Drug-induced, toxic and nutritional myopathies

B. A. Kakulas   F. L. Mastaglia

INTRODUCTION

Skeletal muscle is a ubiquitous and biochemically highly active tissue. This, together with the special physiological demands called for in motor function, contributes to the sensitivity of the tissue to toxins and the side-effects of drugs. The high metabolic rate of muscle is attributable to the need for great energy production and high protein turnover (Daniel et al 1977). Thus, skeletal muscle is prone to damage by a great variety of drugs, chemicals and toxins. Drugs used therapeutically in many branches of medicine, as well as alcohol and other drugs of addiction, may cause muscular symptoms either through a direct effect on the muscles or indirectly by interfering with neuromuscular transmission or with peripheral nerve function. A variety of chemicals, biological toxins and venoms are also known to be myotoxic or neurotoxic.

BASIC MECHANISMS

The mechanisms of action of drugs and toxins on skeletal muscle are diverse (Table 14.1) and have been elucidated by clinicopathological studies in man and by experimental studies. Some agents have a direct toxic effect on muscle while in the case of others muscle damage may be secondary to an immunological process initiated by the drug, to metabolic derangements such as hypokalaemia, to ischaemia or to muscle compression occurring during periods of prolonged unconsciousness and immobility following drug overdose ('crush syndrome'). In the case of certain drugs such as tetrabenazine, phencylidine and acetylcholinesterase inhibitors, muscle fibre necrosis appears to be a consequence of excessive neural driving or of

Table 14.1 Mechanisms of drug-induced muscle damage

Direct toxic effects
Local
Diffuse

Secondary effects
Electrolyte disturbance
Immunological reaction
Ischaemia
Neural activation
ACh accumulation
Compression ('crush syndrome')

the accumulation of acetylcholine at the neuromuscular junction (Wecker et al 1978, Mastaglia 1982).

Many drugs have a direct action on muscle fibres resulting in a widespread necrotizing myopathy with proximal muscle weakness, elevated serum creatine kinase (CK) levels and, at times, myoglobinuria. With the light microscope there is polyfocal necrosis of muscle fibres and associated regeneration which can be expected to be complete and to restore the muscle to normal if the offending agent is withdrawn or neutralized. On the other hand, if the toxic or drug effect continues, a polyphasic and polyfocal process leading to characteristic microarchitectural changes in the muscle will result (Kakulas 1975, 1982).

It is likely that many of the agents which cause a necrotizing myopathy have a primary action on the plasma membrane which, being the outer boundary of the muscle fibres, is exposed to the full extracellular concentration of the toxin and is the most vulnerable component of the cell (Pritchard 1979). A derangement of ionic permeability of the plasma membrane may allow increased entry of calcium ions into muscle fibres leading to myofibrillar contracture and initiating a chain of events which culminates in necrosis (Mastaglia 1982, Steer et al 1986). The myofibre necrosis caused by anticholinesterase inhibitors has been shown to be due to calcium influx at the end-plate region where the degenerative changes commence, and can be prevented in vitro by removing calcium ions from the incubating medium (Leonard & Salpeter 1979). Increased intracellular calcium levels, possibly due to a defective calcium transport function of the sarcoplasmic reticulum, are also thought to be the basis for the myofibrillar contracture and myofibre necrosis which occurs in malignant hyperpyrexia when susceptible individuals are exposed to certain anaesthetic agents or other drugs (Britt 1979, Mastaglia 1982) (see Ch. 15). A change in the electrical properties of the muscle fibre plasma membrane is the basis for the myotonia and may also underlie the myalgia and cramps which may occur during treatment with a variety of drugs (Argov & Mastaglia 1988).

A number of agents may interfere with aerobic or anaerobic pathways of energy metabolism in muscle. An experimental form of mitochondrial myopathy can be induced by 2,4-dinitrophenol and other chemicals which uncouple oxidative phosphorylation (Melmed et al 1975, Sahgal et al 1979). Administration of brominated vegetable oil interferes with β-oxidation of medium and short chain fatty acids and causes a lipid storage myopathy (Brownell & Engel 1978). Iodoacetate, which blocks the glycolytic enzyme glyceraldehyde-3-phosphate dehydrogenase, produces a condition which resembles the naturally occurring disorders of muscle glycolysis and glycogenolysis in man (Brumback et al 1983). Some drugs cause a myopathy by interfering with muscle protein synthesis and degradation. This is the case with the natural and synthetic glucocorticoids which have a dual effect of inhibiting protein synthesis and of enhancing protein degradation (Max et al 1986). The local anaesthetic agent, bupivacaine, also inhibits muscle protein synthesis and increases degradation (Steer & Mastaglia 1986).

Chloroquine and other amphiphilic cationic drugs cause a myopathy characterized by autophagic degeneration and phospholipid accumulation in muscle fibres. These drugs, which are soluble in water and lipids, and are poorly ionized at the pH of plasma, penetrate the cell membrane in the lipid phase and become adsorbed to intracellular membranes, forming inert intra-lysosomal drug–phospholipid complexes which accumulate as membranous and crystalloid structures within autophagic vacuoles (Lullmann et al 1978). Some drugs of this type may also become integrated into the plasma membrane leading to conformational and functional changes in the membrane (Drenckhahn & Lullmann-Rauch 1979).

DRUG-INDUCED DISORDERS

Necrotizing myopathies

A variety of drugs may cause muscle fibre necrosis locally when injected by the intramuscular route, or a more diffuse myopathy in which myofibre necrosis is the most prominent histological change (Lane & Mastaglia 1978, Argov & Mastaglia 1988). The clinical picture is usually that of a proximal myopathy with muscle pain and tenderness in the more rapidly evolving cases. The tendon reflexes are usually preserved unless there is an associated peripheral neuropathy. Serum CK levels are elevated, often markedly. In cases with severe widespread muscle necrosis (*acute rhabdomyolysis*) myoglobinuria may also be present (see below).

Σ-Aminocaproic acid

A myopathy is a well-recognized but uncommon complication of treatment with this antifibrinolytic agent in patients with subarachnoid haemorrhage or hereditary angioneurotic oedema (Lane et al 1979). Muscle biopsy shows disseminated myofibre necrosis and regeneration (Figs 14.1, 14.2). Selective involvement of type 1 fibres has been noted in some cases (Britt et al 1980). It has been suggested that, as Σ-aminocaproic acid is an analogue of lysine, it may replace lysine in cell membranes leading to altered membrane function or may compete with lysine in the synthesis of carnitine (Kane et al 1988). The possibility of an ischaemic basis for the myopathy has been suggested by the finding of capillary occlusions and fibrinogen deposition in some cases (Mastaglia & Argov 1980).

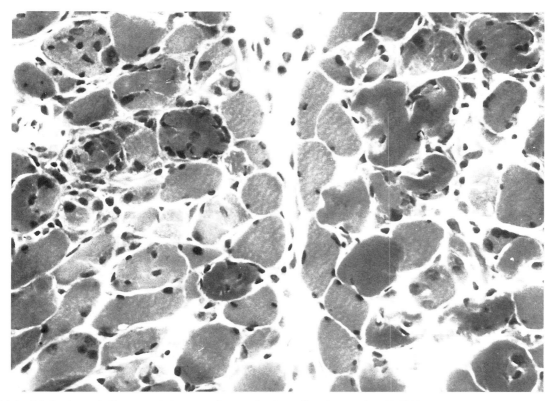

Fig. 14.1   Polyfocal muscle fibre necrosis in a case of myopathy due to Σ-aminocaproic acid. H&E, ×320. (Reproduced from Mastaglia, 1980, with permission of the British Journal of Hospital Medicine)

Clofibrate

A myopathy characterized by severe muscle pain, cramps, tenderness and weakness and markedly elevated serum CK levels develops in some patients with hyperlipidaemia who are treated with clofibrate or one of its congeners bezafibrate, etofibrate or beclofibrate (Afifi et al 1984, Rimon et al 1984, Rumpf et al 1984). The myopathy is more likely to occur in patients with renal failure, nephrotic syndrome or hypothyroidism, situations in which serum levels of the active metabolite chlorophenoxyisobutyric acid are increased. Experimental studies have shown that the drug is both myotoxic and neurotoxic (Teravainen et al 1977, Afifi et al 1984). Metabolic effects of the drug which could be relevant to the development of muscle necrosis are an impairment of glucose and fatty acid oxidation, the latter being due to reduced activity of carnitine acyltransferase (Paul & Adibi

1979), an increase in muscle lipoprotein lipase activity (Lithell et al 1978), and inhibition of branched chain amino acid oxidation (Pardridge et al 1980).

A painful myopathy with myoglobinuria may also occur in patients treated with the new hypocholesterolaemic agent, lovastatin, particularly when administered in combination with cyclosporin or gemfibrozil (Walravens et al 1989, Marais & Larson 1990).

Cardiac glycosides

There have been a number of reports of a proximal myopathy developing in opiate addicts who consume large quantities of the cough suppressant Linctus Codeine, one of the components of which

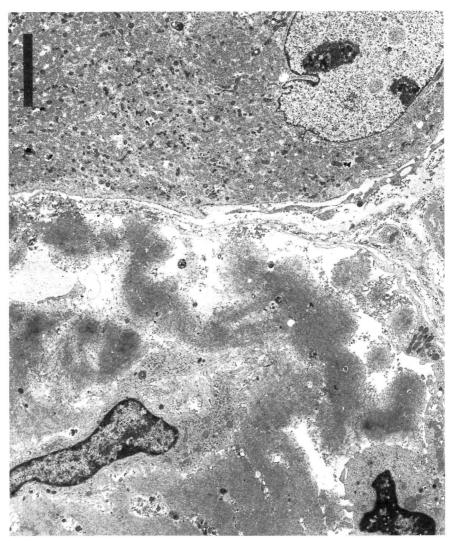

Fig. 14.2   Electron micrograph showing necrotic (bottom) and regenerating muscle fibres (top) in a case of myopathy due to Σ-aminocaproic acid. Bar = 5 μm

is Squill (an extract of the bulb of *Urginea maritama*) which contains the cardiac glycosides scillarin A and B (Kennedy 1981, Kilpatrick et al 1982, Seow 1984). Serum CK levels may be markedly elevated and muscle biopsy shows features of a necrotizing myopathy. The myopathy, and the associated cardiac abnormalities which are present in some cases, have been attributed to the inhibitory effect of cardiac glycosides on the cell membrane Na^+–K^+ pump.

Emetine

A severe myopathy with weakness of neck, bulbar, proximal limb and trunk muscles and elevation of serum CK levels may develop in patients taking emetine for amoebiasis or alcohol aversion therapy, or using ipecac syrup as an emetic (Fewings et al 1973, Brotman et al 1981, Bennett et al 1982, Friedman 1984, Sugie et al 1984, Mateer et al 1985, Palmer & Guay 1985).

Histological changes in biopsied muscles include scattered muscle fibre necrosis and regeneration, type 2 fibre atrophy, and in some cases, focal core–targetoid areas particularly in type 1 fibres (Bennett et al 1982, Sugie et al 1984, Palmer & Guay 1985). Experimental studies have shown that the drug has a pure myotoxic effect leading to mitochondrial and myofibrillar changes followed by necrosis and regeneration, with no evidence of damage to intramuscular nerves or to motor end-plates (Duane & Engel 1970, Bradley et al 1976, Bindoff & Cullen 1978).

Other drugs

The occurrence of a necrotizing myopathy has been reported in heroin (Richter et al 1971) and phencyclidine addicts (Cogen et al 1978). A necrotizing myopathy with prominent mito-chondrial changes may occur in patients with the acquired immunodeficiency syndrome treated with zidovudine (Pinching et al 1989, Panegyres et al 1990). Muscle fibre necrosis may also be an occasional finding in the myopathies induced by a number of other drugs including vincristine, colchicine, plasmocid and other drugs belonging to the amphiphilic cationic group (see below), but is usually relatively inconspicuous in these situations. Muscle fibre necrosis may also occur in severe drug-induced hypokalaemia.

In addition, a variety of drugs may induce localized muscle necrosis following administration by intramuscular injection. These include paral-dehyde, pentazocine, chlorpromazine and a number of antibiotics. Other drugs which have been shown to cause muscle necrosis experi-mentally include corticosteroids, disulfiram, imipramine, pargyline, tetrabenazine, serotonin, marcaine (Fig. 14.3), clonidine, DMSO, p-phenylenediamine, diphenylhydantoin, choline-sterase inhibitors, and azathioprine.

Acute rhabdomyolysis

This most severe form of diffuse necrotizing myopathy is associated with the abrupt onset of severe generalized muscle pain, flaccid areflexic paralysis and myoglobinuria, which may be suffi-ciently severe to lead to acute oliguric renal failure and a fatal outcome in some cases. Serum CK levels are markedly elevated. Muscle biopsy shows widespread necrosis, usually with a mild interstitial inflammatory infiltrate, and, if sufficient time has elapsed, signs of regenerative activity may also be present.

Although a great variety of drugs and toxins have been implicated in causing this syndrome (see Table 14.2), including some of the drugs already discussed above, few have been proven to be intrinsically myotoxic and, in many instances, other factors may have been responsible for causing muscle damage. These include muscle com-pression and ischaemia as a result of prolonged periods of unconsciousness and immobility in cases of alcohol or drug overdose; hypoxia and hypotension (Penn et al 1972); and sustained muscular hyperactivity in patients with drug-induced seizures, dyskinesias or acute dystonic reactions. The occurrence of rhabdomyolysis following general anaesthesia is usually due to malignant hyperthermia (see Ch. 15) although there are certain cases, particularly in children who develop rhabdomyolysis after administration of suxamethonium during anaesthesia, who do not have this condition (Gibbs 1978, Blumberg & Marti 1984). Rhabdomyolysis and myoglobinuria, without other features of malignant hyperthermia, may also occur following anaesthesia in some cases of Duchenne muscular dystrophy (Karpati & Watters 1980, Willner et al 1984).

Mitochondrial myopathy

Dalakas et al (1990) have described a distinctive myopathy characterized by numerous 'ragged-red' fibres containing paracrystalline inclusions in patients with the acquired immunodeficiency syndrome due to HIV infection who had been on long term treatment with zidovudine. Panegyres et al (1990) have also described similar cases in which electron microscopy showed striking mitochondrial enlargement, vacuolation and abnormal cristae (Fig. 14.4). It has been postulated that the drug, which is a nucleoside analogue, interferes with the homeostasis of mitochondrial DNA (Panegyres et al 1990). The myopathy is characterized clinically by myalgia, muscle weakness and elevated serum CK levels and may

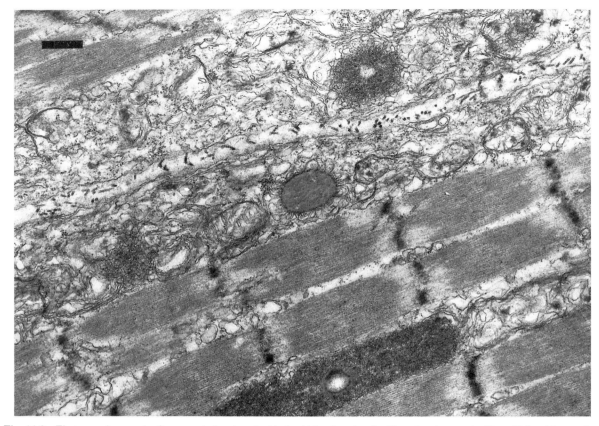

Fig. 14.3 Electron micrograph of rat muscle incubated with 5 mM bupivacaine for 60 m showing patchy Z- and I-band loss and accumulation of abnormal membrane configurations at the periphery of two muscle fibres. Mitochondria are disrupted forming membrane whorls and elements of the sarcoplasmic reticulum are dilated. Bar = 0.5 μm

improve when the drug is withdrawn. All of the patients studied also had an inflammatory myopathy which was thought to be related to the immunodeficiency syndrome (see Ch. 12).

Mitochondrial myopathy has been induced in experimental animals by the administration of a number of chemicals which block aerobic metabolic pathways. These include 2,4-dinitrophenol, β-guanidine propionic acid and diphenyleneiodium (Cooper et al 1988, Gori et al 1988). Mitochondrial abnormalities and reduced cytochrome c oxidase activity were also prominent features of a myopathy induced by germanium (Higuchi et al 1989).

Autophagic myopathies

A large group of drugs with amphiphilic cationic properties have been shown experimentally to interfere with lysosomal digestion and to lead to autophagic degeneration with the accumulation of phospholipids in muscle and other tissues (Drenckhahn & Lullmann-Rauch 1979, Lullmann-Rauch 1979). Three of these drugs, chloroquine, amiodarone and perhexiline, as well as vincristine and colchicine, are also known to cause an autophagic myopathy or neuromyopathy in man.

Chloroquine

This antimalarial and antirheumatic drug may cause a painless proximal myopathy or neuromyopathy with normal or slightly elevated serum enzyme levels and, in some cases, an associated cardiomyopathy (see Mastaglia 1982, Estes et al

Table 14.2 Some of the drugs and toxins that have been implicated in causing the syndrome of acute rhabdomyolysis and myoglobinuria

Drug-induced coma, seizures, dyskinesia (9,11,17,30,38)	*Other drugs*
Barbiturates (30)	Amphetamines (17)
Heroin (28,31)	Phenmetrazine (6)
Methadone (27,40)	Phencyclidine (14)
Glutethimide (30)	Phenylpropanolamine (8,20)
Chlorpromazine (25)	Morphine (7)
Diazepam (9)	Dihydrocodeine (7)
Rohypnol (9)	LSD (17)
Lithium (39)	Salicylates (17)
Amoxapine (1,22)	Clofibrate/Bezafibrate/Fenofibrate (10,17)
Phenelzine	Σ-aminocaproic acid (10,17)
Phenformin/fenfluramine (29)	Isoniazid (40)
Meprobamate (40)	Loxapine (37)
Antihistamines/paracetamol (20,38)	Theophyllin (26)
Oxprenolol (33)	Pentamidine (34)
Ethanol (19)	Vasopressin (2)
Post-anaesthetic	*Toxins*
Suxamethonium	Ethanol (17, 19)
Malignant hyperpyrexia	Isopropyl alcohol (17)
(see Chapter 20)	Carbon monoxide (17)
	Mercuric chloride (12)
Neuroleptic malignant syndrome (15, 23)	Ethylene glycol (17)
Haloperidol	Copper sulphate (13)
Stelazine	Zinc phosphide (13)
Fluphenazine	Strychnine (40)
Other neuroleptics	Metaldehyde (40)
	Chloralose (40)
Hypokalaemia (17)	Paraphenylenediamine (3)
Diuretics	Toluene (paint sniffing) (17)
Carbenoxolone	Gasoline sniffing (24)
Amphotericin B	Lindane/benzene (21)
Liquorice	Snake bite
	Hornet or wasp sting (35)
	Brown spider bite (17)
	Haff disease (4)
	Quail ingestion (?hemlock) (5)

Key to references: 1. = Abreo et al (1982). 2. = Affarah et al (1984). 3. = Baud et al (1983). 4. = Berlin (1948). 5. = Billis et al (1971). 6. = Black & Murphy (1984). 7. = Blain et al (1985). 8. = Blewitt & Siegel (1983). 9. = Briner et al (1986). 10. = Britt et al (1980). 11. = Chaikin (1980). 12. = Chugh et al (1978). 13. = Chugh et al (1979). 14. = Cogen et al (1978). 15. = Eiser et al (1982). 16. = Frendin & Swainson (1985). 17. = Gabow et al (1982). 18. = Gabry et al (1982). 19. = Haller & Knochel (1984). 20. = Jaeger et al (1984). 22. = Jennings et al (1983). 23. = Kleinknecht et al (1982). 24. = Kovanen et al (1983). 25. = Lazarus & Toglia (1985). 26. = Modi et al (1985). 27. = Nanji & Filipenko (1983). 28. = Nicholls et al (1982). 29. = Palmucci et al (1978). 30. = Penn et al (1972). 31. = Richter et al (1971). 32. = Rumpf et al (1984). 33. = Schofield et al (1985). 34. = Sensakovic et al (1985). 35. = Shilkin et al (1972). 36. = Swenson et al (1982). 37. = Tam et al (1980). 38. = Thomas & Ibels (1985). 39. = Unger et al (1982). 40. = Wattel et al (1978).

1987). This complication has been reported in patients treated with doses of the drug of 250 to 750 mg per day for periods of several weeks to four years. The condition is reversible once the drug is withdrawn but recovery is slow. Histologically, there is vacuolar change, which may be more prominent in type 1 or type 2 fibres (Fig. 14.5), and which is shown by electron microscopy to be due to autophagic degeneration of muscle fibres with associated exocytosis and accumulation of lamellated membrane bodies (*myeloid bodies*) and curvilinear bodies (Fig. 14.6) (Neville et al 1979). Myeloid bodies are also present in capillary endothelial cells and other interstitial cells. Quantitative biochemical studies show an abnormal accumulation of phospholipids and to a lesser extent of neutral lipids (Mastaglia et al 1977).

Experimental studies have shown swelling of

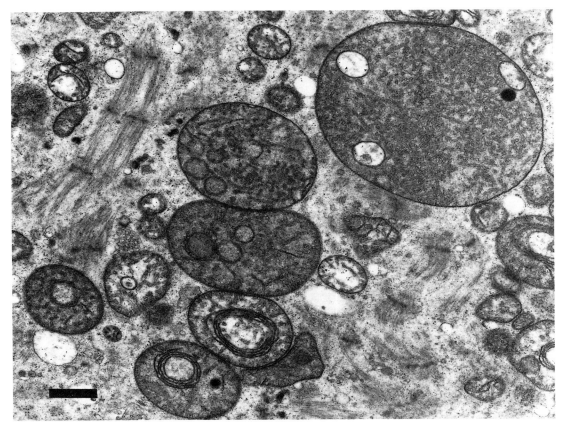

Fig. 14.4 Electron micrograph of a grossly disorganized muscle fibre containing enlarged mitochondria with abnormal cristae and inclusions in a case of AIDS treated with zidovudine. Bar = 1 μm

the sarcoplasmic reticulum in the early stages of the myopathy (Schmalbruch 1980, Trout et al 1981), and a marked increase in the activity of lysosomal enzymes, particularly of acid proteases, as well as an increase in the desmin content of muscle fibres (Stauber et al 1981).

Amiodarone

There have been a number of reports of a demyelinating peripheral neuropathy developing in patients treated with this anti-arrhythmic drug (see Argov & Mastaglia 1988). In some cases biopsies from proximal limb muscles have shown myopathic features including fibre vacuolation, autophagic degeneration, membrane bound dense bodies (Meier et al 1979) and myofibre necrosis (Clouston & Donnelly 1989).

Perhexiline

This drug, which was used to treat angina pectoris, can also cause a demyelinating peripheral neuropathy or neuromyopathy with involvement of proximal muscle groups. Electron microscopy of proximal muscle biopsies from affected patients and of muscle tissue from mice treated with the drug showed numerous membranous and granular inclusions of probable lysosomal origin in muscle fibres as well as endothelial cells and Schwann cells (Fardeau et al 1979).

Vincristine

The alkaloid vincristine, which interferes with RNA and protein synthesis and with the polymerization of tubulin into microtubules, commonly

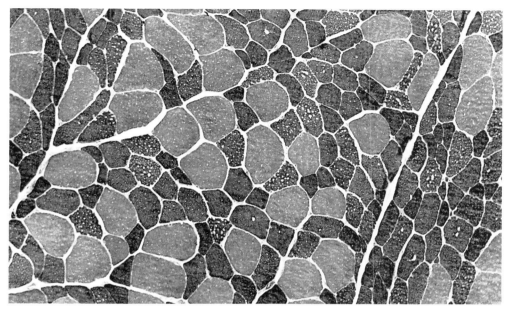

Fig. 14.5 Chloroquine myopathy. Vacuolar change is seen particularly in type 2 fibres. Type 2 fibre atrophy is also present. Myosin ATPase, pH 7.2, ×205

causes an axonal peripheral neuropathy, which is associated with a proximal myopathy in some patients (Bradley et al 1970). Electron microscopic studies in man and in the experimental animal have shown that the drug has a profound effect on membrane systems leading to the formation of complex 'spheromembranous bodies', thought to be derived from the sarcoplasmic reticulum, and autophagic degeneration of muscle fibres (Anderson et al 1967, Bradley 1970).

Colchicine

Like vincristine, this drug prevents the polymerization of tubulin into microtubules and may cause an axonal neuropathy or myopathy in man and in experimental animals (Kontos 1962, Riggs et al 1986, Kuncl et al 1987). A severe neuromyopathy has been reported with prolonged administration of high doses of the drug and may also occur in patients taking conventional doses for the treatment of gout and is more likely to occur in the presence of renal insufficiency. Serum CK levels are usually elevated to 10 to 20 times the upper limit of normal. Prompt recovery occurs on withdrawal of the drug.

Characteristic findings with the light microscope in biopsies from proximal limb muscles comprise excessive variation in fibre size, the presence of small vacuoles in muscle fibres, or of central areas of altered staining on haematoxylin and eosin preparations and loss of enzyme activity resembling cores or core-targetoids in histochemical preparations (Fig. 14.7). Some vacuoles may contain granular haematoxyphilic material. The major features on electron microscopy are the presence of autophagic vacuoles and 'spheromembranous bodies' as in the experimental form of colchicine myopathy. Muscle fibre necrosis and regeneration rarely occur. Denervation changes may also be found in distal limb muscles.

Corticosteroid myopathy

A proximal myopathy is a common complication of prolonged corticosteroid administration. It is most likely to occur in patients taking over 40 mg per day of prednisone but may occur even with lower doses taken for prolonged periods (Bowyer et al 1985). The 9-α-fluorinated steroids triamcinolone, betamethasone and dexamethasone are most likely to cause a myopathy. Diaphragmatic

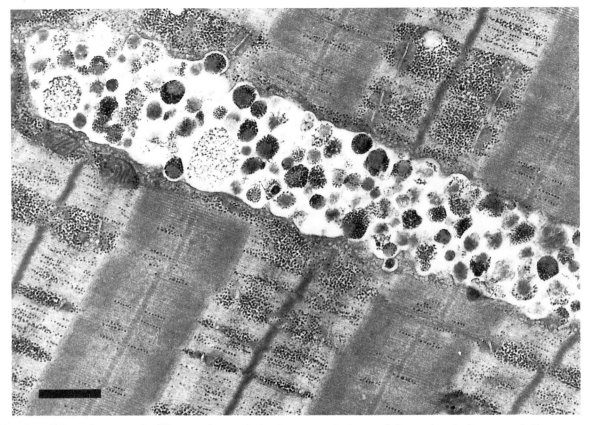

Fig. 14.6 Chloroquine myopathy. Electron micrograph showing an autophagic vacuole in an otherwise intact muscle fibre. Bar = 0.5 μm

weakness may develop in asthmatics on prolonged corticosteroid therapy (Bowyer et al 1985) and a more severe generalized myopathy may occur following the administration of high doses of hydrocortisone in patients with status asthmaticus (MacFarlane & Rosenthal 1977, van Marle & Woods 1980). A localized myopathy of the laryngeal muscles can occur in patients treated with inhaled corticosteroids (Williams et al 1983).

The typical finding in biopsies from proximal limb muscles is of selective atrophy of type 2 fibres (Fig. 14.8A), particularly of the type 2B subgroup which are also severely affected in experimental steroid myopathy (Livingstone et al 1981). Histochemical stains may show accumulation of neutral lipid in muscle fibres. Muscle fibre necrosis, regeneration and other degenerative changes are not usually observed but may occur in the severe generalized form of myopathy developing after high-dose hydrocortisone administration in asthmatics (MacFarlane & Rosenthal 1977, van Marle & Woods 1980) and in some patients treated with high doses of dexamethasone (Ojeda 1982) (Fig. 14.8B). The histological changes in these cases are similar to those found in an experimental form of myopathy induced by high doses of steroids in rabbits (Ellis 1956, Afifi & Bergman 1969).

Experimental studies have shown that corticosteroids have diverse effects on oxidative metabolism, glycogen and lipid metabolism, myofibrillar ATPase activity, protein synthesis and degradation in muscle (see Mastaglia 1982). The basic cellular action of corticosteroids is to inhibit messenger RNA synthesis and thereby reduce protein synthesis (Rannels et al 1978,

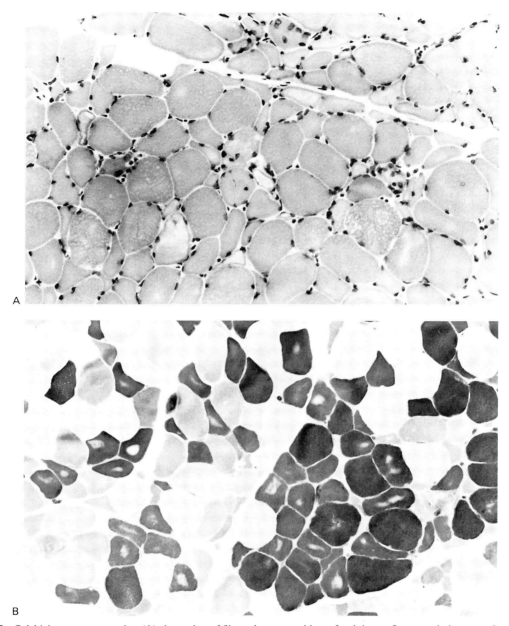

Fig. 14.7   Colchicine neuromyopathy. (A) A number of fibres show central loss of staining or fine vacuolation; occasional necrotic and regenerating fibres are also present. H&E, ×205. (B) Many fibres have central core-like areas lacking enzyme activity. Myosin ATPase, pH 4.6, ×160

Karpati 1984). The atrophic effects of steroids on skeletal muscle are thought to be due to inhibition of synthesis of specific muscle proteins and, in experimental studies are more marked in fast-twitch muscles (with a high content of type 2 muscle fibres) than in slow-twitch muscles (Livingstone et al 1981). The reasons for the differential suscepti-bility of fast-twitch and slow-twitch muscles remains uncertain and it has not been possible to explain it on the basis of differential content of

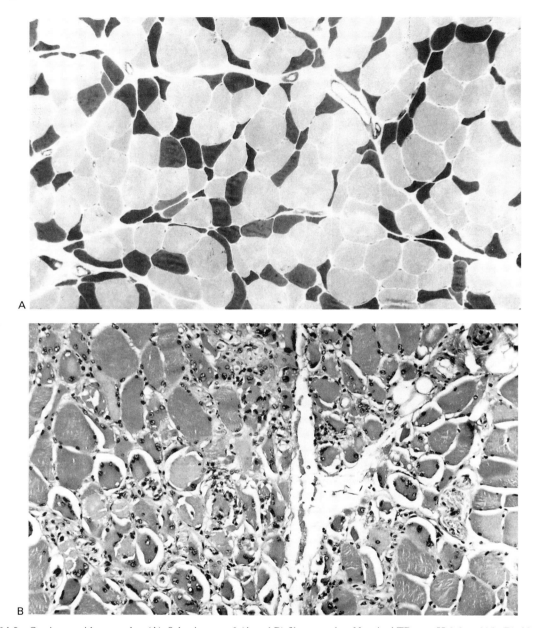

Fig. 14.8   Corticosteroid myopathy. (A) Selective type 2 (A and B) fibre atrophy. Myosin ATPase, pH 9.2, ×205. (B) Muscle fibre necrosis and extensive regeneration in a case of acute corticosteroid myopathy following high-dose parenteral administration of dexamethasone. H&E, ×160

glucocorticoid receptors in the two types of muscle (Mastaglia 1982). Observations in the rat suggest that the particular susceptibility of fast-twitch glycolytic fibres may be linked to the relatively severe reduction in myophosphorylase activity which occurs in these fibres with steroid treatment and their comparative inability to utilize alternative energy sources, especially substrates derived from free fatty acids (Livingstone et al 1981).

Drug-induced myositis

A number of drugs have been implicated in causing an inflammatory myopathy (Mastaglia & Argov 1982). Patients with rheumatoid arthritis, progressive systemic sclerosis or Wilson's disease who are treated with D-penicillamine may develop a necrotizing inflammatory myopathy with the clinical features of polymyositis or dermatomyositis (see Mastaglia & Argov 1982, Doyle et al 1983, Halla et al 1984, Carroll et al 1987). These patients are more likely to be B18, B35 and DR4 positive (Carroll et al 1987). There are also rare reports of the development of polymyositis or dermatomyositis in patients being treated with sulphonamides, penicillin, propylthiouracil or cimetidine (Hayman et al 1956, Watson et al 1983, Shergy and Caldwell 1988). A predominantly interstitial form of myositis may occur as a rare complication of treatment with a number of other drugs including procainamide, hydralazine, phenytoin, mesantoin and levodopa (Mastaglia 1982).

An interstitial form of eosinophilic myositis and fasciitis has recently been recognized in many patients taking preparations containing the naturally occurring amino acid L-tryptophan (the 'eosinophilia-myalgia syndrome') (Hertzman et al 1990, Silver et al 1990, Eidson et al 1990, Medsger 1990, van Garsse and Boeykens 1990). The syndrome is characterized by the abrupt onset of severe myalgia with oedema and induration of the skin of the extremities and a peripheral blood eosinophilia (Varga et al 1990). In some cases there has been an associated ascending polyneuropathy. It is not as yet completely clear as to whether this condition is due to the tryptophan itself or to some contaminant in the preparation (Belongia et al 1990). It is similar in its effects to the 'toxic oil syndrome' (Deighton 1990) and hence a contaminant seems more likely to be the cause.

Hypokalaemic myopathy

Hypokalaemia of sufficient severity to cause a myopathy may develop in patients treated with diuretics, amphotericin B, carbenoxolone, fluoro-prednisolone containing nasal sprays, or in patients with purgative abuse (see Mastaglia 1982, Vita et al 1986). Hypokalaemic myopathy has also been reported in individuals consuming large quantities of liquorice or liquorice extracts which are contained in certain traditional Chinese medicines, and in individuals who use large quantities of snuff or chewing tobacco (Cumming et al 1980, Valeriano et al 1983, Piette et al 1984). The common ingredient which causes hypokalaemia is glycyrrhizinic acid which is a potent mineralocorticoid analogue (Valeriano et al 1983). The clinical picture is that of generalised and sometimes profound hypotonic weakness with depression of tendon reflexes and marked elevation of serum CK levels. Histological changes in muscle are usually relatively inconspicuous with scattered fibres being swollen and vacuolated and in more severe cases fibre necrosis and regeneration (see Ch. 9).

Myotonia

A number of hypocholesterolaemic agents are known to induce myotonia by interfering with the synthesis of cholesterol in the muscle cell membrane (Kwiecinski 1981). That which has been most fully investigated is 20,25-diazacholesterol. The effects are related to the accumulation of desmosterol in the muscle fibre and the serum. Altered permeability of the plasma membrane to chloride ions is believed to be the basis for the myotonia. Clofibrate induces myotonia in animals but not in man (Eberstein et al 1978).

The monocarboxylic acids cause myotonia by blocking chloride conductance (Furman and Barchi 1978). 2,4-dichlorphenoxyacetate has also been used experimentally to induce myotonia. This agent also inhibits glucose-3-phosphate dehydrogenase and produces changes in mitochondria and the sarcotubular systems of muscle fibres resulting in vacuolation and muscle fibre necrosis (Danon et al 1978). Myotonia is also induced by a number of other chemical agents and also occurs in the vitamin E deficient myopathy of the Rottnest Island quokka (Durack et al 1969).

Focal forms of myopathy

Localized muscle damage may occur following the intramuscular administration of various drugs.

This is due to the combined effects of needle insertion ('needle myopathy'), and the local effects of the agent which is injected (Mastaglia 1982). In animals, diazepam, digoxin and lignocaine were shown to cause extensive muscle necrosis and elevation of serum CK levels (Steiness et al 1977, Yagiela et al 1981). In man, chloroquine, opiates, paraldehyde, cephalothin and chlorpromazine may cause severe muscle damage sometimes leading to abscess formation. Repeated injections of drugs into the same muscle may lead to the development of fibrosis and fibrous contracture of the muscle. This complication has been reported particularly following prolonged courses of antibiotic injections into the quadriceps and deltoid muscles in children and in pethidine or pentazocine addicts who may develop contractures of multiple limb muscles (Argov & Mastaglia 1988).

Other drug-induced myopathies

Other drugs which have rarely been implicated in causing a myopathy include β-blockers (Forfar et al 1979), rifampicin (Jenkins & Emerson 1981), mercaptoproprionyl glycine (Sinclair & Phillips 1982), ethchlorvynol (Placidyl) which has been associated with the presence of tubular aggregates in muscle (Petajan et al 1986), and cyclosporin (Goy et al 1989).

Disorders of neuromuscular transmission

A variety of drugs will produce a 'myasthenia gravis-like' syndrome, by interfering with acetylcholine release at the synaptic terminal of the myoneural junction, or by binding with the receptor. Others produce their effect by a direct influence on the post-synaptic membrane (Fig. 14.9). This subject has been fully reviewed elsewhere by Argov and Mastaglia (1979, 1988) and is also discussed in Chapter 17.

Antibiotics

Many antibiotics are known to interfere with neuromuscular transmission (McQuillen et al 1968). These include the aminoglycosides kanamycin, streptomycin, neomycin and gentamicin and the polymyxins colistin and polymyxin B as well as oxytetracycline, rolitetracycline, lincomycin and clindamycin (Argov & Mastaglia 1988). Experimental studies have shown that antibiotics have both a presynaptic action, interfering with transmitter release, and a post-synaptic curariform effect.

Cardiovascular drugs

Quinine, quinidine, procainamide, propranolol and other β-adrenergic blockers all have the potential to interfere with neuromuscular transmission (Argov & Mastaglia 1979).

Anticonvulsants

Phenytoin and trimethadione may rarely produce a myasthenic-like condition. It is believed that phenytoin acts by depressing neurotransmitter release (Yaari et al 1977).

Psychotropic drugs

Lithium carbonate may cause neuromuscular block or prolong the effect of suxamethonium and pancuronium (Argov & Mastaglia 1988). Chlorpromazine may interfere with neuromuscular transmission by depressing transmitter release and also has a post-synaptic curariform action (Argov & Yaari 1979).

Chelating agents

D-Penicillamine may cause a myasthenic disorder which is clinically indistinguishable from myasthenia gravis. This is due to the induction of Ach receptor antibody formation (Argov & Mastaglia 1979, 1988).

Peripheral nerve and spinal cord

A great variety of drugs and toxins will affect the peripheral nerves, producing either a demyelinating neuropathy or an axonopathy. These include various anti-microbial, cytotoxic, anti-rheumatic and cardiovascular drugs (Argov & Mastaglia 1988) as well as many chemical agents. The spinal cord is also vulnerable to a large number of drugs and toxins. Important among these is clioquinol

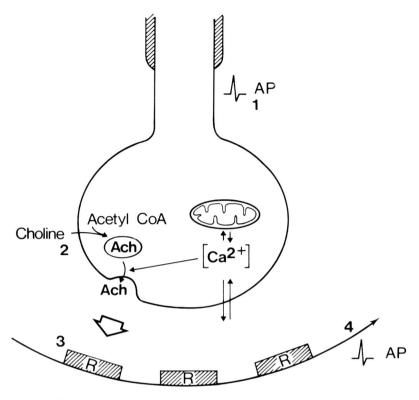

Fig. 14.9 Four sites of action of drugs which may interfere with neuromuscular transmission: 1. presynaptic inhibition of nerve action potential (AP) propogation; 2. impaired release of acetylcholine (ACh) from the nerve terminal; 3. blockade of postsynaptic ACh receptors; 4. impaired generation of muscle action potential. (Reproduced from Walton & Mastaglia (1981) with permission)

which causes subacute myelo-opticoneuropathy (SMON). Triorthocresyl phosphate is also a potent cause of myelopathy as well as of peripheral neuropathy.

Degeneration of motor axons or of spinal motor neurones will lead to denervation and atrophy of muscle fibres in affected motor units. The resulting histological changes in muscle are discussed in detail in Chapter 16. Some drugs (e.g. emetine, vincristine, colchicine and chloroquine) and toxins (e.g. the organophosphates) may produce a neuromyopathy with a combination of neurogenic and myopathic changes in muscle (see above).

TOXIC DISORDERS

Alcoholic myopathy

There is ample clinical and experimental evidence

that ethanol has a direct toxic effect on muscle (Fig. 14.10). Acute, subacute and chronic forms of myopathy may occur in alcoholics and the clinical and myopathological features of these conditions are well documented in the literature (Perkoff et al 1967, Klinkerfuss et al 1967, Martin et al 1982, Haller & Knochel 1984, Charness et al 1989).

Acute alcoholic myopathy

This condition is probably more frequent than is generally appreciated and varies in severity from a transient asymptomatic elevation of serum CK and myoglobin levels to a severe form of rhabdomyolysis characterized by widespread muscle pain, swelling, weakness and myoglobinuria which may lead to acute renal failure. Cases of intermediate severity may have a predominantly

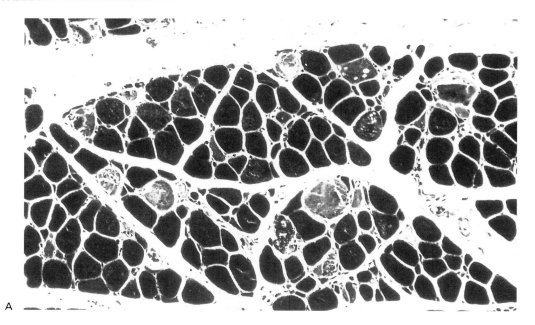

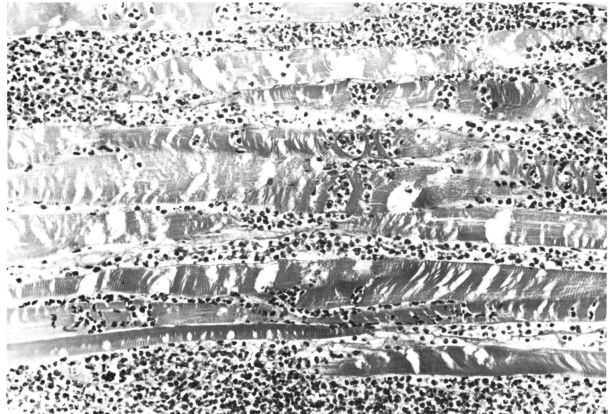

Fig. 14.10 (A) Acute alcoholic myopathy. There is polyfocal necrosis of muscle fibres. PTAH, ×160. (B) Extensive rhabdomyolysis and polymorphonuclear and round cell infiltration induced by intramuscular injection of ethanol (1 ml/d for 10 d) in a rat. H&E, ×260

proximal pattern of muscle weakness. In some alcoholics several episodes may occur following alcoholic binges. In some cases there is focal involvement of the calf muscles and the condition may mimic venous thrombophlebitis (Hed et al 1962, Walsh & Conomy 1977).

Histological changes in muscle biopsies comprise polyfocal muscle fibre necrosis (Fig. 14.10) which is more extensive in patients with the severe acute form of rhabdomyolysis. In addition, there is often also evidence of scattered muscle fibre regeneration. If the biopsy is performed relatively late (e.g. in the second or third weeks after the onset of symptoms) only polyfocal regenerative changes may be found in keeping with a previous (monophasic) toxic insult to the muscle. Other histological changes include a patchy loss of oxidative enzyme activity, especially in type 1 fibres and a mild interstitial mononuclear cellular infiltration in some cases (Kahn & Meyer 1970, Martinez et al 1973).

Experimental observations in humans and in rats have shown acute elevations of serum CK activity of skeletal muscle origin after administration of ethanol with a direct relationship between serum enzyme and blood alcohol levels (Haller & Drachman 1980, Lane & Radoff 1981, Spargo 1984, Haller 1985). In addition, ultrastructural changes in mitochondria and sarcoplasmic reticulum, increase in glycogen, fat and accumulation of osmiophilic particles were found in muscle fibres in human volunteers after regular ingestion of large quantities of ethanol for a period of one month (Song & Rubin 1972).

Chronic alcoholic myopathy

Ekbom et al (1964) first drew attention to a more chronic form of proximal myopathy characterized by progressive painless weakness and atrophy of the muscles of the pelvic and shoulder girdles in long-standing alcoholics who may also have peripheral neuropathy, Wernicke's encephalopathy, hepatic cirrhosis and signs of nutritional deficiency. The serum CK activity is usually normal. Recent studies have shown that there is a generalized decrease in skeletal muscle mass (Duàne & Peters 1988).

The most frequent histological finding in biopsies from proximal limb muscles such as the quadriceps femoris in such cases is of selective type 2 fibre atrophy (Martin et al 1985) (Fig. 14.8A). In addition, histochemical stains and electron microscopy often show evidence of neutral lipid accumulation in muscle fibres and biochemical analysis shows excessive amounts of triglycerides (Sunnasy et al 1983). Type 2 fibre atrophy is also a frequent finding in alcoholics without muscle weakness suggesting that chronic alcoholic myopathy is frequently subclinical (Martin et al 1982). In cases with an associated peripheral neuropathy histological changes of denervation atrophy may be found in proximal lower limb muscles (Faris & Reyes 1971, Urbano-Marquez et al 1985). In some chronic alcoholics tubular aggregates are found in type 2 muscle fibres (Chui et al 1975).

Pathogenesis

The pathogenetic mechanisms involved in the development of alcoholic myopathies are incompletely understood. A number of studies have provided evidence that alcohol interferes with glycolytic and glycogenolytic pathways in muscle. Perkoff et al (1966) found reduced lactic acid production during ischaemic exercise in alcoholics with myoglobinuria and assumed that there was a defect in glycogenolysis. Recent studies have confirmed that there is impaired muscle glycolysis and glycogenolysis in alcoholics with a recent history of rhabdomyolysis as well as in those without such a history, and it has been postulated that these metabolic changes may contribute to the development of acute rhabdomyolysis (Bollaert et al 1989). A reduced activity of glycolytic and glycogenolytic enzyme activity has also been demonstrated in patients with chronic alcoholic myopathy (Langohr et al 1983, Martin et al 1984). In addition experimental studies have shown that ethanol causes marked inhibition of oxidation of palmitic acid and glucose-6-phosphate, two of the major substrates for energy production in skeletal muscle (Anderson & Torrance 1984). In vitro studies have shown that ethanol alters the configuration, fluidity and Na^+,K^+-ATPase activity of cell membranes and inhibits calcium uptake by the sarcoplasmic reticulum (Haller and Knochel

1984). Other factors which may contribute to the development of myopathy in some alcoholics include food deprivation and protein malnutrition (Haller 1985, Duane & Peters 1988), hypokalaemia (Rubenstein & Wainapel 1977), and phosphate depletion (Haller & Knochel 1984).

Chemical poisons

As might be expected, any powerful acid or base or other chemically active compound will produce muscle necrosis at the site of injection. Similarly, powerful organic poisons such as formalin, lysol or turpentine will cause massive necrosis of all tissue, including muscle at the site of injection.

The iodoacetates and fluoroacetates, which block lactate production, cause primary muscle fibre necrosis (Kakulas 1981). Fenichel & Martin (1977) studied an experimental myopathy produced by imidazole in rats which has a similar effect (Martin et al 1977).

Graham et al (1976) demonstrated core formation in the muscles of rats intoxicated with triethyltin sulphate. Ragged-red fibres and mitochondrial inclusions have been produced under experimental conditions by the injection of 2,4-dinitrophenol (Sahgal et al 1979).

Organophosphates will also give rise to muscle fibre necrosis, in addition to the peripheral and spinal cord changes for which they are better known (Ahlgren et al 1979, Vasilescu et al 1984). Mukuno & Imai (1973) produced extra-ocular muscle involvement in beagle dogs by chronic organophosphate intoxication. Tsubaki et al (1977) studied the pathogenesis of central core, multicore, target and cytoplasmic bodies produced by organophosphates. Experimental studies in the rat have shown that organophosphates, which are irreversible cholinesterase inhibitors, produce a progressive dose-related necrosis of muscle fibres which begins in the motor end-plate region (Dettbarn 1984). The myopathy appears to be secondary to increased neurotransmitter release and can be prevented by prior denervation or administration of pyridine-2-aldoxime methiodide (Wecker et al 1978).

Envenomation

Snake venoms

The venoms of a number of snakes have myotoxic properties and may cause rhabdomyolysis in addition to postsynaptic neuromuscular blockade (Meldrum 1965, Tu 1977, Sunderland 1983). Myolysis restricted to the site of the bite may be caused by many venoms but those shown in Table 14.3 have been associated with more widespread rhabdomyolysis and myoglobinuria. The myotoxic components of a number of these venoms have been isolated and found to be polypeptides whose mechanisms of action have been studied in the experimental animal. Those most fully investigated are the venoms of the Australia tiger snake (*Notechis scutatus scutatus*) (Harris et al 1975, Sutherland & Coulter 1977, Pluskal et al 1978, Ng & Howard 1980); the taipan (*Oxyuranus scutellatus*) (Harris & Maltin 1982); the mulga (*Pseudechis australis*) (Fig. 14.11) (Rowlands et al 1969, Papadimitriou & Mastaglia 1973, Leonard et al 1979); the seasnake *Enhydrina schistosa* (Reid 1961, Fohlman & Eaker 1977); the coral snake (*Micrurus nigrocinctus*) (Gutierrez et al 1986); the rattlesnakes of North and South America – the prairie rattlesnake, *Crotalus viridis viridis*, the Western diamondback rattlesnake *Crotalus atrox*

Table 14.3 Snake venoms associated with rhabdomyolysis and their myotoxic components

Elapid	
Notechis scutatus scutatus (Tiger snake)	Notexin Notechis II–5
Oxyuranus scutellatus (Taipan)	Taipoxin
Pseudechis australis (Mulga)	Mulgatoxin a
Enhydrina schistosa (Sea snake)	Phospholipase A
Dendroaspis jamesoni (Jameson's mamba)	–
Crotalid	
Crotalus viridis viridis (Prairie rattlesnake)	Myotoxin a
Crotalus durissus terrificus (South American rattlesnake)	Crotamine Crotoxin
Crotalus atrox (Western diamond-back rattlesnake)	
Bothrops asper	
Bothrops nummifer (Jumping viper of Costa Rica)	

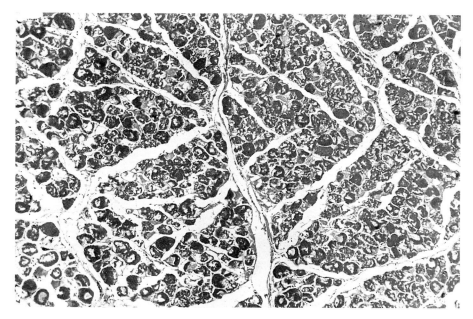

Fig. 14.11   Massive rhabdomyolysis due to envenomation by the mulga snake (*Pseudechis australis*) in a 20-year-old man. H&E, ×40

and the South American rattlesnake *Crotalus durissus terrificus* (Cameron & Tu 1978, Ownby et al 1979, Huang & Perez 1982, Azevedo-Marques et al 1985); and the Costa Rican vipers (*Bothrops nummifer* and *Bothrops asper*) (Gutierrez et al 1984, 1989).

Spider venoms

The venoms of the Arkansas and Honduran tarantulas (*Dugesiella hentzi* and *Aphonophelma* spp.) are intensely myotoxic and cardiotoxic. Both the crude venom and purified necrotoxin (mol. wt 6.7 kDa) cause rapid irreversible injury to the muscle fibre plasma membrane leading to necrosis and marked accumulation of calcium and phosphate in muscle fibres (Ownby & Odell 1983). The brown spider has also been reported to cause rhabdomyolsis (Gabow et al 1982). The venom of the black widow spider (*Lactrodectus*) acts at the neuromuscular junction leading to depletion of ACh from presynaptic terminals and permanent neuromuscular block (Gorio & Mauro 1979, Duchen 1981).

Wasp venoms

There have been reports of severe widespread rhabdomyolysis with associated renal failure following envenomation by the wasp *Vespa cincta* and the hornet *Vespa affinis* (Fig. 14.12) (Shilkin et al 1972, Sitprija & Boonpucknavig 1972). The venom of *Vespa affinis* is known to contain polypeptides and phospholipases but the myotoxic components have not been identified (Shilkin et al 1972). Ishay et al (1975) demonstrated specific involvement of the transverse tubular system by the venom of the oriental hornet (*Vespa orientalis*).

Microbial toxins

Clostridial toxins

Clostridial toxins may have profound effects on the neuromuscular system. *Clostridium perfringens*, which is a cause of gas gangrene, produces a number of toxins. That which is thought to be primarily responsible for the muscle damage is the a-toxin (lecithinase C) which has been shown experimentally to cause focal lysis of the muscle

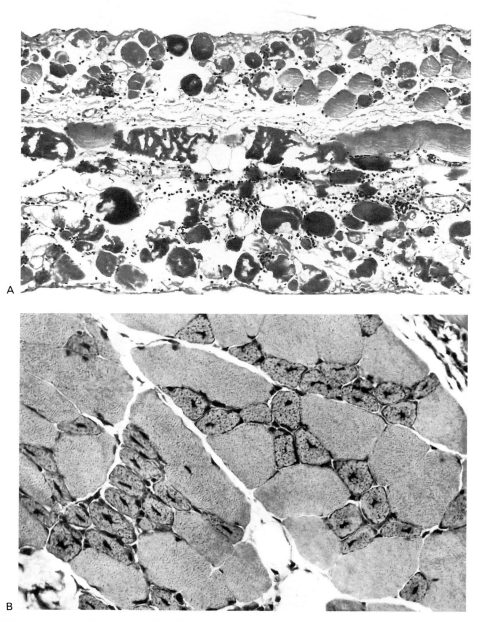

Fig. 14.12 (A) Extensive rhabdomyolysis with mild interstitial inflammatory infiltration in the abdominal wall muscles of a mouse following intraperitoneal injection of mulga snake venom. H&E, ×160. (B) Seven days after the injection of venom there is advanced regeneration with many late myotubes. H&E, ×400

fibre plasma membrane and necrosis (Strunk et al 1967).

Botulinum toxin causes neuromuscular block by preventing acetylcholine release from motor nerve terminals. Experimental studies have shown

degenerative changes in muscle fibres and motor end-plates with prominent sprouting of nerve terminals after intramuscular injection of the toxin (Duchen 1971a, b).

In addition to its central action on inhibitory

spinal cord synapses, tetanus toxin also acts on motor nerve terminals interfering with transmitter release and causing prolonged weakness or paralysis (Duchen 1973). Degenerative changes were found in muscle fibres but not in motor nerve terminals or end-plates in biopsies from patients with tetanus (Agostini & Noetzel 1970). In an experimental study in the mouse, intramuscular injection of tetanus toxin was found to cause sprouting of motor nerve terminals in slow-twitch but not in fast-twitch muscle fibres (Duchen 1973).

Monensin toxicity

Monensin, a polyether antibiotic produced by *Streptomyces cinnamonensis*, is an Na$^+$-selective carboxylic ionophore which can produce cardiac and skeletal muscle necrosis when administered therapeutically in animals. Selective involvement of type 1 fibres has been found in experimental studies (van Vleet & Ferrans 1984).

Toxic plants

Coffee senna (*Cassia occidentalis*) will cause a myopathy in cattle, characterized by widespread muscle fibre necrosis (Montgomery 1978). The animals are soon prostrated and show myoglobinuria. The large muscles of the hind limbs are more involved and appear pale to the naked eye. Microscopic examination shows that the condition is a polyfocal polyphasic necrotising myopathy. The effects of *Cassia occidentalis* on calves were recently studied experimentally. Pulmonary oedema, hepatic necrosis, myocardiopathy and necrosis of skeletal muscle, visible both by light and electron microscopy, were reported (Rogers et al 1979).

The coyotillo plant (*Karwinskia humboldtiana*) is also described as causing muscle fibre necrosis in small ruminants (Jubb & Kennedy 1970).

The seeds of *Ixiolaena brevicompta*, a native herb of New South Wales, cause a severe myopathy and sudden death in sheep (Walker et al 1980). Serum CK activity is increased and there is reduced exercise tolerance. Necrosis of myocardial and skeletal muscles is found at necropsy (Walker et al 1980).

Quail myopathy

On the Greek Island of Lesbos, and to some extent in North Africa, an acute myopathy develops during the period of quail migration from Russia. The myopathy is seasonal and is believed to be due to the feeding habit of the quail during its migration, with hemlock seeds being under suspicion (Hughes 1974). Papapetropoulos (1980) has further described the disorder. Although a necrotizing myopathy would be expected because of the myoglobinuria, muscle biopsies have so far been negative. Creatine kinase activity is increased. Some patients with quail myopathy and myoglobinuria have died, but most survive.

Haff disease

This condition is named from a district in East Prussia where a disease of skeletal muscle reached epidemic proportions in 1924. Those who were affected had consumed a fish meal on the previous day. The disorder was characterized by severe muscle pains and myoglobinuria, with death from renal failure in some cases. Histologically, widespread muscle fibre necrosis was observed. The cause of the condition was never discovered (Hughes 1974).

NUTRITIONAL DISORDERS

Nutritional myopathies are well known in the veterinary and experimental fields (Hadlow 1962, Bradley et al 1988) but are rarely encountered in man in a clinical setting.

Protein–calorie malnutrition

The muscular wasting and weakness which occurs in long-standing protein–calorie malnutrition in children is associated with severe atrophy of muscle fibres and, in some cases, non-specific myopathic changes and fibre type grouping are also found suggesting that there is a combination of neurogenic and myopathic effects (Dastur et al 1982). Electron microscopy shows varying degrees of thinning and disorganization of myofibrillar structure. Similar changes have been found in experimental protein-calorie malnutrition in rhesus monkeys (Chopra et al 1987). A proximal myopathy has been reported following prolonged therapeutic starvation in man (Scobie et al 1980) but the muscle changes in this condition were not investigated. Stewart & Hensley (1981) reported four cases of a painful acute myopathy with elevated serum CK levels occurring in patients on total parenteral nutrition. The myopathy recovered after the administration of intravenous lipid supplements and was postulated to be due to a deficiency of essential fatty acids.

Vitamin E deficiency

Deficiency of vitamin E, which acts as an anti-oxidant in living cells, is known to cause a severe necrotizing myopathy in many species of animals (Nelson 1983, McMurray et al 1983). The pathogenesis of this myopathy has been fully investigated in the Rottnest Island quokka (*Setonix brachyurus*) which develops a naturally occurring myopathy characterized by polyfocal polyphasic myofibre necrosis and regeneration (Fig. 14.14) with myotonia; the myopathy is reversed by administration of α-tocopherol (Kakulas 1981). It has been shown experimentally that the muscles of

vitamin E deficient animals (mice and rats) are more susceptible than normal muscles to peroxidative damage and to damage during contractile activity (Jackson et al 1983).

A human myopathy caused by chronic deficiency of vitamin E is known to occur in patients with chronic cholestatic syndromes and other malabsorptive states, but is rare, and is usually associated with a peripheral neuropathy (Tomasi 1979, Werlin et al 1983, Neville et al 1983, Lazaro et al 1986). In contrast to the necrotizing myopathy in animals, in the human cases the major histopathological finding is the accumulation in muscle fibres of autofluorescent membrane-bound dense bodies with strong acid phosphatase and esterase activity, lying between the myofibrils of otherwise intact muscle fibres (Neville et al 1983). These bodies are thought to represent lipofuscin or ceroid pigment which accumulates in response to disturbed intracellular lipid peroxidation. Type 1 fibre predominance, type 2 fibre atrophy and other non-specific changes in muscle fibres were also present in some reported cases (Neville et al 1983). In other cases, neurogenic atrophy, which is presumably related to the coexisting peripheral neuropathy, was also present (Nelson 1983).

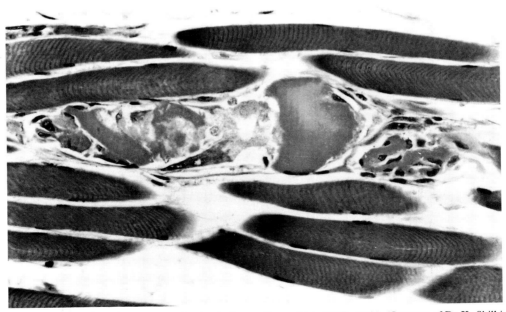

Fig. 14.13 Muscle necrosis following envenomation by the hornet *Vespa affinis*. H&E, ×400. (Courtesy of Dr K. Shilkin)

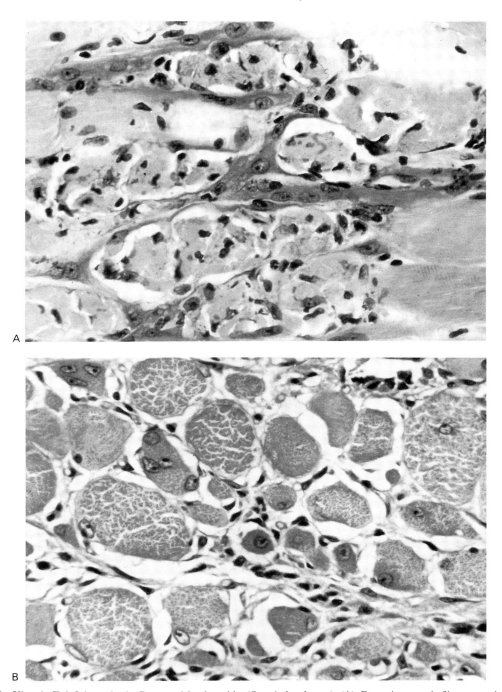

Fig. 14.14 Vitamin E deficiency in the Rottnest island quokka (*Setonix brachyurus*). (A) Extensive muscle fibre necrosis and regeneration. (B) Multiple fibres showing advanced regenerative changes. H&E; A ×400, B ×400

Selenium deficiency

Selenium is also known to be essential for normal muscle function in many farm animals, notably sheep (Swash et al 1957). The lesions of selenium deficiency resemble those of vitamin E deficiency and, in some species, vitamin E and selenium are active prophylactically, together or independently.

REFERENCES

Abreo K, Shelp W D, Kosseff A, Thomas S 1982 Amoxapine-associated rhabdomyolysis and acute renal failure: Case report. Journal of Clinical Psychiatry 43: 426

Affarah H B, Mars R L, Someren A, Smith H W, Heymsfield S B 1984 Myoglobinuria and acute renal failure associated with intravenous vasopressin infusion. Southern Medical Journal 77: 918

Afifi A K, Bergman R A 1969 Steroid myopathy. A study of the evolution of the muscle lesion in rabbits. Johns Hopkins Medical Journal 124: 66

Afifi A K, Hajj G A, Saad S, Tekian A, Bergman R A, Bahuth N B, Abourizk N 1984 Clofibrate-induced myotoxicity in rats. Temporal profile of myopathology. European Neurology 23: 182

Agostini B, Noetzel H 1970 Morphological study of muscle fibres and motor end-plates in tetanus. In: Walton J N, Canal N, Scarlato G (eds) Muscle diseases. Amsterdam, Excerpta Medica, pp 123–127

Ahlgren J D, Manz H J, Harvey J C 1979 Myopathy of chronic organophosphate poisoning: a clinical entity. Southern Medical Journal 72: 555

Anderson T L, Torrance C A 1984 Metabolic mechanisms of acute alcoholic myopathy. Neurology 34: 81.

Anderson P J, Song S K, Slotwiner P 1967 The fine structure of spheromembranous degeneration of skeletal muscle induced by vincristine. Journal of Neuropathology and Experimental Neurology 25: 15

Argov Z, Mastaglia F L 1979 Disorders of neuromuscular transmission caused by drugs. New England Journal of Medicine 301: 409

Argov Z, Mastaglia F L 1988 Drug-induced neuromuscular disorders in man. In: Walton J N (ed) *Disorders of Voluntary Muscle*, 5th ed. Churchill Livingstone, p 981

Argov Z, Yaari Y 1979 The action of chlorpromazine at an isolated cholinergic synapse. Brain Research 164: 227

Ashbury A K, Johnson P C 1978 Pathology of peripheral nerve. In: Bennington J L (ed) Major problems in pathology, vol 9. W B Saunders, Philadelphia

Azevedo-Marques M M, Cupo P, Coimbra T M, Hering S E, Rossi M A, Laure C J 1985 Myonecrosis, myoglobinuria and acute renal failure induced by South American rattlesnake (*Crotalus durissus terrificus*) envenomation in Brazil. Toxicon 23: 631

Baud F, Bismuth C, Galliot M, Garnier R, Peralma A 1983 Rhabdomyolysis in para-phenylenediamine intoxication. Lancet ii: 514.

Belongia E A, Hedberg C W, Gleich G J et al 1990 An investigation of the cause of the eosinophilia–myalgia syndrome associated with tryptophan use. New England Journal of Medicine 323: 357

Bennett H S, Spiro A J, Pollack M A, Zucker P, 1982 Ipecac-induced myopathy simulating dermatomyositis. Neurology (NY) 32: 91

Berlin R 1948 Haff disease in Sweden. Acta Medica Scandinavica 129: 560

Billis A G, Kasyanakis S Giamarellou H, Daikos G K 1971 Acute renal failure after a meal of quail. Lancet i: 702

Bindoff L, Cullen M J 1978 Experimental (−) emetine myopathy. Ultrastructural and morphometric observations. Journal of the Neurological Sciences 39: 1

Black W D, Murphy W M 1984: Nontraumatic rhabdomyolysis and acute renal failure associated with oral phenmetrazine hydrochloride. Journal of Tennessee Medical Association 77: 80

Blain P G, Lane R J M, Bateman D N, Rawlins M D 1985 Opiate-induced rhabdomyolysis. Human Toxicology 4(1): 71

Blewitt G A, Siegel E B 1983 Renal failure, rhabdomyolysis and phenylpropanolamine. Journal of the American Medical Association 249: 3017

Blumberg A, Marti H R 1984 Akute rhabdomyolyse nach succinylcholin. Schweizerische medizinische Wochenschrift 114: 1068

Bollaert P E, Robin-Lherbier B, Escanye J M, Bauer Ph, Lambert H, Robert J, Larcan A 1989 Phosphorus nuclear magnetic resonance evidence of abnormal skeletal muscle k metabolism in chronic alcoholics. Neurology 39: 821

Bowyer S L, LaMonthe M P, Hollister J R 1985 Steroid myopathy: incidence and detection in a population with asthma. Journal of Allergy and Clinical Immunology 76: 234

Bradley W G 1970 The neuromyopathy of vincristine in the guinea pig. An electrophysiological and pathological study. Journal of the Neurological Sciences 10: 133

Bradley W G 1974 Disorders of peripheral nerves. Blackwell Scientific Publications, Oxford

Bradley W G, Lassman L P, Pearce G W, Walton J N 1970 The neuromyopathy of vincristine in man. Clinical, electrophysiological and pathological studies. Journal of the Neurological Sciences 10: 107

Bradley W G, Fewings J D, Harris J B, Johnson M A 1976 Emetine myopathy in the rat. British Journal of Pharmacology 57: 29

Bradley R, McKerrell R E, Barnard E A 1988 Neuromuscular disease in animals. In: Walton J N (ed) Disorders of voluntary muscle, 5th ed. Churchill Livingstone, Edinburgh p 910

Briner V, Colombi A, Brunner W, Truniger B 1986 Die akute rhabdomyolyse. Schweizerische medizinische wochenschrift 116: 198

Britt B A 1979 Etiology and pathophysiology of malignant hyperthermia. Federation Proceedings 38: 44

Britt C W, Light R R, Peters B H, Schochet S S 1980 Rhabdomyolysis during treatment with epsilon-aminocaproic acid. Archives of Neurology 37: 187

Brotman M C, Forbath N, Garfinkel P E, Humphrey J G 1981 Myopathy due to ipecac syrup poisoning in a patient with anorexia nervosa. Canadian Medical Association Journal 125: 453

Brownell A K W, Engel A G 1978 Experimental lipid storage myopathy. A quantitative ultrastructural and biochemical study. Journal of the Neurological Sciences 35: 31

Brumback R A, Gerst J W, Knull H R 1983 High energy

phosphate depletion in a model of defective muscle glycolysis. Muscle and Nerve 6: 52

Cameron D L, Tu A T 1978 Chemical and functional homology of myotoxin a from prairie rattlesnake venom and crotamine from South American rattlesnake venom. Biochimica et Biophysica Acta 532: 147

Carroll G J, Will R K, Peter J B, Garlepp M J, Dawkins R L 1987 Penicillamine induced polymyositis and dermatomyositis. Journal of Rheumatology 14: 995

Chaikin H L 1980 Rhabdomyolysis after drug overdose with coma. Southern Medical Journal 73: 990

Charness M E, Simon R P, Greenberg D A 1989 Ethanol and the nervous system. New England Journal of Medicine 321(7): 442

Chopra J S, Mehta J, Rana S V, Dhand U K, Mehta S 1987 Muscle involvement during postnatal protein calorie malnutrition and recovery in rhesus monkeys Acta Neurologica Scandinavica 75: 234

Chugh K S, Singhal P C, Uberoi H S 1978 Rhabdomyolysis and renal failure in acute mercuric chloride poisoning. Medical Journal of Australia 2: 125

Chugh K S, Nath I V S, Ubroi H S, Singhal P C, Pareek S K, Sarkar A K 1979 Acute renal failure due to non-traumatic rhabdomyolysis. Postgraduate Medical Journal 55: 386

Chui L A, Nevstein H, Munsat T L 1975 Tubular aggregates in sub-clinical alcoholic myopathy. Neurology 25: 405

Clouston P D, Donnelly P E 1989 Acute necrotising myopathy associated with amiodarone therapy Australian and New Zealand Journal of Medicine 19: 483

Cogen F C, Rigg F, Simmons J L, Domino E F 1978 Phencyclidine-associated acute rhbdomyolysis. Annals of Internal Medicine 88: 210

Cooper J M, Petty R K, Hayes D J et al 1988 An animal model of mitochondrial myopathy: a biochemical and physiological investigation of rats treated in vivo with the NAD-Cod reductase inhibitor diphenyleneiodonium. Journal of the Neurological Sciences 83: 335

Cumming A M M, Boddy K, Brown J J, Fraser R, Lever A F, Padfield P L, Robertson J I S 1980 Severe hypokalaemia with paralysis induced by small doses of liquorice. Postgraduate Medical Journal 56: 526

Dalakas M C, Illa I, Pezeshkpour G H, Laukaitis J P, Cohen B, Griffin J L 1990 Mitochondrial myopathy caused by long-term zidovudine therapy. New England Journal of Medicine 322: 1098

Daniel P M, Pratt O E, Spargo E 1977 The metabolic homoeostatic role of muscle and its function as a store of protein. Lancet ii: 446

Danon J M, Karpati G, Carpenter S 1978 Subacute skeletal myopathy induced by 2,4-dichlorophenoxyacetate in rats and guinea pigs. Muscle and Nerve 1: 89

Dastur D K, Gagrat B M, Manghani D K 1979 Fine structure of muscle in human disuse atrophy: significance of proximal muscle involvement in muscle disorders. Neuropathology and Applied Neurobiology 5: 85

Dastur D K, Manghani D K, Osuntokun B O, Sourander P, Kondo K 1982 Neuromuscular and related changes in malnutrition. Journal of the Neurological Sciences 55: 207

Deighton C M 1990 Eosinophilia myalgia syndrome. British Medical Journal 301: 611

Dettbarn W D 1984 Pesticide induced muscle necrosis: mechanisms and prevention. Fundamentals of Applied Toxicology 4: 518

Doyle D R, McCurley T L, Sergent J S 1983 Fatal polymyositis in D-penicillamine-treated rheumatoid arthritis. Annals of

Internal Medicine 98: 327

Drenckhahn D, Lullmann-Rauch R 1979 Experimental myopathy induced by amphiphilic cationic compounds including several psychotropic drugs. Neuroscience 4: 549

Duane D D, Engel A G 1970 Emetine myopathy. Neurology (Minneap) 20: 733

Duane P, Peters T J 1988 Nutritional status in alcoholics with and without chronic skeletal muscle myopathy. Alcohol 23: 271

Duchen L W 1971a An electronmicroscopic study of the changes induced by botulinum toxin in the motor end-plates of slow and fast skeletal muscle fibres of the mouse. Journal of the Neurological Sciences 14: 47

Duchen L W 1971b Changes in the electron microscopic structure of slow and fast skeletal muscle fibres of the mouse after the local injection of botulinum toxin. Journal of the Neurological Sciences 14: 61

Duchen L W 1973 The effects of tetanus toxin on the motor end-plates of the mouse. An electron microscopic study. Journal of the Neurological Sciences 19: 153

Duchen L W 1981 The neuromuscular junction of the mouse after black widow spider venom. Journal of Physiology (London) 316: 279

Durack D T, Gubbay S S, Kakulas B A 1969 Electrophysiological studies in the Rottnest quokka with nutritional myopathy. Australian Journal of Experimental Biology and Medical Science 47: 581

Eberstein A, Goodgold J, Johnston R 1978 Clofibrate-induced myotonia in the rat. Experientia 34: 1607

Eidson M, Philen R M, Sewell C M, Voorhees R, Kilbourne E M 1990 l-tryptophan and eosinophilia-myalgia syndrome in New Mexico. Lancet 335: 645

Eiser A R, Neff M S, Slifkin R F 1982 Acute myoglobinuric renal failure. A consequence of the neuroleptic malignant syndrome. Archives of Internal Medicine 142: 601

Ekbom K, Hed R, Kirstein L, Astrom K-E 1964 Muscular affections in chronic alcoholism. Archives of Neurology 10: 449 treated rabbits.

Ellis J T 1956 Necrosis and regeneration of skeletal muscle in cortisone-treated rabbits. American Journal of Pathology 32: 992

Estes M L, Ewing-Wilson D, Chou S M, Mitsumoto H, Hanson M, Shirey E, Ratliff N B 1987 Chloroquine neuromyotoxicity. American Journal of Medicine 82: 447

Fardeau M, Tomé F M S, Simon P 1979 Muscle and nerve changes induced by perhexiline maleate in man and mice. Muscle and Nerve 2: 24

Faris A A, Reyes M G 1971 Reappraisal of alcoholic myopathy. Journal of Neurology, Neurosurgery and Psychiatry 34: 86

Fenichel G M, Martin J T 1977 An experimental myopathy in rats produced with imidazole. Abstract 331. In: Abstracts of papers presented at the 3rd International Congress on Muscle Diseases, Newcastle upon Tyne. International Congress Series No 334. Excerpta Medica, Amsterdam

Fewings J D, Burns R J, Kakulas B A 1973 A case of acute emetine myopathy. In: Kakulas B A (ed) Clinical studies in myology. Excerpta Medica, Amsterdam, pp 594–598

Fohlman J, Eaker D 1977 Isolation and characterization of a lethal myotoxic phospholipase A from the venom of the common sea snake Enhydrina schistoca causing myoglobinuria in mice. Toxicon 15: 385

Forfar J C, Brown G J, Cull R E 1979 Proximal myopathy during beta-blockade. British Medical Journal 279: 1331

Frendin T J, Swainson C P 1985 Acute renal failure secondary to non-traumatic rhabdomyolysis following amoxapine overdose. New Zealand Medical Journal 98: 690

Friedman E J 1984 Death from ipecac intoxication in a patient with anorexia nervosa. American Journal of Psychiatry 141: 702

Furman R E, Barchi R L 1978 The pathophysiology of myotonia produced by aromatic carboxylic acids. Annals of Neurology 4: 357

Gabow P A, Kaehny W D, Kelleher S P 1982 The spectrum of rhabdomyolysis. Medicine 61: 141

Gabry A L, Pourriat J L, Hoang the Dan P, Cupa M 1982 Acute rhabdomyolysis associated with heroin addiction. Ann Fr Anesth Reanim 1: 179

Gibbs J M 1978 A case of rhabdomyolysis associated with suxamethonium. Anaesthesia and Intensive Care 6: 141

Gori Z, De Tata V, Pollera M, Bergamini E 1988 Mitochondrial myopathy in rats fed with a diet containing beta-guanidine propionic acid, an inhibitor or creatine entry in muscle cells. British Journal of Experimental Pathology 69: 639

Gorio A, Mauro A 1979 Reversibility and mode of action of black widow spider venom on the vertebrate neuromuscular junction. Journal of General Physiology 73: 245

Goy J J, Stauffer J C, Deruaz J P, Gillard D, Kaufmann U, Kuntzer T, Kappenberger L 1989 Myopathy as possible side-effect of cyclosporin. Lancet i: 1446

Graham D I, Bonilla E, Gonatas N K, Schotland D L 1976 Core formation in the muscles of rats intoxicated with triethyltin sulfate. Journal of Neuropathology and Experimental Neurology 35: 1

Gutierrez J M, Ownby C L, Odell G V 1984 Isolation of a myotoxin from Bothrops asper venom: partial characteris-ation and action on skeletal muscle. Toxicon 22: 115

Gutierrez J M, Arrjoyo O, Chaves F, Lomonte B, Cerdas L 1986 Pathogenesis of myonecrosis induced by coral snake (Micrurus nigrocinctus) venom in mice. British Journal of Experimental Pathology 67: 1

Gutierrez J M, Chaves F, Gense J A, Lomonte B, Comacho Z 1989 Myonecrosis induced in mice by a basic myotoxin isolated from the venom of the snake Bothrops nummifer (jumping viper) from Costa Rica. Toxicon 27: 785

Hadlow J J 1962 Diseases of skeletal muscle. In: Innes J R M, Saunders L Z (eds) Comparative neuropathology. Academic Press, New York, p 147

Halla J T, Fallahi S, Koopman W J 1984 Penicillamine-induced myositis: observations and unique features in two patients and review of the literature. American Journal of Medicine 77: 719

Haller R G 1985 Experimental acute alcoholic myopathy — a histochemical study. Muscle and Nerve 8: 195

Haller R G, Drachman D B 1980 Alcoholic rhabdomyolysis. An experimental model in the rat. Science 208: 412

Haller R G, Knochel J P 1984 Skeletal muscle disease in alcoholism. Medical Clinics of North America 68: 91

Harris J B, Maltin C A 1982 Myotoxic activity of the crude venom and the principal neurotoxin, taipoxin, of the Australian taipan, Oxyuranus scutellatus. British Journal of Pharmacology 76: 61

Harris J B, Johnson M A, Karlsson E 1975 Pathological responses of rat skeletal muscle to a single subcutaneous injection of a toxin isolated from the venom of the Australian tiger snake, Notechis scutatus scutatus. Clinical and Experimental Pharmacology and Physiology 2: 383

Hayman L, Abresman C E, Terplan K L 1956 Dermatomyositis following penicillin injections. Neurology 6: 63

Hed R, Lundmark C, Fahlgren H, Orell S 1962 Acute muscular syndrome in chronic alcoholism. Acta Medica Scandinavica 171: 585

Hertzman P A, Blevins W L, Mayer J, Greenfield B, Ting M, Gleich G J 1990 Association of the eosinophilia–myalgia syndrome with the ingestion of tryptophan. New England Journal of Medicine 322: 869

Higuchi I, Izumo S, Kuriyama M et al 1989 Germanium myopathy. Clinical and experimental pathological studies. Acta Neuropathologica (Berl) 79: 300

Huang S Y, Perez J C 1982 A comparative electron microscopic study of myonecrosis induced by Crotalus atrox (Western diamondback rattlesnake) in gray woodrats and mice. Toxicon 20: 443

Hughes J T 1974 Pathology of muscle. In: Bennington J L (ed) Major problems in pathology, vol 4. W B Saunders, Philadelphia, p 151

Ishay J, Lass Y, Sandbank U 1975 A lesion of muscle transverse tubular system by oriental hornet (Vespa orientalis) venom: electron microscopic and histological study. Toxicon 13: 57

Jackson M J, Jones D A, Edwards R H T 1983 Vitamin E and skeletal muscle. In: Biology of vitamin E (Ciba Foundation Symposium 101). Pitman Books, London, pp 224–239

Jaeger U, Prodczeck A, Haubenstock A, Pirich K, Donner A, Hruby K 1984 Acute oral poisoning with lindane-solvent mixtures. Veterinary and Medical Toxicology 26: 11

Jenkins P, Emerson P A 1981 Myopathy induced by rifampicin. British Medical Journal 283: 105

Jennings A E, Levey A S, Harrington J T 1983 Amoxapine-associated acute renal failure. Archives of Internal Medicine 143: 1525

Jubb K V F, Kennedy P C 1970 In: Pathology of domestic animals, vol 2, 2nd edn. Academic Press, New York, p 488

Kahn L B, Meyer J S 1970 Acute myopathy in chronic alcoholism: a study of 22 autopsy cases with ultrastructural observations. American Journal of Clinical Pathology 53: 516

Kakulas B A 1975 Experimental muscle diseases. In: Jasmin G, Cantin M (eds) Methods and achievements in experimental pathology, vol 7. Karger, Basel, p 109

Kakulas B A 1981 Experimental myopathies. In: Walton J N (ed) Disorders of Voluntary muscle, 4th ed. Churchill Livingstone, Edinburgh

Kakulas B A 1982 Drug and toxic myopathies. In: Riddell J (ed) The pathology of drug-induced and toxic disorders. Churchill Livingstone, Edinburgh.

Kane M J, Silverman L R, Rand J H, Paciucci P A, Holland J F 1988 Myonecrosis as a complication of the use of epsilon amino-caproic acid: a case report and review of the literature. American Journal of Medicine 85: 861

Karpati G 1984 Denervation and disuse atrophy of skeletal muscle — involvement of endogenous glucocorticoid hormones? Trends in Neurosciences 61:

Karpati G, Watters G V 1980 Adverse anaesthetic reactions in Duchenne dystrophy. In: Angelini C, Danieli G A, Fontanari D (eds) Muscular dystrophy research: advances and new trends, International Congress Series No 527. Excerpta Medica, Amsterdam, pp 206–217

Kennedy M 1981 Cardiac glycoside toxicity. An unusual manifestation of drug addiction. Medical Journal of Australia 1: 686

Kilpatrick C, Braund W, Burns R 1982 Myopathy with myasthenic features possibly induced by codeine linctus. Medical Journal of Australia 2: 410

Kleinknecht D, Parent A, Blot, Bochereau G, Lasllement P Y,

Pourriat J L 1982 Rhabdomyolysis with acute renal failure and malignant neuroleptic syndrome. Ann Med Interne (Paris) 133: 549

Klinkerfuss G, Bleisch V, Dioso M M, Perkoff G T 1967 A spectrum of myopathy associated with alcoholism. II. Light and electron microscopic observations. Annals of Internal Medicine 67: 493

Kontos H A 1962 Myopathy associated with chronic colchicine toxicity. New England Journal of Medicine 266: 38

Kovanen J, Somer H, Schroder P 1983 Acute myopathy associated with gasoline sniffing. Neurology 33: 629

Kuncl R W, Duncan G, Watson D, Alderson K, Rogawski M A, Peper M 1987 Colchicine myopathy and neuropathy. New England Journal of Medicine 316(25): 1562

Kwiecinski H 1981 Myotonia induced by chemical agents. CRC Critical Reviews in Toxicology 8: 279

Lane R J M, Mastaglia F L 1978 Drug-induced myopathies in man. Lancet ii: 562

Lane R J M, Radoff F M 1981 Alcohol and serum creatine kinase levels. Annals of Neurology 10: 581

Lane R J M, Martin A M, McLelland N J, Mastaglia F L 1979 Epsilon amino-caproic acid (EACA) myopathy. Postgraduate Medical Journal 55: 282

Langohr H D, Wietholter H, Peiffer J 1983 Muscle wasting in chronic alcoholics: comparative histochemical and biochemical studies. Journal of Neurology, Neurosurgery and Psychiatry 46: 248

Lazaro R P, Dentinger M P, Rodichok L D, Barron K D, Satya-Murti S 1986 Muscle pathology in Bassen–Kornzweig syndrome and vitamin E deficiency. American Journal of Clinical Pathology 86: 378

Lazarus A L, Toglia J U 1985 Fatal myoglobinuric renal failure in a patient with tardive dyskinesia. Neurology 35: 1055

Leonard J P, Salpeter M M 1979 Agonist-induced myopathy at the neuromuscular junction is mediated by calcium. Journal of Cell Biology 82: 811

Leonard T M, Howden M E H, Spence I 1979 A lethal myotoxin isolated from the venom of the Australian king brown snake (Pseudechis australis). Toxicon 17: 549

Lithell H, Boberg J, Hellsing K, Lundqvist G, Vessby B 1978 Increase of the lipoprotein–lipase activity in human skeletal muscle during clofibrate administration. European Journal of Clinical Investigation 8: 67

Livingstone I, Johnson M A, Mastaglia F L 1981 Effects of dexamethasone on fibre subtypes in rat muscle. Neuropathology and Applied Neurobiology 7: 381

Lullmann H, Lullman-Rauch R, Wassermann O 1978 Lipidosis induced by amphiphilic cationic drugs. Biochemical Pharmacology 27: 1103

Lullmann-Rauch R 1979 Drug-induced lysosomal storage disorders. In: Dingle J T, Jacques P J, Shaw I H (eds) Lysosomes in applied and therapeutics. North-Holland, Amsterdam, pp 49–130

MacFarlane I A, Rosenthal F D 1977 Severe myopathy after status asthmaticus. Lancet i: 615

McMurray C H, Rice D A, Kennedy S 1983 Experimental models for nutritional myopathy. In: Biology of vitamin E (Ciba Foundation Symposium 101). Pitman Books, London, pp 201–223

McQuillen M P, Cantor H E, O'Rourke J R 1968 Myasthenic syndrome associated with antibiotics. Archives of Neurology (Chicago) 18: 402

Marais G E, Larson K K 1990 Rhabdomyolysis and acute renal failure induced by combination lovastatin and gemfibrozil therapy. Annals of Internal Medicine 112(3): 228

Martin J T, Laskowski M D, Fenichel G M 1977 Imidazole myopathy and its dependence on acetylcholine. Neurology (Minneapolis) 27: 484

Martin F C, Slavin G, Levi A J 1982 Alcoholic muscle disease. British Medical Bulletin 38: 53

Martin F C, Levi A J, Slavin G, Peters T J 1984 Glycogen content and activities of key glycolytic enzymes in muscle biopsies from control subjects and patients with chronic alcoholic skeletal myopathy. Clinical Science 66: 69

Martin F C, Slavin G, Levi J, Peters T J 1985 Alcoholic skeletal myopathy, a clinical and pathological study. Quarterly Journal of Medicine 55: 233

Martinez A J, Hooshmand H, Faris A A 1973 Acute alcoholic myopathy. Journal of the Neurological Sciences 20: 245

Mastaglia F L 1982 Adverse effects of drugs on muscle. Drugs 24: 304

Mastaglia F L, Argov Z 1980 Drug-induced myopathies and disorders of neuromuscular transmission. In: Manzo L et al (eds) Advances in neurotoxicity. Pergamon Press, Oxford, pp 319–328

Mastaglia F L, Argov Z 1982 Immunologically mediated drug-induced neuromuscular disorders. In: Dukor P, Kallos P, Schlumberger H D, West G B (eds) Pseudo-allergic reactions. Involvement of drugs and chemicals, vol 3. Basel, Karger, pp 62–86

Mastaglia F L, Papadimitriou J M, Dawkins R L, Beveridge B 1977 Vacuolar myopathy associated with chloroquine, lupus erythematosus and thymoma. Journal of the Neurological Sciences 34: 315

Mateer J E, Farrel B J, Chou S S M, Gutmann L 1985 Reversible ipecac myopathy. Archives of Neurology 42: 188

Max S R, Konagaya M, Konagaya Y 1986 Drug-induced myopathies: examples of cellular mechanisms. Muscle and Nerve 9: 33

Medsger T A 1990 Tryptophan-induced eosinophilia–myalgia syndrome. New England Journal of Medicine 322(13): 926

Meier C, Kauer B, Muller U, Ludin H P 1979 Neuromyopathy during chronic amiodarone treatment. A case report. Journal of Neurology 220: 231

Meldrum B S 1965 The actions of snake venoms on nerve and muscle. The pharmacology of phospholipase A and of polypeptide toxins. Pharmacological Reviews 17: 393

Melmed C, Karpati G, Carpenter S 1975 Experimental mitochondrial myopathy produced by in vivo uncoupling of oxidative phosphorylation. Journal of the Neurological Sciences 26: 305

Modi K B, Horn E H, Bryson S M 1985 Rhabdomyolysis in theophylline poisoning. Lancet ii: 8447 (161)

Montgomery C A 1978 Muscle diseases. In: Benirschke K, Garner F M, Jones T C (eds) Pathology of laboratory animals, vol 1. Springer, New York, p 853

Mukuno K, Imai H 1973 Study of the effects on extraocular muscles of chronic organophosphate intoxication in beagle dogs. Acta Societatis Ophthalmologicae Japonicae 77: 1246

Nanji A A, Filipenko J D 1983 Rhabdomyolysis and acute myoglobinuric renal failure associated with methadone intoxication. Journal of Toxicology and Clinical Toxicology 20: 353

Nelson J S 1983 Neuropathological studies of chronic vitamin E deficiency in mammals including humans. In: Biology of vitamin E (Ciba Foundation Symposium 101). Pitman Books, London, pp 92–105

Neville H E, Maunder-Sewry C A, McDougall J, Dubowitz V 1979 Chloroquine-induced cytosomes with curvilinear profiles in muscle. Muscle and Nerve 2: 376

Neville H E, Ringel S P, Guggenheim M A, Wehling C A, Starcevich J M 1983 Ultrastructural and histochemical abnormalities of skeletal muscle in patients with chronic vitamin E deficiency. Neurology 33: 483

Ng R H, Howard B D 1980 Mitochondria and sarcoplasmic reticulum as model targets for neurotoxic and myotoxic phospholipases A$_2$. Proceedings of the National Academy of Science of the USA. 77: 1346

Nicholls K, Niall J F, Moran J E 1982 Rhabdomyolysis and renal failure. Complications of narcotic abuse. Medical Journal of Australia 2: 387

Ojeda V J 1982 Necrotizing myopathy associated with steroid therapy. Report of two cases. Pathology 14: 435

Ownby C L, Odell G V 1983 Pathogenesis of skeletal muscle necrosis induced by tarantula venom. Experimental and Molecular Pathology 38: 283

Ownby C L, Woods W M, Odell G V 1979 Antiserum to myotoxin from prairie rattlesnake (Crotalus viridis viridis) venom. Toxicon 17: 373

Palmer E P, Guay A T 1985 Reversible myopathy secondary to abuse of ipecac in patients with major eating disorders. New England Journal of Medicine 313: 1457

Palmucci L, Bertolotto A, Schiffer D 1978 Acute muscle necrosis after chronic overdosage of phenformin and fenfluramine. Muscle and Nerve 1: 245

Panegyres P K, Papadimitriou J M, Hollingsworth P N, Armstrong J A, Kakulas B A 1990 Vesicular changes in the myopathies of AIDS: ultrastructural observations and their relationship to zidovudine treatment. Journal of Neurology, Neurosurgery and Psychiatry 53: 649

Papadimitriou J M, Mastaglia F L 1973 Myopathy induced by mulga snake venom: a model for the study of muscle degeneration and regeneration. In: Basic research in myology, Proceedings of the Second International Congress on Muscle Diseases, Perth, Australia, November 1971, pp 22–26. International Congress Series No. 294, Excerpta Medica, Amsterdam, pp 426–437

Papapetropoulos T A 1980 Myopathies. G K Parisianoss Press, Athens, p 121

Pardridge W M, Casanello-Ertl D, Duduggian-Vartavarian L 1980 Branched chain amino acid oxidation in cultured rat skeletal muscle cells. Selective inhibition by clofibric acid. Journal of Clinical Investigation 66: 88

Paul H S, Abidi S A 1979 Paradoxical effects of clofibrate on liver and muscle metabolism in rats. Journal of Clinical Investigation 64: 405

Penn A S, Rowland L P, Fraser D W 1972 Drugs, coma, and myoglobinuria. Archives of Neurology 26: 336

Perkoff G T, Hardy P, Velez-Garcia E 1966 Reversible acute muscular syndrome in chronic alcoholism. New England Journal of Medicine 274: 1277

Perkoff G T, Dioso M M, Bleisch V, Klinkerfuss G 1967 A spectrum of myopathy associated with alcoholism. 1. Clinical and laboratory features. Annals of Internal Medicine 67: 481

Petajan J H, Townsend J, Currey K M 1986 Ethchlorvynol (Placidyl) may produce tubular aggregates in skeletal muscle. Electroencephalography and Clinical Neurophysiology 64: 54P

Piette A-M, Bauer D, Chapman A 1984 Severe hypokalemia with rhabdomylysis secondary to absorption of an alcohol-free liquorice beverage. Ann Med Interne 135: 296

Pinching A J, Helbert M, Peddle B et al 1989 Clinical experience with zidovudine for patients with acquired immune deficiency syndrome and acquired immune deficiency syndrome-related complex. Journal of Infection 18 (suppl 1): 33

Pluskal M G, Harris J B, Pennington R J, Eaker D 1978 Some biochemical responses of rat skeletal muscle to a single subcutaneous injection of a toxin (notexin) isolated from the venom of the Australian tiger snake Notechis scutatus scutatus. Clinical and Experimental Pharmacology 5: 131

Pritchard J B 1979 Toxic substances and cell membrane function. Federation Proceedings 38: 2220

Rannels S R, Rannels D E, Pegg A E, Jefferson L S 1978 Glucocorticoid effects on peptide-chain initiation in skeletal muscle and heart. American Journal of Physiology 235: E134

Reid H A 1961 Myoglobinuria and sea-snake bite poisoning. British Medical Journal 1: 1284

Richter R W, Challenor Y B, Pearson J, Kagen L J, Hamilton L L, Ramsey W H, 1971 Acute myoglobinuria associated with heroin addiction. Journal of the American Medical Association 216: 1172

Riggs J E, Schochet S S, Gutmann L, Crosby T W, DiBartolomeo A G 1986 Chronic human colchicine neuropathy and myopathy. Archives of Neurology 43: 521

Rimon D, Ludatscher R, Cohen L 1984 Clofibrate-induced muscular syndrome. Case report with ultrastructural findings and review of the literature. Israel Journal of Medical Sciences 20: 1082

Rogers R J, Gibson J, Reichmann K G 1979 The toxicity of Cassia occidentalis for cattle. Australian Veterinary Journal 55: 408

Rowlands J B, Mastaglia F L, Kakulas B A, Hainsworth D 1969 Clinical and pathological aspects of a fatal case of mulga (Pseudechis australis) snakebite. Medical Journal of Australia 1: 226

Rubenstein A E, Wainapel S F 1977 Acute hypokalemic myopathy in alcoholism. A clinical entity. Archives of Neurology 34: 553

Rumpf K W, Barth M, Blech M, Kaiser H, Koop I, Arnold R, Scheler F, 1984 Bezafibrate-induced myolysis and myoglobinuria in patients with impaired renal functions. Klinische Wochenschrift 62: 346

Sahgal V, Subramani V, Hughes R, Shah A, Singh H 1979 On the pathogenesis of mitochondrial myopathies. Acta Neuropathologica (Berlin) 46: 177

Schmalbruch H 1980 The early changes in experimental myopathy induced by chloroquine and chlorphentermine. Journal of Neuropathology and Experimental Neurology 39: 65

Schofield P M, Beath S V, Mant T G K, Bhamra R 1985 Recovery after severe oxprenolol overdose complicated by rhabdomyolysis. Human Toxicology 4(1): 57

Scobie I N, Durward W F, MacCuish A C 1980 Proximal myopathy after prolonged total therapeutic starvation. British Medical Journal 280: 1212

Sensakovic J W, Suarez M, Perez G, Johnson E S, Smith L G 1985 Pentamidine treatment of Pneumocystis carinii pneumonia in the acquired immunodeficiency syndrome. Association with acute renal failure and myoglobinuria. Archives of Internal Medicine 145: 2247

Seow S S W 1984 Abuse of APF linctus codeine and cardiac glycoside toxicity. Medical Journal of Australia 140: 54

Shergy W J, Caldwell D S 1988 Polymyositis after propylthiouracyl treatment. Annals of Rheumatic Diseases 47(4): 340

Shilkin K B, Chen B T M, Khoo O T 1972 Rhabdomyolysis caused by hornet venom. British Medical Journal 1: 156

Silver R M, Heyes M P, Maize J C, Quearry B, Vionnet–Fuasset M, Sternberg E M 1990 Scleroderma, fasciitis and eosinophilia associated with the ingestion of tryptophan. New England Journal of Medicine 322: 874

Sinclair D, Phillips C 1982 Transient myopathy apparently due to tetracycline. New England Journal of Medicine 307: 821

Sitprija V, Boonpucknavig V 1972 Renal failure and myonecrosis following wasp-stings. Lancet i: 749

Song S K, Rubin E R 1972 Ethanol produces muscle damage in human volunteers. Science 175: 327

Spargo E 1984 The acute effects of alcohol on plasma creatine kinase (CK) activity in the rat. Journal of the Neurological Sciences 63: 307

Stauber W T, Hedge A M, Trout J J, Schottelius B A 1981 Inhibition of lysosomal function in red and white skeletal muscles by chloroquine. Experimental Neurology 71: 295

Steer J H, Mastaglia F L 1986 Protein degradation in bupivacaine-treated muscles. The role of extracellular calcium. Journal of the Neurological Sciences 75: 343

Steer J H, Mastaglia F L, Papadimitriou J M, van Bruggen I 1986 Bupivacaine-induced muscle injury. The role of extracellular calcium. Journal of the Neurological Sciences 73: 205

Steinness E, Rasmussen F, Svendsen O, Nielsen P 1977 A comparative study of serum creatine phosphokinase (CPK) activity in rabbits, pigs and humans after intramuscular injection of local damaging drugs. Acta Pharmacologica et Toxicology 42: 357

Stewart P M, Hensley W J 1981 Acute polymyopathy during total parenteral nutrition. British Medical Journal 283: 1578

Strunk S, Smith C W, Blumberg J M 1967 Ultrastructural studies on the lesion produced in skeletal muscle fibers by crude type A Clostridium perfringens toxin and its purified alpha fraction. American Journal of Pathology 50: 89

Sugie H, Russin R, Verity M A 1984 Emetine myopathy: two case reports with pathobiochemical analysis. Muscle and Nerve 7: 54

Sunderland S K 1983 Australian animal toxins. Oxford University Press, Melbourne

Sunnasy D, Cairns S R, Martin F, Slavin G, Peters T J 1983 chronic alcoholic skeletal muscle myopathy: A clinical, histological and biochemical assessment of muscle lipid. Journal of Clinical Pathology 36: 778

Sutherland S K 1983 Australian animal toxins. Oxford University Press, Melbourne

Sutherland S K, Coulter A R 1977 Three instructive cases of tiger snake (Notechis scutatus) envenomation—and how a radioimmunoassay proved the diagnosis. Medical Journal of Australia 2: 177.

Swash K, Schwartz K, Foltz C 1957 Selenium as an integral part of factors against dietary necrotic liver degeneration. Journal of the American Chemical Society 79: 3292

Swenson R D, Golper T A, Bennett W M 1982 Acute renal failure and rhabdomyolysis after ingestion of phenylpropanolamine-containing diet pills. Journal of the American Medical Association 248: 1216

Tam C W, Olin B Y, Ruiz A E 1980 Loxapine-associated rhabdomyolysis and acute renal failure. Archives of Internal Medicine 140: 975

Teravainen H, Larsen A, Hillbom M 1977 Clofibrate-induced myopathy in the rat. Acta Neuropathologica (Berlin) 39: 135

Thomas M A B, Ibels L S 1985 Rhabdomyolysis and acute renal failure. Australian and New Zealand Journal of Medicine 15: 623

Tomasi L G 1979 Reversibility of human myopathy caused by vitamin E deficiency. Neurology 28: 1182

Trout J J, Stauber W T, Schottelius B A 1981 Chloroquine-induced alterations in phasic muscles. II. Sarcoplasmic reticulum. Experimental and Molecular Pathology 34: 237

Tsubaki T, Fukuhara N, Hoshi M, Mori S 1977 The pathogenesis of central core, multicore, target and cytoplasmic bodies. In: Current research in muscular dystrophy, Japan. Proceedings of the Annual Meeting of the Muscular Dystrophy Research Group, Tokyo, p 78

Tu A T 1977 Venoms: chemistry and molecular biology. Wiley, New York, pp 459–526

Unger J, Decaux G, L'Hermite M 1982 Rhabdomyolysis, acute renal failure, endocrine alterations and neurological sequelae in a case of lithium self poisoning. Acta Clinica Belgica 37: 216

Urbano-Marquez A, Estruch R, Grau J M, Fernandez-Huerta J, Sala M 1985 On alcoholic myopathy. Annals of Neurology 17: 418

Valeriano J, Tucker P, Kattah J 1983 An unusual cause of hypokalemic muscle weakness. Neurology (Cleveland) 33: 1242

van Garsse L G M M, Boeykens P P H 1990 Two patients with eosinophilia myalgia syndrome associated with tryptophan. British Medical Journal 301: 21

van Marle W, Woods K L 1980 Acute hydrocortisone myopathy. British Medical Journal 281: 271

van Vleet J R, Ferrans V J 1984 Ultrastructural alterations in skeletal muscle of pigs with acute monensin myotoxicosis. American Journal of Pathology 114: 461

Varga J, Peltonen J, Uitto J, Jimenez S 1990 Development of diffuse fasciitis with eosinophilia during 1-trytophan treatment: demonstration of elevated type I collagen gene expression in affected tissues. Annals of Internal Medicine 112: 344

Vasilescu C, Alexianu M, Dan A 1984 Delayed neuropathy after organophosphorus insecticide (Dipterex) poisoning: a clinical, electrophysiological and nerve biopsy study. Journal of Neurology, Neurosurgery and Psychiatry 47: 543

Vita G, Bartolone S, Santoro M, Toscano A, Carozza G, Girlanda P, Frisina N 1986 Hypokalemic myopathy induced by fluoroprednizolone-containing nasal spray. Acta Neurologica (Napoli) 8: 108

Walker K H, Thompson D R, Seaman J T 1980 Suspected poisoning of sheep by Ixiolaena brevicompta. Australian Veterinary Journal 56: 64

Walravens P A, Greene C, Frerman F E 1989 Lovastatin, isoprenes and myopathy. Lancet ii: 1097

Walsh J C, Conomy A B 1977 The effect of ethyl alcohol on striated muscle: Some clinical and pathological observations. Australian and New Zealand Journal of Medicine 7: 485

Walton J N, Mastaglia F L 1981 In: Davison A N, Thompson R H S (eds) The molecular basis of neuropathology. Arnold, London, p 442

Watson A J S, Dalbrow M H, Stachura I, Fragola J A, Rubin M F, Watson R M, Bourke E 1983 Immunologic studies in cimetidine-induced nephropathy and polymyositis. New England Journal of Medicine 308(3): 142

Wattel F, Chopin C, Dorucher A, Berzin B 1978 Rhabdomyolyses au cours des intoxications aigues. Nouvelle Presse Medicale 7: 2553

Wecker L, Laskowski M B, Dettbarn W-D 1978 Neuromuscular dysfunction induced by acetylcholinesterase inhibition. Federation Proceedings 37: 2818

Werlin S L, Harb J M, Swick H, Blank E 1983 Neuromuscular dysfunction and ultrastructural pathology in children with chronic cholestasis and vitamin E deficiency. Annals of Neurology 13: 291

Williams A J, Baghat M S, Stableforth D E, Layton R M, Shenoi P M, Skinner C 1983 Dysphonia caused by inhaled steroids: recognition of a characteristic laryngeal abnormality. Thorax 38: 813

Willner J, Nakagawa M, Wood D 1984 Drug-induced fiber necrosis in Duchenne dystrophy. Italian Journal of Neurology 5: 117

Yaari Y, Pincus J H, Argov Z 1977 Depression of synaptic transmission by diphenylhydantoin. Annals of Neurology 1: 334

Yagiela J A, Benoit P W, Buoncristiani R D, Peters M P, Fort N F 1981 Comparison of myotoxic effects of lodacaine with epinephrine in rats and humans. Anesthesia Analg 60: 471–480

15. The pathology of malignant hyperthermia

D. G. F. Harriman

INTRODUCTION

Malignant hyperthermia (malignant hyperpyrexia, Denborough's syndrome, MH) is an inherited disorder brought to light when a susceptible member of an affected family undergoes general anaesthesia. The commonly used relaxants and volatile agents may trigger a potentially fatal reaction comprising generalized muscle rigidity and a rapid rise in core temperature threatening cardiac arrest. It was first defined in the early 1960s when Denborough & Lovell (1960) in a letter to the *Lancet* reported a family with a remarkable history. No fewer than 10 members of the sibship had developed hyperthermia during ether or ethyl chloride anaesthesia and had died. Study of that family suggested that susceptibility to MH was inherited as a dominant trait. A flow of case reports followed, and it became apparent that the syndrome was often ushered in by muscular rigidity triggered by the relaxing agent suxamethonium. The commonest volatile anaesthetic associated with the subsequent hyperthermia was the one most frequently used nowadays, namely halothane, although any general anaesthetic (with the probable exception of nitrous oxide) and some local anaesthetics could at times be incriminated. Curiously, a susceptible patient might have one or two anaesthetics without incident before developing MH in the course of a third. The syndrome was not precipitated by anaesthesia of less than 10 minutes' duration. The temperatures attained by many patients were remarkably high, up to 44°C, rising at the rate of 2–6°C per hour. The mortality rate in 1970 was 70%, death often occurring from cardiac arrest, but now with improved management by anaesthe-

tists alert to the condition it has fallen to 30% or lower. In the event of surviving a severe reaction causing rhabdomyolysis and myoglobinuria, death could be caused later by renal failure. At that stage an autopsy would show extensive patchy muscle necrosis and regeneration, more obvious in the lower limbs and clearly attributable to hyperthermia. In ultimate survivors it is interesting to note in follow-up biopsies that recovery from such extensive rhabdomyolysis may be virtually complete in a few months.

When histological investigation of patients suspected of being susceptible to MH began, the myopathic changes found were assumed to be primary, and responsible for the MH reaction. The changes sometimes occurred in susceptible patients who had not been exposed to triggering agents, thus presumably ruling out the attribution of the myopathy to hyperthermia itself.

Muscle changes in MH: early reports

The first report suggesting that MH might be associated with a myopathy was by Isaacs & Barlow (1970a,b) who found raised serum levels of creatine kinase (CK) in some members of affected families. This seemed to indicate that an abnormality of skeletal muscle triggered by anaesthetic agents could account for the considerable heat production during the MH episode. This impression was subsequently supported by the description of a clinical myopathy in an affected family (Steers et al 1970). The propositus was a 16-year-old youth of muscular build, who died following an episode of malignant hyperthermia. His father showed wasting of the lower thighs, and localized areas of hypertrophy in the thighs, sternomastoids, deltoids, rhomboids and biceps. The brother of the propositus was of strikingly muscular build but was otherwise normal. The serum CK in the father was 690 mU/l ($n = 5$–50). A biopsy of the father's muscle showed large fibres with 'central' nuclei, and muscle fibre necrosis and regeneration.

Further experience has shown that a clinically obvious myopathy is rare in MH-susceptible (MHS) patients, but when seen in our series occurred in a similar but more subdued hypertrophic/atrophic form. The hopes that a raised serum CK level could be relied upon to indicate MH susceptibility were dashed when both false-positives and false-negatives were recorded (Ellis et al 1975).

Muscle pathology in MH was described in greater detail after 1970. Harriman et al (1973) made motor-point muscle biopsies in 10 members of five families, of whom six showed susceptibility to MH by an in vitro test. In this, small strips of muscle were placed in a tissue bath at 37°C, and exposed to halothane and other agents. Those patients whose muscle developed contracture were considered to be susceptible to MH. The same patients showed structural changes in their muscle: an increase in the proportion of fibres with internal nuclei, moth-eaten fibres, 'spotted' fibres, partial type 1 fibre atrophy, or regenerating fibres. Despite the myopathic muscle patterns, all the patients were asymptomatic. Only two showed clinical signs of muscle hypertrophy, atrophy or depressed deep-tendon reflexes.

Other workers have made conflicting observations. Reske-Nielsen et al (1975) made motor-point muscle biopsies in 12 healthy relatives of two children who had died of MH. They found collateral re-innervation (a sensitive indicator of neuropathy) in 11 patients, and slight myopathic features in addition. In vitro tests for MH susceptibility were not performed. In a further study, Reske-Nielsen (1978) described 10 patients, one of whom had progressive muscular dystrophy, two of whom had myotonic dystrophy and the remainder of whom showed slight myopathic changes. Heffron & Isaacs (1976) found 'distinct grouping' of atrophic fibres in four patients susceptible to MH, and interpreted this as

neurogenic. Gullotta & Helpap (1975), in contrast, found fibre calibre variation and internal nuclei in four patients. It is difficult to reconcile reports of neurogenic disease with our own extensive material in which susceptible patients have shown either myopathic changes or no significant abnormality, but never neurogenic disease. The reason may be that we have standardized our observations on the vastus medialis as it was found to give the clearest response to the agents used in the in-vitro tests. Using motor-point muscle biopsy it would have been possible to detect even minimal denervation histologically. It is likely that the claims for denervation in MH were based on criteria which by convention were acceptable several years ago but which have now been shown to be inadmissible by data obtained from frozen sections of whole, normal human muscles at autopsy (Lexell et al 1983).

A list of references to the histopathological changes in MH is available elsewhere (Harriman 1988), usually consisting of single or small groups of cases. Most depended for diagnosis on a history, or family history of hyperthermia during anaesthesia and on serum CK levels unsupported by in vitro tests. Unfortunately, histories of hyperthermic reactions are often unreliable for diagnostic purposes unless they are of classical severity. Considering the number of centres throughout the world now investigating MH, there are remarkably few reports of histopathology in MHS subjects.

The most comprehensive of the publications on MH histopathology, unsupported by tests, but based on a carefully scrutinized history was that of Gullota and Spiesz-Kiefer (1983) which described 41 biopsies on MHS patients and relatives. Almost half the biopsies (including those of children) were normal; there was no evidence of denervation; cores and moth-eaten fibres were present, and two MHS patients in fact had central-core disease.

Implicit in the reports quoted so far is the assumption that controls for MH myopathy are provided by normal muscle. It will be shown later that MH insusceptible muscle, the specific controls for MH histopathology, quite often show unsuspected abnormalities which should not be attributed to MH. These range from small numbers of ring and other malformed fibres, aging changes, intercurrent reactions such as type

2B atrophy, or, rarely, asymptomatic neuro-muscular disease.

The aetiology of MH and its presumed association with other muscle disorders

When it was established that a proportion of MH-susceptible (MHS) patients showed myopathic changes, despite the fact that these were not specific and the myopathy was asymptomatic, speculation on the aetiology of MH centred on the histopathology. This was assumed to be the direct manifestation of the genetic disorder, which by an unknown mechanism could raise and maintain at a high level the intracellular calcium concentration when triggered by agents used in anaesthesia.

At that time some other myopathies were thought to be associated with MH and to support the concept of MH as a structural myopathy.

The development of sustained rigidity at the beginning of the MH episode suggested that the patients might be suffering from an incomplete form of myotonia congenita or myotonic dystrophy. Saidman et al (1964) reported MH in a 12-year-old girl who was said to have suffered from myotonia congenita. Anaesthetists are fully aware that patients with myotonic dystrophy require particular care during the induction of anaesthesia, because of the likelihood of a paradoxical reaction to the muscle relaxant, but these patients do not develop hyperthermia nor, in our own experience, do they show MH suscepti-bility by the test in vitro. Moulds & Denborough (1974) tested the muscle of two patients with congenital myotonia, three with dystrophia myotonica and one with hypokalaemic periodic paralysis; none showed susceptibility to MH, although some reacted in an unusual way to anaesthesia. However, Cody (1968) had found in the literature 11 cases of rigidity following the use of a depolarizing relaxant; seven of them developed MH and three had myotonic dystrophy. King et al (1972) described 18 families with MH, and one family also suffered from myotonia congenita. Hypertrophic branchial myopathy was associated in one patient with rigidity during two operations, but without true hyperthermia (Lambert & Young 1976). The relationship of myotonic conditions to MH is thus dubious, and those patients who have

been alleged to suffer from both and whose muscle has been tested in vitro have not been found to be MH susceptible.

Another myopathy reported to be associated with MH is central-core disease (Denborough et al 1973). Their patient's muscle showed cores in over 50% of type 1 fibres, and the in vitro test showed susceptibility to MH. However, cores were begin-ning to be recognized as one of the characteristic, if not specific, features of MH myopathy. We thought that Denborough's patient was more likely to be suffering from MH myopathy than from central-core disease, the latter being a congenital myopathy showing in most, probably all, cases a marked preponderance of type 1 fibres. In our experience this is never present in MH myopathy and was absent in Denborough's patient. It even-tually turned out that central-core disease was the only condition in our series with a highly signi-ficant association with MH: of nine patients with that diagnosis eight were found to be MH-susceptible on testing. It follows that all patients with central-core disease and their families should be warned of the possibility of MH susceptibility and be offered investigation. If surgery is pending the anaesthetist must be informed in advance of the family disease.

The distinction between MH myopathy and central core disease is of more than academic interest. The prognosis is less favourable in central core disease, and inheritance, although usually autosomal dominant, as in MH, may be recessive. Furthermore, sporadic cases have been described (Banker 1986). Most patients with central-core disease show mild proximal weakness, and in a 15-year follow-up we have noted deterioration in a mother.

In some published cases the association of central-core disease with MH appears to have been accepted on insufficient grounds (Isaacs and Bařlow 1974). Two members of a family known to be susceptible to MH were described, one with musculoskeletal abnormalities not uncommon in MH, who survived two episodes of MH during two successive operations. A biopsy showed a moderate number of cores and moth-eaten fibres, similar to those seen in MH myopathy, and without evidence of type 1 fibre preponderance. On the other hand the diagnosis was substantiated in the patient described by Eng et al (1978). This was a 20-month-old baby girl with congenital dislocation of the hips, not uncommon in congenital myopathies. During surgery for this disability the patient suffered an episode of MH which was successfully aborted. A biopsy showed preponderance of type 1 fibres with many cores, and a similar picture was found in the father's muscle, suggesting autosomal dominant inheritance.

In order to distinguish the cores of MH myopathy from those of central-core disease it is necessary to cut longitudinal frozen sections, or to dissect out small bundles of muscle fibres as long as possible, and to stain by a silver method. In MH myopathy the cores are short with NADH staining and do not stain with silver, whereas in central-core disease the cores stain by both methods and nearly always extend the full length of the fibres (Harriman 1990).

In addition to skeletal malformations, various musculoskeletal disorders in which there may be an element of muscle abnormality, have been associated with MH susceptibility on rare occasions. These include strabismus, ptosis, kyphoscoliosis, arthrogryposis, foot deformity and dislocation of the patella and shoulder. A complex of physical abnormalities associated with MH was reported by King & Denborough (1973) in four unrelated boys. They showed cryptorchidism, pectus carinatum, kyphosis, lordosis, webbing of the neck, weakness of serratus muscles, antemongoloid obliquity of the palpebral fissures, crowded lower teeth and sometimes ptosis. These striking signs have since been reported in two further patients (Lenard & Kettler 1975) and more recently by Bergson et al (1978). Bergson's patient was of particular interest in that a muscle biopsy showed variation in fibre size and a total absence of differentiation of muscle fibres. Lack of muscle fibre differentiation has not so far been found in muscle shown by the test in vitro to be susceptible to MH, and may merely indicate an association of two uncommon conditions.

An association between MH and myotonic disorders has not, therefore, been proved, and that between MH and central-core disease is rare. A convincing association will exist between the King and Denborough syndrome and MH, if further biopsies show lack of fibre type differentiation in

the former and a positive in vitro test. The undoubted increased frequency of strabismus and other musculoskeletal disorders in MH patients is of interest but its significance has not yet been revealed. For the most part, MH patients appear to be suffering from a unique and distinctive genetic disorder.

Muscle pathology

Well over 1400 patients have been examined by motor-point biopsy in the Malignant Hyperpyrexia Unit in Leeds, and their susceptibility to MH has been assessed by the Ellis tests in vitro of the muscle reaction to suxamethonium, caffeine, halothane and other agents (Ellis et al 1986).

General anaesthesia is used for the biopsy, modified to reduce the risk of MH as much as possible. The analgesic fentanyl is given first, followed by induction with thiopentone. Anaesthesia is maintained using 50% nitrous oxide in oxygen, with thiopentone and fentanyl administered as required. Full monitoring of core body temperature and cardiac function is maintained throughout the procedure, and all appropriate measures are available for the treatment of MH, should it develop. The advantage of using general anaesthesia rather than local is that it is reassuring to the patient to know that, if he should require surgery, general anaesthesia would be possible. In any case, local anaesthesia is not without risk and the muscle specimen would be rendered inactive for the tests in vitro if it were contaminated even minimally by the local anaesthetic.

The first specimens taken are thin strips 1 mm in diameter for the tests in vitro: these strips should include the innervation zone which lies close to the motor point determined on the exposed muscle. Thereafter, strips of muscle are taken for electron microscopy of motor end-plates and muscle (Harriman 1979), and larger strips for histochemistry and paraffin embedding.

Control muscle, that is from patients whose muscle showed no reaction in the tissue bath to anaesthetic agents, will be described first, as any changes they contain must be 'subtracted' from the findings in patients whose muscle is susceptible to MH. An unexpectedly large number of histopathological changes were encountered in the control muscle, all from healthy people. The findings to be described were in biopsies obtained only from the vastus medialis: some early biopsies were taken from various sites in the search for the most reactive muscle for the in-vitro tests. The results from the first 200 patients investigated were reported in Harriman (1979); they differ in detail only from a further sample of 200 patients described below. Tables 15.1 and 15.2 summarize the main features in MH-insusceptible (control) and MH-susceptible patients.

Table I. Investigation of susceptibility to MH: histopathology (200 patients)

	Insusceptible	Susceptible
Patients	120	80
Normal muscle	59	45
Abnormal muscle	61	35 MH myopathy
fibre splitting	15	internal nuclei
necrosis/regeneration	10	cores
type 2B atrophy	1	moth-eaten fibres

Table II. Investigation of susceptibility to MH: muscle disorders (1000 patients)

Insusceptible		MH-associated	
Central-core disease	1	Central-core disease	8
Limb–girdle dystrophy	2	Ocular myopathy	1
Neurogenic atrophy	2	Congenital myopathy (unclassified)	2

Control patients

The reason for biopsy was either that the patient was a member of a known MH-susceptible family (85), or that he had suffered an MH-like episode under anaesthesia (14), or that a member of the patient's family had suffered an MH-like episode under anaesthesia (21). The biopsies of 59 patients not susceptible to MH were normal by light and electron microscopy. These patients were aged 5–57 years, with a mean age of 22 years. There were, however, abnormalities in the biopsies of 61 insusceptible patients, aged 6–75 years, mean 36 years. One or more of the abnormalities was present in each biopsy. Among these were excess internal nuclei (in eight biopsies), subsarcolemmal rows of nuclei (in one) and nuclear clumps devoid of myoplasm (in three). The internal nuclei had

different characteristics from those in susceptible muscle; they were not diffusely distributed throughout the section, but were focal. Multiple internal nuclei could be found near the insertion of muscle or fascia, or where a fascicle bordered epimysium (Fig. 15.1) but these were not considered to be abnormal. The commonest change (in 15 patients) was a limited degree of fibre splitting (Fig. 15.2A, B). Small round fibres of either main fibre type were even commoner, but were thought to be the tapering ends of normal fibres. One, or sometimes two, flattened fibres were seen in 12 biopsies, similar to those occurring with greater frequency in some neuropathies and myopathies (Fig. 15.3). They may have arisen as a result of oblique section of an atrophied fibre, even though other fibres in the section were cut in an accurate transverse plane, but their pathogenesis remains uncertain. One or two lightly basophilic small angulated fibres, were seen in seven biopsies (Fig. 15.3); while they sometimes accompanied splitting fibres and may have been derived from them, splitting was not always seen in the same biopsy. They are regarded by some as cast-iron evidence of neurogenic disease but in methylene blue preparations there was no other sign of this nor, in particular, of the most sensitive indicator of denervation, which is collateral reinnervation. In this, subterminal nerve fibres branch repeatedly to reinnervate previously denervated muscle fibres.

Segmental regeneration and sometimes necrosis was seen in 10 patients; up to four affected fibres were found in each biopsy. This was a surprisingly large number and raised speculation that wear and tear in this active tissue might be responsible. Lymphorrhages or perivascular collections of lymphocytes were uncommon, occuring in only four patients. A single vacuolated fibre (Fig. 15.4) occurred in each of three biopsies, and a cytoplasmic body in one biopsy. There was one thick epimysial seam separating otherwise normal muscle fascicles, and this was regarded as an anatomical variation.

There was unexpected variability in the proportion of type 1 and type 2 fibres. Although counts were not made on all biopsies, the proportion of type 1 fibres in those analysed varied from 25% to 70%. It is well known that the ratio

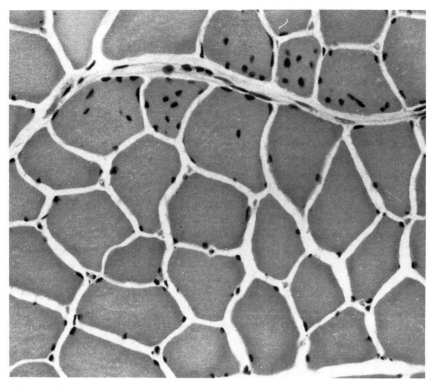

Fig. 15.1   MH 242 Control. Randomly distributed fibres with internal nuclei, often close to tendon insertions, are not abnormal. Cryostat section (CS): H&E ×330

of the two principal fibre types changes from the surface to the limb core, but it was felt that this alone could not account for the figures cited, which probably reflected normal variation. Other changes involving fibre types were type 2B atrophy (Fig. 15.5), unexplained in one biopsy, and type 2 fibre preponderance in two biopsies.

Motheaten fibres and cores (Fig. 15.6) (defined below under *MH myopathy*) were sought in control muscle, but were not found, apart from single examples of each. Early spotted (lobulated) fibres were present in one biopsy, but this finding was later questioned and changed to 'pseudospotted' when it was realized that similar fibres showing mitochondrial proliferation in crescents and clumps could occur during normal human muscle growth in the decade embracing puberty. The pseudospotted fibres shown in figure 15.7A were from a 15-year-old female. The affected type 1 fibres were slightly smaller than average and, curiously, were

reminiscent of the type 1A fibres in the classification proposed by Askanas & Engel (1975). They may be compared with spotted fibres seen in facioscapulohumeral dystrophy in Figure 15.7B.

Three biopsies showed changes at the motor end-plates in the form of distal sprouting (Fig. 15.9). Branches and sprouts developed from axonic expansions at the end-plate, but were not specifically neurogenic. The three biopsies with distal sprouting contained some abnormal fibres, comprising flattened fibres, angular fibres and regenerating fibres respectively.

Quite apart from the sparse abnormalities in the control population described above, four patients were found to be suffering from neurogenic or muscle disease. A woman aged 35 years and an 18-year-old youth showed great variation in fibre calibre and internal nuclei; both patients were asymptomatic but were thought on clinical grounds to be suffering from mild limb-girdle dystrophy

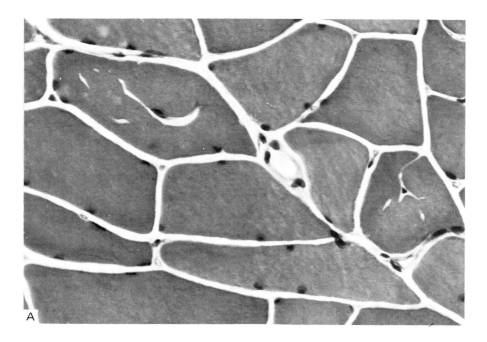

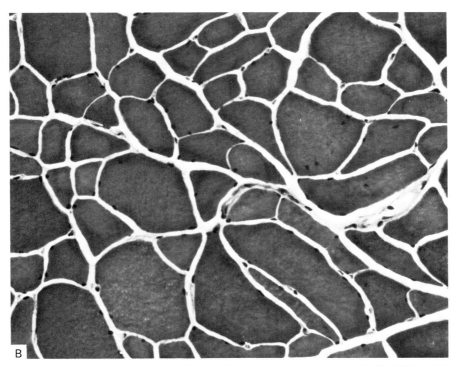

Fig. 15.2 (A) MH 299, control. Splits are appearing within two fibres, related to internal nuclei. CS: H&E, ×450. (B) MH 284, susceptible. At least three fibres show splitting: there is a narrow space between the split-off and the parent fibre, and one often indents the other. CS: H&E, ×270

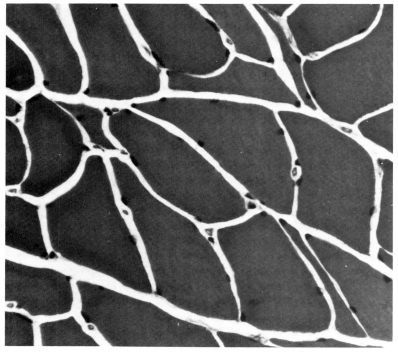

Fig. 15.3   MH 223, susceptible. There are two flattened fibres and one small angulated fibre in the section. CS: H&E, ×450

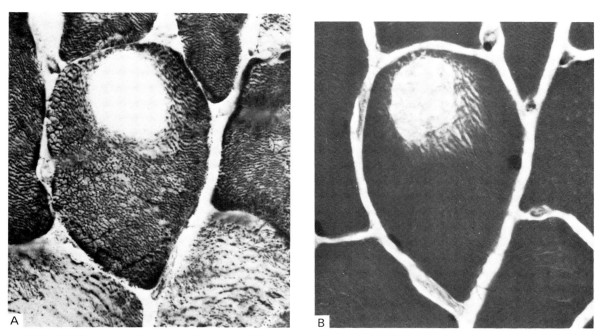

Fig. 15.4   MH 221, control. Large vacuole in a type 1 fibre, apparently empty with NADH (A), but containing pale sinuous structures on staining with H&E (B). CS, ×680

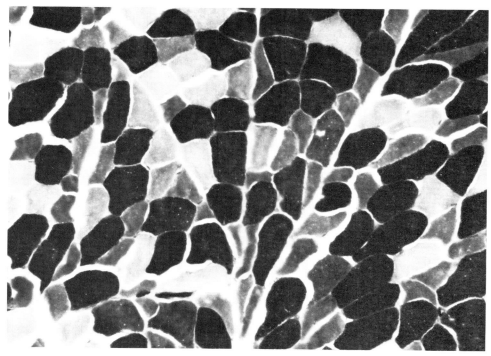

Fig. 15.5   MH 302, control. Black fibres type 1; pale fibres type 2A; intermediately stained fibres type 2B. Most 2B fibres are small or atrophied. CS: ATPase at pH 4.63, ×270

(Fig. 15.10). Both of the patients who were suffering from neurogenic disease (men aged 57 and 58 years) showed collateral re-innervation, but the cause of their neurogenic disease was not discovered (Fig. 15.11). A fifth patient, a 19-year-old youth, had developed exercise-induced myoglobinuria 3 months earlier, but showed no abnormality in the muscle biopsy.

The large variety of structural abnormalities in the muscle of patients found to be MH-insusceptible was unexpected and led to caution in the interpretation of pathological changes in the muscle of MH-susceptible patients. The two control patients with asymptomatic limb–girdle dystrophy showed that this disease does not predispose to MH, but confirms the opinion of some anaesthetists that myopathic patients are not always as tolerant of anaesthesia as is the general population.

MH-susceptible patients

The MH-susceptible (MHS) group consisted of 80 patients, of whom 35 showed myopathic changes at biopsy. Their age range was 14–77 years, mean 38 years, whereas the susceptible but non-myopathic patients were younger (9–72 years, mean 25 years).

The reasons for biopsy were similar to those in the control group: being a member of an MHS family (49), having suffered an MH-like episode under anaesthesia (15), or having a relative who had suffered such an episode (16). Many of the mild changes seen in the control group were again encountered in the MHS group and were excluded from the definition of MH myopathy.

MH MYOPATHY

Tables 15.1 and 15.2 summarize the findings in MH myopathy. Only abnormalities not found in the controls but present in the 35 biopsies from MH-susceptible individuals were ascribed to it. The affected patients were asymptomatic. The most frequent abnormality, present in 18 biopsies, was an increase in the number of internal nuclei.

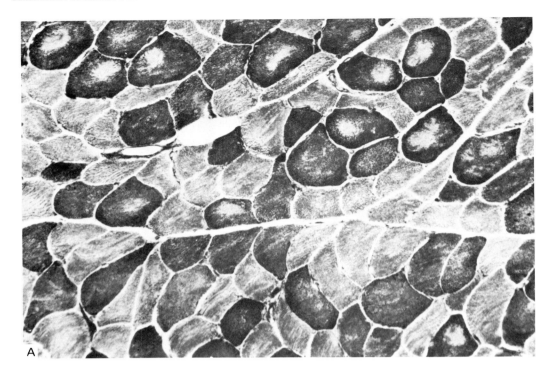

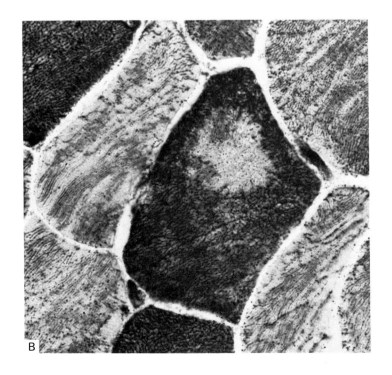

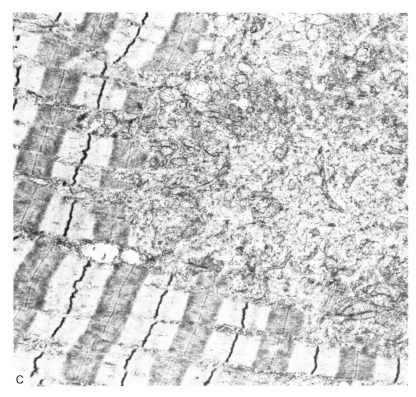

Fig. 15.6 (A) MH 336, susceptible. Cores in many type 1 fibres. CS: NADH, ×180. (B) Detail of core. CS: NADH, ×545. (C) Part of a core. No myofibrils survive in it; there are very few mitochondria but portions of many tubules. EM, ×6400

These were found in from 3 to 25% of muscle fibres which were diffusely distributed in the tissue (Fig. 15.12). In transverse section only one or two internal nuclei were present in each affected fibre, compared with the large number usually found in some other myopathies such as myotonic dystrophy. In longitudinal section they formed short rows.

Moth-eaten fibres (Fig. 15.8A) and cores (Fig. 15.6A, B, C) were also found in significant numbers in MH myopathy. They are not pathognomonic for that condition, as they may be present in small numbers in some other myopathies, and are produced in profusion by experimental tenotomy (Shafiq et al 1969). The fact remains that the myopathy of MH is one of the two important disorders in which they regularly occur. The other is central-core disease which, as already mentioned, is often MH-susceptible when appropriately tested. The differences between these

myopathies may depend on their nature, the one, congenital, causing type 1 fibre preponderance and forming cores of considerable length, the other producing short or medium-length cores well after birth, unaccompanied by fibre type preponderance.

Cores in MH myopathy are, like those in central-core disease, both structured and unstructured (page 241), but are not always sharp-edged. The structured core is recognized in oxidative enzyme stains only, but the fusing Z-line streaming and degeneration of the unstructured core absorb some stains rendering them visible in both frozen and paraffin sections. Both types of core may be bordered by a thin rim of formazan with NADH staining. In the past, cores in MH myopathy were described as core-targetoids when it was difficult to distinguish cores from two-zone targets. In longitudinal section, targets are shaped like short plump spindles; their axial column of

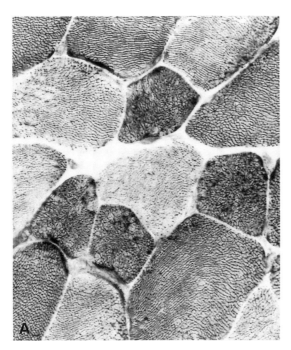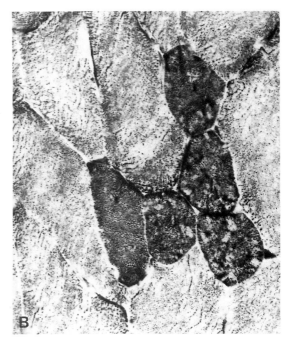

Fig. 15.7 (A) MH 238 Pseudospotted fibres. Type 1 fibres of reduced size contain crescents and small clusters of mitochondria. They suggest early spotted fibre formation but have to be distinguished from fibres of similar appearance which may develop during the final peripubertal stage of human muscle growth. CS NADH ×385 (B) Typical spotted fibres, for comparison. CS NADH ×385

degenerate myofibrils is enclosed by faintly stained dispersed granular material, which forms the middle layer of the target and extends to the poles of the spindle. The axial column does not reach either pole, so that a transverse section of the central region of the structure will produce a conventional three-zone target, but another transverse section nearer one pole will show only two zones. In the absence of longitudinal sections two-zone targets can be distinguished clearly from cores only by electron microscopy. Re-examination of targetoids in MH myopathy has revealed that they are cores, not two-zone targets.

Moth-eaten fibres are also difficult to characterize. They are simple, irregular foci devoid or almost totally devoid of mitochondria, sometimes accompanied by minimal Z-line streaming. By light microscopy they are found only in oxidative enzyme stains, and appear as diffusely outlined, coalescent pale areas. Unfortunately, staining artefact can reproduce this image almost perfectly, and only sharp, high-contrast staining is reliable for diagnosis. The frequent association of moth-

eaten fibres and cores in MH myopathy helps diagnosis. It may be that moth-eaten areas precede core formation, but transitional forms have yet to be identified.

A few single abnormalities were found in the MHS group, but as isolated phenomena were not considered important. Only one lymphorrhage was present (compared with four in the control group), one biopsy showed epimysial thickening between fascicles and there was one fibre with a mulberry inclusion (Fig. 15.13A). Although of no significance in MH myopathy, it was decided to illustrate the inclusion in the first edition of this volume in the hope that a reader would throw light on its nature. Help arrived six years later from Oxford when Dr M. V. (Waney) Squier remembered two relevant muscle biopsies: C177, a female aged 57, in which there was a single mulberry fibre (Fig. 15.13B), and C338, a male aged 64, in which a number of mulberry-like fragments occurred as the only pathological change in a myopathy (Fig. 15.13C).

In electron micrographs the components of the

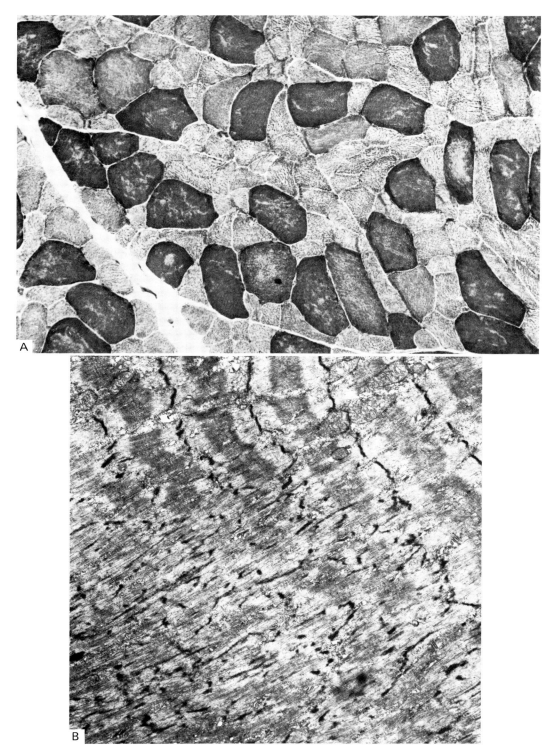

Fig. 15.8 (A) MH 284, susceptible. Moth-eaten fibres, shown as irregular patches of rarefaction in some type 1 fibres. There is also one core fibre. CS: NADH, ×180. (B) core. The lesion consists of Z-band streaming and break-up. EM, ×8000

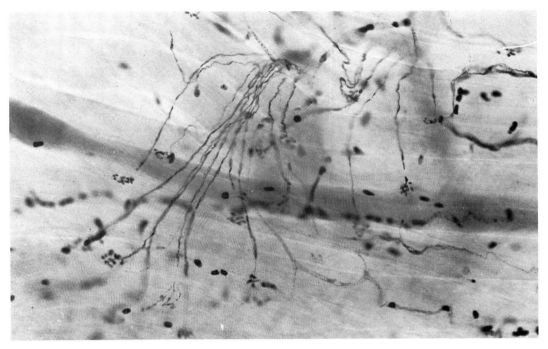

Fig. 15.9   MH 207, susceptible. In this otherwise normal arborization of subterminal nerve fibres and terminals, one motor end-plate (lower left) shows sprouting. Squash: methylene blue, ×270

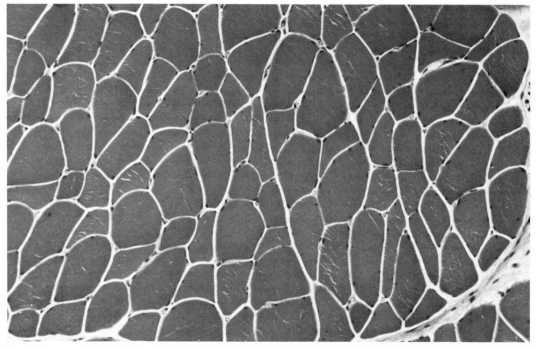

Fig. 15.10   Asymptomatic limb–girdle dystrophy. There is considerable variation in fibre size, found in a histochemical series to be affecting fibre types indiscriminately. CS: H&E, ×180

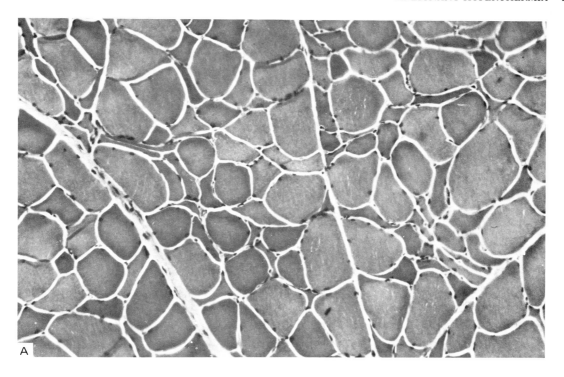

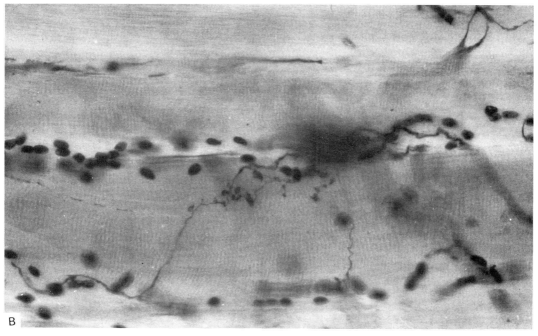

Fig. 15.11   (A) MH 256, control. Neurogenic disease shown by grouping of atrophied fibres. Some of the fibres are flattened or angulated. CS: H&E, ×180. (B) Collateral reinnervation. A single subterminal fibre branches in several places to provide sprouts or new endplates. Methylene blue squash, ×450

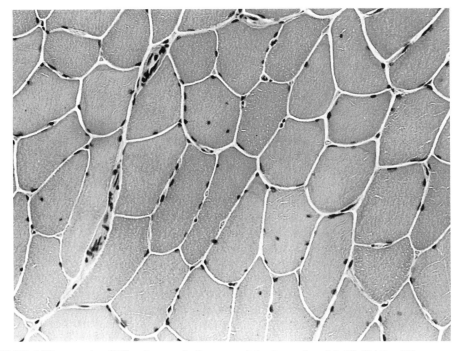

Fig. 15.12   MH 297, MH myopathy. Diffuse increase in fibres containing internal nuclei. CS. H&E ×220

mulberry fragments possessed a core and a halo (Fig. 15.13D). The core was not dense like that of a cytoplasmic body but rather faintly stained and granulofilamentous: the halo consisted of filaments radiating from small dense rod bodies. The mulberry fragments were similar by optical microscopy to some of the clusters of spheroid bodies described by Goebel et al (1978) (Fig. 15.13E), but on electron microscopy the spheroids characteristically were balls of whorling filaments (Fig. 15.13F). Organelles are found around but not within them. As 'mulberry' is no longer appropriate as a descriptive term the inclusions will be renamed *Waney bodies*.

The aetiology of MH and MH myopathy

It is commonly supposed that MH depends upon a persistent rise in sarcoplasmic calcium, although its precise mechanism is not known (Denborough 1979). A great deal of research has been performed using the stress-susceptible pig as an experimental model, but little useful knowledge has emerged by examining this animal's musculature for signs of a structural myopathy. It may be that only young pigs have been used, whereas it is known in humans that myopathy in the MHS subject does not occur earlier than 5 years of age, and is uncommon until the third decade. It is more likely

Fig. 15.13   (A) MH 334. Single 'mulberry' cytoplasmic inclusion in the form of a rounded mass of small pale spherical components. CS H&E ×680
   (B) single mulberry fibre, female aged 57 CS NADH ×680
   (C) Waney body (mulberry fragment): peripheral cytoplasmic inclusion in type 2 fibre. CS NADH ×680
   (D) Waney body: granulofilamentous centre, halo of filaments emanating from rod bodies. Electron micrograph ×17 000
   (E) Peripheral clusters of spheroid bodies, one partly detached. CS NADH ×445
   (F) Spheroid body: filamentous and microtubular material in a whorling pattern. Electron micrograph 17 000 (Figs. 15.13B 15.13C and 15.13D provided by the kindness of Dr M V Squier; Fig. 15.13E and 15.13F provided by the kindness of Professor H. Goebel).

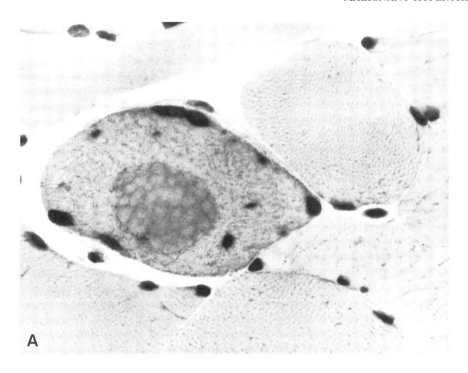

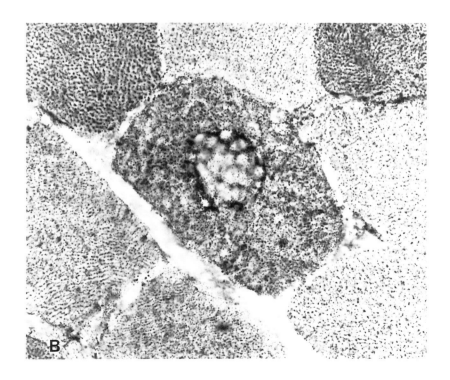

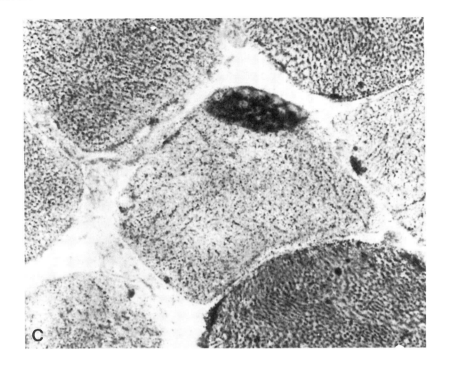

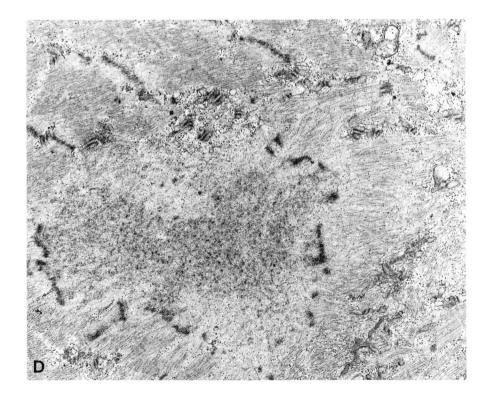

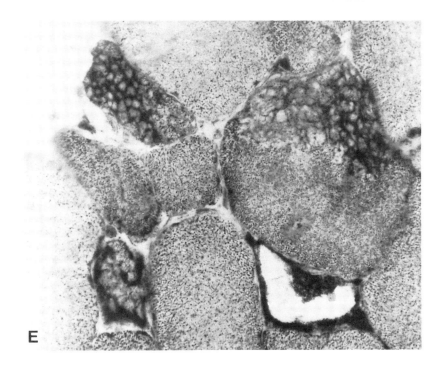

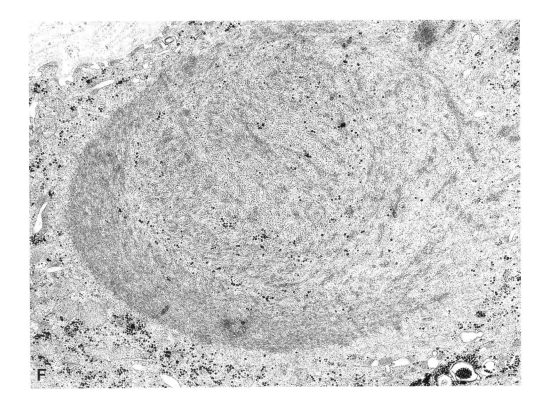

that the primary defect lies in the membrane of the muscle cell, probably in the T-tubule, that it is biochemical, and that it may, but need not, lead eventually to secondary structural changes in muscle fibres. These, in the form of mitochondrial loss, Z band streaming and myofibrillary degeneration, the ingredients of cores and motheaten fibres, could be the result of abnormal, subliminal myofibrillary contraction for which an experimental model is awaited.

On the clinical side, a very large number of cases have been reported, including a remarkable family described by Wingard (1977) recording 630 members over seven generations. There was evidence of MH, unexplained sudden deaths and of numerous episodes of physical and mental stress suggesting that triggers other than anaesthetic agents could exist. Experimental (porcine) research work on muscle dealt with the effects of the MH gene, but recently work has begun on the MH gene itself, thanks to advances in molecular genetics over the last two decades. The investigations are being carried out in collaboration with the Departments of Genetics in the Universities of Leeds, Exeter and Oxford. The MH gene is closely linked to that for central core disease and has been localized on chromosome 19 at 19q12–q13.2 (see Dubowitz 1991).

The neuroleptic malignant syndrome (NMS)

This drug-related disorder was first described by Delay & Deniker (1968) in *Handbook of Clinical Neurology* (vol 6). The syndrome was a life-threatening condition occurring in patients receiving therapeutic doses of chlorpromazine, haloperidol or flupenthixol; it had also been reported during treatment with other drugs which were known to interact with dopaminergic systems (Committee on Safety of Medicines 1986) and had occurred after withdrawal of carbidopa-levodopa therapy (Friedman et al 1985). The main features of the syndrome were hyperthermia, autonomic dysfunction, muscular rigidity, sometimes dystonia and involuntary movements. Most authors accepted that the drugs acted centrally, but interest in the similar condition of MH led others to believe that NMS might also be initiated in

muscle. This was supported by the discovery that dantrolene, the therapeutic agent used in MH, was also of value in the treatment of NMS. The key research showing that NMS differed aetiologically from MH was performed by Adnet et al (1989). They applied the in vitro tests for the detection of MH susceptibility to the muscle of eight NMS, ten MHS and ten control patients. Following the criteria established by the European MH Group the results were clear cut: all eight NMS subjects were insusceptible to MH.

Three papers have been published on the pathology found at autopsy in NMS patients. Martin and Swash (1987) obtained muscle within one hour of death, and found loss of glycogen and of neutral lipid from muscle fibres. This suggested to them that phosphorylation had been uncoupled and could have been responsible for excessive heat production; the primary biochemical abnormality might therefore be muscular rather than hypothalamic. An alternative explanation for the loss of glycogen and lipid is that both fuel muscle contraction and are depleted by excessive muscular activity. In the rat, the glycogen depletion method for establishing type 2 muscle fibre patterns in motor units depends upon this phenomenon.

The second paper on NMS histopathology at autopsy (Jones & Dawson 1989) described gross abnormality in muscle and minor changes only in the brain, in a female aged 70 years. Drugs used included isocarboxazid (a monoamine oxidase inhibitor) and chlorpromazine. NMS developed and was followed by rhabdomyolysis, renal failure and death in a few days. The muscle abnormalities included widespread necrosis and regeneration and a vacuolar myopathy, both findings typical of adverse reactions to a range of drugs. The idea that a gross myopathy could be associated with the prime muscle defect responsible for NMS is not in accord with experience in MH, in which the muscle of the majority of MH-susceptible patients is structurally normal.

The third autopsy (Lee et al 1989) reported for the first time brain damage in the NMS, with survival for 4 months. The patient was 32 years old and had sustained loss of much of the Purkinje cell layer of the cerebellum with resultant gliosis. As this reaction is known to occur in heat stroke, it was attributed to the hyperthermic element of the syndrome. Muscle was examined but appeared normal apart from a few atrophied fibres.

The value of muscle biopsy in MH

It cannot be emphasized too often that a muscle biopsy without in vitro tests for susceptibility to MH is virtually useless for the diagnosis of MH. More MHS patients present with normal morphology than with myopathy. An autopsy is the only occasion when the muscle histology alone could be useful in providing a pointer to the diagnosis by discovering internal nuclei, cores and moth-eaten fibres, now considered to be reasonably characteristic of MH myopathy. Unfortunately, patients who die after a severe MH episode usually develop extensive rhabdomyolysis, capable of obliterating pre-existing pathology.

When a biopsy is taken and the tests are performed it is regrettable if muscle histopathology is not also undertaken. When MH myopathy makes its rare appearance it will have developed in the absence of the anaesthetic trigger; are there other minor triggers which could be responsible for subliminal muscle activity, capable eventually of causing myofibrillar contracture and Z-line streaming? Whether or not speculation promoted by histopathology is useful, the association of MH and other hereditary disorders needs to be investigated and will take much time. Finally, large numbers of muscle biopsies of 'normal' subjects from childhood to old age will provide valuable data not so far available to the neurological sciences.

REFERENCES

Adnet P J Krivosic-Horber R M, Adamantidis M M, Haudecoeur G, Adnet-Bonte C A, Saulnier T, Dupuis B A 1989 The association between the neuroleptic malignant syndrome and malignant hyperthermia. Acta Anaesthesiologica Scandinavica 33: 680

Askanas V, Engel W K 1975 Distinct subtypes of type 1 fibers of human skeletal muscle. Neurology (Minneap) 25: 879

Banker B Q 1986 The congenital myopathies. In: Engel A G, Banker B Q (eds) Myology basic and clinical, vol 2. McGraw Hill, New York, p 1529

Bergson P S, Kaplan A M, Gregg S A, Curless R G 1978 Malignant hyperthermia associated with characteristic findings, myopathy and normal muscle enzymes: a syndrome. In Aldrete J A Britt B A (eds) Second International Symposium on Malignant Hyperthermia Grune and Stratton, New York, p 473

Cody J R 1968 Muscle rigidity following administration of succinyl choline. Anesthesiology 29: 159

Committee on Safety of Medicines 1986 18. Neuroleptic malignant syndrome — an underdiagnosed condition? Pamphlet issued by the Committee on Safety of Medicines, Market Towers, 1, Nine Elms Lane, London SW8 5NQ

Delay J, Deniker P 1968 Drug induced extrapyramidal syndrome. In: Vinken P J, Bruyn G W (eds) Handbook of clinical neurology, vol 6, Disease of the basal ganglia. Elsevier/North Holland, New York, p 248

Denborough M A 1979 Etiology and pathophysiology of malignant hyperthermia. International Anesthesiology Clinics 17 4: 11

Denborough M A, Lovell R R H 1960 Anaesthetic deaths in a family. Lancet ii: 45

Denborough M A, Dennett X, Anderson R MacD 1973 Central core disease and malignant hyperpyrexia. British Medical Journal 1: 272

Dubowitz, V 1991 Neuromuscular disorders; gene location. Neuromuscular Disorders 1: 75

Ellis F R, Clarke I M C, Modgill M et al 1975 Evaluation of creatine phophokinase in screening patients for malignant hyperpyrexia. British Medical Journal 2: 511

Ellis F R, Halsall P J, Harriman D G F 1986 The work of the Leeds malignant hyperpyrexia unit 1971–1984. Anaesthesia 41: 809

Eng G D, Epstein B S, Engel W K McKay R 1978 Malignant hyperthermia and central core disease in a child with congenital dislocating hips. Archives of Neurology (Chicago) 35: 189

Friedman J H, Feinberg S S, Feldman R G 1985 A neuroleptic malignantlike syndrome due to levodopa therapy withdrawal. Journal of the American Medical Association 254: 2792

Goebel H H, Muller J, Gillen H W, Merritt A D 1978 Autosomal dominant 'spheroid body myopathy'. Muscle and Nerve 1: 14

Gullotta F, Helpap B 1975 Histologische histochemische und electronmikroskopische Befunde bei maligner Hyperthermie. Virchows Archiv A Pathological Anatomy and Histology 367: 181

Gullotta F Spiesz-Kiefer C 1983 Muskelbioptische Untersuchungen bei maligner Hyperthermie. Anasthesie Intensivtherapie Notfallmedizin 18: 21

Harriman D G F 1979 Preanesthetic investigation of malignant hyperthermia: microscopy In: Britt B A (ed) International Anesthesiology Clinics 17 4: 97

Harriman D G F 1988 Malignant hyperthermia myopathy — a critical review. British Journal of Anaesthesia 60: 309

Harriman D G F 1990 Muscle In: Weller R O (ed) Systemic pathology, 3rd edn vol 4, Nervous system, muscle and eyes. Churchill Livingstone, Edinburgh, p 580

Harriman D G F, Sumner D W, Ellis F R 1973 Malignant hyperpyrexia myopathy. Quarterly Journal of Medicine New Series 42: 639

Heffron J J A, Isaacs H 1976 Malignant hyperthermia syndrome: evidence for denervation change in human skeletal muscle. Klinische Wochenschrift 54: 865

Isaacs H, Barlow M B 1970a Malignant hyperpyrexia during anaesthesia; possible association with subclinical myopathy. British Medical Journal 1: 275

Isaacs H, Barlow M B 1970b The genetic background to malignant hyperprexia revealed by serum creatine phosphokinase estimations in asymptomatic relatives. British Journal of Anaesthesia 42: 1077

Isaacs H, Barlow M B 1974 Central core disease associated with elevated creatine phosphokinase levels: two members of a family known to be susceptible to malignant hyperprexia. South African Medical Journal 48: 640

Jones E M, Dawson A 1989 Neuroleptic malignant syndrome: a case report with postmortem brain and muscle pathology. Journal of Neurology Neurosurgery and Psychiatry 52: 1006

King J O, Denborough M A 1973 Anesthetic-induced malignant hyperpyrexia in children. Journal of Pediatrics 83: 37

King J O, Denborough M A, Zapf P W 1972 Inheritance of malignant hyperpyrexia. Lancet i: 365

Lambert C D, Young J R B 1976 Hypertrophy of the branchial muscles. A case with unusual features. Journal of Neurology, Neurosurgery and Psychiatry 39: 810

Lee S, Merriam A, Kim T-S, Liebling M, Dickson D W, Moore G R W 1989 Cerebellar degeneration in neuroleptic malignant syndrome: new pathologic findings and review of the literature concerning heat-related nervous system injury. Journal of Neurology Neurosurgery and Psychiatry 52: 387

Lenard H G, Kettler D 1975 Malignant hyperpyrexia and myopathy. Neuropaediatrie 6: 7

Lexell J, Downham D, Sjostrom M 1983 Distribution of different fibre types in human skeletal muscle. Journal of the Neurological Sciences 61: 301

Martin D T, Swash M 1987 Muscle pathology in the neuroleptic malignant syndrome. Journal of Neurology 253: 2

Moulds R F W, Denborough M A 1974 Myopathies and malignant hyperpyrexia. British Medical Journal 3: 520

Reske-Nielsen E 1978 Malignant hyperthermia in Denmark: survey of a family study and investigations into muscular morphology in ten additional cases. In: Aldrete J A Britt B A (eds) Second international symposium on malignant hyperthermia. Grune and Stratton, New York, p 287

Reske-Nielsen E, Haase J, Kelstrup J 1975 Malignant hyperthermia in a family. The neurophysiological and light microscopical study of muscle biopsies of healthy members. Acta Pathologica et Microbiologica Scandinavica, Section A 83: 645

Saidman L J, Havard E S, Egar E I 1964 Hyperthermia during anaesthesia. Journal of the American Medical Association 190: 73

Shafiq S A, Gorycki M S, Asiedu S A, Milhorat A T 1969 Tenotomy. Effect on the fine structure of the soleus of the rat. Archives of Neurology 20: 625

Steers A J W, Tallack J A, Thompson D E A 1970 Fulminating hyperpyrexia during anaesthesia in a member of a myopathic family. British Medical Journal 2: 341

Wingard D W 1977 Malignant hyperthermia — acute stress syndrome of man? In: Henshel E O (ed) Malignant hyperthermia: current concepts. Appleton Century Crofts, New York, p 79

16. Neurogenic disorders of muscle

F. G. I. Jennekens

INTRODUCTION

Experimental investigations have greatly contributed to our knowledge of the disorders to be discussed in this chapter. Three decades ago, grouped fibre atrophy was considered to be the hallmark of neurogenic muscular atrophy. We now know from studies of the organization of the motor unit and from cross-innervation experiments that disseminated fibre atrophy is highly compatible with a neurogenic muscle disorder and that grouped fibre atrophy represents a characteristic phase in the course of the denervation process. Although much remains to be clarified, the findings from experimental studies currently allow a step-by-step analysis of the successive events in denervation atrophy, and this greatly furthers the correct interpretation of histological and histochemical changes in muscle biopsies taken from patients with lower motor neurone diseases or peripheral neuropathies.

The first part of this chapter presents an outline of the consequences of denervation and re-innervation as established by experimental studies. It provides explanations for most of the phenomena described in the second part which deals with diagnostic criteria. The third part is devoted to the changes in muscle biopsies taken from patients with rapidly or gradually progressive and chronic or longstanding neurogenic muscular atrophy. The histological features of a few exceptional forms of neurogenic muscular atrophy are described separately.

EXPERIMENTAL INVESTIGATIONS

Decrease in fibre size as a result of denervation follows a well-defined course. Muscle fibres in the Australian opossum atrophy rapidly in the initial weeks, so that after 60 days the cross-sectional area of the fibres is reduced by 70%. Thereafter, the process slows down and maximal atrophy is reached after approximately 120 days. From this time onwards the cross-sectional area remains at about 10–20% of its initial size and no constant relationship between the degree of atrophy and the duration of denervation can be established (Sunderland & Ray 1950). The course of the atrophying process closely resembles that in other species, although there are apparently some variations. The mean fibre area in the soleus and gastrocnemius muscles of female Sprague–Dawley rats has been reported to be reduced to 20% from the control level 3 weeks after denervation, and a further slow decrease continues over the next 60 days (Stonnington & Engel 1973). Atrophy becomes evident in humans within a few weeks, and in cats after a month (Adams 1975).

Muscle fibre atrophy is accompanied by a decrease in the number of capillaries per muscle fibre (Carpenter & Karpati 1982) and by proliferation of connective tissue in the endomysium and perimysium. The increase is mainly of type I and III collagen and fibronectin in the perimysium and of type III collagen and fibronectin in the endomysium (Salonen et al 1985). Type I collagen is relatively stiff and arranged in bundles; type III collagen tends to form networks and is more apt than type I collagen to adapt to changes in the muscle fibres. Fibronectin may play a role in the adhesion of the newly formed collagen to the muscle fibres (Hynes & Yamada 1982, Salonen et al 1985).

Most authors agree that type 2 fibres tend to

atrophy earlier and more rapidly than type I fibres (Bajusz 1964, Karpati & Engel 1968a, Riley & Allin 1973, Niederle & Mayr 1978). However, the denervation behaviour of the type 1 fibres is not the same in different skeletal muscles. The rat soleus muscle, which consists of 95% red (type 1) fibres, shows a more pronounced degree of atrophy of type 1 fibres than the plantaris muscle (Jaweed et al 1975) and, in the early stages of denervation, changes in the red soleus fibres may be even greater than those in the white (type 2) fibres of the extensor digitorum longus muscle (Pluskal & Pennington 1976, Cullen & Pluskal 1977). The reaction of the different fibre types to denervation seems to depend partly upon the static or phasic character of the muscle concerned (Jaweed et al 1975).

The process of fibre atrophy following denervation can be reversed almost completely by stretching the muscle. Stretch is known to stimulate protein synthesis in innervated and denervated muscle fibres (Goldspink 1977, 1978) and to cause longitudinal growth by the addition of new sarcomeres (Williams & Goldspink 1978). It has been suggested that skeletal growth may cause muscle fibres to stretch and may thus promote their growth (Stewart et al 1972). In adult muscle, apart from longitudinal growth, stretch also induces transient or prolonged hypertrophy of innervated and denervated fibres (Sola et al 1973a,b, Booth 1977, Sarnat et al 1977). As a response to stretch, in denervation models, type 1 fibres are more likely to hypertrophy than are type 2 fibres (Sola et al 1973b). Denervation of the rat hemidiaphragm induces within 10 days an increase in the diameter of red fibres of 35%, of intermediate fibres of 25% and a slight decrease in the diameter of white fibres (Hopkins et al 1983). Hypertrophy is later followed by marked atrophy (Sola & Martin 1953, Turner & Manchester 1972).

Denervation of muscle fibres may be the result of: (i) focal necrosis causing loss of contact of one part of a muscle fibre with its own end-plate area; this occurs in polymyositis and other myopathic disorders; (ii) structural changes in distal parts of preterminal or terminal axons, as in acrylamide and other 'dying back' neuropathies; (iii) loss of one or several motor axons or motor neurones. In the first two instances, one or several fibres in a

motor unit will be denervated; in the last instance whole motor units become denervated simultaneously. When denervation of a few fibres or a single motor unit occurs, the atrophic fibres will be disseminated between others of normal size. In transverse sections the denervated fibres lose their polygonal shape and seem to become compressed in the narrow spaces between other fibres. At first the cross-striations are preserved and the nuclei usually remain in a peripheral position. Some nuclei are enlarged and vesicular in appearance. Authors agree that the number of muscle nuclei does not decrease (for review, see Sunderland 1978). Satellite cells even react by proliferating. Using a light-microscopic technique, Ontell (1974) found that satellite cells accounted for 2% and 0.7% respectively of the total nuclear population in young and adult rats. Three weeks after denervation the proportions had increased to 12% and 5%. Schultz et al (1978) and Snow (1983) found more modest increases in the number of satellite cells. When atrophy proceeds, it gradually becomes apparent that the internal architecture of the muscle fibres is disrupted. The shape of the fibres in transverse section changes to round or oval, the nuclei are small, pyknotic and clumped together, and they are surrounded by little, if any, sarcoplasm without any discernible myofibrillar structure.

Structural abnormalities in denervated fibres, such as vacuolar or granular degeneration, were reported by some of the earlier authors (Stier 1896, Tower 1935), but these observations have not been confirmed (Sunderland & Ray 1950, Karpati & Engel 1968a, Stonnington & Engel 1973). According to Sunderland these changes very rarely occur, at least if the animals are allowed to move about freely in large cages (Sunderland 1978).

For many weeks after denervation, the activity of myosin ATPase remains a highly reliable indicator of the original histochemical type of the muscle fibres (Karpati & Engel 1968b). On denervation many other enzymes react with marked changes in activity, thereby obscuring the original differences between the fibre types (Hogenhuis & Engel 1965, Romanul & Hogan 1965, Smith 1965, Engel et al 1966). The activities of enzymes involved in aerobic metabolism increase, at least for some time. This may be related to the transient, relative increase which occurs in mitochondrial volume and sarcoplasmic membrane surface area (Stonnington & Engel 1973). There is some evidence of dysfunction of mitochondria in denervated muscle. Respiration measured on day 28 after denervation is deficient. The impairment is thought to be localized in complexes I and III of the respiratory chain (Joffe et al 1981). Myophosphorylase activity falls rapidly after denervation and the glycogen content decreases markedly (Pichey & Smith 1979). Increase in lysosomal enzyme activity has been demonstrated biochemically (Romanul & Hogan 1965; Pluskal & Pennington 1973; Stauber & Schottelius 1975; Joffe et al 1981).

The ultrastructure of the denervated muscle fibre

The myofibrillar system

Slight myofibrillar changes are present as early as 3 days after denervation (Cullen & Pluskal 1977) and are initially localized focally in the periphery of the fibre (Pellegrino & Franzini 1963, Miledi & Slater 1969). The alterations spread transversely across several myofibrils. The process of myofibrillar breakdown starts with disruption of the regular alignment of the myofilaments and streaming of Z discs (Fig. 16.1A) (Tomanek & Lund 1973, Cullen & Pluskal 1977). The diameter of the myofibrils and the number of myofibrils per fibre decrease. The shape of the myofibrils becomes irregular. In the periphery, areas devoid of contractile material appear and may cause the sarcolemma to indent (Pellegrino & Franzini 1963). The intermyofibrillar spaces are, however, only slightly enlarged. At this stage myofibrils with normal spatial organization are still present in the centre of the fibre, but as atrophy proceeds total disorganization occurs here as well. The myofibrillar atrophy is proportionate to, or slightly greater than, fibre atrophy (Stonnington & Engel 1973). By 2 to 3 months after denervation, the loss of contractile material has led to extreme reduction in fibre diameter. Because of the focal nature of myofibrillar disorganization and atrophy in the initial stage, the fibres show abrupt variations

along their lengths in the number of remaining myofibrils (Pellegrino & Franzini 1963).

No trace of myofilaments nor their breakdown products in lysosomal structures is found at any stage. For this reason it has been suggested that an extralysosomal mechanism is probably responsible for the depolymerization of the contractile proteins (Schiaffino & Hanzlikova 1972). Loss of proteins in the denervated fibres appears to be the result of increased degradation and decreased synthesis (Margreth et al 1977). Increased activity of neutral proteases and retardation of denervation atrophy by protease inhibitors have been reported (Kar & Pearson 1977, Goldberg et al 1979, Stracher et al 1979). What the signal is for the elevation in neutral protease activity is not known. Experiments on frog muscle, however, have demonstrated an increase in intracellular calcium in denervated fibres (Picken & Kirby 1976), and there is a sarcoplasmic protease which is activated by calcium ions and which degrades certain myofibrillar proteins (Dayton et al 1975, Kar & Pearson 1977). Another mechanism has been suggested by Smith & Appel (1977) and by Smith et al (1978). Protein catabolism in normal skeletal muscles is inhibited by β-adrenergic stimulation of sarcolemmal adenylate cyclase. There is a rapid fall in β-adrenergic response after denervation. According to the authors, this alteration in membrane biochemical function might be responsible for a loss of inhibitory control of muscle protein catabolism.

The mitochondria

The mitochondria undergo a complex series of alterations, beginning within the first 24 hours after denervation (Miledi & Slater 1968) and progressing gradually thereafter. The ring-like mitochondrial expansions which in some rat muscles encircle the myofibrils disappear and, in transverse sections, the mitochondria become small and round. The mitochondria become more aligned along the axis of the myofibrils. It has been suggested that this whole process of change in shape and orientation is related to the loss of contractile activity and, in the later stages of denervation, to less close packing of the myofibrils (Stonnington & Engel 1973, Cullen & Pluskal

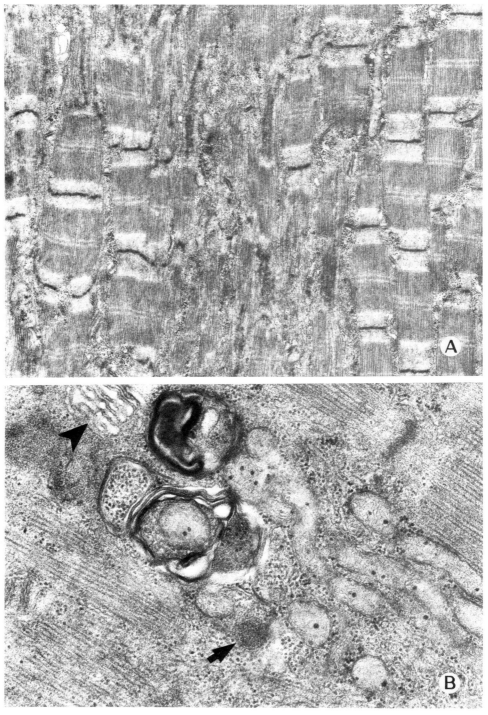

Fig. 16.1 Rat anterior tibial muscle, 10 days after denervation. (A) Focal disorganization of sarcomere structure; ×14 000. (B) Myelinoid figures near mitochondria and between myofibrils, enclosing glycogen granules and undefined material. Note a primary lysosome-like structure (arrow) and a Golgi apparatus (arrowhead); ×42 000

1977). Within 6 days of denervation, many mito-chondria develop structural changes, such as loss of cristae, increase in electron density of the matrix and the appearance of granules or vesicles within the matrix. Such abnormalities are present to a minor extent in mitochondria of normal rat muscle, and it has been suggested that they are ageing phenomena representing stages in the normal turnover of mitochondria (Cullen & Pluskal 1977). As stated, these abnormalities increase in frequency and occasional mitochondria are converted into myeloid structures or become entrapped in auto-phagic vacuoles (Fig. 16.1B) (Stonnington & Engel 1973, Cullen & Pluskal 1977). Morpho-metric studies have shown that during the initial days following denervation the mitochondrial volume increases, only to decrease gradually there-after so that a normal proportion is again reached after about 1 month (Stonnington & Engel 1973, Cullen et al 1975).

T system, sarcoplasmic reticulum and free ribosomes

Denervation leads to a change in orientation of some T tubules from transverse to longitudinal (Gauthier & Dunn 1973, Libelius et al 1979), and to increasing irregularity of the spatial arrangement with focal dilatation of the T system as well as the sarcoplasmic reticulum (Gori 1972, Tomanek & Lund 1973). These systems show an increase in surface area during the first week after denerva-tion. A decrease follows, but less rapidly than that of other elements, thus giving the impression of overdevelopment (Stonnington & Engel 1973). So-called 'pentads', consisting of combinations of the terminal sacs and intermediary elements of triads, and complex structures composed of alternating arrays of tubular and reticular components, have been described (Pellegrino & Franzini 1963, Gori 1972, Stonnington & Engel 1973).

Rough endoplasmic reticulum and free ribo-somes are not prominent in adult muscle fibres. However, soon after denervation they are found consistently in the subsarcolemmal region (Gauthier & Schaeffer 1974). Proliferation of these organelles may be required for the synthesis of acetylcholine receptor proteins and of enzymes involved in the degradation of the muscle fibre.

Lysosomal structures

A few days after denervation, the activity of acid hydrolases increases (Pluskal & Pennington 1973, McLaughlin et al 1974) and organelles fitting the criteria of primary lysosomes appear between the myofibrils at the level of the I bands, or at the periphery close to Golgi systems (Cullen & Pluskal 1977). The Golgi apparatus hypertrophies, increasing in size and complexity, and may be found not only close to nuclei, but also elsewhere in the periphery and even in deeper parts of the muscle fibres (Schiaffino & Hanzlikova 1972). Autophagic vacuoles containing amorphous material or, occasionally, identifiable organelles, appear and other lysosome-derived elements such as myelin figures, multivesicular bodies and dense bodies develop. These structures may already be seen in the first week after denervation. At advanced stages of atrophy, the hypertrophic changes of the Golgi apparatus regress (Schiaffino & Hanzlikova 1972) and many lysosomal structures are present within the atrophic fibres.

Studies by Thesleff's group have shed light on the start of lysosomal activity. In normal muscle fibres, endocytosis occurs at a slow rate and the lysosomal system is poorly developed. It was shown that stimulation of endocytosis by a poly-cationic protein induced lysosomal activation and fibre degeneration (Jirmanová et al 1977). On the second day after denervation, endocytosis is increased as demonstrated by the uptake of [^{3}H] inulin (Libelius et al 1978b). Evidence that the endocytosed material enters the lysosomal structures, via micropinocytosis from T tubules, was inferred from studies on horseradish peroxidase uptake (Libelius et al 1979). The authors suggest that the increased endocytosis is the result of early membrane changes attributable to loss of nerve influence. The enhanced ingestion activates the lysosomal system and the lysosomes become active in autophagic processes which con-tribute to fibre degeneration (Libelius et al 1978a).

Nuclei

Most authors have paid little attention to the ultrastructural changes in myonuclei after denervation. Pellegrino & Franzini (1963) observed that 1–2 months after denervation the nuclei had become extremely irregular in outline and showed deep indentations. Chromatin was distributed irregularly with dense heterochromatin at the periphery.

Several authors have concentrated on changes in satellite cells and, as described previously, it appears that these cells react to denervation with a modest degree of proliferation (Ontell 1974, Schultz et al 1978, Snow 1983). Ultrastructural studies on adult rat muscles 1–3 weeks after denervation, have revealed that some of the satellite cells show signs of activation and structural changes similar to those seen in myoblasts (Ontell 1975). The cells do not succeed, however, in forming myotubes. According to Schultz (1978), the situation is different in growing muscle. In this case, the satellite cells show evidence of increased activity and motility, and some of them separate from their parent muscle fibres. The author suggested that these cells could be the source of the small-diameter immature fibres which were present in the interstitial spaces. Several of these small fibres showed features of degeneration, perhaps attributable to the absence of a viable nerve supply.

Re-innervation

Acetylcholine receptors

Some of the changes which develop in the plasma membrane are relevant with regard to the process of re-innervation. A few days after denervation, the postsynaptic infoldings are slightly decreased in number and in depth (Tachikawa & Clementi 1979). These changes progress slowly but the folds remain identifiable for many weeks (Bowden & Duchen 1976). Freeze–fracture studies have revealed irregular rows of particles on top of the junctional foldings. The particles are thought to represent the acetylcholine receptors (AChRs) and remain almost unchanged during the first weeks after denervation (Ellisman & Rash 1977, Tachikawa & Clementi 1979). The end-plate sensitivity to acetylcholine during this period is main-

tained. Under normal conditions the AChR density falls quite sharply 2 μm from the end-plate. Within 3 days of denervation, however, AChRs appear extrajunctionally and the entire membrane becomes sensitive to acetylcholine (Edwards 1979, Asmark et al 1985).

The receptors are not evenly distributed in the plasma membrane; in some places the density is considerably greater than in others, as shown by studies on the binding of α-bungarotoxin to isolated muscle fibres (Ko et al 1977). It is estimated that the receptor density in these areas is close to that in the postjunctional membrane (Ko et al 1977). As re-innervation of denervated fibres may potentially occur in regions other than the end-plates (Frank et al 1975), it is reasonable to suppose that these patches are possible sites for re-innervation. There is evidence which suggests that extrajunctional AChRs play a part in eliciting motor nerve sprouting. Functional denervation of skeletal muscle causes extrajunctional spread of AChRs and sprouting of motor nerve fibres. Blockade of the new receptors with α-bungarotoxin — a specific blocker of these receptors — prevents sprouting (Pestronk & Drachman 1978, 1985). How this is accomplished is not yet clear, but it demonstrates the significance of the extrajunctional receptors in the process of nerve sprouting.

Three to four weeks after denervation, AChRs are still present in high density at the original junction area. In the extrajunctional membrane, however, a gradual decrease commences and, 6–8 weeks after denervation, extrajunctional AChRs can no longer be demonstrated, at least not at the light-microscopic level using an α-bungarotoxin immunoperoxidase technique (Ringel et al 1976).

Muscle-derived neurotrophic factor

It is now generally accepted that target cells produce neurotrophic factors which influence the survival, maintenance and differentiation of innervating neurons (Snider & Johnson 1989, Walicke 1989). There is little doubt that muscle extract contains a factor which influences lower motor neurone (LMN) survival and stimulates growth of muscle nerves (Slack et al 1983, Brown & Lunn 1988, Oppenheim & Haverkamp 1988, Oppenheim et al 1988, Henderson 1988, Snider & Johnson 1989). Synaptic sites on myotubes and on muscle fibres have been suggested to be areas of release and uptake of muscle-derived neurotrophic factor by nerve terminals (Slack et al 1983, Oppenheim 1989). The sequence of events following denervation might be as follows: denervation activates AChR genes (Tsay & Schmidt 1989) and AChRs are displayed on the entire muscle fibre membrane. AChR up-regulation is accompanied by increased availability of a muscle-derived trophic factor (Slack et al 1983, Oppenheim 1989) which stimulates growth of muscle nerves and re-innervation. The latter is followed by AChR down-regulation, and by restriction of AChRs and trophic factor release to the end-plate area.

The best known neurotrophic factor is 'nerve growth factor' (NGF) which is required by sympathetic and dorsal root ganglion cells and some cells in the central nervous system (Levi-Montalcini 1989). NGF does not influence survival of LMNs in tissue culture conditions and does not stimulate growth of LMN neurites. LMNs are therefore considered NGF-independent. It remains however to be clarified why NGF receptor messenger RNA is expressed during development and after axotomy in rat spinal motor neurons (Ernfors et al 1989) and why NGF receptor is present in developing muscle of the rat (Yan & Eugene 1988). CNTF (ciliary neurotrophic factor) differs in structure and in responsive neurons (in vitro) from NGF. It is expressed by Schwann cells and astrocytes but not by skeletal muscle and has been demonstrated to further survival of damaged LMNs in neonatal rats (Sendtner et al 1990). CDF (choline acetyl transferase development factor) is a 22 kDa polypeptide which has been purified from rat skeletal muscle. This peptide increases choline acetyltransferase activity in LMN-enriched cell cultures and enhances the survival of LMN from naturally occurring cell death in embryonic chickens (McManaman et al 1988, 1990). It has been suggested that CDF may also regulate LMN survival later in life (Oppenheim et al 1990) and it may well prove to be the hypothesized muscle-derived trophic factor.

Nerve–muscle adhesion

Neural cell adhesion molecules (N-CAM) function as ligands in cell–cell interaction (see Rutishauser 1986). Adhesion requires participation of N-CAM molecules in each of the adhering cell membranes. N-CAM consists of a single polypeptide chain with a large carbohydrate moiety and contains sialic acid. In the chicken hindlimb, expression of N-CAM on the muscle membrane precedes growth of intramuscular nerves and formation of synapses. When synaptogenesis is completed N-CAM expression becomes restricted to the synaptic areas. There is evidence suggesting that the same sequence of widespread expression and restriction is seen following denervation and re-innervation. Anti-N-CAM specific antibodies perturb axonal regeneration and cause formation of synaptic contacts at extrasynaptic sites. N-CAM has been localized in the muscle basal lamina and has been found to be concentrated in the synaptic part of the basal lamina (Rieger et al 1985, 1988).

The site of new neuromuscular junctions

New neuromuscular junctions on denervated muscle fibres are generally found at the site of the original end-plates (Birks et al 1960, Saito & Zacks 1969). The high precision of re-innervation may be the result of regrowth of axons within Schwann cell tubes or in fascicles enclosed by perineurium (Miledi 1960, Bennett et al 1973, Brown 1984). This does not explain, however, why sprouts from nearby intact axons also prefer the original end-plate region. Axons regenerating into a region where myofibres are dead and the basal lamina is preserved, contact the latter at the original synaptic sites (Sanes et al 1978, 1986). At the site of contact, the growth cones differentiate into motor nerve terminals (Glicksman & Sanes 1983). Components of the synaptic basal lamina are apparently involved in the regulation of the process of transformation of the growth cones into nerve terminals. Other synaptic basal lamina components influence the differentiation of the postsynaptic membrane (Fallon & Gelfman 1989, Jay & Barald 1989). Most, if not all, of the original subsynaptic membranes become covered by the regenerating axon terminals (Letinsky et al 1976).

If muscle fibres are initially re-innervated by sprouts from nearby intact axons, the regenerating axons which were originally damaged may still succeed in making synaptic contact at the end-plate regions and the sprouts are then eliminated by competition (Bennett & Raftos 1977, Thompson 1978). Elimination of sprouts does not occur after a certain time. A possible explanation for this may be that the sprouts require time before they succeed in occupying the entire synaptic area. Once this has been achieved no innervation target remains because, in the meantime, the extrajunctional acetylcholine receptors have decreased in density or have disappeared.

The length of time during which new neuro-muscular junctions can be formed on denervated muscle fibres is not known precisely. Re-innervation of human muscles may occur even after a period of 12 months (Sunderland 1950, 1978).

Transformation and type grouping

Muscle fibres belonging to the same motor unit are histochemically virtually uniform (Edström & Kugelberg 1968, Mayer & Doyle 1970, Burke et al 1971, Kugelberg 1973). The chemical characteristics are reflected in the physiological properties (Buchthal & Schmalbruch 1970) and these properties are closely related to the discharge patterns of the innervating motor neurones (Grimby et al 1979). Motor neurones innervating type 1 (slow-twitch, aerobic) fibres fire continuously with relatively low frequency. Neurones innervating type 2 fibres (fast-twitch, aerobic-glycolytic or glycolytic) fire phasically at higher rates or in high-frequency bursts (Hannerz 1974, Grimby & Hannerz 1977).

Re-innervation of denervated type 2 units by 'type 1 neurones' converts the units to type 1 and vice versa (Buller et al 1960, Dubowitz 1967, Karpati & Engel 1968c). Continuous low-frequency electrical stimulation of type 2 motor units brings about the same changes as re-innervation by type 1 neurones (Salmons & Vrbová 1969, Sréter et al 1973, Lömo et al 1974, Romanul et al 1974, Salmons & Sréter 1975, Pette & Vrbová 1985). Transformation from slow-twitch (type 1) to fast-twitch (type 2) and from fast-twitch to slow-twitch fibres can be brought about by appropriate stimulation of denervated fibres (Lömo et al 1974, Mommaerts et al 1977, Lömo et al 1980). Prolonged high-intensity endurance training may result in transformation of muscle fibres from fast-twitch to slow-twitch (Schantz et al 1982, 1983, Pette & Staron 1988).

Muscle fibres belonging to one motor unit do not lie in apposition to each other, but are usually intermingled with fibres of other motor units (Edström & Kugelberg 1968, Mayer & Doyle 1970, Kugelberg 1973, 1979). It is only rarely that more than two or three fibres of one motor unit are found side-by-side. This distribution explains the mosaic-like pattern of enzyme activity of the fibres on histochemical staining. In cross-sections of rat soleus and tibialis anterior muscles, fibres belonging to one motor unit may be scattered over areas 2–5 mm in diameter. These fibres are often located in more than one fascicle (Kugelberg 1973, 1979).

Partial denervation leads to collateral sprouting of nearby intact axons (Edds 1953, 1955) and to re-innervation with fibre transformation. This increases the chance that muscle fibres belonging to one histochemical type will lie close together, so that type grouping occurs: i.e. groups of closely packed fibres of the same histochemical type appear (Fig. 16.2). When only a few fibres or motor units are denervated, the type groups will be small. Experimentally, this situation can be attained by sectioning one ventral root. In slowly progressive denervation the type groups may gradually increase in size. Large type groups will also be seen after sectioning and suturing a motor nerve (Karpati & Engel 1968c). With this technique only a percentage of the regenerating nerve fibres will reach the distal portion of the nerve. Nevertheless, many if not all muscle fibres will be re-innervated, but this does not mean that the mosaic pattern will be restored. Many sprouts of regenerating axons leave their Schwann cell tubes and synapse with neighbouring muscle fibres. Thus, fibres of one motor unit are no longer intermingled with other fibres of other units. Instead, they are grouped together, and the overlap between motor units is to a great extent lost. Re-innervation may increase the number of fibres within one unit by a factor of four or even seven (Kugelberg et al 1970, Thompson & Jansen 1977), and the territory of the motor units may

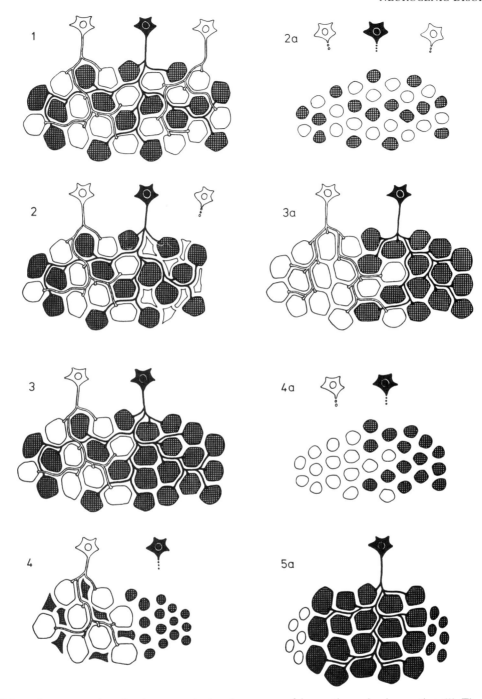

Fig. 16.2 Schematic representation of various stages in chronic processes of denervation and re-innervation. (1) Three motor units, two type 1 units (light) and one type 2 (black). (2) Partial denervation leads to disseminated fibre atrophy. (3) Successful re-innervation by collateral sprouts from a nearby intramuscular axon. The mosaic pattern is replaced in part by a group of histochemically uniform type 2 fibres. (4) The enlarged motor unit is denervated in its turn. There is now a group of histochemically uniform atrophic fibres. Other atrophic fibres belonging to the same motor unit lie disseminated between non-atrophic fibres. (2a) Total denervation. All muscle fibres atrophy. (3a) Two of the original three axons regenerate. All muscle fibres are re-innervated, the mosaic pattern is replaced by type groups. There is some overlap between motor units. (4a) The enlarged motor units are again denervated. (5a) One of the original two axons regenerates. Re-innervation succeeds only partially. Muscle fibres in unfavourable positions remain denervated

become enlarged. Kugelberg (1973) has pointed out that the type groups are often restricted to only one fascicle. This is probably attributable to the barrier which the connective tissue forms for the outgrowing sprouts. Type groups with a uniform activity of one enzyme need not necessarily be uniform for other metabolic parameters (Jennekens et al 1974). There is a twofold explanation for this situation. First, the transformation of some fibres may not yet be completed; secondly, myosin ATPase uniform groups may in fact consist of motor units of different subtypes (Askanas & Engel 1975, Karpati et al 1975).

Early structural changes

It will be clear from the foregoing that, as far as structural changes due to re-innervation are concerned, attention has been concentrated on different aspects of transformation. Observations on other aspects, e.g. the changes occurring when atrophic fibres regain their original size, are fragmentary. Only two phenomena will be discussed here.

Architectural changes in the myofibrillary system such as 'ring' fibres and 'coiled' fibres were observed by Dubowitz (1967) in a study on experimental re-innervation. There is reason to doubt whether these are indeed re-innervation phenomena. They are known to be non-specific and to occur in various conditions, and they have not been reported in other reinnervation experiments (Karpati & Engel 1968c).

With regard to target fibres, the problem is just the opposite. The term 'target' was used by Engel (1961) to denote a concentric change within muscle fibres (see Fig. 16.9). In sections from paraffin-embedded material the targets are easily discerned by a red (Gomori trichrome) discoloration of a central condensed core which is surrounded by a paler area. The targets do not extend over the whole length of the fibres. They may be very small and they are occasionally limited to only a few sarcomeres (De Coster et al 1976).

The targets may be difficult to spot in histologically stained cryostat sections, but they are readily demonstrable by histochemical techniques, and are mostly present in the type 1 fibres (Resnick & Engel 1966). The central zones show no myosin

ATPase or oxidative enzyme activity and they contain no glycogen (Engel 1962, Resnick & Engel 1966). They are surrounded by an area with high myosin ATPase and increased oxidative enzyme activity, which may contain much glycogen. Some targets in which the central zone lacks an area of high enzyme activity have been referred to as 'targetoids'. Targetoids show a close resemblance to unstructured central cores. At the ultrastructural level the central zone of the targets consists of filamentous material, part of which has the same density as Z discs (Shafiq et al 1967, De Coster et al 1976) and mitochondria, sarcoplasmic reticulum and glycogen granules are not present. The ring-like intermediate zone is sometimes narrow and variably structured. Myofilaments are present, and retain their regular orientation. The Z discs are disorganized, and material like that of the Z discs extends from this central zone into the other zones. The intermediate zone may contain many small and electron-dense mitochondria, accumulations of glycogen granules and swollen profiles of sarcoplasmic reticulum.

Target fibres were initially observed in patients with neuropathic disorders (Engel 1962), often in muscle fibres of normal diameter, and for this reason they were considered to be an early denervation phenomenon. This hypothesis has not been confirmed. Most authors have, in fact, experienced great difficulties in producing target fibres by experimental denervation (Hogenhuis & Engel 1965, Engel et al 1966), and some authors have specifically denied their presence (Stonnington & Engel 1973). Target fibres were, however, observed by Dubowitz (1967) in his re-innervation experiments and other workers also reported that they could readily produce targets by reinnervation (De Reuck et al 1977a). A target is a transient phenomenon, which explains why they are often not found in neurogenic muscle disorders (Kovarsky et al 1973). Target fibres are not specific for neurogenic muscle disease: they also appear in muscle fibres after tenotomy (Engel et al 1966, De Reuck et al 1977a,b).

Compensatory hypertrophy and other secondary changes

For a partly denervated muscle, the performance

of a normal task may imply heavy use or functional overloading of the remaining innervated fibres (Schwartz et al 1976). Studies on increased muscle use are, therefore, pertinent to the pathological changes which frequently develop in chronically denervated human muscles (Drachman et al 1967). Two distinct types of exercise stimuli have to be distinguished. Muscle responds to endurance training (long-distance running, rodents on a treadmill) by increasing its capacity for aerobic metabolism and by a tendency for the myosin ATPase activity to change from high to low (for reviews, see Holloszy & Booth 1976, Mendell 1979). Intermittent strenuous exercise (such as weight lifting) induces muscle hypertrophy, but the respiratory capacity need not change. Hypertrophy associated with exercise occurs more frequently in type 2 than in type 1 fibres (Dubowitz & Brooke 1973).

A model which has frequently been used in studies of functional overload is tenotomy, or actual excision of one or two muscles in the posterior or anterior compartment of rodent hind limbs. The procedure causes so-called compensatory hypertrophy in synergistic muscles. This hypertrophy is not, however, necessarily attributable only to functional overload, as excessive stretching of muscle fibres also occurs (Schiaffino & Hanzliková 1970, Gutmann et al 1971). Nevertheless, the model mimics the situation which frequently exists in human neurogenic muscular atrophy, in which agonist and antagonist muscles are usually not affected to the same degree. Whatever the cause, fibre hypertrophy develops in the experimental model and reaches its maximum after approximately 20 days (Hall-Craggs 1970). In some hypertrophic fibres, central nucleation occurs and fissures appear, which in transversely sectioned fibres are seen to extend from the periphery towards the central nucleus. The sarcoplasm bordering the fissures is basophilic and shows high aerobic enzyme activity (Hall-Craggs 1972). It contains glycogen granules, ribosomes, mitochondria and myofibrillar debris (Hall-Craggs 1972, Schwartz et al 1976, Swash et al 1978). The nuclei associated with the clefts are often large and vesicular. The fissures occur most frequently in hypertrophic type 1 fibres.

The mechanism underlying the development of these clefts is disputed. It has been reported that proliferation of satellite cells takes place during the first few days of compensatory hypertrophy (Aloisi et al 1973). In addition, small growing fibres have been observed under the basal lamina. Some of these small fibres seem to have cytoplasmic continuity with the main fibre, and others seem to detach from the main fibres and to extend into the interstitial spaces. The term 'fibre branching' has been used to describe these observations (Schiaffino et al 1979). Schmalbruch (1976, 1979), who has worked on experimentally induced myopathic disorders, has come to the conclusion that the so-called fibre splitting is due to incomplete fusion of multiple fibres regenerating within the same basal lamina tube. Other authors maintain that, in conditions of denervation and 'work hypertrophy', true splitting actually occurs and is likely to be due to mechanical overload (Swash et al 1978, Bradley 1979).

The results of what we now call fibre splitting are complex (Swash & Schwartz 1977). Fibre splitting may lead to forking of individual fibres. The separated parts remain connected to the parent fibre through which they are innervated. Multiple splits in one fibre may cause several forks and in transverse section a small type group may be simulated. Completely separated small fibres may show regenerative activity. When innervated, the small fibres are usually of the same histochemical type as the parent fibre. When multiple fairly small fibres are present around a parent fibre, a small type group may again be simulated. Degenerative changes may occur in a small fibre when it does not become innervated.

The foregoing observations strongly suggest that stretch and functional overload are important complicating factors in chronic neurogenic muscle disease. These factors may initiate the structural abnormalities frequently occurring in fibres which are still innervated. It is possible to explain a number of the secondary changes such as fibre hypertrophy, central nucleation, fibre splitting and regenerative activity in small fibres by the pathophysiological mechanisms described above. These changes are often referred to collectively as 'secondary myopathic change'.

DIAGNOSTIC CRITERIA

The histopathological diagnosis of neurogenic muscular atrophy is usually easy and simple histological staining of paraffin sections may suffice in the chronic disorders. The diagnosis is, however, often greatly facilitated by histochemical staining of cryostat sections which may show type grouping. Ultrastructural examination provides no additional diagnostic information.

The description below will follow the customary sequence of routine diagnostic procedures. Accordingly, the histological and histochemical criteria will be discussed consecutively.

Histological criteria

Fibre size and configuration

The parameter most frequently used to denote the size of a transversely sectioned muscle fibre is the 'diameter', that is the greatest distance between opposite sides of the narrowest aspect of a fibre (Brooke & Engel 1969a). In adolescent and adult men the diameters of fibres in limb muscles are generally 35–80 μm. In women, the muscle fibres are often slightly smaller, varying from 30 to 70 μm (Brooke & Engel 1969a). Denervation causes the fibres to decrease in size, and they ultimately reach a diameter of less than 10 μm. One or several of the normally straight sides of the fibre becomes concave and the angle decreases from 120° or more to much less than 90°. These fibres are termed 'angulated'. Some fibres initially seem to decrease in size in one direction and to increase in the perpendicular direction. Such fibres become 'elongated' in appearance, which means that they are three-dimensionally plate-like (Fig. 16.3). Although highly characteristic for denervation atrophy, angulated and elongated fibres are not diagnostic as similar fibres may be found in conditions such as type 2 fibre atrophy, myotonic dystrophy and facioscapulohumeral dystrophy. When atrophy proceeds, the fibres tend to lose their angulated appearance and eventually become small and round or oval.

Some of the surviving fibres may enlarge and become hypertrophic. The diameter of these fibres increases to more than 100 μm. Increase in

activity is considered to cause preferential hypertrophy of type 2 fibres (Brooke & Engel 1969b, Dubowitz & Brooke 1973); stretch predisposes particularly to hypertrophy of type 1 fibres (Sola et al 1973b). The enlarged fibres may retain their polygonal aspect, or become round.

Brooke & Engel (1969b) devised a method for quantifying the changes in fibre size. The method aims to give information about the number of fibres outside the normal range, and about the degree of changes in size. The diameters of 200 fibres are measured. In men the number of fibres between 30 and 40 μm is counted and multiplied by one. The number of fibres between 30 and 20 μm, 20 and 10 μm, and 10 μm or less are multiplied by two, three and four respectively. The resulting figures are then added, the product is divided by 200 and multiplied by 1000. The value thus obtained is called the 'atrophy factor'. The 'hypertrophy factor' is calculated in the same manner, starting from fibres larger than 80 μm. In women 30 μm and 70 μm are taken as the normal limits. This method is useful in the diagnosis of neurogenic muscular atrophy, but is of greater value in comparing the severity of the changes in different disorders or at different stages of a disease.

Distribution criteria

On the basis of the distribution of denervated atrophic and large fibres, five different situations can be outlined.

1. There are atrophic, angulated or elongated fibres scattered in the sections. The atrophic fibres occur in slightly varying frequency in different fields. This is the classical picture of disseminated neurogenic atrophy caused by partial denervation (Fig. 16.3).

2. Most of the muscle fibres are atrophic and groups of varying numbers of atrophic fibres may be seen without great variation from one field to another. Fibres of normal size or hypertrophic fibres are disseminated between atrophic fibres, and there are small groups of large fibres. The main difference from the previous stage is that many more units are denervated. There are far

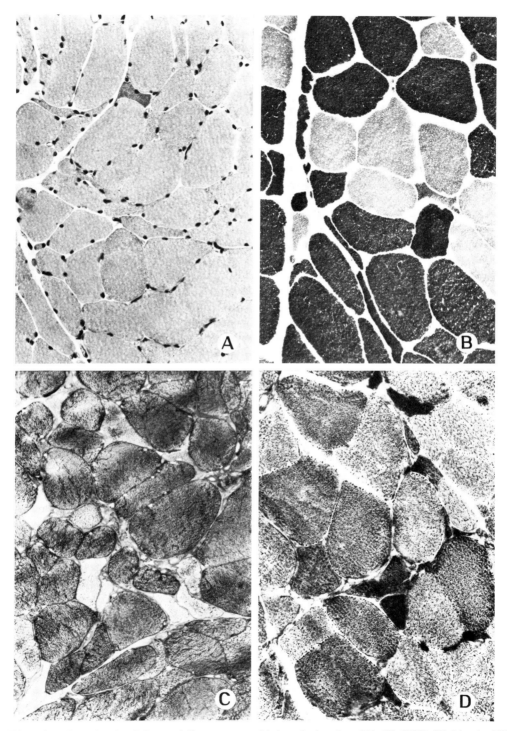

Fig. 16.3 Disseminated angulated and elongated fibres, amyotrophic lateral sclerosis; ×210. (A) H&E. (B) Myosin ATPase pH 9.4. (C) PAS. (D) NADH–TR. Distribution criteria, stage 1 (see text)

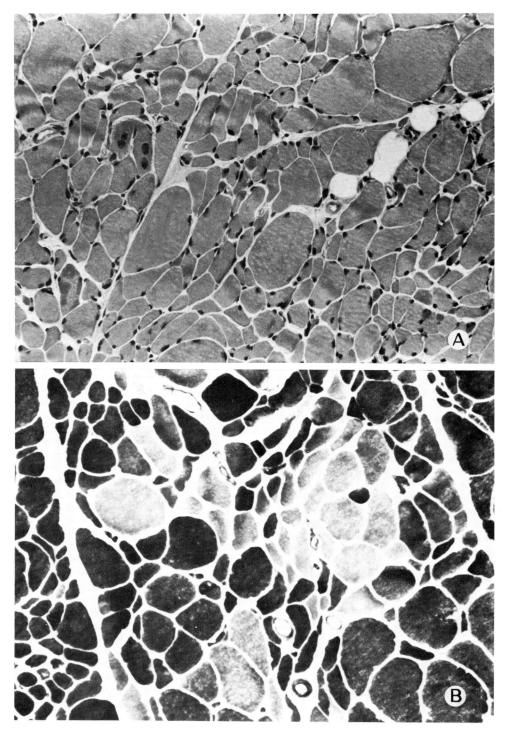

Fig. 16.4.   The majority of the muscle fibres are denervated and atrophic, amyotrophic lateral sclerosis; ×210. (A) H&E; note the two fibres containing enlarged nuclei. (B) Myosin ATPase, pH 9.4; there is a small group of type 2 fibres at the lower left side of the picture. Distribution criteria, stage 2 (see text)

fewer re-innervated fibres than in the following stage (Fig. 16.4).

3. There are clear-cut groups of atrophic fibres, the number of fibres per group varying from less than 10 to more than 100. In between these groups, there are often fields, frequently of large numbers of fibres, mostly normal in size, with some scattered atrophic fibres and some hypertrophic fibres. This situation may develop when the course of the disease allows ample opportunity for re-innervation of denervated fibres. Re-innervation implies a change in the organization of the motor units involved. Fibres belonging to these units are often closely packed, and there is less overlap between motor units than in normal muscle. Subsequent denervation of such closely packed motor units causes groups of atrophic fibres to appear (Fig. 16.5).

4. There are two easily discernible populations of muscle fibres, differing in the location and size of the fibres. Groups of hypertrophic or normal-sized fibres contain few scattered atrophic fibres. Groups of atrophic fibres are often located on the edges of the fascicles, these sites being relatively unfavourable for successful re-innervation. Fibres in the atrophic groups are often extremely small and round or oval. Scattered atrophic fibres are mostly angulated or elongated. This histological picture is seen in slowly progressive disorders, characterized by a process of denervation and re-innervation. Hardly any overlap remains between the motor units. Atrophic and surviving units are almost completely separated (Fig. 16.6).

5. Groups of extremely small atrophic fibres are present within proliferated connective tissue and fat tissue. Surviving fibres are few and mostly packed together in small groups. An end stage has now been reached. Apparently, the surviving motor neurones no longer succeed in re-innervating large numbers of muscle fibres. One possible explanation for this failure may be the proliferation of connective tissue which is likely to hamper the growth of axonal sprouts (Fig. 16.7).

It is clear that the distinction between the various stages has been simplified. In reality there is greater variation and the histological picture is also complicated by structural and degenerative changes in the non-atrophic fibres.

Structural changes in atrophic fibres

One of the most characteristic features of denervated, atrophic fibres is the preservation of a normal cytoarchitecture, at least at the light-microscopic level. It is only in extremely small fibres that the cross-striations are absent. The myonuclei retain their peripheral position. They are often dark and shrunken. Clumping of pyknotic nuclei may be seen (Fig. 16.8). This phenomenon may be attributable in part to crowding of the nuclei in the atrophying fibres. Dark clumps of muscle nuclei are often present in the endomysium and may be considered to be remnants of totally atrophied fibres (Figs 16.7 and 16.8).

Structural and degenerative changes in non-atrophic fibres

Target fibres are seen in only a minority of the muscle biopsies from patients with neurogenic muscle disorders (Fig. 16.9). As they are nearly always associated with diseases involving the lower motor neurones, their diagnostic value is high. Targets are not easy to recognize in sections stained with haematoxylin and eosin, but with Gomori and PTAH stains they are nicely demonstrated as dark reddish zones surrounded by less darkly stained ring-like areas. They may occupy a central or a peripheral position in the fibre. In longitudinal sections the target areas appear to be limited in length; in some cases they are not much longer than a few sarcomeres (De Coster et al 1976). Targetoid fibres are more difficult to spot because of the lack of clear ring-like areas around the central zone.

Several other structural changes occur regularly but are non-specific. They are observed most frequently in chronic disorders in which there are only a limited number of surviving fibres. In transverse sections, internalization of myonuclei may be seen in a high proportion of the non-atrophic fibres (Fig. 16.7) (van Wijngaarden & Bethlem 1973). These nuclei are not pyknotic but are often somewhat vesicular. Fibre splitting occurs most frequently in hypertrophic fibres (Fig. 16.8). Structural changes of the myofibrillar system such as necrosis, phagocytosis and changes indicative of regenerative activity are seen occa-

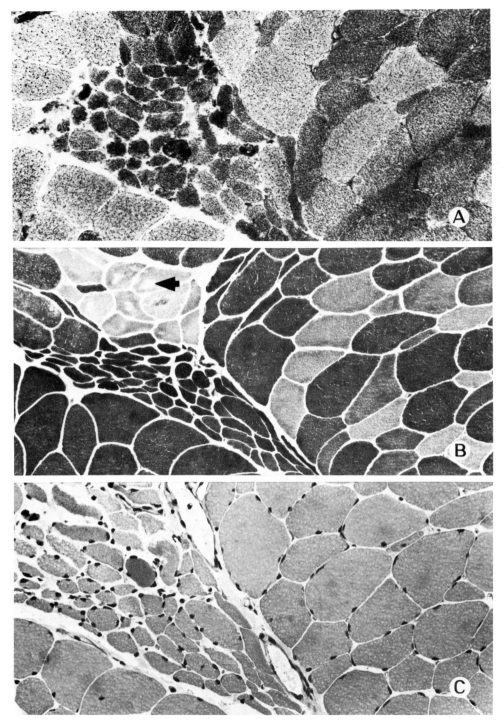

Fig. 16.5   Serial sections, showing a group of atrophic fibres and atrophic fibres in between others of normal size, hereditary motor and sensory neuropathy (HMSN) type I; ×210. (A) NADH–TR. (B) Myosin ATPase, pH 9·4, the activity of this enzyme is uniform in the grouped atrophic fibres. The mosaic pattern at the right side clearly shows that there is overlap between the motor units. There are a few type 1 fibres with target structures (arrow). (C) H&E. Distribution criteria, stage 3 (see text)

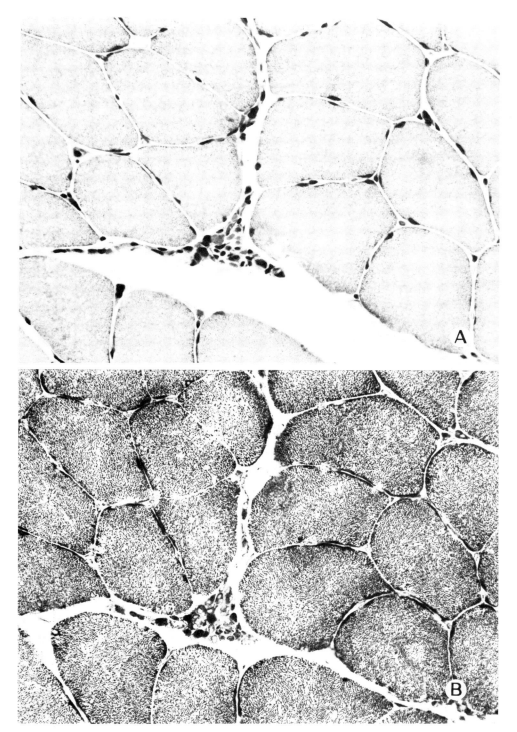

Fig. 16.6 Serial sections showing a group of atrophic fibres in between fascicles composed of large fibres. There is no indication of overlap between the motor units. Disseminated atrophy is lacking and large fibres are histochemically uniform, Kugelberg–Welander disease; ×315. (A) H&E. (B) NADH–TR. Distribution criteria, stage 4 (see text)

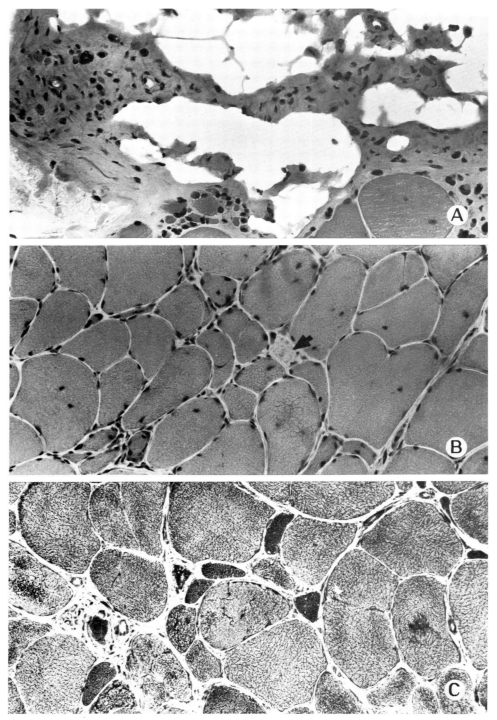

Fig. 16.7 Chronic neurogenic muscular atrophy in a case of progressive spinal muscular atrophy. Fields from different sections of one biopsy are shown. (A) H&E; most muscle fibres are extremely atrophic. Connective tissue and fat tissue have proliferated; ×210. (B) H&E; a number of large fibres have been preserved in one part of the biopsy. Note the variation in fibre size, the frequency of internal nuclei, irregularities in the internal structure of some fibres and the remnants of a necrotic fibre (arrow); ×210. See also Figure 16.8D. (C) NADH–TR; there is no mosaic pattern. Activity is higher in small fibres than in large fibres. Enzyme activity is distributed irregularly in some of the large fibres; ×175. Distribution criteria, stage 5 (see text)

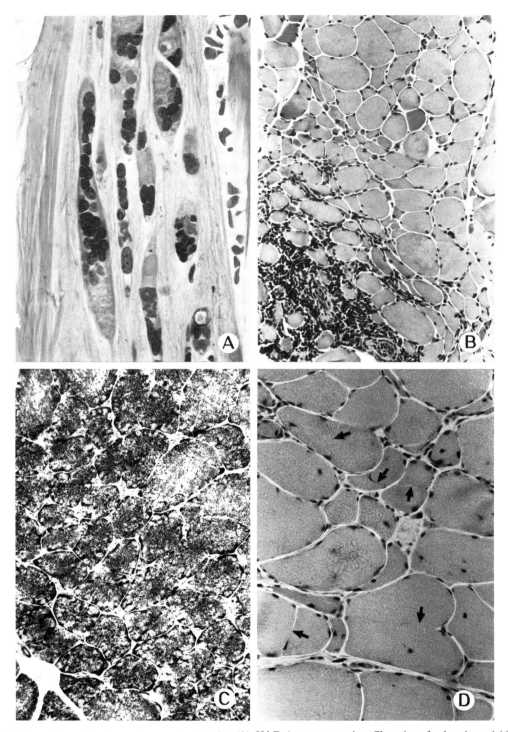

Fig. 16.8   Various changes in neurogenic muscular atrophy. (A) H&E; 1μm epon section. Clumping of pyknotic nuclei in atrophic fibres, progressive spinal muscular atrophy; ×560. (B) Inflammatory cellular infiltrate, amyotrophic lateral sclerosis; ×80. (C) NADH–TR; re-innervated fibres with 'moth-eaten' appearance, following a peripheral nerve lesion; ×245. (D) H&E; same section as in Figure 16.7B. Varying degrees of fibre splitting (arrows); ×210

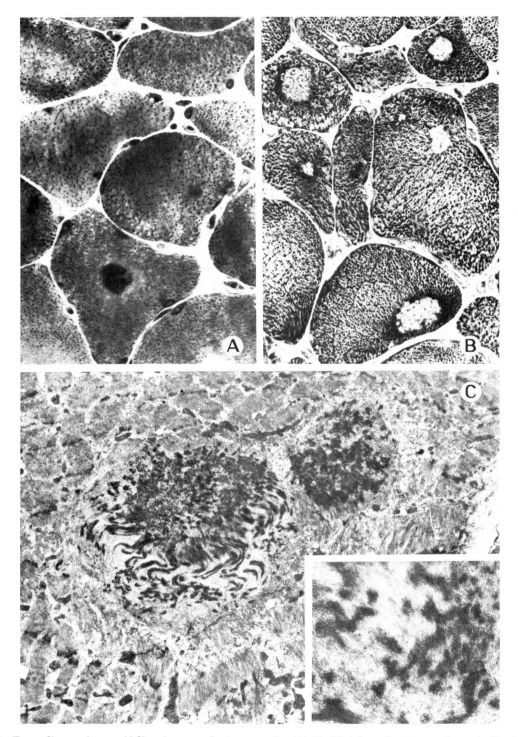

Fig. 16.9   Target fibres and targetoid fibres in a case of polyneuropathy. (A) Modified Gomori trichrome. A muscle fibre located in the lower half of the picture shows a dark (red) spot encompassed by a more lightly stained ring; ×420. (B) NADH–TR; there are round zones devoid of enzyme activity in several fibres; some of these zones are encompassed by a ring of high enzyme activity. (C) Electron micrograph; two targetoid structures in one muscle fibre. No ring-like intermediate zone is discernible; ×7000. Inset: dense filamentous material packed together in the targetoid structure. There are no mitochondria in this zone; ×24 500

sionally and may, to some extent, obscure the typical neurogenic nature of the muscle changes.

Cellular reactions

Inflammatory cell reactions, mainly of lymphocytes and macrophages, are occasionally seen between muscle fibres or perivascularly (Fig. 16.8). These infiltrates are usually small. The significance of this phenomenon is not known. It may be entirely secondary to the pathological changes in the muscle fibres. Whether the infiltrates are in turn harmful to muscle fibres and responsible for some of the degenerative changes is a matter for speculation.

In cases of advanced neurogenic atrophy, a variable degree of proliferation of connective tissue and fat tissue may be observed.

Histochemical criteria

Histochemistry of atrophic fibres

The histochemical type of the atrophic fibres can be established accurately by examination of the myosin ATPase activity (Fig. 16.3). This method may fail, however, in the end stage of fibre atrophy. The activity of aerobic enzymes may be increased in fibres of all types. Phosphorylase activity is decreased and may be absent. An increase of acid phosphatase often cannot be detected by conventional histochemical techniques, probably because of leakage of the enzyme into the incubation medium (Meijer 1978). The glycogen content decreases but neutral fat remains within the normal range.

Histochemistry of non-atrophic fibres

Target fibres are easy to recognize because of the lack of activity of myosin ATPase and aerobic enzymes in their central zone (Fig. 16.9). These enzymes may demonstrate increased activity in the ring-like areas around the central zone. In neurogenic muscle disease, targets occur most frequently in type 1 fibres. Low aerobic enzyme activity is also seen in targetoid structures. Irregular patches of low ('moth-eaten' fibres) or high ('lobulated' fibres) activity of aerobic enzymes may be present

in varying numbers of fibres in some specimens (Fig. 16.8). Fibre splitting is seen mostly in type 1 fibres.

Fibre type grouping

Re-innervation may replace the normal mosaic pattern of types 1 and 2 fibres by groups of histochemically uniform fibres of normal size. Histochemical staining for enzymes is required to detect this change. The presence of large groups of both fibre types is an unmistakable and diagnostic sign of a neurogenic muscular disorder. It may not be easy to distinguish small histochemically uniform groups from normal variations in fibre type distribution in an essentially mosaic pattern. It is in these cases that it is useful to count 'enclosed fibres'. By definition, fibres are enclosed when they are surrounded on all sides by members of their own histochemical type (Jennekens et al 1971). As in transverse section most fibres have six sides, seven fibres are in general required for one fibre to be enclosed (Fig. 16.10). The number of enclosed fibres of one type normally depends on the percentage of fibres of this type in a given population. Johnson et al (1973) calculated the expected number of enclosed fibres for different proportions of fibre types, assuming that the arrangement of the individual fibres was random and confined to a hexagonal lattice (Table 16.1). They compared the actual number of enclosed fibres in a sample of 200 fibres in 36 muscles from six young men, with the expected numbers as calculated in the theoretical model. Only in some distal limb muscles did they find the numbers of enclosed fibres to be frequently higher than expected. These muscles are known to be subject to processes of denervation and reinnervation from an early age in otherwise normal individuals (Jennekens et al 1972). Grouping of only one fibre type because of reinnervation may occur occasionally but must be distinguished from fibre type predominance. It may be helpful in these cases to note the fibre type occurring least frequently. According to the theoretical model, the number of enclosed fibres of any one type is almost negligible if the percentage of fibres of similar type in the population is 40 or less. Even a few enclosed fibres of the minority type may then

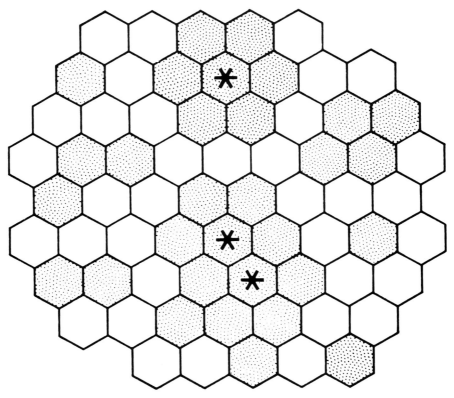

Fig. 16.10 Diagram of a skeletal muscle cross-section. Muscle fibres are often hexagonal and are represented as such. 'Enclosed fibres' (asterisks) are those that are surrounded on all sides by fibres of their own histochemical type. (From Johnson et al 1973)

Table 16.1 The relationship between the observed number of muscle fibres of a particular type and the expected number of 'enclosed' fibres of the same type*. (From Johnson et al 1973)

Number of fibres of a particular fibre type observed	Number of 'enclosed' fibres of that type expected	99.9% Confidence limits
0	0.0	0.0
20	0.0	0.0
40	0.0	0.3
60	0.0	0.7
80	0.3	2.0
100	1.6	4.0
120	5.6	7.6
140	16.5	12.5
160	41.9	18.4
170	64.1	20.7
180	95.7	22.1
190	139.7	20.1
195	167.5	16.1
200	200.0	0.0

*Based on the assumption that the muscle fibres are hexagonal and that the fibres of each type are arranged randomly.

be considered to be indicative of re-innervation. In chronic neurogenic disorders all non-atrophic fibres may eventually become histochemically uniform. A number of other methods for analysis of fibre type distribution have been developed for which the interested reader is referred to the literature (James 1972, Rouques et al 1973, Lexell et al 1983, Lester et al 1983, Howel & Brunsdon 1987, Venema 1988; see also for review Lexell et al 1987).

Small groups of fibres of one type due either to fibre splitting or to degeneration followed by reinnervation must be differentiated from type groups attributable to re-innervation.

MUSCLE PATHOLOGY IN HUMAN DENERVATING DISEASES

The main factor determining the differences in muscle pathology between the various denervating disorders is the time course. Chronic or long-standing disorders offer more opportunity for re-innervation and for the development of structural and degenerative changes than those that are rapidly progressive. Another factor is the time of onset. Denervating diseases affecting the muscle tissue in the neonatal period result in a number of characteristic changes that do not occur in children and adults.

Taking into account the factors just mentioned, we shall first discuss neurogenic muscular atrophy due to rapidly or gradually progressive and chronic denervating diseases, and subsequently consider a number of other forms of neurogenic muscular atrophy.

Rapidly or gradually progressive denervating diseases

Neurogenic muscular atrophy of this type may result from a large number of disorders, for example motor neurone disease and poliomyelitis, inflammatory, metabolic, toxic and ischaemic polyneuropathies and multiple neuropathies, and mononeuropathies caused by compression or traumatic injury. The bulk of the literature has concentrated on the muscle changes in motor neurone disease (MND).

The actual pathological picture in these diseases depends upon the degree of involvement of the LMN and on the time between the onset of the disease and the biopsy. Disseminated atrophy with a variable number of angulated and elongated fibres is seen in the initial stages (distribution criteria stage 1, see p. 574; Fig. 16.3). Atrophy of the type 2 fibres may be more advanced because, in general, these are known to react more rapidly to denervation than type 1 fibres. When the muscle biopsy is taken at a later stage and when the disease has evolved rapidly, the main pathological feature will be the large numbers of atrophic fibres (distribution criteria stage 2, see p. 574; Fig. 16.4). Atrophy of individual fibres will vary from a slight reduction in size to loss of most sarcoplasmic constituents leaving little more than clumps of pyknotic nuclei. Type grouping is usually observed but the number of fibres in the groups is limited. Some of the innervated fibres (usually type 1) may be hypertrophic (Dubowitz & Brooke 1973). Targets and targetoids may be present in a few fibres. Fibres with internal nuclei occur with greater frequency than in normal biopsies. Structural and degenerative changes are present in many biopsies but only in a few fibres (Mumenthaler 1970, Mastaglia & Walton 1971a). Focal, interstitial inflammatory cell infiltrates are seen in a few cases (Mumenthaler 1970, Adams 1975). Usually the infiltrates are small. They may be associated with necrotic fibres or with fibres undergoing phagocytosis.

When the disease has followed a slower progression, scattered fibre atrophy is a less dominant feature. Groups of atrophic fibres and type groups are present which may comprise many fibres (distribution criteria stage 3, see p. 577; Fig. 16.5). Hypertrophy may be seen among the non-atrophic fibres. The hypertrophic fibres belong to types 1 and 2 (Brooke & Engel 1969b, Dubowitz & Brooke 1973). Target and targetoid fibres are often absent but occasionally they are numerous. Internal nuclei may be noted frequently in the surviving fibres. Changes in fibre structure and degenerative changes are present in some cases, probably more frequently than in the rapidly progressive cases. The same holds for 'moth-eaten' and 'lobulated' fibres. In a group of 111 MND cases of mean duration 2.3–2.6 years, Achari & Anderson (1974) observed inflammatory cell infiltrates in 10% of the biopsies.

Ultrastructural findings closely resemble those seen in experimental denervation atrophy (Afifi et al 1966, Shafiq et al 1967).

Chronic or long-standing neurogenic muscular atrophy

This form of denervation atrophy is by no means rare: it occurs in the various types of hereditary motor and sensory neuropathy, in type II (chronic or benign infantile) and type III (Kugelberg–Welander disease) SMA, in some cases of progressive spinal muscular atrophy, and as a natural ageing phenomenon in some distal limb muscles of otherwise healthy people (Jennekens et al 1971). The muscle pathology differs in degree only, and not in any essential aspect, from that in gradually progressive cases.

According to the previously defined distribution criteria, neurogenic muscular atrophy has reached stage 4 or stage 5 (see p. 577; Figs 16.6 and 16.7). Atrophic and non-atrophic fibres are arranged in groups. Fibres in atrophic groups may have acquired a rounded shape (van Wijngaarden & Bethlem 1973). The fibres in these groups usually belong to one histochemical type but it is not always possible to establish this accurately. Frequently the atrophic groups are located at the edges of fascicles (Mastaglia & Walton 1971a). Non-atrophic fibres are also grouped according to histochemical type. Often, they are all histochemically uniform, at least as far as their myosin ATPase activity is concerned. In these cases, some of the fibres with low myosin ATPase activity (type 1 fibres) may show a high activity of enzymes involved in glycolytic metabolism.

Although no strict relationship with the duration of the disease has been demonstrated, structural and degenerative changes are in general most frequent in the chronic or long-standing forms of neurogenic muscular atrophy. To some extent, the real nature of the muscular atrophy may be obscured by these phenomena. When the surviving groups have become reduced, as in stage 5, fibre splitting may increase the number of small fibres in these groups.

Internalization of myonuclei, myofibrillar disorganization and irregular distribution of aerobic enzyme activity are all present with variable frequency. Target and targetoid fibres occur in a minority of the biopsies. Fibre necrosis and phagocytosis are not exceptional; fibre regeneration is observed with approximately the same frequency as fibre necrosis (Mastaglia & Walton 1971a, van Wijngaarden & Bethlem 1973). Inflammatory cell reaction is seen in a few cases, the infiltrates usually being small. Connective tissue and fat tissue proliferate.

Ultrastructural studies of chronic denervating disorders have not revealed any specific features (Roth et al 1965, Mastaglia & Walton 1971b).

Exceptional forms of neurogenic muscular atrophy

Arthrogryposis multiplex congenita due to anterior horn cell dysgenesis or degeneration (AHCD)

The term arthrogryposis multiplex congenita is used for a syndrome characterized by multiple congenital contractures. The contractures are attributable to immobilization of the limbs in the fetal period after the joints have been formed (Banker 1985). In the large majority of the cases the condition is sporadic (see however Fleury & Hageman 1985) and associated with a number of other congenital anomalies (Hall et al 1983). The immobilization of the limbs is either due to a disorder of the developing motor system or to inadequacy of the environment leading to mechanical restriction. Among the disorders of the motor system are congenital myopathies, congenital myasthenia, AHCD and central nervous system (brain or brain and spinal cord) dysgenesis. AHCD is probably the most common cause of multiple congenital contractures.

The changes of the skeletal muscles in AHCD differ in several respects from those in Werdnig–Hoffmann's disease (see below). The most striking feature is the replacement of whole muscles, fascicles, or parts of fascicles by fat tissue (Banker 1986a,b). The muscle fibres, such as are present may be entirely normal and may show a perfect mosaic pattern of type 1 and 2 fibres or, less often, there may be fibre type predominance or grouping. In exceptional cases the distinction from infantile spinal muscular atrophy may be difficult but will be possible when attention is given to the replacement of parts of fascicles by fat tissue.

The pathogenetic mechanisms underlying AHCD have not yet been established. Most authors believe however that the cause is in the spinal cord (Clarren & Hall 1983, Banker 1986a, Hageman et al 1988). The observations of Banker (1985) in a child with a spinal cord terminating at the T 12 segment are in this regard of interest. In the lower limbs of this child the typical picture of 'amyoplasia congenita' was observed with fat tissue replacing muscle as described in the foregoing. The case demonstrates that a primary spinal cord lesion can indeed produce the changes in the musculature which are seen in AHCD. Clarren & Hall (1983) examined the spinal cord in cases of AHCD and reported that the numbers of alpha motor neurons were reduced.

Spinal muscular atrophy (SMA) type I or Werdnig–Hoffmann disease

Two types of infantile spinal muscular atrophy must be distinguished (Emery 1971). The onset of the first type usually stems from the neonatal or intrauterine period. Mothers questioned about fetal movements acknowledge in one-third of the cases that these have weakened during the later months of pregnancy (Pearn 1973). The symptoms are always manifest by 3–6 months of age (Pearn et al 1973), by which time the musculature is already weak or very weak, the lower limbs being affected more severely. In type II SMA, weakness may also be present in the neonatal period, but in most children the disease becomes noticeable between 6–12 months of age.

Although acute and severe infantile SMA has often been considered to be a pure lower motor neurone disease, histopathological studies of biopsy and necropsy material have shown that the nerve fibres of the peripheral sensory neurones are not entirely free of change (Chou & Nonaka 1978). Abnormalities of the CNS have been reported, and it has been suggested that these are particularly likely to be present in the most rapidly progressive cases, which succumb within the first year of life (Nieves & Castello 1970). The cause of the LMN

degeneration is not known but several hypotheses have been proposed; these include proximal axonopathy (Hogenhuis et al 1967), radicular compression by glial bundles invading the anterior roots and to a lesser degree the posterior roots (Chou & Fakaday 1971), defective synaptogenesis in motor neurones (Chou et al 1979), and a functional defect of Schwann cells during early development (Ohama & Ikuta 1979). Whatever the cause, investigations at necropsy have shown that the number of anterior horn cells is markedly reduced, and that the cells which are still present are shrunken or chromatolytic (Chou & Fakaday 1971). According to Coërs et al (1973), the loss of motor neurones is accompanied by sprouting of remaining intramuscular nerves.

Muscle biopsies show fascicles composed of small fibres and a scattering of strikingly large fibres (Fig. 16.11). The small fibres are polygonal or round, and are differentiated into two fibre types, which demonstrates that they have been innervated. The large fibres are round, occur either singly or in small groups, and according to their myosin ATPase activity, are nearly always of type 1. The large fibres are innervated or re-innervated, their hypertrophy being a compensatory phenomenon (Dubowitz & Brooke 1973). Estimations of aerobic and glycolytic metabolism in these fibres may indicate high or low levels of either pathway. In some hypertrophic fibres both NADH–TR and phosphorylase or menadione-linked α-GPD show high activity, while myosin ATPase activity is low (Dubowitz 1966). According to Fenichel & Engel (1963) who performed quantitative studies on muscle biopsies from infantile spinal muscular atrophy patients, the hypertrophic fibres may measure up to 80 μm. When compared with fibre size in control material, type 1 fibres are more atrophic than type 2 fibres (Fenichel & Engel 1963). Many of the light microscopic changes found in other denervating diseases, are slight or absent in acute and severe infantile SMA. There is no clumping of muscle nuclei in the small fibres and there are no targets or targetoids.

Studies of the ultrastructure of skeletal muscle in this disease did reveal features characteristic of denervation atrophy (Fig. 16.12A) (Shafiq et al 1967, Hughes & Brownell 1969, Roy et al 1971). Two authors reported an increase in the number

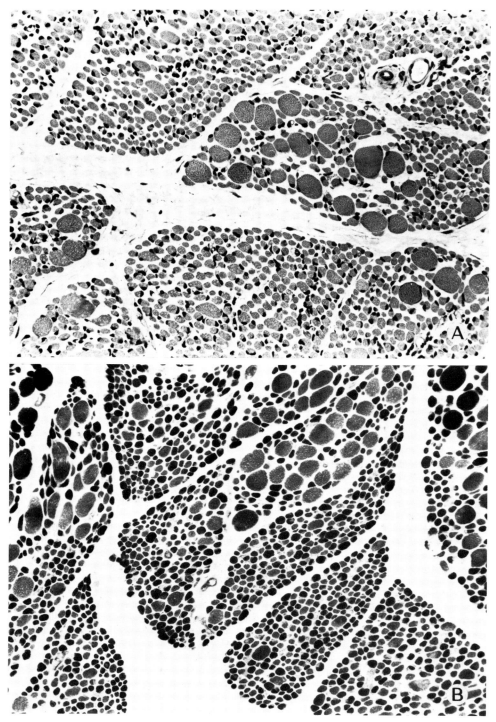

Fig. 16.11 Werdnig–Hoffmann disease. Large groups of small fibres and small groups of large fibres; ×210. (A) H&E. (B) Myosin ATPase, pH 9.4; small fibres are either type 1 or type 2; most·large fibres are of type 1

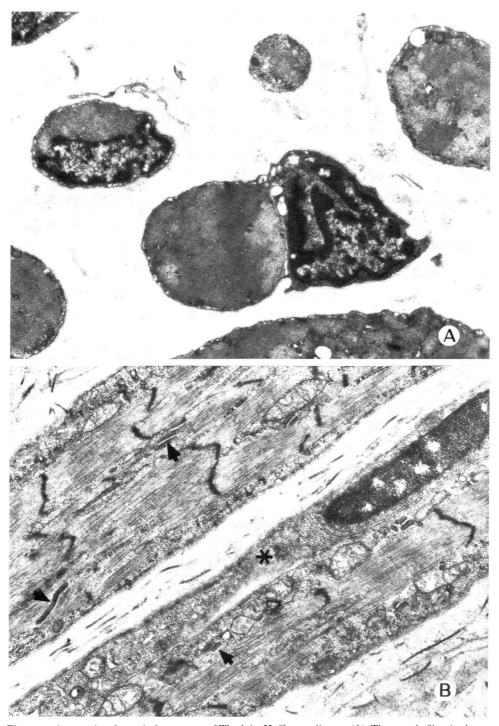

Fig. 16.12 Electron micrographs of muscle from a case of Werdnig–Hoffmann disease. (A) The muscle fibre in the centre of the picture contains a satellite cell; the nucleus of this cell is shaped irregularly. In the upper half of the picture a small fibre (diameter 1 μm) is present. The basal lamina of this fibre shows many loose foldings; ×14 000. (B) Two longitudinally cut muscle fibres, one containing a satellite cell (asterisk) with many organelles. The internal structure of the fibres shows evidence of disorganization, i.e. streaming of Z discs, disruption of sarcomeres, triads (arrows) frequently orientated longitudinally; ×18 200

of satellite cells, many of which contained abundant cytoplasm with numerous organelles (Fig. 16.12B) (van Haelst 1970, Fidziánska 1974). In two biopsies from children with acute infantile SMA aged 5 months and 3 months respectively, we counted 25 and 35 nuclei of satellite cells per 200 muscle nuclei. In a control biopsy from a child aged 8 days, 15 satellite cell nuclei per 200 muscle nuclei were counted (Jennekens & Veldman, unpublished observation). Hausma-nowa–Petrusewicz et al (1975) and Fidziánska (1974, 1976) contend that maturation of muscle fibres in Werdnig–Hoffmann disease is retarded by a fetal defect in innervation. This would explain the presence of fetal-like muscle fibres with round shape (in transverse sections), extremely small diameter, single nucleus, and normal architecture, of myoblast-like cells (Shafiq et al 1967) and small fibres containing two or three unfused cells within one basal lamina. The pattern of myosin isoform expression in Werdnig–Hoffmann disease is not however in support of a maturational arrest

(Sawchak et al 1990). Only a low percentage of small fibres express myosin heavy chain isoforms of prenatal type and these fibres may be regenerating and derived from satellite cells (Schiaffino et al 1988). The observation of Schultz (1978) on experimentally denervated growing muscle supports this suggestion.

Spinal muscular atrophy types II and III

Neurogenic atrophy in the intermediate form of SMA (type II) cannot be distinguished from that in type I. The characteristics of type III (Kugelberg–Welander) SMA have been delineated in the section on chronic denervating disease. One single point deserves attention here. Hausmanowa-Petrusewicz et al (1980) advocate that a fetal defect in innervation is also involved in Kugelberg–Welander disease and is responsible for the very small round muscle fibres of normal architecture which are also seen in SMA type III though much less frequently than in SMA type I.

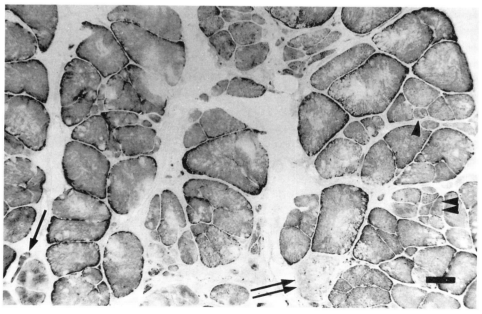

Fig. 16.13 Post-poliomyelitis muscular atrophy. Transverse cryostat section. Succinic dehydrogenase. Bar = 100 μm. All muscle fibres belong to the same histochemical type and show irregular distribution of mitochondrial enzyme activity. Atrophic fibres are often due to fibre splitting and are lying in small groups (double arrowhead) or isolated (arrowhead) in between fibres of normal size. Other atrophic fibres are not obviously related to fibre splitting and are probably denervated (arrow). One fibre has largely lost its enzyme activity, which is compatible with necrosis (double arrow).

Denervation in myasthenia gravis

Block of neuromuscular transmission may result in functional — and in the long run histological — denervation. Denervation is due to a postsynaptic process and is accompanied by enlargement of end-plates and sprouting of intramuscular nerve fibres. Denervation does not involve 'whole motor units' as in most neurogenic disorders but muscle fibres within motor units. Histologically, the condition is characterized by disseminated muscular atrophy, with angulated and elongated fibres without grouping of histochemically uniform fibres. Severe muscular atrophy in myasthenia gravis has been observed notably in tongue and extra-ocular muscles (Oosterhuis & Bethlem 1973, Hoogenraad et al 1978, Oosterhuis 1984). Denervation in myasthenia gravis resembles electromyographically a myopathic condition (affliction of some muscle fibres of motor units, not accompanied by re-innervation).

Post-poliomyelitis muscular atrophy

Following partial or complete recovery from poliomyelitis, slowly progressive muscular weakness may develop after periods of clinical stability varying from 20 to 40 years (Mulder et al 1972, Cashman et al 1987, Klingman et al 1988). Biopsies from previously not clinically involved, or clinically recovered newly affected muscles, show type grouping and disseminated muscle fibre atrophy of neurogenic type (Fig. 16.13). This form of atrophy has been hypothesized to be the outcome of degeneration of single nerve terminals. The initial recovery from partial denervation after the attack of poliomyelitis is effected by sprouting of intact intramuscular nerve fibres and re-innervation. Muscle fibres which survive belong to type groups and remnants of denervated fibres disappear. The metabolic demands of the enlarged motor units are thought to overstrain gradually the capacity of the motor neurone cell bodies which are not able to maintain the increased number of sprouts. This might be the cause of slowly progressive deterioration and death of some nerve terminals with disseminated atrophy of muscle fibres (Weichers and Hubbell 1981, Dalakas et al 1986).

ACKNOWLEDGEMENTS

The author is grateful to Dr A. Jennekens-Schinkel, for helpful discussions and for reading the manuscript. The figures were prepared by Mr H. Veldman.

REFERENCES

Achari A N, Anderson M S 1974 Myopathic changes in amyotrophic lateral sclerosis. Neurology (Minneapolis) 24: 477

Adams R D 1975 Diseases of muscle. A study in pathology, 3rd edn. Harper & Row, Hagerstown, p 114, 419

Afifi A K, Aleu F P, Goodgold J, MacKay B 1966 Ultrastructure of atrophic muscle in amyotrophic lateral sclerosis. Neurology (Minneapolis) 16: 475

Aloisi M, Mussini I, Schiaffino S 1973 Activation of muscle nuclei in denervation and hypertrophy. In: Kakulas B A (ed) Basic research in myology. Excerpta Medica, Amsterdam, p 338

Askanas V, Engel W K 1975 Distinct subtypes of type I fibers of human skeletal muscle. Neurology (Minneapolis) 25: 879

Askmark H, Gilberg P G, Aquilonius S M 1985 Autoradiographic visualization of extrajunctional acetylcholine receptors in whole human biceps brachii muscle. Changes in amyotrophic lateral sclerosis. Acta Neurologica Scandinavica 72: 344

Bajusz E 1964 'Red' skeletal muscle fibres: relative independence of neural control. Science 145: 938

Banker B 1985 Neuropathologic aspects of arthrogryposis multiplex congenita. Clinical Orthopaedics 194: 30

Banker B Q 1986a Arthrogryposis multiplex congenita. Human Pathology 17: 656

Banker B Q 1986b Congenital deformities. In: Engel A G, Banker B Q (eds) Myology. McGraw Hill, New York, p 2109

Bennett M R, Raftos J 1977 The formation and regression of synapses during the re-innervation of axolotl striated muscles. Journal of Physiology 265: 261

Bennett M R, McLachlan E M, Taylor R S 1973 The formation of synapses in reinnervated mammalian striated muscle. Journal of Physiology 233: 481

Birks R, Katz B, Miledi R 1960 Physiological and structural changes at the amphibian myoneural junction in the course of nerve degeneration. Journal of Physiology 150: 145

Booth F W 1977 Time course of muscular atrophy during immobilization of hind limbs in rats. Journal of Applied Physiology 43: 656

Bowden R E M, Duchen L W 1976 The anatomy and pathology of the neuromuscular junction. In: Zaimis E (ed) Neuromuscular junction. Handbook of experimental pharmacology 42. Springer, Berlin, p 23

Bradley W 1979 Muscle fiber splitting. In: Mauro A (ed) Muscle regeneration. Raven, New York, p 215

Brooke M H, Engel W K 1969a The histographic analysis of

human muscle biopsies with regard to fiber types. 1. Adult male and female. Neurology (Minneapolis) 19: 221

Brooke M H, Engel W K 1969b The histographic analysis of human muscle biopsies with regard to fiber types. 2. Diseases of the upper and lower motor neuron. Neurology (Minneapolis) 19: 378

Brown M C 1984 Sprouting of motor nerves in adult muscles: a recapitulation of ontogeny. Trends in Neuroscience 7: 10

Brown M C, Lunn E R 1988 Mechanism of interaction between motoneurons and muscle. In: Evered D, Whelan J (eds) Plasticity of the neuromuscular system. John Wiley, Chichester, p 78

Buchthal F, Schmalbruch H 1970 Contraction times and fibre types in intact human muscles. Acta physiologica scandinavica 79: 435

Buller A J, Eccles J C, Eccles R M 1960 Interactions between motor neurones and muscles in respect to the characteristic speeds of their responses. Journal of Physiology 150: 417

Burke R E, Levine D M, Zajac F E, Tsaris P, Engel W K 1971 Mammalian motor units: physiologic–histochemical correlation in three fibre types in cat gastrocnemius. Science 174: 709

Carpenter S, Karpati G 1982 Necrosis of capillaries in denervation atrophy of skeletal muscle. Muscle and Nerve 5: 250

Cashman N R, Maselli R, Wollmann R L, Roos R, Simon R, Antel J P 1987 Late denervation in patients with antecedent paralytic poliomyelitis. New England Journal of Medicine 317: 7

Chou S M, Fakaday A V 1971 Ultrastructure of chromatolytic motoneurons and anterior spinal roots in a case of Werdnig-Hoffmann disease. Journal of Neuropathology and Experimental Neurology 30: 368

Chou S M, Nonaka I 1978 Werdnig-Hoffmann disease: proposal of a pathogenetic mechanism. Acta neuropathologica (Berlin) 41: 45

Chou S M, Miike T, Davis G J 1979 Experimental induction of Werdnig-Hoffmann-type neuroglial peninsulas by prenatal PCB intoxication. In: Tsubaki T, Toyokura Y (eds) Amyotrophic lateral sclerosis. University Park, Baltimore, p 239

Clarren S K, Hall J G 1983 Neuropathologic findings in the spinal cords of 10 infants with arthrogryposis. Journal of Neurological Science 58: 89

Cullen M J, Pluskal M G 1977 Early changes in the ultrastructure of denervated rat skeletal muscle. Experimental Neurology 56: 115

Cullen M J, Harris J B, Marshall M W, Ward M R 1975 An electrophysiological and morphological study of normal and denervated chicken latissimus dorsi muscles. Journal of Physiology 245: 371

Dalakas M C, Elder G, Hallet M, Ravits J, Papadopoulos N, Albrecht P, Sever J 1986 A long-term follow up study of patients with post-poliomyelitis neuromuscular symptoms. New England Journal of Medicine 314: 959

Dayton W R, Goll D E, Stromer M H, Reville W J, Zeece M G, Robson R M 1975 Some properties of a Ca^{2+}-activated protease that may be involved in myofibrillar protein turnover. In: Reich E, Rifkin D B, Shaw E (eds) Proteases and biological control. Cold Spring Harbor, New York, p 551

De Coster W, De Reuck J, Van der Eecken H 1976 The target phenomenon in human muscle. A comparative light microscopic, histochemical and electron microscopic study. Acta neuropathologica (Berlin) 34: 329

De Reuck J, De Coster W, Van der Eecken H 1977a The target phenomenon in rat muscle following tenotomy and neurotomy. A comparative light microscopic and histochemical study. Acta neuropathologica (Berlin) 37: 49

De Reuck J, De Coster W, Van der Eecken H 1977b Development and inhibition of the target phenomenon in tenotomized rat muscle. Acta neuropathologica (Berlin) 40: 179

Drachman D B, Murphy S R, Nigam M P, Hills J R 1967 'Myopathic' changes in chronically denervated muscle. Archives of Neurology (Chicago) 16: 14

Dubowitz V 1966 Enzyme histochemistry of skeletal muscle. 3. Neurogenic muscular atrophies. Journal of Neurology, Neurosurgery and Psychiatry 29: 23

Dubowitz V 1967 Pathology of experimentally re-innervated skeletal muscle. Journal of Neurology, Neurosurgery and Psychiatry 30: 99

Dubowitz V 1968 The floppy infant. Clinics in developmental medicine 31. Spastics International in association with Heinemann, London

Dubowitz V, Brooke M H 1973 Muscle biopsy: a modern approach. Saunders, London

Edds M V Jr 1953 Collateral nerve regeneration. Quarterly Review of Biology 28: 260

Edds M V Jr 1955 Collateral regeneration in partially denervated muscles of the rat. Journal of Experimental Zoology 129: 2

Edström L, Kugelberg E 1968 Histochemical composition, distribution of fibres and fatiguability of single motor units. Anterior tibial muscle of the rat. Journal of Neurology, Neurosurgery and Psychiatry 31: 424

Edwards C 1979 The effect of innervation on the properties of acetylcholine receptors in muscle. Neuroscience 4: 565

Ellisman M H, Rash J E 1977 Studies of excitable membranes 3. Freeze-fracture examination of the membrane specializations at the neuromuscular junction and in the non-junctional sarcolemma after denervation. Brain Research 137: 197

Emery A E H 1971 The nosology of the spinal muscular atrophies. Journal of Medical Genetics 8: 481

Engel W K, 1961 Muscle target fibers, a newly recognized sign of denervation. Nature 191: 389

Engel W K, Brooke M H, Nelson P G 1966 Histochemical studies of denervated or tenotomized cat muscle: illustrating difficulties in relating experimental animal conditions to human neuromuscular diseases. Annals of the New York Academy of Sciences 138: 160

Ernfors P, Henschen A, Olsen L, Persson H 1989 Expression of nerve growth factor receptor messenger RNA is developmentally regulated and increased after axotomy in rat spinal cord motoneurons. Neuron 2: 1605

Fallon J R, Gelfman C E 1989 Agrin-related molecules are concentrated at acetylcholine receptor clusters in normal and aneural developing muscle. Journal of Cell Biology 108: 1527

Fenichel G M, Engel W K 1963 Histochemistry of muscle in infantile spinal muscular atrophy. Neurology (Minneapolis) 13: 1059

Fidziánska A 1974 Ultrastructural changes in muscle in spinal muscular atrophy — Werdnig-Hoffmann's disease. Acta neuropathologica (Berlin) 27: 247

Fidziánska A 1976 Morphological differences between the atrophied small muscle fibres in amyotrophic lateral sclerosis and Werdnig-Hoffmann disease. Acta neuropathologica (Berlin) 34: 321

Fleury P, Hageman G 1985 A dominantly inherited lower

motor neuron disorder presenting at birth with associated arthrogryposis. Journal of Neurology Neurosurgery and Psychiatry 48: 1037

Frank E, Jansen J K S, Lömo T, Westgaard R H 1975 The interaction between foreign and original nerves innervating the soleus muscles of rats. Journal of Physiology 247: 725

Gauthier G F, Dunn R A 1973 Ultrastructural and cytochemical features of mammalian skeletal muscle fibres following denervation. Journal of Cell Science 12: 525

Gauthier G F, Schaeffer S F 1974 Ultrastructural and cytochemical manifestations of protein synthesis in the peripheral sarcoplasm of denervated and newborn skeletal muscle fibres. Journal of Cell Science 14: 113

Glicksman M A, Sanes J A 1983 Differentiation of motor nerve terminals formed in the absence of muscle fibres. Journal of Neurocytology 12: 661

Goldberg A L, DeMartino G N, Libby P 1979 Influence of thyroid hormones and protease-inhibitors on protein degradation in skeletal muscle. In: Aguayo A J, Karpati G (eds) Current topics in nerve and muscle research. Excerpta Medica International Congress Series 455, Amsterdam, p 53

Goldspink D F 1977 The influence of immobilization and stretch on protein turnover of rat skeletal muscle. Journal of Physiology 264: 267

Goldspink D F 1978 The influence of passive stretch on the growth and protein turnover of the denervated extensor digitorum longus muscle. Biochemical Journal 174: 595

Gori A 1972 Proliferations of the sarcoplasmic reticulum and the T system in denervated muscle fibres. Virchows Archiv; Abteilung B: Zellpathologie 11: 147

Grimby L, Hannerz J 1977 Firing rate and recruitment order of toe extensor motor units in different modes of voluntary contraction. Journal of Physiology 264: 865

Grimby L, Hannerz J, Hedman B 1979 Contraction time and voluntary discharge properties of individual short toe extensor motor units in man. Journal of Physiology 289: 191

Gutmann E, Schiaffino S, Hanzlikova V 1971 Mechanism of compensatory hypertrophy in skeletal muscles of the rat. Experimental Neurology 31: 451

Hageman G, Ippel P F, Beemer F A, DePater J M, Lindhout D, Willemse J 1988 The diagnostic management of newborns with congenital contractures. American Journal of Medical Genetics 30: 883

Hall J G, Reed S D, Driscoll E P 1983 Amyoplasia: a common sporadic condition with congenital contractures. American Journal of Genetics 15: 571

Hall-Craggs E C B 1970 The longitudinal division of fibres in overloaded rat skeletal muscle. Journal of Anatomy 107: 459

Hall-Craggs E C B 1972 The significance of longitudinal fibre division in skeletal muscle. Journal of the Neurological Sciences 15: 27

Hannerz J 1974 Discharge properties of motor units in relation to recruitment order in voluntary contraction. Acta physiologica scandinavica 91: 374

Hausmanowa-Petrusewicz I, Fidzianska A, Dobosz I, Drac H, Rijniewicz B 1975 The focal character of the lesion in the acute form of Werdnig–Hoffmann disease. In: Bradley W G, Gardner-Medwin D, Walton J N (eds) Recent advances in myology. Excerpta Medica, Amsterdam, p 546

Hausmanowa-Petrusewicz I, Fidzianska A, Niebroj-Dobosz I, Strugalska M H 1980 Is Kugelberg–Welander spinal muscular atrophy a fetal defect. Muscle and Nerve 3: 389

Henderson C E 1988 The role of muscle in the development and differentiation of spinal motoneurons: in vitro studies. In: Evered D, Whelan J (eds) Plasticity of the neuromuscular system. John Wiley, Chichester, p 172

Hogenhuis L A, Engel W K 1965 Histochemistry and cytochemistry of experimentally denervated guinea pig muscle. 1. Histochemistry. Acta anatomica 60: 39

Hogenhuis L A H, Spaulding S W, Engel W K 1967 Neuronal RNA metabolism in infantile spinal muscular atrophy (Werdnig-Hoffmann's disease) studied by radioautography: a new technic in the investigation of neurological disease. Journal of Neuropathology and Experimental Neurology 26: 335

Holloszy J O, Booth F W 1976 Biochemical adaptations to endurance exercise in muscle. Annual Review of Physiology 38: 273

Hoogenraad Tj U, Jennekens F G I, Tan K E W P 1978 Ophthalmoplegia due to myasthenia gravis. Histological and histochemical observations in the inferior oblique muscle. Documenta Ophthalmologica Proceedings Series 17: 27

Hopkins D, Manchester K L, Gregory M 1983 Histochemical and biochemical characteristics of the transient hypertrophy of the denervated rat hemidiaphragm. Experimental Neurology 81: 279

Howel D and Brunsdon C 1987 A simple test for the random arrangement of muscle fibres. Journal of the Neurological Science 77: 49

Hughes J T, Brownell B 1969 Ultrastructure of muscle in Werdnig-Hoffmann disease. Journal of the Neurological Sciences 8: 363

Hynes R O, Yamada K M 1982 Fibronectins: multifunctional modular glycoproteins. Journal of Cell Biology 95: 369

James N T 1972 A quantitative study of the clumping of muscle fibre types in skeletal muscles. Journal of the Neurological Science 17: 41

Jaweed M M, Herbison G J, Ditunno J F 1975 Denervation and reinnervation of fast and slow muscles. A histochemical study in rats. Journal of Histochemistry and Cytochemistry 23: 808

Jay J C, Barald K F 1989 Denervated single myofibres: neurite interactions and synaptic molecules. Muscle and Nerve 12: 981

Jeffrey P L, Appel S H 1978 Denervation alterations in surface membrane glycoprotein glycosyltransferase of mammalian skeletal muscle. Experimental Neurology 61: 432

Jennekens F G I, Tomlinson B E, Walton J N 1971 Data on the distribution of fibre types in five human limb muscles. An autopsy study. Journal of the Neurological Sciences 14: 245

Jennekens F G I, Tomlinson B E, Walton J N 1972 The extensor digitorum brevis: histological and histochemical aspects. Journal of Neurology, Neurosurgery and Psychiatry 35: 124

Jennekens F G I, Meijer A E F H, Bethlem J, Van Wijngaarden G K 1974 Fibre hybrids in type groups. An investigation of human muscle biopsies. Journal of the Neurological Sciences 23: 337

Jirmanová I, Libelius R, Lundquist I, Thesleff S 1977 Protamine induced intracellular uptake of horseradish peroxidase and vacuolation in mouse skeletal muscle in vitro. Cell and Tissue Research 176: 463

Joffe M, Savage N, Isaacs H 1981 Biochemical functioning of mitochondria in normal and denervated mammalian skeletal muscle. Muscle and Nerve 4: 514

Johnson M A, Polgar J, Weightman D, Appleton D 1973 Data on the distribution of fibre types in 36 human muscles. An autopsy study. Journal of the Neurological Sciences 18: 111

Kar N C, Pearson C M 1977 Hydrolytic enzymes and human muscular dystrophy. In: Rowland L P (ed) Pathogenesis of human muscular dystrophies. Excerpta Medica International Congress Series 404, Amsterdam, p 387

Karpati G, Engel W K 1968a Correlative histochemical study of skeletal muscle after suprasegmental denervation, peripheral nerve section and skeletal fixation. Neurology (Minneapolis) 18: 681

Karpati G, Engel W K 1968b Histochemical investigation of fiber type ratios with myofibrillar ATPase reaction in normal and denervated skeletal muscles in guinea pig. American Journal of Anatomy 122: 145

Karpati G, Engel W K 1968c 'Type grouping' in skeletal muscles after experimental reinnervation. Neurology (Minneapolis) 18: 447

Karpati G, Eisen A W, Carpenter S 1975 Subtypes of the histochemical type I muscle fibres. Journal of Histochemistry and Cytochemistry 23: 89

Klingman J, Chui H, Corgiat M, Perry J 1988 Functional recovery. A major risk factor for the development of postpoliomyelitis muscular atrophy. Archives of Neurology 45: 645

Ko P K, Anderson M J, Cohen M W 1977 Denervated skeletal muscle fibres develop discrete patches of high acetylcholine receptor density. Science 196: 540

Kovarsky J, Schochet S S, McCormick W F 1973 The significance of target fibres: a clinico-pathologic review of 100 patients with neurogenic atrophy. American Journal of Clinical Pathology 59: 790

Kugelberg E 1973 Histochemical composition, contraction speed and fatiguability of rat soleus motor units. Journal of the Neurological Sciences 20: 177

Kugelberg E 1979 Anatomy and histochemistry of normal and reinnervated rat motor units: aspects of spinal muscular atrophy. In: Tsubaki T, Toyokura Y (eds) Amyotrophic lateral sclerosis. University Park, Baltimore, p 365

Kugelberg E, Edström L, Abbruzzese M 1970 Mapping of motor units in experimentally reinnervated rat muscle. Journal of Neurology, Neurosurgery and Psychiatry 33: 319

Lester J M, Silber D I, Cohen M H, Hirsch R P, Bradley W G, Brenner J F 1983 The co-dispersion index for the measurement of fiber type distribution patterns. Muscle and Nerve 6: 581

Letinsky M S, Fischbeck K H, McMahan U J 1976 Precision of reinnervation of original postsynaptic sites in frog muscle after a nerve crush. Journal of Neurocytology 5: 691

Levi-Montalcini R 1987 The nerve growth factor 35 years later. Science 237: 1154

Lexell J, Downham D, Sjöström M 1983 Distribution of different fibre types in human skeletal muscles. A statistical and computational model for the study of fibre type grouping and early diagnosis of skeletal muscle fibre denervation and reinnervation. Journal of the Neurological Sciences 6: 301

Lexell J, Downham D, Sjöström M 1987 Morphological detection of neurogenic muscle disorders: how can statistical methods aid diagnosis. Acta Neuropathologica (Berlin) 75: 109

Libelius R, Lundquist I, Thesleff S 1978a Endocytosis as inducer of degenerative conditions in skeletal muscle. Physiologia bohemoslovenica 27: 415

Libelius R, Lundquist I, Templeton W, Thesleff S 1978b Intracellular uptake and degradation of extracellular tracers in mouse skeletal muscle in vitro. The effect of denervation. Neuroscience 3: 641

Libelius R, Josefsson J-O, Lundquist I 1979 Endocytosis in chronically denervated mouse skeletal muscle. A biochemical and ultrastructural study with horseradish peroxidase. Neuroscience 4: 283

Lömo, T, Westgaard R H, Dahl H A 1974 Contractile properties of muscle: control by pattern of muscle activity in the rat. Proceedings of the Royal Society of London; B: Biological Sciences 187: 99

Lömo T, Westgaard R H, Engebretsen L 1980 Different stimulation patterns affect contractile properties of denervated rat soleus muscles. In: Pette D (ed) Plasticity of muscle. W de Gruyter, Berlin, p 297

McLaughlin J, Abood L G, Bosmann H B 1974 Early elevations of glycosidase, acid phosphatase and acid proteolytic enzyme activity in denervated skeletal muscle. Experimental Neurology 42: 541

McManaman J L, Crawford P G, Scott Stewart S, Appel S H 1988 Purification of a skeletal muscle polypeptide which stimulates choline acetyltransferase activity in cultured spinal cord neurons. Journal of Biological Chemistry 263: 5890

McManaman J L, Oppenheim R W, Prevette D, Marchetti D 1990 Rescue of motoneurons from cell death by a purified skeletal muscle polypeptide: effects of the ChAT development factor, CDF. Neuron 4: 891

Margreth A, Carraro V, Salviati G 1977 Effects of denervation on protein synthesis and on properties of myosin of fast and slow muscles. In: Rowland L P (ed) Pathogenesis of human muscular dystrophies. Excerpta Medica International Congress Series 404, Amsterdam, p 161

Mastaglia F L, Walton J N 1971a Histological and histochemical changes in the skeletal muscle from cases of chronic juvenile and early adult spinal muscular atrophy (the Kugelberg-Welander syndrome). Journal of the Neurological Sciences 12: 15

Mastaglia F L, Walton J N 1971b An electron microscopic study of skeletal muscle from cases of the Kugelberg-Welander syndrome. Acta neuropathologica (Berlin) 17: 201

Mayer R F, Doyle A M 1970 Studies of the motor unit in the cat. Histochemistry and topology of anterior tibial and extensor digitorum longus muscle. In: Walton J N, Canal N, Scarlato G (eds) Muscle diseases. Excerpta Medica International Congress Series 199, Amsterdam, p 159

Meijer A E F H 1978 Skeletal muscle diseases with disordered oxidative phosphorylation in the isolated muscle mitochondria. Cellular and Molecular Biology 23: 257

Mendell J R 1979 Experimental myopathies. A review of experimental models and their relationship to human neuromuscular diseases. In: Vinken P J, Bruyn G W (eds) Diseases of muscle. 1. Handbook of clinical neurology 40. North Holland, Amsterdam, p 133

Miledi R 1960 Properties of regenerating neuromuscular synapses in the frog. Journal of Physiology 154: 190

Miledi R, Slater C R 1968 Some mitochondrial changes in denervated muscle. Journal of Cell Science 3: 49

Miledi R, Slater C R 1969 Electron microscopic structure of denervated skeletal muscle. Proceedings of the Royal Society of London B: Biological Sciences 174: 253

Mommaerts W F H M, Seraydarian K, Suh M, Kean C J C, Buller A J 1977 The conversion of some biochemical properties of mammalian skeletal muscles following cross-reinnervation. Experimental Neurology 55: 637

Mulder D W, Rosenbaum R A, Layton D Q 1972 Late progression of poliomyelitis or forme fruste of amyotrophic lateral sclerosis. Mayo Clinic Proceedings 47: 756

Mumenthaler M 1970 Myopathy in neuropathy. In: Walton

J N, Canal N, Scarlato G (eds) Muscle diseases. Excerpta Medica International Congress Series 199, Amsterdam, p 585

Murphy R A, Singer R H, Pantaris N J, Soide J D, Arnason B W G, Young M 1979 Muscle production of nerve growth factor. In: Mauro A (ed) Muscle regeneration. Raven, New York, p 443

Niederle B, Mayr R 1978 Course of denervation atrophy in type I and type II fibres of rat extensor digitorum longus muscle. Anatomy and Embryology 153: 9

Nieves M G, Castello C J 1970 Pathological findings in Werdnig-Hoffmann's disease with special remarks on diencephalic lesions. European Neurology 3: 231

Ohama E, Ikuta F 1979 Pathological investigation of the peripheral nerves in Werdnig–Hoffmann disease. In: Tsubaki T, Toyokura Y (eds) Amyotrophic lateral sclerosis. University Park, Baltimore, p 263

Ontell M 1974 Muscle satellite cells: a validated technique for light microscopic identification and a quantitative study of changes in their population following denervation. Anatomical Record 178: 211

Ontell M 1975 Evidence for myoblastic potential of satellite cells in denervated muscle. Cell and Tissue Research 160: 345

Oosterhuis H J G H 1984 Myasthenia gravis. Churchill Livingstone, Edinburgh p 93

Oosterhuis H J G H, Bethlem J 1973 Neurogenic muscle involvement in myasthenia gravis. Journal of Neurology, Neurosurgery and Psychiatry 36: 244

Oppenheim R W 1989 The neurotrophic theory and naturally occurring motoneuron death. Trends in Neuroscience 12: 252

Oppenheim R W, Haverkamp L J 1988 Neurotrophic interactions in the development of spinal cord motoneurons. In: Evered D, Whelan J (eds) Plasticity of the neuromuscular system. John Wiley, Chicester, p 152

Oppenheim R W, Haverkamp L J, Prevette D, McManaman J L, Appel S H 1988 Reduction of naturally occurring motoneuron death in vivo by a target-derived neurotrophic factor. Science 240: 919

Oppenheim R W, McManaman J L, Haverkamp L, Prevette D 1990 Neurotrophic regulation of motoneuron survival during development. Journal of the Neurological Sciences 98 (suppl): 26

Pearn J H 1973 Fetal movements and Werdnig–Hoffmann's disease. Journal of the Neurological Sciences 18: 373

Pearn J H, Carter C O, Wilson J 1973 The genetic identity of acute infantile spinal muscular atrophy. Brain 96: 463

Pellegrino C, Franzini C 1963 An electron microscope study of denervation atrophy in red and white skeletal muscle fibres. Journal of Cell Biology 17: 327

Pestronk A, Drachman D B 1978 Motor nerve sprouting and acetylcholine receptors. Science 199: 1223

Pestronk A, Drachman D B 1985 Motor nerve terminal outgrowth and acetylcholine receptor antibodies. Journal of Neuroscience 5: 751

Pette D, Staron R S 1988 Molecular basis of the phenotypic characteristics of mammalian muscle fibres. In: Evered D, Whelan J (eds) Plasticity of the neuromuscular system. John Wiley, Chicester, p 22

Pette D, Vrbová G 1985 Invited review: neural control of phenotypic expression in mammalian muscle fibres. Muscle and Nerve 8: 676

Pichey E L, Smith P B 1979 Denervation and developmental alterations of glycogen synthase and glycogen phosphorylase in mammalian skeletal muscle. Experimental Neurology 65: 118

Picken J R, Kirby A C 1976 Denervated frog skeletal muscle: calcium content and kinetics of exchange. Experimental Neurology 53: 64

Pluskal M G, Pennington R J 1973 Peptide hydrolase activities in denervated muscles. Biochemical Society Transactions 1: 1307

Pluskal M G, Pennington R J 1976 Protein synthesis by ribosomes from normal and denervated red and white muscle. Experimental Neurology 51: 574

Resnick J S, Engel W K 1966 Target fibres: structural and cytochemical characteristics and their relationship to neurogenic muscle disease and fibre types. In: Milhorat A T (ed) Exploratory concepts in muscular dystrophy and related disorders. Excerpta Medica International Congress Series 147, Amsterdam, p 255

Rieger F, Grunet M, Edelman G M 1985 N-CAM at the vertebrate neuromuscular junction. Journal of Cell Biology 101: 285

Rieger F, Nicolet M, Pinçon-Raymond M, Murawsky M, Levi G, Edelman G M 1988 Distribution and role in regeneration of N-CAM in the basal laminae of muscle and Schwann cells. Journal of Cell Biology 107: 707

Riley D A, Allin E F 1973 The effects of inactivity, programmed stimulation and denervation on the histochemistry of skeletal muscle fibre types. Experimental Neurology 40: 391

Ringel S P, Bender A N, Engel W K 1976 Extrajunctional acetylcholine receptors. Archives of Neurology (Chicago) 33: 751

Romanul F C, Hogan E L 1965 Enzymatic changes in denervated muscle 1. Histochemical studies. Archives of Neurology (Chicago) 13: 263

Romanul F C A, Sréter F A, Salmons S, Gergely J 1974 The effect of a changed pattern of activity on histochemical characteristics of muscle fibres. In: Milhorat A T (ed) Exploratory concepts in muscular dystrophy 2. Excerpta Medica International Congress Series 333, Amsterdam, p 344

Roth R G, Graziani L J, Terry R D, Scheinberg L C 1965 Muscle fine structure in the Kugelberg-Welander syndrome (chronic spinal muscular atrophy). Journal of Neuropathology and Experimental Neurology 24: 444

Rouques C, Jarmot J, Cathala H P, Castaigne P 1973 Analyse de la distribution des fibres musculaire au sein du muscle squelettique; Intérêt clinique. Resultats préliminaires. Revue Neurologique (Paris) 129: 300

Roy S, Dubowitz V, Volman L 1971 Ultrastructure of muscle in infantile spinal muscular atrophy. Journal of the Neurological Sciences 12: 219

Ruthishauser U, 1986 Differential cell adhesion through spatial and temporal variations of N-CAM. Trends in Neuroscience 9: 374

Saito A, Zacks S I 1969 Fine structure observations of denervation and reinnervation of neuromuscular junctions in mouse foot muscle. Journal of Bone and Joint Surgery 51A: 1163

Salmons S, Sréter F A 1975 The role of impulse activity in the transformation of skeletal muscle by cross innervation. Journal of Anatomy 120: 413

Salmons S, Vrbová G 1969 The influence of activity on some contractile characteristics of mammalian fast and slow muscles. Journal of Physiology 201: 535

Salonen V, Lehto M, Kalimo H, Penttinen R, Aro H 1985
   Changes in intramuscular collagen and fibronectin in
   denervation atrophy. Muscle and Nerve 8: 125

Sanes J R 1986 The extracellular matrix. In: Engel A G, Banker
   B Q (eds) Myology. Basic and clinical, vol 1. McGraw-Hill,
   New York, p 155

Sanes J R, Marshall L M, McMahan U J 1978 Reinnervation of
   muscle fiber basal lamina after removal of myofibers.
   Differentiation of regenerating axons at original synaptic
   sites. Journal of Cell Biology 78: 176

Sarnat H B, Portnoy J M, Chi D Y K 1977 Effects of
   denervation and tenotomy on the gastrocnemius muscle in
   the frog: a histological and histochemical study. Anatomical
   Record 187: 335

Sawchak J A, Benaff B, Sher J H, Shafic S A 1990 Werdnig–
   Hoffmann disease: myosin isoform expression not arrested at
   prenatal stage of development. Journal of the Neurological
   Sciences 95: 183

Schantz P, Billeter R, Henriksson J, Jansson E 1982 Training
   induced increase in myofibrillar ATPase intermediate fibres
   in human skeletal muscle. Muscle and Nerve 5: 628

Schantz P, Henriksson J, Jansson E 1983 Adaptation of human
   skeletal muscle to endurance training of long duration.
   Clinical Physiology 3: 141

Schiaffino S, Hanzlikova V 1970 On the mechanism of
   compensatory hypertrophy in skeletal muscle. Experientia
   26: 152

Schiaffino S, Hanzlikova V 1972 Studies on the effect of
   denervation in developing muscle 2. The lysosomal system.
   Journal of Ultrastructure Research 39: 1

Schiaffino S, Bormioli S P, Aloisi M 1979 Fibre branching and
   formation of new fibres during compensatory muscle
   hypertrophy. In: Mauro A (ed) Muscle regeneration. Raven,
   New York, p 177

Schiaffino S, Gorza L, Pitton G, Saggin L, Simonetta A,
   Sartore S, Lömo T 1988 Embryonic and neonatal myosin
   heavy chain in denervated and paralyzed rat skeletal muscle.
   Developmental Biology 127: 1

Schmalbruch H 1976 Muscle fibre splitting and regeneration in
   diseased human muscle. Neuropathology and Applied
   Neurobiology 2: 3

Schmalbruch H 1979 Manifestations of regeneration in
   myopathic muscles. In: Mauro A (ed) Muscle regeneration.
   Raven, New York, p 201

Schultz, E 1978 Changes in the satellite cells of growing muscle
   following denervation. Anatomical Record 190: 299

Schultz E, Gibson M C, Cohen J 1978 Mitotic activity of
   satellite cells in normal and denervated adult rat muscle as
   visualized by radioautography after injection of
   ^{3}H-thymidine. Anatomical Record 190: 535

Schwartz M S, Sargeant M, Swash M 1976 Longitudinal fibre
   splitting in neurogenic muscular disorders — its relation to
   the pathogenesis of 'myopathic change'. Brain 99: 617

Sendtner M, Kreutzberg G W, Thoenen H 1990 Ciliary
   neurotrophic factor prevents the degeneration of motor
   neurons after axotomy. Nature 345: 440

Shafiq S A, Milhorat A T, Gorycki M A 1967 Fine structure of
   human muscle in neurogenic atrophy. Neurology
   (Minneapolis) 17: 934

Slack J R, Hopkins W G, Pockett S 1983 Evidence for a motor
   nerve growth factor. Muscle and Nerve 6: 243

Smith B 1965 Changes in the enzyme histochemistry of skeletal
   muscle during experimental denervation and reinnervation.
   Journal of Neurology, Neurosurgery and Psychiatry 28: 99

Smith P B, Appel S H 1977 Development of denervation
   alterations in surface membranes of mammalian skeletal
   muscle. Experimental Neurology 56: 102

Smith P B, Grefrath S P, Appel S H 1978 β-adrenergic
   receptor adenylate cyclase of denervated sarcolemmal
   membrane. Experimental Neurology 59: 361

Snider W D, Johnson E M 1989 Neurotrophic molecules.
   Annals of Neurology 26: 489

Snow M H 1983 A quantitative ultrastructural analysis of
   satellite cells in denervated fast and slow muscles of the
   mouse. Anatomical Record 207: 593

Sola O M, Martin A W 1953 Denervation hypertrophy and
   atrophy of the hemidiaphragm of the rat. American Journal
   of Physiology 172: 324

Sola O M, Christensen D L, Martin A W 1973a Hypertrophy
   and hyperplasia of adult chicken anterior latissimus dorsi
   muscles following stretch with and without denervation.
   Experimental Neurology 41: 76

Sola O M, Christensen D L, Khan M A, Kakulas B A, Martin
   A W 1973b Post-denervation muscle hypertrophy. A review
   with evaluation. In: Kakulas B A (ed) Clinical studies in
   myology. Excerpta Medica International Congress Series
   295, Amsterdam, p 310

Sréter F A, Gergely J, Salmons S, Romanul F C A 1973
   Synthesis by fast muscle of myosin light chain characteristics
   of slow muscle in response to long-term stimulation. Nature
   New Biology 241: 17

Stauber W T, Schottelius B A 1975 Enzyme activities and
   distributions following denervation of anterior and posterior
   latissimus dorsi muscles. Experimental Neurology 48: 524

Stewart D M, Sola O M, Martin A W 1972 Hypertrophy as a
   response to denervation in skeletal muscle. Zeitschrift für
   vergleichende Physiologie 76: 146

Stier S 1896 Experimentelle Untersuchungen über das
   Verhalten der quergestreiften Muskeln nach Läsionen des
   Nervensystems. Archiv für Psychiatrie und
   Nervenkrankheiten 29: 249

Stonnington H H, Engel A G 1973 Normal and denervated
   muscle. A morphometric study of fine structure. Neurology
   (Minneapolis) 23: 714

Stracher A, McGowan E B, Hedrych A, Shafiq S A 1979 In
   vivo effect of protease inhibitors in denervation atrophy.
   Experimental Neurology 66: 611

Sunderland S 1950 Capacity of reinnervated muscle to function
   efficiently after prolonged denervation. Archives of
   Neurology and Psychiatry (Chicago) 64: 755

Sunderland S 1978 Nerve and nerve injury. Churchill
   Livingstone, Edinburgh, p 312

Sunderland S, Ray L J 1950 Denervation changes in
   mammalian striated muscle. Journal of Neurology,
   Neurosurgery and Psychiatry 13: 159

Swash M, Schwartz M 1977 Implications of longitudinal
   muscle fibre splitting in neurogenic and myopathic
   disorders. Journal of Neurology, Neurosurgery and
   Psychiatry 40: 1152

Swash M, Schwartz M S, Sargeant M K 1978 Pathogenesis of
   longitudinal splitting of muscle fibres in neurogenic
   disorders and in polymyositis. Neuropathology and Applied
   Neurobiology 4: 99

Tachikawa T, Clementi F 1979 Early effects of denervation on
   the morphology of junctional and extrajunctional
   sarcolemma. Neuroscience 4: 437

Thompson W 1978 Reinnervation of partially denervated rat
   soleus muscle. Acta physiologica scandinavica 103: 81

Thompson W, Jansen J K S 1977 The extent of sprouting of remaining motor units in partly denervated immature and adult rat soleus muscle. Neuroscience 2: 523

Tomanek R J, Lund D D 1973 Degeneration of different types of skeletal muscle fibres 1. Denervation. Journal of Anatomy 117: 395

Tower S S 1935 Atrophy and degeneration in skeletal muscle. American Journal of Anatomy 56: 1

Tsay H-J, Schmidt J 1989 Skeletal muscle denervation activates acetylcholine receptor genes. Journal of Cell Biology 108: 1523

Turner L V, Manchester K L, 1972 Effects of denervation on the glycogen content and on the activities of glucose and glycogen metabolism in rat diaphragm muscle. Biochemical Journal 128: 789

van Haelst V 1970 An electron microscopic study of muscle in Werdnig–Hoffmann's disease. Virchows Archiv; Abteilung A: Pathologische Anatomie 351: 291

van Wijngaarden G K, Bethlem J 1973 Benign infantile spinal muscular atrophy. A prospective study. Brain 96: 163

Venema H W 1988 Spatial distribution of fiber types in skeletal muscle: test for a random distribution. Muscle and Nerve 11: 301

Walicke P A 1989 Novel neurotrophic factors, receptors, and oncogenes. Annual Reviews of Neuroscience 12: 103

Weichers D O, Hubbell S L 1981 Late changes in the motor unit after acute poliomyelitis. Muscle and Nerve 4: 11

Williams P E, Goldspink G 1978 Changes in sarcomere length and physiological properties in immobilized muscle. Journal of Anatomy 127: 459

Yan Q, Eugene M J 1988 An immunohistochemical study of the nerve growth factor receptor in developing rats. Journal of Neuroscience 1988; 8: 3481

17. Pathology of the neuromuscular junction

S. M. Chou

INTRODUCTION

The past two decades have witnessed remarkably rapid progress in our understanding of the pathogenesis and ultrastructural pathology of myasthenia gravis and the Lambert–Eaton myasthenic syndrome (LEMS). However, various factors continue to hamper further advances in understanding of the pathology of motor end-plates in human diseases. They include: (i) the unavailability of motor end-plates in routine muscle biopsy material unless a muscle with the shortest possible muscle fibres is selected (e.g. the external intercostal muscles), or a motor point biopsy is performed (Coërs & Woolf 1959); (ii) marked morphological variation of normal motor end-plates from muscle to muscle, and between type 1 and type 2 (or red, white and intermediate) muscle fibres (Padykula & Gauthier 1970, Duchen 1971a, Santa & Engel 1973); (iii) ultrastructural variation of motor end-plates according to the angle and plane of sectioning or whether the myofibre is stretched or contracted (Harriman 1976); (iv) the age of the patient; senile changes occur in nerve terminals (Tuffery 1971), and axonal sprouting in developing or immature myofibres (Teräväinen 1968); (v) effects of various drugs, e.g. long-term anticholinesterase therapy (Bickerstaff & Woolf 1960, Engel et al 1973) or corticosteroids; and (vi) the degree of muscle activity or inactivity (Pachter & Eberstein 1983, 1984).

In order to overcome the problem of marked variation in the ultrastructure of the motor end-plate and consequent bias in interpretation, Engel & Santa (1971) advocated morphometric analysis using planimetry and line-and-point sampling techniques. The measurements they used included: (i) nerve terminal area; (ii) mitochondrial percentage of the nerve terminal area; (iii) synaptic vesicle concentration; (iv) postsynaptic area of clefts and folds per nerve terminal; (v) postsynaptic membrane length per nerve terminal, and (vi) postsynaptic membrane profile concentration. Such a morphometric analysis of individual motor end-plates does not entirely overcome the problems mentioned above because such a quantitative assessment may be greatly biased by the type of motor end-plate (type 1 or type 2 fibre) (Ogata & Murata 1973, Ogata 1988) (Fig. 17.1), by the individual muscle concerned, or by the age of the patient (Oda 1984). A second set of statistical analyses was proposed to correct bias from other variables by determining the frequency of certain non-specifics. Because the gleaning of sufficient motor end-plates for statistical analysis from routine muscle biopsies is already exceedingly difficult, even if one applies the motor point biopsy technique, the proposed two-step quantitative analysis (Engel et al 1975) remains unfeasible for practising pathologists or neurologists wishing to make a diagnosis based upon examination of very few motor end-plates. Furthermore, control motor end-plates from the same muscle of a subject in the same age group are not usually available. The difficulty is therefore not only technical but also interpretative for morphological studies on motor end-plates. Correlation of light and electron microscopic findings has in general been unfruitful.

It is, therefore, a great relief to learn that some qualitative studies are now applicable to end-plates in both light and electron microscopic preparations in order to assist in making certain diagnoses. As reviewed in the following sections, the techniques

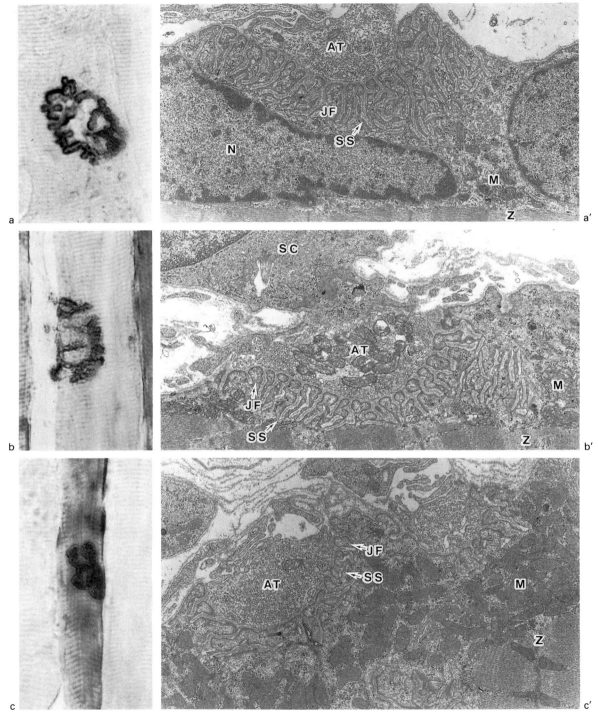

Fig. 17.1 Motor end-plates of mouse triceps muscle showing large AChE (+) end-plate (a) with more numerous and longer secondary synaptic (ss) clefts in the white (fast) fibre (a'). In contrast to small and compact AChE (+) end-plate (c) of red (slow) fibre (c and c'). Intermediate (slow-fatigue resistant) fibre showing intermediate length and numbers of secondary synaptic clefts (ss) and junctional folds (JF) (b and b'). a–c: ×1080, a'–c'. ×9000. (Reproduced with permission from Ogata 1988)

of localizing the acetylcholine receptor (AChR) or immune complexes at end-plates by the immuno-peroxidase method or localizing active zone particles at the presynaptic membranes by freeze–fracture electron microscopy have opened up new vistas for future research and for practical diagnostic approaches in motor end-plate diseases.

AGING OF MOTOR END-PLATES

For understanding the pathology of motor end-plates, a knowledge of non-specific changes related to functional plasticity and aging of end-plates is essential (Pestronk et al 1980, Rosenheimer & Smith 1985). Such changes differ both quantitatively and qualitatively between type 1 and 2 end-

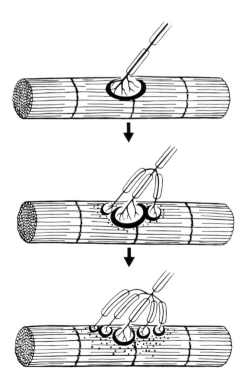

Fig. 17.2 Schematic illustration of age changes in human skeletal muscle end-plates depicting an increase in numbers of preterminal axons small AChR end-plates (in black circle) and prejunctional AChR in dots with aging (revised from Oda 1984)

plates and are influenced also by the degree of muscle activity and inactivity (Pachter & Eberstein 1983, 1984, Malathi & Batmanabane 1983). Type 2 end-plates appear to be more susceptible than type 1 end-plates to physiological and pathological processes in general. An increase in the average number of myelinated as well as intrasynaptic branches of terminal axons was reported in aged cats (Tuffrey 1971), mice (Fahim et al 1983), and rats (Smith & Rosenheimer 1982). At the same time, broken and fragmented patterns of acetyl-choline esterase (AChE) and acetylcholine receptor (AChR) distribution were described in aged rats.

Having studied human intercostal muscle end-plates from 12 non-neurological patients (age 32 to 76 years), Oda (1984) concluded that aging of motor end-plates in man is characterized by an increase in (i) the number of preterminal axons entering an end-plate, (ii) the length of end-plates as revealed by AChE staining, (iii) the presence of prejunctional AChRs (absent in the younger), and (iv) the number of small conglomerates of AChRs as depicted in the diagram (Fig. 17.2).

MYASTHENIA GRAVIS

Myasthenia gravis (MG) is a disease characterized clinically by muscle weakness and fatiguability due to impaired neuromuscular transmission secondary to severe depletion of AChRs. Walker's observation (1934), that both parenteral and oral physostigmine were capable of relieving the muscle weakness temporarily in a MG patient, led her to the supposition that the site of its anticholinesterase action might be the AChR at the neuromuscular junction. Simpson (1960) noted that MG was sometimes associated with autoimmune diseases (in 25% of cases according to Oosterhuis 1989) and speculated that an autoimmune process might underlie the disorder. Attention was focused for a while on the possibility of a presynaptic defect, for Elmqvist et al (1964) demonstrated a marked decrease in miniature end-plate potentials (m.e.p.p.) in MG patients and attributed this to decreased release of acetylcholine. Others realized, however, that a decrease in postsynaptic AChRs could also account for a reduction in m.e.p.p. values; indeed, Fambrough et al (1973) demonstrated that MG patients had only 11–30% of the

AChRs present in normal controls. This reduction in AChR number is apparently due to the presence of antibodies to the AChR which are found in the serum of about 90 percent of MG patients (Lindstrom et al 1976, Lindstrom & Lambert 1978). IgG isolated from the serum of MG patients and injected into experimental animals induces a decremental response to repetitive nerve stimulation and a reduction in the number of AChRs as well as in m.e.p.p. amplitudes (Toyka et al 1975). Thus the crucial role of the humoral immune response in MG appears established; however, there has been a lack of correlation between the density of AChR loss and the transmission defect in mice following transfer of MG IgG (Mossman et al 1988).

Elias & Appel (1979) summarized four possible mechanisms which might produce a decreased concentration of functional AChRs: (i) antibodies block the AChR; (ii) antibodies stimulate lysis of postsynaptic membranes; (iii) antibodies increase the rate of degradation of AChR, and (iv) antibodies decrease the rate of synthesis of AChR. Of these, antibody-mediated breakdown of postsynaptic membranes appears to be an important mechanism which leads to physiological dysfunction. The demonstration (Engel et al 1977b, Sahashi et al 1980) of immune complexes (C3, C9 and IgG) on postsynaptic membranes and of degenerate material in synaptic clefts in MG endplates indicates a complement-mediated destruction of postsynaptic membranes (Lennon et al 1978). More direct evidence of an antibody-dependent complement-mediated injury to AChRs has recently been provided by Fazekas et al (1986) and Engel & Arahata (1987) by demonstrating the neoantigenic determinants of the C5b–9 complement membrane attack complex (MAC) in MG endplates. The evidence concerning the accelerated rate of degradation of receptors is well summarized by Drachman (1979) who noted that IgG from myasthenic patients in the absence of complement causes a two- to three-fold increase in the normal rate of AChR degradation in tissue culture. This has also been shown to occur in-vivo at intact neuromuscular junctions in animals with experimental autoimmune myasthenia gravis (EAMG) (Stanley & Drachman 1978). Lindstrom (1979) cites evidence which suggests that the increased

rate of AChR degradation is the primary mechanism in chronic EAMG and probably also in human MG. In the latter, both receptor synthesis and incorporation of receptors into membranes may also be decreased (Elias & Appel 1979).

When one attempts to correlate antibody levels with the actual clinical state of the patient, one finds both severely weak patients with no detectable antibodies (Mossman et al 1986) and patients in clinical remission with high antibody levels. Recently, Tsujihata et al (1989) advocated that detection of immune complexes on motor endplates is a more sensitive and confirmatory method for diagnosing minimal or atypical MG when serum AChR antibodies are non-detectable. Indeed, in 26 (17%) of 153 validated MG cases AChR antibody was undetectable in the serum (Vincent & Newsom-Davis 1985). Questions remain as to the factors controlling this antibody response and why it arises in the first place. Immunological studies on MG patients reviewed by Penn (1979) have shown no increase in the numbers of B-lymphocytes, plasma cells, or T-lymphocytes.

The thymus is the organ most often implicated as the initiator of the pathological process in MG. Thymectomy has been for many years a recognized form of treatment of the disease (see review by Gutmann & Chou 1976) and may lead to clinical improvement and even complete remission (Genkins et al 1975, Buckingham et al 1976). Examination of glands from MG patients has revealed that about 15% have thymomas and 70% have thymic hyperplasia in which germinal centres not normally present in the thymus are seen (Castleman 1966). Cuenoud et al (1980) have shown that three of eleven patients with thymoma, but without MG, had low titres of antibody to AChR. There is evidence that B-lymphocytes may be present in normal thymus and might produce antibody to AChR. Thus, part of the benefit of thymectomy may stem from the removal of an abnormal population of B-lymphocytes in the thymus. Another benefit apparently lies in the removal of thymic hormone which has been shown to be capable of inducing T-lymphocyte maturation and perpetuating the immune response to AChR (Shore et al 1979, Twomey et al 1979, Dalakas et al 1983). The fact that muscle-like ('myoid') cells with AChRs and immunocompetent cells exist together in the thymus (Kao & Drachman 1977) makes it appear very probable that this organ is the site at which the pathogenetic process originates. A certain virus, e.g. the rabies virus, has a specific high affinity for the AChRs of motor end-plates (Lentz et al 1982) and could potentially trigger the immunopathic process against AChR. A search for viral antigens in myasthenic thymus glands showed that herpes simplex antigen is more common in myasthenic than in normal thymus (Penn 1979). However, multiple approaches for identification and isolation of virus from thymus homogenate and cell suspensions from many MG patients have failed to detect any evidence for persistent viral infection (Aoki et al 1985, Klarinskis et al 1986).

In summary, the antibody to AChR is clearly established as the immediate cause of the clinical disease in MG. The possible roles of the thymus and of the T-lymphocyte systems in inciting and modulating the production of antibodies are fascinating areas for future research.

Light microscopy

Focal clusters of lymphocytes in skeletal muscle described as lymphorrhages (Russell 1953) are observed in a small number of MG patients (one-third of cases, according to Fenichel 1966). With both methylene blue and acetylcholinesterase stains, two major types of abnormal end-plate are described (Coërs & Desmedt 1958). They are: (i) a 'dystrophic' type characterized by abnormally profuse ramifications and the formation of multiple end-plates, and (ii) a 'dysplastic' type characterized by marked elongation of the end-plate in one direction with few side branchings or sproutings. The authors implied that the dysplastic change is more characteristic than the dystrophic change, as the latter is often seen in association with lymphorrhages or with degeneration or atrophy of myofibres (Woolf & Coërs 1974). As in the acute phase of EAMG (Lennon et al 1976, Corey et al 1985), a mononuclear cell reaction directed at end-plates has been described in biopsied muscles (Fig. 17.3) from MG patients (Wiesendanger & D'Alessandri 1963, Pascuzzi & Campa 1988). Among 45 myasthenic biopsies

studied, elongated motor end-plates were noted in 26 biopsies from younger patients, whereas all seven biopsies from patients over the age of 50 years showed abnormal collateral branching (Coërs & Telerman-Toppet 1976). While the former may represent an effort by terminal axons to increase the synaptic area (Bickerstaff & Woolf 1960), the latter is more suggestive of a non-specific aging change.

Electron microscopy

The early electron microscopy of MG end-plates was marred by preparative artifacts and yielded few positive findings (Bickerstaff et al 1959, 1960). Zacks (1964) classified the abnormal ultra-structural findings of motor end-plates from six MG patients into two major types. The first type was characterized by focal rarefaction in the sarcolemma within the secondary synaptic clefts, and the second type, by changes in the terminal axons and the secondary synaptic clefts. Attenuation of secondary synaptic clefts was particularly emphasized as the unique finding which would decrease the available number of postsynaptic AChRs and would simulate the effect of decreased quantities of acetylcholine. Subsequent studies by others (Woolf 1966, Fardeau & Godet-Guillain 1970, Sakimoto & Cheng-Minoda 1970) also described poorly developed or simplified junctional folds and widened primary synaptic clefts. Changes in the secondary synaptic clefts such as greatly widened, less numerous, or shortened clefts filled with acid mucopolysaccharide spheres were observed in six MG cases and were considered to be the 'only consistent abnormality' by Edwards (1970).

Morphometric analysis of 68 motor end-plates from 18 MG cases (Engel & Santa 1971, Santa et al 1972) showed a significant decrease in the mean terminal area and the mean postsynaptic membrane profile concentration; secondary synaptic clefts were widened, sparse and shallow or sometimes absent. These abnormalities were apparently unrelated to the duration of the disease or the duration of treatment. Essentially similar findings were observed in motor end-plates of external intercostal muscle biopsies from six MG patients studied

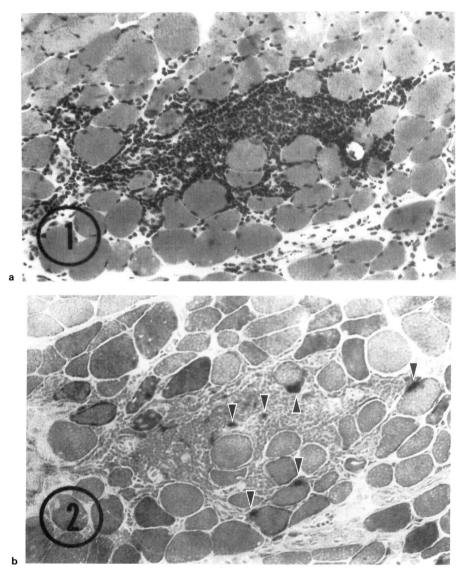

Fig. 17.3 (a) Triceps muscle from a MG patient showing lymphocytic infiltrate ('lymphorrhage') (H&E stain). (b) Multiple motor end-plates demonstrated with esterase stain in the neighbouring section counterstained with haematoxylin. ×100. (Reproduced with permission from Pascuzzi & Campa 1988)

in our laboratory (Fig. 17.4) (Gutmann & Chou 1976). The neuromuscular junctions of seven myasthenics reported by Korényi-Both et al (1973) also demonstrated dilated synaptic gaps and increased amounts of basement membrane material. The authors considered that these changes might eventually lead to 'intersynaptic denervation'.

Retraction of the terminal axon, or postsynaptic regions denuded of their nerve terminals, were also described (Santa et al 1972, Korényi-Both et al 1973) in advanced cases and were apparently not secondary to terminal neuropathy. With the immunoperoxidase method (Daniels & Vogel 1975) for localizing the AChRs with α-bungarotoxin

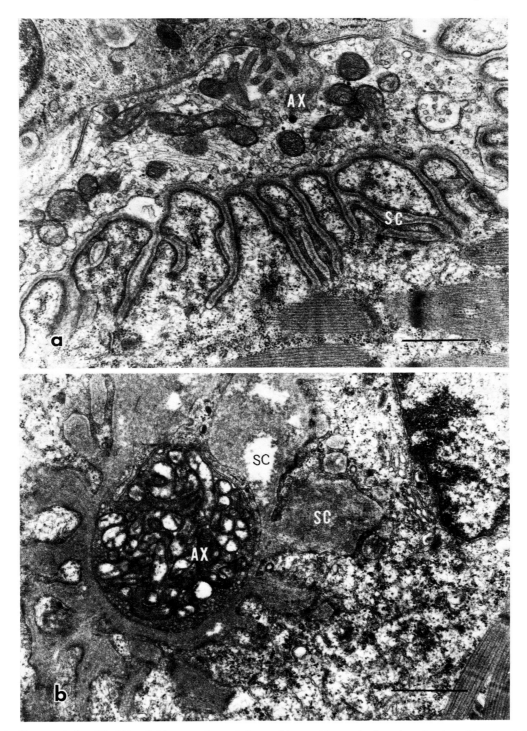

Fig. 17.4   Motor end-plate (b) of biopsied intercostal muscle from a 64-year-old myasthenic patient showing widened and shallow synaptic clefts (SC) containing amorphous granular material with little alteration within the terminal axon (AX). Secondary synaptic clefts are thinner and more numerous and elongated in motor end-plates from control intercostal muscle (a). Bar = 1 μm. (Reproduced with permission from Gutmann & Chou 1976 by courtesy of *Archives of Pathology and Laboratory Medicine*)

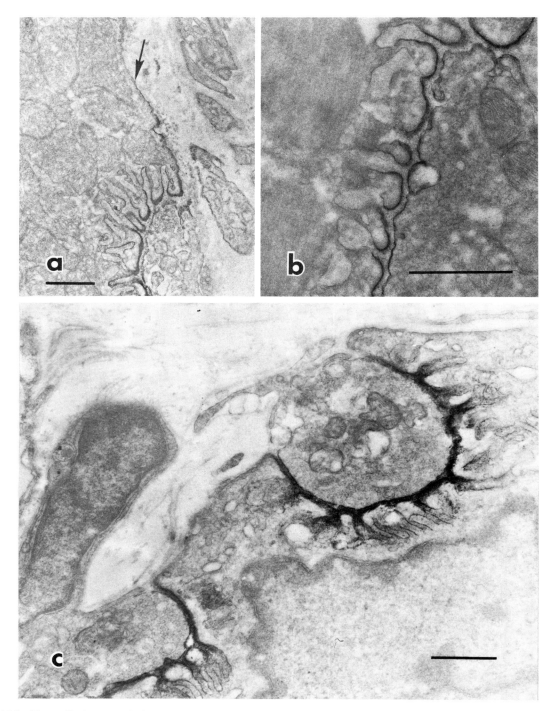

Fig. 17.5 Mouse diaphragm end-plates (a,b) stained by the αBT-immunoperoxidase method. Note that the nearby muscle plasma membrane (arrow) and other structures are not stained. Sections were not stained with lead or uranium salts. Reproduced from Daniels & Vogel (1975) by courtesy of *Nature*. Mouse extensor digitorum brevis muscle end-plates (c) stained by erabtoxin-b immunoperoxidase method. Note reduction of staining product at the periphery of secondary clefts. Bar = 1 μm. (Reproduced with permission from Dr T. Sato)

(α-BT) (Fig. 17.5) or with erabtoxin and cobro-toxin (Fig. 17.5c, 17.6) (Sato et al 1977), which bind specifically to the nicotinic AChR (Lee et al 1967), distinction between denervated end-plates and myasthenic-denuded end-plates has become possible (Tsujihata et al 1980, 1981).

The MG end-plates, which structurally may resemble those seen in denervation, show no extrajunctional spread of AChRs (Bender et al 1976). In fact, the synaptic folds and postsynaptic membranes of myasthenic end-plates display only faint segmental staining for AChR, especially in simplified and degenerated end-plates (Engel et al 1977c). Marked reduction in the numbers of AChRs as measured by the AChR index (length of AChR-positive postsynaptic membrane divided by length of presynaptic membrane) can thus be demonstrated (Fig. 17.6a,b), and has also been shown by quantitative autoradiographic studies using isotope-labeled α-BT (Fambrough et al 1973, Pestronk et al 1985a). Loss of AChRs is attributed to autoimmune attack and subsequent complement-mediated lysis of segments of the junctional membranes (Rash et al 1976). The evidence has been elegantly provided by localizing immune complexes (IgG and C3) at the post-synaptic region and on degenerate material within the synaptic spaces both in MG (Engel et al 1977b) and EAMG (Engel et al 1976, Lennon et al 1978, Sahashi et al 1978a, Engel et al 1979). Binding of immune complexes to well-preserved end-plate postsynaptic membranes was more prominent in mild than in more severely affected patients. Evidence of activation of the lytic phase of the complement reaction was indirectly demonstrated by localizing the C9 component on degenerate material in the synaptic space and on the simpli-fied postsynaptic membrane (Sahashi et al 1980). More direct evidence of antibody-dependent complement-mediated injury to AChRs in MG has been provided recently by Fazekas et al (1986) and Engel & Arahata (1987), who demonstrated the presence of the membrane attack complex (MAC) of complement at the motor end-plates in the thyro-hyoid muscle in 11 MG patients who under-went thymectomy. Although the exact mechanism of the autoimmune attack on AChRs leading to impairment of neuromuscular transmission remains to be elucidated, the evidence is convincing that complement-mediated lysis of the postsynaptic membrane is the cause of AChR deficiency and of the accumulation of 'granular' or 'globular' AChR-enriched membrane fragments within widened clefts (Engel 1984) so frequently described by previous investigators. Such membrane debris with immune complexes may eventually be phago-cytosed and removed by monocytes as well illustra-ted in EAMG, although such a phenomenon has seldom been described in human MG end-plates (Albuquerque et al 1976, Wiesendanger & D'Alessandri 1963, Pascuzzi & Campa 1988).

THE LAMBERT–EATON MYASTHENIC SYNDROME

The Lambert–Eaton myasthenic syndrome (LEMS), is characterized by proximal muscle weakness which differs clinically and pathophysio-logically from MG. The first descriptions were of proximal muscle weakness and diminished or absent deep tendon reflexes in patients who often (60%, according to O'Neil et al 1988) had a small cell carcinoma of the lung (Lambert et al 1956, Eaton & Lambert 1957). Unlike MG, which is characterized by a decrease in the number of AChRs and a diminution in the size of m.e.p.p., in LEMS, the number of postsynaptic AChRs (Engel et al 1977a) and the m.e.p.p. amplitude (Lambert & Elmqvist 1971) are normal. Fewer quanta of acetylcholine are released in response to a single nerve action potential but repetitive stimulation results in an increase in excitatory end-plate potentials which is usually sufficient to depolarize the muscle (Lambert & Elmqvist 1971). The physiological defect in the LEMS is therefore analogous to that caused by botulinum toxicity, elevated magnesium and neomycin in high concentration — i.e the net release of a diminished amount of acetylcholine from the terminal axon by the nerve action potential (Lambert & Rooke 1965). The fact that the condition is palliated by calcium and guanidine hydrochloride, which promote acetylcholine release from nerve terminals, is in accord with this concept. Dis-organization and paucity of active zone particles at the presynaptic membrane of motor end-plates in LEMS was demonstrated by freeze-fracture elec-

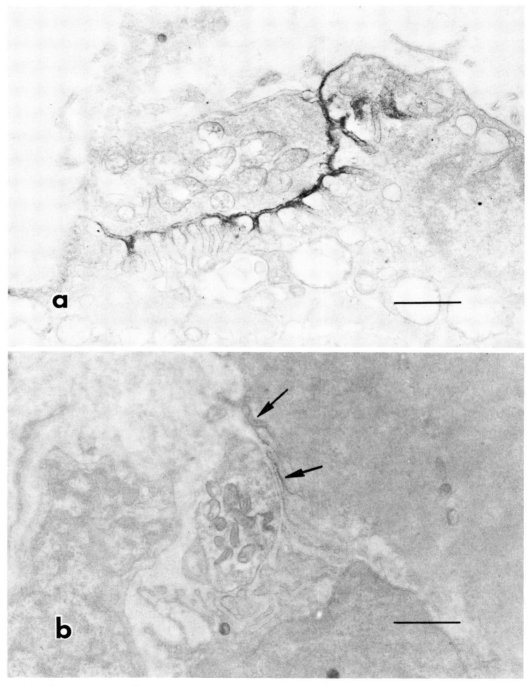

Fig. 17.6   Control mouse extensor digitorum brevis end-plate (a) and external intercostal end-plate from a patient with myasthenia gravis (b) both stained by the cobrotoxin immunoperoxidase method. Note a faint staining reaction of AChR (arrows) in postsynaptic folds in (b). Sections were not stained with lead or uranium salts. Bar = 1 μm. (Reproduced with permission from Dr T. Sato)

tron microscopy by Fukunaga et al (1982). Those particles appear to represent the putative voltage-sensitive calcium channel. Hence the reduced ingress of calcium into the nerve terminal was suspected. An autoimmune pathogenesis was established by passive transfer of the disease to mice by injecting IgG molecules or plasma from LEMS patients which blocked voltage-dependent calcium channels (Lang et al 1981, 1983, 1987, Fukunaga et al 1983, Kim 1987, Kim & Neher 1988) and morphological changes in active zone particles appeared similar in these mice (Fukuoka et al 1987a,b). In fact, a comparison of LEMS IgG with control IgG supported the contention that IgG auto-antibodies from LEMS patients blocked voltage-dependent calcium flux and the flux correlated with disease severity (Lang et al 1987).

Light microscopy

No characteristic features have been observed in muscle biopsies. Engel & Santa (1971) examined biopsies from five patients and concluded that no clear abnormalities in motor end-plates could be seen on light microscopy. The study by Lambert & Rooke (1965) on 20 biopsies showed that 11 were normal and nine had only non-specific alterations in muscle fibres. Fukuhara et al (1972) studied motor end-plates in four cases with acetylcholinesterase staining and found no significant abnormalities. Large and complex end-plates in LEMS, often showing degenerative changes and increased preterminal axon branching, have been considered by Wise & MacDermot (1962) to suggest a mild terminal neuropathy. Four patients with LEMS studied by Tsujihata et al (1987) all showed type 2 myofibre atrophy, normal AChRs as visualized by peroxidase-labeled α-bungarotoxin binding, and absence of immune complexes (including IgG, C3 and C9) at the motor end-plates.

Electron microscopy

The most characteristic finding on electron microscopy is proliferation and enlargement of the secondary synaptic clefts (Fig. 17.7) (Engel & Santa 1971, Fukuhara et al 1972). Engel & Santa (1971) performed morphometric analysis on 42 end-plates from five cases of LEMS and found a significant increase in: (i) the mean area of secondary postsynaptic clefts and folds per nerve terminal, and (ii) the postsynaptic/presynaptic membrane length ratio. Presynaptic terminal axons did not show any significant change in mean nerve terminal area or mean synaptic vesicle count; there was a slight but significant decrease in mean mitochondrial area. Fukuhara et al (1972), however, found atrophy of presynaptic nerve terminals in 40% of 63 neuromuscular junctions from four patients studied. Atrophy of the terminal axons was characterized by aggregates of glycogen granules, increased neurofilaments and occasional myelin figures. Many vesicles 30–50 nm in diameter resembling caveolae were found subjacent to the proliferative and hypertrophic postsynaptic membranes (Fig. 17.7). These changes were considered to be secondary to repeated degeneration and regeneration of the presynaptic membranes and not specific for LEMS. However, no ultrastructural changes, including hypertrophy of junctional folds, were noted in four LEMS patients' motor end-plates, although postsynaptic area, postsynaptic membrane length, and membrane density all appeared decreased (Tsujihata et al 1987). By localization of AChR with the αBT-immunoperoxidase method in 196 end-plates from seven patients with LEMS, Sahashi et al (1978b) concluded that the AChR index was normal, in contrast to myasthenia gravis, in which the mean AChR index and m.e.p.p. amplitude are reduced.

By freeze–fracture electron microscopy of presynaptic membranes (protoplasmic [p] membrane leaflet) in nine patients with LEMS (227 end-plates) and in 14 controls (148 end-plates), a marked decrease in active zones and active zone particles per unit area as well as clusters of large active zone particles (Fig. 17.8) were observed (Fukunaga et al 1982, Engel et al 1989). Those particles were thought to represent voltage-gated calcium channels and LEMS IgG was localized to the zone of those particles by immunoelectron microscopic methods in mice injected with LEMS IgG (Fukuoka et al 1987b, Nagel et al 1988, Engel et al 1989).

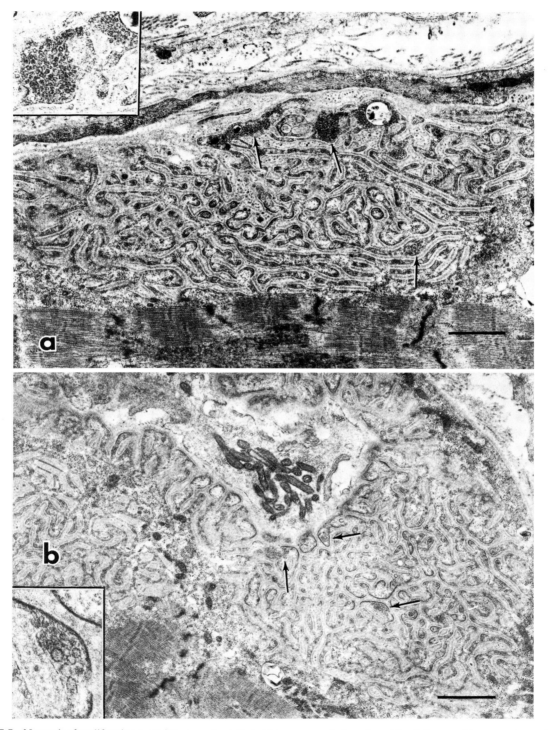

Fig. 17.7   Network of proliferative secondary synaptic clefts (a,b) in motor end-plates from biopsied external intercostal muscle from a patient with Lambert–Eaton syndrome. Note streaming of Z-bands (a) and marked proliferation of caveolae, 30–50 nm in diameter, subjacent to postsynaptic membrane (arrows) in insets (top inset, ×35 200 and bottom inset ×66 000). Bar = 1 μm. (Reproduced with permission from Fukuhara et al (1972) by courtesy of *Archives of Neurology* (Chicago))

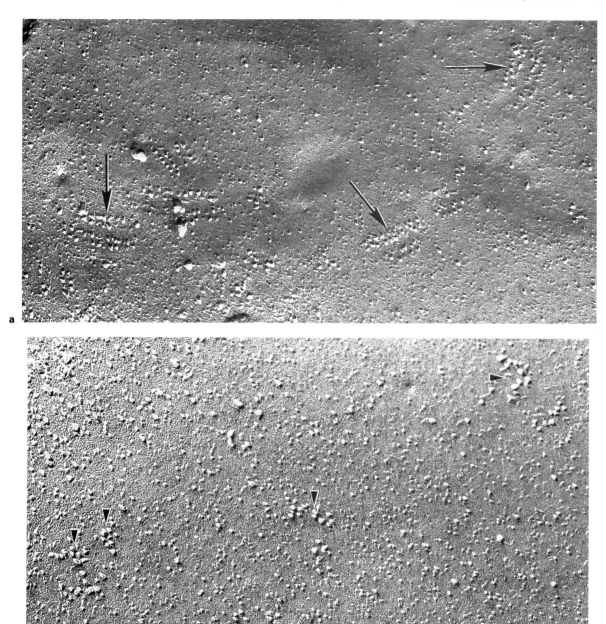

Fig. 17.8 (a) Control presynaptic membrane P-face with the active zones displaying characteristic four rows of particles (arrows). ×90 160. (b) Portion of LEMS presynaptic membrane P-face with few active zones showing several clusters (arrowheads) of large intramembranous particles. ×132 480. (Reproduced with permission from Fukunaga et al 1982)

CONGENITAL MG AND MYASTHENIC SYNDROMES

While MG and LEMS are the most frequent and best characterized clinical disorders of neuro-muscular transmission of adulthood, a variety of similar conditions also occur from the neonatal period through to adulthood as summarized by Albers et al (1984) and Engel (1984). Some of these syndromes are hereditary, with either autosomal recessive or dominant transmission. The underlying pathological features reflect whether they have a presynaptic or postsynaptic defect of neuromuscular transmission. At least five subtypes of congenital disorder of neuromuscular transmission have been described:

(a) Transient neonatal MG

This occurs in infants born to mothers with MG. Transitory muscle weakness is presumably related to passive transfer of maternal AChR antibody (Fenichel 1978). However, it is not clear why only a small proportion of infants born to MG mothers is afflicted. Among 17 infants born to 15 mothers, only 2 developed transient neonatal MG, while 16 of them had AChR antibodies probably transferred from the mothers (Lefvert & Osterman 1983). It was postulated that only those infants who produce AChR antibodies of their own develop transient neonatal MG. Ultrastructural changes in motor end-plates are similar to those in adult MG.

(b) Synaptic vesicle defect syndrome

The so-called familial infantile myasthenia (FIM), an autosomal recessive disorder, is characterized by fluctuating ophthalmoparesis, feeding difficulty, easy fatiguability and attacks of apnea from birth (Conomy et al 1975, Robertson et al 1980, Seybold & Lindstrom 1981, Gieron & Korthals 1985). No circulating AChR antibody is found. The electromyographic findings suggest a defect in either the synthesis or packaging of ACh quanta into synaptic vesicles (Hart et al 1979, Engel et al 1981). Motor end-plates reveal increased numbers of synaptic vesicles but normal synaptic junctions; AChR is normally distributed on the junctional folds and immune complexes are absent. A recent morphometric study of end-plates in three FIM patients showed abnormally small synaptic vesicles supporting the notion of a defect in synthesis or packaging of ACh quanta (Mora et al 1987).

(c) AChE deficiency syndrome

In the single case reported to date there was severe weakness and fatiguability of all muscles from birth (Engel et al 1977a). The condition was refractory to anticholinesterase therapy and AChE was completely absent from all motor end-plates which showed some postsynaptic degeneration. Morphometry of end-plates revealed a decrease in nerve terminal size with a 50% increase in synaptic vesicle density and normal AChRs. Though the average number of ACh quanta released on nerve stimulation was reduced, the prolonged end-plate potential (e.p.p.) and m.e.p.p. were considered to be secondary to persistence of ACh in the synaptic clefts due to absence of AChE.

(d) Slow channel syndrome

This is an autosomal dominant myasthenic syndrome due to an abnormally prolonged open time of the ACh-induced ion channel. The onset of selective weakness primarily of the shoulder girdle muscles with variable involvement of ocular, facial and masticatory muscles occurs either in infancy or adulthood. Marked prolongation of e.p.p., m.e.p.p. and miniature end-plate current, despite normal quantum content of the e.p.p., is considered to be due to a prolonged opening of the ACh-induced ion channel (Engel et al 1982). Muscles show type 1 fibre predominance, small group atrophy, and tubular aggregates and vacuoles near end-plates. Ultrastructure of junctional folds with focal degeneration and loss of AChRs is consistent with reduced amplitude of the m.e.p.p.

(e) CPSC syndrome

Congenital myasthenia which is characterized by 'congenital paucity of secondary synaptic clefts (CPSC)' occurs in both children and adults who present clinically with proximal muscle weakness, ophthalmoparesis, ptosis, and some contractures since birth (Smit et al 1984, 1988). While end-plate AChE is present, the number of end-plates per myofibre is increased but secondary synaptic clefts and AChRs are markedly deficient (Fig. 17.9) resembling those in human fetal muscle, consistent with electrophysiologically small m.e.p.p.s. The cases reported by Vincent et al (1981) and Lecky et al (1986) may belong to this syndrome. AChR antibodies are absent. Recently, two elderly adults with ptosis since early childhood

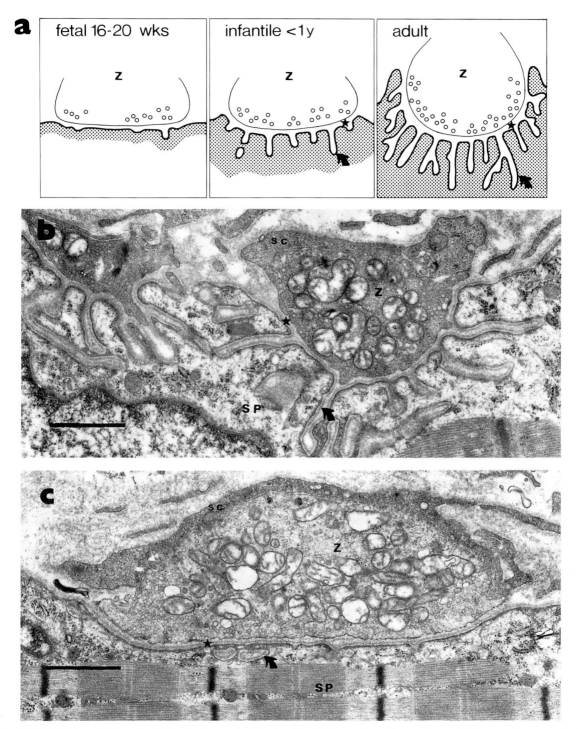

Fig. 17.9 (a) Schematic drawing of the development and maturation of the postsynaptic membrane. (b) A normal motor end-plate from a control subject aged 4 years. (c) Developmental arrest of the secondary synaptic clefts in a child aged 4 years with congenital myasthenia (the CPSC syndrome). Z = nerve terminal; sc = Schwann cell; SP = muscle sarcoplasm; asterisk = primary synaptic cleft. Bar = 1 μm. (Reproduced with permission from Smit et al 1984)

have been reported (Wokke et al 1989), suggesting that the CPSC syndrome may be a developmental disorder of clustering or insertion of AChRs, and the increased number of end-plates per myofibre is thought to be a compensatory mechanism. Patients with the CPSC syndrome apparently have a normal life expectancy.

LOSS OF AChRs SECONDARY TO TREATMENT WITH ANTICHOLINESTERASE DRUGS

Fambrough et al (1973) demonstrated a decrease in the number of AChRs at the postsynaptic area of the neuromuscular junction in rats after administration of neostigmine for 14–34 days. The authors pointed out that, on a weight basis, the dose used was 10–20 times the human dose. Engel et al (1973) performed a morphometric analysis on 77 motor end-plates from 13 rats treated with neostigmine for 42–149 days and demonstrated a decrease in m.e.p.p. amplitude and postsynaptic atrophy, predominantly of type 1 fibre endplates, whereas MG affects all fibre types equally. They noted no significant change in synaptic vesicle count per unit area, mean nerve terminal area, or mean postsynaptic area. There is no clear evidence to indicate that this type of change occurs as a side effect of chronic anticholinesterase treatment in human myasthenia, but Elias & Appel (1979) do point out the occasional beneficial effect of temporarily stopping anticholinesterase treatment while a MG patient is in the hospital.

THE MYASTHENIC STATE ASSOCIATED WITH LONG-TERM D-PENICILLAMINE TREATMENT

Argov & Mastaglia (1979) reviewed the data on the myasthenic state which has been reported in over 40 patients on long-term treatment with D-penicillamine. Elevated titres of antibody to AChR are found in many patients, though they are often lower and less frequently elevated than in MG patients, and the titres fall and weakness improves after withdrawal of D-penicillamine. The condition is rare, occurring in less than 1% of patients with rheumatoid arthritis or other conditions who had

received D-penicillamine (Albers et al 1980, Argov et al 1980, Burres et al 1984, Vincent and Newsom-Davis 1982, Bever et al 1984). It has been concluded that myasthenia seems to develop only in certain susceptible individuals treated with D-penicillamine. The mechanism of AChR antibody induction is unknown; a recent detailed case study of Kuncl et al (1986) suggested that D-penicillamine produces MG by initiating a new autoimmune response rather than enhancing ongoing autoimmunity. No ultrastructural evidence of degeneration or simplification of motor end-plates was found in rats which received daily intramuscular injections of D-penicillamine for 33–37 days (Aldrich et al 1979); anti-AChR antibodies were not detected in these animals.

MYASTHENIC SYNDROME ASSOCIATED WITH SYSTEMIC FUNGAL INFECTION

Gutmann et al (1975) reported a case of systemic infection with the fungus *Fusarium oxysporum* in a patient who exhibited aplastic anaemia and muscle weakness. This fungus produces a mycotoxin which is known to cause aplastic anaemia and which may also have been the cause of the muscle weakness. The myasthenia had the same electrophysiological characteristics as the LEMS and improved with guanidine therapy. The ultrastructural changes in endplates were also similar to those seen in the LEMS (Fig. 17.10). No neoplasm was found in the lungs or elsewhere in the body. Thus the intriguing possibility arises that those cases of LEMS in which no tumour is found may be attributable to a toxin produced by certain infectious agents.

BOTULISM

Botulism is a disease characterized by weakness or paralysis of the limbs, external ophthalmoplegia, dysphagia and dysarthria. These clinical manifestations are secondary to blockade of neuromuscular transmission by an exotoxin produced by the causative organism, *Clostridium botulinum*. The binding of the toxin is irreversible, and clinical recovery occurs only with the formation of new neuromuscular junctions. The toxin interferes with acetylcholine release from the presynaptic

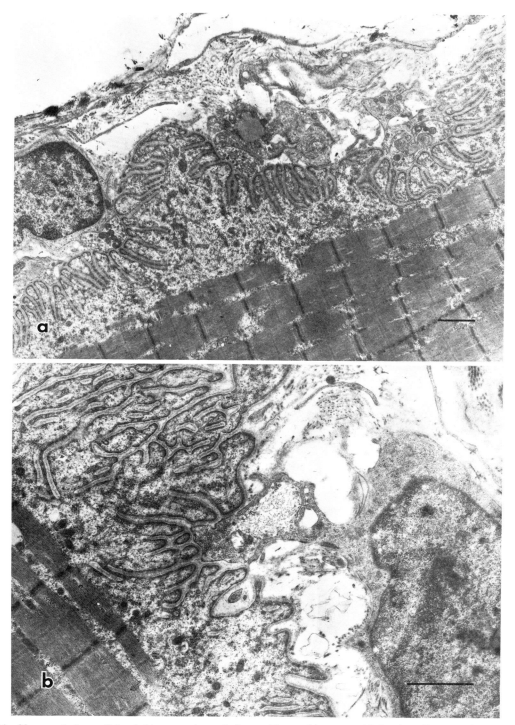

Fig. 17.10   Motor end-plates of biopsied intercostal muscle from a 66-year-old woman with Lambert–Eaton syndrome concurrent with fusariosis. Prominent secondary synaptic clefts despite retracted terminal axons and invading Schwann cell cytoplasmic processes (a) Note proliferative secondary synaptic clefts, atrophic terminal axon and infiltration of collagen fibrils in the primary cleft (b). Bar = 1 μm

nerve terminal (Burgen et al 1949). The binding of botulinum toxin to the area of the neuromuscular junction is now well established (Zacks 1964, Zacks et al 1968, Hirokawa & Kitamura 1975). Binding occurs specifically to the synaptosome fraction of rat brain but does not involve gangliosides as tetanus toxin does (Habermann & Heller 1975).

The exact mechanism by which botulinum toxin interferes with acetycholine release is still debated. The strongest evidence at present appears to support the concept that the toxin interferes with the exocytosis of synaptic vesicles which release acetylcholine (Kao et al 1976, Pumplin & Reese 1977, Simpson 1978, Hanig & Lamanna 1979). Interestingly, Black Widow spider venom which, in normal tissue, causes massive release of acetylcholine from nerve terminals, is best able to antagonize the effect of botulinum toxin in experimental animals (Kao et al 1976, Simpson 1978).

Any discussion of botulinum toxin must refer to the similarities of its actions to those of tetanus toxin. As will be discussed fully in the next section, tetanus toxin is able, in some circumstances, to induce blockade of the neuromuscular junction. Using a cholinergic system in primary nerve cell cultures, Bigalke et al (1978) demonstrated that the physiological characteristics of the inhibition of acetylcholine release by tetanus toxin were similar to those of botulinum toxin; however, the latter was unable to inhibit glycine and γ-aminobutyric acid release. Botulinum toxin was 1000 times more potent than tetanus toxin in inhibiting acetycholine release. Other investigators have demonstrated that botulinum toxin is transported by retrograde axonal flow to the cell bodies of the α-motor neurons (Wiegand et al 1976), as was also demonstrated for tetanus toxin.

Light microscopy

Duchen (1970) has delineated the sequence of events at the neuromuscular junction in mice treated with botulinum toxin. He noted that nerve sprouting originated from nerve terminals in the end-plate region four days after a dose of toxin in slow muscle (soleus) and four weeks after the toxin in fast muscle (gastrocnemius). The new sprouts did not re-innervate old end-plates but formed new connections elsewhere on the muscle fibre.

Spread of AChRs over the entire muscle surface due to neuromuscular block is best demonstrated directly by the ^{125}I-labelled αBT method or indirectly by measuring the amount of sprouting and the size of each end-plate as outlined by the cholinesterase stain (Pestronk et al 1976a). Pestronk et al (1976b) and Pestronk & Drachman (1978) also demonstrated marked sprouting in botulinum-poisoned muscles in association with an increase of extrajunctional AChRs.

Electron microscopy

Duchen (1971b) studied the neuromuscular junctions in 65 mice after they had received local injections of botulinum toxin, and found no degenerative changes in presynaptic nerve terminals. No ultrastructural abnormalities were noted in the junctional folds or presynaptic vesicles of acutely poisoned guinea pig, frog or cat muscles (Thesleff 1960). In 22 motor end-plates from the intercostal muscle of a patient studied 20 days after the onset of wound botulism (Gutmann et al 1973) we found that most terminal axons were retracted and detached from the primary synaptic folds (Fig. 17.11). Degenerated material was seen in both primary and secondary synaptic clefts. Schwann cell cytoplasm often invaded the enlarged primary cleft after nerve terminal retraction, and redundant Schwann cell basement membranes were seen in degenerating end-plates. Streaming of Z-disc and rod-body formation were found in the vicinity of altered junctional folds (Fig. 17.11). Kao et al (1976) demonstrated that clusters of synaptic vesicles collected at the release site across the postjunctional folds when muscle preparations were treated with botulinum toxin and then with spider venom. This strongly suggests that the toxin interferes with the exocytotic process of vesicle release at the presynaptic membrane and blocks release of acetylcholine from the nerve terminals. This contention was supported by the experimental finding that frog muscles treated with toxin showed a decreased number of exocytotic vesicle sites but not of active zone particles at the presynaptic membrane as visualized

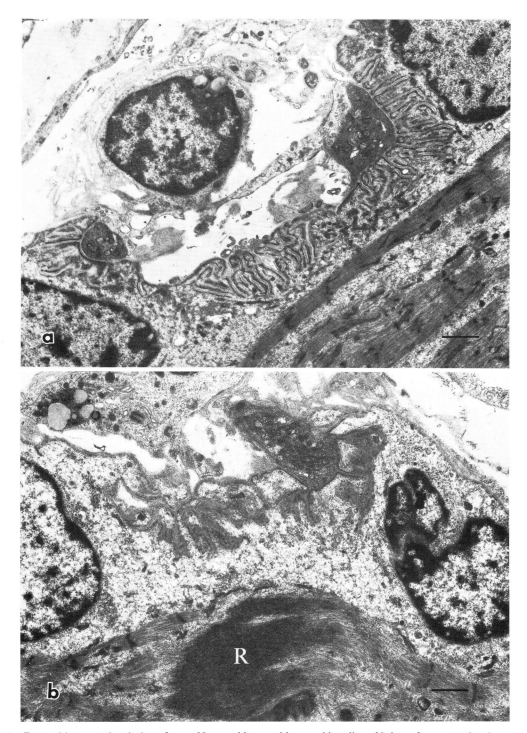

Fig. 17.11   External intercostal end-plates from a 38-year-old man with wound botulism, 20 days after onset, showing retracted terminal axons forming retraction space with some degenerated membranous and granular substance. Note Z disc streaming (a) and rod (R) formation (b) in the vicinity of the end-plates; note also densely packed synaptic vesicles in the terminal axons. Bar = 1 μm

by freeze–fracture electron microscopy (Hirokawa & Heuser 1981).

While the changes in skeletal muscle in the acute phase of human botulism have not been documented, in the chronic phase neurogenic atrophy has been described (Korényi-Both 1983). In a study of three patients with type A botulism, Tsujihata et al (1987) reached the conclusion that at the chronic stage, the nerve terminal zone demonstrated decreased area and significantly more denuded postsynaptic regions than controls, the findings being similar to those in motoneurone disease.

TETANUS

Tetanus is a disease characterized clinically by persistent muscle spasms which occur as a result of overactivity of motor neurones. The infectious organism, *Clostridium tetani*, produces an exotoxin which has both central and peripheral actions. The central actions which result in a diminution of inhibitory input to motor neurones have recently been well-reviewed (Habermann 1978, Bizzini 1979); the peripheral action of the toxin at the neuromuscular junction will be considered in this section. Tetanus toxin has been shown to inhibit release of acetylcholine in cell culture and is similar in molecular weight and structure to botulinum toxin (Bigalke et al 1978). An autoradiographic study (Price et al 1977, Wernig et al 1977) localized tetanus toxin at the motor end-plates, probably in terminal axons. It is now known that the toxin binds to ganglioside in the axon and is transported retrogradely to the spinal cord (Stockel et al 1975). Nerve terminal activity is not necessary for binding. Tetanus toxin is transported to cell somas even from inactivated nerve terminals previously treated with botulinum toxin (Habermann & Erdmann 1978). The toxin appears to be much more potent in its central than its peripheral actions; thus peripheral manifestations of the disease are difficult to evaluate and are often overlooked.

The induction of local tetanus by intramuscular injection of a dose of toxin sufficient to induce focal but not generalized tetanus provides the best means of studying the peripheral action of tetanus toxin. Thorough investigations of motor end-plate changes induced by local tetanus in the mouse were carried out by Duchen et al (1972a) and Duchen (1973a). Slow muscle fibres (soleus) were much more sensitive than fast fibres (peripheral gastrocnemius) to the peripheral action of tetanus toxin. Local tetanus was induced by 48 hours, and the first morphological changes indicating axonal sprouting were seen at 10–12 days after injection. The soleus underwent atrophy, was reinnervated by new axonal sprouts, and had returned to a fairly normal appearance by about four weeks. This sequence of events is similar to that in botulinum-toxin-treated muscle, as discussed in the previous section. These morphological changes were correlated with electrophysiological changes by Duchen et al (1972b) and Duchen & Tonge (1973). Four days after injection of tetanus toxin, the soleus (slow) muscle demonstrated acetycholine supersensitivity and spontaneous fibrillations with no response to nerve stimulation. These changes had reverted to normal by four weeks and were never found in the extensor digitorum longus (fast) muscle. Hofmann & Feigen (1971) studied local tetanus in rats, which were injected with colchicine before receiving tetanus toxin, in order to retard retrograde axonal transport and thus diminish the amount of toxin delivered to motor neurone cell bodies. Colchicine-treated animals developed only mild local tetanus or were completely unaffected.

The toxin may block acetylcholine release presynaptically at the neuromuscular junctions of type 1 fibres as indicated by Duchen (1973a), or it may impair motor neurone activity to cause neuromuscular junction dysfunction as suggested by Hofmann & Feigen (1977).

Light microscopy

Changes in experimental animals with local tetanus, as observed by light microscopy, include (type 1) muscle fibre atrophy and sprouting of axons (Duchen 1973a). Studies in our laboratory revealed a variety of interesting changes in muscle fibres including the formation of central cores, rods and fibre atrophy with various doses of toxin; cholinesterase staining of these fibres has shown no clear abnormality of motor end-plates (Miike et al 1980).

Electron microscopy

A study of muscle biopsies from human cases of tetanus (Eyrich et al 1967, Agostini & Noetzel 1970) revealed no abnormality of motor nerve terminals but did show gross degeneration of muscle fibres with Z-line alterations accompanied by many calcium-containing vesicles. The pronounced muscle fibre damage was also noted by Barua et al (1976) who described swollen fibres, oedema and sarcolemmal damage in each of 25 cases of human tetanus; no mention was made of neuromuscular junctions in this study. Zacks et al (1966) studied muscle from five cases of human tetanus but did not mention the neuromuscular junction. Thus, no study of human tetanus has yet demonstrated any clear abnormality of the neuromuscular junction, whereas several have shown muscle fibre atrophy and degeneration.

During the first week of local tetanus in mice (Duchen 1973a) type 1 nerve terminals were sometimes enlarged and had an increased number of synaptic vesicles. Accumulation of synaptic vesicles was the only visible ultrastructural change in motor end-plates of rat diaphragm injected with tetanus toxin (Kryzhanovsky 1973). By day 10–12, axonal sprouts were seen near the end-plates. Formation of new end-plates with small terminal axons and small primary or secondary synaptic clefts with occasional dense granules was observed to begin three weeks after injection. Thus, the basic picture was one of axonal sprouting and reinnervation. Between days 7 and 12, severe atrophy of the soleus was also noted (Duchen 1973b) with Z-line degeneration similar to that seen by Eyrich et al (1967) in human cases. Muscle fibres were relatively normal 6–7weeks after reinnervation. Fast muscle end-plates remained normal throughout the observation period.

DUCHENNE MUSCULAR DYSTROPHY

Duchenne muscular dystrophy is a sex-linked recessive disease characterized clinically by the onset of proximal muscle weakness during childhood. The basic biochemical defects responsible for both Duchenne and Becker muscular dystrophy have recently been identified as absence or deficiency of dystrophin, a component of the sarcolemmal cytoskeleton (Hoffman et al 1987, Monaco et al 1986). At present, involvement of the motor neurone, axon or neuromuscular junction is not considered to play any crucial part in the pathogenesis of the disease. There is no loss of anterior horn motor neurones in the spinal cord in patients with Duchenne dystrophy (Tomlinson et al 1974). Morphological studies have repeatedly failed to reveal any abnormality of intramuscular nerves in this disease (Jerusalem et al 1974, Engel et al 1977d); the same studies also revealed normal preterminal axons but focal degeneration of postsynaptic folds. As this latter finding raised the question of loss of AChRs and impaired neuromuscular transmission, appropriate studies were performed (Sakakibara et al 1977) and revealed no decrease in the number of AChRs on the postsynaptic membrane, no spread of extrajunctional AChRs and intact neuromuscular transmission. The focal postsynaptic atrophy is apparently a consequence of some pathological change in the muscle cell itself rather than being the result of abnormal nerve transmission or loss of AChRs.

Light microscopy

Coërs et al (1973) studied 14 muscle samples and described small irregular motor endings without excessive ramification of axons. Many myofibres demonstrate normal esterase staining of end-plates on light microscopy. Other degenerating or regenerating fibres sometimes demonstrate varying degrees of esterase staining over the entire sarcolemma. This is probably secondary to 'myogenous mal-innervation' of fibres which have undergone segmental necrosis, longitudinal splitting, or of regenerating fibres which have not yet been reinnervated (Engel et al 1977d).

Electron microscopy

Morphometric analysis by Jerusalem et al (1974) on 36 peroneus brevis motor end-plates from three patients with Duchenne dystrophy revealed focal degeneration of postsynaptic folds with a significant decrease in mean postsynaptic profile concentration and post- to presynaptic membrane length ratio. Electron-dense deposits, basement membrane remnants, and sometimes Schwann cell processes were seen in widened primary or secondary synaptic clefts. No changes indicating acute denervation were seen. Mean nerve terminal area, mean synaptic vesicle count and mean synaptic vesicle diameter did not differ significantly from aged-matched controls. Some apparently immature neuromuscular junctions with shallow secondary clefts and widened primary clefts sometimes containing Schwann cell processes were seen. A later study (Engel et al 1975) revealed that 47% of end-plate regions in Duchenne dystrophy exhibited focal degeneration of postsynaptic folds and an increased incidence of simplified postsynaptic regions; this percentage is much higher than that seen in other forms of muscular dystrophy or in polymyositis. Sakakibara et al (1977) confirmed the preservation of AChRs at normal, degenerated and simplified end-plates with no extrajunctional AChRs in intercostal muscle from two patients. A slight but significant increase in the AChRs index was recorded. Harriman (1976) studied 42 end-plates from 13 patients with Duchenne dystrophy and found that many did not differ from those seen in control specimens. In three end-plates the sole plate appeared to retract from the nerve terminal; Schwann cell cytoplasm and redundant basement membrane occupied the newly created space. Other infrequent findings included sprouting from nerve terminals, newly formed end-plates, and dense packing of neurofilaments in the terminal axons.

Fukuhara et al (1985), who studied 105 end-plates from three patients with Becker-type muscular dystrophy, also found a significant decrease in mean post- to presynaptic membrane length ratio and mean postsynaptic profile concentration (Fig. 17.12), and concluded that a neural factor might participate in the cause of this type of muscular dystrophy.

MYOTONIC DYSTROPHY

Traditionally, myotonic dystrophy is classified as a form of myopathy (see Chapter 8) and it is thought that primary dysfunction of the muscle cell is part of a multisystem disorder. An alternative theory is that the muscle dysfunction is secondary to some dysfunction of the motor neurone, resulting in impairment of some trophic influence normally exerted by motor neurones on muscle (Engel 1971). The frequent occurrence of type 1 fibre atrophy or 'hypotrophy', in myotonic dystrophy led Engel to advance his neurogenic theory (Engel & Warmolts 1973). Conversely, the fact that atrophic fibres have morphologically normal innervation (Engel et al 1975) leads one to suspect that the atrophy arises as a result of a primary muscle fibre abnormality. Morphological evidence suggestive of 'sick' spinal motor neurons (McComas et al 1971) has been lacking. For example, Walton et al (1977) were unable to find any significant decrease in number or alteration in distribution of lumbosacral limb motor neurones in five myotonic dystrophy patients compared with five controls. It is possible, however, that the hypothetical neuronal involvement could be of a functional nature. Signs of neuropathy are sometimes seen in patients with myotonic dystrophy but are absent in many others. Borenstein et al (1977) evaluated the relationship between neuropathy and myotonic dystrophy and concluded that there may be some association; they suggested that EMG screening of myotonic dystrophy patients may confirm a subclinical neuropathy. The neuronal dysfunction and peripheral neuropathy seen in some cases of myotonic dystrophy probably represent additional manifestations of the genetic defect in myotonic dystrophy rather than the actual cause of muscle dysfunction.

Light microscopy

The investigation of 17 cases by Coërs & Woolf (1959) showed an increased size of motor end-plates and some terminal axons. Marked axonal sprouting was seen; the sprouts sometimes formed multiple end-plates on a single fibre with occasional formation of miniature synapses. A later study confirmed the finding of increased numbers of double or multiple end-plates on single muscle fibres and an increase in mean maximum diameter of end-plates in eight cases of myotonic dystrophy (Allen et al 1969). However, in the study of 10 cases by MacDermot (1961), the majority of the end-plates were abnormally small in transversely cut myofibres, but were unusually elongated in longitudinal sections.

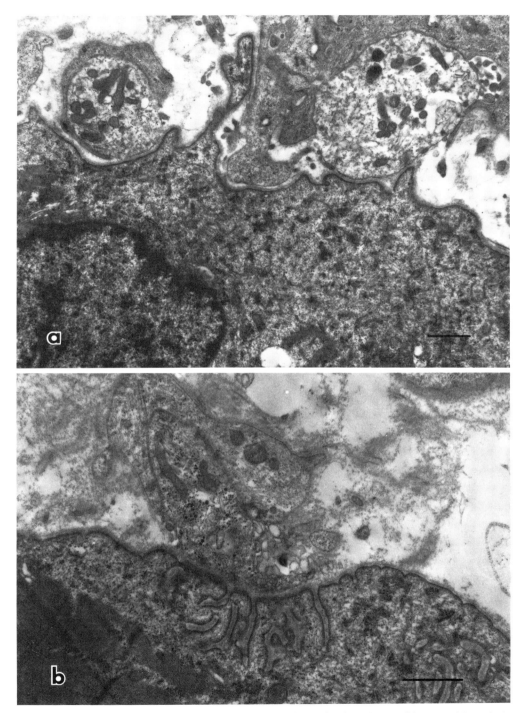

Fig. 17.12 Biceps end-plate from a 14-year-old boy, with Becker-type dystrophy since the age of 5 years, with marked pseudohypertrophy of calf muscles and 50-fold increase in serum CK, showing a marked decrease in the postsynaptic membrane profile concentration and in the synaptic vesicle density in the axon terminal (a). The postsynaptic regions are partly denuded and the secondary synaptic clefts are simplified. Marked collection of glycogen granules is seen in terminal axons (b). Bar = 1 μm. (Courtesy of Drs Fukuhara et al)

Electron microscopy

An electron-microscopic study by Allen et al (1969), of motor end-plates from seven cases of myotonic dystrophy, showed that most terminal axons were unremarkable although they demonstrated hypertrophy of secondary synaptic folds in some junctions, normal postsynaptic areas in others, and rarely a decrease in size and number of secondary synaptic folds. A later study of 16 biopsy specimens (Casanova & Jerusalem 1979) showed that there was postsynaptic atrophy in one neuromuscular junction while the others were normal. In another study (Karpati et al 1973) of four cases of infantile myotonic dystrophy, all motor end-plates except one were found to be normal. Morphometric analysis by Engel et al (1976) on 230 nerve terminals from four patients demonstrated a mild but significant increase in the mean mitochondrial density; no abnormalities were observed in the postsynaptic regions.

In summary, the postsynaptic area in myotonic dystrophy usually appears normal on electron microscopy and shows no consistent pathological pattern when it is altered; the slight presynaptic alterations are of uncertain significance and appear inadequate to support the neurogenic theory.

POLYMYOSITIS

The salient clinical and pathological features of polymyositis are presented in Chapter 12. The pathological changes at the neuromuscular junction are minor and appear to be secondary to the myopathic changes in this disease.

Light microscopy

Coërs & Woolf (1959) used vital staining to study 14 cases of polymyositis and found frequent swelling of terminal axons and preterminal areas of the nerve fibre. They felt that these swellings were probably caused by oedema. They were sometimes seen in regions without inflammatory cell infiltration or muscle fibre degeneration. In other areas, nerve fibres appeared to be shrunken. Occasional areas of axonal sprouting and multiple, enlarged end-plates were seen; changes indicative of collateral reinnervation were also encountered in some areas.

Electron microscopy

Disorganized end-plates with dilated primary synaptic clefts containing vesicular, floccular or granulovacuolar necrotic material, and similarly disorganized secondary clefts containing granular material were described by Stoebner et al (1970) in five cases of chronic polymyositis. Morphometric analysis on 64 end-plates from five patients with polymyositis (Engel et al 1975) revealed several alterations of uncertain significance. A small but significant increase in mean mitochondrial content of presynaptic nerve terminals occurred, together with a small but significant decrease in synaptic vesicle density. Distension of nerve terminals by neurofilaments was seen in controls, in polymyositis cases, and in several other conditions. There were no postsynaptic abnormalities. In 24 motor end-plates from four adult polymyositis patients, we saw conspicuous collections of amorphous granular material around terminal axons, Schwann cells and over the sarcolemma (Fig. 17.13) instead of synaptic clefts as observed in myasthenia gravis. Swelling of terminal axons with marked loss of synaptic vesicles and attenuated secondary synaptic clefts were frequent in two cases of childhood dermatomyositis. The attenuated secondary synaptic clefts may be related to reduction of AChRs as demonstrated by Pestronk and Drachman (1985) in a study with 19 polymyositis patients. They postulated that circulating IgG from polymyositis patients caused accelerated rates of AChR degradation.

NEMALINE MYOPATHY

Nemaline myopathy is characterized by the presence of rod bodies in muscle fibres. As the name implies, it is traditionally classified as a myopathic disease although a primary neuropathic lesion has been suggested by electromyographic (EMG) findings suggestive of denervation and the finding of depressed deep tendon reflexes. This has recently been called into question by the study of Fukuhara et al (1978) on motor end-plates in this disease. These authors found features of degeneration in terminal axons and a decrease in number and length of secondary synaptic clefts in the absence of actual fragmentation of axons or reinnervation. These findings led them to speculate

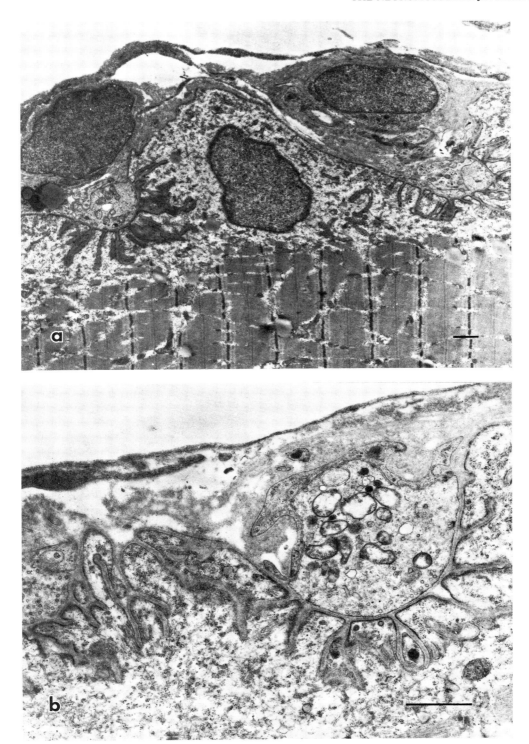

Fig. 17.13 Biceps end-plate from a 40-year-old patient with chronic polymyositis with marked deposits of amorphous ground substance around Schwann cell or fibroblast (a). The reduplicated basal membranes and amorphous material surround terminal axons (b); the secondary synaptic clefts appear normal in width and shape. Bar = 1 μm

that loss of some trophic influence of nerve on muscle might be responsible for the disease. Studies in our laboratory, in which local tetanus was induced in laboratory rats, revealed the presence of rods, multicores, and central cores in affected muscles (Miike et al 1980). Combinations of rods, cores and miniature cores also occur in some human myopathies (Bethlem et al 1978). All of this invites speculation that some derangement of neuromuscular transmission or trophic neural influence on muscle may underlie nemaline myopathy and possibly central core and multicore disease.

Light microscopy

Type 1 fibre grouping and predominance were seen in many cases of nemaline myopathy (Bender & Willner 1978, Fukuhara et al 1978) suggesting a defect in innervation or neurotrophic influence. Light microscopy of motor end-plates in nemaline myopathy has not been well-documented.

Electron microscopy

Fukuhara et al (1978) examined 255 neuromuscular junctions in 64 blocks from three biopsy specimens (gastrocnemius and/or biceps brachii) of patients with nemaline myopathy. In 27% of the junctions, abundant myelin figures, mitochondria, and glycogen granules were seen in swollen terminal axons (Fig. 17.14) indicating degeneration, although actual atrophy of terminal axons was absent. Secondary synaptic clefts demonstrated statistically significant decreases in number and length, although width remained normal. This is in contrast to myasthenia gravis and Duchenne dystrophy, where all three parameters are decreased. No evidence of re-innervation was seen.

DISTAL MYOPATHY

Welander (1951) provided a detailed description of the clinical, electrophysiological and morphological findings in 249 cases of a disease which she termed 'myopathia distalis tarda hereditaria' and which is now commonly referred to as distal myopathy. The investigation, which involved autopsy studies on three patients, showed that the spinal cord and

peripheral nerves were normal. This finding, in conjunction with myopathic changes seen on muscle biopsy, led her to classify the disease as a myopathy. Necropsy studies of two other patients (Markesbery et al 1974) revealed no peripheral nerve or spinal root changes in one case and mild changes in the other, which the authors attributed to the patient's coincident diabetes. Markesbery et al (1977) studied three additional patients and concluded that the histochemical and electron-microscopic findings made a neurogenic process unlikely. Some evidence that a neurogenic process may play a part in distal myopathy comes from the electrophysiological demonstration of slight fibrillations in five of six patients in one study (Stålberg & Ekstedt 1969) and of fibrillations in 'most investigated muscles' in 13 patients with the disease in another study (Edström 1975); other studies (Markesbery et al 1974, 1977) failed to denervation, the fact that only one patient was nerve terminals over postsynaptic regions, seen by Engel et al (1976), suggests focal functional denervation, the fact that only one patient was studied makes it difficult to extrapolate these findings to all cases of distal myopathy.

Light microscopy

There has been no systematic light microscopic study of motor end-plates. The pattern seen in muscle specimens is generally one of myopathic change (Welander 1951, Markesbery et al 1974, 1977, Edström 1975). Occasional small angular fibres were seen in one of three cases, and mild fibre type grouping in two of three cases by Markesbery et al (1977). Edström (1975) reported type 1 fibre atrophy in 13 patients with the disease.

Electron microscopy

Engel et al (1975) examined six end-plates from one patient with distal myopathy and found a large number of denuded postsynaptic regions, a finding similar to those in amyotrophic lateral sclerosis. Markesbery et al (1977) did not report on motor end-plate alterations in their study of three patients. They did find structures resembling autophagic vacuoles in the subsarcolemmal region, which they assumed were derived from the sarco-

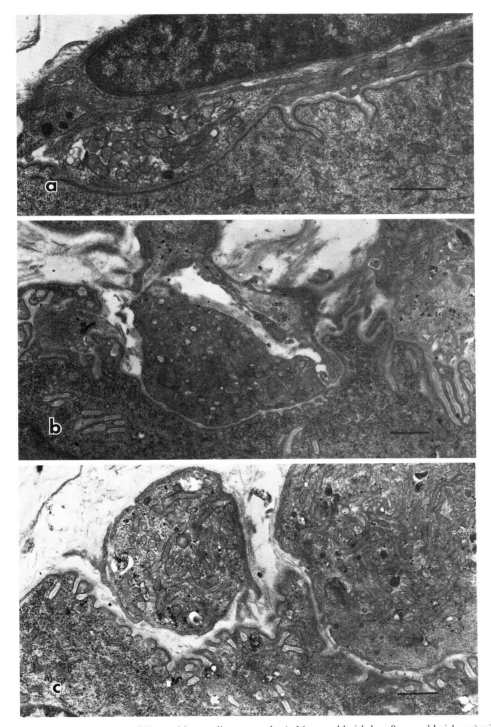

Fig. 17.14   Motor end-plates from two siblings with nemaline myopathy (a 14-year-old girl, b; a 9-year-old girl, a,c) with very poorly developed synaptic clefts, and the terminal axon filled with glycogen granules, electron-dense multimembranous bodies, and increased mitochondria. Bar = 1 μm. (Courtesy of Drs Fukuhara et al)

plasmic reticulum. These structures were also observed frequently in five patients from the same family pedigree studied in our laboratory. It is possible that such structures may represent engulfed postsynaptic areas of motor end-plates, because remnants of synaptic clefts are frequently encountered around such subsarcolemmal autophagosomes which are always lined by a basement membrane.

MOTOR END-PLATES IN DENERVATING DISORDERS

Changes in the neuromuscular junction occur in a variety of human diseases of the motor neurones or peripheral nerves. Diseases of motor neurones include amyotrophic lateral sclerosis (ALS) (usually called motor neurone disease in Britain), Werdnig–Hoffmann disease (WHD) and poliomyelitis. Three common forms of peripheral neuropathy are the alcoholic, diabetic and carcinomatous types. The basic pathological process with respect to the neuromuscular junction is denervation in all of these conditions, although the causes of neuronal or axonal damage in the given diseases vary. The common feature which can be seen is the spread of extrajunctional AChRs (Lee et al 1967, Ringel et al 1975, Bender et al 1976).

Light microscopy

There appears to be a basic pattern of motor end-plate pathology among the diseases causing denervation (Coërs & Woolf 1959). Studies of diabetic neuropathy (Reske-Nielsen et al 1970), carcinomatous neuropathy (Awad 1968) and vitamin B1 deficiency diseases or alcoholic polyneuropathy as well as the Guillain-Barré syndrome (Coërs & Woolf 1959) all described swollen, fused and degenerated preterminal and terminal axons, collateral sprouting and regenerating end-plates. In agreement with the findings previously summarized by Coërs & Woolf (1959), Bjornskov et al (1975, 1984) reported increased numbers of segmented and enlarged end-plates in 19 of 22 patients. In WHD, tangles of terminal fibres consisting of fine, beaded, branching fibres with little distal sprouting are the characteristic features which are also found in rapidly progessive cases of

ALS. Motor end-plates in WHD may appear larger than normal on both hypertrophic and atrophic myofibres (Fig. 17.15a,b) as described by Coërs & Woolf (1959). After measuring the terminal innervation ratio (TIR) in 251 neuromuscular biopsies, Coërs et al (1973) suggested that an increased TIR is a reliable early indicator of denervation, because it is within normal limits in familial muscular dystrophies and myasthenia.

Electron microscopy

Over the last 40 years, numerous experiments have clearly established the sequence of changes which occur in laboratory animals after peripheral nerve section or other injury to the nerve. These findings are thoroughly reviewed by Sandbank & Bubis (1974) and provide a framwork for evaluating the motor end-plate pathology in human denervation. The sequence of events is recapitulated in the studies of Pulliam & April (1979) on motor end-plates of the basic muscle fibre types (red, white, intermediate) in the rat. Degeneration begins with a decrease in size of the terminal axon and a loss of the close axon/sole-plate relationship. White muscle shows these changes first, followed by the intermediate type. The nerve ending then withdraws from the primary synaptic cleft and becomes rounded. The Schwann cell cytoplasm surrounds the shrinking axon and gradually fills the primary synaptic cleft. When the axon terminal has disappeared, the Schwann cell occupies the primary cleft completely. The primary cleft is flattened, but little alteration occurs in the secondary clefts. Several days after disappearance of the axon terminal, mild degenerative changes occur in the subsynaptic sarcoplasm of the muscle cell. Similar motor end-plate changes were described by Tsujihata et al (1974) in acrylamide-poisoned rats.

The findings in human denervation are well summarized by Harriman (1976), who studied 134 end-plates from 50 patients with various types of neuropathy, motor neurone disease, chronic spinal muscular atrophy and peroneal muscular atrophy. As no attempt was made to differentiate morphological changes according to disease, one may assume that the changes were similar in all diseases. The withdrawal and separation of the

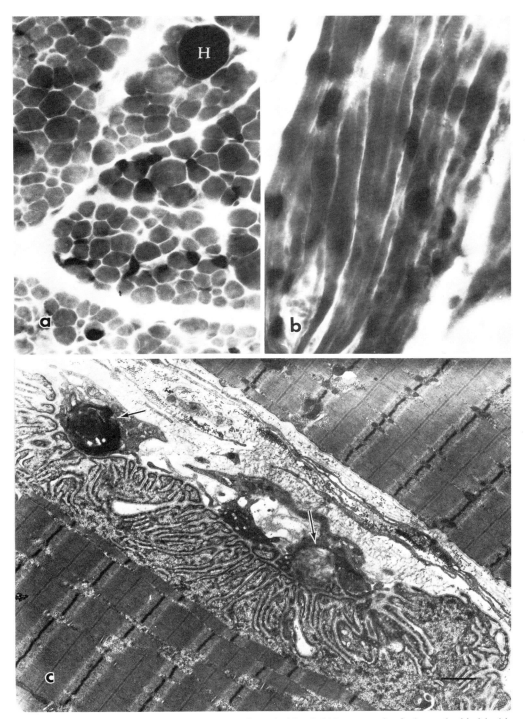

Fig. 17.15   Motor end-plates stained for acetylcholinesterase from the biopsied biceps muscle of a 2-month-old girl with Werdnig–Hoffmann disease, demonstrating end-plates even in small atrophic fibres both in cross- (a) and longitudinal- (b) section; note a hypertrophic fibre (H) characteristic of WHD. ×630. Myelin figures in terminal axons (arrows) in biopsied external intercostal muscle from a 47-year-old woman with ALS (c). Note well-preserved secondary synaptic clefts and sarcomeres near the end-plate. Bar = 1 μm

nerve terminal from the primary groove by Schwann cell cytoplasm was a characteristic early finding, as it is in the animal model. Formation of myelin bodies (Fig. 17.15c), dense bodies and mitochondrial aggregations, as well as dense packing of neurofilaments, were also seen. Break-up and disappearance of many nerve terminal elements often left electron-dense membranous profiles and debris engulfed by Schwann cell cytoplasm. Increased activity of caveolae can be readily seen in lanthanum-stained denervated motor end-plates (Fig. 17.16a). Internalization of separated terminal axons or Schwann cell cytoplasm in the sole-plate may be seen (Fig. 17.16b,c). Marked attenuation of the presynaptic membranes, and atrophied as well as rarefied clefts in the postsynaptic membranes have been described in motor end-plates in Charcot–Marie–Tooth disease (de Recondo 1970).

It is well-known that denervation of muscle results in the spread of extrajunctional AChRs over the entire sarcolemma. This phenomenon was studied by Ringel et al (1975) and Bender et al (1976) in rats, 2–40 days after denervation, by labelling AChRs with α-BT. Extrajunctional AChRs first appeared at 7 days, peaked at 2–3 weeks, and had almost disappeared by day 40. Bender et al (1976) found extrajunctional receptors on the sarcolemma of some small angulated fibres from 19 biopsies from patients with peripheral neuropathy, ALS or infantile spinal muscular atrophy. Engel et al (1975) emphasized the frequent presence of denuded postsynaptic regions in ALS, suggesting lack of regeneration and reinnervation.

In 22 motor end-plates of external intercostal muscle biopsies from four ALS patients, we too observed a denuded postsynaptic region covered with Schwann cell cytoplasm and reduplicated basal lamina (Fig. 17.17). Marked disarray of Z-discs around atrophied end-plates is frequently noted in denervated myofibres (Fig. 17.17). Motor end-plates found in two of six patients with WHD appeared to be ultrastructurally normal (Szliwowski & Drochmans 1975). Morphometry on the ultrastructure and AChRs of 74 end-plates from 10 ALS patients shows over one-third of the end-plates being denuded. Postsynaptic folds, however, are well-preserved at the denuded region,

as are the AChRs, suggesting that re-innervation by axonal sprouting may occur (Tsujihata et al 1980, 1981, 1984).

Re-innervation

In many denervating diseases, re-innervation of denervated fibres occurs from remaining viable motor axons. This process results initially in simplified, and later in apparently normal, neuromuscular junctions on denervated fibres. Sandbank & Bubis (1974) summarized the details in their review. When new motor end-plates are being formed, a double innervation (Reznik 1975) or multiple sprouting axons may share the same motor end-plates. The presence of more than one end-plate on individual myofibres with ensuing 'hyperneurotization' in various human neuromuscular diseases is described by Coërs et al (1973). Motor end-plates of target fibres indicative of post-denervation–reinnervation from a case of tourniquet paralysis during recovery show no significant morphometric differences from control end-plates and no sign of active denervation (Hazama et al 1982).

CONCLUSIONS

The documented morphological changes in motor end-plates in various neuromuscular diseases might lead one to suppose that no specific or pathognomonic alteration exists in any given disease. Such an erroneous supposition is analogous to what one may expect from light microscopic studies of end-stage diseased muscle. For example, atrophied and retracted terminal axons, denuded primary synaptic clefts and simplified secondary clefts characteristic of denervated end-plates are frequently encountered in Duchenne (or Becker-type) muscular dystrophy. Potentially, diagnostic ultrastructural parameters for specific pathological processes involving the end-plates are often obscured by other variables related to the chronicity of the disease. Had one studied the early stage of denervated end-plates, the secondary synaptic clefts would have been seen in a well-preserved state. Similarly, retraction atrophy of terminal axons should not occur in end-plates at the early stage of a myopathic disease.

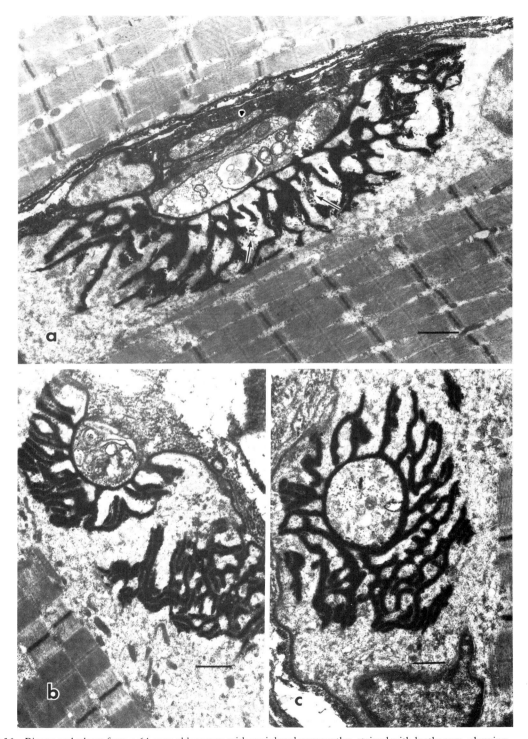

Fig. 17.16 Biceps end-plates from a 64-year-old woman with peripheral neuropathy, stained with lanthanum, showing invagination of atrophic terminal axons into the sole-plates (a,b) as well as internalization of terminal axon (c). Note active caveola (arrow) formation around secondary synaptic clefts. Bar = 1 μm

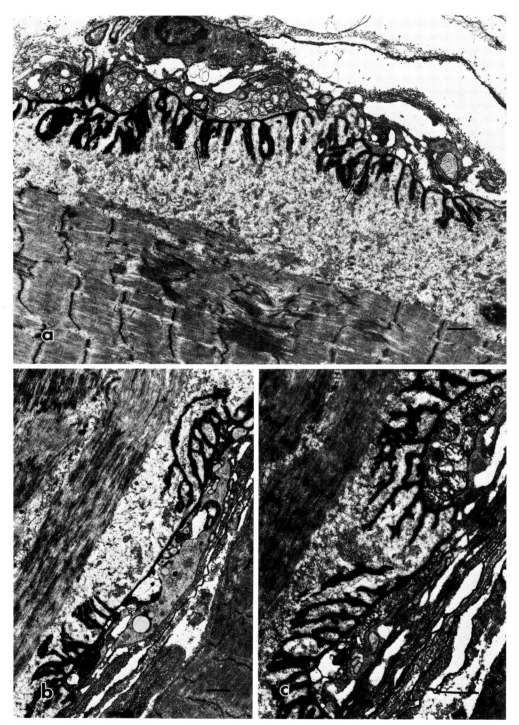

Fig. 17.17 Motor end-plates of biopsied external intercostal muscle, stained with lanthanum, from a 51-year-old man with ALS showing well-preserved secondary clefts with active caveola formation (arrow), associated with atrophic terminal axons and retraction spaces. Note streaming of Z discs in the sole-plate zone (a) and marked sarcomere disorganization with Z disc streaming (b,c); note also multiple layers of basement membrane covering the end-plate region. Bar = 1 μm

Once secondary changes are established, no matter how elaborate or extensive the morphometric analysis one applies, the data obtained for various parameters may not lead to a correct diagnosis. Furthermore, it is clearly impractical to seek age- and sex-matched as well as fibre type-matched control end-plates in order to avoid statistical bias, even when one disregards critical clinical data such as the duration of the illness, the extent of muscle activities or the drugs given. It is therefore useful to recognize the current trend towards qualitative studies, especially with various immunoperoxidase methods for observing AChRs or specific immune complexes localized at the end-plates. Together with workable experimental models, recent studies of neuromuscular junctions in MG, LES and congenital myasthenic syndromes have provided a prime example of such a fruitful approach in unravelling the enigma of the complex pathogenetic process involved. For other neuromuscular diseases, more data about the early ultrastructural changes in end-plates are needed. In addition, more descriptions are required of the accompanying findings, specific to the given end-plate lesions, in the surrounding subcellular structures including the sarcomeres immediately around the sole plate, caveolae and transverse tubules along the synaptic clefts, basal lamina and autophagosome activity.

At the moment, neuromuscular pathology alone is rarely, if ever, sufficient to determine the exact cause of a given neuromuscular disease. At the same time, one must examine muscle fibres and peripheral nerve, as well as using clinical and EMG findings to make a definite diagnosis.

ACKNOWLEDGEMENT

The author wishes to express gratitude to Drs S. Shymansky and K. Madalin for their discussion and review of the manuscript and to Mrs Sharon Sminchak for her efficient secretarial assistance.

REFERENCES

Agostini B, Noetzel M 1970 A morphological study of muscle fibers and motor endplates in tetanus. In: Walton J N, Canal N, Scarlato G (eds) Muscle diseases. Proceedings of an International Congress, Milan, 1969. Excerpta Medica, Amsterdam, p 123

Albers J W, Hodach R J, Kimmel D W, Treacy W L 1980 Penicillamine-associated myasthenia gravis. Neurology 30: 1246

Albers J W, Faulkner J A, Dorovini-Zis K, Barald K F, Must R E, Ball R D 1984 Abnormal neuromuscular transmission in an infantile myasthenic syndrome. Annals of Neurology 16: 28

Albuquerque E X, Rash J E, Mayer R F, Satterfield J R 1976 An electrophysiologic and morphological study of the neuromuscular junction in patients with myasthenia gravis. Experimental Neurology 51: 536

Aldrich M S, Kim Y I, Sanders D B 1979 Effect of D-penicillamine on neuromuscular transmission in rats. Muscle and Nerve 1: 180

Allen D E, Johnson A G, Woolf A L 1969 The intramuscular nerve endings in dystrophia myotonica. Journal of Anatomy 105: 1

Aoki T, Drachman D B, Asher D M, Gibbs C J Jr, Bahamanyar S, Wolinsky J S 1985 Attempts to implicate viruses in myasthenia gravis. Neurology 35: 185

Argov Z, Mastaglia F L 1979 Disorders of neuromuscular transmission caused by drugs. New England Journal of Medicine 301: 409

Argov Z, Nicholson L, Fawcett P R W, Mastaglia F L, Hall M 1980 Neuromuscular transmission and acetylcholine receptor antibodies in rheumatoid arthritis patients on D-penicillamine. Lancet i: 203

Awad E A 1968 Motor-point biopsies in carcinomatous neuropathology. Archives of Physical Medicine and Rehabilitation 49: 643

Barua A R, Pal N C, Ghose B P 1976 Tetanus myopathy. Indian Journal of Medical Research 64: 673

Bender A N, Willner J P 1978 Nemaline (rod) myopathy: the need for histochemical evaluation of affected families. Annals of Neurology 4: 37

Bender A N, Ringel S P, Engel W K 1976 The acetylcholine receptor in normal and pathologic states. Neurology (Minneapolis) 26: 477

Bethlem J, Arts W F, Dingemans K P 1978 Common origin of rods, cores, miniature cores, and focal loss of cross-striations. Archives of Neurology (Chicago) 35: 555

Bever C T, Dretchen K L, Blake G T et al 1984 Augmented anti-acetylcholine receptor response following longterm penicillamine administration. Annals of Neurology 16: 9

Bickerstaff E R, Woolf A L 1960 The intramuscular nerve endings in myasthenia gravis. Brain 83: 10

Bickerstaff E R, Evans J V, Woolf A L 1959 Ultrastructure of the myoneural junction in myasthenia gravis. Nature 184: 1500

Bickerstaff E R, Evans J V, Woolf A L 1960 The ultrastructure of human myasthenia and non-myasthenic motor end-plates. Brain 83: 638

Bigalke H, Dimpfel W, Habermann E 1978 Suppression of 3H-acetylcholine release from primary nerve cell cultures by tetanus and botulinum-A toxin. Naunyn-Schmiedebergs

Archiv für experimentelle Pathologie und Pharmakologie 303: 133

Bizzini B 1979 Tetanus toxin. Microbiological Reviews 43: 224

Bjornskov E J, Dekker N P, Norris F H, Stuart M E 1975 End-plate morphology in amyotrophic lateral sclerosis. Archives of Neurology (Chicago) 32: 711

Bjornskov E J, Norris F H, Mower–Kuby G 1984 Quantitative axon terminal and endplate morphology in amyotrophic lateral sclerosis. Archives of Neurology (Chicago) 32: 711

Borenstein S, Noel P, Jacquy J, Flament–Durand J 1977 Myotonic dystrophy with nerve hypertrophy. Journal of the Neurological Sciences 34: 87

Buckingham J M, Howard F M Jr, Bernatz P E, Payne W S, Harrison E G Jr, O'Brien P C, Weiland L H 1976 The value of thymectomy in myasthenia gravis. Annals of Surgery 184: 453

Burgen A S V, Dickens F, Zatman L J 1949 The action of botulinum toxin on the neuromuscular junction. Journal of Physiology 109: 10

Burres C T, Dretchen K L, Blake G J et al 1984 Augmented anti-acetylcholine receptor response following long-term penicillamine administration. Annals of Neurology 16: 9

Casanova G, Jerusalem F 1979 Myopathology of myotonic dystrophy. Acta Neuropathologica (Berlin) 45: 231

Castleman B 1966 The pathology of the thymus gland in myasthenia gravis. Annals of the New York Academy of Sciences 135: 496

Coërs C, Desmedt J E 1958 Abnormal end-plates in myasthenic muscle. Lancet ii: 1124

Coërs C, Telerman–Toppet N 1976 Morphological and histochemical changes of motor units in myasthenia. Annals of the New York Academy of Sciences 274: 6

Coërs C, Woolf A L 1959 The innervation of muscle. Blackwell, Oxford

Coërs C, Telerman–Toppet N, Gerard J M 1973 Terminal innervation ratio in neuromuscular disease II. Disorders of lower motor neuron, peripheral nerve and muscle. Archives of Neurology (Chicago) 29: 215

Conomy J P, Levinsohn M, Fanaroff A 1975 Familial infantile myasthenia gravis: a cause of sudden death in young children. Journal of Pediatrics 87: 428

Corey A L, Richman D P, Shuman C A, Gomez C M, Arnason B G W 1985 Use of monoclonal anti-acetylcholine receptor antibodies to investigate the macrophage inflammation of acute experimental myasthenia gravis: refractoriness to a second episode of acute disease. Neurology 35: 1455

Cuenoud S, Feltkamp T E W, Fulpius B W, Oosterhuis H J G H 1980 Antibodies to acetylcholine receptor in patients with thymoma but without myasthenia gravis. Neurology (Minneapolis) 30: 201

Dalaka M C, Rose J W, Paul J et al 1983 Increased circulation of T-lymphocytes bearing surface thymosin-d1 in patients with myasthenia gravis: effects of thymectomy. Neurology (Cleveland) 34: 144

Daniels M P, Vogel Z 1975 Acetylcholine receptor staining: immunoperoxidase visualization of α-bungarotoxin binding sites in muscle endplates. Nature 253: 339

de Recondo J 1970 Amyotrophie de Charcot–Marie–Tooth: Étude ultra-structurale du nerf sensitif et de la junction myoneurale. In: Proceedings of the 6th International Congress of Neuropathology. Masson, Paris, p 721

Drachman D B 1979 Acetylcholine receptors and myasthenia gravis. Proceedings of the Society for Experimental Biology and Medicine 162: 26

Duchen L W 1970 Changes in motor innervation and cholinesterase localization induced by botulinum toxin in skeletal muscles of the mouse: differences between fast and slow muscles. Journal of Neurology, Neurosurgery and Psychiatry 33: 40

Duchen L W 1971a An electron microscopic comparison of motor endplates of slow and fast skeletal muscle fibers of the mouse. Journal of the Neurological Sciences 14: 47

Duchen L W 1971b An electron microscopic study of the changes induced by botulinum toxin in the motor endplates of slow and fast skeletal muscle fibers of the mouse. Journal of the Neurological Sciences 14: 47

Duchen L W 1973a The effects of tetanus toxin on the motor end-plates of the mouse. Journal of the Neurological Sciences 19: 153

Duchen L W 1973b The local effects of tetanus toxin on the electron microscopic structure of skeletal muscle fibres of the mouse. Journal of Neurological Sciences 19: 169

Duchen L W, Tonge D A 1973 The effects of tetanus toxin on neuromuscular transmission and on the morphology of motor end-plates in slow and fast skeletal muscle of the mouse. Journal of Physiology 228: 157

Duchen L W, Stolkin C, Tonge D A 1972a Light and electron microscopic changes in slow and fast skeletal muscle fibers and their motor endplates in the mouse after the local injection of tetanus toxin. Journal of Physiology 222: 136

Duchen L W, Stolkin C, Tonge D A 1972b Changes in neuromuscular transmission in slow and fast skeletal muscles of the mouse after local injection of tetanus toxin. Journal of Physiology 222: 147

Eaton L M, Lambert E H 1957 Electromyography and electric stimulation of nerves in diseases of motor unit: observations in the myasthenic gravis syndrome associated with malignant tumors. Journal of the American Medical Association 163: 1117

Edstrom L 1975 Histochemical and histopathological changes in skeletal muscle in late-onset hereditary distal myopathy (Welander). Journal of the Neurological Sciences 26: 147

Edwards W 1970 Ultrastructural changes in the human motor endplate in myasthenia gravis. In: Proceedings of the 6th International Congress of Neuropathology. Masson, Paris, P 751

Elias S B, Appel S H 1979 Current concepts of pathogenesis and treatment of myasthenia gravis. Medical Clinics of North America 63: 745

Elmqvist D, Hoffman W W, Kugelberg J, Quastel D M J 1964 An electrophysiological investigation of neuromuscular transmission in myasthenia gravis. Journal of Physiology 174: 417

Engel W K 1971 Myotonia — a different point of view. California Medicine 114 (2): 32

Engel A G 1984 Myasthenia gravis and myasthenic syndrome. Annals of Neurology 16: 519

Engel A G, Arahata K 1987 The membrane attack complex of complement at the endplate in myasthenia gravis. Annals of the New York Academy of Sciences 505: 326

Engel A G, Santa T 1971 Histometric analysis of the ultrastructure of the neuromuscular junction in myasthenia gravis and in the myasthenic syndrome. Annals of the New York Academy of Sciences 83: 46

Engel W K, Warmolts J R 1973 The motor unit. In: Desmedt J E (ed) New developments in electromyography and clinical neurophysiology, vol 1. Karger, New York, p 141

Engel A G, Lambert E H, Santa T 1973 Study of longterm anticholinesterase therapy. Neurology (Minneapolis) 23: 1273

Engel A G, Tsujihata M N, Jerusalem F 1975 Quantitative assessment of motor endplate ultrastructure in normal and diseased human muscle. In: Dyck P J, Thomas P K, Lambert E H (eds) Peripheral neuropathy, vol 2. Saunders, Philadelphia p 1404

Engel A G, Tsujihata M N, Lambert E H, Lindstrom J M, Lennon V A 1976 Experimental autoimmune myasthenia gravis. A sequential and quantitative study of the neuromuscular junction: ultrastructural and electrophysiological correlations. Journal of Neuropathology and Experimental Neurology 35: 569

Engel A G, Lambert E H, Gomez M R 1977a A new myasthenic syndrome with endplate acetylcholinesterase deficiency, small nerve terminals and reduced acetylcholine release. Annals of Neurology 1: 4

Engel A G, Lambert E H, Howard F M 1977b Immune complexes (IgG and C3) at the motor endplate in myasthenia gravis: ultrastructural and light microscopic localization and electrophysiologic correlations. Proceedings of Staff Meetings of the Mayo Clinic 52: 267

Engel A G, Lindstrom J M, Lambert E H, Lennon V A 1977c Ultrastructural localization of acetylcholine receptor in myasthenia gravis and its experimental autoimmune model. Neurology (Minneapolis) 27: 307

Engel A G, Mokri B, Jerusalem F, Sakakibara H, Paulson O B 1977d Ultrastructural clues in Duchenne dystrophy. In: Rowland L P (ed) Pathogenesis of human muscular dystrophies. Excerpta Medica, Amsterdam, p 310

Engel A G, Sakakibara H, Sahashi K, Lindstrom J M, Lambert E H, Lennon V A 1979 Passively transferred experimental autoimmune myasthenia gravis. Neurology (Minneapolis) 29: 179

Engel A G, Lambert E H, Mulder D M et al 1981 Recently recognized myasthenic syndromes: (A) Endplate acetylcholine (ACh) esterase deficiency, (B) Putative abnormality of the ACh induced ion channel, (C) Putative defect of ACh, resynthesis or mobilization. Clinical features, ultrastructure and cytochemistry. Annals of the New York Academy of Sciences 377: 614

Engel A G, Lambert E H, Mulder D M et al 1982 A newly recognized congenital myasthenic syndrome attributed to a prolonged open time of the acetylcholine induced ion channel. Annals of Neurology 11: 553

Engel A G, Fukuoka T, Lang B, Newsom–Davis J, Vincent A, Wray D 1987 Lambert–Eaton myasthenia gravis syndrome IgG: early morphologic effects and immunolocalization at the motor endplates. Annals of the New York Academy of Sciences 505: 333

Engel A G, Nagel A, Fukuoka T et al 1989 Motor nerve terminal calcium channels in Lambert–Eaton myasthenic syndrome. Morphologic evidence for depletion and that the depletion is mediated by autoantibodies. Annals of the New York Academy of Sciences 560: 278

Eyrich K, Agostini B, Schultz A, Muller E, Noetzel M, Reichenmiller H E, Wieniers K 1967 Klinische und morphologische beobactungen von skeletmuskel-veranderinger beim tetanus. Deutsche medizinische Wochenschrift 92: 530

Fahim M A, Holley J A, Robbins N 1983 Scanning and light microscopic study of age changes at a neuromuscular junction in the mouse. Journal of Neurocytology 12: 13

Fambrough D M, Drachman D B, Satyamurti S 1973 Neuromuscular junction in myasthenia gravis. Science 172: 293

Fardeau M, Godet–Gullain J 1970 Étude ultrastructurale des

plaques motrices du muscle squelettique humain et de leurs modifications pathologiques. Proceedings of the 6th International Congress of Neuropathology. Masson, Paris p 746

Fazekas A, Komoly S, Bozsik B, Szobor A 1986 Myasthenia gravis: demonstration of membrane attack complex in muscle endplates. Clinical Neuropathology 5: 78

Fenichel G M 1966 Muscle lesions in myasthenia gravis. Annals of the New York Academy of Sciences 153: 60

Fenichel G M 1978 Clinical syndromes of myasthenia in infancy and childhood. Archives of Neurology (Chicago) 35: 97

Fukuhara N, Takamori M, Gutmann L, Chou S M 1972 Eaton–Lambert syndrome: ultrastructural study of the motor endplates. Archives of Neurology (Chicago) 27: 67

Fukuhara N, Yuaasa T, Tsubaki T, Kushiro S, Takasawa N 1978 Nemaline myopathy: histological, histochemical and ultrastructural studies. Acta Neuropathologica (Berlin) 42: 33

Fukuhara N, Suzuki M, Tsubaki T, Kushiro S, Takasawa N 1985 Ultrastructural studies on the neuromuscular junctions of Becker's muscular dystrophy. Acta Neuropathologica (Berlin) 66: 283

Fukunaga H, Engel A G, Osame M, Lambert E H 1982 Paucity and disorganization of presynaptic membrane active zones in the Lambert–Eaton myasthenic syndrome. Muscle and Nerve 5: 686

Fukunaga H, Engel A G, Lang B, Newsom–Davis J, Vincent A 1983 Passive transfer of Lambert–Eaton myasthenic syndrome with IgG from man to mouse depletes the postsynaptic membrane active zones. Proceedings of National Academy of Science 80: 7636

Fukuoka T, Engel A G, Lang B, Newsom–Davis J, Prior C, Wray D W 1987a Lambert–Eaton myasthenic syndrome: I. Early morphological effects of IgG on the presynaptic membrane active zones. Annals of Neurology 22: 193

Fukuoka T, Engel A G, Lang B, Newsom–Davis J, Vincent A 1987b Lambert–Eaton myasthenic syndrome: II. Immunoelectron microscopy localization of IgG at the mouse motor endplate. Annals of Neurology 22: 200

Genkins G, Papatestas A E, Horowitz S H, Kornfeld P 1975 Studies in myasthenia gravis: early thymectomy. American Journal of Medicine 58: 517

Gieron M A, Korthals J K 1985 Familial infantile myasthenia gravis: report of three cases with follow-up until adult life. Archives of Neurology 42: 143

Gutmann L, Chou S M 1976 Myasthenia gravis current concepts. Archives of Pathology and Laboratory Medicine 100: 401

Gutmann L, Oguchi K, Chou S M 1973 Neuromuscular junction in human botulism. Neurology (Minneapolis) 23: 424

Gutmann L, Chou S M, Pore R S 1975 Fusariosis, myasthenic syndrome and anaplastic anemia. Neurology (Minneapolis) 25: 922

Habermann E 1978 Tetanus. In: Vinken P J, Bruyn G W (eds) Handbook of clinical neurology, vol 41. North Holland, Amsterdam, p 491

Habermann E, Erdmann G 1978 Pharmacokinetic and histoautoradiographic evidence for the intra-axonal movement of toxins in the pathogenesis of tetanus. Toxicon 16: 611

Habermann E, Heller I 1975 Direct evidence for the specific fixation of Cl botulism A neurotoxin to brain matter. Naunyn–Schmiedebergs Archiv für experimentelle Pathologie und Pharmakologie 287: 97

Hanig J P, Lamanna C 1979 Toxicity of botulism toxin. Journal of Theoretical Biology 77: 107

Harriman D G F 1976 A comparison of the fine structure of motor endplates in Duchenne dystrophy and in human neuromuscular diseases. Journal of the Neurological Sciences 28: 233

Hart Z H, Sahashi K, Lambert E H, Engel A G, Lindstrom J M 1979 A congenital familial myasthenic syndrome caused by a presynaptic defect of transmitter resynthesis or mobilization. Neurology 29: 556

Hazama R, Tsujihata M, Mori M, Yoshimura T, Takamori M 1982 Ultrastructural observations of target fibers and their motor endplates in tourniquet paralysis. Clinical Neurology 22: 1

Hirokawa N, Kitamura M 1975 Localization of radioactive ^{125}I-labeled botulinus toxin at the neuromuscular junction of the mouse diaphragm. Naunyn–Schmiedebergs Archiv für experimentelle Pathologie und Pharmakologie 287: 117

Hirokawa N, Heuser 1981 Structural evidence that botulinum toxin blocks neuromuscular transmission by impairing the calcium influx that normally accompanies nerve depolarization. Journal of Cell Biology 88: 160

Hoffman E P, Brown R H, Kunkel L M 1987 Dystrophin: the protein product of the Duchenne muscular dystrophy locus. Cell 51: 919

Hofmann W W, Feigen G A 1977 Attenuation of local tetanus by treatment of ipsilateral sciatic nerve with colchicine. Experimental Neurology 54: 77

Jerusalem F, Engel A G, Gomez M R 1974 Duchenne dystrophy II. Morphometric study of motor endplate fine structure. Brain 97: 123

Kao I, Drachman D B 1977 Thymic muscle cells bear acetylcholine receptors possible relation to myasthenia gravis. Science 195: 74

Kao I, Drachman D B, Price D L 1976 Botulinum toxin mechanism of presynaptic blockade. Science 193: 1256

Karpati G, Carpenter S, Watters G V, Eisen A A, Andermann F 1973 Infantile myotonic dystrophy. Neurology (Minneapolis) 23: 1066

Kim Y I 1987 Lambert–Eaton myasthenic syndrome: evidence of calcium channel blockade. Annals of the New York Academy of Sciences 505: 377

Kim Y I, Neher E 1988 IgG from patients with Lambert–Eaton syndrome blocks voltage-dependent calcium channels. Science 239: 405

Klarinskis L S, Willcox H N A, Richmond J E, Newsom–Davis J 1986 Attempted isolation of viruses from myasthenia gravis thymus. Journal of Neuroimmunology 11: 287

Korényi–Both A L 1983 Botulism in muscle pathology in neuromuscular disease. Charles C Thomas, Springfield, IL, pp 368–369

Korényi–Both A L, Szobor A, Lapis K, Szathmary I 1973 Fine structural studies in myasthenia gravis. II. Lesions of the neuromuscular junction. European Neurology 10: 311

Kryzhanovsky G N, 1973 The mechanism of action of tetanus toxin: effect on synaptic processes and some particular features of toxin binding by the nervous tissue. Naunyn–Schmiedebergs Archiv für experimentelle Pathologie und Pharmakologie 276: 247

Kuncl R W, Pestronk A, Drachman D B, Rechthand E 1986 The pathophysiology of penicillamine induced myasthenia gravis. Annals of Neurology 20: 740

Lambert E H, Elmqvist D 1971 Quantal components of endplate potentials in the myasthenic syndrome. Annals of the New York Academy of Sciences 183: 183

Lambert E H, Rooke E D 1965 Myasthenic state and lung cancer. In: Brain L, Norris F M (eds) The remote effects of cancer on the nervous system. Grune and Stratton, New York, p 67

Lambert E H, Eaton L M, Rooke E D 1956 Defect of neuromuscular conduction associated with malignant neoplasms. American Journal of Physiology 187: 612

Lang B, Newsom-Davis J, Wray D et al 1981 Autoimmune etiology for myasthenic (Lambert–Eaton) syndrome. Lancet ii: 224

Lang B, Newsom–Davis J, Prior C, Wray 1983 Antibodies to motor nerve terminals: and electrophysiological study of a human myasthenic syndrome transferred to a mouse. Journal of Physiological 344: 335

Lang B, Newsom–Davis J, Peers C et al 1987 The effect of myasthenic syndrome antibody on presynaptic calcium channels in mouse. Journal of Physiology 390: 257

Lecky B R, Morgan–Hughes J A, Murray N M, Landon D N, Wray D 1986 Congenital myasthenia: further evidence of disease heterogeneity. Muscle and Nerve 9: 233

Lee Cy, Tseng L F, Chiu T H 1967 Influence of denervation on localization of neurotoxin from celapid venoms in rat diaphragm. Nature 215: 1177

Lefvert A K, Osterman P O 1983 Newborn infants to myasthenic mothers: a clinical study and an investigation of acetylcholine receptor antibodies in 17 children. Neurology 33: 133

Lennon V A, Lindstrom J M, Seybold M E 1976 Experimental autoimmune myasthenia gravis: cellular and humoral immune responses. Annals of the New York Academy of Sciences 274: 283

Lennon V A, Seybold M E, Lindstrom J M 1978 Role of complement in the pathogenesis of experimental autoimmune myasthenia gravis. Journal of Experimental Medicine 147: 973

Lentz T L, Burrago T G, Smith A L, Crick J, Tignor G H 1982 Is the acetylcholine receptor a rabies virus receptor? Science 215: 182

Lindstrom J M 1979 Experimental autoimmune myasthenia gravis. In: Aguayo A J, Karpati G (eds) Current topics in nerve and muscle research. Excerpta Medica, Amsterdam, p 104

Lindstrom J M, Lambert E H 1978 Content of acetylcholine receptors and antibodies bound to receptor in myasthenia gravis, experimental autoimmune myasthenia gravis, and Eaton–Lambert syndrome. Neurology (Minneapolis) 28: 130

Lindstrom J M, Seybold M E, Lennon V A, Whittingham S, Duane D D 1976 Antibody to acetylcholine receptor in myasthenia gravis. Neurology (Minneapolis) 26: 1054

McComas A J, Sica R E P, Campbell M J 1971 'Sick' motor neurones — a unifying concept of muscle disease. Lancet i: 321

MacDermot D 1961 The histology of the neuromuscular junction in dystrophia myotonica. Brain 84: 75

Malathi S, Batmanabane M 1983 Alterations in the morphology of the neuromuscular junctions following experimental immobilization in cats. Experimenta 39: 547

Markesbery W R, Griggs R C, Leach R P, Lapham L W 1974 Late onset hereditary distal myopathy. Neurology (Minneapolis) 24: 127

Markesbery W R, Griggs R C, Herr B 1977 Distal myopathy: electron microscopic and histochemical studies. Neurology (Minneapolis) 27: 727

Miike T, Chou S M, Payne W N 1980 Formation of rods,

central cores/targetoids and multicores in experimental local tetanus. Neurology (Minneapolis) 30: 402

Monaco A P, Neve R L, Colletti–Feener C, Bertelson C J, Kurnit D M, Kunkel L M 1986 Isolation of candidate cDNA's for portions of the Duchenne muscular dystrophy gene. Nature 323: 644

Mora M, Lambert E H, Engel A G 1987 Synaptic vesicle abnormality in familial infantile myasthenia. Neurology 37: 206

Mossman S, Vincent A, Newsom–Davis J 1986 Myasthenia gravis without acetylcholine receptor antibody: a distinct disease entity. Lancet i: 116

Mossman S, Vincent A, Newsom–Davis J 1988 Passive transfer of myasthenia gravis by immunoglobulins: lack of correlation between AChR with antibody bound, acetylcholine receptor loss and transmission defect. Journal of the Neurological Sciences 84: 15

Nagel A, Engel A G, Lang B, Newsom–Davis J, Fukuoka T 1988 Lambert–Eaton syndrome IgG depletes presynaptic membrane active zone particles by antigenic modulation. Annals of Neurology 24: 552

Oda K 1984 Age changes of motor innervation and acetylcholine receptor distribution on human skeletal muscle fibers. Journal of the Neurological Sciences 66: 327

Ogata T 1988 Structure of motor endplates in the different fiber types of vertebrate skeletal muscles. Archives of Histology and Cytology 51: 385

Ogata T, Murata F 1973 Cytological features or red, white and intermediate muscle fibers and their motor end-plates. In: Kakulas B A (ed) Basic research in myology. Excerpta Medica, Amsterdam, p 469

O'Neil J H, Murray N M F, Newsom–Davis J 1988 Lambert–Eaton syndrome: a review of 50 cases. Brain 11: 577

Oosterhuis H J G H 1989 The natural course of myasthenia gravis: a long-term follow-up study. Journal of Neurology, Neurosurgery and Psychiatry 52: 1121

Pachter B R, Eberstein A 1984 Neuromuscular plasticity following limb immobilization. Journal of Neurocytology 13: 1013

Pachter B R, Eberstein A 1983 Endplate postsynaptic structure dependent upon muscle activity. Neuroscience Letter 43: 277

Padykula H A, Gauthier G F 1970 The ultrastructure of the neuromuscular junctions of mammalian red, white and intermediate skeletal muscle fibers. Journal of Cell Biology 46: 27

Pascuzzi R M, Campa J F 1988 Lymphorrhage localized to the muscle and endplate in myasthenia gravis. Archives of Pathology and Laboratory Medicine 112: 934

Penn A S 1979 Immunological features of myasthenia gravis. In: Aguayo A J, Karpati G (eds) Current topics in nerve and muscle research. Excerpta Medica, Amsterdam, p 123

Pestronk A, Drachman D B 1978 Motor nerve sprouting and acetylcholine receptors. Science 199: 1123

Pestronk A, Drachman D B 1985 Polymyositis: Reduction of acetylcholine receptors in skeletal muscle. Muscle and Nerve 8: 233

Pestronk A, Drachman D B, Griffin J W 1976a Effects of muscle disuse on acetylcholine receptors. Nature 260: 352

Pestronk A, Drachman D B, Griffin J W 1976b Effect of botulinum toxin on trophic regulation of acetylcholine receptors. Nature 264: 787

Pestronk A, Drachman D B, Griffin J W 1980 Effects of aging on nerve sprouting and regeneration. Experimental Neurology 70: 65

Pestronk A, Drachman D B, Self S G 1985 Measurement of junctional acetylcholine receptors on myasthenia gravis: clinical correlates. Muscle and Nerve 8: 245

Price D L, Griffin J W, Peck K 1977 Tetanus toxin evidence for binding at presynaptic nerve endings. Brain Research 121: 379

Pulliam D L, April E W 1979 A degenerative change at the neuromuscular junctions of red, white and intermediate muscle fibers. 1. Response to short stump nerve section. 2. Response to long stump nerve section and colchicine treatment. Journal of the Neurological Sciences 43: 205

Pumplin D W, Reese T S 1977 Action of brown widow spider venom and botulinum toxin on the frog neuromuscular junction examined with the freeze fracture technique. Journal of Physiology 273: 443

Rash J E, Albuquerque E X, Hudson C S 1976 Studies of human myasthenia gravis: electrophysiological and ultrastructural evidence compatible with antibody attachment to acetylcholine receptor complex. Proceedings of the National Academy of Sciences of the United States of America 73: 4584

Reske–Nielsen E, Gregersen G, Harmsen A, Lundback K 1970 Morphological abnormalities of the terminal neuromuscular apparatus in recent juvenile diabetics. Diabetologia 6: 104

Reznik M 1975 Histochemical aspects of regenerating myofibres before and after reinnervation. In: Bradley W (ed) Recent advances in myology: Third International Congress in Muscle Diseases 1974. Excerpta Medica Amsterdam, p 330

Ringel S P, Bender A N, Festhoff B W, Vogel Z, Daniels M P 1975 Ultrastructural demonstration and analytical application of extrajunctional receptors of denervated human and rat skeletal muscle fibers. Nature 255: 730

Robertson W C, Chun R W M, Kornguth S E 1980 Familial infantile myasthenia. Archives of Neurology 37: 117

Rosenheimer J L, Smith D O 1985 Differential changes in the endplate architecture of functionally diverse muscles during aging. Journal of Neurophysiology 53: 1567

Russell D S 1953 Histological changes in the striped muscles in myasthenia gravis. Journal of Pathology 65: 270

Sahashi K, Engel A G, Lindstrom J M 1978a Ultrastructural localization of immune complexes (IgG and C3) at the endplate in experimental autoimmune myasthenia gravis. Journal of Neuropathology and Experimental Neurology 37: 212

Sahashi K, Engel A G, Lambert E H, Sakakibara H 1978b Ultrastructural location and quantitation of the acetylcholine receptor (AChR) in Lambert–Eaton myasthenic syndrome and electrophysiological correlation. Journal of Neuropathology and Experimental Neurology 37: 684

Sahashi K, Engel A G, Lambert E H, Howard F M Jr 1980 Ultrastructural localization of the terminal and lytic ninth complement component (C9) at the motor endplate in myasthenia gravis. Journal of Neuropathology and Experimental Neurology 39: 160

Sakakibara H, Engel A G, Lambert E H 1977 Duchenne dystrophy: ultrastructural localization of the acetylcholine receptor and intracellular microelectrode studies of neuromuscular transmission. Neurology (Minneapolis) 27: 741

Sakimoto T, Cheng–Minoda K 1970 Fine structure of neuromuscular junctions in myasthenic extraocular muscles. Investigative Ophthalmology 9: 316

Sandbank U, Bubis J J 1974 The morphology of motor end-plates. Brain Information Service/Brain Research Institute, Los Angeles, p 21

Santa T, Engel A G 1973 Histometric analysis of neuromuscular junction ultrastructure in red, white and intermediate muscle fibers. In: Desmedt J E (ed) New developments in electromyography and clinical neurophysiology, vol 1. Karger, Basel, p 41

Santa T, Engel A G, Lambert E H 1972 Histometric study of neuromuscular junction ultrastructure, I. Myasthenia gravis. Neurology (Minneapolis) 22: 71

Sato T, Tamiya N, Yang C C 1977 Ultracytochemical localization of acetylcholine receptor in myasthenia gravis in nude mice transplanted with thymoma. Muscular Dystrophy Group, Tokyo, Japan, p 36

Seybold M E, Lindstrom J M 1981 Myasthenia gravis in infancy. Neurology (NY) 31: 476

Shore A, Limatibul S, Dosch H-M, Gelfand E W 1979 Identification of two serum components regulating the expression of T-lymphocyte function in childhood myasthenia gravis. New England Journal of Medicine 301: 625

Simpson J A 1960 Myasthenia gravis: a new hypothesis. Scottish Medical Journal 5: 419

Simpson L S 1978 Pharmacological studies on the subcellular site of action of botulinum toxin type A. Journal of Pharmacology and Experimental Therapeutics 206: 661

Smit L M E, Jennekens F G, Veldman H, Barth P G 1984 Paucity of secondary synaptic clefts in a case of congenital myasthenia with multiple contractures: ultrastructural morphology of a developmental disorder. Journal of Neurology, Neurosurgery and Psychiatry 47: 1091

Smit L M E, Hageman G, Veldman H, Molenar P C, Oen B S, Jennekens F G I 1988 A myasthenic syndrome with congenital paucity of secondary synaptic clefts: CPSC syndrome. Muscle and Nerve 11: 337

Smith D O, Rosenheimer J L 1982 Decreased sprouting and degeneration of nerve terminals of active muscles in aged rats. Journal of Neurophysiology 48: 100

Stålberg E, Ekstedt J 1969 Signs of neuropathology in distal hereditary myopathy (Welander). Electroencephalography and Clinical Neurophysiology 26: 338

Stanley E F, Drachman D B 1978 Effect of myasthenic immunoglobulin on acetylcholine receptors intact mammalian neuromuscular junctions. Science 200: 1285

Stockel K, Schwab M, Thoenen 1975 Comparison between the retrograde axonal transport of nerve growth factor and tetanus toxin in motor, sensory and adrenergic neurons. Brain Research 99: 1

Stoebner P, Sengel A, Gesel M, Isch F 1970 Ultrastructure de certains polymyosites myastheniforme. Proceedings of the 6th International Congress of Neuropathology. Masson, Paris, p 1078

Szliwowski H B, Drochmans P 1975 Ultrastructural aspects of muscle and nerve in Werdnig–Hoffman disease. Acta Neuropathologica (Berlin) 31: 281

Teräväinen H 1968 Development of the myoneural junction in the rat. Zeitschrift für Zellforschung und mikroskopische Anatomie 79: 198

Thesleff S 1960 Supersensitivity of skeletal muscle produced by botulinum toxin. Journal of Physiology 151: 598

Tomlinson B E, Walton J N, Irving D 1974 Spinal cord limb motor neurons in muscular dystrophy. Journal of the Neurological Sciences 22: 305

Toyka K V, Drachman D B, Pestronk A, Kao I 1975 Myasthenia gravis: passive transfer from man to mouse. Science 190: 397

Tsujihata M, Engel A G, Lambert E H 1974 Motor end-plate fine structure in acrylamide dying-back neuropathy: a sequential morphometric study. Neurology (Minneapolis) 24: 849

Tsujihata M, Hazama R, Ishii N, Yoshihiko I, Takamori M 1980 Ultrastructural localization of acetylcholine receptor at the motor endplate: myasthenia gravis and other neuromuscular diseases. Neurology 30: 1203

Tsujihata M, Hazama R, Yoshimura T, Akira S 1981 The motor endplate in human neuromuscular disorders: a quantitation study. Journal of Clinical Electron Microscopy 14: 5

Tsujihata M, Hazama R, Yoshimura T, Satoh A, Mori, Nagasaki S 1984 The motor endplate fine structure and ultrastructural localization of acetylcholine receptors in amyotrophic lateral sclerosis. Muscle and Nerve 7: 243

Tsujihata M, Kinohsita I, Mori M, Mori K, Shirabe S, Satoh A, Nagasaki S 1987 Ultrastructural study of the motor endplate in botulism and Lambert–Eaton myasthenic syndrome. Journal of the Neurological Sciences 81: 197

Tsujihata M, Yoshimura T, Satoh A et al 1989 Diagnostic significance of IgG, C3 and C9 at the limb muscle motor endplate in minimal myasthenia gravis. Neurology 39: 1359

Tuffery A R 1971 Growth and degeneration of motor end-plates in normal cat hind limb muscles. Journal of Anatomy 110: 221

Twomey J J, Lewis V M, Patten B M, Goldstein G, Good R A 1979 Myasthenia gravis, thymectomy and serum thymic hormone activity. American Journal of Medicine 66: 639

Vincent A, Newsom–Davis J 1982 Acetylcholine receptor antibody characteristics in myasthenia gravis: II. Patients with penicillamine-induced myasthenia or idiopathic myasthenia of recent onset. Clinical and Experimental Immunology 49: 1982

Vincent A, Newsom–Davis J 1985 Acetylcholine receptor antibody as a diagnostic test for myasthenia gravis: results in 153 validated cases and 2967 diagnostic assays. Journal of Neurology, Neurosurgery and Psychiatry 48: 1246

Vincent A, Cull–Candy S G, Newsom–Davis J et al 1981 Congenital myasthenia: endplate acetylcholine receptors and electrophysiology in five cases. Muscle and Nerve 4: 306

Walker M B 1934 Treatment of myasthenia gravis with physostigmine. Lancet i: 1200

Walton J N, Irving D, Tomlinson B E 1977 Spinal cord limb motor neurons in dystrophica myotonica. Journal of the Neurological Sciences 34: 199

Welander L 1951 Myopathia distalis tarda hereditaria. Acta Medica Scandinavica 141 (supplement 265): 1

Wernig A, Stover H, Tonge D 1977 The labeling of motor end-plates in skeletal muscle of mice with ^{125}I tetanus toxin. Naunyn-Schmiedebergs Arch für experimentelle Pathologie und Pharmakologie 298: 37

Wiegand H, Erdmann G, Wellhoner H H 1976 ^{125}I-labeled botulinum A neurotoxin: pharmacokinetics in cats after intramuscular injection. Naunyn–Schmiedebergs Archiv für experimentelle Pathologie und Pharmakologie 292: 161

Wiesendanger M, D'Alessandri A 1963 Myasthenia gravis mit fokaler infiltration der Endplattenzone. Acta Neuropathologica 2: 246

Wise R P, MacDermot V 1962 A myasthenic syndrome associated with bronchial carcinoma. Journal of Neurology, Neurosurgery and Psychiatry 25: 31

Wokke J H J, Jennekens F G I, Molenaar P C, Van den Oord C J M, Oen B S, Busch H F M 1989 Congenital paucity of secondary synaptic clefts (CPSC) syndrome in two adult sibs. Neurology 39: 648

Woolf A L 1966 Morphology of the myasthenic neuromuscular junction. Annals of the New York Academy of Sciences 135: 35

Woolf A L, Coërs C 1974 Pathological anatomy of the intramuscular nerve endings. In: Walton J N (ed) Disorders of voluntary muscle, 3rd edn, Churchill Livingstone, Edinburgh, p 274

Zacks S I (ed) 1964 The motor endplate. W B Saunders, Philadelphia

Zacks S I, Hall J A S, Scheff M F 1966 Intramitochondrial disease granules in skeletal muscle from human case of tetanus intoxication. American Journal of Pathology 48: 811

Zacks S I, Rhoades M V, Sheff M F 1968 The localization of botulinum A toxin in the mouse. Experimental and Molecular Pathology 9: 77

18. Pathology of intramuscular nerves and nerve terminals

C. Coërs

INTRODUCTION

Increasing experience with muscle biopsies stained by conventional methods has shown that the classical criteria for the diagnosis of denervation and myopathy are often misleading. Myopathic changes in the muscle fibres occur frequently in chronic denervation (Haase & Shy 1960, Drachman et al 1967, Mumenthaler 1970). Conversely, grouped fibre atrophy, which is considered to be the hallmark of denervation, may occasionally also be observed in myopathy (Dastur & Razzak 1973, Dubowitz & Brooke 1973, Adams 1974), and is frequently missing in biopsies from patients with neurogenic disorders (Coërs & Telerman-Toppet 1978).

Histochemical typing of muscle fibres provided new morphological criteria of denervation. A striking change, probably related to collateral reinnervation and enzymatic conversion of muscle fibres has been described as type grouping (Brooke & Engel 1966). It has also been assumed that denervated fibres undergoing atrophy become angulated and darkly stained in oxidative enzyme preparations (Dubowitz & Brooke 1973). Indeed, type grouping is a reliable index of denervation but not a very sensitive one as it has been found in only about one-fifth of biopsies in some studies (Coërs & Telerman-Toppet 1978). Moreover, this change is occasionally seen in myopathy and has been related to longitudinal splitting or regeneration of muscle fibres ('myopathic type grouping') (Karpati et al 1974, Carpenter et al 1978).

Small fibres stained darkly for oxidative enzymes are present in any kind of muscular atrophy, and become angulated only when closely surrounded and apparently compressed by other fibres (Coërs

& Telerman-Toppet 1978). This situation is common in denervation, but is also seen in the myopathies in which compact bundles of muscle fibres are preserved, as in facioscapulohumeral and oculopharyngeal dystrophy (Dubowitz & Brooke 1973), Becker dystrophy (Bradley et al 1978) and limb-girdle dystrophy (Coërs & Telerman-Toppet 1979). Small dark angular fibres are numerous in these conditions, as they are in type 2 fibre atrophy (Telerman-Toppet & Coërs 1975) and in some cases of myasthenia gravis (Brody & Engel 1964). If there is a loss of muscle fibres and endomysial fibrosis, small fibres remain rounded, as in Duchenne muscular dystrophy and also in infantile spinal muscular atrophy (Dubowitz & Brooke 1973). Therefore, small angular dark fibres are by no means a reliable histological indication of denervation.

Some myologists have been misled by certain muscle fibre changes, attributing them specifically to denervation or to myopathy, and creating a state of confusion by blurring the boundaries of neuromuscular diseases without improving our understanding of their pathophysiology. Accuracy of histological diagnosis of neuromuscular disorders requires, in addition to conventional histology and histochemistry, the investigation of intramuscular nerves. This task has been made possible through the demonstration of the zonal distribution of intramuscular nerve endings and the electrical localization of this region, and by the introduction into the muscle biopsy technique of vital staining with methylene blue, and histochemical demonstration of the (acetyl)-cholinesterase activity of the subneural apparatus of the motor end-plate (Coërs 1952, 1953a,b, 1955). A combined silver and acetylcholinesterase method has also been described (Beerman & Cassens 1976, Pestronk and Drachman 1978).

TECHNIQUE OF SAMPLING AND STAINING OF THE INTRAMUSCULAR INNERVATION

Most limb muscles have only one band of terminal motor innervation which, in some of them, corresponds closely to the motor point (Fig. 18.1 a,b). These muscles are therefore particularly suitable for biopsy of intramuscular nerves. They are palmaris longus and flexor carpi radialis in the upper limb, and vastus medialis in the lower limb. The biceps brachii, deltoid and rectus femoris may also be used but the localization of the innervation band is less accurate in these muscles.

Sampling

A careful determination of the motor point of the muscle selected is carried out using an electrical stimulator. After local anaesthesia of the subcutaneous tissue, the skin and fascia are incised across the motor point, parallel to the long axis of the muscle fibres. An opening of 4–5 cm only is necessary. The terminal innervation area can be localized accurately on the exposed muscle with a sterile metallic electrode connected to the cathode of the stimulator. This localization is important because the band of terminal innervation is very narrow and usually not broader than 2 mm (Fig. 18.1c). Stimuli 0.1 ms in duration are delivered at a frequency of 1/s. The nerve endings will be found at the points where a single fascicle, and not the whole muscle, contracts when stimulated by a current too weak to produce contraction when applied to any other part of that fascicle. The current should usually be of the order of 0.1–0.5 mA with a stabilized current stimulator, or 1–10 V with a stabilized voltage apparatus. The accuracy of this localization can be blurred in partly denervated muscles or in myopathy when the innervation zone is enlarged (see below). On the whole, the yield of the method is about 95%. Confirmation that localization of the terminal innervation zone was correct can usually be obtained by passing a scalpel along the fascicle. A muscle twitch results when the innervation zone is crossed.

Staining

Before staining the selected fascicle with methylene blue, specimens are removed for muscle fibre histology and histochemistry outside the innervation zone. If electron microscopy is to be performed, a strip, not wider than 2 mm, is removed with a biopsy forceps across the innervation zone. Another strip may be removed within the same area for the cholinesterase reaction, if needed.

Vital staining with methylene blue

The selected fascicle is injected with an 0.05% sterile solution of methylene blue in physiological saline, using the finest needle available. The needle is introduced parallel to the long axis of the fascicle and just below its surface, and the solution is injected gently as the needle is being withdrawn. This is repeated on the length to be removed (2–3 cm), during a period of 3–5 min, using 10–30 ml of solution. The patient sometimes experiences an aching pain during the injection, and when the muscle sample is cut. This pain may be prevented without interfering with the vital staining by injecting 1% xylocaine solution before the methylene blue injection. Two or three strips, no more than a few millimetres thick, are removed and placed on gauze moistened with physiological saline in a Petri dish and oxygenated for 1 h. For this purpose a suitable sized funnel is inverted over the specimen, and oxygen is passed at the rate of 1 l/min for 1 h. A flowmeter, in which the oxygen is bubbled through water, is of great value as otherwise the specimens must be moistened by drops of saline every 10–15 min to avoid drying. This oxygenation converts the leucoderivative of methylene blue into the blue form. If oxygenation is insufficient, the nerve endings will not appear stained. Excessive oxygenation causes the subneural apparatus to appear stained and confuses the picture. Immediately after oxygenation has been completed, the muscle is placed in a filtered, cold, aqueous, saturated solution of ammonium molybdate in the refrigerator at 4°C for 24 h. It is then thoroughly washed in three changes of distilled water. This is also important as insufficient washing may result in crystals of ammonium molybdate forming when frozen sections are cut.

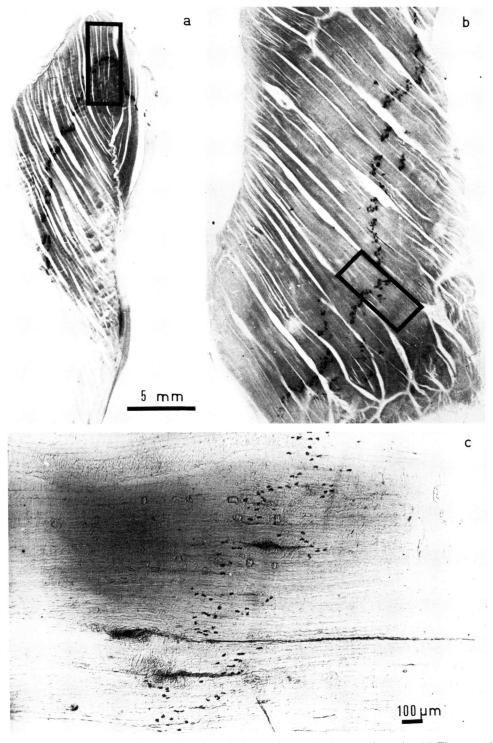

Fig. 18.1 Modified thiocholine method. Topography of terminal motor innervation in normal muscles. (a) Flexor carpi radialis of a 3-month-old child. (b) Vastus internus of an 8-month-old child. The site for biopsy of the intramuscular innervation across the motor point is indicated. (c) Localization of motor nerve endings in vastus internus of a 9-year-old child

After washing, the muscle is placed in 10% formol saline for 24 h, after which frozen longitudinal sections are cut at 75–100 nm. Sections from infants are cut thinner, e.g. 30 nm. Too long a period in formol saline leads to fading of the stain. The sections are washed in distilled water, placed in a 50% solution of alcohol, mounted and dried on albuminized slides, dehydrated in acetone (absolute alcohol produces fading), cleared in toluol and mounted in a neutral medium (Harleco synthetic resin).

Cholinesterase staining

The strip removed across the innervation zone for this purpose is placed in 10% formol saline for 4–5 h, and then cut as frozen longitudinal sections 50–75 nm thick. The sections are rinsed in three changes of distilled water and placed in the incubating solution (formula below) at 37°C. Not more than 10 sections should be placed in 10 ml of this solution. After incubation for 30 min, a section is taken out, washed in distilled water, placed for 5 min in 5% aqueous ammonium sulphide and examined under the low-power microscope. If the staining of the subneural apparatus is satisfactory, the remaining sections are taken out and treated in the same way. If staining is too weak, incubation may be prolonged for up to 45 or 60 min. To prevent fading of the brown coloration of the subneural apparatus, a further 24 h period of fixation in 10% formalin is recommended. The sections are then mounted in the same way as the methylene blue preparations.

The incubating solution is prepared according to the method of Koelle & Friedenwald (1949) modified by Couteaux (1951) and by Coërs (1953b).

Solution 1: Aminoacetic acid 3.75 g
Distilled water 100 ml

Solution 2: CuSO$_4$ 0.1 M (24.9g/l)

Solution 3: Buffer at pH5
Acetic acid 0.1 mol/l (6ml/l) 6 ml
Na acetate 0.1 mol/l (13.6g/l) 2 ml

Solution 4: Acetyl thiocholine freshly prepared by taking the supernatant fluid after centrifuging the following mixture at 2000 r.p.m.:

Acetyl thiocholine iodide 30 mg
Distilled water 1.4 ml
Solution 2 0.6 ml

The incubating solution is made up as follows:

Solution 1 0.4 ml
Solution 2 0.4 ml
Solution 3 10.0 ml
Distilled water 7.6 ml
Solution 4 0.8 ml, added immediately before use

MOTOR INNERVATION IN NORMAL MUSCLES

The innervation zone contains small nerves which give rise to individual nerve fibres, or break up into a group of such fibres, which run only a short course in isolation before they reach the muscle fibres and form their terminal arborization (Fig. 18.2). These fibres, which can be followed individually from the intramuscular nerve up to the motor ending, are defined as subterminal axons because occasional branching of these fibres can occur at collateral, terminal or ultraterminal level. The two arborizations resulting from such a branching usually subserve the same muscle fibre (Fig. 18.2b) and less frequently two different muscle fibres (Fig. 18.2c). This branching can be quantitatively estimated as the terminal innervation ratio (TIR).

In order to give a functional significance to this ratio, we must count double end-plates on single muscle fibres as single units, and should only consider, in arriving at the functional or true TIR, the formation by subterminal nerve fibres of end-plates on more than one muscle fibre (Fig. 18.3). Thus the true TIR can be defined as the number of muscle fibres innervated by a given number of subterminal axons. Measurements are made only on the subterminal axons that can be traced from an intramuscular nerve up to the motor arborization, or that can be followed for a distance exceeding 200 μm to their endings. An average of 50 subterminal axons meet these criteria in each biopsy. Occasionally 100–200 axons are available. Branching within intramuscular nerves is not included in measurements. In most instances the neuromuscular junction is clearly seen, making it easy to decide whether a branching axon supplies

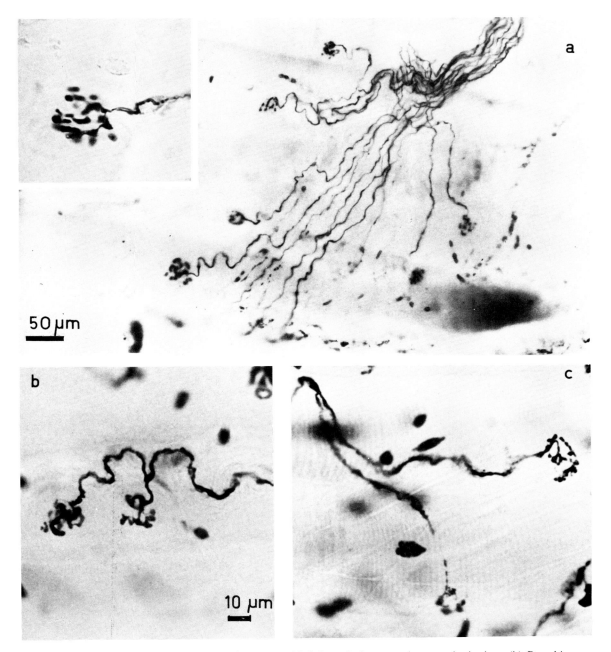

Fig. 18.2 Vital methylene blue. Normal innervation pattern. (a) Subterminal axons and motor arborizations. (b) Branching axon forming two motor arborizations on the same muscle fibre. (c) Branching axon innervating two muscle fibres. Reproduced from Arch. Neurol. 1973, 29: 210–222 with kind permission of Coërs C, Telerman-Toppet N and Gerard J M.

only one muscle fibre through two or more terminal arborizations, or innervates more than one muscle fibre. Occasionally, however, because of superimpositions, the borders of the muscle fibres are blurred, and tracing the actual distri-bution of a branching nerve fibre is impossible. In that case, assuming that distant motor arborizations have more chance of innervating different muscle

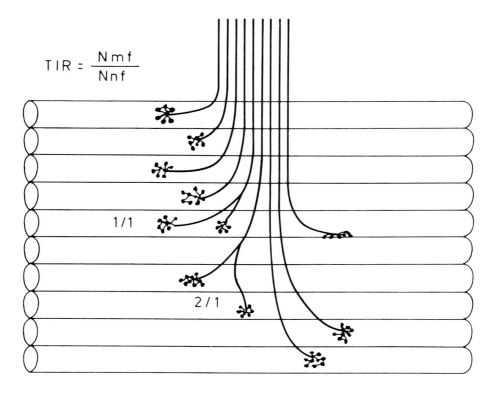

$$TIR = \frac{Nmf}{Nnf}$$

1/1

2/1

$$TIR = 10/9 = 1.11$$

Fig. 18.3 Diagrammatic representation of the pattern of terminal motor innervation, and formula for calculating the terminal innervation ratio (TIR). Nmf: number of muscle fibres; Nnf: number of terminal motor axons

fibres than have arborizations close to each other, we have adopted the arbitrary rule that a branching axon supplies two muscle fibres when the distance between the two motor arborizations resulting from this branching exceeds the diameter of the larger arborization (Coërs et al 1973b).

The TIR was measured in a control group including 13 volunteer university students (Coërs et al 1973a) and 43 patients with no clinical or electromyographic indication of neuromuscular diseases and without histological changes in muscle stained by conventional methods (Coërs 1955, Coërs et al 1973b). The mean TIR in this group was 1.11 ± 0.05, the range of individual values being 1.01–1.20. There are no significant differences in the TIR between the more frequently biopsied muscles and no apparent changes with age. It can be stated that values exceeding 1.21

(mean + 2 s.d.) are probably abnormal, and values exceeding 1.26 (mean + 3 s.d.) are certainly abnormal, and indicate a compensatory collateral re-innervation in response to partial denervation.

At the level of the neuromuscular junction (motor end-plate), the axoplasmic enlargements of terminal arborizations (telodendrion) lie in grooves on the surface of the sarcoplasm, forming the primary synaptic clefts (see Ch. 1). At these grooves, or gutters, the sarcoplasmic plasma membrane undergoes a profuse folding (secondary synaptic clefts, or junctional folds) (de Harven & Coërs 1959; Fig. 18.4), which in histochemical preparations for cholinesterase appear as stripes, more or less parallel to each other and perpendicular to the surface of the gutters. This palisade-like structure (subneural apparatus) represents the postsynaptic part of the neuromuscular junction

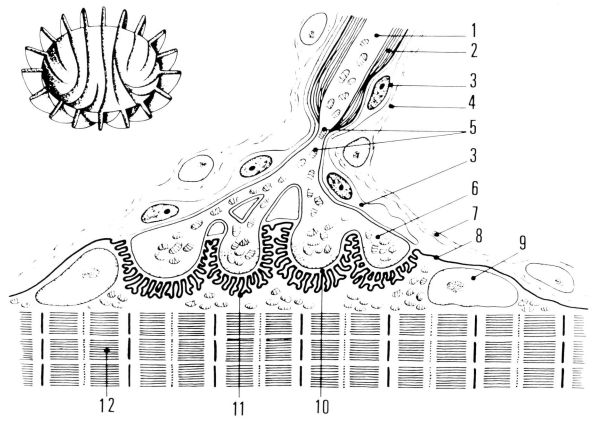

Fig. 18.4 Diagram of the neuromuscular junction. 1—axis clinder; 2—myelin; 3—Schwann cell; 4—Henle sheath; 5—mitochondria; 6—motor arborization; 7—endomysium; 8—sarcolemma; 9—muscle fibre nucleus; 10—primary synaptic cleft; 11—secondary synaptic clefts (junctional folds); 12—myofibrils. Upper left, tridimensional representation of a unit of the subneural apparatus

(Couteaux 1947). In man, the subneural apparatus is formed by separate elements or units and accommodates only the axoplasmic enlargements of the telodendrion and not the whole terminal arborisation (Fig. 18.5), as is the case in other animal species (Coërs 1955, Coërs & Woolf 1959). Its shape is fairly constant and only its size shows variations which were estimated in our control material by the measurement of either the diameter or the surface area of the subneural apparatus. The mean diameter was 32.2 μm ± 10.5, the observed values ranging from 10 μm to 80 μm (Coërs 1955). The mean value for the surface area of the motor end-plates ranged from 177 μm² to 314 μm² (Coërs & Hildebrand 1965, Reske-Nielsen et al 1970). The histograms of motor end-

plate diameter and surface area corresponded to a unimodal normal or logarithmic-normal distribution curve and did not indicate that more than one population of motor nerve endings was present which might be related to the enzymatic and functional heterogeneity of muscle fibres. The only correlation found was that the size of the motor endings is proportional to the diameter of the muscle fibres they supply (Coërs 1955, Anzenbacher & Zenker 1963, Nyström 1968, Witalinski & Loesch 1975).

In addition to marked variations in size, some motor arborizations in biopsies from healthy young adults show marked irregularity of the size of the axoplasmic expansions of the telodendrion (Reske-Nielsen et al 1970), a feature that was

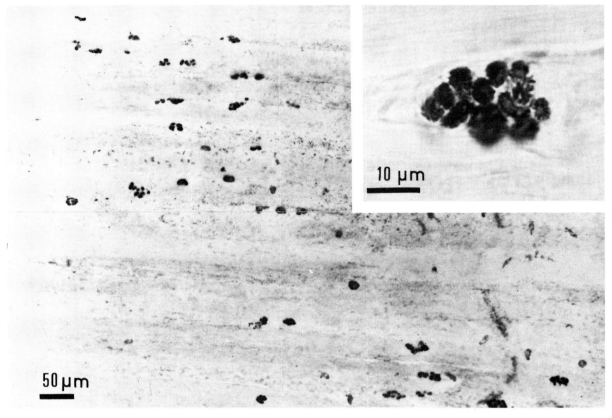

Fig. 18.5   Subneural apparatus in normal human muscle (modified thiocholine method)

previously considered to indicate a regressive or dystrophic state (Coërs 1962). The presence of a few apparently abnormal end-plates in muscle from healthy subjects must therefore be taken into account in the interpretation of pathological material.

PATHOLOGICAL REACTIONS IN INTRAMUSCULAR MOTOR NERVES AND ENDINGS

Marked changes in the rather simple and uniform pattern of intramuscular motor innervation are observed in neuromuscular diseases. Most of these are non-specific, being found both in myopathy and in denervation. However, our accumulated experience has established that denervation produces characteristic regressive and reactive

alterations of the motor nerve and nerve endings which may be useful in histological diagnosis.

Regressive changes

The histological expression of an acute injury of the lower motor neurone or its axonal process is the well-known Wallerian degeneration. Actually, the process of axonal fragmentation is seldom visible in biopsy material obtained in cases of acute denervation, for example, in poliomyelitis or after nerve injury. The disintegration that starts at the terminal arborization and spreads proximally, proceeds so rapidly that within a few days the axonal debris, initially in the form of pale globules (when stained by methylene blue), will have disappeared from the intramuscular nerve bundles. In contrast, the postsynaptic component undergoes changes that persist for a longer time, as revealed in histochemical preparations. The lamellated layer of the units of the subneural apparatus becomes pale (poorly stained) and irregular, and the stained products accumulate within the cuplets, which are normally unstained (Fig. 18.6a). This change could be related to electron microscopic observations of denervated myoneural junctions in which the cytoplasm of the Schwann cell tends to flow into space vacated by the degenerating terminal axoplasmic expansions, thereby usurping their synaptic position (Birks et al 1960, Johnson & Woolf 1965).

In slowly progressive denervation, the motor nerve fibres may show localized swellings or take on a reticulated appearance. The localized swellings consist of spherical or elongated enlargements along the course of axis cylinders which otherwise appear normal (Fig. 18.6b). They are occasionally observed in chronic neuropathies and more rarely in motor neurone diseases. They could represent the earliest morphological expression of an axonal disturbance. The reticulated axons are networks of very fine beaded nerve fibres wandering among the muscle fibres without making visible contact with them (see Fig. 18.8d). These formations are often seen in motor neurone disorders, particularly in Werdnig–Hoffmann disease and in hereditary neuropathies of the Charcot–Marie–Tooth type. One may assume that they reflect an incapacity of growing diseased fibres to make a proper neuromuscular contact.

Non-specific changes

These changes may be observed in motor endplates and in intramuscular nerve fibres. In many biopsies one frequently encounters slender and beaded axons (see Fig. 18.8c) which could either be regenerating nerve fibres, such as are seen in muscle recovering after a nerve injury, or unemployed fibres coursing through degenerated or atrophic muscle tissue, as in myopathies (see Fig. 18.10b). In chronic involvement of the lower motor neurone or peripheral nerve, such finely beaded nerve fibres could be either regenerating or degenerating axis cylinders.

Some motor end-plates may present abnormally large junctional swellings (Fig. 18.6e). These changes are reflected in the structure of the sub-neural apparatus (irregular end-plates), the units of which show marked variations in size (Fig. 18.6f). The motor endings may also be abnormally small and reduced to a few or even to one large terminal expansion (reduced end-plates), as if the arborization had fused into a single mass (Fig. 18.6c). The corresponding subneural apparatus is formed by a single large unit with a well-preserved laminated border (Fig. 18.6d). Such changes are particularly conspicuous in diabetic neuropathy (Woolf & Malins 1957), although they have also been observed in other conditions, for example in alcoholic neuropathy (Coërs & Hilderbrand 1965) and coeliac disease (Cooke et al 1966). This reduction in the size of end-plates seems to represent the earliest morphological indication of a disease process affecting motor nerve fibres. However, it must be pointed out that this apparently regressive change closely resembles the first stage of differentiation of the motor end-plate, either in normal development or in regeneration, at a time when the axoplasmic growth cone reaches the sarcoplasm and before it starts its ramification. In addition, the possibility exists that the reduction and simplification of motor end-plates is merely related to the atrophy of the muscle fibre occurring in any neuromuscular disease, in keeping with the principle that there is a correlation between the size of a muscle fibre and its motor nerve ending. For example, it is difficult to decide whether diminutive end-plates found in nemaline and centronuclear myopathy and in familial focal loss of cross-striations (see Fig. 18.14) are related to a delayed maturation of the myoneural junction or to the small size of muscle fibres (Coërs et al 1976, van Wijngaarden et al 1977).

Changes related to axonal sprouting

Excessive branching of intramuscular nerve fibres may occur at various levels, collateral, terminal or ultraterminal. The result of terminal and ultraterminal ramification taking place distally is usually the formation of expanded motor endings or of several motor arborizations on the same muscle fibre, and this may be observed either in denervation or myopathy, usually on hypertrophic muscle fibres (Fig. 18.7). In some instances, however,

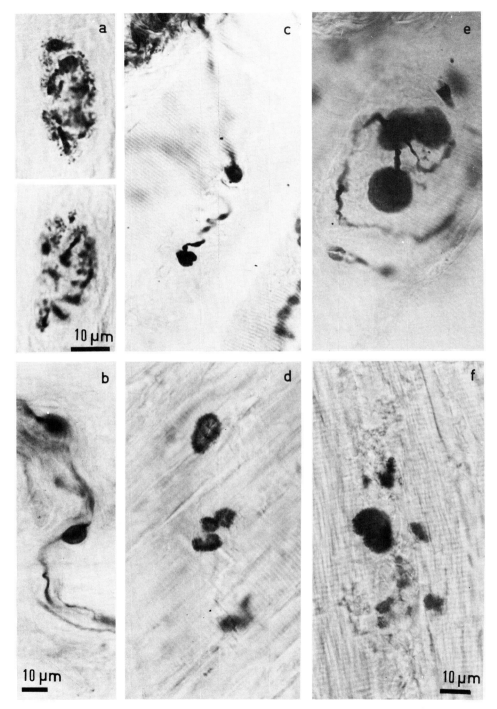

Fig. 18.6 Pathological changes. (a) Denervated subneural apparatus in subacute polyneuropathy (modified thiocholine method). (b) Localized axonal swellings in chronic neuropathy (vital methylene blue). (c) Motor endings reduced to one terminal expansion (diabetic neuropathy) (vital methylene blue). (d) Corresponding subneural apparatus (diabetic neuropathy) (thiocholine method). (e) Abnormally large terminal expansions (myasthenia gravis) (methylene blue). (f) Irregular subneural apparatus in chronic neuropathy (thiocholine method)

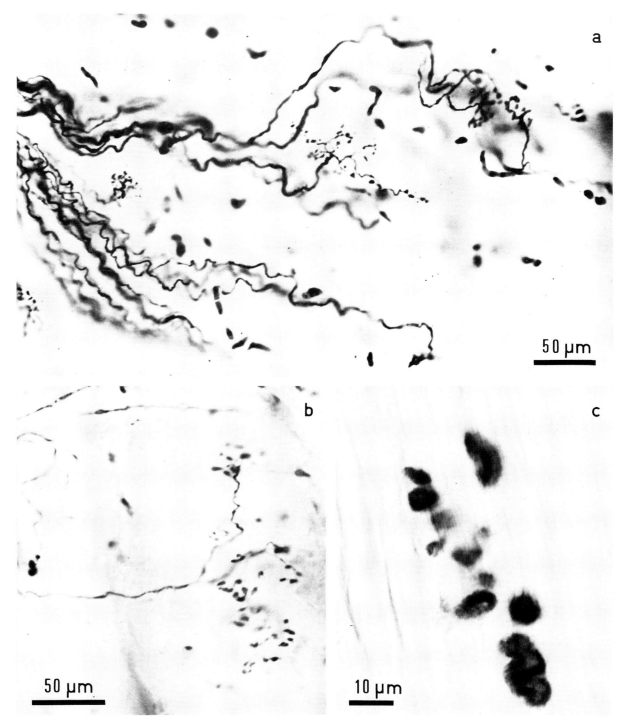

Fig. 18.7 Expanded motor endings. (a) In myasthenia gravis. (b) In limb girdle myopathy (vital methylene blue). (c) Expanded subneural apparatus in chronic neuropathy (modified thiocholine method)

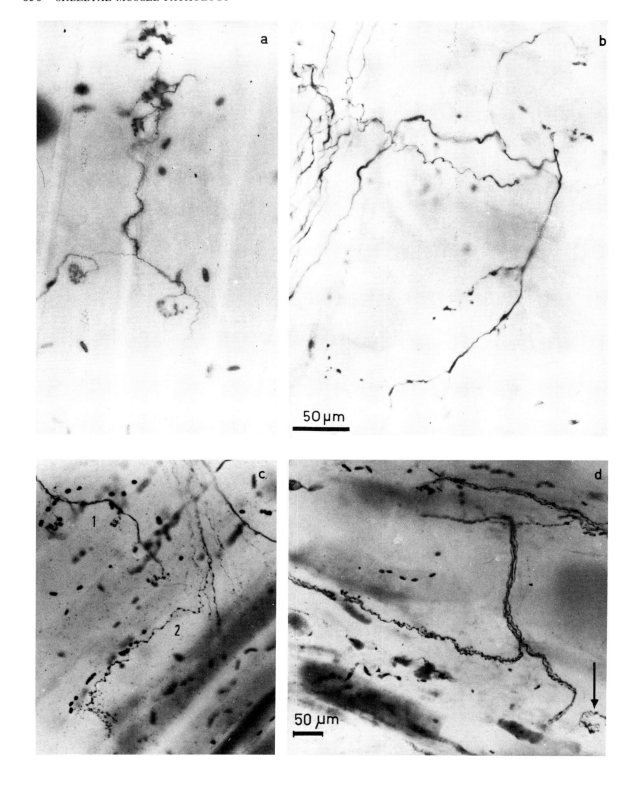

50 µm

50 µm

such expanded motor endings may be seen on normal-sized or small muscle fibres, and this is particularly the case in myotonic dystrophy, myasthenia gravis and polymyositis (Coërs 1965).

Collateral ramification of the proximal part of the subterminal axons, and occasionally ultra-terminal ramification, results in the innervation of different muscle fibres and an increase of this process is mainly observed in denervation (Fig. 18.8). Collateral sprouting has been noted both in experimental material (Edds 1950, Hoffman 1950, Hildebrand et al 1968a,b) and in human diseases (Coërs 1955, Wohlfart 1957, 1960, Coërs & Woolf 1959, Coomes 1960, Harriman 1962, Hatsuyama 1964). This sprouting results in an increase of the functional (true) TIR and therefore in an extension of the territory of the motor unit by inclusion of muscle fibres from denervated units.

The functional significance of axonal sprouting appears to be different in neurogenic and myogenic conditions. In denervation, sprouting attempts to compensate for the loss of nerve fibres and ensures the reinnervation of denervated muscle fibres. In other diseases, the result of axonal ramification is the formation of expanded or multiple motor arborizations on the same muscle fibre, without extension to adjacent fibres. This terminal branching may be a response to disturbed function of the muscle, as in muscular dystrophy, or to impaired neuromuscular transmission, as in myasthenia. It can also be an adaptation of the size of the myoneural junction to that of the muscle fibre in situations of hypertrophy.

SPECIAL PATHOLOGY OF INTRAMUSCULAR INNERVATION

This section will be mainly concerned with the changes in motor nerve fibres and endings which can contribute to histological diagnosis of the various muscular atrophies, including disorders of the motor neurone and peripheral nerve, genetic and acquired myopathies, myotonic dystrophy, myasthenia gravis, congenital myopathies and disuse atrophy.

Neurogenic disorders

Characteristic changes in the motor innervation are seen particularly in the more chronic conditions. In acute neuropathy, a biopsy taken within the first week may show a normal terminal motor innervation pattern. On the other hand, after nerve injury, or in acute anterior poliomyelitis in its early stages there may be a complete absence of motor nerve fibres and endings (Coërs & Woolf 1959).

In chronic disorders, including acquired neuropathies of various aetiologies, hereditary neuropathy (Charcot–Marie–Tooth disease) and motor neurone diseases (amyotrophic lateral sclerosis and spinal muscular atrophy), the TIR was found to be normal in only 15% of biopsies, from clinically unaffected muscles in which conventional histology did not demonstrate grouped atrophy of muscle fibres. It is worth pointing out that 75% of these normal muscles had an increased TIR (Coërs et al 1973c). In clinically affected muscles (atrophy and weakness) and in muscles with grouped atrophy of muscle fibres, the TIR was increased in nearly all biopsies in which motor axons and endings persisted.

Axonal sprouting seems to occur first as an outgrowth of fine beaded fibres ending as an axonal dilatation (growth cone) which eventually reaches a muscle fibre and forms a terminal arborization. The result of this process may be a well-established collateral re-innervation in which the branching axons and motor arborizations appear normal (Fig. 18.8a). However, the collaterals may remain fine and beaded and the motor endings small or attenuated with unduly slender branches (Fig. 18.8b). Occasionally, the intramuscular axons have the appearance of

Fig. 18.8 Specific changes of motor innervation in neurogenic disorders (vital methylene blue). (a) Well-established collateral re-innervation in hereditary neuropathy (Dejerine–Sottas). (b) Increased collateral ramification forming slender terminal arborizations (chronic neuropathy). (c) Chronic polyradiculoneuritis: (1) Collateral re-innervation; (2) Slender axon ending as a plexiform network. Reproduced from Arch. Neurol. 1973, 29: 210–222 with kind permission of Coërs C, Telerman-Toppet N and Gerard J M. (d) Reticulated axons in Charcot–Marie–Tooth disease. Arrow: terminal network

ramified reticulated fibres wandering among the muscle fibres and ending as growth cones or as a plexiform network without forming a visible neuromuscular junction (Fig. 18.8d). Frequently these changes are seen in the distal part of the axon, the proximal part having a normal appearance and giving rise to healthy collateral branches ending as normal end-plates. This pattern can be interpreted as 'dying back' of the neurone (Coërs & Woolf 1959), or as an abortive attempt to form end-plates, impaired regenerative activity first appearing at the end of the neural tree (Coërs et al 1973c).

Comparison between the functional state of the muscle, the histological changes in muscle fibres, and the changes in the motor innervation, has unravelled the evolution of the denervating process. In the first stage the TIR is increased, even though there is no weakness of the muscle or histological change in the muscle fibres themselves; the collateral re-innervation has fully compensated for the loss of motor axons and the denervation remains latent. In the second stage, the disease process exceeds the capacity of collateral sprouting which eventually becomes exhausted, resulting in weakness and atrophy of muscle fibres. Collateral re-innervation from rarefied motor axons is still seen in the bundles of large muscle fibres, but most motor endings are poorly developed and reticulated nerve fibres ending blindly are observed. At the ultimate stage, a few wandering motor axons not visibly connected to muscle fibres are seen and the TIR can no longer be measured.

Obviously, this evolution is quite variable in the different pathological conditions, according to the efficiency of collateral reinnervation. The correlation between the TIR and the severity of the disease has been demonstrated by comparing Charcot–Marie–Tooth disease (CMT) and amyotrophic lateral sclerosis (ALS), the former having a much slower and milder evolution. The process of collateral ramification was found to be significantly more marked in CMT, the mean TIR measured in 12 cases being 2.16 ± 0.56, whereas its mean value in 18 cases of ALS was 1.66 ± 0.30 (Telerman-Toppet & Coërs 1978). This difference indicates that the unaffected motor neurones in CMT have a greater capacity for re-innervation of adjacent denervated muscle fibres than their

counterparts in ALS. The high TIR value is reflected by an increased degree of fibre type grouping in CMT as compared with ALS (Dubowitz & Brooke 1973, Jennekens et al 1974, Telerman-Toppet & Coërs 1978). Electromyographic estimation of fibre density (Schwarz et al 1976) has produced results in agreement with these morphometric data, which provide evidence that both increased collateral branching and type grouping are the expression of a compensatory increase in the size of residual motor units in chronic denervation. Similarly, the formation of muscle fibre groups with the same enzymatic profile (type 1 or type 2) suggests that reinnervation of muscle fibres by collaterals from motor neurones of a different type may lead to full conversion on their metabolic characteristics, as has also been demonstrated by experimental cross-re-innervation (Close 1972; Fig. 18.9).

Muscular dystrophies

Duchenne muscular dystrophy

Methylene blue vital staining of biopsy specimens demonstrated that there was no re-innervation through collateral sprouting in this disease, as assumed by Desmedt & Borenstein (1973, 1976). The mean TIR was 1.12 ± 0.06, not significantly different from controls, and the individual values ranged from 0.01 to 1.23 (Coërs & Telerman-Toppet 1977).

It seems likely that the end result of collateral sprouting is to compensate for the loss of motor axons that characterizes lower motor neurone and peripheral nerve disorders. In muscular dystrophy, such an axonal loss does not take place. On the contrary, a very dense innervation persists in muscles which have been deprived of many muscle fibres and there is apparently an excess of motor axons. It is easy in methylene blue preparations to follow unemployed nerve fibres running in connective tissue parallel to the longitudinal axis of the muscle and ending freely (Fig. 18.10b). Eventually, these fibres make contact with a muscle fibre as a diminutive motor arborization, sometimes several millimetres from the intramuscular nerve (Fig. 18.10a). These nerve fibres are often abnormally thin and beaded, but do not

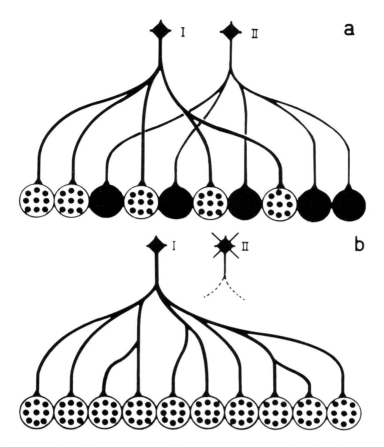

Fig. 18.9 Diagrammatic representation of the mechanism of fibre type grouping through collateral re-innervation of adjacent denervated muscle fibres. (a) Normal distribution of type 1 and type 2 motor units; (b) Type 1 motor neurone has reinnervated muscle fibres previously innervated by the damaged type 2 motor neurone and has induced their enzymatic conversion

branch excessively. This distorted pattern of motor innervation results in a very marked enlargement of the terminal innervation area and a longitudinal scatter of motor end plates that may reach 10 mm (Fig. 18.10c) whereas the terminal innervation area in muscles of normal children does not exceed 1 mm (Fig. 18.1c).

This dispersion of motor endings may be explained in two ways. According to Desmedt & Borenstein (1973), focal necrosis can produce a transection of muscle fibres with the formation of denervated segments. It may be assumed that unemployed axons available in the vicinity of the denervated segments could be accepted and form ectopic end-plates. They could also be used to innervate regenerated muscle fibres (Desmedt &

Borenstein 1976), for regeneration is known to take place particularly in the early stages of the disease. Another possibility could be that the dispersion of the motor end-plate is merely related to the longitudinal displacement of transected muscle fibres resulting from focal necrosis.

In any case, there is apparently no need for collateral sprouting in muscles with a redundant innervation, and this is in agreement with morphological evidence. On the other hand, this evidence indicates that if a 'neural factor' were involved in Duchenne dystrophy, as was postulated by McComas et al (1970), it does not involve denervation in the conventional sense of an axonal degeneration.

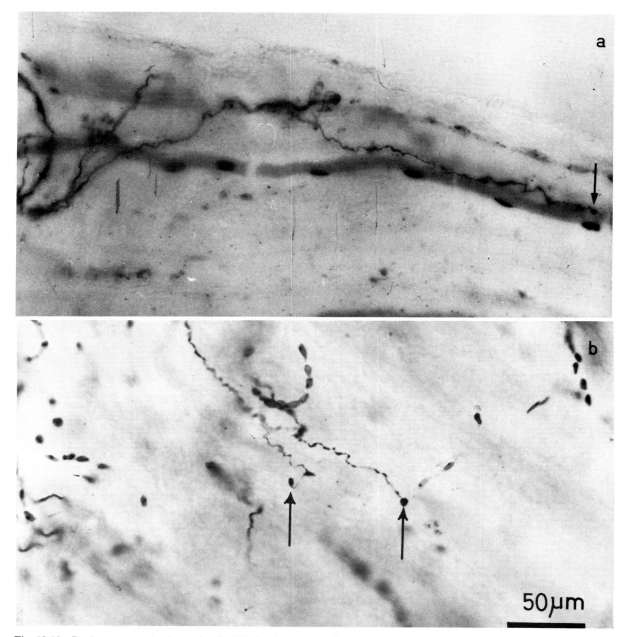

Fig. 18.10   Duchenne muscular dystrophy. (a) Diminutive motor ending on an atrophic muscle fibre (arrow). Reproduced from Arch. Neurol. 1973, 29: 210–222 with kind permission of Coërs C, Telerman-Toppet N and Gerard J M. (b) Unemployed motor axons (arrows). Reproduced with permission from Arch. Neurol. 1977, 34: 396–402. (c) Enlargement of the terminal innervation area (arrows). Reproduced with permission from Arch. Neurol. 1977, 34: 396–402. Compare with Fig. 18.1c. (a, b) Vital methylene blue. (c) Modified thiocholine method

Limb–girdle muscular dystrophy

Measurement of the TIR has been particularly useful for the differential diagnosis between limb–girdle myopathy (LGM) and juvenile spinal muscular atrophy (SMA) (Coërs & Telerman-Toppet 1979). The clinical picture of these two conditions may be very similar, and the myopathic

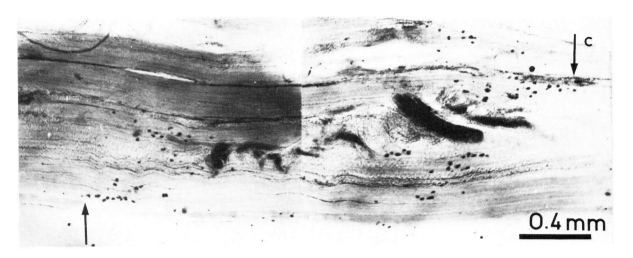

Fig. 18.10 *Cont'd*

changes of the muscle fibres may be so prominent in SMA that its neurogenic nature may be overlooked (Gardner-Medwin et al 1967, Mastaglia & Walton 1971). We studied 18 patients with a progressive proximal muscular atrophy and weakness without fasciculation. Only two cases could be safely diagnosed as having spinal muscular atrophy according to classical criteria. Both had large group fibre atrophy and a neurogenic electromyogram (EMG), and also had a very high TIR (respectively 2.0 and 3.1). A firm diagnosis of muscular dystrophy could be made in two other cases in which myopathic changes alone were found in the biopsy and EMG, and both had a normal TIR. In the other cases, the diagnosis remained uncertain on the basis of histology and EMG, because of discrepancies or inconclusive data. Some had a predominantly neurogenic EMG with marked myopathic histological changes; others had a myopathic EMG with histological changes suggesting denervation, or a mixture of neuropathic and myopathic signs in both the EMG and the biopsy. In such ambiguous situations, measurement of the TIR settled the diagnosis. In one case, an increased TIR (2.2) conformed to the EMG pattern of denervation despite a myopathic biopsy. In one other case, a normal value of TIR confirmed the diagnosis of myopathy suggested by the EMG, although there were numerous small dark angular fibres and small groups of atrophic fibres with a bimodal distribution of fibre diameters. In a third case, in which neither histology nor EMG were conclusive, an increased TIR suggested denervation.

On the whole, the TIR was more closely correlated with the EMG than with muscle fibre changes, particularly small group atrophy and small angular dark fibres, and appeared to be the most reliable morphological index of denervation.

Myotonic dystrophy

A marked distortion of the terminal motor innervation pattern takes place in this disease. Sub-terminal axons are intermingled and at times twisted around muscle fibres and difficult to follow individually (Fig. 18.11a). There is a striking axonal sprouting leading to the formation of several end-plates on the same muscle fibre, sometimes along a length of several millimetres (Coërs & Woolf 1959), or to the innervation of several muscle fibres, thus increasing the functional TIR in some cases (Coërs et al 1973c). Because of this distal proliferation of axons, individual end-plates tend to cover a larger area than normal, while the size of terminal expansions is very irregular (Fig. 18.11b).

A neural disorder in myotonic dystrophy was postulated by MacDermot (1961) because of the very marked changes in the intramuscular inner-

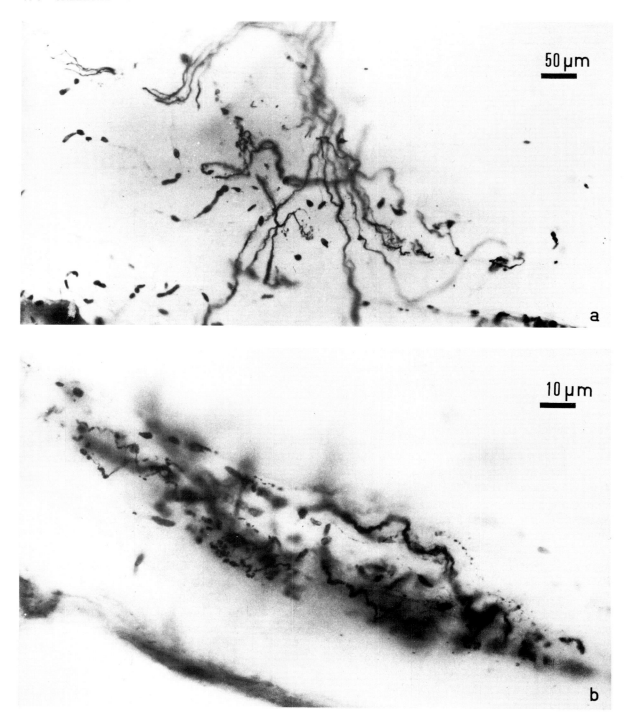

Fig. 18.11 Myotonic dystrophy. Vital methylene blue. (a) Distorted pattern of terminal innervation. (b) Extremely expanded motor ending

vation contrasting with the relative integrity of the muscle fibres, and by McComas et al (1971) from electromyographic data. Caccia et al (1972) also found clinical and EMG evidence of peripheral nerve involvement in two cases of myotonic dystrophy. According to Panayiotopoulos & Scarpalezos (1976, 1977) this peripheral nerve involvement takes place in addition to the muscle disorder in some cases of myotonic dystrophy. Therefore the increased TIR found in five out of 13 cases (Coërs et al 1973c) does not necessarily imply that myotonic dystrophy is due to denervation, but rather that this polysystemic disease can occasionally be associated with a neuropathy.

Myasthenia gravis

Investigations of the intramuscular innervation have demonstrated characteristic changes in this disease. Methylene blue preparations showed remarkably elongated, almost filamentous motor endings. Cholinesterase preparations disclosed a ribbon-like appearance of the subneural apparatus corresponding to the elongated motor arborizations (Fig. 18.12; Coërs & Woolf 1954). Later studies (Woolf et al 1956, Coërs & Desmedt 1959, Coërs & Woolf 1959, Bickerstaff & Woolf 1960, MacDermot 1960) indicated that, in addition to elongated end-plates, myasthenic muscles contained enlarged and irregular end-plates similar to those seen in other neuromuscular disorders (Figs. 18.6e, 18.7a) whereas the elongated appearance was quite different from that seen in any other disease.

In a series of 45 cases (Coërs & Telerman-Toppet 1976), elongated end-plates were found in 26 biopsies, more frequently in younger patients, and consequently in women who in general are distributed within a younger age group. There was no correlation between the incidence of this change and the severity of the disease or changes in the histological or histochemical pattern of the muscle fibres. Non-specific changes in motor endings were present in 38 biopsies without correlation with clinical data, age or histochemical pattern of the muscle fibres. In addition, a TIR exceeding the upper normal limit and suggesting denervation was found in seven biopsies, all from patients over the age of 50 years. Denervation in myasthenia has

been postulated from histological and histochemical changes in the muscle fibres (Fenichel & Shy 1963, Brody & Engel 1964). However, there is a discrepancy between the small proportion of biopsies with increased TIR and the high incidence of histochemical changes suggesting denervation, found by Engel & McFarlin (1966).

The reciprocal relationship between the increased TIR in elderly patients and the presence of elongated end-plates, which tend to be more frequent in younger patients, suggests a chronological evolution of the changes in innervation pattern in myasthenic muscles. Elongation and simplification of the motor endings could be the primary change, related to the autoimmune attack on the postsynaptic region (Engel et al 1976). This change is followed by distal branching of motor axons forming expanded or multiple motor arborizations, that could represent a form of compensation to impaired neuromuscular transmission, similar to the axonal changes which occur after the local application of botulinum toxin (Duchen & Strich 1968). Collateral branching with re-innervation of adjacent muscle fibres appears as a late and infrequent feature in myasthenia, occurring only in some elderly patients, irrespective of the apparent duration or severity of the disease. Another possibility is that the presence of elongated motor endings characterizes a type of myasthenia which occurs preferentially in a younger age group, and that other types of myasthenic syndrome, some of which are associated with denervation, occur in older subjects. Anticholinesterase therapy could contribute to the changes in motor endings, but the importance of this factor is still unsettled as far as elongated end-plates are concerned, as this change has been observed in undiagnosed and untreated as well as in treated cases (Coërs & Telerman-Toppet 1976).

Acquired myopathies

A morphometric study of the intramuscular innervation was performed in 16 cases of dermatomyositis, nine cases of polymyositis and six cases of muscle sarcoidosis (granulomatous myopathy according to Coërs & Carbone 1966 and Coërs 1967) (Coërs et al 1973c). In some biopsies, the

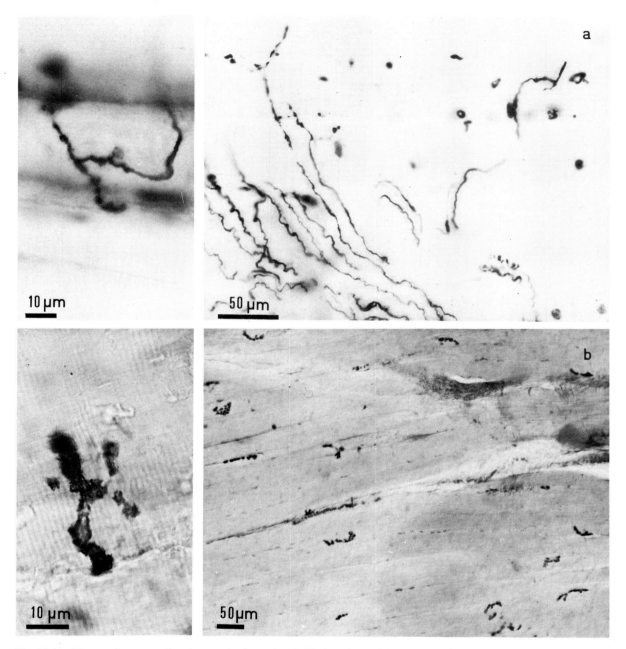

Fig. 18.12 Elongated motor endings in myasthenia gravis. (a) Vital methylene blue. (b) Modified thiocholine method

changes in motor innervation were similar to those found in other myopathies and involved the more distal parts of the nerve fibres, forming small and irregular motor endings or abnormally expanded or multiple terminal arborizations through distal branching (Fig. 18.13a). In other samples, marked collateral ramification increased the TIR. Usually the axonal branching occurred in the vicinity of, or within foci of cellular infiltration (Fig. 18.13b), so that the degree of ramification differed from

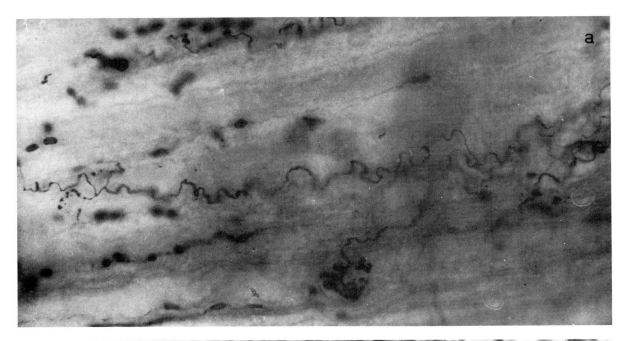

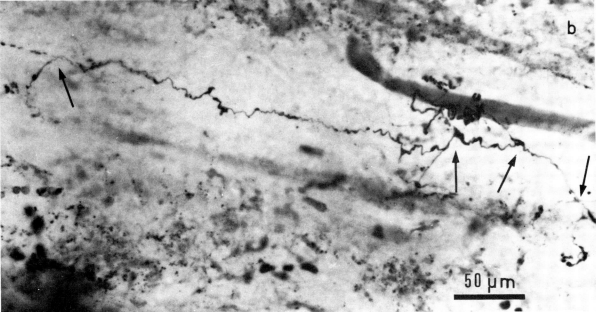

Fig. 18.13   Terminal motor innervation in acquired myopathy (vital methylene blue). (a) In polymyositis. Irregular and expanded motor endings. No increased collateral branching. (b) In granulomatous myopathy. Very marked collateral ramification (arrows)

one part of the specimen to another. In one case of granulomatous myopathy, the TIR was 1.73 in regions with granulomatous infiltration and 1.17 elsewhere, with a mean of 1.44. The mean TIR was significantly increased in dermatomyositis and granulomatous myopathy but did not exceed the normal level in polymyositis. It was concluded that this abnormal collateral branching occurred as a reaction to axonal breakdown in the vicinity of, or within, the foci of inflammatory cells (intramuscular denervation). The higher incidence of increased TIR in dermatomyositis and granulomatous myopathy, in which the cellular infiltration was more marked than in polymyositis, supports this interpretation.

Congenital myopathies

In some of these diseases, a neural defect has been suspected, particularly in central core disease (Resnick & Engel 1967), in nemaline myopathy (Karpati et al 1971) and in myotubular and centronuclear myopathy (Engel et al 1968, Munsat et al 1969). Investigation of the intramuscular innervation in these conditions (Coërs et al 1976) showed evidence of collateral reinnervation in one case of central core disease only. In all other biopsies, no structural abnormality of motor axons, myelin sheaths or neuromuscular junctions suggesting denervation were observed. The only relevant change found in centronuclear myopathy and in

one case of familial focal loss of cross-striations (van Wijngaarden et al 1977), and also to a lesser extent in nemaline myopathy, was an unusual smallness and simplification of motor endings, suggesting delayed or impaired maturation (Fig. 18.14).

Type 2 fibre atrophy

Disuse atrophy, as well as joint diseases, cachexia and corticosteroid therapy produce a selective atrophy of type 2 muscle fibres. This change is also occasionally observed in neurogenic disorders, and similar electronmicroscopic changes have been reported in type 2 fibres following disuse and denervation (Mendell & Engel 1971). From these observations, type 2 atrophy was considered to be evidence of a neural disorder (Engel 1965). Motor innervation studies (Telerman-Toppet & Coërs 1975) showed that the TIR was increased in all cases in which type 2 atrophy was associated with an overt denervation, but remained normal in more than half the cases without clinical indication

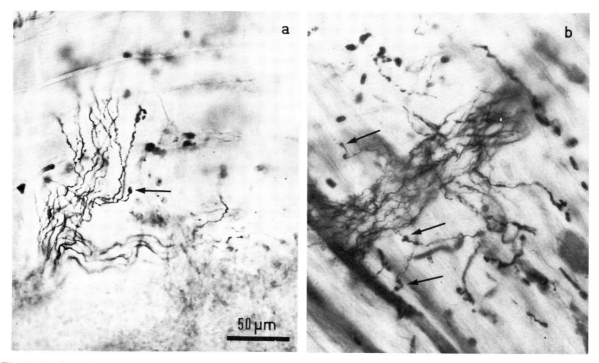

Fig. 18.14 Congenital myopathies. Vital methylene blue. (a) Myotubular myopathy. (b) Familial focal loss of cross-striations. Small and poorly ramified motor endings (arrows)

of neuropathy. This result indicates that type 2 atrophy may occur without any neurogenic participation.

CONCLUSIONS

The investigation of intramuscular motor nerves and nerve endings must be regarded as complementary to the conventional histological and histochemical examination of muscle. With the utilization of both approaches, a fairly good approximation to the correct diagnosis may be attained. The following may be taken as diagnostic guide-lines.

1. Collateral ramification producing a significant increase of TIR is a clear indication of a neurogenic process even if 'myopathic' changes in the muscle fibres are present, as is frequently the case in the benign form of spinal muscular atrophy. The TIR has been found to be significantly increased in nearly all cases of long-standing denervation, whereas it remains normal in myopathies. This increase appears to be a very sensitive morphological index of denervation, for it has been observed in a high proportion of clinically normal muscles in neurogenic disorders, even in the absence of grouped atrophy or type grouping of muscle fibres. Rarefaction of intramuscular nerve fibres and a reticulated appearance of these fibres provides additional evidence of denervation.

2. In addition to genuine peripheral nerve and motor neurone disorders, an increased TIR may indicate involvement of intramuscular nerves in myositis. In that case, a marked inflammatory reaction will usually be found in the muscle biopsy. The TIR may be increased in some cases of myotonic dystrophy, suggesting the association of a muscular and a neural disorder. It is also increased in some elderly patients with myasthenia gravis.

3. The neurogenic nature of small dark angular fibres, of small group atrophy and even of type grouping cannot be safely accepted if the density of intramuscular nerves is not reduced and the TIR is normal. Fibre type predominance or type 2 atrophy cannot be related to denervation if the TIR is not increased.

4. Marked variation in size and irregularity of motor nerve endings, and slender beaded axons wandering along muscle fibres have a limited diagnostic value, being found in all neuromuscular diseases. However, the pattern of intramuscular innervation is particularly distorted in myotonic dystrophy and sometimes in polymyositis and myasthenia gravis.

5. In myasthenia gravis, these non-specific changes are frequently associated with simplification and a characteristic elongation of motor arborizations, particularly in younger patients.

ACKNOWLEDGEMENTS

I acknowledge with thanks the permission of the authors, editors and publishers to reproduce Figures 18.2, 18.8c and 18.10a from Coers et al (1973b), and Figure 10b and c from Coers & Telerman-Toppet (1977).

Research work reported in this chapter was supported by the Muscular Dystrophy Association of America Inc., the Muscular Dystrophy Group of Great Britain, the Free University of Brussels and the Fonds de la Recherche Scientifique Médicale of Belgium.

REFERENCES

Adams R D 1974 Pathological reaction of the skeletal muscle fibre in man. In: Walton J N (ed) Disorders of voluntary muscle, 3rd edn. Churchill Livingstone, Edinburgh, p 168

Anzenbacher H, Zenker W 1963 Uber die Grössenbezichung der Muskelfasern zu ihren motorischen Endplatten und Nerven. Zeitschrift für Zellforschung und miroskopische Anatomie 60: 860

Beerman D H, Cassens R G 1976 A combined silver and acetylcholinesterase method for staining intramuscular innervation. Stain Technology 51: 173

Bickerstaff E R, Woolf, A L 1960 The intramuscular nerve endings in myasthenia gravis. Brain 83: 10

Birks R, Katz B, Miledi R 1960 Physiological and structural changes at the amphibian myo-neural junction, in the course of nerve degeneration. Journal of Physiology 150: 145

Bradley W G, Jones M Z, Mussini J M, Fawcett P R W 1978 Becker-type muscular dystrophy. Muscle and Nerve 1: 111

Brody I A, Engel W K 1964 Denervation of muscle in myasthenia gravis. Archives of Neurology (Chicago) 11: 350

Brooke M H, Engel W K 1966 The histologic diagnosis of neuromuscular diseases: a review of 79 biopsies. Archives of Physical Medicine and Rehabilitation 47: 99

Caccia M R, Negri S, Pretoparvis V 1972 Myotonic dystrophy with neural involvement. Journal of the Neurological Sciences 16: 253

Carpenter S, Karpati G, Heller I, Eisen A 1978 Inclusion body myositis. A distinct variety of idiopathic inflammatory myopathy. Neurology (Minneapolis) 28: 8

Close R 1972 Dynamic properties of mammalian skeletal muscles. Physiological Reviews 52: 129

Coërs C 1952 The vital staining of muscle biopsies with methylene blue. Journal of Neurology, Neurosurgery and Psychiatry 15: 211

Coërs C 1953a Topographie zonale de l'innervation motrice terminale dans les muscles striés. Archives de biologie (Liège) 64: 495

Coërs C 1953b La détection histochimique de la cholinestérase au niveau de la jonction neuromusculaire. Revue belge de pathologie et de médecine expérimentale 22: 306

Coërs C 1955 Les variations structurelles normales et pathologiques de la jonction neuromusculaire. Acta neurologica belgica 55: 741

Coërs C 1962 Analyse critique et essai d'interprétation des anomalies morphologiques de la jonction neuromusculaire en pathologie. Mémoires de l'Académie Royale de la Médecine de Belgique 4: 71

Coërs C 1965 Histology of the myoneural junction in myopathies. In: Paul W M, Daniel E E, Kay C M, Monckton G (eds) Muscle. Pergamon Press, Oxford, New York, p 453

Coërs C 1967 The histological features of muscle sarcoidosis. Acta neuropathologica (Berlin) 7: 242

Coërs C, Carbone F 1966 La myopathie granulomateuse. Acta neurologica belgica 66: 353

Coërs C, Desmedt J E 1959 Mise en évidence d'une malformation caractéristique de la jonction neuromusculaire dans la myasthénie. Acta neurologica belgica 59: 539

Coërs C, Hildebrand J 1965 Latent neuropathy in diabetes and alcoholism: electrophysiological and histological study. Neurology (Minneapolis) 15: 19

Coërs C, Telerman-Toppet N 1976 Morphological and histochemical changes of motor units in myasthenia. Annals of the New York Academy of Sciences 274: 6

Coërs C, Telerman-Toppet N 1977 Morphological changes of motor units in Duchenne's muscular dystrophy. Archives of Neurology (Chicago) 34: 396

Coërs C, Telerman-Toppet N 1978 Fact and fancy in the histological diagnosis of denervation. In: Pozza G, Canal N (eds) Peripheral neuropathies. Elsevier, Amsterdam, p 25

Coërs C, Telerman-Toppet N 1979 Differential diagnosis of limb girdle muscular dystrophy and spinal muscular atrophy. Neurology (Minneapolis) 29: 957

Coërs C, Woolf A L 1954 Etude histologique et histochimique de la jonction neuromusculaire dans deux cas de myasthénie. C R Congres médecins aliénistes et neurologistes de langue française, Masson, Paris, p 1

Coërs C, Woolf A L 1959 The innervation of muscle, a biopsy study. Blackwell, Oxford

Coërs C, Reske-Nielsen E, Harmsen A 1973a The pattern of terminal motor innervation in healthy young adults. Journal of the Neurological Sciences 19: 351

Coërs C, Telerman-Toppet N, Gerard J M 1973b Terminal innervation ratio in neuromuscular disease. I. Methods and controls. Archives of Neurology (Chicago) 29: 210

Coërs C, Telerman-Toppet N, Gerard J M 1973c Terminal innervation ratio in neuromuscular disease. II. Disorders of lower motor neuron, peripheral nerve and muscle. Archives of Neurology (Chicago) 29: 215

Coërs C, Telerman-Toppet N, Gerard J M, Szliwowski H, Bethlem J, Van Wijngaarden, G K 1976 Changes in motor innervation and histochemical pattern of muscle fibres in some congenital myopathies. Neurology (Minneapolis) 26: 1046

Cooke W T, Johnson A G, Woolf A L 1966 Vital staining and electron microscopy of the intramuscular nerve endings in the neuropathy of adult coeliac disease. Brain 89: 663

Coomes E N 1960 A correlated study of intensity duration curves and terminal neuronal reinnervation of muscle. Annals of Physical Medicine 5: 243

Couteaux R 1947 Contribution á l'étude de la synapse myoneurale. Therien, Montréal

Couteaux R 1951 Remarque sur les méthodes actuelles de détection histochimique des activitiés cholinestérasiques. Archives internationales de physiologie 59: 526

Dastur D K, Razzak Z A 1973 Possible neurogenic factor in muscular dystrophy: evidence from muscle biopsy. In: Kakulas B (ed) Clinical studies in myology. International Congress Series no. 295. Excerpta Medica, Amsterdam, p 186

De Harven E, Coërs C 1959 Electron microscope study of the human neuromuscular junction. Journal of Biophysical and Biochemical Cytology 6: 7

Desmedt J E, Borenstein S 1973 Collateral innervation of muscle fibres by motor axons of dystrophic motor units. Nature 264: 500

Desmedt J E, Borenstein S 1976 Regeneration in Duchenne dystrophy. Archives of Neurology (Chicago) 33: 642

Drachman D B, Murphy S, Nigam N P, Hills J R 1967 'Myopathic' changes in chronically denervated muscles. Archives of Neurology (Chicago) 16: 14

Dubowitz V, Brooke M H 1973 Muscle biopsy: a modern approach. 2. Major problems in neurology. W B Saunders, Philadelphia

Duchen L W, Strich S J 1968 The effect of botulinum toxin on the pattern of innervation of skeletal muscle in the mouse. Quarterly Journal of Experimental Physiology 53: 84

Edds V 1950 Collateral regeneration of residual motor axons in partially denervated muscles. Journal of Experimental Zoology 122: 498

Engel W K 1965 Histochemistry of neuromuscular diseases. Significance of muscle fibre types. In: Neuromuscular diseases. (Proceedings of the 8th International Congress of Neurology. Vienna, Austria), vol 2, p 67

Engel W K, McFarlin D E 1966 Discussion of paper by G M Fenichel. Annals of the New York Academy of Sciences 135: 68

Engel W K, Gold G N, Karpati G 1968 Type I fibre hypotrophy and central nuclei. A rare congenital muscle abnormality with a possible experimental model. Archives of Neurology (Chicago) 18: 435

Engel A G, Tsujihata M, Lindström J, Lennon V A 1976 End-plate fine structure in myasthenia gravis and the experimental autoimmune myasthenia. Annals of the New York Academy of Sciences 274: 60

Fenichel G M, Shy G M 1963 Muscle biopsy experience in myasthenia gravis. Archives of Neurology (Chicago) 9: 237

Gardner-Medwin D, Hudgson P, Walton J N 1967 Benign spinal muscular atrophy arising in childhood and adolescence. Journal of the Neurological Sciences 5: 121

Haase G R, Shy G M 1960 Pathological changes in muscle biopsies from patients with peroneal muscular atrophy. Brain 83: 631

Harriman D 1962 Histology of the motor end-plate (motor point muscle biopsy). In: Licht S (ed) Electrodiagnosis and electromyography. Licht, New Haven, p 134

Hatsuyama Y 1964 Histological studies on the reinnervation of denervated muscle with special reference to collateral branching. Journal of the Japanese Orthopedic Association 38: 375

Hildebrand J, Joffroy A, Coërs C 1968a Myoneural changes in experimental isoniazid neuropathy. Archives of Neurology (Chicago) 19: 60

Hildebrand J, Joffroy A, Graff G, Coërs C 1968b Neuromuscular changes with alloxan hyperglycemia. Archives of Neurology (Chicago) 18: 633

Hoffman H 1950 Local reinnervation in partially denervated muscle: a histopathological study. Australian Journal of Experimental Biology and Medical Science 28: 383

Jennekens F G I, Meijer A E F H, Bethlem J, Van Wijngaarden G K 1974 Fibre hybrid in type groups. An investigation of human muscle biopsies. Journal of the Neurological Sciences 23: 337

Johnson A G, Woolf A L 1965 Replacement at the neuromuscular synapse of the terminal axonic expansion by the Schwann cell. Acta neuropathologica (Berlin) 4: 436

Karpati G, Carpenter S, Andermann F 1971 A new concept of childhood nemaline myopathy. Archives of Neurology (Chicago) 24: 291

Karpati G, Carpenter S, Melmed C 1974 Experimental ischemic myopathy, Journal of the Neurological Sciences 23: 129

Koelle G B, Friedenwald J S 1949 A histochemical method for localizing cholinesterase activity. Proceedings of the Society for Experimental Biology and Medicine 70: 617

McComas, A J, Campbell M J, Sica R E P 1971 Electrophysiological study of dystrophia myotonica. Journal of Neurology, Neurosurgery and Psychiatry 34: 132

McComas A J, Sica R E P, Currie S 1970 Muscular dystrophy, evidence for a neural factor. Nature 226: 1263

MacDermot V 1960 The change in the motor end-plate in myasthenia gravis. Brain 83: 24

MacDermot V 1961 The histology of the neuromuscular junction in dystrophia myotonica. Brain 84: 75

Mastaglia F L, Walton J N 1971 Histological and histochemical changes in skeletal muscles from cases of chronic juvenile and early adult spinal muscular atrophy (the Kugelberg-Welander syndrome). Journal of the Neurological Sciences 12: 15

Mendell J R, Engel W K 1971 The fine structure of type II muscle fiber atrophy. Neurology (Minneapolis) 21: 358

Mumenthaler M 1970 Myopathy in neuropathy. In: Walton J N, Canal N, Scarlato G (eds) Muscle diseases, International Congress Series no. 199. Excerpta Medica, Amsterdam, p 585

Munsat T L, Thompson L R, Coleman R F 1969 Centronuclear ('myotubular') myopathy. Archives of Neurology (Chicago) 20: 120

Nyström B 1968 Postnatal development of motor nerve terminals in 'slow-red' and 'fast-white' cat muscles. Acta neurologica scandinavica 44: 363

Panayiotopoulos C P, Scarpaleos S 1976 Dystrophia myotonica. Peripheral nerve involvement and pathogenetic implications. Journal of the Neurological Sciences 27: 1

Panayiotopoulos C P, Scarpalezos S 1977 Dystrophia myotonica. A model of combined neural and myopathic muscle atrophy. Journal of the Neurological Sciences 31: 261

Pestronk A, Drachman D B 1978 A new stain for quantitative measurement of sprouting at neuromuscular junctions. Muscle and Nerve 1: 70

Reske-Nielsen E, Coërs C, Harmsen A 1970 Qualitative and quantitative histological study of neuromuscular biopsies from healthy young men. Journal of the Neurological Sciences 10: 369

Resnick J S, Engel W K 1967 Target fibres—structural and cytochemical characteristics and their relationship to neurogenic muscle disease and fiber type. In: Milhorat A T (ed) Exploratory concepts in muscular dystrophy and related disorders, International Congress Series no. 147. Excerpta Medica, Amsterdam, p 255

Schwarz M S, Stalberg E, Schiller H H, Thiele B 1976 The reinnervated motor unit in man. Journal of the Neurological Sciences 27: 303

Telerman-Toppet N, Coërs C 1975 Motor innervation in type II atrophy of skeletal muscle. Journal of the Neurological Sciences 25: 449

Telerman-Toppet N, Coërs C 1978 Motor innervation and fiber type pattern in amyotrophic lateral sclerosis and in Charcot-Marie-Tooth disease. Muscle and Nerve 1: 133

van Wijngaarden G K, Bethlem J, Dingemans K P, Coërs C, Telerman-Toppet N, Gerard J M 1977 Familial focal loss of cross-striations. Journal of Neurology 216: 163

Witalinski W, Loesch A 1975 Structure of muscle fibres and motor end plates in extraocular muscles of the Grass snake, Natrix natrix L. Zeitschrift für Zellforschung und mikroskopische Anatomie 89: 1133

Wohlfart G 1957 Collateral regeneration from residual motor nerve fibres in amyotrophic lateral sclerosis. Neurology (Minneapolis) 7: 124

Wohlfart G 1960 Clinical significance of collateral sprouting of remaining motor nerve fibres in partially denervated muscles. Journal of the Experimental Medical Sciences 3: 128

Woolf A L, Malins J M 1957 Changes in intramuscular nerve endings in diabetic neuropathy. Journal of Pathology and Bacteriology 73: 316

Woolf A L, Bagnal H T, Bauwens P, Bickerstaff E R 1956 A case of myasthenia gravis with changes in the intramuscular nerve endings. Journal of Pathology and Bacteriology 71: 173

19. Pathology of the muscle spindle

Michael Swash

INTRODUCTION

Muscle spindles (Fig. 19.1) are sensory receptors which signal information concerning the degree of stretch applied to a muscle and the velocity of the applied stretch; that is, they signal length and rate of change of length. They are found in all human striated muscles except the facial muscles (Cooper 1960, 1966) and the intrinsic muscles of the larynx (Raman & Devanandam 1989). The muscles of mastication contain spindles grouped together in certain portions of these muscles (Rowlerson et al 1989). Skeletal muscles contain other sensory receptors in addition to spindles. Occasionally a spindle may insert into a tendon near Golgi tendon organs (Fig. 19.2), which signal tension; and Pacinian corpuscles (Fig. 19.3), which signal pressure, are often found near muscle spindles. Freely ending unmyelinated C fibres, probably important in the perception of muscle pain, are also a feature of skeletal muscles (Stacey 1969).

Muscle spindles were first recognized by Hassall in 1849 (see Ruffini 1898), but the first description of the intrafusal muscle fibres was given by Weissmann (1860) in a study of frog muscle. Weissmann suggested that the intrafusal muscle fibres were immature fibres in the process of differentiation and Kölliker (1862), who referred to them as a 'muscle bud', reinforced this concept which was widely accepted until Kerschner (1888) found similar numbers of spindles in fetal and adult biceps muscles. The work of Onanoff (1890), Christomanos & Strossner (1891), Sherrington (1894) and Ruffini (1898) established the role of the spindles as sensory receptors. The term muscle spindle was introduced by Kuhne (1863) to describe the morphological resemblance

of the intrafusal muscle bundle to the stem of the spindle plant.

Human muscle spindles consist of a group of intrafusal muscle fibres, separated from each other by thin strands of connective and elastic tissue, and surrounded by a fibrous capsule (Fig. 19.4). The capsule is expanded in the central or equatorial region of the spindle, to form the periaxial space (Fig. 19.5). In this region the spindle may reach 100–300 μm in diameter. Spindles are situated in parallel with muscle fascicles, often in close relation to a neurovascular bundle (Fig. 19.1).

The intrafusal muscle fibres, 3–14 in number, are of two major types, *nuclear bag* and *nuclear chain* fibres (Boyd 1962, Cooper & Daniel 1963, Swash & Fox 1972a). In cat, rabbit and human, and probably also in other mammals, there are two subtypes of the nuclear bag fibres, based on certain histochemical and ultrastructural features that represent functional specializations (Ovalle & Smith 1972). The nuclear bag$_1$ intrafusal fibre mediates the sensitivity of the primary afferent sensory ending to the rate of change in muscle length (the dynamic response), and the nuclear bag$_2$ and nuclear chain fibres mediate the response of spindle afferents to changes in length itself of the muscle (the static response) (Boyd et al 1977). The nuclear bag fibres project from their capsular investment at the spindle poles before inserting into extrafusal connective tissue or tendon. In the cat most spindles contain one bag$_1$ fibre, one bag$_2$ fibre and several chain fibres, but in humans there are often three bag fibres, at least one of which is a bag$_1$ fibre. Nuclear chain fibres usually arise and insert within the investing spindle capsule, which is itself closely adherent to nearby interfascicular

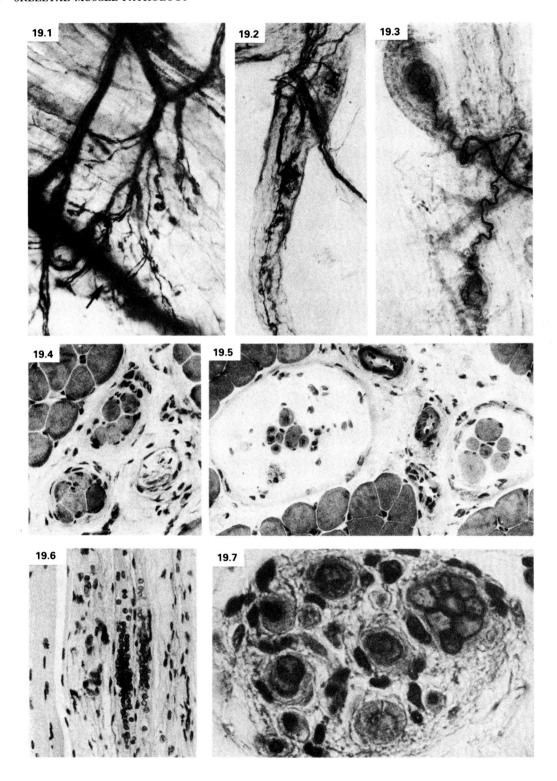

connective tissue planes. Several spindles may be found arranged in tandem within a muscle; this is an anatomical arrangement characteristic of as many as a third of the spindles in some muscles in the cat, and it is common also in humans. A single nuclear bag$_1$ fibre may extend through the length of two or more such spindles. In addition, several spindles may be found closely spaced in parallel with each other, occasionally sharing a common capsule, and innervated by branches from a single neighbouring nerve trunk.

Spindles vary in length from 2 to 6 mm (Voss 1937, Cooper & Daniel 1963). Human muscle spindles receive a complex motor and sensory nerve supply. Several capillaries (see Figs. 19.12, 19.20, 19.22 traverse the periaxial space (Cooper & Daniel 1963), a feature also of rabbit (Banks & James 1973) and baboon spindles (Fox et al 1974), but not of cat spindles. Before discussing the changes found in muscle spindles in neuromuscular disorders the features of the normal human muscle spindle will be described in more detail.

MUSCLE SPINDLE ANATOMY

Distribution of muscle spindles

In man, muscle spindles are found in *all* skeletal muscles, except the facial muscles and the intrinsic muscles of the larynx (Dogiel 1902, Cooper 1960, 1966, Raman & Devanandam 1989). Even the stapedius and the external anal sphincter muscle contain spindles. Spindles are particularly numerous in muscles capable of fine postural adjustments, such as the small muscles of the hands, in the supinator and pronator teres muscles and in the small deep muscles of the neck (Voss 1937, 1958, Cooper & Daniel 1963), but the large proximal muscles contain relatively few spindles (Cooper 1966, Swash & Fox 1972a). There are probably about 20 000 muscle spindles in the human body.

The precise location of muscle spindles within individual muscles has been studied in man by Voss (1937, 1958). In most muscles the spindles are concentrated in the belly of the muscle, and particularly near its motor point. In some muscles, however, especially the external ocular, spindles are located only in certain parts of the cross-sectional area of the muscle (Cooper & Daniel 1957, Bach-y-Rita 1971). Moreover, spindles are not evenly distributed in the bellies of limb muscles. For example, the medial head of the quadriceps near its insertion into the patella contains more spindles than other parts of this muscle. Neck muscles, and intrinsic hand muscles, contain relatively large numbers of muscle spindles commensurate with the roles of these muscles in posture and fine movement respectively (Cooper 1966).

Fig.19.1 Teased preparation. The nerve bundle entering the spindle (arrow) is one of several small nerves supplying motor end-plates situated on nearby extrafusal muscle fibres. Ranvier's gold chloride impregnation, ×75

Fig. 19.2 Teased preparation. Golgi tendon organ. Ranvier's gold chloride, ×90

Fig. 19.3 Pacinian corpuscles. These are sometimes found in muscle situated close to a muscle spindle. Barker and Ip silver impregnation, ×68

Fig. 19.4 Frozen section. Two spindles, sectioned in their polar regions. The capsules are thin. The intrafusal fibres are nearly as large as the extrafusal fibres in this biopsy of a child aged 14 years. H&E, ×68

Fig. 19.5 Frozen section. The same two spindles as in Figure 19.4, sectioned near their equatorial region. The periaxial spaces are large, containing a few thin strands of inner capsular cells and several nerve fibres, in addition to the intrafusal muscle fibres. H&E, ×68

Fig. 19.6 Longitudinal section of a normal muscle spindle. Two nuclear bag fibres, containing the aggregation of nuclei characteristic of the primary sensory region are seen. H&E, ×188

Fig. 19.7 Transverse section of a normal muscle spindle in the primary sensory (equatorial) region. The nuclear bag and nuclear chain fibres can be clearly seen. The intrafusal muscle fibres are surrounded by tissue of the inner capsule, in which several nerve fibres can be seen. H&E, ×900

It will be apparent from this discussion that the muscles commonly chosen for biopsy in pathological work, especially the biceps brachii, quadriceps and deltoid, contain relatively few spindles. Indeed, retrospective studies of spindles in biopsy material have yielded only small numbers of spindles for study (Lapresle & Milhaud 1964, Cazzato & Walton 1968, Patel et al 1968).

The intrafusal muscle fibres

The intrafusal muscle fibres show different structural characteristics at their polar and equatorial regions. In their poles subsarcolemmal nuclei are present, as in extrafusal muscle fibres, but in the capsular regions of the intrafusal fibres central nucleation is found. In a zone immediately adjacent to the equatorial region, the myotube region (Barker 1948), the nuclei lie in single file in a central core within the muscle fibre, and in the equatorial region itself, which is 300–500 μm long, these central nuclei are clustered together to form either a bag-like collection of several hundred vesicular nuclei (the *nuclear bag*, Figs 19.6, 19.7) or a closely applied chain of nuclei (the *nuclear chain*, Fig. 19.7; Boyd 1962).

In their equatorial regions the diameters of the intrafusal muscle fibres, especially of the nuclear bag fibres, may increase slightly, although the myofilaments passing around the nuclear bags themselves are reduced to a thin layer at the edges of the fibres (Fig. 19.6). The nuclear chain fibres show less attenuation of their myofilamentous content in this region. Human spindles contain 3–14 (mean 7) intrafusal muscle fibres (Cooper & Daniel 1963, Swash & Fox 1972a); 1–3 of these fibres are nuclear bag fibres and the remainder are nuclear chain fibres. Nuclear bag fibres are somewhat larger in diameter (median 14 μm) than nuclear chain fibres (median diameter 10 μm) and are longer, extending beyond the encapsulated part of the spindle. These diameters (see Fig. 19.25) are less than those recorded in cat muscle spindles by Boyd (1962).

Nuclear bag fibres show other structural differences from nuclear chain fibres and, in addition, two types of nuclear bag fibres have been identified; these are termed the dynamic bag_1 and static bag_2 fibres (Barker 1974, Barker & Laporte 1974).

Enzyme histochemical studies have shown that intrafusal muscle fibres have a different profile of reactions in the standard series of enzyme histochemical techniques (Dubowitz & Brooke 1973) than extrafusal muscle fibres (Spiro & Beilin 1969, Sahgal & Morgen 1976). All intrafusal muscle fibres react strongly in the PAS technique for glycogen (Fig. 19.8). The static bag_2 fibre reacts darkly with acid-preincubated myosin ATPase, while bag_1 fibres react lightly (Harriman et al 1974, Kucera & Dorovini-Zis 1979). With alkali-stable myosin ATPase, however, some of the encapsulated portions of the bag_2 fibres react as lightly as the dynamic bag_1 fibre (Kucera & Dorovini-Zia 1979). Nuclear chain fibres react darkly both with acid- and alkali-stable myosin ATPase (Fig. 19.9). All the intrafusal muscle fibres react more strongly than extrafusal muscle fibres for NADH–TR (Fig. 19.10), but the reaction product is coarser and more variable in static bag_2 and nuclear chain fibres than in dynamic bag_1 fibres. In the adult rat soleus muscle slow tonic and neonatal myosin heavy-chain isoforms are expressed only in intrafusal muscle fibres. Regional variability in staining reactivity to slow and fast myosins is evident in all three fibre types (Pedrosa et al 1989).

The ultrastructural features of dynamic bag_1 and static bag_2 fibres vary along the lengths of individual fibres, but nuclear chain fibres show more constant characteristics. The nuclear chain fibres show well-developed M bands in the H zones of their myofilaments, but M bands are found only in the extracapsular, polar parts of dynamic bag_1 and static bag_2 fibres. In these parts of the nuclear bag fibres, the static bag_2 fibres show more prominent intermyofibrillar material, containing larger, clustered mitochondria than dynamic bag_1 fibres. Leptomeres may occur in all three types of intrafusal muscle fibre, particularly at the periphery of fibres near motor and sensory nerve terminals. These histochemical and ultrastructural features of human intrafusal muscle fibres are similar to those found in the cat, rat and rabbit (Banks et al 1977, Kucera et al 1978).

Cooper & Gladden (1974) demonstrated differences in the amount of elastic tissue surrounding the two types of bag fibre in human lumbrical muscle spindles. The nuclear chain fibres are more closely applied to one another than are the nuclear bag fibres, so that it is difficult to tease them apart in studies of their innervation in whole silver-impregnated spindles. Ultrastructurally, adjacent nuclear chain fibres are often apparently attached to one another by their sensory innervation (see Fig. 19.17). Specialized zones of apposition between nuclear chain fibres, at the polar regions, called zonulae adherentes, that are devoid of basal lamina, are frequent. Nuclear chain fibres often contract as a single unit (Boyd 1976), reflecting their close anatomical relationships. These differences in the three types of intrafusal muscle fibre are summarized in Table 19.1.

In strap muscles, intrafusal muscle fibres generally insert into the intramuscular connective tissue, but in pennate muscles they more frequently insert into tendon. Some intrafusal muscle fibres insert into the capsular investment of the spindle. The largest intrafusal muscle fibre is usually the static bag$_2$ fibre.

The spindle capsule

The spindle capsule varies in length. It encloses the periaxial space of the equatorial and juxta-equatorial regions of the spindle, which are the site of the sensory innervation, and is thinner and more closely applied at the polar regions, becoming gradually less clearly defined as the poles are reached (Fig. 19.4, 19.5). The nuclear chain fibres sometimes seem to originate from the capsule in the polar regions. The capsule is pierced by entering nerve fibre bundles and arterioles. It contains a gel-like substance, consisting of mucopolysaccharide (Fig. 19.8) (von Brzezinski 1961). Strands of capsular cells, collagen and elastic tissue traverse the periaxial space and an inner layer of these cells encloses the intrafusal muscle fibre bundle (Fig. 19.7). The periaxial space often contains a separate neurovascular bundle. Normal spindles may reach 350 μm in diameter in their equatorial regions. The capsule itself consists of lamellae of capsular or perineurial cells (Shantha

Table 19.1 Some morphological characteristics of human intrafusal muscle fibres

| Characteristic | Type of human intrafusal muscle fibre | | |
	Nuclear dynamic bag$_1$	Nuclear static bag$_2$	Nuclear chain
Number	1 or 2	0 or 1	4–10
Length	Extend out of spindle capsule	Extend out of spindle capsule	Usually intracapsular only
Median diameter	14 μm	14 μm	10 μm
Elastic tissue	Marked investment in equatorial region	Less marked investment in equatorial region	Tend to be bound together by elastic tissue
Histochemical typing			
(ATPase) pH 4.3	Light	Dark	Dark
pH 9.4	Light	Variably light	Dark
(NADH)	Very dark	Coarsely dark	Coarsely dark
Ultrastructure	M bands only in extracapsular portions Thick Z bands Mitochondria inconspicuous	Prominent M band except in equatorial region Prominent clusters of mitochondria	M bands prominent Mitochondria inconspicuous
Innervation:			
Sensory	Prominent primary ending Inconspicuous secondary endings		Minimal primary ending Well-developed secondary endings, usually on both poles, shared between adjacent chain fibres
Motor (see text)	Dynamic P$_2$ endings P$_1$ ending (β innervation)	Static γ axons	Static P$_1$ endings γ-trail endings

et al 1968) together with a meshwork of longitudinally and circumferentially arranged elastic tissue.

The outer layers of the capsule (see Fig. 19.17) consist of 6–8 concentric layers of basement membrane-covered flat cells whose elongated processes contain many pinocytotic vesicles. Collagen fibres lie between the layers. These cells resemble, and are continuous with, perineurial cells. The inner layers of the capsule, which are continuous with the inner capsular layers covering the intrafusal muscle fibres themselves, are devoid of basement membrane and of pinocytotic vesicles, and resemble fibroblasts (Kennedy & Staley 1973). The capsule cells constitute a functional barrier that regulates the internal environment of the spindle (Dow et al 1980). Fukami and Schlesinger (1989) have shown that the spindle capsular cells are active in endocytosis and transport of both small molecules and macromolecules into the capsular space.

It is not uncommon for part of the spindle capsule to invest some 6–20 adjacent extrafusal fibres, but no functional connection is apparent between the intrafusal and extrafusal muscle fibres or their innervation in this relationship (Cooper & Daniel 1963, Swash & Fox 1972a,b) and the functional significance of this relationship is unknown.

Innervation of intrafusal muscle fibres

Extensive, and often controversial, studies of the motor and sensory innervation of muscle spindles have been carried out in amphibian and in cat and rabbit spindles (see Barker 1948, Boyd 1962, Barker 1974). The pattern of innervation of human spindles is similar to that of other mammalian species (Kennedy 1970, Swash & Fox 1972a, Fox et al 1974). The innervation is complex, consisting of motor and sensory components, representing a polyneuronal innervation. Unlike extrafusal muscle fibres, intrafusal fibres are innervated by multiple motor axons, supplying many motor end-plates of differing morphology. Direct observation has shown that these end-plates excite contraction by a graded response occurring locally, and that twitch contractions do not occur (Boyd 1976). A diagrammatic representation of the innervation of an idealised human muscle spindle is shown in Figure 19.16.

The sensory and motor innervation of nuclear bag and nuclear chain fibres differs. In cat and rat spindles the nuclear bag_1 and bag_2 fibres receive slightly different motor innervations (Barker et al 1976, 1978) and similar differences probably also occur in human spindles, although these have not yet been established. No differences in the pattern of spindle innervation in different muscles are known (Swash & Fox 1972a).

Fig. 19.8 The periaxial space is filled with a gelatinous material which contains mucopolysaccharide (diastase-resistant). PAS, ×188

Fig. 19.9 Polar section. Dark, intermediate and lightly reacting fibres can be identified. ATPase, pH 4.3; ×300

Fig. 19.10 The intrafusal muscle fibres react more intensely than the extrafusal muscle fibres. NADH–TR, ×68

Fig. 19.11 The primary sensory ending consists of a series of loops, with a dense network of beaded terminal enlargements on the surface of the nuclear bag fibre. Barker and Ip silver impregnation, ×263

Fig. 19.12 The entering nerve bundle (e.n.b.) supplies group I (I) innervation to the two primary sensory endings and group II (II) innervation to the secondary sensory endings. The nuclear chain intrafusal muscle fibres receive only a small branch from the group I afferent fibres and do not form well-developed primary sensory endings. The periaxial space contains several capillaries (c). Ranvier gold impregnation, ×68

Fig. 19.13 A juxta-equatorial secondary sensory ending, consisting of several discrete clusters of sensory terminals (2), arises from the two major branches of a secondary afferent fibre (II). The primary sensory ending can also be seen (I). Ranvier gold impregnation, ×188

Fig. 19.14 P_2 plate motor ending. These endings are usually discrete. Barker and Ip silver impregnation, ×263

Fig. 19.15 This P_2 plate motor ending has a more diffuse form than that shown in Figure 19.14. Barker and Ip silver impregnation, ×263

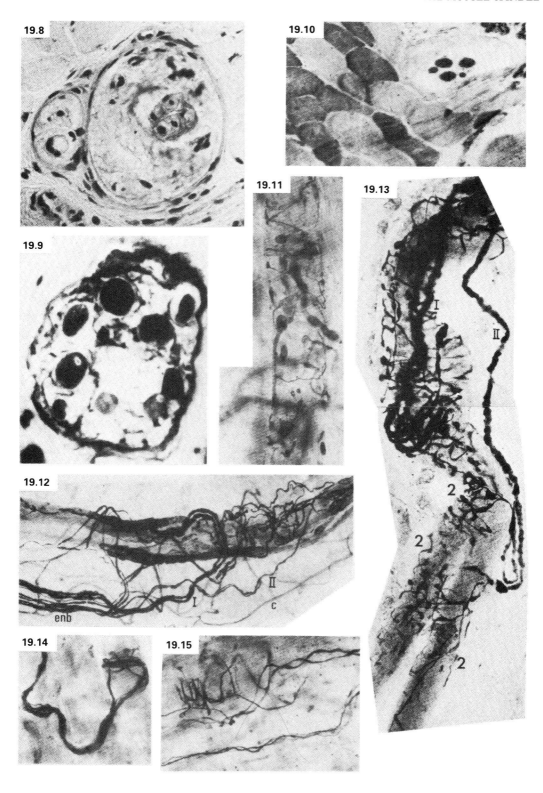

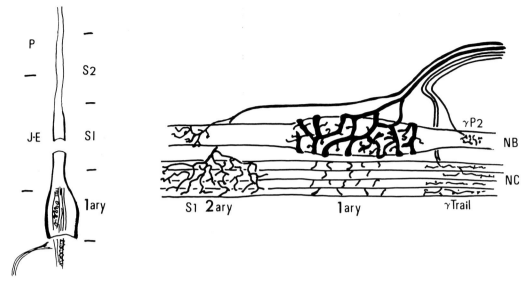

Fig. 19.16 Diagrammatic representation of motor and sensory innervation of a human muscle spindle. Note the notation of intrafusal muscle fibre segments according to polar (P), equatorial (E) and juxta-equatorial (J–E) regions or according to the regions of secondary sensory innervation (S1, S2) or to the primary sensory innervation (1ary). NB: nuclear bag, NC: nuclear chain, P2 plate innervation and gamma trail innervation also shown

Sensory innervation

The nuclear bag region is the site of the *primary sensory* ending (Figs. 19.11–19.13). In humans, each spindle receives a single group 1a afferent nerve fibre which branches within the periaxial space to supply each primary sensory ending. Only one primary ending is found on each intrafusal nuclear bag fibre, and the nuclear chain fibres receive a less rich primary ending consisting of a few short unmyelinated spirals. The nuclear bag primary ending consists of complex, loosely wrapped, single or double spirals of unmyelinated nerve terminals which slightly indent the surface of the fibre. Very fine unmyelinated terminal branches ending in flat, plate-like expansions arise from these spirals (Fig. 19.11). The ending occupies a length of 150–250 μm (Swash & Fox 1972a).

The *secondary sensory endings* (Figs. 19.13, 19.17, 19.20) are situated in the periaxial space in the juxta-equatorial region, predominantly on nuclear chain fibres (Fig. 19.13). They are about 300–500 μm in length, and are usually found on both sides of the equatorial primary region.

Occasionally they are found on one pole only and some spindles are devoid of secondary sensory endings (Boyd 1962). Each is innervated by a separate group II afferent nerve fibre. Secondary endings on the S1 region, nearest the primary ending, often have a rather spiral form (Fig. 19.13) and are supplied by larger diameter group II afferent fibres, but those situated at a distance from the primary region, in the S2 or S3 regions have a more typical flower-spray form, with multiple fine branches ramifying over the nuclear chain fibres (Fig. 19.20). These flower-spray secondaries are innervated by group II afferents of smaller diameter (Fox et al 1974). Secondary sensory endings are also often found on the static bag$_2$ fibre, but less commonly on the dynamic bag$_1$ fibre (Banks et al 1982, Swash & Fox 1972a).

The primary and secondary sensory endings have a similar ultrastructural appearance (Adal 1969, Landon 1972). In both types of ending, the sensory terminals are separated from the plasma membrane of the adjacent muscle fibre only by the plasma membrane of the nerve terminal itself. A single layer of basement membrane encloses both muscle fibre and nerve terminal (Fig. 19.17). The cytoplasm of the sensory terminal contains prominent mitochondria, microtubules, dense bodies and clear vesicles, some dense-cored. The secondary sensory terminals tend to lie in a gutter-like depression in the surface of the muscle fibre (Fig. 19.18), but the primary sensory terminals form a bulge on the surface of the fibre, in which the characteristic nuclear bag can be seen (Fig. 19.19). Cross-terminals formed from secondary endings connect adjacent nuclear chain fibres (Fig. 19.17), so that they form a single functional unit.

Motor innervation

Functionally, muscle spindles contain a discrete dynamically responsive system consisting of the dynamic bag$_1$ fibre and its dynamic motor innervation, and a statically responsive system consisting of the chain fibres and the static bag$_2$ fibre, and their static motor innervation. The former dynamic response is largely signalled through primary sensory endings, and the latter, static response is largely signalled through secondary sensory endings. Correlation of these functional characteristics with the morphology of the motor innervation of intrafusal muscle fibres has proved a complex and controversial problem (Barker et al 1973, Boyd et al 1977). Motor end-plates are found in the juxta-equatorial and polar regions of intrafusal muscle fibres, on both sides of the equatorial sensory region. The distribution of these motor endings is best demonstrated in cholinesterase preparations (see Coërs & Woolf 1959, Kucera 1980). Most of these endings are innervated by γ-motor nerve fibres. They have been classified according to the terminology introduced by Barker et al (1970) in their study of the fusimotor innervation in de-afferented cat spindles.

P_2 *end plates* are located in the mid-polar region occupying a zone 300–600 μm in length on both sides of the equatorial region. These motor endings are often intermingled with the secondary sensory endings. They consist of several loops or rings from which fine terminal branches ending in knobs, tapers or round end-plates, closely applied to the surface of the muscle fibre, are derived (Figs. 19.14, 19.15, 19.22). The muscle fibre in this region may be somewhat expanded in diameter

(Swash & Fox 1972a). Ultrastructurally, these P$_2$ plate, gamma endings are substantially indented and show only shallow post-synaptic folds (Arbuthnott et al. 1982). These endings have a lower acetycholinesterase content than other fusimotor endings (Kucera 1982). These P$_2$ plate endings terminate on dynamic bag$_1$ intrafusal muscle fibres (Barker et al 1976, 1978).

Gamma-trail motor endings are diffuse multi-terminal endings extending over several hundred micrometres (Fig. 19.21). They are usually most prominent in the S1 juxta-equatorial region and are found predominantly, but not exclusively, on nuclear chain fibres. Indeed, nuclear chain fibres rarely receive additional motor innervation (Barker et al 1970, Swash & Fox 1972a). Fine unmyelinated nodal branches of the γ-fibres innervating these endings run for long distances before ending in a leash of multibranched axons bearing synaptic knobs or beads. Sometimes these endings are relatively more discrete (Swash & Fox 1972a). Gamma-trail endings show few, if any, synaptic folds and no sole-plate eminence (Barker et al 1970).

P_1 *plate endings* resemble the motor end-plates of extrafusal muscle. There is a prominent Doyère eminence with sole-plate nuclei, and the ending is found at the pole of a nuclear bag fibre (Fig. 19.23). Not all spindles receive this form of motor innervation, which is derived by branching from α-motor fibres to extrafusal muscle (β-innervation).

The ultrastructural features of P$_1$ plate endings resemble those of extrafusal end-plates. The synaptic folds are complex and lined with basement membrane, and the sole-plate is prominent. Sympathetic nerve fibres innervate arterioles in the periaxial space (Swash & Fox 1985) but reports of catecholaminergic endings in the equatorial regions of mammalian spindles (Banker & Girvin 1971) are unconfirmed (see Barker & Saito 1979).

This classification of the morphology of the motor innervation of intrafusal muscle fibres, which is derived from light microscopy of the silver-impregnated whole mount preparations (Barker et al 1970, Swash & Fox 1972a,b) has been superseded by direct functional/anatomical correlations. These more recent studies suggest that the dynamic and static functions of the motor

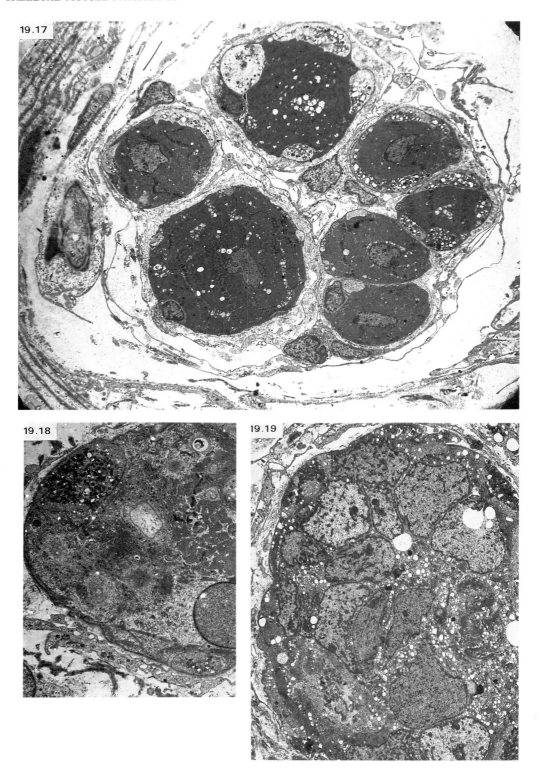

innervation are conferred by a combination of location of the ending and degree of folding of its postjunctional folds. More polar endings are more likely to be static (Arbuthnott et al 1982). Confusion regarding the motor innervation of intrafusal muscle fibres can be resolved by considering the motor innervation of the three types of intrafusal fibres in relation to the morphology of the motor end plates found on these fibres (Arbuthnott et al 1982, 1989). The dynamic bag$_1$ fibre receives gamma innervation from P_2 plates and beta innervation from P_1 plates. These motor end plates are morphologically indistinguishable in ultrastructural studies, having m_b characteristics according to the criteria of Arbuthnott et al (1982). M_b plate endings indent muscle fibres, have shallow post-synaptic folds and a lower AChE content than other fusimotor endings (Kucera 1981). Motor endings on the static bag$_2$ fibre do not indent the fibres, are smooth and unfolded, and probably represent part of the trail endings identified by Barker and his colleagues. These terminals are m_a endings in the Arbuthnott et al (1982) classification. Nuclear chain fibres receive three types of fusimotor innervation. The majority of chain fibres are innervated by m_a plates that typically imply static innervation. Some nuclear chain plates receive m_c plates, endings situated in raised indentations, that show shallow folds. Long chain fibres receive a single plate ending, probably of beta origin, located in the extracapsular region that resembles extrafusal motor endings, and was termed m_d by Arbuthnott et al (1989). The apparent simplicity of this classification is, nonetheless, belied by the observation that the degree of post-synaptic folding of end plates can vary along their length (Arbuthnott et al 1982).

AGE EFFECTS ON SPINDLE MORPHOLOGY

Age effects on skeletal muscle are well recognized (Adams et al 1962, Tomlinson et al 1969) and the effect of age on muscle spindles must be recognized in any description of their pathology. Aging is associated with increased amounts of collagen and fibrous tissue in muscle, as in other tissues. In addition, loss of muscle bulk may be a striking feature of apparently normal aged subjects. This reflects loss of muscle fibres, a phenomenon which probably results mainly from changes in the innervation of muscle. The number of nerve fibres in the ventral roots declines in aged subjects; Gardner (1940) found a 27% reduction in the ventral roots of subjects in their eighth decade, compared with others in their second decade. Wohlfart (1939, 1957) and Tomlinson et al (1969) found grouped denervation atrophy and disseminated neurogenic atrophy in skeletal muscles of subjects older than 65 years, while Tomlinson and Irving (1977) found a progressive diminution in anterior horn cell numbers in the spinal cord after the age of 60 years.

In a quantitative study of the effect of increasing age on muscle spindles, Swash & Fox (1972b) found that there was a gradual increase in the mean thickness of the spindle capsule in both proximal and distal muscles (Fig. 19.24). This effect was generally more marked in distal than in proximal muscles, but it was also prominent in the quadriceps muscles. The spindle capsules in aged subjects contained increased numbers of outer and inner capsular lamellae, so that the latter often seemed to encroach on the periaxial space (Fig. 19.24). Collagen was present in increased amounts

Fig. 19.17   De-afferented baboon muscle spindle sectioned in region of S1 secondary ending. Note the secondary sensory endings closely applied to the surface of the intrafusal muscle fibres and tending to bridge the gaps between neighbouring nuclear chain fibres. The nuclear bag fibres receive only scanty innervation from secondary endings. Electron micrograph, ×1875

Fig. 19.18   Secondary sensory ending. The sensory terminals lie in depressions in the surface of the muscle fibre and contain densely packed mitochondria. The sensory ending is separated from its muscle fibre only by plasma membrane. The intrafusal muscle fibre in this micrograph is abnormal, showing degenerative features as part of the changes found in myotonic dystrophy. Electron micrograph, ×3000

Fig. 19.19   Primary sensory endings. The nuclear bag and the sensory terminals can be seen. There is an excess of lipid droplets in this fibre, studied in a biopsy from a patient with myotonic dystrophy. Electron micrograph, ×2475

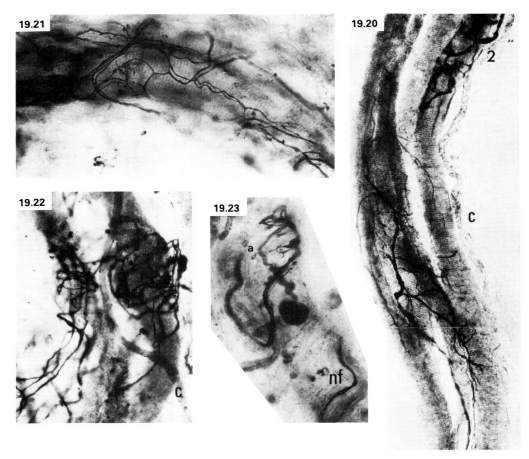

Fig. 19.20 This midpolar secondary sensory ending consists of a spray of widely distributed fine branching axons arising from a thin secondary afferent nerve fibre. Part of the juxta-equatorial (S1) secondary ending, consisting of a spray of sensory terminals, can also be seen (2). (c: capillary). Barker and Ip silver impregnation, ×188

Fig. 19.21 Trail-ending γ-motor fibres end in scattered clusters of motor end-plates. Sole plate nuclei cannot be identified. Barker and Ip silver impregnation, ×263

Fig. 19.22 Two P$_2$ motor endings are supplied by γ motor fibres. End-plates can be seen in the larger of these two endings, and the muscle fibre in the region of each ending is slightly expanded. (c: capillary). Barker and Ip silver impregnation, ×263

Fig. 19.23 P$_1$ motor ending showing the thickly myelinated nerve fibre (n.f.) supplying the ending. A fine axonal sprout leading to an accessory end-plate (a) is present. Barker and Ip silver impregnation, ×263

between these capsular lamellae. The elastic fibres found in the capsule and near the intrafusal fibres appeared normal. There was a slight decrease in the mean number of intrafusal muscle fibres in the spindles in each muscle studied, and sometimes a granular or vacuolated fibre could be seen. The two-peaked distribution of fibre diameter found in normal spindles was less prominent in subjects older than 60 years (Fig. 19.25). The histochemical heterogeneity of intrafusal muscle fibres is maintained with aging (Ishihara 1988).

Studies of the innervation of muscle spindles in aged subjects showed no change in the distribution of motor and sensory endings, but increased terminal branching of motor axons was noted, and both large myelinated nerve fibres and small

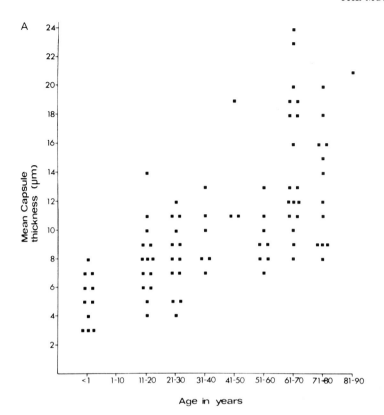

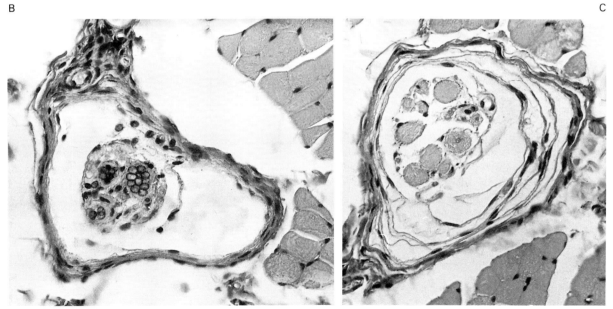

Fig. 19.24 (A) The thickness of the spindle capsule increases with increasing age. Each point represents the mean thickness of all the spindle capsules measured in a single muscle; 629 spindles were measured (see Swash & Fox 1972b). (B) Spindle from a 16-year-old subject; ×350. (C) Spindle from a 65-year-old subject. The capsule is thickened and its lamellae seem to encroach on the periaxial space; ×350

Number intrafusal muscle fibres

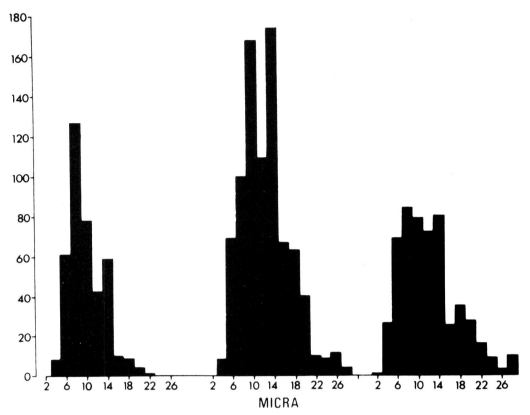

Fig. 19.25 The three histograms represent the distribution of intrafusal muscle fibre diameter according to age; from left to right: newborn; aged 16–33 years; and aged 64–73 years respectively (1782 fibres in 10 subjects (Swash & Fox 1972b))

thinly myelinated fibres showed spherical axonal swellings near their termination. In many of the aged subjects examined in this study, disseminated neurogenic atrophy was found in the extrafusal muscle, and some of the changes found in the muscle spindles might thus represent the effect of partial damage to their nerve supply. De Reuck (1973) has described similar changes in spindle morphology with increasing age.

METHODS FOR STUDY OF MUSCLE SPINDLE PATHOLOGY

Muscle spindles are usually recognized in transverse sections of muscle, but they can also be found in longitudinal sections, especially in autopsy material when muscles rich in spindles, such as pronator teres or small hand muscles, may be available for study. Spindles are not commonly found in muscle biopsies because the muscles usually selected for biopsy, the deltoid, biceps brachii and quadriceps muscles, contain relatively few spindles (Cooper & Daniel 1963, Swash & Fox 1972c).

In paraffin-embedded material, haematoxylin and eosin and elastic van Gieson stains are useful for routine use, and the Glees and Marsland silver technique can be used to demonstrate the innervation in thick (20–30 μm) sections (Swash & Fox 1972c). Biopsy specimens allow enzyme histochemical reactions to be studied (Dubowitz & Brooke 1973) but these do not contribute greatly to studies of the pathological reactions of the muscle spindle. If fresh unfixed and unfrozen muscle is available, metallic block-impregnation methods, using gold chloride or silver nitrate, enable teased preparations of whole muscle spindles to be obtained for detailed study of the pattern of innervation (Barker & Ip 1963, Swash & Fox 1972c). It is difficult to study the innervation in serially sectioned material (see Barker 1948, Cooper & Daniel 1963, Kucera 1986).

DENERVATION

The abnormalities observed in human muscle spindles after sensorimotor, sensory and motor denervation are characteristic, and are recognizable from case to case. Difficulties experienced by earlier workers (Lapresle & Milhaud 1964, Jedrzejowska & Fidziańska 1966, Cazzato & Walton 1968, Patel et al 1968) were probably due to their reliance on biopsied material and to confusion regarding the effects of aging. Experimental studies of spindle morphology after denervation have been reported by Onanoff (1890), Tower (1932, 1939), Boyd (1962), Barker et al (1970) and by Schröder (1974a,b). Onanoff's studies established the dual nature of the sensory and motor innervation of muscle spindles. Tower (1932, 1939) noted increased thickness of the spindle capsules and of the fibrous tissue in the periaxial space, derived from internal capsular tissue, after sensorimotor denervation and after ventral root section of prolonged duration, but not after sensory root section or dorsal ganglionectomy, although in the latter experiment the spindle capsule seemed to invest the intrafusal muscle fibres more closely than normal. A similar abnormality occurs in man in tabes dorsalis (Swash & Fox 1974).

The innervation is important in determining spindle differentiation and maturation in utero and even in early post-natal life. For example, no spindles form in hind-limb muscles denervated in utero by section of the sciatic nerve (Zelena 1957). Sciatic nerve crush causes arrest of spindle development up to the first postnatal week in the rat (Zelana & Hnik 1960), but the full complement of encapsulated and differentiated intrafusal muscle fibres persists in de-efferented muscles (Zelena and Soukup 1974), illustrating the

importance of the sensory innervation (Kucera & Walro 1987).

In man, sensorimotor denervation, whether due to mononeuropathy, diabetes mellitus, drug-induced neuropathy or carcinomatous polyneuropathy, results in striking capsular thickening, consisting of increased numbers of lamellae of perineurial capsular cells and increased amounts of collagen (De Reuck 1974, Swash & Fox 1974). These changes occur both in equatorial and in polar sections and are much greater than expected for age. In addition, the periaxial space in the equatorial region becomes fibrosed. These changes are most prominent in long-standing sensorimotor denervation, probably becoming evident within several months of denervation, as shown in studies of vincristine polyneuropathy (Swash & Fox 1974). Elastic tissue surrounding the intrafusal muscle fibres appears fragmented in these abnormal spindles. In *sensory denervation* due to tabes dorsalis, or to carcinomatous sensory neuropathy (Croft et al 1965) deposition of collagen in the periaxial space is prominent only in the equatorial and juxta-equatorial regions, but in *motor denervation* capsular thickening is marked only in polar sections (Swash & Fox 1974). The marked reaction of the spindle capsule to denervation is consistent with the similar change that occurs in perineurial cells in peripheral nerves (see Shantha et al 1968). In equatorial sections of denervated spindles a prominent 'balloon-like' enlargement of the periaxial space, with separation of the capsular layers, is sometimes seen (see Fig. 19.34). This was first observed by Amersbach (1911) and was reported by Cazzato & Walton (1968) in one spindle in a case of dermatomyositis. In our material this abnormality has occurred only in muscles denervated for many years, for example in poliomyelitis, motor neurone disease, diabetic neuropathy, syringomyelia and meningomyelocele, and in all these cases there was extensive fatty replacement of extrafusal muscle. This abnormality may result from absence of the usual physical forces which normally result from muscular contraction.

In both sensorimotor and motor denervation, the nuclear chain fibres undergo earlier and more severe degenerative changes than the nuclear bag fibres so that, in some spindles, only nuclear bag fibres remain detectable by light microscopy. After sensorimotor denervation of a year or more, all the intrafusal muscle fibres show degenerative changes, becoming clumped together in a poorly defined mass in the centre of the periaxial space. After prolonged motor denervation, however, although polar sections show similar atrophy of the intrafusal fibres, in equatorial sections normal primary sensory endings can be found on nuclear bag fibres of only slightly reduced diameter. Secondary sensory endings are difficult to identify in sectioned material, but these are usually also identifiable in the juxta-equatorial region. Schröder (1974a) found an increase in intrafusal muscle fibres, up to twice the normal number, in 20% of spindles studied in rat muscles re-innervated after sciatic nerve crush performed 2 years previously. In some spindles, in muscles in which re-innervation had been prevented, a similar increase in number of intrafusal muscle fibres was observed, suggesting that this abnormality was due to denervation, rather than to re-innervation. However, an increase in number of intrafusal muscle fibres (normal <15) has not been observed after denervation in human spindles (Swash & Fox

1974). Sahgal & Morgen (1976) reported target-fibre formation and 'splitting' of a nuclear bag fibre in acute denervation, but their illustration of fibre splitting seems to show only nuclear chain and nuclear bag fibres in a spindle with a thickened capsule. Kucera (1977), however, noted two bag_1 fibres in re-innervated spindles in the soleus muscle of the rat and suggested that the second of these was derived by splitting from a single parent bag_1 fibre.

Intrafusal muscle fibres, like external ocular muscle fibres (see Peachey 1971), are hyper-neurotized and their reaction to denervation would not be expected, therefore, to mimic that of ordinary skeletal extrafusal muscle fibres. Boyd (1962), in experimental work in the cat, found that nuclear chain fibres showed degenerative changes before nuclear bag fibres, and Barker et al (1970) have shown that the γ-trail fusimotor endings, which are distributed to nuclear chain fibres and to the static bag_2 fibres, are more resistant to degeneration after nerve section than the γ-plate (P_2) endings, but that the β-endings, which chiefly innervate the poles of nuclear bag fibres, degenerate even more quickly after nerve

---

Fig. 19.26 Motor neurone disease. The primary and secondary sensory endings are clearly demonstrated. Only one fusimotor axon can be seen, entering the spindle with the group Ia afferent fibre, and the juxta-equatorial regions are devoid of motor endings and axons. Ranvier gold impregnation, ×45 approx

Fig. 19.27 Werdnig–Hoffmann disease. The primary ending and its nuclear bag nuclei, and the secondary sensory ending (below) are normal. Glees and Marsland silver, ×263

Fig. 19.28 Motor neurone disease. The equatorial nuclei and the primary sensory ending are normal. Glees and Marsland silver, ×263

Fig. 19.29 Vincristine neuropathy. A single large diameter axon approaches the intrafusal muscle fibres, but the sensory and motor endings themselves are destroyed. Ranvier gold impregnation, ×68

Fig. 19.30 Motor neurone disease. The two muscle spindles are prominent because their capsules are thickened and because there is marked denervation atrophy of nearby extrafusal muscle. The nuclear chain fibres are thinner than normal. Elastic van Gieson, ×68

Fig. 19.31 Werdnig–Hoffman disease. There are three muscle spindles, two of which contain intrafusal fibres larger than extrafusal fibres. One spindle shows 'spindle oedema' and its intrafusal muscle fibres are atrophic; these are features of motor denervation. Elastic van Giesen, ×68

Fig. 19.32 Poliomyelitis. In these polar sections the capsule is thickened, but expanded (compare Fig. 19.4), and only one intrafusal fibre remains. These are features of long-standing motor denervation. Elastic van Gieson, ×188

Fig. 19.33 Carcinomatous sensory neuropathy. The intrafusal muscle fibres, sectioned in a near-equatorial plane, are atrophic and surrounded by a dense mass of collagen. The capsule is not unduly thickened. There is a striking absence of nerve fibres. These features are consistent with predominantly sensory denervation. Glees and Marsland, ×68

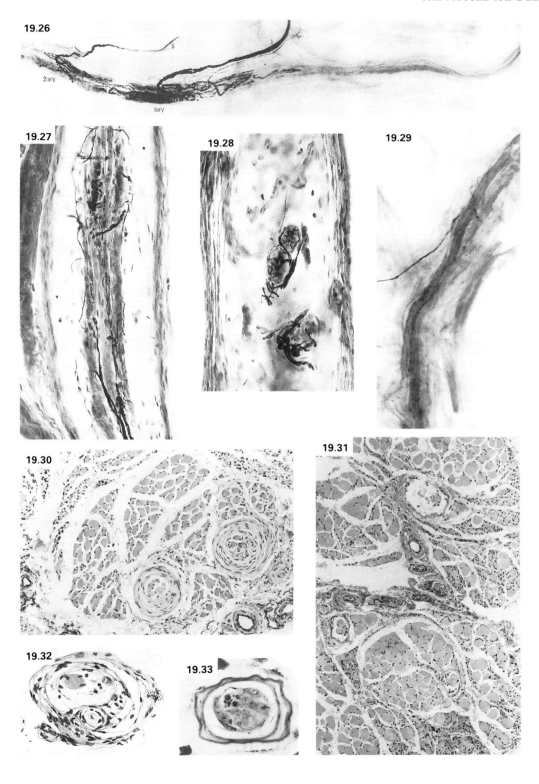

19.26

2ary

II

Iary

19.27

19.28

19.29

19.30

19.31

19.32

19.33

section. These conflicting observations suggest that the more rapid atrophy of nuclear chain than of nuclear bag fibres reflects structural differences in the muscle fibres themselves, rather than in their innervation. The nuclear chain fibres have several histochemical and ultrastructural features in common with type 2 extrafusal fibres (Matthews 1972, Smith & Ovalle 1972, Kucera & Dorovini-Zis 1979), and this might be an important factor in determining their response to motor denervation. Type 2 atrophy, for example, is an early feature of experimental denervation (Engel et al 1973).

Motor neurone disease

In motor neurone disease the tendon reflexes are characteristically preserved, or exaggerated, even when there is severe muscular atrophy; it is clear, therefore, that the primary sensory endings remain functional. These endings, and the secondary sensory endings, are morphologically normal in this disease, in Werdnig–Hoffman disease, and also in poliomyelitis (Figs. 19.26–19.28) (Swash & Fox 1974). In these disorders, however, the γ-innervated fusimotor endings are abnormal. Swash & Fox (1974) found that there was a marked reduction in the number of fusimotor nerve fibres and of motor endings, and were unable to locate any α-P_1 plate endings. Some spindles were devoid of motor innervation (Fig. 19.29). Kennedy (1971) reported that increased tortuosity of fusimotor axons was a characteristic feature of motor neurone disease, but this is a non-specific age-related effect (Swash & Fox 1972b). Indeed, Kennedy (1969) earlier reported a similar abnormality in teased spindles in polyneuropathies. The few surviving fusimotor endings generally show simplification of their terminals, but in motor neurone disease and in some polyneuropathies fine terminal and preterminal axonal sprouts occur. Thus the γ- and α-fusimotor innervation is abnormal in both motor neurone disease and poliomyelitis. However, Saito et al (1978) noted from their studies of the distribution of acetylcholinesterase on intrafusal muscle fibres in motor neurone disease that the intermediate polar zones seemed to be less denuded of enzyme activity than the poles themselves,

suggesting that the γ-trail fibres and endings were more resistant to degeneration than the P_1 or P_2 plate fibres and endings.

The spindle capsules are thickened in their polar regions (Figs 19.31, 19.32) and, because of atrophy of the extrafusal fibres, may appear to be more prominent and closer together than in normal muscle (Figs 19.30, 19.31). This appearance led to the suggestion at one time that there was an increase in the number of spindles in muscles in motor neurone disease (see Adams et al 1962). There may be marked 'spindle oedema' (see above) in long-standing motor denervation, e.g. poliomyelitis (Figs 19.34, 19.37).

Mixed neuropathies

In diabetic neuropathy and in entrapment neuropathies the larger diameter sensory and motor fibres and their endings are more severely affected than the fine, thinly myelinated, γ-fusimotor fibres, an observation consistent with the relative susceptibility of these fibres in these disorders observed by Thomas & Fullerton (1963) and by Thomas & Lascelles (1965). Kennedy (1969) studied the innervation of muscle spindles in biopsies of small hand muscles in patients with the Guillain–Barré syndrome, Charcot–Marie–Tooth disease, alcoholic neuropathy and chronic progressive idiopathic polyneuropathy. He found reduced numbers, only 1–3 rather than 6–15, of fusimotor axons entering the spindles, with increased complexity of their ramification on the intrafusal muscle fibres. Many of these axons showed sphere-like deformation (simplification) of their synaptic terminals. The primary sensory axon and ending was often absent, especially in severe acute polyneuropathies, but in some this ending seemed to have more complex branching than normal. Secondary sensory endings were not reliably identified. These findings proved difficult to interpret in the absence of age-matched controls, but they are consistent with the later findings of Swash & Fox (1974).

Later, Kennedy (1974) reported that the abnormally innervated spindles in a case of hypertrophic neuropathy seemed to receive as many as 2–4 group Ia afferent fibres. However, it is unlikely that any disease of nerve cells or Schwann

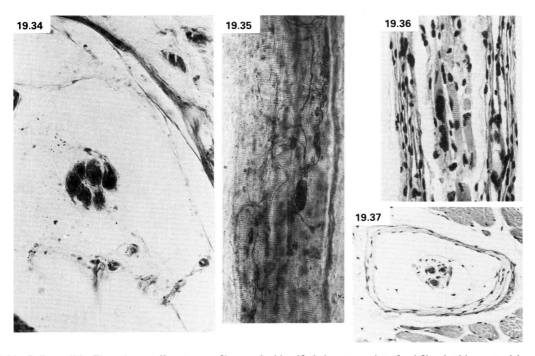

Fig. 19.34 Poliomyelitis. The primary afferent nerve fibre can be identified close to one intrafusal fibre in this equatorial section. Note the dilated periaxial space ('spindle oedema'). Glees and Marsland, ×188

Fig. 19.35 Tabes dorsalis. The primary sensory ending (see Figs. 17.11, 17.13, 17.26, 17.28) consists of a thin, irregularly and prominently beaded, tortuous unmyelinated axon. Only two or three sensory enlargements remain. Barker and Ip silver impregnation, ×263

Fig. 19.36 Tabes dorsalis. The nuclear bag nuclei are poorly defined, unusually basophilic and situated in a fibre which appears granular. The neighbouring fibres are nuclear chain fibres. H&E, ×263

Fig. 19.37 Diabetic neuropathy. Spindle oedema, atrophy of intrafusal muscle fibres and slight thickening of the capsule are features of denervation in this juxta-equatorial section. Elastic van Gieson, ×188

cells could lead to the formation of entirely new sensory axons, other than by branching, because this would presuppose the existence of an additional population of cells in the posterior root ganglia, and it is more likely that Kennedy (1974) misidentified secondary afferent fibres as primaries. The identification of primary and secondary afferents in primate spindles is difficult (Swash & Fox 1972a, 1974) because of overlap in diameter of their afferent fibres (Fox et al 1974) and in the morphology of the primary endings and the S1 juxta-equatorial sensory endings (Ruffini 1898, Swash & Fox 1972a, Fox et al 1974).

Changes in the permeability of the spindle capsule in leprosy may be important in the patho-genesis of this disease, providing a possible means of access of *Mycobacterium leprae* to the peripheral nervous system (Edwards 1975).

Sensory neuropathies

In sensory denervation, abnormalities can always be observed in the primary sensory endings, but the recognition of abnormalities in the secondary sensory innervation is more difficult. In carcinomatous sensory neuropathy, primary sensory endings and their afferent nerve fibres and equatorial nuclear aggregations could not be identified; the intrafusal muscle fibres were atrophic in these regions and the periaxial space contained excess amounts of collagen (Fig. 19.33) (Swash & Fox 1974). The sensory innervation of muscle spindles is also abnormal in tabes dorsalis (Swash & Fox 1974). Although this disorder is not usually classified as a sensory neuropathy, the tendon reflexes are absent in the legs, and Greenfield (1963) noted loss of large myelinated fibres in the posterior spinal roots, especially in the root entry zone, with a variable loss of nerve cells in the posterior root ganglia. Batten (1897) noted that the equatorial nuclei in the muscle spindles appeared pyknotic in this disorder (Fig. 19.36), an observation which was confirmed by Swash & Fox (1974). In later experimental work, Batten (1898) noted degenerative changes in the equatorial nuclei, 5 days after dorsal rhizotomy. He compared these findings with those in tabes dorsalis (see Tower 1932) but the rapid appearance of these abnormalities is unlike the incomplete equatorial nuclear degeneration found even in well-established cases of that condition (Swash & Fox 1974). Further, the axonal swellings and attenuations found on the terminal parts of the primary and secondary sensory nerve fibres and in the simplifed endings of tabetic spindles suggest that terminal sprouting and reinnervation occur during the course of the disease (Fig. 19.35), the causative lesion lying in the sensory nerves themselves or in the neurones of the posterior root ganglia, as in the proximal and distal axonopathies.

It is, perhaps, somewhat unexpected that sensory denervation should produce degenerative changes in a muscle fibre (Fig. 19.37). Experimental work, however, clearly indicates the importance of the trophic role of the sensory innervation in spindle morphogenesis (Zelena 1957, Landon 1972, Milburn 1973). Furthermore, experimentally denervated spindles in adult animals do not usually receive functionally competent reinnervation (Tower 1932, 1939, Zelena 1964). Systematic ultrastructural observations on denervated human muscle spindles are not yet available.

Certain toxic neuropathies may selectively damage the sensory innervation of muscle spindles, e.g. pyridoxine and acrylamide poisoning, an observation perhaps accounting for the ataxia found so prominently in these toxic neuropathies (Krinke et al 1978, Lowndes et al 1978).

MYOPATHIES AND DYSTROPHIES

Myotonic dystrophy

In 1964, Daniel & Strich described changes in the muscle spindles in five cases of myotonic dystrophy examined at autopsy, but three subsequent surveys of spindle pathology, based on biopsies because the few spindles examined in these latter studies did not form a representative sample (Lapresle & Milhaud 1964, Cazzato & Walton 1968, Patel et al 1968). More recent studies (Swash 1972, Heene 1973, Swash & Fox 1975a, 1975b, Maynard et al 1977, Stranock & Newson Davis 1978a,b) have confirmed the characteristic nature of this spindle abnormality in myotonic dystrophy.

The principal feature of the spindle abnormality is longitudinal splitting or fragmentation of the intrafusal muscle fibres (Figs 19.39, 19.40). This process is much more marked in the polar regions of affected intrafusal muscle fibres than in the equatorial sensory regions. Indeed, the equatorial regions are often unaffected (Fig. 19.41) even when the poles are very abnormal. Not all spindles are affected in any individual patient with myotonic dystrophy, and in some spindles only a few intrafusal muscle fibres may show fragmentation (Swash & Fox 1975a). In seven patients with myotonic dystrophy, in whom muscle spindles were studied at autopsy in samples of both proximal and distal muscles, Swash (1972) found that 40% of 198 spindles examined showed the abnormality (Fig. 19.38). The spindle abnormality was far more prominent, and far more frequently found in distal limb muscles than in proximal muscles, although spindles in the suboccipital muscles seemed also to be markedly affected. The abnormality was patchily distributed within individual muscles, and many muscles contained both normal and abnormal muscle spindles. However, in muscles with only slight dystrophic changes the spindle abnormality was less prominent and less severe than in more severely dystrophic muscles.

With the light microscope the tiny (<1–3 μm) intrafusal muscle fibres are usually arranged in 4–10 groups, each group bounded by a thin, irregular, and often incomplete layer of elastic fibres. These groups probably represent the

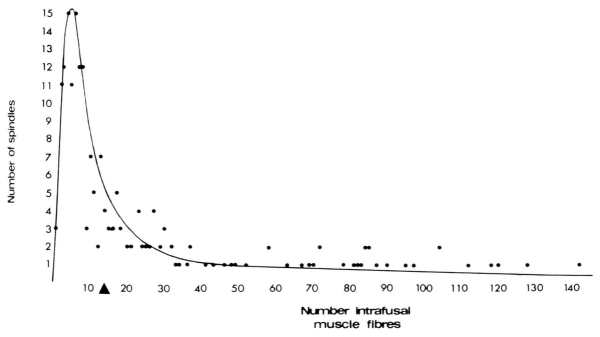

Fig. 19.38 The points on the graph represent the numbers of spindles containing a given number of intrafusal muscle fibre fragments in myotonic dystrophy. The arrow, on the abscissa, marks the maximum number of intrafusal muscle fibres (14) found in normal human spindles (Cooper & Daniel 1963, Swash & Fox 1972b)

original number of intrafusal muscle fibres in the spindle, the elastic tissue forming part of the tissue of the inner capsule. Silver preparations show that the intrafusal nerve fibres ramify around these groups of intrafusal muscle fibre fragments (Fig. 19.42). Each fragment is usually surrounded by a thin layer of reticulin, enabling the numbers of fragments in the spindle to be counted. In the more severely abnormal spindles, studied in severely affected muscles, the grouped arrangement of the intrafusal muscle fibre fragments is lost so that they become clumped together in the centre of the periaxial space. In some spindles the intrafusal muscle fibres are even more abnormal, having become aggregated into a central mass of eosinophilic, vacuolated sarcoplasm surrounded by fragmented elastic fibres and fibrous tissue. However, in the equatorial regions the nuclear bags are relatively unaffected, and in plastic-embedded sections the sensory innervation can be recognized (Figs 19.39, 19.41). Fibre fragmentation is largely a phenomenon of the polar regions of the intrafusal muscle fibres.

The capsules of abnormal spindles are usually thicker than normal, and contain increased amounts of collagen (Fig. 19.39). In some spindles the periaxial space is entirely filled with disorganized intrafusal muscle fibres, and with capsular tissue.

In serial transverse sections, the number of fibre fragments found in individual spindles varied greatly, even in sections only 10 μm apart (Swash & Fox 1975a), indicating that the abnormality represents both longitudinal splitting and fusion of individual intrafusal fibres. The poles of both nuclear bag and nuclear chain fibres appear equally susceptible to fragmentation. Each fragment is therefore separated from adjacent fragments for only a few micrometres of the length of the spindle. Some fragments are nucleated but many are not; the latter are presumably non-viable but the former might possess the potential for regeneration by de-differentiation and myoblast formation. In the early stages of the process only one intrafusal muscle fibre may be fragmented (Swash & Fox 1975a). The first demonstrable abnormality,

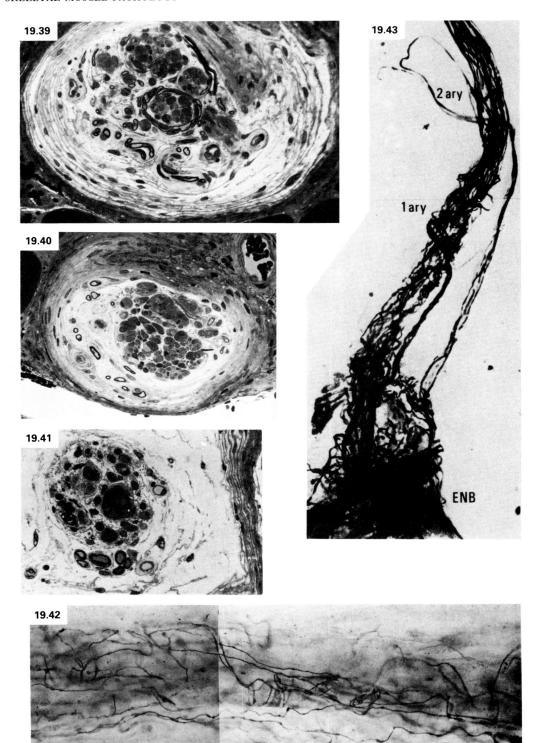

however, may be the presence of peripheral sites of excess acid phosphatase activity (Karpati et al 1973). Sahgal et al (1983) thought that in the preterm infant with myotonic dystrophy the intrafusal muscle fibres were simply immature.

Heene (1973) noted that the fibre fragments in two abnormal spindles in myotonic dystrophy showed homogeneous reactivity to NADH, PAS and ATPase at acid and alkaline pre-incubation, in contrast to the well-defined histochemical types of normal intrafusal muscle fibres in man (see above).

With the electron microscope, the process of fragmentation and fusion of intrafusal muscle fibres appears even more complex. Individual fragments, defined by their limiting layers of plasma membrane, are closely apposed (Fig. 19.44), and some show desmoplasmic regions of attachment to each other. In others the process of fibre fragmentation can be observed (Fig. 19.45). Pinocytotic vesicles are prominent beneath the plasma membrane of the fibre fragments (Figs. 19.44, 19.45). Clusters of fragments are bounded by a layer of basement membrane (Fig. 19.44). The fragments themselves show marked variation in their electron density, because of degeneration and loss of myofibrils to varying degrees within them, and of the presence of sarcoplasmic masses at the edges of some. Some fibre fragments, in which myofibrillar degeneration is particularly marked, contain rod bodies and lamellated lipid bodies. In these fragments, autophagic vacuoles and other degenerative features are found (Fig. 19.46).

Other fibre fragments contain small groups of well-formed myofilaments in a granular cytoplasm in which polysomes, free ribosomes, glycogen granules and small mitochondria are abundant. Rough endoplasmic reticulum and tubules of the Golgi apparatus are frequent features of these fibres. These features are consistent with the basophilia observed in some fibre fragments with the light microscope. The most abnormal fragments in a cluster are situated at the periphery, and it has been suggested that these degenerate fragments are extruded into the periaxial space (Swash & Fox 1975b). Satellite cells are present in increased numbers in nuclear bag and nuclear chain fibres in myotonic dystrophy, but the nucleated fibre fragments described above do not have the features of satellite cells (Maynard et al 1977, Stranock & Newsom Davis 1978a,b).

The pattern of innervation of muscle spindles in myotonic dystrophy is also disturbed. Daniel & Strich (1964) recognized that the innervation was more complex than in normal spindles but in their sectioned material they could not investigate this abnormality further. In teased preparations of silver- (Fig. 19.42) or gold-impregnated (Fig. 19.43) whole spindles the abnormality in the spindle innervation is shown to consist of a dense meshwork of sprouted, tortuous nerve fibres, often obliterating the normal pattern of innervation (Swash 1972). In these spindles it may be difficult even to discern the motor and sensory nerve fibres, and the characteristic helical pattern

---

Fig. 19.39 Myotonic dystrophy. The intrafusal muscle fibres are fragmented but retain, in part, their arrangement in clusters indicating their origin from individual intrafusal muscle fibres. One such cluster of tiny fragments is enclosed by branches of the secondary sensory innervation in this juxta-equatorial section. Note the thickened inner and outer capsular layers which have encroached on the periaxial space. Plastic embedded semi-thin, toluidine blue, ×188

Fig. 19.40 Myotonic dystrophy. In this polar section of the same spindle as Figure 19.39, the variable morphology and staining intensity of the fragmented intrafusal fibres can be seen. Plastic-embedded semi-thin, toluidine blue, ×188

Fig. 19.41 Myotonic dystrophy. Equatorial section to show the relative preservation of the intrafusal fibres in their primary sensory regions (nuclear bag fibres). Compare with Figures 19.18 and 19.19 in which the ultrastructure of the equatorial and juxta-equatorial regions are shown. Plastic-embedded semi-thin, toluidine blue, ×188

Fig. 19.42 Myotonic dystrophy. The normal pattern of fusimotor innervation is replaced by a tangle of fine γ-axons from which many branches arise. Barker and Ip silver impregnation, ×263

Fig. 19.43 Myotonic dystrophy. In this severely abnormal spindle the pattern of innervation is disorganized. Both motor and sensory innervation are disturbed and even the primary sensory ending is unrecognizable. (1ary: primary afferent nerve fibre; 2ary: secondary afferent nerve fibre; ENB: entering nerve bundle). Ranvier gold impregnation, ×188

of the primary sensory ending cannot be recognized (Fig. 19.43). The fusimotor innervation is abnormal, even in spindles containing intrafusal muscle fibres which themselves appear normal; the abnormality of the fusimotor innervation consisting of increased branching, strikingly tortuous ramification of terminal axons, and incomplete or poorly formed motor end-plates, without the normal specialization into P_1 and P_2 plates, and trail endings (Fig. 19.42). This end-plate abnormality may also be recognized with the electron microscope (Fig. 19.47) (Swash & Fox 1975b, Stranock & Newsom Davis 1978b). Although Swash (1972) suggested that the fusimotor abnormality preceded fragmentation of intrafusal muscle fibres, later studies suggest that fibre fragmentation is the primary abnormality (Swash & Fox 1975a, Stranock & Newsom Davis, 1978a).

The pathogenesis of the spindle abnormality in myotonic dystrophy is not fully understood. The spindle abnormality occurs in muscles in which the extrafusal muscle fibres show only minor changes and, indeed, it has been observed in a 2-year-old child with the disease (Dubowitz 1977, personal communication). The histological features have led to the suggestion that fragmentation of the poles of the intrafusal muscle fibres results from excessive mechanical stresses, perhaps due to myotonia, or to myotonic after-discharges causing overloading of the intrafusal fibres. The polar regions exhibit graded contraction in response to fusimotor discharges, rather than an all-or-none twitch contraction, and this may account for the particularly severe midpolar involvement. It is not known, however, whether or not intrafusal muscle fibres themselves are affected by myotonia. The equatorial sensory region is relatively spared. The response of extrafusal muscle fibres to overload also includes splitting, and even fragmentation (Hall–Craggs & Lawrence 1970, Schwartz et al 1976), and this provides analogous support for this suggestion. The abnormality in the motor, and in the sensory innervation, is probably secondary to the deformity of the intrafusal muscle fibre surface produced by fragmentation. The end-stage of the process is loss of intrafusal muscle fibres, and fibrosis of the spindle capsule and of the periaxial space. The observation that muscle spindle morphology is normal in myotonia congenita (Swash & Schwartz 1983) must also be taken into account in understanding the abnormality in myotonic dystrophy.

Duchenne muscular dystrophy

In earlier reports the fate of muscle spindles in progressive muscular dystrophy was controversial (see Batten 1897, Sala 1915, Adams et al 1962), but Lapresle & Milhaud (1964) and Cazzato & Walton (1968) illustrated spindles showing swelling of their periaxial spaces and of their capsules, and destruction of their intrafusal muscle fibre bundle. Swash & Fox (1976a), in a quantitative study of 230 muscle spindles studied at autopsy in seven cases of Duchenne dystrophy, found a number of abnormalities.

The spindle capsule is thickened, but the increase in capsular thickness found in Duchenne dystrophy is not as great as that found in denervated spindles (Figs. 19.48, 19.49). There is a slight decrease in intrafusal muscle fibre diameter,

Fig. 19.44   Myotonic dystrophy. Fibre fragmentation results in membrane-bound fragments of variable size, shape and electron density surrounded as a group by a layer of basement membrane. The latter represents the basal lamina surrounding individual intrafusal muscle fibres in normal spindles. Electron micrograph, ×11 250

Fig. 19.45   Myotonic dystrophy. Fibre splitting occurs before plasma membrane is formed. The latter seems to be related to membrane acquisition from 'pinocytotic' vesicles close to the developing clefts. Electron micrograph, ×22 500

Fig. 19.46   Myotonic dystrophy. Degenerative features include lipid droplets and displaced leptomeres. Myofilament regeneration is probably in progress in this fibre. Electron micrograph, ×4500

Fig. 19.47   Myotonic dystrophy. This motor end-plate shows no junctional folds and is probably simplified trail innervation. Electron micrograph, ×13 500

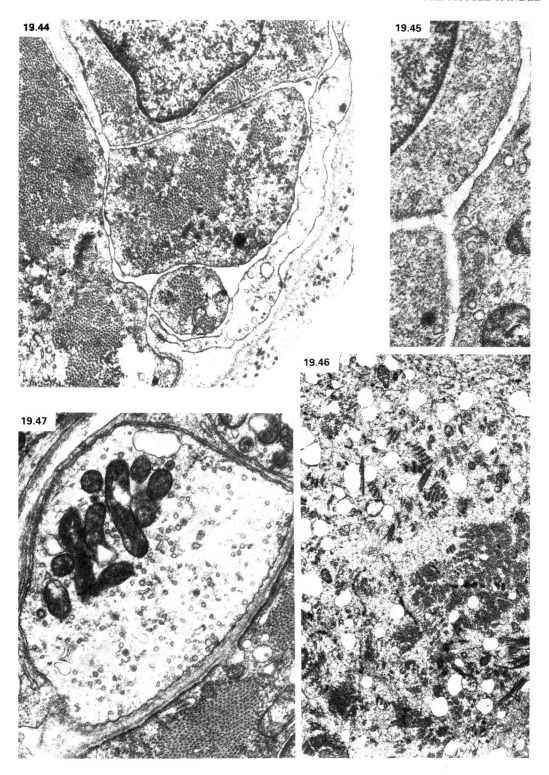

the twin-peaked distribution of fibre diameter found in normal muscle spindles being replaced by a unimodal distribution with a peak at about 9 μm. In addition, the mean number of intrafusal muscle fibres found in dystrophic spindles is slightly reduced.

In some spindles the intrafusal muscle fibres are abnormal, consisting of a degenerate mass of centrally placed amorphous material. In a few spindles, the intrafusal muscle fibres and the intrafusal nerve fibres have disappeared, and in these there is marked fibrosis of the periaxial space (Fig. 19.49). The most abnormal spindles were found isolated in a fibrous scar devoid of intrafusal fibres and of nearby extrafusal fibres. The intrafusal muscle fibres in spindles situated close to a group of relatively well-preserved extrafusal fibres, however few, are usually less abnormal, but hyaline or granulovacuolar change is common, often accompanied by peripherally placed clear eosinophilic zones of sarcoplasm free of myofibrillar material (Fig. 19.50). Basophilia was never observed. The equatorial nuclear bag and nuclear chain regions are normal in some spindles (Fig. 19.51), but atrophic, with reduced numbers of pyknotic nuclei, in others. The equatorial elastic tissue is fragmented in these abnormal spindles. In some spindles the periaxial space is considerably enlarged ('spindle oedema') but this is always more apparent in near-equatorial sections (Fig. 19.50) than in other parts of the spindle (Fig. 19.52). In silver-impregnated longitudinal sections the pattern of motor and sensory innervation appeared normal (Swash & Fox 1976a).

These observations suggest that some intrafusal muscle fibres atrophy and are destroyed during the course of the disease, and that eventually the spindles themselves may be replaced by a fibrous scar, as in the case of extrafusal muscle fibres. No increase in the number of intrafusal muscle fibres has been observed in this disease (Swash & Fox 1976a). These spindle abnormalities in Duchenne dystrophy may explain the relatively early loss of the tendon reflexes often found in this condition.

Other muscular dystrophies

Cazzato & Walton (1968) observed abnormalities in 23 spindles found in biopsies of five cases of congenital muscular dystrophy, and in 11 spindles found in five cases of limb–girdle dystrophy. In some of these spindles it was thought that the spindle capsule was thickened, and that there was atrophy or degeneration of intrafusal muscle fibres. In addition, collagenous thickening of the inner capsular lamellae, and of the periaxial spaces of these spindles was noted. However, so few spindles have been studied in these conditions that it is difficult to draw firm conclusions as to the specificity or otherwise of these observations.

In two cases of facioscapulohumeral dystrophy, Swash (1973) found evidence that spindles were

---

Fig. 19.48 Duchenne dystrophy. Increased capsular thickness and enlargement of the periaxial space are evident, but the intrafusal muscle fibres are relatively well preserved, and several groups of extrafusal muscle fibres remain nearby. The spindle is situated near an intramuscular nerve. Phosphotungstic acid–haematoxylin, ×68

Fig. 19.49 Duchenne dystrophy. This spindle is fibrosed and its capsule is thickened. Only the remains of intrafusal fibres can be discerned. H&E, ×263

Fig. 19.50 Duchenne dystrophy. The intrafusal muscle fibres are abnormal; some have an irregular myofibrillar margin. The eosinophilic, viscous, mucopolysaccharide of the periaxial space is visible. Note the 'spindle oedema'. H&E, ×263

Fig. 19.51 Duchenne dystrophy. The equatorial nuclei associated with the primary sensory ending are preserved. H&E, ×263

Fig. 19.52 Duchenne dystrophy. The intrafusal muscle fibres are atrophic and embedded in collagen and thickened inner capsular tissue. H&E, ×263

Fig. 19.53 Myasthenia gravis. Axonal sprouting in motor endings of undetermined type. Barker and Ip silver impregnation, ×188

Fig. 19.54 Myasthenia gravis. Two P₂ plate endings and a number of γ-trail fusimotor fibres are present. The trail fibres and their endings are tortuous and some of them give rise to fine axonal sprouts. Barker and Ip silver impregnation, ×188

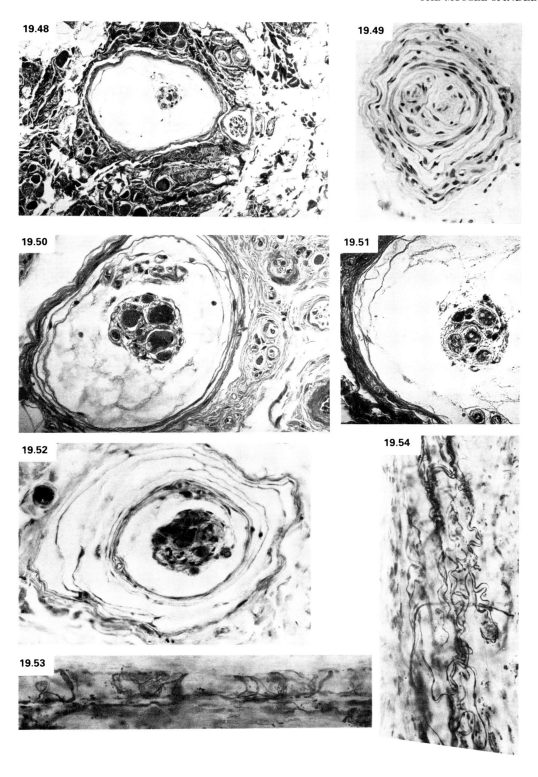

destroyed in the course of the disease, the remaining spindles showing capsular thickening, degenerate changes in intrafusal muscle fibres and collagen deposition in the periaxial space. These changes were similar to those found in Duchenne dystrophy. In teased silver preparations, however, the pattern of innervation appeared to be normal, although there was some increased complexity of the motor innervation in some spindles.

In murine muscular dystrophy Ovalle & Dow (1986) found atrophy and vacuolation of intrafusal muscle fibres with a variety of non-specific ultrastructural abnormalities, and thickening of the spindle capsule.

Congenital myopathies

Few spindles have been studied in the congenital myopathies. Bethlem et al (1969) noted the occurrence of myotube-like changes in the intra-

fusal muscle fibres in a single spindle in a patient with type 1 fibre atrophy associated with central nuclei and myotube-like structures (myotubular myopathy), and nemaline bodies are occasionally observed in the intrafusal fibres in nemaline (rodbody) myopathy. The intrafusal muscle fibres show changes comparable with those of extrafusal muscle fibres in the glycogen storage myopathies (Figs 19.55, 19.56) (van der Walt et al 1987), including McArdle's disease. The intrafusal fibres are thus similarly susceptible to the morphological changes associated with the congenital and metabolic myopathies, but no specific features have been reported in these disorders.

Polymyositis, polyarteritis nodosa and scleroderma

No specific abnormalities in spindle morphology occur in these disorders, other than those due to

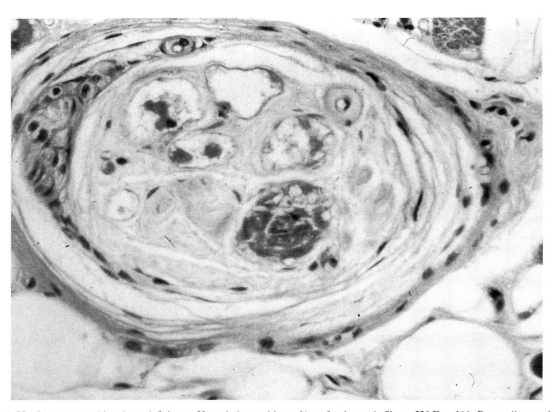

Fig. 19.55   Late-onset acid maltase deficiency. Vacuolation and loss of intrafusal muscle fibres. H&E, ×300. Pectoralis muscle (autopsy specimen)

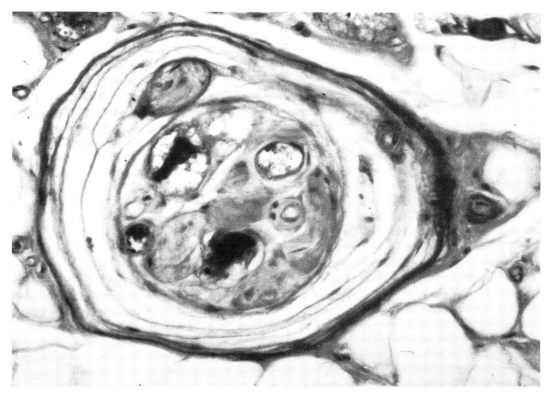

Fig. 19.56   Late-onset acid maltase deficiency. Glycogen accumulation in remaining intrafusal muscle fibres. PAS, ×300

patchy denervation and to occasional infiltration of spindles by mononuclear cells (Banker & Victor 1966). In rheumatoid arthritis, Magyar et al (1973) reported thickening of the spindle capsule, with degenerative changes in the intrafusal muscle fibres; these workers suggested that the changes might be due to a generalized vasculitis, but the descriptions are consistent with denervation rather than with infarction.

Myasthenia gravis

Muscle spindle morphology in myasthenia gravis has been studied by Cazzato & Walton (1968), Swash & Fox (1975c) and Saito et al (1978). Saito et al (1978) studied the distribution of motor nerve endings with the acetylcholinesterase technique and found that the P_1 and P_2 plate endings were atrophic at the spindle poles, whereas the trail endings were normal. However, their findings, based on serial transverse sections, differ from those of studies of the pattern of spindle inner-

vation carried out on silver-impregnated teased whole spindles. The latter revealed terminal and ultraterminal sprouts arising both in abnormally long and complex P_1 and P_2 plate endings, and in γ-trail endings (Figs 19.53, 19.54); the sensory innervation was normal (Swash & Fox 1975c). In addition, some spindles showed atrophy of their intrafusal muscle fibres, especially of the nuclear chain fibres, increased capsular thickness and deposition of collagen in the periaxial space in the polar regions due to fibrosis of the internal capsule (Swash & Fox 1975c). Rarely, marked dilatation of the periaxial space associated with degeneration of the intrafusal muscle fibres has been noted (Cazzato & Walton 1968, Swash & Fox 1974, 1976a), an appearance probably due to denervation.

Long-term anticholinesterase therapy may contribute to the ultrastructural and light microscopical changes found in motor end-plate morphology in extrafusal muscle in myasthenia gravis (Engel et al 1973, Schwartz et al 1977) and the abnormalities found in the motor innervation of the intrafusal muscle fibres thus probably represent a combination of the effects of the disease itself and of prolonged, high-dose anticholinesterase drug treatment. In advanced intractable cases, denervation atrophy may occur in extrafusal muscles (Brownell et al 1972).

In two spindles in a single case of the myasthenic (Eaton–Lambert) syndrome, Saito et al (1978) reported abnormalities in acetylcholinesterase localization similar to those noted in myasthenia gravis.

Parkinson's disease and torsion dystonia

Byrnes (1926) described abnormalities in spindles teased from biopsies taken from the thenar eminences of patients with Parkinson's disease, consisting of degeneration of the nerve supply to the spindles, but Swash & Fox (1974) suggested from similar observations in three patients with Parkinson's disease that these changes were due to denervation associated with a coincidental carpal tunnel syndrome. Saito et al (1978) noted enlargement of the area of acetylcholinesterase activity associated with γ-trail endings, but atrophy of P_1 and P_2 plate endings, and suggested that this might be correlated with increased static sensitivity to stretch in this disease. These observations require further analysis.

In an autopsy study of a patient with torsion dystonia, Swash & Fox (1976b) found no abnormality in the morphology or innervation of the muscle spindles.

REFERENCES

Adal M N 1969 The fine structure of the sensory region of cat muscle spindles. Journal of Ultrastructure Research 26: 332

Adams R D, Denny-Brown D E, Pearson C M 1962 Diseases of muscle, 2nd edn. Hoeber, New York

Amersbach K 1911 Beiträge zur normalen und pathologischen Histologie der Muskelspindeln des Menschen. Beiträge zur pathologischen Anatomie und zur allgemeinen Pathologie 51: 56

Arbuthnott E R, Ballard K J, Boyd I A, Gladden M H, Sutherland F 1982 The ultrastructure of cat fusimotor endings and their relationship to foci of sarcomere convergence in intrafusal fibres. Journal of Physiology 331: 285

Arbuthnott E R, Gladden M H, Sutherland F I 1989 The selectivity of fusimotor innervation in muscle spindles of the rat studied by light microscopy. Journal of Anatomy 163: 183

Bach-y-Rita P (ed) 1971 Neurophysiology of eye movements. In: The control of eye movements. Academic Press, New York, p 7

Banker B Q, Girvin J P 1971 The ultrastructural features of the mammalian muscle spindle. Journal of Neuropathology and Experimental Neurology 30: 155

Banker B Q, Victor M 1966 Dermatomyositis of childhood. Medicine (Baltimore) 45: 261

Banks R W, James N T 1973 The blood supply of rabbit muscle spindles. Journal of Anatomy 114: 7

Banks R W, Barker D W, Stacey M J 1982 Form and distribution of sensory terminals in cat hind-limb muscle spindles. Philosophical Transactions of the Royal Society (London) B. 229: 329

Banks R W, Harker D W, Stacey M J 1977 A study of mammalian intrafusal muscle fibres using a combined histochemical and ultrastructural technique. Journal of Anatomy 123: 783

Barker D 1948 The innervation of the muscle spindle. Quarterly Journal of Microscopical Science 89: 143

Barker D 1974 The morphology of muscle receptors. In: Hunt C C (ed) Muscle receptors. Springer-Verlag, New York, p 1

Barker D, Ip M C 1963 A silver method for demonstrating the innervation of mammalian muscle in teased preparations. Journal of Physiology 169: 73P

Barker D, Laporte Y 1974 Introduction to symposium on muscle spindles. Journal of Anatomy 119: 183

Barker D, Saito M 1979 Autonomic innervation of cat muscle spindles. Journal of Physiology 301: 240

Barker D, Stacey M J, Adal M N 1970 Fusimotor innervation in the cat. Philosophical transactions of the Royal Society of London, series B, 258: 315

Barker D, Emonet-Dénand F, Harker D W, Jami L, Laporte Y 1976 Distribution of fusimotor axons to intrafusal muscle fibres in cat tenuissimus spindles as determined by the glycogen-depletion method. Journal of Physiology 261: 49

Barker D, Bessou P, Jankowska E, Pagès B, Stacey M J 1978 Identification of intrafusal muscle fibres activated by single fusimotor axons and injected with fluorescent dye in cat tenuissimus spindles. Journal of Physiology 275: 149

Barker D, Emonet-Denand F, Laporte Y, Proske V, Stacey M J 1973 Morphological identification and intrafusal distribution of the endings of static fusimotor axons in the cat. Journal of Physiology 230: 405

Batten F E 1897 The muscle spindle under pathological conditions. Brain 20: 138

Batten F E 1898 Experimental observations on early degenerative changes in the sensory end organs of muscles. Brain 21: 388

Bethlem J, Van Wijngaarden G K, Hugo Meijer A E F, Hulsmann W C 1969 Neuromuscular disease with Type 1 fiber atrophy, central nuclei and myotube-like structures. Neurology (Minneapolis) 19: 705

Boyd I A 1962 The structure and innervation of the nuclear bag muscle fibre system and the nuclear chain muscle fibre system in mammalian muscle spindles. Philosophical Transactions of the Royal Society of London, series B, 245: 81

Boyd I A 1976 The response of fast and slow nuclear bag fibres and nuclear chain fibres in isolated cat muscle spindles to fusimotor stimulation, and the effect of intrafusal contraction to the sensory endings. Quarterly Journal of Experimental Physiology 61: 203

Boyd I A, Gladden M H, McWilliam P N, Ward J 1977 Control of dynamic and static nuclear bag fibres and nuclear chain fibres by gamma and beta axons in isolated cat muscle spindles. Journal of Physiology 265: 133

Brownell B, Oppenheimer D R, Spalding J M K 1972 Neurogenic muscle atrophy in myasthenia gravis. Journal of Neurology, Neurosurgery and Psychiatry 34: 311

Byrnes C M 1926 A contribution to the pathology of paralysis agitans. Archives of Neurology and Psychiatry (Chicago) 15: 407

Cazzato G, Walton J N 1968 The pathology of the muscle spindle: a study of biopsy material in various muscular and neuromuscular diseases. Journal of the Neurological Sciences 7: 15

Christomanos A A, Strossner E 1891 Beitrag zur Kentniss der Muskelspindeln. Sitzungsberichte der Akademie der Wissenschaften in Wien. Math. Nat. Kl. 100: 417

Coërs C, Woolf A L 1959 The innervation of muscle: a biopsy study. Blackwell, Oxford

Cooper S 1960 Muscle spindles and other muscle receptors. In: Bourne G H (ed) The structure and function of muscle. Academic Press, New York, vol 1, p 381

Cooper S 1966 Muscle spindles and other muscle receptors. In: Andrew B L (ed) Control and innervation of skeletal muscle. University of St. Andrews' Press, Dundee, p 9

Cooper S, Daniel P M 1957 Responses from the stretch receptors of the goat's extrinsic eye muscles with an intact motor innervation. Quarterly Journal of Experimental Physiology 42: 222

Cooper S, Daniel P M 1963 Muscle spindles in man: their morphology in the lumbricals and in the deep muscles of the neck. Brain 86: 563

Cooper S, Gladden M H 1974 Elastic fibres and reticulin of mammalian muscle spindles and their functional significance. Quarterly Journal of Experimental Physiology 59: 367

Croft P B, Henson R A, Urich H, Wilkinson M 1965 Sensory neuropathy with bronchial carcinoma: a study of four cases showing serological abnormalities. Brain 88: 501

Daniel P M, Strich S J 1964 Abnormalities in the muscle spindles in dystrophia myotonica. Neurology (Minneapolis) 14: 310

De Reuck J 1973 Biometric analyses of spindles in normal human skeletal muscles. Acta neurologica belgica 73: 339

De Reuck J 1974 The pathology of the human muscle spindle — a light microsopic, biometric and histochemical study. Acta neuropathologica (Berlin) 30: 43

Dogiel A S 1902 Die Nervenendigungen im Bauchfell, Sehnen Muskelspindeln und den Centrum tendineum des Menschen und der Saugetiere. Archivs für die mikrokopische Anatomie 59: 1

Dow P R, Shinn S L, Ovalle W K 1980 Ultrastructural study of a blood-muscle spindle barrier after systemic administration of horse-radish peroxidase. American Journal of Anatomy 157: 375

Dubowitz V, Brooke M H 1973 Muscle biopsy — a modern approach. W B Saunders, Philadelphia

Edwards R P 1975 An ultrastructural study of neuromuscular spindles in normal mice with reference to mice and men injected with M. leprae. Journal of Anatomy 120: 149

Engel A G, Lambert E H, Santa T 1973 Study of long-term anticholinesterase therapy — effects on neuromuscular transmission and on motor end-plate fine structure. Neurology (Minneapolis) 23: 1273

Fox K P, Koeze T H, Swash M 1974 Sensory innervation of baboon muscle spindles. Journal of Anatomy 119: 557

Fukami Y, Schlesinger P H 1989 Endocytosis and transcytosis by the capsule cell of vertebrate muscle spindles. Brain Research 499: 249

Gardner E 1940 Decrease in human neurones with age. Anatomical Record 77: 529

Greenfield J G 1963 Infectious diseases of the central nervous system. In: Greenfield J G, Mayer A, Norman R M, McMenemy W H, Blackwood W (eds) Neuropathology. Arnold, London, p 173

Hall–Craggs E C B, Lawrence C A 1870 Longitudinal division in skeletal muscle: a light and electron microscopic study. Zeitcheift für Zellforschung und Mikroskopische Anatomie 109: 481

Harriman D G F, Parker P L, Elliott B J 1974 The histochemistry of human intrafusal muscle fibres. Journal of Anatomy 119: 206

Heene R 1973 Histological and histochemical findings in muscle spindles in dystrophia myotonica. Journal of the Neurological Sciences 18: 369

Ishihara A 1988 Histochemical properties of intrafusal muscle fibres in the soleus muscle of the aged rat. Japanese Journal of Physiology 38: 747

Jedrzejowska H, Fidziańska A 1966 Zmiany we wrzecionach miesniowych w charobach miesni. Neuropatologi Polska 4: 218

Karpati G, Carpenter S, Watters G V, Eisen A A, Andermann F 1973 Infantile myotonic dystrophy. Neurology (Minneapolis) 23: 1066

Kennedy W R 1969 Innervation of human muscle spindles in patients with polyneuropathy. Transactions of the American Neurological Association 94: 59

Kennedy W R 1970 Innervation of normal human muscle spindles. Neurology (Minneapolis) 20: 463

Kennedy W R 1971 Innervation of muscle spindles in amyotrophic lateral sclerosis. Proceedings of Staff Meetings of the Mayo Clinic 46: 245

Kennedy W R 1974 The innervation of muscle spindles in a case of hypertrophic polyneuropathy. Neurology (Minneapolis) 24: 788

Kennedy W R, Staley N 1973 Find structure of the human muscle spindle: primary sensory region. Electroencephalography and Clinical Neurophysiology 34: 802

Kerschner C 1888 Bewerkungen über ein besonderes Muskelsystem in willkurlichen Muskel. Anatomische Anzeiger 3: 126

Kölliker A 1862 On the termination of nerves in muscles, as observed in the frog, and on the disposition of the nerves in the frog's heart. Proceedings of the Royal Society (London) series B 12: 65

Krinke G, Heid J, Bittinger H, Hess R 1978 Sensory denervation of the plantar lumbrical muscle spindles in pyridoxine neuropathy. Acta Neuropathologica 43: 213

Kucera J 1977 Intrafusal muscle fiber biochemistry following its motor reinnervation. Journal of Histochemistry and Cytochemistry 25: 1260

Kucera J 1980 Motor nerve terminals of cat nuclear chain fibers studied by the cholinesterase technique. Neuroscience 5: 403

Kucera J 1981 Histochemical profiles of cat intrafusal muscle fibres and their motor innervation. Histochemistry 73: 397

Kucera J 1982 A quantitative study of motor nerve terminals on cat nuclear bag$_1$ intrafusal muscle fibres using the CRE staining technique. Anatomical Record 202: 407

Kucera J 1986 Reconstruction of the nerve supply to a human muscle spindle. Neuroscience Letters 63: 180

Kucera J, Durovini–Zis K 1979 Types of human intrafusal muscle fibers. Muscle and Nerve 2: 437

Kucera J, Dorovini–Zis K, Engel W K, Flye M W 1978 Correlation of ultrastructure and histochemistry in the same human intrafusal muscle fiber: differences between bag$_1$ and bag$_2$. Neurology (Minneapolis) 28: 387

Kucera J, Walro J M 1987 Postnatal maturation of spindles in deafferented rat soleus muscles. Anatomy and Embryology 176: 449

Kuhne W 1863 Die Muskelspindeln. Ein beitrag zur Lehre von der Entwickelung der Muskeln und Nerven fasern. Virchows Archiv: Abteilung A: Pathologisch Anatomie 28: 528

Landon D N 1972 The fine structure of the equatorial regions of developing muscle spindles in the rat. Journal of Neurocytology 1: 189

Lapresle J, Milhaud M 1964 Pathologie du fuseau neuromusculaire. Revue neurologique 110: 97

Lowndes H E, Baker T, Cho E-S, Jortner B S 1978 Position sensitivity of de-afferented muscle spindles in experimental acrylamide neuropathy. Journal of Pharmacology and Experimental Therapeutics 250: 40

Magyar E, Talerman A, Wouters H W 1973 Histological abnormalities in the muscle spindles in rheumatoid arthritis. Annals of the Rheumatic Diseases 32: 143

Matthews P B C 1972 Mammalian muscle receptors and their central actions. Arnold, London

Maynard J A, Cooper J R, Ionasescu V V 1977 An ultrastructure investigation of intrafusal muscle fibers in myotonic dystrophy. Virchows Archiv. A: Pathological Anatomy and Histology 373: 1

Milburn A 1973 The early development of muscle spindles in the rat. Journal of Cell Science 12: 175

Onanoff J G 1890 Sur la nature des faisceaux neuromusculaires. Comptes rendus des séances de la Société de biologie 42: 432

Ovalle W K, Dow P R 1986 Alterations in muscle spindle morphology in advanced stages of murine muscular dystrophy. Anatomical Record 216: 111

Ovalle W K, Smith R S 1972 Histochemical identification of three types of intrafusal muscle fibres in the cat and monkey based on the myosin ATPase reaction. Canadian Journal of Physiology and Pharmacology 50: 195

Patel A N, Lalitha V S, Dastur D K 1968 The spindle in normal and pathological muscle: an assessment of the histological changes. Brain 91: 737

Peachey C D 1971 The structure of the extraocular muscles of mammals. In: Bach-y-Rita P (ed) The control of eye movements. Academic Press, New York, p 47

Pedrosa F, Butler-Browne G S, Ghost G K, Fischman D A, Thorwell I E 1989 Diversity in expression of myosin heavy chain isoforms and M-band proteins in rat muscle spindles. Histochemistry 92: 185

Raman R, Devanandam M S 1989 Muscle receptors: content of some of the extrinsic and intrinsic muscles. The larynx in the bonnet monkey (M radiata). Anatomic Record 223: 433

Rowlerson A, Mascarello F, Barker D, Saed H 1989 Muscle spindle distribution in relation to the fibre type distribution of masseter in mammals. Journal of Anatomy 161: 37

Ruffini A 1898 On the minute anatomy of the neuromuscular spindles of the cat, and on their physiological significance. Journal of Physiology 23: 190

Sahgal V, Morgen C A 1976 Histochemical and morphological changes in human muscle spindle in upper and lower motor neurone lesions. Acta neuropathologica (Berlin) 34: 41

Sahgal V, Sahgal S, Barnes S, Subramani V 1983 Ultrastructure of muscle spindle in congenital myotonic dystrophy: a study of preterm infant muscle spindles. Acta Neuropathologica 61: 207

Saito M, Tomonago H, Narabayashi H 1978 Histochemical studies of the muscle spindle in Parkinsonism, motor neuron disease and myasthenia. Journal of Neurology 219: 261

Sala G 1915 Die pseudohypertrophische Paralyse — Klinische und histopathologische Betrachtungen. Archiv für Psychiatrie und Nervenkrankheiten 55: 389

Schröder J M 1974a The fine structure of de- and reinnervated muscle spindles. I. The increase, atrophy and 'hypertrophy' of intrafusal muscle fibers. Acta neuropathologica (Berlin) 30: 109

Schröder J M 1974b The fine structure of de- and reinnervated muscle spindles. II. Regenerated sensory and motor terminals. Acta neuropathologica (Berlin) 30: 129

Schwartz M S, Sargeant M K, Swash M 1976 Longitudinal fibre splitting in neurogenic muscular disorders — its relation to the pathogenesis of 'myopathic' change. Brain 99: 617

Schwartz M S, Sargeant M K, Swash M 1977 Neostigmine-induced end-plate proliferation in the rat: a study using supra-vital methylene blue. Neurology (Minneapolis) 27: 289

Shantha T R, Golarz M N, Bourne G H 1968 Histological and histochemical observations on the capsule of the muscle spindle in normal and denervated muscle. Acta anatomica 69: 632

Sherrington C S 1894 On the anatomical constitution of nerves of skeletal muscles; with remarks of recurrent fibres in the ventral spinal nerve roots. Journal of Physiology 17: 211

Smith R S, Ovalle W K 1972 The structure and function of intrafusal muscle fibres. In: Cassens R G (ed) Muscle biology. Marcel Dekker, New York, vol 1, p 147

Spiro A J, Beilin R L 1969 Human muscle spindle histochemistry. Archives of Neurology (Chicago) 20: 271

Stacey M J 1969 Free nerve endings in skeletal muscle of the cat. Journal of Anatomy 105: 231

Stranock S D, Newsom-Davis J 1978a Ultrastructure of the muscle spindle in dystrophia myotonica. I. The intrafusal muscle fibres. Neuropathology and Applied Neurobiology 4: 393

Stranock S D, Newsom-Davis J 1978b Ultrastructure of the muscle spindle in dystrophia myotonica. II. The sensory and motor nerve terminals. Neuropathology and Applied Neurobiology 4: 407

Swash M 1972 The morphology and innervation of the muscle spindle in dystrophia myotonica. Brain 95: 357

Swash M 1973 Histopathological studies of human muscle spindles. MD Thesis, University of London

Swash M, Fox K P 1972a Muscle spindle innervation in man. Journal of Anatomy 112: 61

Swash M, Fox K P 1972b The effect of age on human skeletal muscles: studies of the morphology and innervation of muscle spindles. Journal of the Neurological Sciences 16: 417

Swash M, Fox K P 1972c Techniques for the demonstration of human muscle spindle innervation in neuromuscular disease. Journal of the Neurological Sciences 15: 291

Swash M, Fox K P 1974 The pathology of the muscle spindle: effect of denervation. Journal of the Neurological Sciences 22: 1

Swash M, Fox K P 1975a Abnormal intrafusal muscle fibres in myotonic dystrophy: a study using serial sections. Journal of Neurology, Neurosurgery and Psychiatry 38: 91

Swash M, Fox K P 1975b The fine structure of the spindle abnormality in myotonic dystrophy. Neuropathology and Applied Neurobiology 1: 171

Swash M, Fox K P 1975c The pathology of the muscle spindle in myasthenia gravis. Journal of the Neurological Science 26: 39

Swash M, Fox K P 1976a The pathology of the muscle spindle in Duchenne muscular dystrophy. Journal of the Neurological Sciences 29: 17

Swash M, Fox K P 1976b Normal muscle spindles in idiopathic torsion dystonia. Journal of the Neurological Sciences 27: 525

Swash M, Fox K P 1985 Adrenergic innervation of baboon and human muscle spindles. In: Boyd I A, Gladden M H (eds) The Muscle Spindle. MacMillan, London p 121

Swash M, Schwartz M S 1983 Normal muscle spindle morphology in myotonia congenita: the spindle abnormality in myotonic dystrophy is not due to myotonia alone. Clinical Neuropathology 2: 75

Thomas P K, Fullerton P M 1963 Nerve fibre size in the carpal tunnel syndrome. Journal of Neurology, Neurosurgery and Psychiatry 26: 520

Thomas P K, Lascelles R G 1965 Schwann cell abnormalities in diabetic neuropathy. Lancet 1: 1355

Tomlinson B E, Walton J N, Rebeiz J J 1969 The effects of aging and cachexia upon skeletal muscle: a histopathological study. Journal of the Neurological Sciences 9: 321

Tower S S 1932 Atrophy and degeneration in the skeletal muscle. Brain 55: 77

Tower S S 1939 The reaction of muscle to denervation. Physiological Reviews 19: 1

van der Walt J D, Swash M, Leake J, Cox E L 1987 The pattern of involvement of adult-onset acid maltase deficiency at autopsy. Muscle and Nerve 10: 271

von Brezezinski D K 1961 Untersuchungen zur Histochemie der Muskelspindeln. II. Mitteilung (Topochemie der Polysaccharide). Acta histochemica (Jena) 12: 72

Voss H 1937 Untersuchungen über Zahl, Anordnung und Länge der Muskelspindeln in den Lumbrical muskeln des Menschen und einiger Tiere. Zeitschrift für mikroskopisch-anatomische Forschung 42: 509

Voss H 1958 Zahl und Anordnung der Muskelspindeln in der unteren Zungen beinmuskeln, der M. Sternocleiodomastoideus und den Branch und tiefen Nacken muskeln. Anatomische Anzeiger 105: 265

Weissmann A 1860 Ueber des Wachsen der quergestreiften Muskeln nach Beobachtungen am Frosch. Zeitschrift rationalische Medicin 10: 263

Wohlfart G 1939 Histopathological studies on muscular atrophy. In: Winther K, Krabbe K H (eds). Proceeding of the 3rd Congress of International Neurology. Munksgaard, Copenhagen, p 465

Wohlfart G 1957 Collateral regeneration from residual nerve fibres in amyotrophic lateral sclerosis. Neurology (Minneapolis) 7: 124

Zelena J 1957 The morphogenetic influence of innervation on the autogenetic development of muscle spindles. Journal of Embryology and Experimental Morphology 5: 283

Zelena J 1964 Development, degeneration and regeneration of receptor organs. In: Singer M, Schade J P (eds) Mechanisms of neural regeneration (Progress in brain research, vol 13). Elsevier, Amsterdam, p 175

Zalena J, Hnik P 1960 Absence of spindles in muscles of rats reinnervated during development. Physiologica Bohemoslovensko 9: 373

Zelena J, Soukup T 1974 The differentiation of intrafusal fibre types in rat muscle spindles after motor denervation. Cell Tissue Research 153: 115

20. Circulatory disorders and pathology of intramuscular blood vessels

F. Jerusalem

INTRODUCTION

Adequate perfusion is essential for muscle function because storage of carbohydrates and lipids, the main energy sources, is only minimal in muscle fibres and these stores are rapidly exhausted during exercise. The oxygen requirement of skeletal muscle in a subject at rest is, on average, only 0.16 ml/100 g per min. With vigorous exercise the oxygen consumption rises to 12 ml/100 g per min (Milnor 1974). This enormous adaptation to work with a 75-fold increment in oxygen use is maintained by an abundant vascularization of muscle tissue and efficient regulation of the blood flow. Mechanical conditions inside the muscle can influence flow, and nervous factors play an important part in its regulation (Hudlicka 1973, Koller & Kaley 1990). The vascular bed can be influenced by a vast number of metabolic products and substrates: 5-hydroxytryptamine (5-HT), α-adrenergic agents, endothelin (ET-1) and angiotensin are vasoconstrictive, while β-adrenergic and cholinergic agents, cyclic AMP, potassium, lactic acid, and a reduced tissue oxygen tension are vasodilatory. Prostaglandins and kinins probably also take part in the regulation of muscle blood flow (Bevan & Su 1973, Quastel & Hackett 1973, Bohr et al 1978, Vanhoutte 1990). Recent investigations have shown that there are at least three main classes of 5-HT receptors, and further subclasses can be distinguished on the basis of their pharmacological properties (Göthert 1990). Depending on the circumstances, 5-HT induces not vasoconstrictor and pressor but vasodilator and depressor responses. In addition, interactions between 5-HT$_2$ receptor and α-adrenoreceptor activation and between endothelium-derived vasoactive factors and effects of serotonin have been found (van Neuten & Janssens 1990).

Pathological alteration of the blood supply leads to serious metabolic consequences, disturbs function and may destroy muscle structure. On the other hand, it is to be expected that primary disorders of the muscle fibres or motor neurones may induce secondary structural changes in intramuscular blood vessels.

ANATOMY

The macroscopic pattern of arteries and veins in human skeletal muscle varies considerably from muscle to muscle. Blomfield (1945) differentiated five main patterns of intramuscular vascularization:

1. A longitudinal anastomotic chain formed by a succession of separate nutrient vessels entering the muscle throughout most of its length, e.g. in the soleus and peroneus longus.

2. A longitudinal pattern of vessels derived from a single group of arteries arising from a common stem and entering one end of the muscle, e.g. in the gastrocnemius.

3. A radiating pattern of collaterals arising from a single vessel entering the middle part of the muscle, e.g. in the biceps brachii.

4. A pattern formed by a series of anastomotic loops extending throughout the length of the muscle and derived from a succession of entering vessels, e.g. in the tibialis anterior, extensor hallucis longus and the long flexors of the leg.

5. An open quadrilateral pattern with sparse anastomotic connections, e.g. in the extensor hallucis longus.

Considerable branching of arteries takes place in the perimysial space. From there, arterioles, terminal arterioles and capillaries enter the endomysium and are located close to the muscle fibres. Capillaries run parallel to these and there are many cross-anastomoses.

The outer diameters of arterioles range from 50–100 μm; of terminal arterioles from 15–50 μm; of precapillary sphincters from 10–15 μm; and of capillaries from 4–15 μm (Fig. 20.1) (Rhodin 1967, 1968). Arterioles of about 100 μm in diameter possess a media composed of two or three layers of smooth muscle cells while vessels of about 50 μm usually have only one smooth muscle layer (Fig. 20.2). The smooth muscle cells have on average a length of about 30–40 μm and width of about 5 μm, and are surrounded by a basement membrane. Neighbouring muscle cells frequently establish contacts in the form of a close junction or nexus. The smooth muscle cells contain myofilaments and microtubules, and various organelles and dense bodies which form long bar-like structures along the surface membrane. The endothelial cells are separated from the smooth muscle cells of the media by at least two basement membranes, and

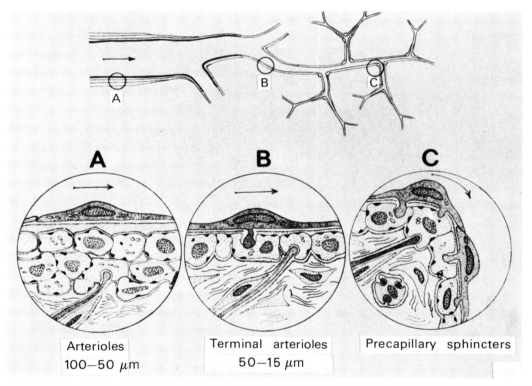

Fig. 20.1 These diagrams summarize the analysis of dilated mammalian arterioles and precapillary sphincters by electron microscopy with particular reference to the location, frequency, and general organization of the myoendothelial junctions, (A) In arterioles with an inner diameter of 50–100 μm, continuous elastica interna, and several smooth muscle cell layers in the media, there are generally no myoendothelial junctions. Non-myelinated nerves terminate in the most superficial smooth muscle layer. (B) Terminal arterioles are classified as those vessels which have an inner diameter of 15–50 μm, an elastica interna which gradually disappears distally, and only one smooth muscle layer but peripherally increasing number of myoendothelial junctions, established by endothelial protrusions which make membranous contacts and membranous fusions with the smooth muscle cells of the media. Free nerve axons, invested by a thin basement membrane and containing both granulated and non-granulated vesicles, accompany the terminal arterioles in close proximity. They establish myoneural junctions. (C) Precapillary sphincters are part of the smooth muscle cells of the media and surround the orifices of those terminal arterioles which have an inner diameter of less than 15 μm. There are frequent myoendothelial junctions within the precapillary sphincter area and also nerve endings. (From Rhodin J A G 1967 with permission)

in places by elastic components. The adventitial layer is represented by occasional spindle-shaped fibroblasts which are not surrounded by a basement membrane, and by loosely arranged bundles of collagen fibrils. Non-myelinated nerves accompany arterioles, of all sizes, and precapillary sphincters (Fig. 20.2). In terminal arterioles, foot-like processes occur between the smooth muscle cells and the endothelium (Figs. 20.2, 20.3). These myoendothelial junctions are more numerous in precapillary sphincters than in terminal arterioles. The nerves are particularly abundant near the precapillary sphincters.

The capillary bed of muscle differs from that of most other organs in possessing a relatively small number of open capillaries at rest. However, during muscle contraction the number of open capillaries increases considerably (Renkin et al 1966). The muscle fibres receive oxygen by diffusion from capillaries across a distance that averages some 50 μm during rest and only a few μm during work (Milnor 1974). Internalized myofibre capillaries do not occur in normal muscle but are occasionally seen in association with neurogenic or myopathic muscle alterations (Gutmann et al 1989). A significant difference in capillary density exists in different muscles of the human body and between trained and untrained individuals (Ingjer 1979, Mizuno & Secher 1989). Damaged muscle tissue releases a factor which stimulates revascularization (Phillips & Knighton 1990).

In cross-sections, a single muscle fibre is surrounded by 1.7 ± 0.6 capillaries (see Figs. 20.11–20.13). The number of capillaries per muscle fibre in a whole section is 0.7 ± 0.3 (mean $\pm$s.d). The mean muscle fibre area per capillary in 10 non-weak adults was 1363 ± 363 μm^2 (Jerusalem et al 1980). Data on the ultrastructural morphometric analysis of the dimensions and organelles of normal capillaries (Fig. 20.4) are shown in Tables 20.1 and 20.2. In the rabbit there are statistically significant differences in size and structure of the capillaries of muscle spindles and those associated with the extrafusal muscle fibres (Tasuku et al 1979). The intrafusal capillaries are larger in diameter and their endothelial cells contain fewer vesicles but have higher mitochondrial counts.

Mukai et al (1980) demonstrated factor VIII-related antigen in endothelial cells and in a variety of tumours known to be related to the endothelial cell. A monoclonal antibody which decorates the endothelial cells of normal and lymphatic vessels in formalin-fixed, paraffin-embedded tissue was isolated by Matsuo et al (1990). These immuno-histochemical methods improve the examination of the microcirculation. Ulex europaeus agglutinin I has already become established as a marker for microvascular changes in muscle biopsies (Emslie-Smith & Engel 1990).

POLYARTERITIS NODOSA (PERI-, PANARTERITIS NODOSA)— NECROTIZING VASCULITIDES

Polyarteritis nodosa is an inflammatory disease of the arterial system with a predilection for medium-sized and smaller arteries and arterioles. The characteristic findings are necrosis of the muscular media with oedema, fibrinoid exudation and a cellular infiltration. Nodule formation is often lacking and necrotizing features prevail. In the later stages of the disease, granulation tissue forms. Aneurysmal dilatation with occasional haemorrhages may occur. Finally, occlusions of the vascular lumen may cause small infarcts. Because of the recurrent course of the disorder, acute and chronic alterations may coexist.

Peripheral neuropathy is by far the most common neurological manifestation of polyarteritis nodosa but muscle involvement does occur. Myalgia is a common complaint in patients with arteritis and muscle weakness with proximal accentuation may be the result of an inflammatory myopathy. Rarely, leg swelling simulating deep-vein thrombosis is due to a necrotizing arterial vasculitis (Leib et al 1979). Untreated, polyarteritis nodosa was a progressive disease with a five-year survival of only 13%. Treatment with corti-costeroids improved this survival to 48–55% (Frohnert & Sheps 1967, Cohen et al 1980). The early use of cyclophosphamide was associated with five-year survival rates of 80% (Leib et al 1979).

The pathogenetic mechanisms involved in this disease are unknown, but several observations have pointed to a significant role of arterial hyper-tension and the occurrence of immunological

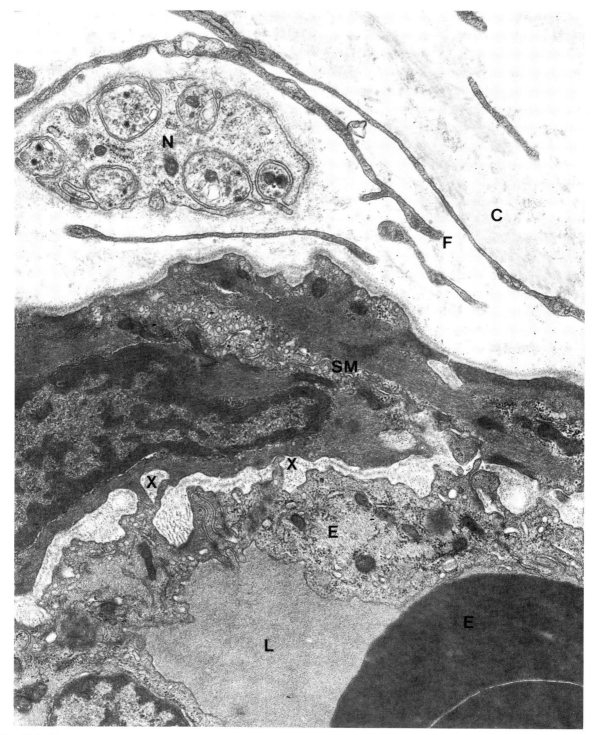

Fig. 20.2 Transverse electron-microscopic section of a terminal arteriole with approaching unmyelinated nerve (N) of normal skeletal muscle. Several foot-like processes (X) with myoendothelial junctions between the smooth muscle cell (SM) and the endothelial cell (E) are demonstrated. The vessel lumen (L) contains an erythrocyte (E). In the adventitial space, slender processes of fibroblasts (F), which are not surrounded by a basement membrane, and rather loosely arranged bundles of collagenous fibrils (C) can be seen. ×12 240

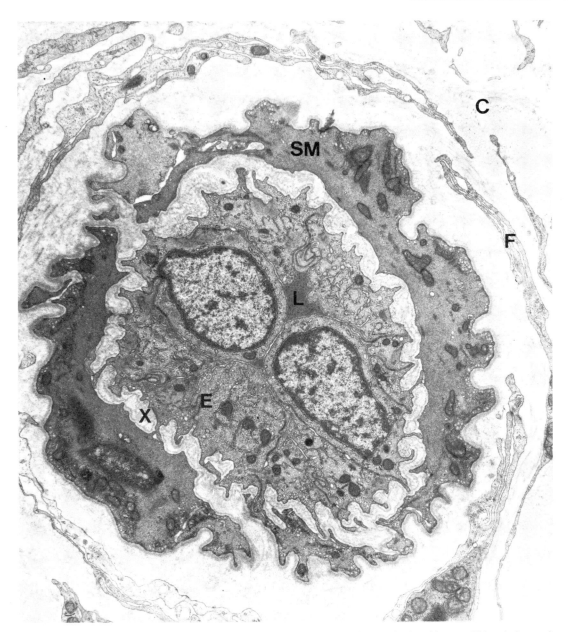

Fig. 20.3 Transverse electron-microscopic section of a precapillary sphincter with a nearly closed lumen. Abbreviations as in Figure 20.2. ×7400

phenomena. These include the finding of hyper-gammaglobulinaemia, rheumatoid factor, and hypocomplementaemia in some patients; the clinical response to high-dose corticosteroid and/or immunosuppressive treatment; and the fact that some patients with hepatitis B-related necrotizing angiitis or rheumatoid arthritis appear to have a polyarteritis nodosa-like disease (Alarcon-Segovia 1977).

Site of biopsy

Although polyarteritis nodosa more often involves the kidneys, heart, liver and gastrointestinal tract,

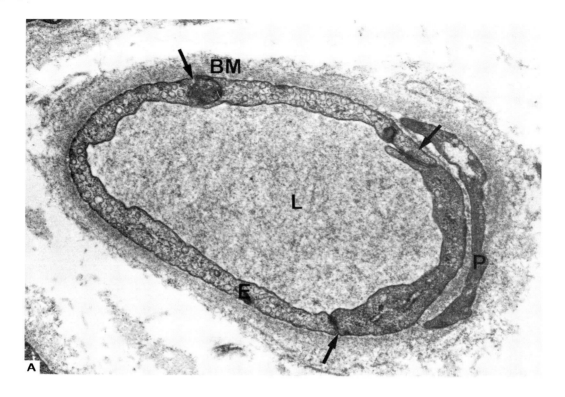

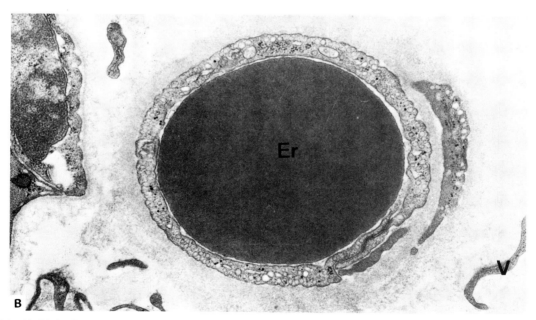

Fig. 20.4   (A, B) Capillaries from normal muscle. Arrows indicate tight junctions between endothelial cells. BM = basement membrane; E = endothelial cell; P = pericyte; V = veil cell; Er = erythrocyte; L = lumen. (A) ×20 900; (B) ×12 700

Table 20.1 Morphometric analysis of capillary dimensions[a]

	Capillary area (μm^2)[b]	Endothelial fraction of capillary area (%)	Basement membrane area as fraction of capillary area (%)	Pericyte area as fraction of capillary area (%)
Control capillaries (n = 41)	12.50 ± 1.31	34.00 ± 2.00	18.00 ± 1.40	7.10 ± 0.75
Scleroderma (n = 23)	26.38 ± 3.47 $P < 0.001$	47.55 ± 4.18 $P < 0.01$	10.22 ± 0.83 $P < 0.001$	14.49 ± 2.75 $P < 0.05$
Polymyositis (n = 30)	12.13 ± 1.48 N.S.	46.35 ± 2.76 $P < 0.001$	16.06 ± 1.06 N.S.	14.72 ± 2.04 $P < 0.01$
Dermatomyositis (n = 40)	21.08 ± 2.28 $P < 0.01$	51.02 ± 3.06 $P < 0.001$	13.49 ± 0.72 $P < 0.01$	21.01 ± 3.91 $P < 0.01$
Lupus erythematosus (n = 50)	17.29 ± 1.36 $P < 0.05$	44.56 ± 2.35 $P < 0.01$	16.98 ± 0.95 N.S.	12.75 ± 2.03 $P < 0.05$

[a]Values indicate mean ± standard error.
[b]Capillary area represents sum of endothelial and luminal area. N.S.: Not significant.
Reproduced, with permission, from Jerusalem et al (1974b).

Table 20.2 Morphometric analysis of endothelial cell organelles[a]

	Vesicles no. (μm^2)	Mitochondrial area (%)	Endoplasmic reticulum area (%)
Control capillaries (n = 41)	37.32 ± 1.71	1.70 ± 0.37	1.94 ± 0.10
Scleroderma (n = 23)	19.90 ± 1.70 $P < 0.001$	2.80 ± 0.39 $P < 0.05$	3.55 ± 0.25 $P < 0.01$
Polymyositis (n = 30)	30.31 ± 1.73 $P < 0.01$	2.41 ± 0.42 N.S.	3.73 ± 0.32 $P < 0.001$
Dermatomyositis (n = 40)	19.25 ± 1.25 $P < 0.001$	3.84 ± 0.46 $P < 0.001$	4.27 ± 0.22 $P < 0.001$
Lupus erythematosus (n = 50)	22.29 ± 1.07 $P < 0.001$	2.90 ± 0.32 $P < 0.05$	3.29 ± 0.17 $P < 0.001$

[a]Values indicate mean ± standard error.
N.S.: Not significant.
Reproduced, with permission, from Jerusalem et al (1974b).

it is, for obvious reasons, muscle that is usually chosen first for biopsy. The gastrocnemius or deltoid muscles are favourite sites. If possible, we take the gastrocnemius and part of the sural nerve through the same incision, or choose a tender spot in the muscle, or any suspected skin lesion with a sample of the underlying muscle.

The frequency of muscle involvement in polyarteritis nodosa is not precisely known. Only 13% of biopsies from patients in whom the disease was suspected on clinical grounds and 35–37% of biopsies from patients with proved polyarteritis nodosa, showed typical arterial changes (Maxeiner et al 1952, Wallace et al 1958). Diagnostic abnormalities were demonstrated in approximately 50% of cases even in the absence of clinically detectable muscle abnormality by Cohen et al (1980). If the first series of sections yields negative results, further sections must be cut and examined.

Light-microscopic findings

The primary structural alteration is fibrinoid exudation and necrosis of the media. This may involve the entire circumference or only a segment, producing a homogeneous pink staining with eosin (Fig. 20.5) and a red staining with Gomori trichrome. The acid phosphatase reaction is positive in macrophages in the affected areas. Veins and lymphatics are not seriously involved. Occasionally there is slight adventitial infiltration of veins. The arterial lesions are usually situated at the bifurcations. It has been shown (Lendrum et al 1962) that the substance which was termed fibrinoid is actually fibrin.

The next step is the appearance of leukocytes and other inflammatory cells in the fibrinoid and necrotic regions of the vessel wall (Fig. 20.5). The nuclei of the smooth muscle cells stain poorly, if at all. There remains a fibrinoid degeneration which was formerly called hyaline-like medial necrosis. At this stage cellular infiltration throughout the entire vessel wall, but especially in the adventitia, is maximal. Polymorphonuclear leukocytes, lymphocytes, plasma cells and large mononuclear cells prevail. In addition, eosinophils are common and giant cells are often present. In rare instances, fibrinoid necrosis occurs without any cellular reaction (Zeek et al 1948).

During the inflammatory stage, swelling and desquamation of the endothelial cells occurs. This is followed by proliferation which, in the granulation stage, leads to partial or total occlusion of the lumen. Recent thrombi in the vessels are a common finding. Occasionally, aneurysms of the medium-sized arteries can be seen. The Weigert elastic stain usually demonstrates a partial disappearance, or splitting and fragmentation, of the internal elastic lamina. The final granulation tissue formation (Fig. 20.5) is characterized by the replacement of leukocytes and lymphocytes by fibroblasts, which invade the necrotic media forming a connective tissue scar here and in the perivascular mantles.

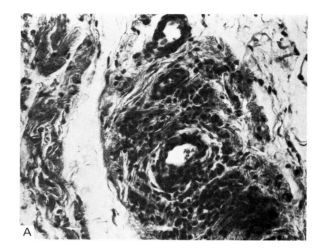

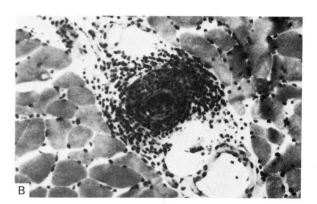

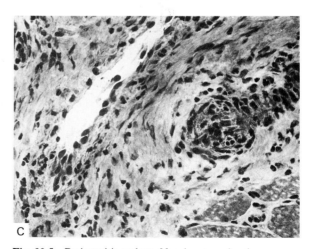

Fig. 20.5 Periarteritis nodosa. Muscle artery showing fibrinoid necrosis of the vessel wall (top picture), mural and adventitial inflammatory invasion (middle picture), and granulation tissue formation (bottom picture). H&E, ×180

The histological lesions observed in muscle are of four types:

1. Extension of the vascular inflammation into the adjacent muscle tissue
2. Ischaemic infarction
3. Haemorrhagic infarction
4. Neurogenic atrophy caused by ischaemic neuritis resulting from arteritic lesions in motor nerves or spinal roots.

The myopathologist has to consider that inflammatory disease of small and/or medium-sized intramuscular vessels with fibrinoid necrosis of the vascular wall and surrounding inflammatory infiltrates can occur in a variety of diseases — the polyarteritis nodosa group, the immunological vasculitides and the giant-cell arteritides (Alarcon-Segovia 1977). It therefore seems more appropriate to restrict the morphological diagnosis to that of a necrotizing vasculitis.

POLYMYALGIA RHEUMATICA

Muscular pain, stiffness and wasting, predominantly in the region of the axial skeleton, a raised erythrocyte sedimentation rate and increased serum α-globulins in a middle-aged or older patient are the cardinal features of polymyalgia rheumatica. As many as 50% of these patients can be shown to have underlying giant-cell arteritis of cranial and other vessels (Ettlinger et al 1978, Gerber 1984), but the striated muscles are unaffected. Nevertheless, muscle biopsy is important in some cases of polymyalgia rheumatica because differentiation from polymyositis and other neuromuscular disorders can be difficult without examination of muscle tissue.

In 1972, Brooke & Kaplan reported on seven muscle biopsies from patients suffering from this condition. Three showed type 2B and two others type 2A and B fibre atrophy. The remaining two had atrophy of all three fibre types. Four of the seven biopsies demonstrated moth-eaten and whorled fibres, and one had numerous cytoplasmic bodies. Five of our own seven cases also showed type 2 atrophy, and two of these showed a slight lipid storage in type 1 fibres (Fig. 20.6). One seldom sees central nuclei or small endomysial round-cell infiltrations. The phase-microscopic

analysis of semi-thin cross-sections of four biopises showed that capillary density was normal. Roux et al (1975) found only slight muscle changes. In contrast to these observations, 14 biopsies reported by Miller & Stevens (1978) were normal. So far, no alterations of the intramuscular vessels and microvasculature have been reported.

FIBROMYALGIA

Biopsies of tender points from 12 primary fibromyalgia syndrome patients showed type II fibre atrophy in 7 and a moth-eaten appearance of type I fibres in 5. Electron microscopy revealed segmental muscle fibre necrosis with lipid and glycogen deposition as well as subsarcolemmal mitochondrial accumulation in all cases (Kalyan-Raman et al 1984). Alterations of muscle capillaries with swelling of endothelial cells as reported by Fassbender (1975) were not observed. The histological findings are non-specific (Yunus & Kalyan-Raman 1989).

EFFECTS OF ISCHAEMIA ON MUSCLE

Although metabolic activity of working muscle is possible under anaerobic conditions for a short period, prolonged oligaemia or ischaemia causes muscle damage. In human disorders, vascular muscular injury is due to arterial or venous stenosis or occlusion, and less often to haemorrhage. This occurs especially in atherosclerosis with thrombosis, bland or septic embolism, trauma (Volkmann's contracture), polyarteritis nodosa, giant-cell arteritis, and some other types of vasculitis or phlebitis.

The effects of ischaemia on muscle have been studied experimentally in animals more thoroughly than in spontaneous human disorders.

Experimental ischaemic myopathy

In 150 rats the acute and chronic morphological changes in ischaemic solei and gastrocnemii produced by abdominal aortic ligation were studied at intervals from 2 h to 4 months after ligation, using histochemical and electron-microscopic techniques, by Karpati et al (1974). Lesions visible with the light microscope occurred earlier in the type 2C

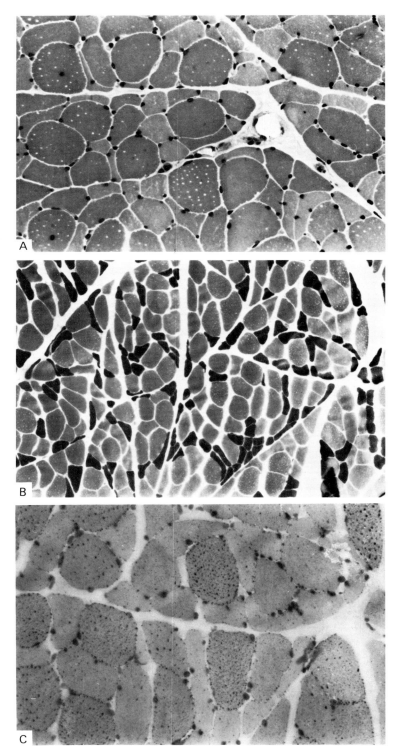

Fig. 20.6 Muscle biopsy cross-sections of a patient suffering from polymyalgia rheumatica. Multiple atrophic fibres (A), in particular type 2, are present (B). The fibres with normal diameters contain many small empty spaces (A), which are positive in Oil red O (C). H&E, ×240; (B) myofibrillar ATPase pH 9.3; ×120; (C) Oil red O, ×280

than in the type 1 fibres. The intermyofibrillar network became disorganized and large clumps of diformazan deposits were seen with oxidative enzyme reactions. Acid phosphatase activity was positive before phagocyte invasion occurred. PAS-staining and phosphorylase activity were completely lost in affected fibres after 6 hours. Myofibrillar ATPase activity was not lost in these muscle fibres until invasion of phagocytes had occurred. The fully developed lesions, 4–7 days after aortic ligation, consisted of grouped or scattered single necrotic fibres undergoing phagocytosis, as well as regenerating fibres. On longitudinal view, the necrosis appeared to be segmental, involving a variable length (up to 1 cm) of the muscle fibre. Alkaline phosphatase activity in many intra-muscular capillaries was lost in the necrotic regions, but without any change in the patency of these capillaries. Intramuscular nerves and muscle spindles appeared to be intact. About 30% of the soleus and only 3% of the gastrocnemius muscle fibres were necrotic.

From 1–4 months after aortic ligation, no necrotic fibres were present. There were many groups of small fibres with central nuclei ('nesting fibres'). With the myofibrillar ATPase reaction (pH 9.3), moderately large groups of up to 18 fibres (of a single histochemical type) were found scattered throughout the muscle. The endomysial connective tissue was not significantly increased. The earliest lesions were seen on electron micro-scopy 2 hours after aortic ligation. They consisted of trilaminar plates in the intracristal space of mitochondria, and muscle-cell necrosis as shown by interruption of the plasma membrane and dissolution of the Z discs. After 18 hours, Z disc streaming was also present.

Aortic ligation in rats followed by treatment with vasoactive amines, and vascular embolization in rabbits, both induced focal muscle fibre necrosis and regeneration (Selye 1965, Hathaway et al 1970, Mendell et al 1971, Mendell et al 1972).

In chronically ischaemic skeletal muscle the diameters of the arterioles increased, the capillary density decreased during the first 7 days, while capillary RBC-velocity was reduced (Menger et al 1988). Luminal narrowing and endothelial cell swelling in skeletal muscle capillaries occurs during hemorrhagic shock (Mazzoni et al 1989). Menger et al (1989) introduced a new model, permitting quantitative intravital microscopic analysis of microvascular perfusion after prolonged ischaemia in skeletal muscle.

Ischaemic myopathy in man

Scully & Hughes (1956) studied formalin-fixed muscle samples from limbs of 30 soldiers who had sustained an arterial injury. The muscle changes during the first 2 days after arterial injury con-sisted of degeneration and necrosis of muscle fibres, congested small vessels, focal haemorrhages and neutrophil infiltration in a few cases. Many fibres were normal in appearance. Four to 26 days after injury, the changes varied widely, from more or less completely or focally necrotic muscle, to normal muscle. A reparative response with little or no inflammation was also present. The gastroc-nemius muscles were consistently less affected than the solei.

In a study of formalin-fixed muscles from 21 and 38 amputated limbs respectively (Boehme et al 1966, Harriman 1977), degeneration of isolated fibres was found with, in some biopsies, regenera-tion and haemosiderosis. Grouped atrophic fibres were common, probably reflecting co-existing denervation secondary to ischaemic or diabetic neuropathy. Electron microscopy showed several non-specific features in 11 biopsies (Boehme et al 1966). Some of the changes mentioned above are illustrated in Figures 20.7 and 20.8.

The light-microscopic appearance of major infarcts of the thigh muscles in two diabetics, secondary to occlusive vascular disease, was described by Banker & Chester (1973). Prominent features were interference with muscle regeneration by proliferating connective tissue, denervation within the infarct zone, repeated haemorrhages into the area undergoing repair, and insufficiency of the intramuscular arterial anastomoses.

Particularly in traumatology, organ trans-plantation, plastic and reconstructive surgery, prolonged ischaemia and incomplete reperfusion prevent a successful outcome from surgical inter-ventions. In both human skeletal muscle and animal tissues the luminal endothelial cell membrane of the microvascular bed is most reactive following periods of ischaemia and reper-fusion. The observed fine structural alterations include swelling of endothelial cells, endothelial

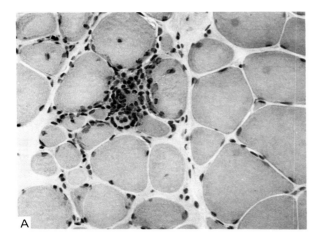

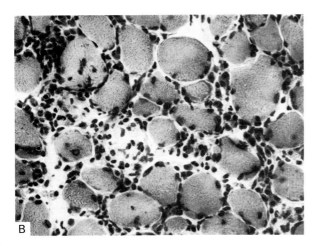

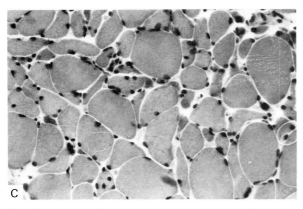

Fig. 20.7 Ischaemic muscle changes in a patient suffering from arteriosclerotic occlusion and stenosis. Scattered necrotic fibres undergoing phagocytosis (A), endomysial round-cell infiltration (B) and atrophic muscle fibres (C) are present. H&E; (a) ×252 (b) ×216, (c) ×198

breaks, widening of the intercellular gap between endothelial cells, capillary plugging by leukocytes and interactions between thrombocytes and the endothelium (Hammersen et al 1989). It is assumed that the revascularization of regenerating muscle tissue is stimulated by a factor released by the damaged muscle (Phillips & Knighton 1990).

BLOOD VESSELS AND CAPILLARIES IN DIFFERENT NEUROMUSCULAR DISORDERS

Duchenne dystrophy

The structure of intramuscular blood vessels as well as the PO_2 values of the muscle and the muscle blood flow in Duchenne dystrophy have been investigated (Kunze 1969, Jerusalem et al 1974a, Paulson et al 1974, Koehler 1977) because it has been suggested that a circulatory abnormality might have a role in the pathogenesis of this disorder (for references see Engel 1975). Although this hypothesis has not been substantiated, it is obvious that there are structural alterations of the vascular bed. These were previously observed by Erb in 1891. He described thickening of the walls of small blood vessels, mononuclear infiltrates and narrowing of the vessel lumens. Indeed, such vascular alterations can easily be demonstrated (Fig. 20.9), but identical changes also occur in other neuromuscular disorders (see Fig. 20.16).

Occlusion of small blood vessels in Duchenne dystrophy has not been convincingly demonstrated by histochemical methods or by electron microscopy. Occasionally, 'occluded' blood vessels occur in normal muscle biopsies and in several neuromuscular disorders; in some instances these probably represent an artefact. A few of these 'occluded' blood vessels have been shown by us to be normal precapillary sphincters on electron microscopy (Fig. 20.3). In cross-sections of epon-embedded blocks examined with the phase microscope, the mean muscle fibre area per capillary in five patients with Duchenne dystrophy was 930 ± 147 μm² (mean ± s.e.) (range 608–1420 μm²). In four control children the corresponding value was 951 ± 125 μm² (range 745 ± 1314 μm²). The two means were not significantly different (Jerusalem et al 1974a).

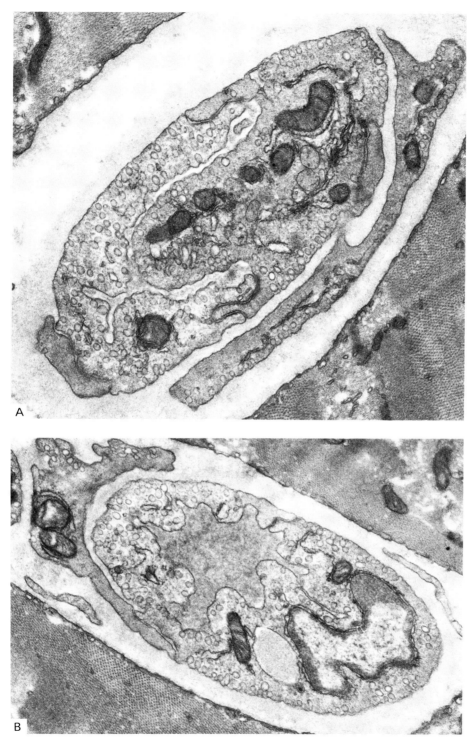

Fig. 20.8 Cross-sections of capillaries from a patient with ischaemic myopathy attributable to arteriosclerotic occlusions. Variation in size of lumen and endothelial area in comparison to normal capillaries (Fig. 20.4) can be noted. (A) ×20 400, (B) ×17765

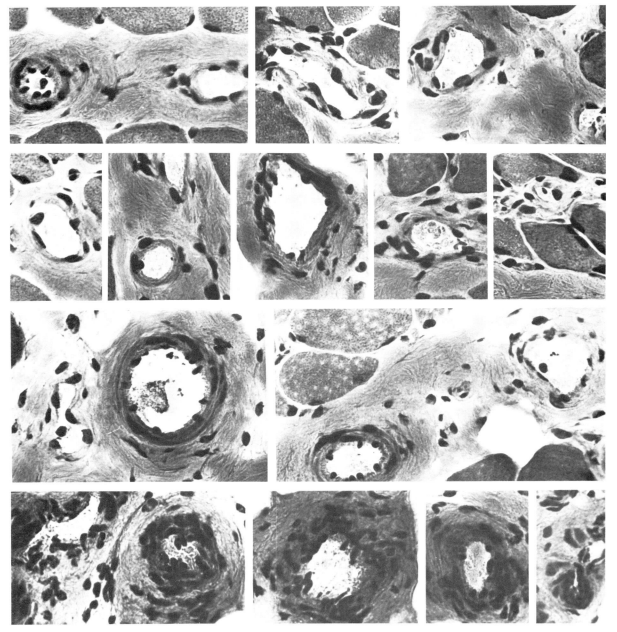

Fig. 20.9 Collection of small arteries and arterioles from muscle biopsies of patients with Duchenne muscular dystrophy. Several of the blood vessels demonstrate thickening of the walls with an increase in peri-adventitial connective tissue and number of nuclei. H&E, ×460

Replication of the basement membrane was found in relation to small venules, arterioles, precapillary sphincters and in two-thirds of the capillaries (Fig. 20.10b). The basement membrane was replicated in only one of 30 capillaries of control children. The same abnormality is found in polymyositis, dermatomyositis, and scleroderma with a frequency comparable to that in Duchenne

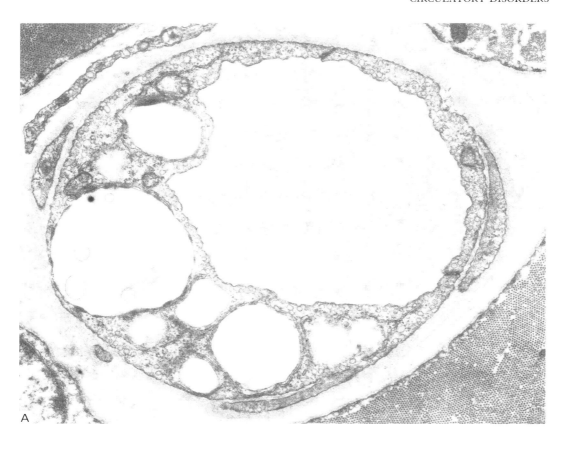

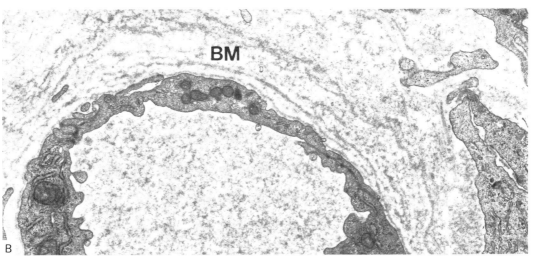

20.10 (A) Capillary with vacuolation of the endothelium in muscle biopsy of a patient suffering from Churg–Strauss disease. (B) Capillary with replication of the basement membrane (BM) in Duchenne dystrophy. (B) ×17 800, (B) ×12 400

dystrophy and in systemic lupus erythematosus, infantile and childhood spinal muscular atrophy, and in other types of muscular dystrophy with significantly lower frequency. The cause and significance of the basement membrane alteration in Duchenne dystrophy and in the other disorders mentioned has not yet been established. Experimentally, replication of capillary basement membrane can be observed after capillary necrosis and subsequent regeneration induced by cold or by ischaemia (Vracko & Benditt 1972). Pale swelling of endothelial cells in Duchenne dystrophy may be indicative of repeated cycles of degeneration and regeneration, but direct evidence of capillary necrosis and repair is lacking.

Electron-microscopic morphometric analysis of 71 capillaries from nine patients with Duchenne dystrophy and 30 capillaries from control children (Jerusalem et al 1974a) gave the following results. The mean capillary area was significantly larger in children with Duchenne dystrophy than in normal children. The dimensions of the endothelial cells and pericytes were also increased, but these increases were proportional to the overall increases in the capillary area. Analysis of the organelles in endothelial cells and pericytes showed that the cytoplasmic fractions occupied by mitochondria and by endoplasmic reticulum, as well as the number of tight junctions per capillary, were not significantly different in Duchenne dystrophy and control capillaries. However, the concentration of pinocytotic vesicles in the capillary endothelial cells was 22% less in Duchenne dystrophy than in the controls (32.9 ± 2.3 vesicles per μm^2 in the controls; 25.6 ± 1.2 vesicles per μm^2 in Duchenne dystrophy; $P < 0.01$).

Further ultrastructural studies also failed to demonstrate evidence for a primary vascular factor in the pathogenesis of muscular dystrophy (Musch et al 1975, Koehler 1977).

Polymyositis, dermatomyositis and other collagen vascular diseases

One cardinal feature of polymyositis and dermatomyositis in muscle biopsies is the presence of mononuclear cells. These are often situated near blood vessels, especially venules, in the perimysial and endomysial space, and quite often around capillaries of degenerating and even normal-appearing muscle fibres. In the chronic stages, an increase of perivascular connective tissue can be demonstrated. Very occasionally a proliferation of endothelial cells, a thrombosed lumen, or a few inflammatory round cells in the vessel wall are present in arteries, arterioles or pre-capillary sphincters. With the alizarin red stain, calcium deposits can be demonstrated in arterial vessel walls, and these deposits may be more extensive than those found in normal muscle and in other disorders.

The light- and electron-microscopic demonstration of capillary abnormalities (Banker & Victor 1066, Jerusalem et al 1974b, Carpenter et al 1976), the observation of IgG, IgM and C3 deposits in the walls of veins and small arteries in 44% of patients, especially those with childhood dermatomyositis, and the demonstration of a significantly reduced muscle blood flow, indicate participation of the muscle vasculature in inflammatory myopathies (Whitaker & Engel 1972, Paulson et al 1974). In fact, capillary necrosis and significant capillary loss, which generally starts at the periphery of muscle fascicles, thickened small arteries in which the endothelial cells are prominent, intimal hyperplasia in medium-sized arteries, segmental inflammation of vessel walls, fibrin thrombi and small muscle infarctions have been found in childhood dermatomyositis (Banker 1975, Carpenter et al 1976). Sequential in vivo nail-fold microscopy confirms the frequency and degree of vasculopathy in children with dermatomyositis (Silver & Maricq 1989). In dermatomyositis of children and adults, the effector mechanism appears to be predominantly humeral and directed against intramuscular blood vessels (Emslie-Smith and Engel 1990). Capillary abnormalities precede other changes is muscle in adult dermatomyositis (De Visser et al 1989). In six biopsies examined by these authors, the endothelial cells harboured microtubular inclusions and microvacuoles in all cases; pale swollen endothelial cells were observed in three specimens. In all cases, a small proportion of muscle capillaries were immunoreactive for complement membrane attack complex neoantigens. Our study (Jerusalem et al 1980) consisted of nine muscle biopsies from adults with polymyositis, and 10 from controls. Five transversely orientated blocks were taken at

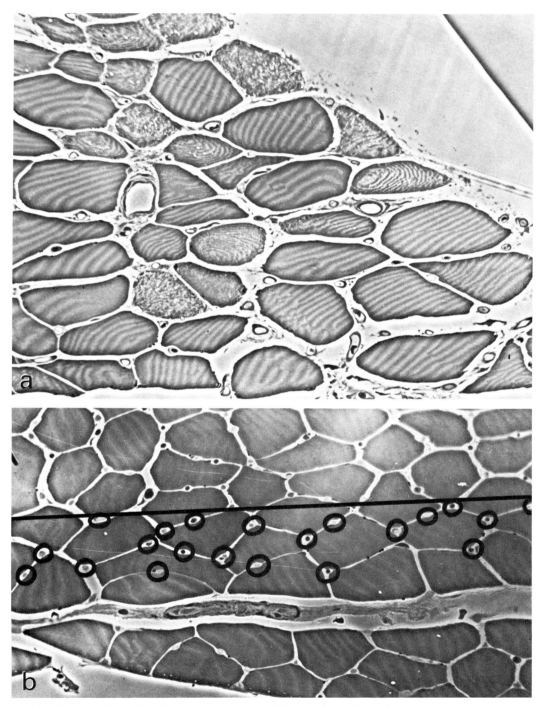

Fig. 20.11 Muscle cross-sections viewed in the phase microscope from a patient suffering from polymyositis. Capillaries in the endomysial space can be counted to determine muscle fibre area per capillary (A). In (B) the number of capillaries in a perifascicular area 60 μm wide is demonstrated. (A) ×304, (B) ×224. From Jerusalem et al (1980), with permission.

random from each biopsy; semi-thin sections were taken and photographed with the phase microscope (Fig. 20.11, 20.12), the final magnification being ×480. In each biopsy, 200–600 fibres were counted. The total fibre area was determined by the point-sampling technique and the number of capillaries and muscle fibres was counted. The mean muscle fibre area per capillary was 1615 ± 318 μm² (mean ± s.e.) (range 1353–2370) in polymyositis and 1363 ± 363 μm² (range 990–2044) in controls. The value for the polymyositis biopsies was higher, which might indicate a slight capillary loss, but the difference was not statistically significant. Because phase-microscopic identification of capillaries in polymyositis is often difficult or impossible, we checked our results using the electron microscope with a low magnification of ×1200. These pictures allow a very precise identification of capillaries (Fig. 20.13), but again no significant differences could be detected. In fact, the values for the polymyositis and control patients were closer than mentioned above.

It is of interest to analyse the perifascicular area separately (Fig. 20.11b). Again, the mean muscle fibre area per capillary in the perifascicular region was higher than in controls, but the two means

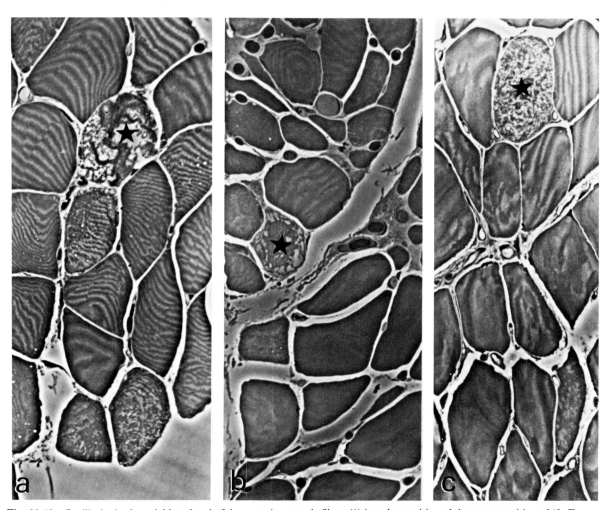

Fig. 20.12 Capillaries in the neighbourhood of degenerating muscle fibres (*) in polymyositis and dermatomyositis. ×342. From Jerusalem et al (1980), with permission

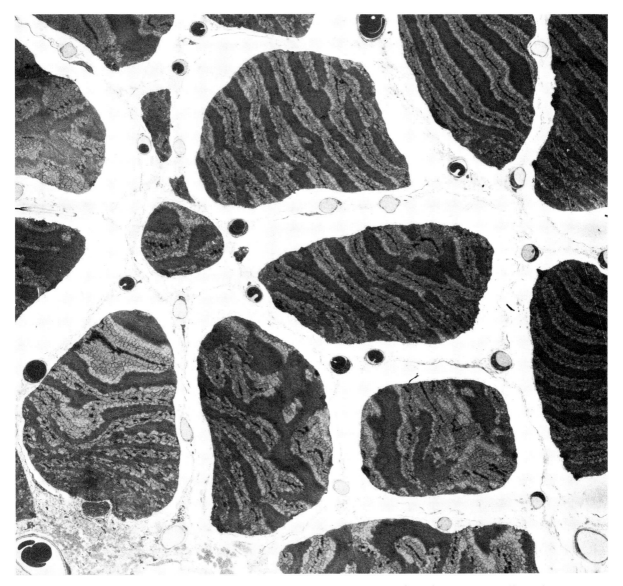

Fig. 20.13 Low-power electron-microscopic magnification of cross-sectioned muscle fibres from a patient suffering from polymyositis. The capillaries of the interstitial space can be identified more accurately than by phase microscopy. ×720. From Jerusalem et al (1980), with permission

were not significantly different. Finally, we estimated the number of capillaries adjacent to single degenerating muscle fibres (n = 119) in seven patients with polymyositis and five control patients (n = 171) (Fig. 20.12). The mean number of capillaries per degenerating muscle fibre in polymyositis was 1.53 ± 0.63; in controls, 1.73 ±

0.66 capillaries were in close proximity to a single muscle fibre. Again, these values are not significantly different.

Although no consistent numerical loss was detected in adults with polymyositis, the fact remains that a high percentage of capillaries show ultrastructural abnormalities. In polymyositis,

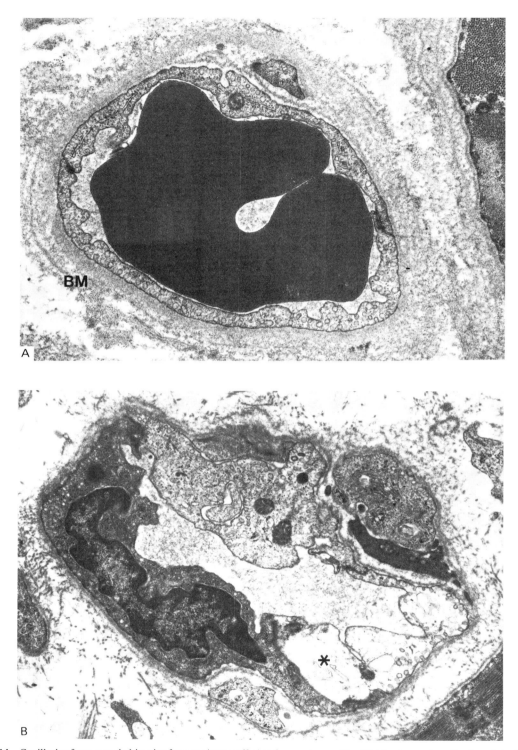

Fig. 20.14 Capillaries from muscle biopsies from patients suffering from polymyositis. Thickening and replication of the basement membrane (BM) is evident (A). Pale swelling (*) of an endothelial cell can be seen in (B). (A) ×17 440, (B) ×14 240

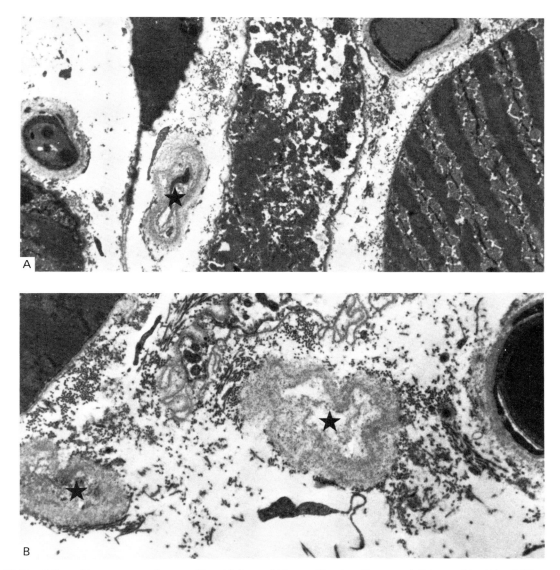

Fig. 20.15   Collapsed basement membrane residues (*) from which a capillary has disappeared. Polymyositis. (A) ×6600, (B) ×3600

dermatomyositis and also in scleroderma and systemic lupus erythematosus (SLE), the capillary basement membrane is thickened and replicated, forming two or more continuous or discontinuous layers around a portion of the vessel (Table 20.3; Fig. 20.14a) (Shafiq et al 1967, Gonzalez-Angulo et al 1968, Norton et al 1968, Mastaglia & Walton 1971). The control capillaries only rarely showed this alteration. In each disease, collapsed basement membrane residues, presumably corresponding to regions in which capillaries have undergone complete necrosis, were occasionally encountered (Fig. 20.15). Pale swollen capillary endothelial cells were observed in all the connective tissue disorders (Fig. 20.14b). Twenty per cent of the capillaries in dermatomyositis, 10% in polymyositis, 4% in scleroderma and 3% in SLE, and nine of the control capillaries showed this alteration. It

Table 20.3 Frequency of capillary basement membrane abnormalities[a]

	No. of cases	Capillaries	
		No.	% abnormal
Controls	5	41	0
Scleroderma	5	23	74
Polymyositis	4	30	47
Dermatomyositis	6	40	45
Lupus erythematosus	5	50	24

[a]Abnormality refers to presence of two or more layers of basal lamina around vessel.
Reproduced with permission, from Jerusalem et al (1974b).

is possible that, in the inflammatory myopathies, these basement membrane and endothelial cell abnormalities (replication, empty tubes and pale swelling) are indicative of repeated cycles of degeneration and regeneration. In addition, there may be other pathogenetic factors that contribute to this change.

Endothelial microtubular inclusions were observed in two of six patients with dermatomyositis and in two of five patients with SLE. While the inclusions appear to be highly specific for these diseases, their nature and pathogenetic significance remains undetermined (Hashimoto et al 1970, Norton et al 1970, Tisher et al 1971, Landry & Winkelmann 1972, Carpenter et al 1976, De Visser et al 1989).

The fine structure of muscle capillaries was analysed morphometrically in five normal controls (41 capillaries), five patients with scleroderma (23 capillaries), four patients with polymyositis (30 capillaries), six patients with dermatomyositis (40 capillaries) and five patients with systemic lupus erythematosus (SLE) (50 capillaries). In all four connective tissue disorders there was hypertrophy of the endothelial cells and of the pericytes. The mean capillary area was also significantly increased in scleroderma, dermatomyositis and SLE, but not in polymyositis (Table 20.1). In all four diseases the number of pinocytotic vesicles per unit endothelial cell area was significantly reduced, while the mitochondrial and endoplasmic reticulum fractions of the endothelial area were significantly increased (Table 20.2). The data of the pericyte organelles are listed in Table 20.4. In scleroderma and SLE, the muscle capillaries are also decreased in number (Norton et al 1968).

The light-microscopic pathology of intramuscular blood vessels in scleroderma and SLE is poorly documented. In scleroderma, the perifascicular and endomysial proliferation of connective tissue with strongly positive acid phosphatase reactions may be accentuated around intramuscular blood vessels and may be associated with round-cell infiltrates. About 20% of biopsies in SLE demonstrate slight perivascular or endomysial round-cell collections.

Table 20.4 Morphometric analysis of pericyte organelles[a]

	Vesicles no. (μm[a])	Mitochondrial area (%)	Endoplasmic reticulum area (%)
Control capillaries (n = 41)	12.35 ± 1.93	6.30 ± 1.34	1.50 ± 0.21
Scleroderma (n = 23)	13.37 ± 1.35 N.S.	4.70 ± 0.80 N.S.	2.13 ± 0.31 N.S.
Polymyositis (n = 30)	15.15 ± 1.04 N.S.	5.16 ± 0.94 N.S.	2.22 ± 0.27 $P < 0.05$
Dermatomyositis (n = 40)	11.91 ± 1.13 N.S.	5.64 ± 0.84 N.S.	3.84 ± 0.53 $P < 0.001$
Lupus erythematosus (n = 50)	8.34 ± 0.94 $P < 0.01$	3.47 ± 0.56 N.S.	2.32 ± 0.27 $P < 0.05$

[a]Values indicate mean ± standard error.
N.S.: Not significant.
Reproduced, with permission, from Jerusalem et al (1974b).

Perivascular lymphohistiocytic infiltrations are often found in viral, bacterial and parasitic myositis.

Motor neurone disease

The myopathological criteria for the diagnosis of a neurogenic syndrome, for example spinal muscular atrophy, is based on alterations of the muscle fibres and their type pattern but not on blood vessel changes. Nevertheless, thickening of vessel walls, an increase in the number of nuclei, and narrowing of the vessel lumen may be found occasionally (Fig. 20.16), but these are non-specific

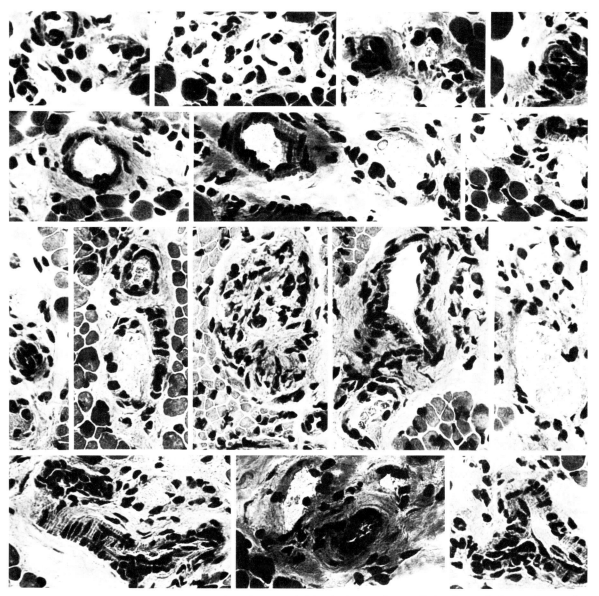

Fig. 20.16 Collections of small arteries and arterioles from muscle biopsies from patients suffering from spinal muscular atrophy. Several of the blood vessels demonstrate thickening of the walls, with an increase of peri-adventitial connective tissue and number of nuclei. The vessel in the centre of the picture is occluded. H&E, ×437

changes. On the other hand, there are a few experimental observations which indicate a neurogenic influence on capillary density in the muscles. Long-term stimulation of fast muscles, at a frequency which normally occurs in a nerve supplying a slow muscle, causes a transformation of muscle fibres towards the 'slower' type, with an increased activity of oxidative enzymes and an increase in the number of capillaries (Cotter et al 1973). Experimental denervation induces a decrease in capillary density (Chernukh & Alekseeva 1976). Kunze (1969) reported a reduced intramuscular PO_2 value in chronic neurogenic atrophies in humans.

With these observations in mind, we measured the capillary density in cross-sections of muscle biopsies from 11 patients with chronic neurogenic atrophy and 10 controls. The mean muscle fibre area per capillary was 1611 ± 848 μm^2 (mean $\pm$ s.d.) in the patients and 1363 ± 363 μm^2 in the controls. These values indicate a tendency towards decreased capillary density in these neurogenic disorders, but statistically the results were not significantly different. In addition, we measured the muscle fibre area per capillary in the vicinity of single hypertrophic muscle fibres ($n = 50$; calibre 110 μm and over) in five biopsies from patients with chronic spinal muscular atrophy and in normal muscle fibres ($n = 50$) in five controls. The values were 1505 ± 174 μm^2 in the muscles of the patients and 724 ± 147 μm^2 in the controls. This difference, which is statistically significant, indicates a reduced capillary density in hypertrophic muscle fibres. It is possible that hypoxia of hypertrophic muscle fibres plays a part in causing degenerative changes in these fibres, and in causing the early exhaustion and myalgia which is experienced by some patients with chronic spinal muscular atrophy.

Malik et al (1989) assessed capillary abnormalities in simultaneous nerve, muscle and skin biopsies from 21 diabetic patients and control subjects. Nerve capillaries demonstrated markedly greater pathology than skin and muscle capillaries. A microvascular lesion characterized by extensive platelet aggregation, thrombosis, and vascular damage with haemorrhages was found in the muscle of a 2-month-old boy with a myopathic form of the arthrogryposis syndrome (Fidzianska et al 1989).

REFERENCES

Alarcon-Segovia D 1977 The necrotizing vasculitides. A new pathogenetic classification. Medical Clinics of North America (Philadelphia) 61: 241

Banker B Q 1975 Dermatomyositis of childhood. Ultrastructural alterations of muscle and intramuscular blood vessels. Journal of Neuropathology and Experimental Neurology 34: 46

Banker B Q, Chester C S 1973 Infarction of thigh muscle in the diabetic patient. Neurology (Minneapolis) 23: 667

Banker B Q, Victor M 1966 Dermatomyositis (systemic angiopathy) of childhood. Medicine 45: 261

Bevan J A, Su Che 1973 Sympathetic mechanisms in blood vessels: nerve and muscle relationships. Annual Review of Pharmacology 13: 269

Blomfield L B 1945 Intramuscular vascular pattern in man. Proceedings of the Royal Society of Medicine 38: 617

Boehme D, Themann H, Gold J 1966 Structural and ultrastructural changes in striated human muscle caused by chronic ischemia. American Journal of Pathology 49: 569

Bohr D F, Greenberg S, Bonaccorsi A 1978 Mechanisms of action of vasoactive agents. In: Kaly G, Altura B M (eds) Microcirculation. University Park Press, Baltimore, ch 7, p 311

Brooke M H, Kaplan M D 1972 Muscle pathology in rheumatoid arthritis, polymyalgia rheumatica, and polymyositis. Archives of Pathology 94: 101

Carpenter S, Karpati G, Eisen A 1975 A morphologic sutdy of muscle in polymyositis: clues to pathogenesis of different types. In: Bradley W G, Gardner-Medwin D, Walton J N (eds) Recent advances in myology. Excerpta Medica, Amsterdam, American Elsevier, New York, p 374

Carpenter S, Karpati G, Rothman, S, Watters G 1976 The childhood type of dermatomyositis. Neurology (Minneapolis) 26: 952

Chernukh A M, Alekseeva N N 1976 Changes in capillary bed of skeletal muscle at various times after nerve section. Bulletin of Experimental Biology and Medicine 80: 1009

Cohen R D, Conn D L, Ilstrup D M 1980 Clinical features, prognosis and response to treatment in polyarteritis. Mayo Clinic Proceedings 55: 146

Cotter M, Hudlicka O, Pette D, Staudte H, Vrbovà G 1973 Changes of capillary density and enzyme pattern in fast rabbit muscles during long-term stimulation. Journal of Physiology 230: 34

De Visser M, Emslie-Smith A M, Engel A G 1989 Early ultrastructural alterations in adult dermatomyositis. Capillary abnormalities precede other structural changes in muscle. Journal of Neurological Science 94: 181

Emslie-Smith A M, Engel A G 1990 Microvascular changes in early and advanced dermatomyositis: a quantitative study. Annals of Neurology 27: 343

Engel W K 1975 The vascular hypothesis. In: Bradley W G,

Gardner-Medwin D, Walton J N (eds) Recent advances in myology. Excerpta Medica, Amsterdam. American Elsevier, New York, p 166

Erb W H 1891 Dystrophia muscularis progressiva. Klinische und pathologisch-anatomische Studien. Deutsche Zeitschrift für Nervenheilkunde 1: 173

Ettlinger R E, Hunder G G, Ward L E 1978 Polymyalgia rheumatica and giant cell arteritis. Annual Review of Medicine 29: 15

Fassbender H G 1975 Pathology of rheumatic disease. Springer Verlag, New York p 304

Fidzianska A, Goebel H H, Burck-Lehmann U 1989 Myopathic form of arthrogryposis and microcirculation lesion. Journal of Neurological Science 92: 337

Frohnert P P, Sheps S G 1967 Long-term follow-up study of periarteritis nodosa. American Journal of Medicine 43: 8

Gerber N J 1984 Giant cell arteritis and its variants. European Neurology 23: 410

Gonzalez-Angulo A, Fraga A, Mintz G 1968 Submicroscopic alterations in capillaries of skeletal muscles in polymyositis. American Journal of Medicine 45: 873

Göthert M 1990 Pharmacological, biochemical and molecular classification schemes of serotonin (5-HT) receptors with special reference to the $5-HT_2$ class. Progress in Pharmacology and Clinical Pharmacology 7: 3

Gutmann, L, Wolf R, Nix W, Goebel H H, Schochet S S, Hopf H C, Kramer G 1989 Internalized myofiber capillaries: observations on their origin and clinical features. Muscle and Nerve 12: 191

Hammersen F, Barker J H, Gidlöf A, Menger M D, Hammersen E, Messmer K 1989 The ultrastructure of microvessels and their contents following ischemia and reperfusion. Progress in Applied Microcirculation 13: 1

Harriman D G F 1977 Ischaemia of peripheral nerve and muscle. Journal of Clinical Pathology supplement 11: 94

Hashimoto K, Robinson L, Velayos E 1970 Dermatomyositis. Electron microscopic, immunologic, and tissue culture studies of paramyxovirus-like inclusions. Acta dermatologica 103: 120

Hathaway P W, Engel W K, Zellweger H 1970 Experimental myopathy after microarterial embolization. Archives of Neurology (Chicago) 22: 365

Hudlickà O 1973 Muscle blood flow. Swets & Zeitlinger B V, Amsterdam

Ingjer F 1979 Effects of endurance training on muscle fibre ATPase activity, capillary supply and mitochondrial content in man. Journal of Physiology 294: 419

Jerusalem F, Engel A G, Gomez M R 1974a Duchenne dystrophy. I. Morphometric study of the muscle microvasculature. Brain 97: 115

Jerusalem F, Rakusa M, Engel A G, MacDonald R D 1974b Morphometric analysis of skeletal muscle capillary ultrastructure in inflammatory myopathies. Journal of the Neurological Sciences 23: 391

Jerusalem F, Simona F, Fontana A 1980 Myopathologische und immunologische Befunde zur Diagnose und Pathogenese der Polymyositis und Dermatomyositis. Nervenarzt 51: 255

Kalyan-Raman U P, Kalyan-Raman K, Yunus M B, Masi A T 1984 Muscle pathology in primary fibromyalgia syndrome: a light microscopic, histochemical and ultrastructural study. Journal of Rheumatology 11: 808

Karpati G, Carpenter S, Melmed C, Eisen A A 1974 Experimental ischemic myopathy. Journal of the Neurological Sciences 23: 129

Koehler J 1977 Blood vessel structure in Duchenne muscular dystrophy. I. Light and electron microscopic observations in resting muscle. Neurology (Minneapolis) 27: 861

Koller A, Kaley G 1990 Endothelium regulates skeletal muscle microcirculation by a blood flow velocity-sensing mechanism. American Journal of Physiology 258: 916

Kunze K 1969 Das Sauerstoffdruckfeld im normalen und pathologisch veränderten Muskel. Schriftenreihe Neurologie, vol 3. Springer-Verlag, Heidelberg

Landry M, Winkelmann R K 1972 Tubular cytoplasmic inclusions in dermatomyositis. Proceedings of Staff Meetings of the Mayo Clinic 47: 479

Leib E S, Restivo C, Paulus H E 1979 Immunosuppressive and corticosteroid therapy of polyarteritis nodosa. American Journal of Medicine 67: 941

Lendrum A C, Fraser D S, Slidders W, Henderson R 1962 Studies on the character and staining of fibrin. Journal of Clinical Pathology 15: 401

Malik R A, Newrick P G, Sharma A K et al 1989 Microangiopathy in human diabetic neuropathy: relationship between capillary abnormalities and the severity of neuropathy. Diabetologia 32: 92

Mastaglia F L, Walton J N 1971 An ultrastructural study of skeletal muscle in polymyositis. Journal of the Neurological Sciences 12: 437

Matsuo S, Penneys N S, Fine J D, Gay S, Nadji M 1990 A monoclonal antibody which identifies an antigen in endothelial cell and epithelial basement membrane. Blood Vessels 27: 35

Maxeiner S R, McDonald J R, Kirklin J W 1952 Muscle biopsy in the diagnosis of periarteritis nodosa. Surgical Clinics of North America 32: 1225

Mazzoni M C, Borgstrom P, Intaglietta M, Arfors K E 1989 Lumenal narrowing and endothelial cell swelling in skeletal muscle capillaries during hemorrhagic shock. Circulatory Shock 29: 27

Mendell J R, Engel W K, Derrer E C 1971 Duchenne dystrophy: functional ischemia reproduces its characteristic lesions. Science 172: 1143

Mendell J R, Engel W K, Derrer E C 1972 Increased plasma enzyme concentrations in rats with functional ischaemia of muscle provide a possible model of Duchenne muscular dystrophy. Nature 239: 522

Menger M D, Hammersen F, Barker J, Feifel G, Messmer K 1988 Tissue PO_2 and functional capillary density in chronically ischemic skeletal muscle. Advances in Experimental Medicine and Biology 222: 631

Menger M D, Hammersen F, Barker J H, Feifel G, Messmer K 1989 Ischemia and reperfusion in skeletal muscle: experiments with tourniquet ischemia in the awake syrian golden hamster. Progress in Applied Microcirulation 13: 93

Miller L D, Stevens M B 1978 Skeletal manifestations of polymyalgia rheumatica. Journal of the American Medical Association 240: 27

Milnor W R 1974 Capillaries and lymphatic vessels. Regional circulations. In: Mountcastle V B (ed) Medical physiology. C V Mosby, Saint Louis, p 984

Mizuno M, Secher N H 1989 Histochemical characteristics of human expiratory and inspiratory intercostal muscles. Journal of Applied Physiology 67: 592

Mukai L, Rosai J, Bergdorf W 1980 Localization of factor VIII-related antigen in vascular endothelial cells using an immunoperoxidase method. American Journal of Surgery and Pathology 4: 273

Musch B C, Paparetropoulos T A, McQueen D A, Hudgson P, Weightman D 1975 A comparison of the structure of small blood vessels in normal, denervated and dystrophic human muscle. Journal of the Neurological Sciences 26: 221

Norton W L, Hurd E R, Lewis D C, Ziff M 1968 Evidence of vascular injury in scleroderma and systemic lupus erythematosus: quantitative study of the microvascular bed. Journal of Laboratory and Clinical Medicine 71: 919

Norton W L, Velayos E, Robinson L 1970 Endothelial inclusions in dermatomyositis. Annals of the Rheumatic Diseases 29: 67

Paulson O B, Engel A G, Gomez M R 1974 Muscle blood flow in Duchenne type muscular dystrophy, limb-girdle dystrophy, polymyositis, and in normal controls. Journal of Neurology, Neurosurgery and Psychiatry 37: 685

Phillips G D, Knighton D R 1990 Angiogenic activity in damaged skeletal muscle. Proceedings of the Society of Experimental Biology and Medicine 193: 197

Quastel D M, Hackett J T 1973 Effects of drugs on smooth and striated muscle. In: Bourne G H (ed) The structure and function of muscle, 2nd edn. Academic Press, New York, vol 4

Renkin E M, Hudlickà O, Shechan R M 1966 Influence of metabolic vasodilatation on blood–tissue diffusion in skeletal muscle. American Journal of Physiology 211: 87

Rhodin J A G 1967 The ultrastructure of mammalian arterioles and precapillary sphincters. Journal of Ultrastructure Research 18: 181

Rhodin J A G 1968 The ultrastructure of mammalian venous capillaries, venules and small collecting veins. Journal of Ultrastructure Research 25: 452

Roux H, Serratrice G, Aguaron R, Cartouzou G, de Bisshop G, Gambarelli D, Baret J, Recordier A M 1975 Les atteintes musculaires de la pseudopolyarthrite rhizomélique (PPR). Rheumatology 5: 511

Scully R E, Hughes C W 1956 The pathology of ischemia of skeletal muscle in man. American Journal of Pathology 32: 805

Selye H 1965 A muscular dystrophy induced by cold following restriction of the arterial blood supply. Experientia 21: 610

Shafiq S A, Milhorat A T, Górycki A 1967 An electron-microscopic study of muscle degeneration and vascular changes in polymyositis. Journal of Pathology and Bacteriology 94: 139

Silver R M, Maricq H R 1989 Childhood dermatomyositis: serial microvascular studies. Pediatrics 83: 278

Tasuku M, Kennedy W R, Yoon K S 1979 Morphometric comparison of capillaries in muscle spindles, nerve, and muscle. Archives of Neurology (Chicago) 36: 547

Tisher C C, Kelso H B, Robinson R R 1971 Intra-endothelial inclusions in kidneys of patients with systemic lupus erythematosus. Annals of Internal Medicine 75: 537

van Nueten J M, Janssens W J 1990 Interactions between $5-HT_2$-receptors and α_1-adrenoceptors in vascular tissues. Progress in Pharmacology and Clinical pharmacology 7: 35

Vanhoutte P M 1990 Vascular effects of serotonin. Progress in Pharmacology and Clinical Pharmacology 7: 17

Vracko Benditt E P 1972 Basal lamina: the scaffold for orderly cell replacement. Journal of Cell Biology 55: 406

Wallace S L, Lattes R, Ragan C 1958 Diagnostic significance of the muscle biopsy. American Journal of Medicine 25: 600

Whitaker J N, Engel W K 1972 Vascular deposits of immunoglobulin and complement in idiopathic inflammatory myopathy. New England Journal of Medicine 286: 333

Yunus M B, Kalyan-Raman U P 1989 Muscle biopsy findings in primary fibromyalgia and other forms of nonarticular rheumatism. Rheumatic Disease Clinics of North America 15: 115

Zeek P M, Smith C C, Weeter J C 1948 Studies on periarteritis nodosa. III. The differentiation between the vascular lesions of periarteritis nodosa and of hypersensitivity. American Journal of Pathology 24: 889

21. Tumours of striated muscle

J. T. Hughes

INTRODUCTION

True tumours derived from striated muscle are uncommon, and the early literature is confused by a descriptive nomenclature in which terms such as muscle sarcoma have been used for a variety of soft tissue tumours (Geschikter 1934). The paper by Stout (1946) began the careful separation on morphological grounds of benign and malignant tumours, truly derived from striated muscle cells, and hence called rhabdomyomas and rhabdomyosarcomas. The advent of electron microscopy has added a new dimension of morphological precision to tumour classification, which has benefitted the study of many groups of tumours, including muscle tumours (Kastendieck et al 1976, Cori et al 1977). The use of specific antibodies, either polyclonal or monoclonal, directed against muscle components and used either on paraffin sections from formalin-fixed tissues, or on fresh snap-frozen sections is now playing a prominent part in tumour classification, including this group of tumours. One relatively common tumour formerly thought to arise from muscle was the so-called myoblastoma (Cappell & Montgomery 1937), a variety of which was called, from a prominent cytological feature, the granular-cell myoblastoma. The exclusion of this tumour from the group of muscle tumours directly followed the study of its ultrastructure (Sobel et al 1973). Another example of reclassification is the so called cardiac rhabdomyoma (Batchelor & Maun, 1945), frequently associated with tuberose sclerosis, and now considered to be a malformation arising from elements of cardiac and not striated muscle (Moran & Enterline 1964, Silverman et al 1976, Fenoglio et al 1976).

The account which follows begins with some remarks on the morphology of the striated muscle fibre and its precursors, as seen by light microscopy, electron microscopy, and immunohistochemistry. This introduction will simplify the subsequent descriptions of the various benign and malignant tumours of striated muscle, as seen with these techniques.

MORPHOLOGY OF THE DEVELOPING MUSCLE CELL

The precursors of muscle cells arise in the mesodermal somites at the embryonal disc stage of about 2–3 weeks development. These primitive mesodermal cells develop not only into the striated muscle of our current interest, but also into smooth muscle, and a whole range of other mesodermal tissues. This plurality of possible differentiation of these cells explains some curious sites in which tumours of striated muscle may arise. These tumours are seen, for example, in the middle ear, the bile ducts, bladder, and brain, all very strange locations for striated muscle, but possible sites where nests of primitive mesenchyme may develop into tumours. The occurrences of muscle tumours within mixed tumours have a similar explanation.

Some of these primitive mesenchymal cells elongate and develop bipolar tapering processes of granular cytoplasm extending the cell body. These cells are called myoblasts, whilst the presence of myofilaments and myofibrils confers the name of myocyte, by which stage groups of cells are fusing longitudinally to form the myotube which later develops into the adult multinucleated muscle fibre. At this adult stage, DNA synthesis and nuclear division normally cease. The electron microscope has revealed the ultrastructural details of this development. Actin filaments are the first to form followed by myosin filaments of greater diameter. The alignment of groups of these two filaments produces the striated myofibrils with the distinctive band structure of I and A bands, bisected by the Z lines and M bands. Recognition of muscle tumours is greatly aided by seeing components of this band structure, sometimes by light microscopy, but more readily by electron microscopy. Ultrastructural features to be sought are parallel thick and thin myofilaments arranged in alternating or hexagonal patterns, Z-band material, and myosin–ribosome complexes, in which ribosomes are aligned in single rows alongside myosin filaments. Other more general features of muscle tumours, seen both by light and electron microscopy are indentations of nuclei, prominent nucleoli, and intracytoplasmic glycogen granules.

HISTOCYTOCHEMISTRY

The development of specific antibody/antigen markers for certain components of cells has greatly helped tumour identification, and naturally several have been examined in muscle tumours. The list includes desmin, myoglobin, the MM isoenzyme of creatine kinase, myosin, fast myosin, Z-protein, specific muscle actin, β-enolase, and anti-muscle antibody. These names identify the antigen marked, but the interpretation of results with muscle tumours requires caution. Specificity of reaction may be less than claimed and varies with the source of the antibody. The methods of preparation of tissue sections and whether and how the tissue is fixed alters the intensity of reaction, as does the immunological technique, of which even minor variations are important. If a tumour infiltrates muscle or invades adjacent muscle this 'substrate' muscle may be revealed and thought to be part of the tumour. More subtly, in the invasion of muscle by tumour, tissue macrophages within the tumour may contain elements of muscle, of no direct relationship to the tumour, and which may be not a muscle tumour but, for example, a carcinoma or lymphoma.

Despite these serious reservations, these immunohistological markers are of great assistance in the identification of muscle tumours and may be positive in tumours in which light and electron microscopy fail to show myogenic elements. Myoglobin and desmin have been most generally used with variable but useful results. Current practice is to use a group of antibodies with many controls and to assess positive results by a consensus of the most reliable of the reactions.

CLASSIFICATION

Our classification of these tumours truly derived from the striated muscle cell is based on a nomenclature of rhabdomyomas for the benign tumours and rhabdomyosarcomas for the malignant examples. Certain special histological and clinical features of these tumours prompt further subdivisions. The rhabdomyomas are divided into adult rhabdomyomas and fetal rhabdomyomas, although, as we shall see, the age incidence is not strictly according to this nomenclature. The rhabdomyosarcomas are subdivided into pleomorphic rhabdomyosarcomas (also called adult rhabdomyosarcomas), embryonal rhabdomyosarcomas, and alveolar rhabdomyosarcomas, these last two mentioned forms being sometimes grouped as juvenile rhabdomyosarcomas. The sarcoma botyroides, usually embryonal in histological type, may be added as a familiar type of tumour with a typical gross appearance. This classification is imperfect, as are most working classifications of groups of tumours, but serves both clinician and pathologist well enough to deserve retention, and in summary is as follows:

Rhabdomyomas
    Adult
    Fetal

Rhabdomyosarcomas
    Adult (pleomorphic)
    Juvenile
        Embryonal
        Alveolar
        Sarcoma botyroides

ADULT RHABDOMYOMAS (Fig. 21.1)

The benign rhabdomyomas are rare tumours, of which probably less than 100 cases have been

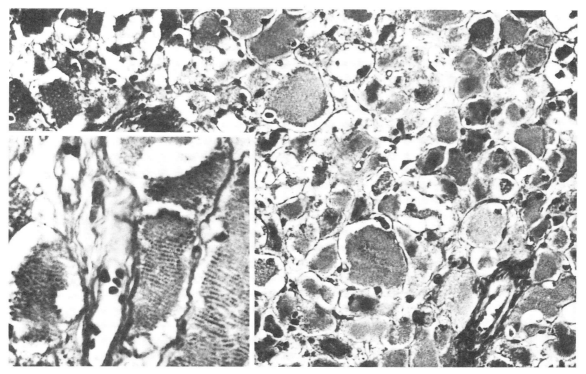

Fig. 21.1 Adult type rhabdomyoma. The large picture shows abnormal striated muscle fibres, round, polygonal or oval, and cut in cross section. The inset shows striated muscle fibres cut obliquely at higher magnification. Phosphotungstic acid haematoxylin stain, ×300; inset ×800. (From Lattes (1982), with permission)

described (Gale et al 1984), and about half are of this 'adult' type, the distinction however being histological. All the rhabdomyomas, adult and fetal, form only some 1–2% of striated muscle tumours, the remaining tumours being the much commoner rhabdomyosarcomas (Tuazon 1969, Dehner et al 1972, Solomon Tolete-Velcek 1979, Weitzner et al 1979). The adult tumour commonly occurs in the mouth, pharynx, and larynx but occasionally has been reported from other parts of the body. Most cases occur in middle-aged males, the sex incidence in males being 4–5 times that in females, but a few cases, of the same histological type, have been described in children.

The macroscopic appearance is that of a medium-sized mass, which, because of its place of origin, usually presents as a tumour bulging into the cavity of the mouth or pharynx, or expanding some other of the many rarer sites (lip, tongue, orbit, submandibular region, tissues of the mediastinum (Miller et al 1978) and retroperi-

toneum, and muscles of the neck, chest wall and abdominal wall). The presenting symptoms are due to expansion of the tissue of origin. The consistency of the tumour is firm and the cut surface has a pink fleshy appearance.

The microscopic appearance of this group of tumours is distinctive. The tumour cells are large, and either round, oval or polygonal. They pack closely together with very little stroma separating each tumour cell from its neighbour. The nuclei are vesicular, medium in size, and are usually placed eccentrically in the cell. Mitotic figures are rarely seen. The cytoplasm is eosinophilic and often contains prominent vacuoles situated at the cell margin, very evident in paraffin sections, and due to the presence of glycogen. Frozen sections stained by PAS demonstrate the glycogen, which is also readily seen with the electron microscope. The cytoplasm may also contain rod-shaped crystalline bodies, 1–5 μm in diameter, which stain darkly with phosphotungstic acid haematoxylin; with the electron microscope these bodies are seen to be parts of abnormally formed Z-band protein. Thick and thin myofilaments are present, and cross-striations, though uncommon, may be found. Antibodies to muscle proteins such as myosin, myoglobin and desmin are often positive.

The striking histological appearance of this benign tumour is a cellular resemblance, by light microscopy, electron microscopy and immunocytochemistry, to the adult striated muscle cell.

FETAL RHABDOMYOMAS (Fig. 21.2)

This name is given to a group of benign rhabdomyomas, differing in histology from the adult type, and with an age incidence from birth to young adult life, and occurring equally in males and females. The tumours often arise in the subcutaneous tissues of the head and neck, the posterior auricular region being a common site. There are many other rarer sites such as tongue, palate, larynx, nose, orbit (Knowles & Jakobiec 1975), parotid, chest and abdominal wall, and the female genital tract.

The histological appearances are more variable than the previous type, with cells suggesting the precursor forms of the striated muscle cell (Stout & Lattes 1967, Dehner et al 1972, Walter & Guerbaoui 1976, Meehan & Davie 1979). The predominant cells in this tumour are spindle-shaped cells resembling myoblasts. These cells have oval or elongated nuclei which are seldom in mitosis, and which are located centrally in thin tapering cells with an indistinct cell border. The degree of resemblance to primitive muscle cells varies, but more mature cells with prominent cross-striations (which should be termed 'myocytes') are common. The cellular differentiation may be greater at the periphery of the tumour, where there are many well-differentiated myocytes, whilst centrally there are undifferentiated tumour cells which are less readily recognized as being derived from muscle. The tumour cells resembling myoblasts are surrounded by a stroma which is often oedematous and contains primitive mesenchymal cells.

The central parts of this tumour may be mistaken for an embryonal rhabdomyosarcoma or some other form of soft tissue sarcoma, although the infrequency of mitotic figures should guide the

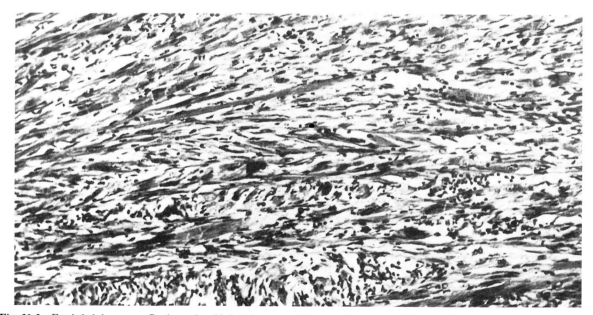

Fig. 21.2 Fetal rhabdomyoma. Benign polypoid rhabdomyoma of the nasopharynx in a 12-year-old boy. The tumour consists of interdigitating fascicles of striated muscle fibres. There is no pleomorphism and no mitotic activity. H&E, ×100. (From Lattes (1982, with permission.)

pathologists away from a diagnosis of a malignant tumour. Electron microscopy and immunocytochemistry are particularly valuable in confirming the origin of this tumour from muscle. Correct diagnosis of these tumours is important as they are benign and do not metastasize. After local excision, many cases have been followed for many years without recurrence.

The benign fetal rhabdomyoma occurs rarely as a polypoid growth projecting into the vagina of middle-aged women (Ceremsak 1969, Leone & Taylor 1973, Gad & Eusebi 1975, Norris & Taylor 1966, Gold & Bossen 1976), and may rarely occur in this form in some other sites (Smith 1959). The histological features are similar to the tumours in other locations except that the tumour cells show more maturity in differentiation towards muscle and the stroma may resemble adult fibrous tissue rather than primitive mesenchyme. Ultrastructural and antibody studies give good results in these tumours although the diagnosis may often be made by light microscopy.

ADULT (PLEOMORPHIC) RHABDOMYOSARCOMAS (Fig. 21.3A, B, C)

The most comprehensive review of these tumours is by Kyriakos (1990). They occur in the lower limb, upper limb, and trunk (Keyhani & Booher 1968, Ariel & Briceno 1975) in descending order of incidence with occasional cases arising in the head and neck. A few cases have been described in the urinary and biliary systems.

Macroscopically, the tumour is usually deep-seated, either embedded in muscle or situated between muscle bundles (Fig. 21.3A). At later stages of growth or after recurrences it may be widely and densely infiltrative. Whilst at first the tumour does not ulcerate through the skin, this may occur, later, especially after local recurrences after surgical excision. The tumour is usually soft rather than firm with a cut surface which is pink or red but is often discoloured by yellowish areas of necrosis and dark red areas of haemorrhage. This tumour is highly malignant and metastases are common, most frequently by the bloodstream, but also by lymphatics to local lymph nodes. Shimada et al (1987) reported the experience of the USA Intergroup Rhabdomyosarcoma Study

(IRS-1 and IRS-11) examining clinicopathological and post mortem data on 274 deaths from these tumours. The alveolar histological type had the highest number of distant metastases. The lung was the most common site of metastasis followed by regional lymph nodes, bone, liver and brain. The principal cause of death was progressive tumour growth, followed by infections, toxicity of therapy including bone marrow suppression, and pulmonary complications.

Microscopically, these tumours appear as anaplastic pleomorphic neoplasms derived from primitive mesenchyme (Figs. 21.3B, C). In most instances, their origin from primitive striated muscle cells, using conventional light microscopy, can be determined only by prolonged careful scrutiny. Well-fixed tissue, embedded in paraffin, and thin sections, stained with haematoxylin and eosin and also with phosphotungstic acid haematoxylin, are still the best means of diagnosis since many large sections are required for an extensive histological survey. These may be supplemented by frozen sections and the 'thick' 1 μm sections from araldite-embedded blocks. Electron microscopy and antibody reactions will clearly be of value.

Much of the tissue will consist of primitive mesenchymal cells, oval or elongated in shape and resembling the cells of a fibrosarcoma. The cells however are generally rather eosinophilic, more so than other mesodermal tumours, and this should encourage a search for the typical rhabdomyoblasts. These are rounded in cross section, but more typically in longitudinal orientation they are oval, sometimes with a 'handle' giving a resemblance to a racquet. The nuclei of these cells are round or elongated, and in the racquet-shaped cells may be in the expanded part of the cell. Two or more nuclei may be present in a cell often arranged serially. Mitoses are frequent, especially in the more undifferentiated areas of the tumour. When well-differentiated, the tumour cell looks like the ribbon of a primitive muscle cell. It is in these ribbon-shaped cells, which are strongly eosinophilic, that myofibrils directed longitudinally, and with cross-striations may be found, most readily with the PTAH stain. To identify cross-striations is less frequent — Linscheid et al (1965) found them in 6 out of 87 cases — than demonstrating longitudinal myofibrils, which are essential to the diagnosis. The electron microscopic and immunocytochemical features described earlier are very important in diagnosis, although the small sample examined by these techniques is a drawback, not evident in the large sections cut from paraffin blocks, and examined by light microscopy.

JUVENILE RHABDOMYOSARCOMAS (Figs. 21.4, 21.5, 21.6A, B)

Rhabdomyosarcomas occur in children and more rarely in young adults (Jenkins 1972, Bale & Reye 1975). They have been subdivided into various types on the basis of certain microscopic and macroscopic appearances. These histological appearances give us the embryonal or alveolar forms of the tumour. The gross appearances are peculiar in those tumours which present from a mucosal surface and a separate description will be added of this tumour, which is usually called the 'sarcoma botyroides'. This botyroid sarcoma commonly has the histological appearance of the embryonal type.

Embryonal rhabdomyosarcomas

These tumours arise in infancy and early childhood, most cases presenting before the age of 12 years. The commonest sites in children are the orbit, other sites in the head and neck (Miller & Dalager 1974, Tefft et al 1978), the urogenital tract, and the retro-peritoneal tissues (Fig. 21.4). In the rarer cases in young adults the tumours are found more often in the limbs, limb girdles, and trunk than in the sites mentioned above for young children (Moore & Grossi 1959, Lawrence et al 1964, Liebner 1976, Maurer 1979).

The precise origin of these tumours is curious, since, where the location can be readily studied, as in the limb muscles or trunk, the tumour seems to arise in deep subcutaneous tissues or between muscle fascicles rather than in actual muscle tissue. The gross appearance is that of a bulging mass in the site concerned. Growth is rapid and patients come under observation less than a year from the onset of symptoms.

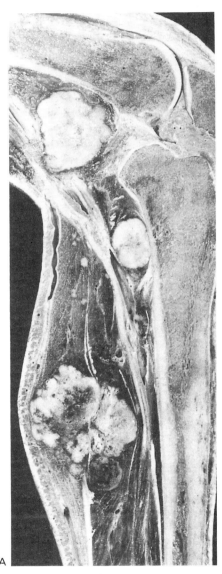

A

Fig. 21.3 (A) Rhabdomyosarcoma. Amputation specimen sawn longitudinally to show tumour in gastrocnemius with secondary nodules elsewhere. Twenty-one-year-old man who died three months after the amputation. (From Lattes (1982), with permission.) (B) Rhabdomyosarcoma. Section from a deep-seated malignant tumour of the lower limb. The tumour cells are variable in size and shape but most have a spindle-like form. There are scanty multinucleated tumour cells resembling muscle fibres. H&E, ×60. (From Hughes (1974), with permission.) (C) Rhabdomyosarcoma. Photomicrograph showing one of the multinucleate cells in (B) at higher magnification. H&E, ×220. (From Hughes (1974), with permission)

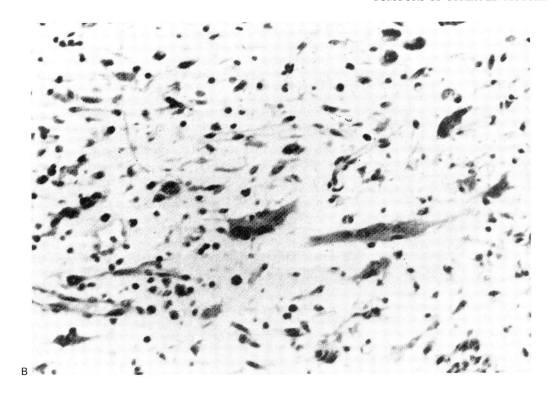

B

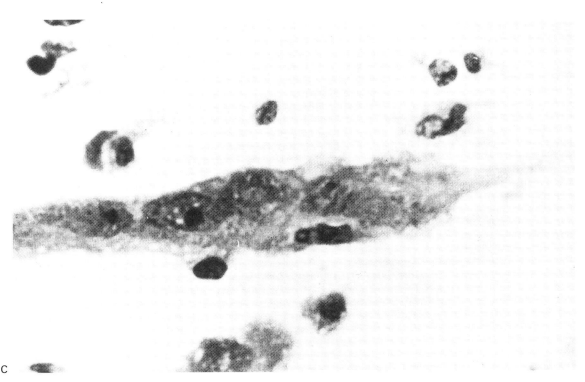

C

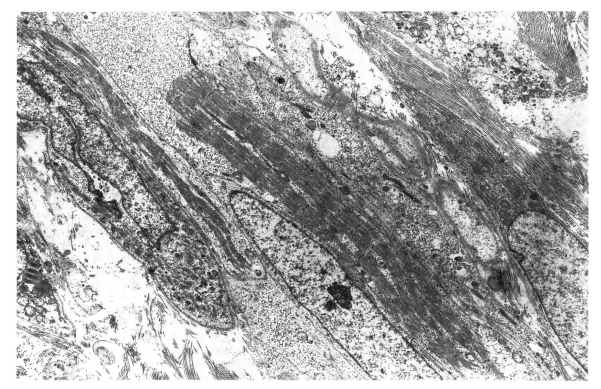

Fig. 21.4 Rhabdomyosarcoma arising in the testicle of a young boy. The electron micrograph shows part of a well-formed striated muscle fibre within the tumour; ×23 250. Case of Dr A. R. Skinner, with electron microscopy by Dr D. Ferguson, Electron Microscopy Unit, John Radcliffe Hospital, Oxford

The microscopic appearances, although varied, have a strong resemblance to the early stages of myogenesis. The tumour cells may be small round cells with medium-sized nuclei and scanty cytoplasm and very similar to adult lymphocytes or small monocytes. Other tumour cells, probably more differentiated, are oval, spindle-shaped, racquet-shaped, or strap-shaped, the last mentioned form being very suggestive of muscle. The undifferentiated cells are the most common but the other forms must be sought for diagnosis, as the cytoplasm is eosinophilic and granular or fibrillar and contains glycogen. Electron microscopy and antibody reactions confirm the muscle elements in the cell body.

Mitotic figures are common in these highly malignant tumour cells which are surrounded by a loose myxoid stroma. Without treatment the tumour spreads widely, locally and by metastasis.

The recent success of modern therapies including cytotoxic drugs in these cases is most gratifying (Gutjahr et al 1976).

Alveolar rhabdomyosarcomas

This is a histological variant of these juvenile muscle sarcomas and is commonest in the younger age group, being seen in older children, and young adults (Gutjahr et al 1976, Enzinger & Shiraki 1969). It is rare in persons older than 50 years. In contrast to the embryonal form, these alveolar rhabdomyosarcomas have most often been described arising in the muscles of the limbs and trunk, being rarer in the head and neck. They also seem to develop precisely within the belly of a muscle, again a distinction from the embryonal form. They form rapidly-growing masses expanding greatly the site of origin.

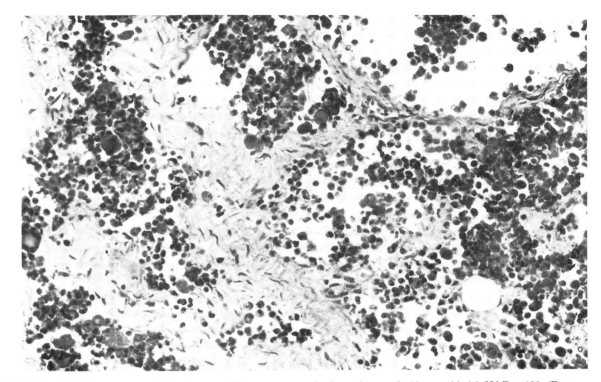

Fig. 21.5 Rhabdomyosarcoma of alveolar type. This tumour arose in the perineum of a 12-year-old girl. H&E, ×130. (From Lattes (1982), with permission)

Histologically the characteristic form of this tumour variant is an arrangement of the tumour cells into loosely arranged groups of small to medium-sized rounded or polygonal cells arranged in cell nests. The large, rounded, periphery of the cell nest has a framework of reticulin and connective tissue, giving the outer border to the nest. Centrally the cells are looser, and there may appear to be a lumen due to the hypocellularity of the centre of the nest. These are the histological appearances giving rise to the name 'alveolar', although 'solid' tumour is also common. There are many mitoses, and all the indications are those of an aggressive infiltrating sarcoma. There is no resemblance to a sarcoma but rather to the patterns seen in malignant tumours of lymphatic, neural, or vascular tissue. The diagnosis of rhabdomyosarcoma is suggested by strongly eosinophilic cytoplasm in which elements of muscle can be identified by ultrastructure (Churg & Ringus 1978) or antibody reactions. As with all these tumours, extensive search is made in large paraffin sections for occasional tumour cells with differentiation towards recognizable muscle cells.

Sarcoma botyroides (Fig. 21.6A, B)

This well-known tumour is an embryonal rhabdomyosarcoma which arises from a muscosal surface or a body cavity unlined by mucosa. The place of origin allows the tumour to grow in a pedunculated form, and a fancied resemblance of these smooth, covered, lobulated tumours to bunches of grapes gave rise to the name 'botyroides'. This tumour most frequently arises in the urogenital tract, but also occurs in the nasal cavity, nasopharynx, cranial sinuses, common bile duct, orbit, and auditory canal.

The histological appearances are those of an embryonal rhabdomyosarcoma with prominent myxomatous degeneration, particularly in the

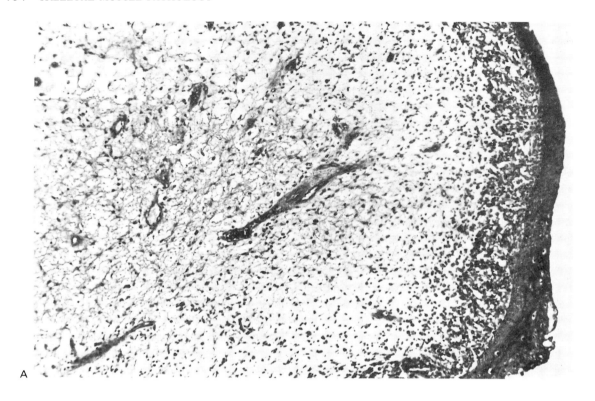

A

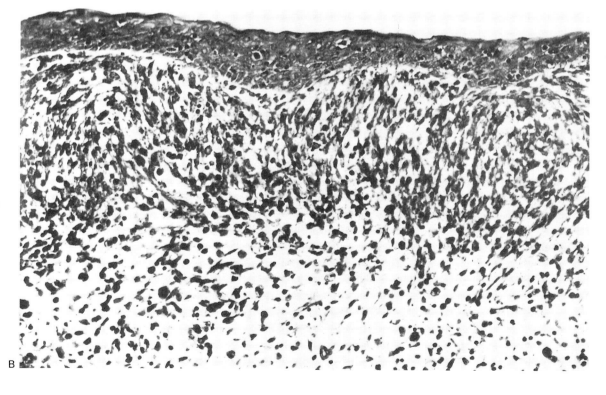

B

centre of the tumour lobules. This histological feature gives rise to a distinctive appearance of hypocellular central areas with more cellular tumour cells beneath the mucosa of the body cavity in which the tumour lies. This layered arrangement of cells gives rise to the botanical term 'cambium', by which this submucosal layering is known.

REFERENCES

Ariel M, Briceno M 1975 Rhabdomyosarcoma of the extremities and trunk: analysis of 150 patients treated by surgical resection. Journal of Surgical Oncology 7: 269

Bale P M, Reye R D K 1975 Rhabdomyosarcoma in childhood. Pathology 7: 101

Batchelor T M, Maun M E 1945 Congenital glycogenic tumors of the heart. Archives of Pathology 39: 67

Cappell D F, Montgomery G L 1937 On rhabdomyoma and myoblastoma. Journal of Pathology and Bacteriology 44: 517

Ceremsak R J 1969 Benign rhabdomyoma of the vagina. American Journal of Clinical Pathology 52: 604

Churg A, Ringus J 1978 Ultrastructural observations on the histogenesis of alveolar rhabdomyosarcoma. Cancer 41: 1355

Cori G, Faraggiana T, Grandi C, Nardi F 1977 The diagnostic usefulness of electron microscopy. Investigation of orbital embryonal rhabdomyosarcomas. Tumori 63: 205

Dehner L P, Enzinger F M, Font P L 1972 Fetal rhabdomyoma: an analysis of nine cases. Cancer 30: 160

Enzinger F M, Shiraki M 1969 Alveolar rhabdomyosarcoma: an analysis of 110 cases. Cancer 24: 18

Fenoglio J J, McAllister H A Jr, Ferrans V J 1976 Cardiac rhabdomyoma: a clinicopathological and electron microscopic study. American Journal of Cardiology 38: 241

Gad A, Eusebi V 1975 Rhabdomyoma of the vagina. Journal of Pathology 115: 179

Gale N, Rott T, Kambic V 1984 Nasopharyngeal rhabdomyoma. Path Res Pract 178: 454

Geschickter C F 1934 Tumours of muscle. American Journal of Cancer 22: 378

Gold J H, Bossen E H 1976 Benign vaginal rhabdomyoma: a light and electron microscopic study. Cancer 37: 2283

Gutjahr P, Hutteroth H, Meyer W W 1976 Das primar generalisierte alveolare Rhabdomyosarkom. Klinische Padiatrie 188: 372

Hughes J T 1974 Pathology of muscle. Saunders, Philadelphia

Jenkin R D T 1972 Rhabdomyosarcoma in childhood. In: Godden J O (ed) Cancer in childhood. The Ontario Cancer Treatment and Research Foundation, Toronto, p 157

Kastendieck H, Bocker W, Husselmann H 1976 Zur Ultrastruktur und formalen Pathogenese des embryonalen Rhabdomyosarkoms. Zeitschrift fur Krebsforschung und Klinische Oncologie 86: 55

Keyhani A, Booher R J 1968 Pleomorphic rhabdomyosarcoma. Cancer 22: 956

Knowles D W, Jakobiec F A 1975 Rhabdomyoma of the orbit. American Journal of Ophthalmology 88: 1011

Kyriakos, M 1990 Tumors and tumorlike conditions of the soft tissue. In: Kissane J M (ed) Anderson's pathology, vol 2, ch 37. C V Mosby, St Louis

Lattes R 1982 Tumors of the soft tissues. In: Atlas of tumor pathology. Armed forces Institute of Pathology, Washington DC

Lawrence W, Jegge G, Foote F W Jr 1964 Embryonal rhabdomyosarcoma: a clinicopathological study. Cancer 17: 361

Leone P G, Taylor H B 1973 Ultrastructure of a benign polypoid rhabdomyoma of the vagina. Cancer 31: 1414

Liebner E J 1976 Embryonal rhabdomyosarcoma of head and neck in children: correlation of stage, radiation dose, local control and survival. Cancer 37: 2777

Linscheid R L, Soule E H, Henderson E D 1965 Pleomorphic rhabdomyosarcomata of the extremities and limb girdles. Journal of Bone and Joint Surgery 47A: 715

Maurer H M 1979 Rhabdomyosarcoma. Pediatric Annals 8: 35

Meehan S E, Davie R M 1979 Foetal rhabdomyoma. Journal of the Royal College of Surgeons of Edinburgh 24: 234

Miller R W, Dalager N A 1974 Fatal rhabdomyosarcoma among children in the United States, 1960–69. Cancer 34: 1987

Miller R, Kurtz S M, Powers J M 1978 Mediastinal rhabdomyoma. Cancer 42: 1983

Moore D, Grossi C 1959 Embryonal rhabdomyosarcoma of the head and neck. Cancer 12: 69

Moran J J, Enterline H T 1964 Benign rhabdomyoma of the pharynx: a case report, review of the literature, and comparison with cardiac rhabdomyoma, American Journal of Clinical Pathology 42: 174

Norris H J, Taylor H B 1966 Polyps of the vagina: a benign lesion resembling sarcoma botryoides. Cancer 19: 227

Shimada H, Newton W A, Soule E H, Beltangady M S, Maurer H M 1987 Pathology of fatal rhabdomyosarcoma. Cancer 59: 459

Silverman J F, Kay S, McCue C M, Lower R R, Brough A J, Chang C H 1976 Rhabdomyoma of the heart: ultrastructural study of three cases. Laboratory Investigation 35: 596

Smith H W 1959 Skeletal muscle rhabdomyoma of the larynx: report of a case. Laryngoscope 69: 1528

Sobel H J, Schwarz R, Marquet E 1973 Light and electron microscopic study of the origin of granular cell myoblastoma. Journal of Pathology 109: 101

Solomon M P, Tolete-Velcek, F 1979 Lingual rhabdomyoma (adult variant) in a child. Journal of Pediatric Surgery 14: 91

Fig. 21.6   (A) Sarcoma botyroides. Embryonal rhabdomyosarcoma presenting as a polypoid mass in the vagina of an 11-month-old girl. The loose tissue contains embryonal rhabdomyoblasts. The distinction of this tumour from a harmless adenomatous polyp is most important. H&E, ×60. (B) Sarcoma botyroides. Higher magnification of (A). The picture shows the subepithelial cellular zone (cambium), an important feature of these tumours. H&E, ×130. (A and B from Lattes (1982), with permission)

Stout A P 1946 Rhabdomyosarcoma of the skeletal muscle. Annals of Surgery 123: 447

Stout A P, Lattes R 1967 Tumors of the soft tissue. In: Atlas of tumor pathology, series 2, fasc 1. Armed Forces Institute of Pathology, Washington DC, p 66

Sutow W W, Sullivan M P, Ried H L, Taylor H G, Griffith K M 1970 Prognosis in childhood rhabdomyosarcoma. Cancer 25: 1384

Tefft M, Fernandez C, Donaldson M, Newton W, Moon T E 1978 Incidence of meningeal involvement by rhabdomyosarcoma of the head and neck in children: a report of the intergroup rhabdomyosarcoma study (IRS). Cancer 42: 253

Tuazon R 1969 Rhabdomyoma of the stomach: report of a case. American Journal of Clinical Pathology 52: 37

Walter P, Guerbaoui M 1976 Rhabdomyome foetal: étude histologique et ultrastructural d'une nouvelle observation. Virchows Archiv A: Pathological Anatomy and Histology 371: 59

Weitzner S, Lockery M L, Lockard V G 1979 Adult rhabdomyoma of soft palate. Oral Surgery 47: 70

22. Muscle trauma

Byron A. Kakulas

INTRODUCTION

Skeletal muscle would be expected to be injured frequently for no reason other than its mass. Although much is said about clinical and therapeutic aspects of sports injuries it is a surprise to find so little written on the pathology of muscle trauma. This situation contrasts with the vast literature on bony injuries, consideration of which forms a major part of orthopaedic practice. This apparent paradox is at least partly explained by the great ability of skeletal muscle to compensate for the loss of a substantial part of its bulk as a result either of injury or of surgical removal. Improvement of muscle function is achieved by hypertrophy of the remaining normal muscle tissue and, to a lesser degree, by regeneration. Muscle is also able to resorb large extravasations of blood and to heal with relatively little scar tissue formation. Serious bacterial infections of muscle are uncommon, except in tropical countries; this is probably a reflection of its rich blood supply. Such resistance may also be contributed to by intrinsic biological factors which are at present little understood. A similar phenomenon is the relative resistance of muscle to the establishment within it of metastases of malignant neoplasms.

The crush syndrome is an exception to the rule that muscle injures are usually less important than the bony fracture which they often accompany. The crush syndrome may cause death from renal failure secondary to myoglobinuria. Sports injuries, although not a serious matter in terms of threat to life, also deserve attention because of their effect on athletic performance.

A classification of muscle trauma is given in Table 22.1. Listed separately are the experimental muscle injuries and the traumatic disorders of muscle which form clinical entities.

Table 22.1 A classification of traumatic disorders of skeletal muscle

---

Experimental
Regeneration after crush
Transplantation
Other methods

Clinical
The crush syndrome
Penetrating and non-penetrating injuries without fracture
Muscle injuries in association with bony fracture
Muscle hernia
Muscle and tendon rupture
The anterior tibial syndrome
The over-use syndrome
Birth trauma
Myositis ossificans
Pseudotumour and proliferative myositis
Denervation atrophy
Miscellaneous (pressure necrosis, disuse atrophy and needle myopathies)

Muscle pain, in contrast to the relative un-importance of muscle injuries, is a clinical problem which concerns and preoccupies every medical practitioner. Pain referred to various muscles of the body is an extremely common symptom. Pain is often the result of a visceral lesion which is referred to a muscle served by the same or a contiguous neural segment as is the diseased organ in question. Referred pain may also result from disease in the central nervous system or from peripheral nerve or nerve root irritation or compression. Myalgia is also part of the clinical syndrome of many infective illnesses. Sometimes muscle pain is caused by drugs (Ch. 14). In a small proportion of patients the muscle pain is due to a defined rheumatological syndrome such as rheumatoid arthritis, non-articular rheumatism, polymyalgia rheumatica, polymyositis or myalgic encephalomyelitis.

However, in many patients, the cause of muscle pain is obscure. Without real proof, popular medical opinion holds that such pain is caused by muscle tension resulting from 'psychological tension' in these individuals. In some cases spasm or, more often, tearing of muscle fibres causing local pain results from a minor injury as may happen when an untrained individual undertakes unaccustomed exercise, particularly when this involves forceful eccentric muscle contractions (Clarkson & Tremblay 1988). Spasm and muscle fatigue may also be due to reflex stimulation of motor nerves resulting from compression or irritation of a sensory peripheral nerve or nerve root. It is also believed that the painful nodules which can be palpated in some patients with persistent muscle pain are focal points of muscle spasm. Pain may be relieved in these instances by the injection of local anaesthetic or of corticosteroids into the tender nodule.

Injury to muscle may occur 'post-traumatically' by iatrogenic intervention. One instance is when the blood supply is restricted as occurs in some forms of 'Volkmann's ischaemic contracture' which is usually due to a too-tight plaster cast or to spasm of the brachial artery following supracondylar humeral fracture. Another indirect effect of trauma on muscle is the disuse atrophy which follows tendon or muscle rupture. The same applies to nerve injuries causing denervation atrophy of muscle.

Myopathologists believe that normal muscle may be injured by physiological contraction under strenuous conditions. The consequent minor muscle tear is reflected by a transient rise in the serum creatine kinase (CK) activity in the 24 hours following such vigorous exercise. Microscopic injuries of this type are liable to occur particularly during unaccustomed exercise.

In diseased muscle, injuries resulting from physical exertion may be much more severe. This is particularly the case in denervated muscle. It is assumed that under such circumstances, increases in CK activity reflect polyfocal muscle necrosis secondary to the metabolic 'stress' associated with the unaccustomed exercise, or may simply be due to mechanical rupture of muscle fibres. In the Meyer–Betz syndrome of paroxysmal myoglobinuria there is an inherited predisposition to massive rhabdomyolysis which may be precipitated by sudden exertion. It is also believed that persons susceptible to the malignant hyperthermia syndrome may occasionally develop rhabdomyolysis on violent exertion.

The introduction of magnetic resonance imaging provides a new method for the assessment of muscle injuries. Fleckenstein et al (1989) report their experience with sports-related muscle injuries evaluated with this technique. It has been possible to document structural changes such as fascial herniation, fibrosis, fatty infiltration, while pain associated with strain has been found to be associated with prolongation of muscles T1 and T2. The use of magnetic resonance spectroscopy also promises to provide insights into muscle pain and strain syndromes.

EXPERIMENTAL INJURIES

Experimental injuries of skeletal muscle are mainly used to study regeneration. Post-traumatic regeneration is often of the *heteromorphic* type and is therefore incomplete. Loss of the supporting connective tissues and vascular framework with haemorrhage caused by the experimental trauma leads to healing by scar tissue and to architecturally disorganized regeneration. This eventuality is in contrast to those experimental techniques which injure sarcoplasm alone and which leave the 'scaffolding' of the muscle fibres intact. In this case *isomorphic* regeneration ensues and continues so that muscle restoration is architecturally complete.

Many of the early, pre-1961, experimental studies of muscle regeneration which employed physical methods of damage resulted in the heteromorphic type of response. This probably accounts for the views expressed by some workers who suggested that skeletal muscle possesses only limited powers of regeneration. This myth is still commonly perpetuated outside the field of myology.

Certainly it was not until more recent techniques were introduced which preserve the endomysial framework, e.g. partial ischaemia (Adams 1975), or when experience with various experimental myopathies was used in order to study muscle responses to injury, that the full powers of regeneration of the muscle fibre were demonstrated. Much of this work was based on the experimental studies of the nutritional myopathy of the Rottnest Island quokka (*Setonix brachyurus*) (Kakulas 1961, 1966, 1975).

Regeneration after crush

Volkmann (1893) first studied the effects of crush on muscle. Much later, similar experiments were undertaken by Clark (1946) and Clark & Wajda (1947). Reznik (1973) more recently studied regeneration following muscle injury using a variety of agents including trauma. Post-traumatic necrosis of muscle manifests initially as a disintegration and fragmentation of sarcoplasm and of supporting tissue elements. Phagocytosis of muscle debris and of red cells by macrophages begins within 24 hours.

Young myoblasts soon appear and multiply and join to form multinucleated myotubes. Although some regeneration continues, complete restoration is prevented by the loss of the endomysial and sarcolemmal sheaths. Fibrous scar tissue admixed with muscle fibres is characteristic of heteromorphic regeneration. However, in other experiments Clark (1946) demonstrated that partial ischaemia caused necrosis with preservation of the sarcolemma and endomysium. In this case regeneration was more complete.

Transplantation

The behaviour of skeletal muscle when transplanted is an active area of recent research. This subject is fully reviewed by Mauro (1979) and by Sloper & Partridge (1980). Included among the many studies recorded in Mauro's monograph are many interesting experiments using normal and dystrophic mice. Although regeneration under these conditions is sometimes almost complete, the question concerning the possible 'dystrophic influence' when normal muscle is transplanted into dystrophic host animals, and vice versa, is still not totally resolved. In a study of regeneration of rabbit muscle following freezing, ischaemia and in situ autografting, Vracko & Benditt (1972) concluded that preservation of the basal lamina provided a scaffold for orderly cell replacement.

Other methods

Coagulative necrosis caused by temperature change is fully described by Adams (1975). When frostbite and immersion foot were common in the First World War, degeneration of muscle fibres and fibrosis was reported to result from such injuries. Experimental studies of immersion foot were undertaken by Freidman et al (1950) in animals. They found early coagulative necrosis with hyaline and granular changes of muscle fibres and regeneration in the day succeeding the injury.

Gutmann & Guttmann (1942) studied the effects of electrical stimulation on muscle especially from the point of view of preventing changes secondary to denervation.

Nageotte (1937) studied the shredding effect of electrical stimulation in vitro. AC and DC electrical discharges were studied experimentally in dogs by Smith et al (1965). In these experiments skin and subcutaneous tissue were not injured but the muscle fibres were frankly necrotic with loss of architectural detail. Regardless of the specific type of injury, the end result was the same.

The response of skeletal muscle to X-irradiation was studied by Warren (1943) and Khan (1974). Muscle fibre necrosis secondary to vascular changes was described along with aminoaciduria by Goyer & Yin (1967) following muscle injury induced by X-irradiation.

McGeachie & Grounds (1989) have studied myogenesis in denervated mouse skeletal muscle after injury. They concluded in their study that the onset of myogenesis at 30 hours was essentially the same in denervated and innervated muscle, despite the increased turnover of muscle nuclei and connective tissue cells known to occur in denervation. Carpenter & Karpati (1989) demonstrated that demarcation of segmental necrosis following experimental micropuncture occurs rapidly, the stumps from necrotic segments being covered by a membrane within 7 hours.

With regard to healing following muscle trauma, Lehto & Alanen (1987) correlated sonographic and histological findings 1–21 days in muscle-injured rats. Haematoma was visualized in the first 5 days followed by regenerating muscle which was sonographically better defined than scar tissue, demonstrated histologically. Ultrasonography was therefore shown to be an adequate method for assessing progress.

The effects of microwave radiation on living tissues have been investigated by Surrell et al (1987) who were interested in comparing the changes with those noted in an alleged case of child abuse. Anaesthetized piglets were exposed to radiation in a standard household microwave for varying lengths of time. Characteristic burn patterns were identified in a layered pattern with tissue sparing and burned layers in between. This finding was characteristic of burnt skin and muscle.

In the past several years, experimental cardiac assist operations using latissimus dorsi muscle in dogs, have been applied to patients. Sola et al (1989) have recently reviewed this topic, demonstrating that the technique is feasible in selected patients.

CLINICAL ASPECTS

The crush syndrome

This serious and life-threatening condition arises from massive injuries to muscle usually as part of extensive body trauma. It was common in air-raid casualties in the Second World War due to crush injuries in collapsing buildings. Very high concentrations of myoglobin in the serum are soon reached in these circumstances. However, because of its low renal threshold the myoglobin concentrates and precipitates in the renal tubules and this blockage may cause renal failure. Although the renal failure is at least partly due to this mechanism it has also been attributed to the severe shock associated with injuries of this type as there is always much blood loss into the soft tissues. Cardiac complications with conduction disorders also occur because of the flood of potassium into the bloodstream from the injured muscle.

Penetrating and non-penetrating injuries without fracture

Penetrating injuries are due to sharp instruments, e.g. stab wounds, bullets or any other hard object which might enter the muscle such as often occurs in motor vehicle collisions and in war. Standard surgical treatment usually ensures quick healing of such wounds by scar tissue formation. Even when large quantities of muscle are lost, the amount of residual limb weakness is surprisingly much less than would be expected a first sight.

Demetriades et al (1988) reviewed their experience with 163 patients who suffered penetrating injuries of the diaphragm (knife wounds 139, bullet wounds 24). The diagnosis was missed initially in 10 patients who turned up at a later stage with diaphragmatic hernia. They therefore advocate a high index of suspicion in such circumstances.

Muscle injuries in association with bony fracture

Muscle is always injured in limb fractures but this aspect usually attracts little clinical attention because of its relatively benign nature. Large pieces of muscle may also be removed during surgical procedures when restoring a fracture, e.g. during internal fixation. This is especially true in comminuted fractures.

In a study of muscle injuries associated with bony fractures Anastas & Kakulas (1968) gave particular attention to the regenerative response. Human muscle was obtained from patients undergoing internal fixation for fractures.

A surprisingly wide spectrum of changes was found on histological examination. In seven patients with injuries to the radius and ulna, three showed muscle necrosis and regeneration, two necrosis, one simple atrophy and one was normal. In 33 patients with fractures of the femur and hip, seven showed simple atrophy, two denervation atrophy, three necrosis, six necrosis and regeneration, three scar tissue, six haemorrhage, two inflammation and four were normal. In eight patients with fractures of the tibia and fibula, four showed necrosis, one necrosis and regeneration, two inflammation and one simply atrophy.

In this study an isolated traumatic episode was found to have the ability to induce many of the

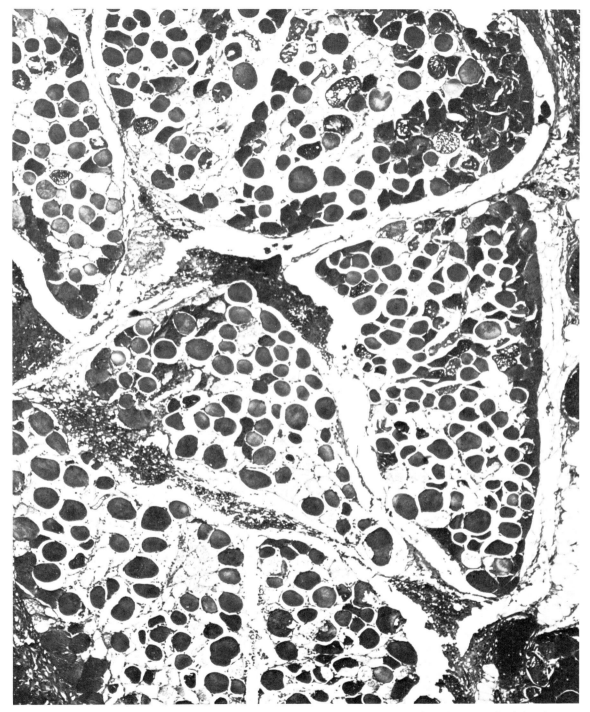

Fig. 22.1   Tibialis anterior muscle in cross-section, removed from the vicinity of a fracture of the tibia 12 h after injury in a 36-year-old man. There is acute swelling and necrosis of muscle fibres with oedema and leucocytic infiltration and haemorrhage. H&E; ×240

recognized forms of myopathological reaction. In individual cases it was possible to select microscopic fields which showed necrosis, acute inflammation, infarction, 'dystrophy-like' changes and severe atrophy. Some of the findings are shown in Figures 22.1, 22.2 and 22.3.

The results of the survey underline the stereotyped nature of skeletal muscle reactions to injury as well as the wide variety of myopathological changes which occur in association with bony injuries.

An important conclusion of the study was the discovery of prominent muscle regeneration even well into old age. Five patients over 70 years of age showed active regeneration of muscle. Both the isomorphic and heteromorphic types of regeneration were observed in the series.

Muscle hernia

The tearing of the epimysium by trauma may give rise to a gap in the sheath through which the muscle belly then protrudes on muscle contraction. Muscle herniae, which are not uncommon, become maximal some days after injury. They are usually asymptomatic but occasionally a hernia may cause pain. Strangulation with consequent necrosis is unusual.

Muscle and tendon rupture

Tendon and muscle rupture are common among athletes or when sudden and unaccustomed violent exercise is undertaken, especially in middle life. The tear may occur in the muscle belly or it may be at the junction of the tendon and muscle. In other cases it is at the point of tendinous insertion into the bone. Traction of digits may also cause muscle rupture (Ponnampalam 1974). These indirect muscle injuries are associated with severe pain and bruising with haemorrhage. If they involve tendons, considerable time is required for healing.

The muscles most frequently ruptured are the biceps, triceps and adductor longus (Peterson & Stener 1976). The rectus abdominis may also rupture, especially in toxaemic states. Kretzler & Richardson (1989) report their experience with surgical repair of pectoralis major muscle in 16 cases as compared with 3 patients in whom repair was not performed. In those operated upon, pain relief was prompt and deformity minimal. No comment is made about those treated conservatively. The topic of Achilles tendon rupture was recently reviewed in a Lancet editorial (Lancet 1989).

The anterior tibial syndrome

Pain and swelling of the anterior tibial compartment is frequent in athletes, for which the term 'shin splints' is used (Adams 1975). More severe degrees of this phenomenon cause massive necrosis of the muscles of the anterior tibial compartment.

The pathogenesis of the condition is not totally clear but it is probably due to muscle swelling as a result of exercise. The swelling leads to impairment of blood supply because of the complete enclosure of the muscle within the anterior tibial fascial sheath. The syndrome is most commonly seen after a prolonged march. The pathological changes are those of ischaemia and variable necrosis of muscle fibres with regeneration. A subacute or chronic syndrome with recurring pain on repeated moderate exercise is recognized. Holden (1974), in an experiment on an amputated limb, showed that increasing interstitial pressure significantly reduced blood flow to the muscles. On this basis he strongly advocated early fasciotomy in appropriate cases. Rorabeck & Macnab (1975) reviewed 45 patients with the anterior tibial compartment syndrome and explored the pathophysiology experimentally. In addition to rising pressure interfering with blood flow they concluded that the concept of 'critical closing pressure' was important in the pathogenesis.

The over-use syndrome

The over-use syndrome or repetitive strain injury has caused a great deal of morbidity among keyboard operators in recent years, especially in Australia. Objective evidence of muscle damage in such individuals has been difficult to demonstrate. However Dennett & Fry (1988) in a muscle biopsy study, showed that in 28 women with painful chronic over-use syndrome, structural differences were in evidence compared with the findings in 8

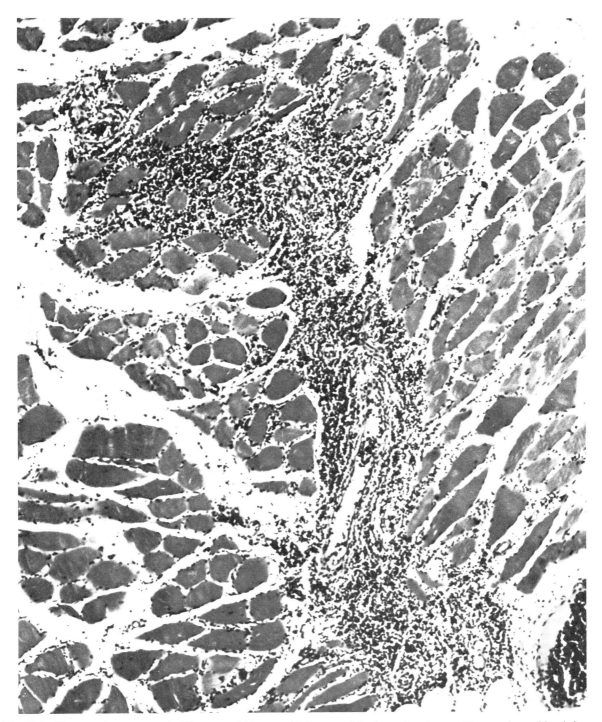

Fig. 22.2 Obturator internus muscle. Woman aged 83 years with fracture of the femoral trochanter. The muscle was biopsied on the day after injury and shows a large number of lymphocytes and polymorphs. H&E; ×240

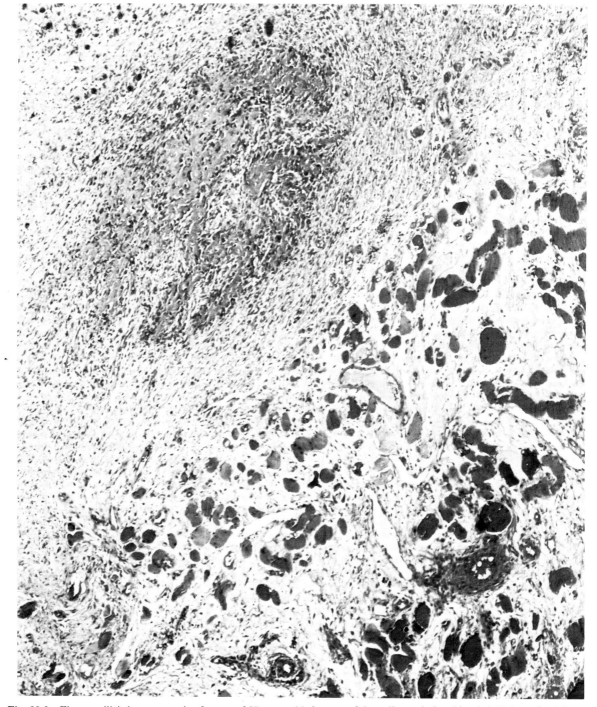

Fig. 22.3 Flexor pollicis longus muscle of a man of 57 years with fracture of the radius and ulna, biopsied 17 days after injury. There is excessive variation in size of muscle fibres, prominent centrally placed nuclei, hyaline changes in sarcoplasm and increase in interstitial connective tissue. In addition, on the left there is osteoid tissue formation representing early traumatic myositis ossificans. H&E; ×240

volunteer controls. The over-use syndrome changes included increased type 1 fibres with type grouping, decreased type 2 fibres and type 2 fibre hypertrophy, increased internal nuclear count, mitochondrial changes and various ultrastructural abnormalities. The changes were related to clinical severity and in the view of the authors, indicated an organic cause of the syndrome.

Birth trauma

Muscle injuries are particularly common in breech delivery. Ralis (1975) examined the muscle of 86 babies who died after breech delivery and of 38 who died after vertex presentation. The most common injury observed in the breech delivery group was injury to the muscles and soft tissues of the back and lower limbs. He concluded that muscle trauma contributed significantly to the death of those infants.

Myositis ossificans

Myositis ossificans is well recognized as a late complication of acute muscle injury (Wilson 1976). In these cases scar tissue, calcification and later ossification result. The inflammatory infiltrate is minor and usually confined to round cells, while the osteoblasts are believed to be derived from the periosteum which has also been traumatized in these individuals.

Calcification of tendons and myotendinous junctions is also a well-known post-traumatic complication. Similar changes in the thigh adductor muscles are not infrequent in patients with spastic paraparesis.

Chronic and repeated injury to muscle may also give rise to ossification and this may be associated with a particular occupation — for instance 'rider's bone' in horse-riders who have developed local ossification in the adductors of the thighs.

In infantrymen, the deltoid or pectoral muscle may ossify. These have been called 'drill bones' (Foster 1988). Fencers and other athletes may develop ossification of the biceps, brachialis or brachioradialis of the arm involved.

Lipscomb et al (1976) advocate conservative management of these cases but good results with reasonable restoration of function have been achieved with surgical excision in long-standing cases where the ossification is restrictive or disabling.

Pseudotumour and proliferative myositis

Localized injury to muscle, especially if repeated, may give rise to a tumour mass. Such masses are believed to originate from muscle regeneration and fibrosis continuing to progress as a result of the stimulation of repeated injury. The mass is contributed to by the very active associated proliferation of connective tissue (Fig. 22.4A, B). Such a localized mass has many features in common with a desmoid tumour (Ramsey 1955) and is akin to a traumatic neuroma of a peripheral nerve. The muscle fibres within the pseudotumours are enlarged and may show polyfocal necrosis and regeneration. Round cell foci in the vicinity of blood vessels are common. In the acute phase of localized injuries of muscle of this type the inflammatory infiltrate is polymorphonuclear. With hyperaemia and oedema these may present clinically as painful lumps.

This finding has given rise to the term 'proliferative myositis' (Fig. 22.5). Although there is a high recurrence rate, the lesions are always benign (Enzinger & Dulcey 1967).

Denervation atrophy

Nerve injuries are also common in association with muscle and bone injury. In this case, denervation atrophy occurs in the muscle supplied by the injured motor nerve. Muscle biopsy undertaken later will reveal histochemical muscle fibre-type grouping. In the later stages, grouped atrophy and hypertrophy will be observed as a result of collateral reinnervation. In those patients in whom regeneration of the nerve occurs, the muscle may also be expected eventually to return to normal but the histochemical fibre-type grouping will persist. Tell-tale nuclear clumps will mark those muscle fibres which were not reinnervated and were thus lost altogether.

Miscellaneous

Pressure necrosis of muscle occurs in patients who lie unconscious for long periods. The calf muscles

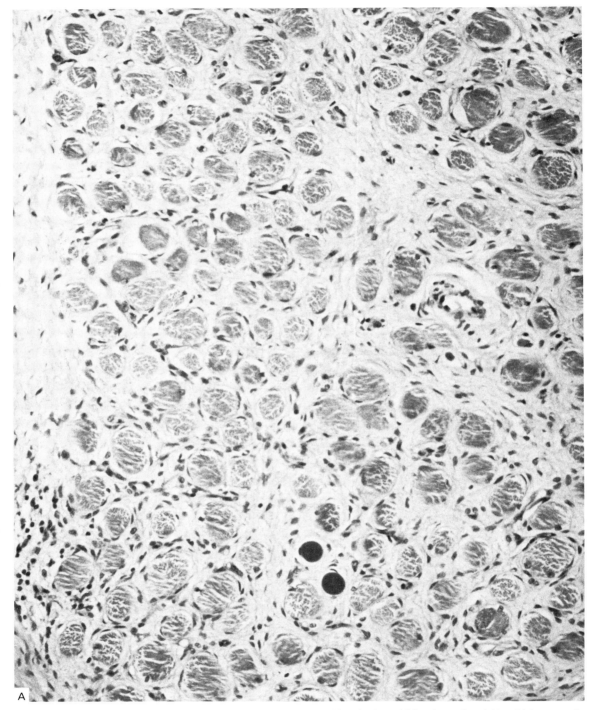

Fig. 22.4 (A) Muscle 'pseudotumour' in a 76-year-old woman with proliferative 'myositis' or 'myosclerosis' in which trauma is believed to be the initiating factor. The muscle in cross-section shows each individual muscle fibre to be surrounded by a thick and cellular fibrous tissue sheath. H&E; ×240

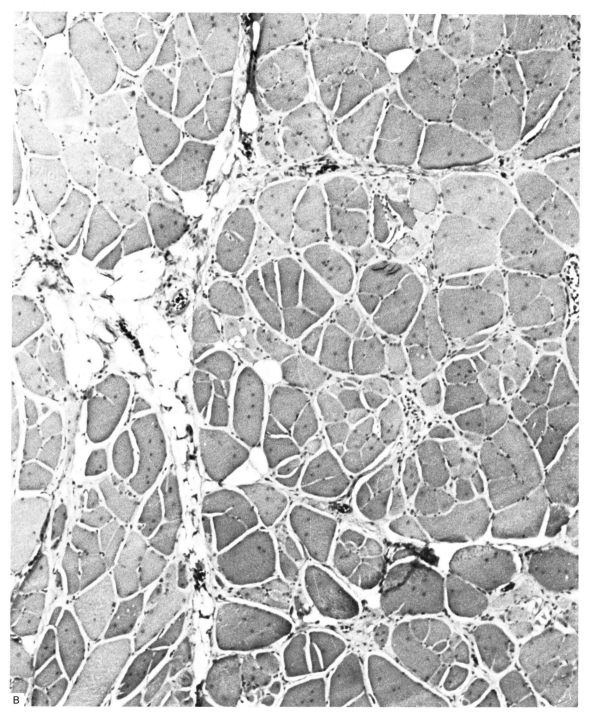

(B) In another field there are pseudomyopathic changes. Muscle fibres are irregular in size and shape. There are split muscle fibres with central nucleation and fibrous tissue and fat increase.

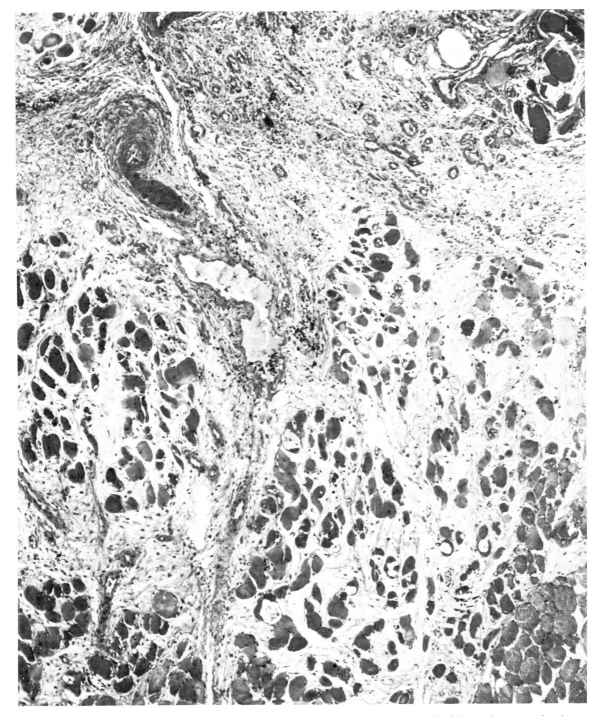

Fig. 22.5 Biopsy of a localized muscle mass in a 35-year-old man showing proliferative myositis with vascular connective tissue infiltrating atrophic and disorganized muscle fascicles. H&E; ×240

are mainly affected in this way. This complication may be associated with myoglobinuria and is clinically signalled by an increase of serum CK activity.

Disuse atrophy is observed in limbs immobilized in plaster casts. Myostatic contracture will also occur when joints are immobilized. In this event the muscle fibre length approximates to the extent to which it is stretched on a daily basis. Chronic and repeated injury to muscle will give rise to *polyphasic monofocal* muscle fibre necrosis. Eventually, pseudomyopathic changes appear in such areas, there is loss of a number of muscle fibres and fibrous tissue proliferation results. At the same time, surviving muscle fibres show disorganization of architecture with variation in size, irregular nuclear distribution and muscle fibre splitting.

Needle myopathy is of some interest because it may give rise to spurious elevations of CK activity after intramuscular injections or electromyography (Hathaway et al 1969, Paakkari & Mumenthaler 1974).

Sjostrom et al (1988) obtained muscle biopsies of a vastus lateralis in five male marathon runners and five sprinters. The biopsy specimens from the sprinters were overall normal in morphology; however, in the marathon runners structural deviations were in evidence. There was irregular size and shape of muscle fibres with increased connective tissue. Central nuclei were also a feature. In some, evidence of fibre type grouping was found. The authors believe that the changes were an expression of a repeated muscle fibre injury. Ahrenholz et al (1988) report serum creatine kinase (CK) elevation as a prognostic indicator in patients who suffered electrical injury. Higher levels were associated with longer hospitalization and a greater risk of skin grafting or amputation than with levels less than 400 U/L.

CONCLUSION

In this review of muscle trauma the known clinical entities within surgical practice have been brought together and reference is made to experimental lesions involving muscle injury.

The relative unimportance of muscle trauma in clinical practice is a reflection of the great power of regeneration and repair inherent in skeletal muscle. It is a maxim of experimental myopathology that, when the cause of focal muscle injury is removed, regeneration goes on to reconstitute the muscle. This potential is observed in human muscle even in the very latest years of life, as indicated in the study of muscle lesions associated with bony injuries described above.

The exception to this rule is observed when injuries of muscle are so severe that vascular damage and endomysial sheath disruption occurs in association with haemorrhage and tearing of the muscle. In these cases, proliferation of fibroblasts leads to scar tissue formation, while the breakdown of the supporting framework of the muscle fibre interferes with its full regenerative potential. The term 'heteromorphic regeneration' is used in this situation. The early experiments on muscle regeneration were hampered by this phenomenon, in that the physical injury caused disruption of the structural and supporting tissues and thus led to scar tissue formation. The popular but false assumption that muscle possesses limited powers of regeneration was based on this observation.

On the other hand, the study of metabolic myopathies demonstrates the great powers of muscle regeneration. In these conditions the supporting framework is preserved. This principle was well demonstrated in the Rottnest Island quokka (*Setonix brachyurus*) and is now known to hold for skeletal muscle generally, regardless of species (Kakulas 1975).

Trauma to previously diseased muscle is of special interest. In the early stages of denervation the myopathologist is constantly reminded of the appearance of regeneration because of the presence of features such as basophilia (due to an increase in the number of ribosomes) and the enlargement of muscle nuclei with prominent nucleoli. In these cases the regenerative changes may have been due to preceding necrosis caused by injury and associated clinically with elevation of the serum CK activity. When stretch is applied to denervated muscle it may show sustained hypertrophy and even hyperplasia (Sola et al 1973).

In the Meyer–Betz syndrome of paroxysmal rhabdomyolysis or myoglobinuria, massive breakdown of muscle with consequent myoglobinuria is precipitated by sudden or extreme exercise. The cause of this phenomenon is unknown. However, there is a parallel in the veterinary field when farm animals (especially horses) which have been placed in barns for the winter are suddenly exercised. The condition is thought to be due to a relative deficiency of vitamin E which produces an acute myopathy on sudden exertion in the spring.

Trauma may play a part in the pathogenesis of some human diseases of muscle, such as polymyositis and myalgic encephalomyelitis. It is postulated that in these conditions a virus enters the muscle after minor trauma and remains dormant. The infection may then become active due to a recurrence of the trauma some years later. Antigens may than be produced which contain molecules common to the virus and the host tissues. Such antigens may then stimulate an immune reaction against host tissue and virus and may bring about the presumptive autoimmune disorder.

ACKNOWLEDGEMENT

The photomicrographs were prepared by Mr Philip J. Morling BSc.

REFERENCES

Adams R D 1975 Diseases of muscle. A study in pathology, 3rd edn. Harper & Row, New York

Ahrenholz D H, Schubert W, Solem L D 1988 Creatine kinase as a prognostic indicator in electrical injury. Surgery 104: 741

Anastas N C, Kakulas B A 1968 Muscle lesions associated with bony injuries. Proceedings of the Australian Association of Neurologists 5: 545

Carpenter S, Karpati G 1989 Segmental necrosis and its demarcation in experimental micropuncture injury of skeletal muscle fibres. Journal of Neuropathology and Experimental Neurology 48: 154

Clark W E Le Gros 1946 An experimental study of the regeneration of mammalian striped muscle. Journal of Anatomy 80: 24

Clark W E Le Gros, Wajda H S 1947 The growth and maturation of regenerating striated muscle fibres. Journal of Anatomy 81: 56

Clarkson P M, Tremblay I 1988 Exercise-induced muscle damage. Journal of Applied Physiology 65: 1

Demetriades D, Kakoyiannia S, Parekh D, Hazitheofilou C 1988 Penetrating injuries of the diaphragm. British Journal of Surgery 75: 824

Dennett X, Fry H J 1988 Overuse syndrome: a muscle biopsy study. Lancet i: 905

Enzinger F M, Dulcey F 1967 Proliferative myositis — report of 33 cases. Cancer 20: 2213

Fleckenstein J L, Weatherall P T, Parkey R W, Payne J A Peshock R M 1989 Sports-related muscle injuries: evaluation with MR imaging. Radiology 172: 793

Foster J B 1988 The clinical features of some miscellaneous neuromuscular disorders. In: Walton J N (ed) Disorders of voluntary muscle, 5th edn. Churchill Livingstone, Edinburgh, p 891

Freidman N B, Lange H, Wiener D 1950 Pathology of experimental immersion foot. Archives of Pathology 49: 21

Goyer R A, Yin N W 1967 Taurine and creatine excretion after X-irradiation and plasmocid-induced muscle necrosis in the rat. Radiation Research 30: 301

Gutmann E, Guttman L 1942 Effect of electrotherapy on denervated muscles in rabbits. Lancet i: 169

Hathaway P W, Dahl D P, King Engel W 1969 Myopathic changes produced by local trauma. Archives of Neurology (Chicago) 21: 355

Holden C E A 1974 Traumatic tension ischaemia in muscle injury. British Journal of Accident Surgery 5: 223

Kakulas B A 1961 Myopathy affecting the Rottnest quokka (Setonix brachyurus) reversed by α-tocopherol. Nature 191: 402

Kakulas B A 1966 Regeneration of skeletal muscle in the Rottnest quokka. Australian Journal of Experimental Biology and Medical Science 44: 673

Kakulas B A 1975 Experimental muscle diseases. Methods and achievements in experimental pathology, vol 7. S Karger, Basel, p 109

Kakulas B A 1981 Drug and toxic myopathies. In: Riddell R H (ed) The pathology of drug and toxic disorders. Churchill, London

Khan M Y 1974 Radiation-induced changes in skeletal muscle: an electron-microscopic study. Journal of Neuropathology and Experimental Neurology 33: 42

Kretzler H H Jnr, Richardson A B 1989 Rupture of the pectoralis major muscle. American Journal of Sports Medicine 17: 453

Lancet (editorial) 1989 Achilles tendon rupture. Lancet i: 1427

Lehto M, Alanen A 1987 Healing of a muscle trauma. Correlation of sonographical and histological findings in an experimental study in rats. Journal of Ultrasound in Medicine 6: 425

Lipscomb A B, Thomas E D, Johnston R K 1976 Treatment of myositis ossificans traumatica in athletes. American Journal of Sports Medicine 4: 111

Mauro A (ed) 1979 Muscle regeneration. Raven Press, New York

McGeachie J K, Grounds M D 1989 The onset of myogenesis in denervated mouse skeletal muscle regenerating after injury. Neuroscience 28: 509

Nageotte J 1937 Sur la contraction extrème des muscles squeletiques chez les vertébrés. Zeitschrift für Zellforschung und Mikroskopische Anatomie 26: 603

Paakkari J, Mumenthaler M 1974 Needle myopathy — an experimental study. Journal of Neurology 208: 133

Peterson L, Stener B 1976 Old total rupture of the adductor longus muscle. A report of seven cases. Acta Orthopedica Scandinavica 47: 653

Ponnampalam M S 1974 Rupture of muscles by traction. Injury 5: 237

Ralis Z A 1975 Birth trauma to muscles in babies born by breech delivery and its possible fatal consequences. Archives of Disease in Childhood 50: 4

Ramsey R H 1955 The pathology, diagnosis and treatment of extra-abdominal desmoid tumours. Journal of Bone and Joint Surgery 37A: 1012

Reznik M 1973 Regeneration experimentale de la fibre musculaire squelettique adulte. Annales de l'Anatomie Pathologique 108: 91

Rorabeck C H, Macnab I 1975 The pathophysiology of the anterior tibial compartmental syndrome. Clinical Orthopaedics and Related Research 113: 52

Sjostrom M, Johansson C, Lorentzon R 1988 Muscle pathomorphology in m. quadriceps of marathon runners. Early signs of strain disease or functional adaptation? Acta Physiologica Scandinavica 132: 537

Sloper J C, Partridge T A 1980 Skeletal muscle: regeneration and transplantation studies. British Medical Bulletin 36: 153

Sola O M, Christensen D L, Martin A W 1973 Hypertrophy and hyperplasia of adult chicken anterior latissimus dorsi muscles following stretch with and without denervation. Experimental Neurology 41: 76

Sola O M, Kakulas B A, Dillard D H, Ivey T D, Thomas R, Martin A W, Shoji Y, Fujiyama H 1989 The stretch factors in muscle transformation: gross and cytoarchitectural changes. In: Chiu R, Bourgeois I (eds) Transformed muscle for cardiac assist and repair, ch 6. Future, New York

Smith G T, Beeuwkes R, Tomkiewicz Z M, Tadaaki A, Town B 1965 Pathological changes in skin and skeletal muscle following alternating current and capacitor discharge. American Journal of Pathology 47: 1

Surrell J A, Alexander R C, Cohle S D, Lovell F R Jr, Wehrenberg R A 1987 Effects of microwave radiation on living tissues. Journal Traumatization 27: 935

Volkmann R 1893 Ueber die Regeneration des quergstreiften Muskelgewebes beim Menschen und Saugethier. Beitrage zue pathologischen Anatomie und zue allgemeinen Pathologie 12: 233

Vracko R, Benditt E P 1972 Basal lamina: the scaffold of orderly cell replacement. Journal of Cell Biology 55: 406

Warren S 1943 Effects of radiation on normal tissues. XIV. Effects on striated muscle. Archives of Pathology 35: 347

Wilson J N 1976 Myositis and traumatic ossification. In: Wilson J N (ed) Watson-Jones' fractures and joint injuries. Churchill Livingstone, Edinburgh, p 81

23. Disuse, cachexia and aging

F. G. I. Jennekens

INTRODUCTION

It is for practical reasons that disuse, cachexia and old age will be discussed in one chapter. The main histopathological feature of these diverse conditions is atrophy of muscle fibres. Disuse causing muscular weakness may be present in patients who have been immobilized for prolonged periods. Interest in this condition has been stimulated by theoretical issues, one of these being whether atrophy of denervated fibres should be considered to be a consequence of inactivity. Cachexia is a major problem in many patients in underdeveloped countries. It is seen occasionally in patients with cancer and in the elderly. Aging implies a decrease in locomotor activity, in motor performance and in muscle volume.

DISUSE

The size of muscle fibres is determined multi-factorially. Influence is exerted by such factors as activity and innervation, hormones, growth, stretch and nutrition. Disuse in the sense of inactivity leads to muscle atrophy as is well known from clinical experience. The morphological and histochemical changes underlying this atrophy have been studied in human muscle biopsies and in experimental animal models.

Investigations of human muscle biopsies

Investigations of disuse in human muscles are sparse, probably because of the difficulty of obtaining adequate material. The muscle atrophy which occurs with inactivity may be considerable.

In a group of patients examined by Gibson et al (1987) the cross-sectional area of the quadriceps muscle at mid-thigh level fell by 17% in a period of 6 weeks of immobilization following a fracture of the distal third of the tibia. The mean fibre size in the same muscle decreased in a period of 8 weeks' immobilization by approximately 50% (Dastur et al 1979).

One of the main issues in the research on disuse has been whether there is a preferential atrophy of one of the major fibre types. Selective or preferential atrophy of type 1 as well as of type 2 fibres has been reported. Engel (1965) was the first to specify that disuse caused a greater degree of atrophy of type 2 than of type 1 fibres. In transverse sections the atrophic fibres were slightly elongated and angulated. He suggested that type 2 fibre atrophy in this and in other conditions reflected a preferential susceptibility of type 2 fibres to loss of neural trophic influence (Engel 1970). In accordance with this contention, the ultrastructural findings in four patients with type 2 fibre atrophy due to cachexia and disuse were found to resemble those in the early stages of denervation atrophy (Mendell & Engel 1971). The Z discs showed smearing but there were no core or target formations. The loss of myofilaments was greatest at the periphery of the fibres, and scattered areas of myofibrillar loss were observed in the interior. In the atrophic fibres the sarcoplasmic reticulum was more prominent than usual. The numerical decrease in mitochondria approximately paralleled the loss of myofibrils. No striking increase of lysosomes or residual bodies was observed (Mendell & Engel 1971, Dastur et al 1979).

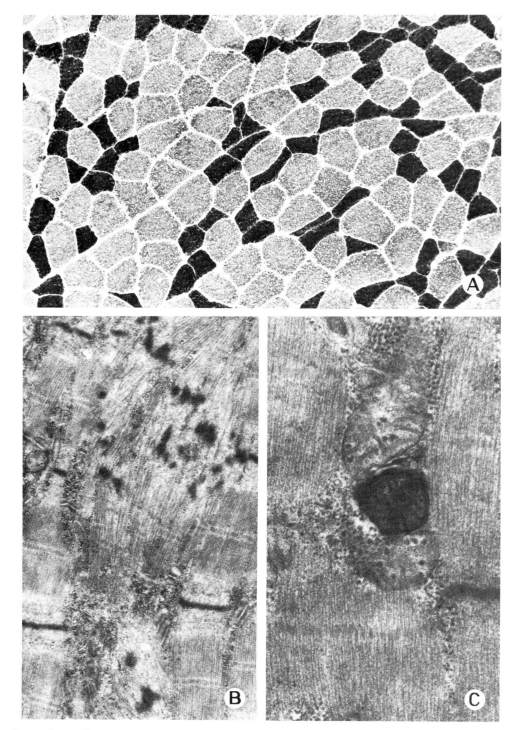

Fig. 23.1   A case of type 2 fibre atrophy. (A) Myosin ATPase, pH 9.4: there is little variation in size of the type 1 fibres. Type 2 fibres are smaller than type 1 fibres and some type 2 fibres are obviously atrophic; ×210. (B) Electron micrograph: focal disorganization of sarcomere structure in one of the atrophic fibres; ×19 600. (C) Darkly stained mitochondrion enwrapped by a membrane in another small fibre, probably a secondary lysosome; ×51 450

Type 2 atrophy was reported by several authors in conditions of decreased activity caused by various forms of arthritis. Brooke & Kaplan (1972) studied muscle biopsies from patients with non-painful rheumatoid arthritis. They noted atrophy of the type 2B fibres in particular, which they considered to be a specific effect of inactivity (Fig. 23.1). Preferential atrophy of type 2 fibres was also observed in large series of patients with degenerative arthritis of the hip (Bundschu et al 1973, Širca & Sušec-Michieli 1980). Comparison with control biopsies showed that this was not purely an age-related effect (Širca & Sušec-Michieli 1980)

Type 1 fibre atrophy was seen in patients with long-standing injuries of the anterior cruciate ligament of the knee. These fibres are thought to be engaged in the maintenance of muscle tone. It was postulated that the instability in the knee joint was physiologically comparable to a tendinous injury and would interfere with spindle activity. This would lead to loss of activity of red (type 1) fibres and to disuse atrophy (Edström 1970). Tenotomy is known to cause preferential atrophy of red fibres (Engel et al 1966). Immobilization of the lower limb in cases of fracture of the tibia caused in the quadriceps muscle atrophy mainly of type I fibres (Young et al 1982, Gibson et al 1987).

A change in muscle protein turnover was found to be responsible for muscle atrophy during disuse; protein synthesis was reduced whilst protein breakdown remained approximately at the same level. Daily, low-intensity electrical stimulation prevented lowering of protein synthesis and decrease in quadriceps muscle cross-sectional area (Gibson et al 1988).

Muscle activity influences not only fibre sizes but also fibre type proportions. Investigations on this subject were initially concentrated on the effect of training and of electrical stimulation (Gollnick et al 1973, Munsat et al 1976). Subsequently it was demonstrated that immobilization or lack of training increases the ratio of type 2B:2A fibres (Andersen & Henriksson 1977, Jansson & Kayser 1977). Sudden immobilization of a well-trained individual was reported to result in a marked decrease in the percentage of type 1 fibres (Jansson et al 1978).

Animal models

Experimental investigations have for long been hampered by the fact that no satisfactory disuse model was available. Spinal cord transection, spinal cord isolation (cordotomy and dorsal root sectioning), tenotomy, immobilization, compression of a peripheral nerve by a pneumatic cuff, local anaesthesia of a peripheral nerve, and other pharmacological methods have been used and have been criticized for various reasons (Guth & Albuquerque 1979). Immobilization in plaster casts or by placing pins in knee and ankle joints, has been used by many authors. It does not result in complete disuse but it is a relatively simple method with the additional advantage that it mimics the situation in patients treated for lower limb fractures (Dastur et al 1979).

An almost ideal animal model has been available for some time. Local application of tetrodotoxin (TTX) to a peripheral nerve blocks axonal conduction by specific blockage of sodium channels in the axolemma. It does not damage the nerve structurally and does not interfere with fast axonal transport nor with spontaneous acetylcholine release. If locally applied to a nerve, it does not act systemically on muscle fibre membranes. The effect of TTX is therefore considered to be attributable to impulse blockade (Lavoie et al 1976, Pestronk et al 1976, Stanley & Drachman 1979).

Disuse induced by one of the older methods may lead to four kinds of change: decrease in fibre size, changes in fibre lengths and in fibre type, and architectural changes in occasional fibres. As the latter type of change is non-specific and considered to be due to unwanted complications, it will not be discussed here. Decrease in fibre size has been reported to develop equally in the two fibre types (Karpati & Engel 1968), preferentially in white, fast glycolytic fibres (Riley & Allin 1973, Herbison et al 1978, Lindboe & Presthus 1985) and preferentially in red, slow oxidative fibres (Maier et al 1972, see also Jaffe et al 1978). The experiments provide no ready explanation for these discrepancies. Herbison et al (1978) suggested that the activity of the fibre types might differ, depending upon the specific function of the muscle concerned. In muscles used predominantly for phasic activity, fast glycolytic fibres may be recruited more often than other fibres. Disuse might then cause preferential atrophy of fast glycolytic fibres. In muscles used predominantly for static functions, atrophy might develop preferentially in oxidative fibres. The ultrastructural changes in experimental disuse atrophy are similar to those in the initial stages of denervation atrophy (Klinkerfuss & Haugh 1970, Cooper 1972).

The time course of the development of atrophy in immobilized limbs varies depending upon the degree of stretch that is applied to the muscle (Booth 1977). Stretch stimulates protein synthesis (Goldspink 1977); fixation of a muscle in a lengthened position delays atrophy and may even cause hypertrophy of the fibres. The number of sarcomeres in the lengthened fibre increases until maximal tension can again be developed (Williams & Goldspink 1978). Immobilization in a shortened position leads to a decrease in the number of sarcomeres. It increases the percentage of white fibres in rat soleus (Herbison et al 1978), but does not affect the number of muscle fibres (Cardenas et al 1977).

TTX-induced disuse of the gastrocnemius muscle produces a more marked degree of atrophy than joint fixation (St-Pierre & Gardiner 1985). TTX-disused soleus muscle has a distinctly higher percentage of fast-oxidative-glycolytic (type 2A) and a lower percentage of slow-twitch-oxidative (type 1) fibres than normal (Spector 1985). Apparently inactivity causes some type I fibres to transform into IIA fibres.

Disuse versus denervation

In recent years the question of the difference between denervation and disuse in the sense of the inactivity which each induces has attracted considerable interest. Two approaches have been used to tackle this problem. First, by means of TTX and other advanced techniques, the effects of disuse and denervation have been analysed and compared. Secondly, attempts have been made to counteract the effects of denervation by direct electrical stimulation of the muscle.

It has already been pointed out in previous paragraphs that the morphological changes caused by disuse show a close resemblance to those

following denervation. Disuse as well as denervation leads to a decreased resting membrane potential (Albuquerque & McIsaac 1970, Stanley & Drachman 1979), decreased protein synthesis and increased protein breakdown (Goldspink 1977, Margreth et al 1977), decreased muscle acetylcholinesterase (Butler et al 1978), the appearance of extrajunctional acetylcholine receptors (see Edwards 1979 for review), and sprouting of intramuscular nerve fibres (Brown & Ironton 1977, Snider & Harris 1979). On the other hand, muscle activity induced by electrical stimulation prevents many of the changes following denervation (Pestronk & Drachman 1978, see Lömo 1976 for review).

Despite all the similarities between disuse and denervation, a number of subtle differences remain. There is less sprouting in conditions of disuse than after denervation (Brown & Ironton 1977). The decrease in resting membrane potential begins later and reaches a peak later in disuse than in denervation (Stanley & Drachman 1979). The density of extrajunctional acetylcholine receptors produced by disuse is less than that caused by denervation (Lavoie et al 1976, Pestronk et al 1976, Gilliatt et al 1978). One possible explanation for the dissimilarities in the two conditions is spontaneous (that is, not nerve-impulse evoked) release of acetylcholine or of another specialized but as yet unidentified trophic factor (Stanley & Drachman 1979). Denervation-related changes are not however influenced by miniature end-plate potentials (Deshpande et al 1980). Oh & Markelonis (1979) have isolated a protein from peripheral nerve that exerts a trophic effect on cultured muscle in the absence of innervation. Davis et al (1985) reported that mammalian peripheral nerve contains a trophic factor which ameliorates denervation atrophy. Cangiano & Lutzemberger (1979) suggested that the difference between disuse and denervation might be caused by a specific effect of nerve fibre degeneration products on the muscle fibre membrane.

CACHEXIA

Anyone involved in the microscopic examination of muscle tissue obtained at biopsy or necropsy is confronted regularly with the histopathology of this condition. The causes of cachexia are multi-tudinous, undernutrition still being the most frequent. Experimental investigations of the consequences of food deprivation and chronic undernutrition have produced some interesting data. Food deprivation in rats or monkeys leads to loss of body weight and loss of muscle volume (Lindboe & Presthus 1985, Chopra et al 1987). Biochemical investigations have shown that the muscle DNA content remains unchanged; however, food deprivation causes a decrease in the muscle RNA level, a marked decrease in protein synthesis and a variable degree of increase in protein breakdown (Goldspink 1978, Li et al 1979). In terms of histopathology this means that food deprivation causes atrophy of muscle fibres. The magnitude of the changes depends to some extent on the anatomical location of the muscle (Spence & Hansen-Smith 1978). In rats the trunk muscles tend to change most, while the distal forelimb muscles change least. There is evidence that white muscle fibres atrophy more than red fibres (Walsh et al 1971). Ultrastructural studies have revealed focal or generalized disorganisation or dissolution of myofibrils, apparently without lysosomal stimulation (Hansen-Smith et al 1978). Of particular interest is the effect of undernutrition in the neonatal period upon subsequent muscle growth. This problem has been investigated by Williams & Hughes (1978) in rats. The authors compared the growth of pups from large and control litters. The degree of muscle growth retardation due to large litter size and consequent undernutrition was about 20 per cent. Catch-up growth took many months. At the end of the experiment (after 228 days) female rats had caught up to normal, but muscle width in male rats was still below the normal limit.

The histopathological features of muscle cachexia in adult humans have been described in reports based on investigations at necropsy (Tomlinson et al 1969, Rebeiz et al 1972). In mild cases the muscle fibres in various limb muscles are normal in appearance but smaller than usual. Single fibres are sharply angulated. Type 2 fibres are more atrophic than type 1 fibres (Engel 1970). When cachexia is severe, the decrease in fibre size is marked and large groups of atrophic fibres are often seen. The changes are generally more severe in the lower limbs than in the upper limbs. Protein malnutrition in infants may reduce the muscle fibres to a size comparable to that of fetal muscle fibres (Montgomery 1962). The proportion of satellite cells in skeletal muscles of malnourished children is significantly below that of well-nourished children of the same age (Hansen-Smith et al 1979).

AGING

Skeletal muscle performance

In comparison with that in young people, muscle volume is decreased in elderly subjects (Tzankoff & Norris 1977) and muscle strength is diminished. The latter contention is not only supported by general experience but has been demonstrated and analysed in studies of muscle function. In men, muscle strength is highest in the third decade (Kamon & Goldfuss 1978). Although it may decrease a little, this level is generally maintained until approximately 50 years of age. In the sixth decade, maximal dynamic and isometric strength declines slightly but unmistakably and this trend continues in senescence (Burke et al 1953, Larsson et al 1979, Aniansson et al 1986). Contraction velocity and speed of movement decrease as well, at least in muscles which have been examined in this respect (Campbell et al 1973, Larsson et al 1979, Davies et al 1986). If the decline in maximal strength is taken into account, it transpires that, up to 65 years of age, muscle endurance does not diminish and even a tendency to increase has been shown (Petrofsky & Lind 1975, Larsson & Karlsson 1978). Exercise can, however, produce improvement in strength and aerobic power (Young 1986). The results of these physiological investigations can be explained on the basis of what is now known about the histological and histochemical changes in muscle.

Pathology

Aging is a continuous process. In successive decades more age-related changes appear and new types of change develop. Aging is not expressed in the same manner and to the same degree in different skeletal muscles. Until now few data are available on aging of the external eye muscles and laryngeal muscles and this holds to a lesser extent for intercostal and other trunk muscles. The following account therefore deals primarily with skeletal limb muscles.

Four kinds of alteration may be discerned in aged limb muscles: a decrease in numbers of fibres, a shift in the proportions of fibre types, neurogenic muscular atrophy, and structural and histochemical changes within muscle fibres.

Fibre numbers, fibre type proportions and sizes

The assessment of total numbers of fibres in large limb muscles has become feasible through the introduction of new techniques. Lexell et al (1983, 1988) studied cross-sections of whole vastus lateralis muscle and found significantly fewer fibres in aged subjects than in young adults. As myopathic changes in muscles of aged individuals are rare, and neurogenic changes very common, the loss of fibres was attributed to denervation. A decrease in the number of fibres was also found in the human vocalis muscle (Sato & Tauch 1982) and in animal muscles (Caccia et al 1979).

Larsson et al (1978) examined muscle tissue obtained by needle biopsy from 55 healthy untrained sedentary men 22–65 years old. In the third decade the proportion of type 1 fibres in the vastus lateralis was approximately 40%. Other investigators found an almost similar percentage at this age (Gollnick et al 1972, Johnson et al 1973). No marked changes were observed until the sixth decade. Between 50 and 60 years, however, the proportion of type 1 fibres increased to 50% and between 60 and 65 years to 55%. No change could be demonstrated in the proportions of the subtypes of type 2 fibres. Lexell et al (1988) however found a slightly higher proportion of type 1 fibres in young adults than did Larsson et al (1978) and no obvious change in fibre type proportions with age. Studies in rats have demonstrated marked differences between muscles. In the rat extensor digitorum longus the percentage of slow oxidative and fast oxidative/glycolytic fibres increased markedly in old age. In the rat soleus, which contains almost exclusively slow oxidative fibres at middle age, the percentage of slow fibres decreased in old age whereas the proportion of fast oxidative

glycolytic fibres increased to about 45% (Caccia et al 1979).

Several authors have reported a decrease in the shortest diameter or cross-sectional area of type 2 fibres with age, whereas there is little, if any, reduction in the size of type 1 fibres (Jennekens et al 1971, Tauchi et al 1971, Tomonaga 1977, Larsson et al 1978, Širca & Sušec-Michieli 1980, Aniansson et al 1986, Poggi et al 1987, Lexell et al 1988). A reduction in level of activity has been put forward as the explanation for this change.

Neurogenic muscular atrophy and type grouping

The variation in size of the muscle fibres is often larger in senescent subjects than in young or middle-aged adults. This is partly attributable to selective atrophy of type 2 fibres, but in some cases the atrophic fibres are of both types and all of the characteristic features of denervation and re-innervation may then be encountered. Neurogenic muscle changes are most frequent and severe in distal limb muscles, particularly in the lower limbs (Tomlinson et al 1969, Jennekens et al 1971, Moore et al 1971, Adams 1975, Tomonaga 1977) but are also seen in the vastus lateralis muscle (Lexell et al 1986, Poggi et al 1987), the biceps brachii and deltoid muscles (Aniansson et al 1986, Oertel 1986) and the external intercostal muscles (Wokke et al 1990) and should therefore be considered as a general feature of the skeletal musculature in old age. Differences between adjacent muscles may be marked. In a comparative investigation of four distal lower limb muscles, it was observed that atrophy of muscle fibres and fibre type grouping were present in all specimens of the extensor digitorum brevis muscle which were examined, from young adults and older subjects (Jennekens et al 1972). Neurogenic changes in the flexor digitorum brevis were less striking and appeared later. The results suggested further that neurogenic changes were more frequent and more extensive in the flexor digitorum brevis than in the tibialis anterior and gastrocnemius muscles. Neurogenic muscular atrophy in the latter two muscles is not usually present before the eighth decade. Obvious evidence of type grouping is present frequently in proximal limb muscles in the eighth and ninth decades (Fig. 23.2).

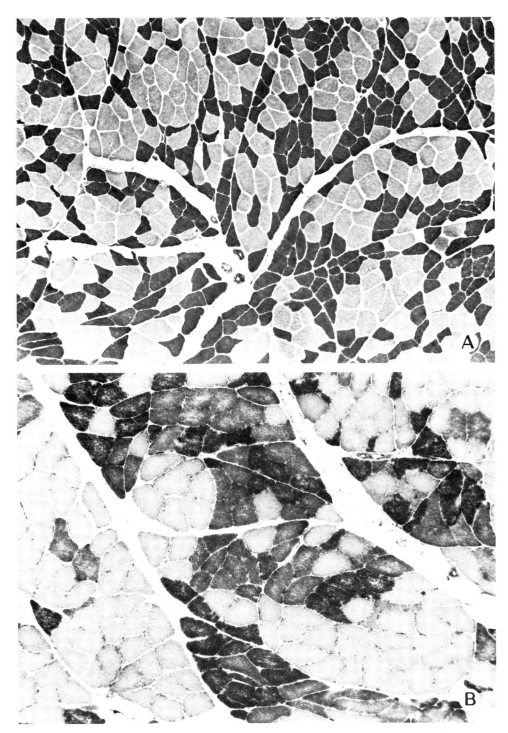

Fig. 23.2 Sections from two consecutive biopsies of proximal lower limb muscles from women aged 86 and 83 years respectively. (A) Myosin ATPase, pH 9.4: the mosaic pattern is replaced in part by small histochemically uniform groups of type 1 and type 2 fibres. There is disseminated atrophy of type 2 fibres and of some type 1 fibres; ×84. (B) Menadione-linked α-GPD showing type grouping; ×84

There is little difficulty in explaining these neurogenic changes. It is well known that the number of myelinated nerve fibres decreases and that the frequency of structural changes in the myelin sheaths and axons increases from about middle age (Ochoa & Mair 1969). Tomlinson & Irving (1977) have demonstrated that the number of motor neurones in the lumbosacral cord decreases by about 25% between youth and old age. The loss is slight until 60 years and is variable but often marked thereafter.

Structural changes in muscle fibres

At the light-microscope level, structural changes are inconspicuous up to about the eighth decade, at least in limb muscles of healthy active old people (Shafiq et al 1978). Even after the age of 70 years, muscle fibres are nearly all normal but occasional structural and degenerative changes may appear. These include internal nuclei, cytoplasmic bodies, rods, ring fibres, ragged-red fibres, necrosis and phagocytosis (Fig. 23.3) (Jennekens et al 1971, Tomonaga 1977, Shafiq et al 1978, Aniansson et al 1986). Tomonaga (1977) states that these changes develop predominantly in the trunk and proximal limb muscles. Massive necrobiosis in the triceps surae, apparently due to disturbance of the vascular supply, has been observed incidentally on necropsy (Tomlinson et al 1969, Jennekens et al 1972).

Attempts have been made to elucidate the basis for the decrease in muscle function which occurs with age, by investigation of specific organelles; although these studies do not allow definite conclusions to be reached, the results are of interest. Up to at least 70 years of age, the nucleocytoplasmic ratio (the relationship between fibre size and the number and sizes of the myonuclei) remains constant (Vassilopoulos et al 1977). According to Tomonaga (1977) some myonuclei in senile muscles are abnormally small and deformed. Deformation of the nuclear membrane was observed also by Fujisawa (1975) in aged rats. Myonuclei of aged mice and rats have varying amounts of heterochromatin (Snow 1977). It should be added here that in aged laboratory animals the rate of RNA synthesis in muscle nuclei and the rate of protein turnover in muscle

fibres are diminished in comparison with adult animals (Britton et al 1972, Florini 1978, Millward 1978). Satellite cells in old animals appear to be dormant, like those in adult animals. Heterochromatin is a typical feature of the nucleus, nucleoli are observed rarely (Schultz 1976, Snow 1977), and there is a paucity of cytoplasmic organelles in these cells. Basal lamina material may occupy part of the satellite cell–myofibre interspace or may wholly separate the satellite cell from the muscle fibre. The basal lamina which envelops the muscle fibre usually does not thicken with age (Snow 1977, Vracko 1979). The proportion of satellite cell nuclei to the total number of nuclei in myofibres in the soleus muscle in mice is 4.6% in young animals and 4.3% in middle-aged animals. In old age — if cells fully separated by basal lamina material are excluded — the proportion drops to 2.4% (Snow 1977). A decline of satellite cell proportions with advancing age was also found in rat muscles (Gibson & Schultz 1983). Schmalbruch & Hellhammer (1976) examined human muscle tissue from nine subjects, aged 7–45 years. Four per cent (range 2.5–6.7) of the nuclei within the basal laminae of the muscle fibres belonged to satellite cells. In the extensor digitorum longus of a 73-year-old man the proportion was 0.6%. It is clear that further investigations concerning a possible loss of satellite cells with aging are necessary.

Reports on age-related changes of the contractile units are few and do not allow any useful conclusions to be drawn. Shafiq et al (1978) noted only occasional changes in myofibrils in biopsy specimens from unspecified muscles from eight subjects (aged 70–83 years) and referred to rare streaming of Z discs or accumulation of Z-disc like material in irregular dense structures. Tomonaga (1977) observed frequent disorganization of sarcomere structure, thinning or streaming of Z discs and occasional nemaline rods in biopsy specimens from various muscles taken from 79 subjects (aged 60–90 years). According to Fujisawa (1975), myofibrillar degeneration occurs frequently in aged rat skeletal muscle. Myosin ATPase activity has been reported not to undergo any significant alterations (Ermini 1976).

Comments upon morphological changes of the sarcoplasmic reticulum and the sarcotubular

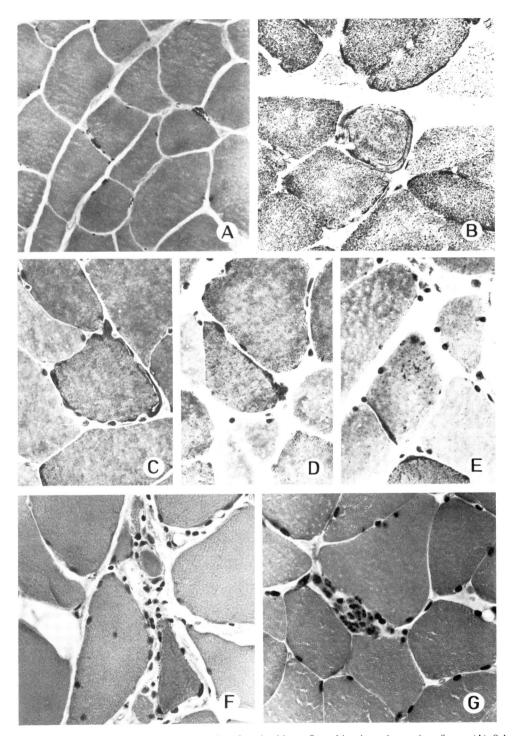

Fig. 23.3 Various changes in proximal lower limb muscles of aged subjects. Same biopsies as in previous figure. (A) Schmorl's method; subsarcolemmal accumulations of lipofuscin granules; ×280. (B) NADH–TR: ring fibre; ×315. (C) Modified Gomori trichrome: ragged red fibre; ×315. (D) Modified Gomori trichrome: rods located perinuclearly; ×350. (E) Modified Gomori trichrome; transversely sectioned rod-like structures dispersed in a fibre; ×350. (F) H&E: slight mononuclear cell reaction in between a few small fibres; ×280. (G) H&E: phagocytosis of a muscle fibre; ×315

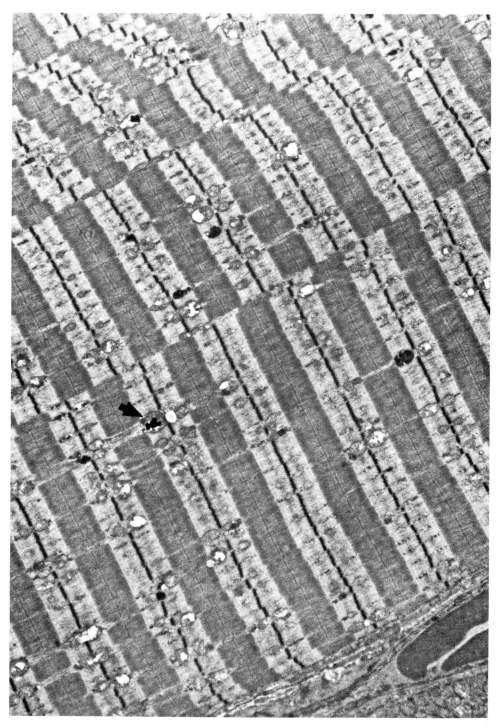

Fig. 23.4   Electron micrograph of a muscle fibre from the vastus lateralis muscle of an 86-year-old woman. Same case as in Figure 23.2A. In several places dense structures instead of mitochondria are present between I bands. Lipid material is enclosed in some mitochondria (arrow). Note that, unlike the situation in type 2 fibre atrophy and denervation, the sarcomere structure is preserved; ×6300

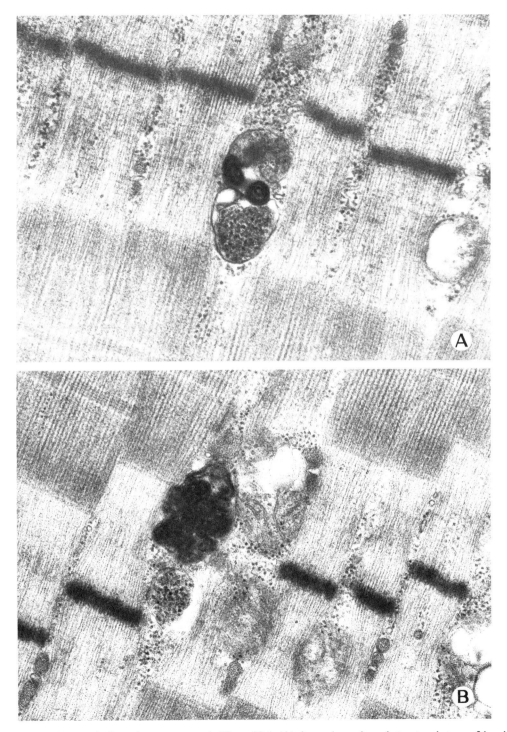

Fig. 23.5 Electron micrographs from the same case as in Figure 23.4. (A) A membrane-bound structure between I bands contains lipid material and glycogen granules. The location of this structure suggests that it is an abnormal mitochondrion; ×41 650.
(B) There is a dense structure between I bands with features of a secondary lysosome; ×51 450

system are few (Inesi 1978). Stereological investigation of rat muscle showed a reduction in volume and surface densities of sarcoplasmic reticulum and of the T-tubular system in old animals which was thought to influence excitation–contraction coupling (De Coster et al 1981). Dilatation of these structures has been observed occasionally (Tomonaga 1977, Shafiq et al 1978), sometimes in association with myofibrillar degeneration (Fujisawa 1975). More work has been done on the energy supply systems and processes. The number of mitochondria in middle-aged men is equal to, or higher than, that in young adults (Kiessling et al 1974, Örlander et al 1978). The mean volume, however, tends to become smaller. In the seventh decade, mean volume, total volume as well as number are significantly decreased (Örlander et al 1978, Poggi et al 1987). The changes are more marked in subsarcolemmal than in intermyofibrillar mitochondria, which is another indication that these two mitochondrial populations have different functions within the muscle fibre (Hülsmann 1970, Palmer et al 1977). The mitochondria do not fully escape from ultrastructural alterations (Figs 23.4, 23.5). Apparently these changes occur late and only in occasional fibres of some individuals (Tomonaga 1977, Örlander et al 1978). Biochemical investigation of state III (activated) respiration rates in isolated intact mitochondria from vastus lateralis muscle showed a significant decline with age which was thought to be related to error accumulation in mitochondrial DNA (Trounce et al 1989). These findings have not yet been confirmed by other authors.

Lipofuscin is invariably present in muscle tissue from elderly subjects and is usually accumulated in subsarcolemmal regions near myonuclei (Fig. 23.3). It is occasionally present in satellite cells (Snow 1977). Exactly how the granules originate in the muscle fibres is unknown (Shafiq et al 1978). The lipofuscin granules are to be considered as lysosomal residual bodies and accordingly they possess acid phosphatase activity. It is generally assumed that the formation of lipofuscin is due to peroxidation of unsaturated fatty acids. An age-related fluorescent substance has been shown to accumulate particularly in tissues classified as aerobic (Shimasaki et al 1977). There is some evidence that lipofuscin occurs more frequently in type 1 than in type 2 fibres (Örlander et al 1978). Acid phosphatase activity is relatively high in fibres which also have high activity of aerobic enzymes, but no clear-cut relation with the level of myosin ATPase activity could be demonstrated (Lojda & Gutmann 1976). Gutmann et al (1976) suggested that there might be a relationship between acid phosphatase activity and the relatively high rate of protein breakdown in slow ('red') muscle fibres.

ACKNOWLEDGEMENTS

The author is grateful to Mrs A. Jennekens–Schinkel for stimulating interest and helpful discussions. The photographs were prepared by Mr H. Veldman and Mr H. J. W. Eelderink.

REFERENCES

Adams R D 1975 Diseases of muscle: a study in pathology, 3rd edn. Harper & Row, Hagerstown
Albuquerque E X, McIsaac R J 1970 Fast and slow mammalian muscles after denervation. Experimental Neurology 26: 183
Andersen P, Henriksson J 1977 Training-induced changes in the subgroups of human type II skeletal muscle fibres. Acta physiologica scandinavica 99: 123
Aniansson A, Hedberg M, Henning G-B, Grimby G 1986 Muscle morphology, enzymatic activity and muscle strength in elderly men: a follow-up study. Muscle and Nerve 9: 585
Booth F W 1977 Time course of muscular atrophy during immobilization of hind limbs in rats. Journal of Applied Physiology 43: 656
Britton V J, Sherman F G, Florini J R 1972 Effect of age on RNA synthesis by nuclei and soluble RNA polymerases from liver and muscle of C 57 BL/6 J mice. Journal of Gerontology 27: 188
Brooke M H, Kaplan H 1972 Muscle pathology in rheumatoid arthritis, polymyalgia rheumatica and polymyositis. Archives of Pathology 94: 101
Brown M C, Ironton R 1977 Motor neurone sprouting induced by prolonged tetrodotoxin block of nerve action potentials. Nature 265: 459
Bundschu H D, Suchenwirth R, D'Avis W 1973 Histochemical changes in disuse atrophy of human skeletal muscle. In: Kakulas B A (ed) Basic research in myology, part I, Proceedings of the 2nd International Congress on Muscle Diseases. Excerpta Medica International Congress Series no. 294, Amsterdam, p 108
Burke W E, Tuttle W W, Thompson C W, Janney C D, Weber R J 1953 The relation of grip strength and grip-strength

endurance to age. Journal of Applied Physiology 5: 628

Butler I J, Drachman D B, Goldberg A M 1978 The effect of disuse on cholinergic enzymes. Journal of Physiology 274: 593

Caccia M R, Harris J B, Johnson M A 1979 Morphology and physiology of skeletal muscle in aging rodents. Muscle and Nerve 2: 202

Campbell M J, McComas A J, Petito F 1973 Physiological changes in ageing muscles. Journal of Neurology, Neurosurgery and Psychiatry 36: 174

Cangiano A, Lutzemberger L 1979 Effects of afferent nerve fibre degeneration on membrane properties of skeletal muscle fibres. Neuroscience Letters supplement 3, p 18 (abstract)

Cardenas D D, Stolov W C, Hardy R 1977 Muscle fiber number in immobilization atrophy. Archives of Physical and Medical Rehabilitation 10: 423

Chopra J S, Metha J, Rana S V, Dhand U K, Mehta S 1987 Muscle involvement during postnatal protein calorie malnutrition and recovery in rhesus monkeys. Acta Neurologica Scandinavica 75: 234

Cooper R R 1972 Alterations during immobilization and regeneration of skeletal muscle in cats. Journal of Bone and Joint Surgery 54A: 919

Dastur D K, Gagrat B M, Manghani D K 1979 Human muscle in disuse atrophy. Neuropathology and Applied Neurobiology 5: 85

Davies C T M, Thomas D O, White M J 1986 Mechanical properties of young and elderly human muscle. Acta Medica Scandinavica Suppl 711: 219

Davies H L, Heinicke E A, Cook R A, Kiernan J A 1985 Partial purification from mammalian peripheral nerve of a trophic factor that ameliorates atrophy of denervated muscle. Experimental Neurology 89: 159

DeCoster W, DeReuck J, Sieben G, VanDerEecken H 1981 Early ultrastructural changes in aging rat gastrocnemius muscle: a stereologic study. Muscle and Nerve 4: 111

Deshpande S S, Warnicke J E, Guth L, Albuquerque E X 1980 Quantal release of acetylcholine does not regulate the resting membrane potential of mammalian skeletal muscle: evidence from in vivo experiments. Experimental Neurology 70: 122

Edström L 1970 Selective atrophy of red muscle fibres in the quadriceps in long-standing knee-joint dysfunction. Injuries to the anterior cruciate ligament. Journal of the Neurological Sciences 11: 551

Edwards C 1979 The effects of innervation on the properties of acetylcholine receptors in muscle. Neuroscience 4: 565

Engel W K 1965 Histochemistry of neuromuscular disease — significance of muscle fiber types. In: Proceedings of the 8th International Congress of Neurology 2. Excerpta Medica Foundation, Amsterdam, p 67

Engel W K Selective and nonselective susceptibility of muscle fibre types. Archives of Neurology (Chicago) 22: 97

Engel W K, Brooke M H, Nelson P G 1966 Histochemical studies of denervated or tenotomized cat muscle. Annals of the New York Academy of Sciences 138: 160

Ermini M 1976 Ageing changes in mammalian skeletal muscle. Biochemical studies. Gerontology 22: 301

Florini J R 1978 Biosynthesis of contractile proteins in normal and aged muscle. In: Kaldor G, DiBattista W J (eds) Aging in muscle. Raven Press, New York, ch 3, p 49

Fujisawa K 1975 Some observations on the skeletal musculature of aged rats, 2. Fine morphology of diseased muscle fibres. Journal of the Neurological Sciences 24: 447

Gibson M C, Schultz E 1983 Age-related differences in absolute numbers of skeletal muscle satellite cells. Muscle and Nerve 6: 574

Gibson J A, Halliday D, Morrison W L et al 1987 Decrease in human quadriceps muscle protein turnover consequent upon leg immobilization. Clinical Science 72: 503

Gibson J N A, Smith K, Rennie M J 1988 Prevention of disuse muscle atrophy by means of electrical stimulation: maintenance of protein synthesis. Lancet ii: 767

Gilliatt R W, Westgaard R H, Williams I R 1978 Extrajunctional acetylcholine sensitivity of inactive muscle fibres in the baboon during prolonged nerve pressure block. Journal of Physiology 280: 499

Goldspink D F 1977 The influence of immobilization and stretch on protein turnover of rat skeletal muscle. Journal of Physiology 264: 267

Goldspink D 1978 The effects of food deprivation on protein turnover and nuclei acid concentrations of active and immobilized extensor digitorum longus muscle of the rat. Biochemical Journal 176: 603

Gollnick P D, Armstrong R B, Saubert C W, Piehl K, Saltin B 1972 Enzyme activity and fiber composition in skeletal muscle of untrained and trained men. Journal of Applied Physiology 33: 312

Gollnick P D, Armstrong R B, Saltin B, Saubert C W, Sembrowich W L, Shepherd R E 1973 Effect of training on enzyme activity and fiber composition of human skeletal muscle. Journal of Applied Physiology 34: 107

Guth L, Albuquerque E X 1979 The neurotrophic regulation of resting membrane potential and extrajunctional acetylcholine sensitivity in mammalian skeletal muscle. In: Mauro A (ed) Muscle regeneration. Raven Press, New York, p 405

Gutmann E, Lojda Z, Teisinger J 1976 Changes of acid phosphatase activity of fast and slow muscles during ontogenetic development. Histochemistry 49: 227

Hansen-Smith F M, van Horn D L, Maksud M G 1978 Cellular response of rat quadriceps muscle to chronic dietary restrictions. Journal of Nutrition 108: 248

Hansen-Smith F M, Picou D, Golden A M H 1979 Muscle satellite cells in malnourished and nutritionally rehabilitated children. Journal of the Neurological Sciences 41: 207

Herbison G J, Jaweed M M, Ditunno J F 1978 Muscle fiber atrophy after cast immobilization in the rat. Archives of Physical and Medical Rehabilitation 59: 301

Hülsmann W C 1970 Two types of mitochondria in heart muscle from euthyroid and hyperthyroid rats. Biochemical Journal 116: 32P

Inesi G 1978 The sarcoplasmic reticulum: structure, function and development. In: Kaldor G, DiBattista W J (eds) Aging in muscle. Raven Press, New York, ch 8, p 159

Jaffe D M, Terry R D, Spiro A J 1978 Disuse atrophy of skeletal muscle. A morphometric study using image analysis. Journal of the Neurological Sciences 35: 189

Jansson E, Kayser L 1977 Muscle adaptation to extreme endurance training in man. Acta physiologica scandinavica 100: 315

Jansson E, Sjödin B, Tesch P 1978 Changes in muscle fibre type distribution in man after physical training. A sign of fibre type transformation? Acta physiologica scandinavica 104: 235

Jennekens F G I, Tomlinson B E, Walton J N 1971 Histochemical aspects of five limb muscles in old age. An autopsy study. Journal of the Neurological Sciences 14: 259

Jennekens F G I, Tomlinson B E, Walton J N 1972 The extensor digitorum brevis: histological and histochemical aspects. Journal of Neurology, Neurosurgery and Psychiatry 35: 124

Johnson M A, Polgar J, Weightman D, Appleton D 1973 Data on the distribution of fibre types in 36 human muscles. An autopsy study. Journal of the Neurological Science 18: 111

Kamon E, Goldfuss A J 1978 In-plant evaluation of the muscle strength of workers. American Industrial Hygiene Association Journal 39: 801

Karpati G, Engel W K 1968 Correlative histochemical study of skeletal muscle after suprasequential denervation, peripheral nerve section and skeletal fixation. Neurology (Minneapolis) 18: 681

Kiessling K-H, Pilström L, Bylund A-Ch, Saltin B, Piehl K 1974 Enzyme activities and morphometry in skeletal muscle of middle-aged men after training. Scandinavian Journal of Clinical and Laboratory Investigations 33: 63

Klinkerfuss G H, Haugh M J 1970 Disuse atrophy of muscle. Histochemistry and electron microscopy. Archives of Neurology (Chicago) 22: 309

Larsson L, Karlsson J 1978 Isometric and dynamic endurance as a function of age and skeletal muscle characteristics. Acta physiologica scandinavica 104: 129

Larsson L, Sjödin B, Karlsson J 1978 Histochemical and biochemical changes in human skeletal muscle with age in sedentary males, age 22–65 years. Acta physiologica scandinavica 103: 31

Larsson L, Grimby G, Karlsson J 1979 Muscle strength and speed of movement in relation to age and muscle morphology. Journal of Applied Physiology 46: 451

Lavoie P A, Collier B, Tenenhouse A 1976 Comparison of α-bungarotoxin binding to skeletal muscle after inactivity or denervation. Nature 260: 349

Lexell J, Henriksson-Larsen K, Winblad B, Sjostrom M 1983 Distribution of different fiber types in human skeletal muscles: effects of aging studied in whole muscle cross sections. Muscle and Nerve 6: 588

Lexell J, Downham D, Sjostrom M 1986 Distribution of different fibre types in human skeletal muscle. Fibre type arrangement in m. vastus lateralis from three groups of healthy men between 15 and 83 years. Journal of the Neurological Sciences 72: 211

Lexell J, Taylor C C, Sjostrom M 1988 What is the cause of the ageing atrophy? Total number, size and proportion of different fiber types studied in whole vastus lateralis muscle from 15 to 83 year-old men. Journal of the Neurological Sciences 84: 275

Li J B, Higgins J E, Jefferson L S 1979 Changes in protein turnover in skeletal muscle in response to fasting. American Journal of Physiology 236: E222

Lindboe C F, Presthus J 1985 Effects of denervation, immobilization and cachexia on fibre size in the anterior tibial muscle of the rat. Acta Neuropathologica (Berlin) 66: 42

Lojda Z, Gutmann E 1976 Histochemistry of some acid hydrolases in striated muscles of the rat. Histochemistry 48: 1

Lömo T 1976 The role of activity in the control of membrane and contractile properties of skeletal muscle. In: Thesleff S (ed) Motor innervation of muscle. Academic Press, London, p 289

Maier A, Eldred E, Edgerton V R 1972 The effects on spindles of muscle atrophy and hypertrophy. Experimental Neurology 37: 100

Margreth A, Carraro U, Salviati G 1977 Effects of denervation on protein synthesis and on properties of myosin in fast and slow muscles. In: Rowland L P (ed) Pathogenesis of human muscular dystrophies. Proceedings of the 5th International Scientific Conference of the Muscular Dystrophy Association. Excerpta Medica International Congress Series no. 404, Amsterdam, p 161

Mendell J R, Engel W K 1971 The fine structure of type II muscle fibre atrophy. Neurology (Minneapolis) 21: 358

Millward D J 1978 The regulation of muscle-protein turnover in growth and development. Biochemical Society Transactions 6: 494

Montgomery R D 1962 Muscle morphology in infantile protein malnutrition. Journal of Clinical Pathology 15: 511

Moore M J, Rebeiz J J, Holden E M, Adams R D 1971 Biometric analysis of normal skeletal muscle. Acta neuropathologica (Berlin) 19: 51

Munsat T L, McNeal D, Waters R 1976 Effects of nerve stimulation on human muscle. Archives of Neurology (Chicago) 33: 608

Ochoa J, Mair W G P 1969 The normal sural nerve in man. 2. Changes in the axons and Schwann cells due to ageing. Acta neuropathologica (Berlin) 13: 217

Oertel G 1986 Changes in human skeletal muscle due to ageing. Histological and histochemical observations on autopsy material. Acta Neuropathologica (Berlin) 69: 309

Oh T H, Markelonis G J 1979 Neurotrophic effects of a protein fraction isolated from peripheral nerves on skeletal muscle in culture. In: Mauro A (ed) Muscle regeneration. Raven Press, New York, p 417

Örlander J, Kiessling K-H, Larsson L, Karlsson J, Aniansson A 1978 Skeletal muscle metabolism and ultrastructure in relation to age in sedentary men. Acta physiologica scandinavica 104: 249

Palmer J W, Tandler B, Hoppel C L 1977 Biochemical properties of subsarcolemmal and interfibrillar mitochondria isolated from rat cardiac muscle. Journal of Biological Chemistry 252: 8731

Pestronk A, Drachman D B 1978 Motor nerve sprouting and acetylcholine receptors. Science 199: 1223

Pestronk A, Drachman D B, Griffin J W 1976 Effect of muscle disuse on acetylcholine receptors. Nature 260: 352

Petrofsky J S, Lind A R 1975 Aging, isometric strength and endurance and cardiovascular responses to static effort. Journal of Applied Physiology 38: 91

Poggi P, Marchetti C, Seels R 1987 Automatic morphometric analysis of skeletal muscle fibres in the aging man. Anatomical Record 217: 30

Rebeiz J J, Moore M J, Holden E M, Adams R D 1972 Variations in muscle status with age and systemic diseases. Acta neuropathologica (Berlin) 22: 127

Riley D A, Allin E F 1973 The effects of inactivity, programmed stimulation and denervation on the histochemistry of skeletal muscle fiber types. Experimental Neurology 40: 391

Sato T, Tauch H 1982 Age changes in human vocal muscle. Mechanisms of Ageing and Development 18: 67

St-Pierre D, Gardiner P F 1985 Effect of disuse on mammalian fast-twitch-muscle: joint fixation compared with neurally applied tetrodotoxin. Experimental Neurology 90: 635

Schmalbruch H, Hellhammer U 1976 The number of satellite cells in normal muscle. Anatomical Record 185: 279

Schultz E 1976 Fine structure of satellite cells in growing skeletal muscle. American Journal of Anatomy 147: 49

Shafiq S A, Lewis S G, Dimino L C, Schutta H S 1978 Electron microscopic study of skeletal muscle in elderly subjects. In: Kaldor G, DiBattista W J (eds) Ageing in muscle. Raven

Press, New York, ch 4, p 65

Shimasaki H, Nozawa T, Privett O S, Anderson W R 1977 Detection of age-related fluorescent substances in rat tissues. Archives of Biochemistry and Biophysics 183: 443

Širca A, Sušec-Michieli M 1980 Selective type II fibre muscular atrophy in patients with osteoarthritis of the hip. Journal of the Neurological Sciences 44: 149

Snider W D, Harris G L 1979 A physiological correlate of disuse-induced sprouting at the neuromuscular junction. Nature 281: 69

Snow M H 1977 The effects of ageing on satellite cells in skeletal muscles of mice and rats. Cell and Tissue Research 185: 399

Spector S A 1985 Effects of elimination of activity on contractile and histochemical properties of rat soleus muscle. Journal of Neuroscience 5: 2177

Spence C A, Hansen-Smith F M 1978 Comparison of the chemical and biochemical composition of thirteen muscles of the rat after dietary protein restriction. British Journal of Nutrition 39: 647

Stanley E F, Drachman D B 1979 Effect of disuse on the resting membrane potential of skeletal muscle. Experimental Neurology 64: 231

Tauchi H, Yoshioka T, Kobayashi H 1971 Age changes of skeletal muscles of rats. Gerontologia 17: 219

Tomlinson B E, Irving D 1977 The number of limb motor neurons in the human lumbosacral cord throughout life. Journal of the Neurological Sciences 34: 213

Tomlinson B E, Walton J N, Rebeiz J J 1969 The effects of ageing and of cachexia upon skeletal muscle. A histopathological study. Journal of the Neurological Sciences 9: 321

Tomonaga M 1977 Histochemical and ultrastructural changes in senile human skeletal muscle. Journal of the American Geriatric Society 25: 125

Trounce I, Byrene E, Marzuki S 1989 Decline in skeletal muscle mitochondrial respiratory chain function: possible factor in ageing. Lancet i: 637

Tzankoff S P, Norris A H 1977 Effect of muscle mass decrease on age-related BMR changes. Journal of Applied Physiology 43: 1001

Vassilopoulos D, Lumb E M, Emery A E H 1977 Karyometric changes in human muscle with age. European Neurology 16: 31

Vracko R 1979 Basal lamina scaffold. In: Créteil L R (ed) Frontiers of matrix biology 7. Karger, Basel, p 78

Walsh G, DeVivo D, Olson W 1971 Histochemical and ultrastructural changes in rat muscle. Archives of Neurology (Chicago) 24: 83

Williams P E, Goldspink G 1978 Changes in sarcomere length and physiological properties in immobilized muscle. Journal of Anatomy 127: 459

Williams J P G, Hughes P C R 1978 Muscle growth during neonatal undernutrition and subsequent rehabilitation in the rat. Acta anatomica 101: 249

Wokke J H J, Jennekens F G I, van den Oord C J M, Veldman H, Smit L M E, Leppink G J 1990 Morphological evidence of remodelling in the human endplate with age. Journal of the Neurological Sciences 95: 291

Young A 1986 Exercise physiology in geriatric practice. Acta Medica Scandinavica Suppl 711: 227

Young A, Hughes I, Round J M, Edwards R H T 1982 The effect of knee injury on the number of muscle fibres in the human quadriceps femoris. Clinical Science 62: 227

24. Myositis ossificans, myosclerosis and other miscellaneous disorders

Eijiro Satoyoshi   Ikuya Nonaka

MYOSITIS (FIBRODYSPLASIA) OSSIFICANS

Calcareous deposition in the subcutaneous tissue and skeletal muscle may occur in various diseases (Wheeler et al 1952) such as calcinosis universalis (Davis & Moe 1959), dermatomyositis (Muller et al 1959), tumours, hypercalcaemia and myositis ossificans. Myositis ossificans is characterized clinically by ectopic bone formation in skeletal muscle and subcutaneous tissue and has been classified into two major forms, circumscribed (myositis ossificans circumscripta and pseudo-malignant osseous tumour of soft tissue) and progressive. Because the muscle fibre is thought to be secondarily affected in this disorder, the term 'myositis' has occasionally been substituted for 'fibrodysplasia' or 'fibrositis'. Although a connective tissue abnormality seems to play a part in the ectopic bone formation, the basic pathogenetic mechanism remains unknown.

Myositis (fibrodysplasia) ossificans progressiva

This inherited, congenital disorder affects not only the muscle, but also the subcutaneous tissue, fascia, and aponeuroses, with the formation of strips and masses of bone in these tissues. While the term myositis ossificans progressiva was coined by Dusch in 1868, a number of cases had been noted since 1692 when Patin first described the symptoms of this unique disorder (Rosenstirn 1918). Rosenstirn (1918) reviewed 120 cases (including his own case) from the literature, and Lutwak (1964) estimated that approximately 260 cases had been reported in the world literature from 1700 to 1963.

The disease is probably inherited as an autosomal dominant trait, though almost all of the reported cases have been sporadic, with a few familial cases (Lutwak 1964). An effect of advanced paternal age on the incidence may reflect a high mutation rate in the dominant condition (Tünte et al 1967, Rogers & Chase 1979, Conner & Evans 1982). Although this disorder was initially thought to be limited to the Anglo-Saxon race, recent reports indicate that all races may be involved. More than 60 cases have been described in Japan, and several cases in Indians (Grewal & Dass 1953, Sastri & Yadav 1977) and Africans (Ebrahim et al 1966, Conner & Beighton 1982). The earlier reports suggested that the disorder occurred more commonly in males, in a ratio of 4:1 (Ryan 1945), but in larger groups of patients in cumulative studies the incidence was approximately the same in males and females (Lutwak 1964, Rogers & Geho 1979).

The disease usually becomes manifest in early childhood, usually before the age of 4 years, and almost all patients have various congenital anomalies involving the toes and fingers. The most commonly recognized anomaly is microdactyly or adactyly of the great toes which may be seen in 75–90% of cases and may be the hallmark of the disorder before muscle symptoms appear. In addition, almost half of the patients have short thumbs and clinodactyly, and there may also be deformity of the ears, deafness and absence of teeth (Lutwak 1964, Ludman et al 1968, Rogers & Geho 1979). The presence of these various anomalies reflects the congenital nature of the disorder and the onset of the disease state in fetal life. Similar anomalies have also been described in relatives without muscle and connective tissue involvement (Sympson 1886, Stonham 1892, Knoots 1927, Creveld & Soeters 1941).

The initial hot and tender swelling or soft tissue nodule tends to localize over the neck and in the proximal portions of the extremities and dorsal regions. The lesion may appear at the site of trauma, but usually the injury itself does not play a major part. The swellings disappear as days or weeks go by, and the affected areas then become indurated. The tumours may be cystic and contain bloody fluid which may at times be extruded from the skin.

After repeated episodes of swelling and induration, columns, masses or plates of bone appear in the soft tissues and may replace tendon, fascia and skeletal muscles (Fig. 24.1). Wry neck is a common symptom attributable to the lesions in the sternocleidomastoid muscles, and the spine may become rigid, with or without kyphoscoliosis. The masseter is occasionally involved, but the tongue, diaphragm, sphincter muscles and the heart are not affected. Although death from respiratory failure or pneumonia may occur in early adult life, a number of patients have survived to fairly advanced ages but have been severely disabled.

Laboratory examination may not help to clarify the underlying pathogenetic mechanism. Serum calcium, alkaline phosphatase and creatine kinase levels are within normal limits or slightly increased. The electromyogram shows either a myopathic pattern (Smith et al 1966, Chaco 1967), or non-specific changes.

Pathology

Although the initial pathological changes are still not clear, the main pathogenetic process seems to take place in the connective tissue around the muscle. As indicated by the alternative label of fibrocellulitis ossificans progressiva which was proposed by Rosenstirn (1918), the early affected area is occasionally inflammatory with haemorrhage and connective tissue proliferation. The interstitial haemorrhage may lead to abnormal collagen outgrowth followed by cartilage and bone formation encircling the haemorrhagic mass (Rosenstirn 1918, Magruder 1926, Fairbank 1950).

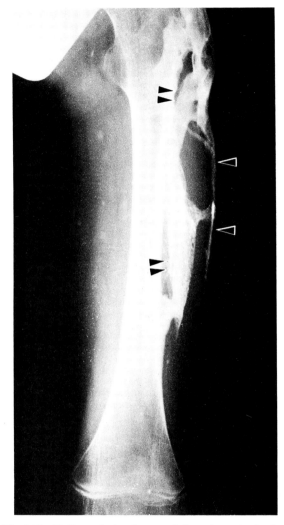

Fig. 24.1 Radiograph showing ectopic bone formation in the subcutaneous tissue (arrowheads) and muscle (double arrowheads) of the left femur. An 11-year-old Japanese girl with myositis ossificans progressiva. (Courtesy of Dr Y. Une, Kitakyushu, Fukuoka. Figs. 24.1 and 24.3 from same case)

The areas of the proliferated connective tissue occasionally resemble a fibroma or fibrosarcoma (Paul 1925, Geschickter & Masteritz 1938) and the cytoplasm of the cells contains mannose-rich glycoprotein as demonstrated by the concanavalin A and horseradish peroxidases methods (Maxwell et al 1977). On electron microscopy the tumour-like cells show a hyperplastic granular endoplasmic

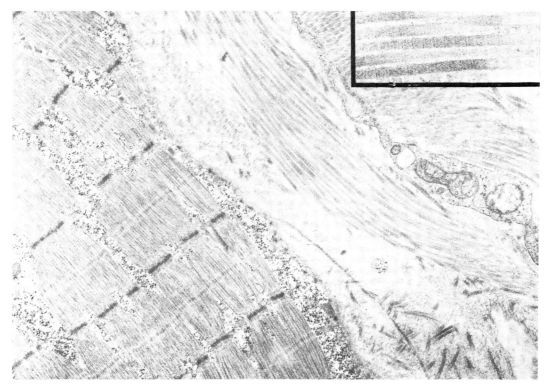

Fig. 24.2 Electron micrograph of the left rectus femoris muscle representing densely proliferated collagen tissue in the endomysium, and an adjacent intact muscle fibre. Collagen fibrils have normal axial periodicity of 64–65 nm (inset). ×16 000, ×45 000 (inset)

reticulum and a well-developed Golgi apparatus suggesting active synthesis and secretion of protein (Maxwell et al 1977, Hentzer et al 1977). Both electron-microscopic and histochemical observations suggest that in the interstitial tissue there is an accumulation of glycoproteins and proteoglycans which are known to be capable of binding calcium and phosphate (Bonnuchi 1971, Hentzer et al 1977). Hentzer et al (1977) found that the collagen fibrils in the lesions had a normal axial periodicity and diameter, whereas Maxwell et al (1977) found a periodicity of 50–53.5 nm, which is shorter than the expected 64.0 nm periodicity seen in areas of uninvolved skin. If the latter finding is a constant feature of this disorder, a genetically determined abnormality of collagen could possibly be the basis of the pathological ossification. There is no evidence of a systemic collagen abnormality and it is possible that abnormal collagen may exist only in the advanced

tumour-like lesions. Our personal observations in a case showed collagen fibrils with a normal periodicity of 63–65 nm (Fig. 24.2). The newly formed bone in the lesions is metaplastic without accompanying osteoblasts, but microscopic and chemical observations have shown no significant differences from normal bone.

Many authors have concluded that the muscle involvement is secondary to compression and/or invasion by proliferated connective tissue and newly formed bone. In the lesions, the individual muscle fibres are embedded in dense collagen and are occasionally atrophic with excessive variation in fibre size (Fig. 24.3A, B), and may show focal loss of band structure and fibre necrosis (Creveld & Soeters 1941, Eaton et al 1957, Lutwak 1964, Frame et al 1972, McKusick 1974). On the other hand, on the basis of histological findings, Smith et al (1966), Smith (1975) and Smith et al (1976) suggested that the muscle fibres were involved

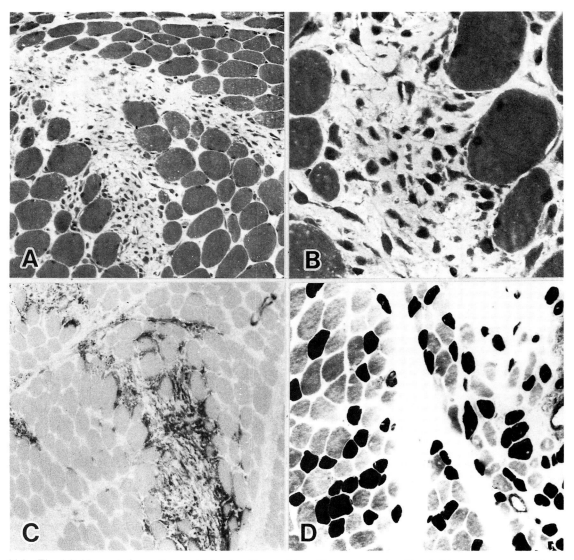

Fig. 24.3 The deltoid muscle from a 7-year-old female with myositis ossificans progressiva. Muscle fibres are compressed by abnormally proliferated endomysial and perimysial connective tissue and some are atrophic (A), where spindle-shaped mononuclear cells are numerous (B). Away from the lesion, the muscle fibres are atrophic with mild variation in fibre size but with no structural changes. On alkaline phosphatase staining (C), the proliferated connective tissue has high enzyme activity. The type 1 and 2 fibres are distributed in a normal mosaic pattern (D). A, B, H&E; C, alkaline phosphatase; D, routine ATPase A ×250, B ×700, C ×180, D ×180

before the phase of collagen invasion. Because of a variation in muscle fibre size even in areas without fibrous tissue proliferation, and decreased ATPase reactions in the muscle fibres, Smith et al (1966) thought that the muscle abnormality was primarily responsible for producing the lesions. As shown in Figure 24.3D, however, ATPase reactions in or around the affected areas show a normal checkerboard distribution of type 1 and 2 fibres, and the muscle fibres seem to be affected by the connective tissue proliferation.

The significance of an increase in alkaline phosphatase activity in acute pre-ossified lesions is still controversial. The enzyme activity was high in samples of muscle and fibrous tissue biochemically (Wilkins et al 1935), and in muscle fibres (Smith et al 1966) and in the cytoplasm of tumour cells (Miller et al 1977) histochemically. Although the enzyme activity in tumour cells from an acute lesion was also elevated (Miller et al 1977), it was within normal limits in cultured skin fibroblasts from unaffected sites (Beratis et al 1976, Conner & Evans 1981). On histochemical examination of muscle biopsies from the acute lesions, alkaline phosphatase activity is demonstrated to be markedly increased in the interstitium (Fig. 24.3C). Since a similar finding is commonly recognizable in polymyositis and dermatomyositis (Engel 1977), an increase in enzyme activity in acute lesions may not be a pathognomonic finding for the disease. There is no supporting evidence that the muscle defect has a primary role in the pathogenesis of the connective tissue proliferation and bone formation.

Myositis ossificans circumscripta (traumatica)

This condition of localized ectopic cartilage and bone formation may be induced by trauma, as in the thigh adductor muscles in habitual horse-riders (Caulet et al 1969, Plezia et al 1977, Mahmud et al 1978) or tetanus (Walter et al 1974, Mitra et al 1976). It may also occur in the lower limbs, in patients with paraplegia. The pathological findings in the affected areas are similar to those seen in myositis ossificans progressiva. Caulet et al (1969), who examined a 62-year-old man with this condition, found short collagen fibrils with a periodicity of 28–35 nm and considered that the condition was possibly genetic and familial in origin.

MYOSCLEROSIS

This condition, characterized by progressive joint contractures, was described by Löwenthal (1954) who thought that intramuscular connective tissue proliferation was probably responsible for the contracture. The disorder seems to be inherited as an autosomal dominant trait, but more than one genotype may be involved, as three females and one male were affected in one family, and four patients in three generations in another family. The clinical symptoms are somewhat similar to

those of Ullrich's disease, although the latter is inherited as an autosomal recessive trait. Further studies are necessary to determine whether or not the disorder is a distinct clinical entity caused by an abnormality of the connective tissue.

It should also be pointed out (Bradley et al 1973) that myosclerosis with diffuse proliferation of connective tissue in muscle and consequential strangulation of muscle fibres may be a long-term consequence of chronic polymyositis or of chronic spinal muscular atrophy. In such cases there is evidence that, when the primary process is inflammatory, steroids may be helpful, and when the sclerosis is of undetermined cause, treatment with penicillamine is worthy of a trial.

Localized fibrosis with muscle contracture (see below) can also result from repetitive intramuscular injection of drugs such as pethidine (Mastaglia et al 1971).

MUSCLE CONTRACTURE

Loss of muscle fibres and interstitial fibrosis are mainly responsible for the muscle contractures and joint rigidity which occur in the advanced stages of muscular dystrophy and of other neuromuscular disorders. In the conditions caused by immobility of the fetus (arthrogryposis multiplex congenita) or with congenital anomalies such as Marfan's disease, the contracture may result from absence, or discrepancy in development, of some muscle groups. Because the pathology of arthrogryposis multiplex congenita (see Ch. 5) and other neuromuscular disorders has been considered elsewhere, several different clinical syndromes with common features will be described here.

Rigid spine syndrome

The term rigid spine syndrome was coined by Dubowitz (1971, 1973) to refer to a condition in which progressive limitation of flexion of the spinal column occurs, and which is probably attributable to a systemic myopathic process. All reported cases have been sporadic and the disease was initially thought to be limited to males. However, a number of female cases have been reported more recently (Dubowitz 1978, Colver et al 1981, Vogel et al 1982, Mussini et al 1982,

Poewe et al 1985, Bertini et al 1986, van Munster et al 1986). A somewhat similar condition with X-linked inheritance was described by Rotthauwe et al (1972).

There is still controversy as to whether the rigid spine syndrome is a distinct clinical entity or is part of the Emery–Dreifuss form of muscular dystrophy which is typically-X-linked, and rarely autosomal recessive or dominant in inheritance (Rowland et al 1979, Bertini et al 1986, van Munster et al 1986, Goto et al 1986). Because there are some common clinical and pathological features between the two conditions, Rowland et al (1979) suggested that younger patients with the rigid spine syndrome may in fact be cases of Emery–Dreifuss dystrophy with the potential to develop other characteristic manifestations such as heart block at a later stage. Since the gene for X-linked Emery–Dreifuss dystrophy is now known to be located at the distal end of the long arm of the X-chromosome (Thomas et al 1986, Yates et al 1986) linkage analysis may allow a definitive diagnosis to be made in such cases.

The symptom of rigid spine becomes manifest in infancy or early school life, and may occasionally be associated with a gait disturbance suggesting a generalized muscle disorder. In the cases with early onset, the parents may notice a delay in motor developmental milestones, a waddling gait, and difficulty in climbing stairs when the child starts to walk (Dubowitz & Brooke 1973, Dubowitz 1978).

Although the limitation of flexion of the spine is slowly progressive, leading to kyphoscoliosis and associated deformities including flexion contractures of the elbow joints, the weakness of the truncal and limb muscles seems to be non-progressive. The myopathic electromyogram and mildly to moderately elevated serum CK level are suggestive of a systemic myopathy.

Cardiomyopathy may be an associated feature in the rigid spine syndrome (Colver et al 1981, Thery et al 1981, Mussini et al 1982, Poewe et al 1985). One patient died from cardiac failure at the age of $7\frac{1}{2}$ years (Colver et al 1981).

Pathology

The muscle pathology may be different in degree in the truncal and limb muscles. For example, in one case the truncal muscles showed severe endomysial fibrosis and marked variation in fibre size, whereas in the biceps and thigh abductors there was only a slightly increased fibre diameter spectrum (Goebel et al 1977, Uehara et al 1982) (Fig. 24.4). Muscle fibre degeneration, necrosis and phagocytosis are not constant features, but may be encountered especially in truncal (Goebel et al 1977, van Munster et al 1986) and proximal limb muscles (Dubowitz 1978). Rimmed vacuole formation was described in some biopsies (Goto et al 1981, Uehara et al 1982, Bertini et al 1986, van Munster et al 1986), suggesting an active autophagic phenomenon after focal myofibrillar degeneration. Since there is no evidence of muscle fibre necrosis with phagocytosis in most muscle biopsies, this focal degenerative process may, at least in part, play an important role in causing muscle fibre atrophy and fibrosis in this disorder (Fig. 24.4B).

On histochemical examination, most biopsies showed variation in both type 1 and 2 fibres with no selective fibre type involvement. A variation in fibre size with a selective type 1 fibre atrophy (hypotrophy) was demonstrated in some biopsies from the limb muscles which showed neither fibrosis nor fibre necrosis (Goebel et al 1977, Seay et al 1977, Vogel et al 1982) (Fig. 24.5). Because the selective type 1 fibre atrophy seemed to precede other myopathic changes in these cases, the authors considered that the type 1 fibre involvement played an important part in the pathogenesis of the disorder. Type 1 fibre predominance (Mussini et al 1982, Bertini et al 1986, van Munster et al 1986) and type 2B fibre deficiency (Goebel et al 1977, Mussini et al 1982, Vogel et al 1982, Bertini et al 1986) are additional histochemical abnormalities.

Selective atrophy of type 1 fibres is relatively uncommon in children's biopsies, but is seen in various neuromuscular disorders including myotonic dystrophy, type 1 fibre atrophy with central nuclei (Engel et al 1968), in most cases of nemaline myopathy (Kinoshita & Satoyoshi 1974), congenital fibre type disproportion (Brooke 1973), immobility, and rheumatoid arthritis (Dubowitz & Brooke 1973). Congenital fibre type disproportion may advance to severe myopathic change with

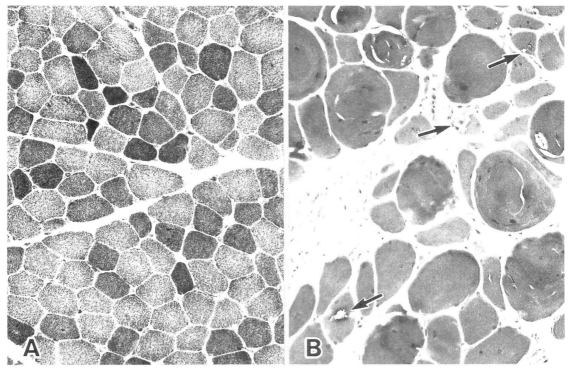

Fig. 24.4   The biceps brachii (A) and trapezius (B) muscles from a 12-year-old boy with the rigid spine syndrome. There is a moderate size variation in type 1 and 2 fibres in the former (A), while the latter shows more advanced changes, including marked variability of muscle fibre size with hypertrophic fibres, occasional snake-coiled structures and rimmed vacuole formation (arrow), and marked interstitial fibrosis (B). A, NADH–TR, B, H&E. A and B ×200

marked variation in size of both fibre types and increased endomysial connective tissue (Cavanagh et al 1979). Further study is necessary to determine whether the small type 1 fibres in all of these conditions reflect the same basic pathogenetic process or are a non-specific finding secondary to immobility of the proximal joints.

At any rate, the muscle pathology in the rigid spine syndrome points to a systemic myopathic disorder with preferential involvement of the truncal muscles. There have been no descriptions of grouped fibre atrophy, type grouping, or small angular fibres suggesting a neuropathic process. An autopsy case (Dubowitz 1978) demonstrated no pathological changes in the peripheral or central nervous system on conventional neuropathological examination.

Ullrich's disease (congenital atonic–sclerotic muscular dystrophy)

Ullrich's disease is characterized by severe proximal joint contractures and muscle weakness, and hyperflexible distal joints manifesting from birth or early infancy and remaining stationary or following a slowly progressive course. Ullrich (1930a,b) described the following 12 clinical characteristics for this disorder: (i) the presence of symptoms since birth; (ii) acroatonia, or markedly thin, not easily palpable, moderately functional musculature of distal extremities with marked joint looseness and hyperflexibility; (iii) truncal contracture, i.e. shortened, hardened and non-elastic trunk musculature together with torticollis and kyphoscoliosis, restricted mobility especially of large proximal joints, because of contracted flexor and abductor muscles; (iv) relative sparing of muscles innervated by cranial nerves; (v) taille

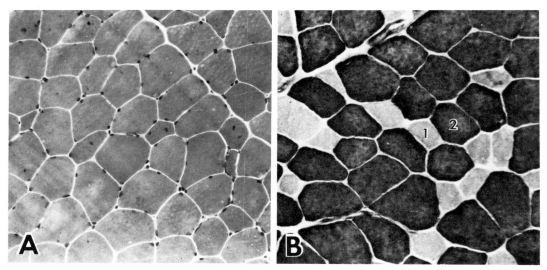

Fig. 24.5 The biceps brachii muscle obtained from a 24-year-old woman with the rigid spine syndrome. Note a variation in fibre size with a bimodal distribution and an increased number of fibres with central nuclei, especially in the atrophic fibres (A) The type 1 fibres (1) are significantly small in comparison with the type 2 fibres (2) (B) A: H&E, ×160. B: routine ATPase, ×200. (Courtesy of Drs Y. Toyokura and M. Takatsu, Department of Neurology, Brain Research Institute, Faculty of Medicine, University of Tokyo)

de guêpe (slender figure); (vi) spur-like protrusion of the calcaneus; (vii) high-arched palate; (viii) normal to hyperactive tendon and periosteal reflexes and intact sensorium; (ix) strongly positive facial sign; (x) hyperhidrosis; (xi) good intellectual development; and (xii) no noticeable progression, but with improvement of motility.

Twenty-nine similar cases, including Ullrich's two male patients, have been reported in the literature from Germany, France, Italy and Japan (Ullrich 1930a,b, Stoeber 1939, Gött & Josten 1954, Schneider 1957, Toyokura et al 1966, Sato & Sannomiya 1970, Segawa et al 1973, Naito et al 1974, Nonaka et al 1974, Joh et al 1976, Nakano et al 1976, Furukawa & Toyokura 1977, Nihei et al 1979, Nonaka et al 1981, Serratrice & Pellissier 1983, Sasaki et al 1985, Ricci et al 1988, de Paillette et al 1989, Santoro et al 1989). Twenty patients were male and nine were female. Consanguineous marriage of the parents was noted in eight of 24 parents, and affected siblings were described in two families (Gött & Josten 1954, Furukawa & Toyokura 1977). The disease seems to be inherited as an autosomal recessive trait (Nonaka & Chou 1979).

The symptoms become manifest at birth or in early infancy with muscular hypotonia and weakness in association with marked contractures of proximal joints involving the neck, shoulder, elbow, spine, hip and knee joints. On the other hand, distal joints such as those of the hand, ankle, fingers and toes are hyperflexible and hyperextensible. There is occasional looseness of cutaneous tissue, somewhat mimicking that of the Ehlers–Danlos syndrome. The muscle wasting and weakness are generalized but the facial muscles are spared. In almost all cases, developmental milestones were delayed and only seven of 23 reported cases had learned to walk by the age of 2–6 years. However they usually became non-ambulant several years later, which suggests that the disease is progressive. The patients have a predisposition to repeated upper respiratory tract infections, probably because of deficient cellular immunity (Furukawa & Toyokura 1977).

Pathology

The muscle pathology in previously reported cases has varied in severity from case to case. With the exception of one case in which no pathological changes were found (Sato & Sannomiya 1970), the

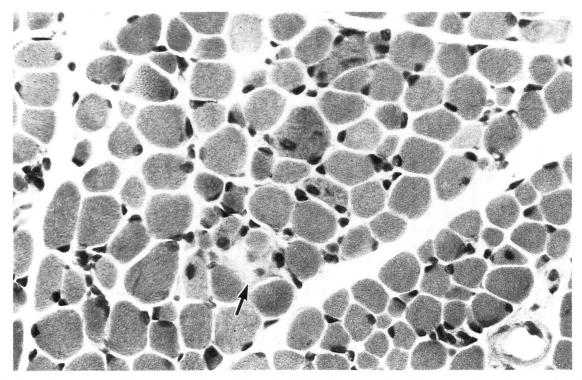

Fig. 24.6   The biceps brachii muscle from a 2-year-old female with Ullrich's disease. The findings of marked variation in fibre size with scattered necrotic (arrow) and regenerating fibres, and interstitial fibrosis are consistent with the pathology of progressive muscular dystrophy. Fibres with centrally placed nuclei are increased in number. H&E, ×400

remaining cases have shown myopathic changes with mild variation in fibre size and small calibre fibres in some (Joh et al 1976, Nihei et al 1979) and more marked variation in fibre size, loss of striations, fibre necrosis and striking fibrosis in others (Fig. 24.6) (Ullrich 1930a, Gött & Josten 1954, Rotthauwe et al 1969, Segawa et al 1973, Naito et al 1974, Nonaka et al 1976, Furukawa & Toyokura 1977, Serratrice & Pellissier 1983, Ricci et al 1988, de Paillette et al 1989, Santro et al 1989). The clinical symptoms were usually described as being slowly progressive or stationary. Observations in five cases over a period of several years suggested that the disease was slowly progressive, leading to severe disability in young adulthood (Nonaka et al 1981). When the histology of the right rectus femoris muscle from a 9-year-old boy was compared with that of the left rectus femoris muscle at subsequent autopsy at the age of 11 years (Mishima et al 1973, Nonaka et al 1974), the latter demonstrated more advanced myopathic

changes with severe endomysial fibrosis, a number of degenerating and regenerating muscle fibres and occasional hypertrophic fibres, evidently reflecting the clinical progression.

Histochemical examination was carried out in several cases (Segawa et al 1973, Nihei et al 1979, Nonaka et al 1981, de Paillette et al 1989) and demonstrated involvement of both fibre types 1 and 2. Except for occasional rod-like bodies in a case demonstrated by the Gomori trichrome stain and by electron microscopy (Segawa et al 1973), specific intracytoplasmic changes have not been documented. In a histological study of five patients (Nonaka et al 1981) the muscles in all cases showed advanced myopathic changes with occasional necrotic fibres and marked endomysial fibrosis. On histochemical examination in three cases, there were no specific cytoplasmic inclusions such as nemaline rods, central cores, or myotube-like structures. The striking finding was that the fibre type proportion with ATPase staining differed

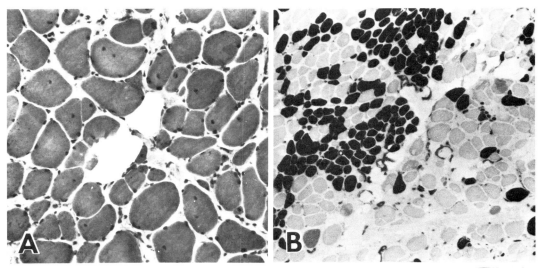

Fig. 24.7 The biceps brachii muscle from an 11-year-old boy with Ullrich's disease. A remarkable variation in fibre size, endomysial fibrosis, and a number of fibres with central nuclei are seen (A). An equivocal finding of fibre type grouping in the left half and type 1 fibre predominance in the right half of the figure are seen in (B). A: H&E, ×160. B: routine ATPase, ×40

from case to case and from muscle fascicle to fascicle. In relatively well-preserved fascicles, both type 1 and 2 fibres were normally distributed in a checkerboard pattern, while type 1 fibre predominance (type 2 fibre deficiency) was recognized in the advanced fascicles where type 2 fibres were significantly atrophic. In addition, there was equivocal fibre type grouping as shown in Figure 24.7, suggesting the possibility of a neuropathic process occurring in association with a primary myopathic process. Although no evidence of a neuropathic process has been found on the basis of clinical symptoms, EMG findings and three autopsy examinations (Ullrich 1930a, Mishima et al 1973, Ricci et al 1988), some evidence of dysgenesis of the central nervous system, including disorganized gyral formation and glial bundles in the proximal part of the oculomotor nerve roots, was suggested in an autopsy case (Sasaki et al 1985).

REFERENCES

Beratis N G, Kaffe S, Aron A M, Hirschhorn K 1976 Alkaline phosphatase activity in cultured skin fibroblasts from fibrodysplasia ossificans progressiva. Journal of Medical Genetics 13: 307

Bertini E, Marini R, Sabetta G, Palmieri G P, Spagnoli L G, Vaccario M L, de Barsy T 1986 The spectrum of the so-called rigid spine syndrome: nosological considerations and report of three female cases. Journal of Neurology 233: 248

Bonnuci E 1971 The locus of initial calcification in cartilage and bone. Clinical Orthopaedics 78: 108

Bradley W G, Hudgson P, Gardner-Medwin D, Walton J N 1973 The syndrome of myosclerosis. Journal of Neurology, Neurosurgery and Psychiatry 36: 651

Brooke M H 1973 Congenital fiber type disproportion. In: Kakulas B A (ed) Clinical studies in myology. Excerpta Medica, Amsterdam, p 147

Caulet T, Adnet J J, Pluot M, Gougeon J, Hopfner C 1969 Myosite ossifiante circonscrite. Etude histochimique et ultrastructurale d'une observation. Virchows Archiv; Abteilung A: Pathologische Anatomie 348: 16

Cavanagh N P C, Lake B D, McMeniman P 1979 Congenital fibre type disproportion myopathy. A histological diagnosis with an uncertain clinical outlook. Archives of Disease in Childhood 54: 735

Chaco J 1967 Myositis ossificans progressiva. Acta rheumatologica scandinavica 13: 235

Colver A F, Steer C R, Godman M J, Uttley W S 1981 Rigid spine syndrome and fatal cardiomyopathy. Archives of Disease in Childhood 56: 148

Conner J M, Beighton P 1982 Fibrodysplasia ossificans progressive in South Africa. Case reports. South African Medical Journal 61: 404

Conner J M, Evans D A P 1981 Quantitative and qualitative studies on skin fibroblast alkaline phosphatase in fibrodysplasia ossificans progressiva. Clinica chimica Acta 117: 355

Conner J M, Evans D A P 1982 Genetic aspects of fibrodysplasia ossificans progressiva. Journal of Medical Genetics 19: 35

Creveld S, Soeters J M 1941 Myositis ossificans progressiva. American Journal of Diseases of Children 62: 1000

Davis H, Moe P J 1959 Favorable response of calcinosis universalis to edathamil disodium. Pediatrics 32: 780

de Paillette L, Aicardi J, Goutières F 1989 Ullrich's congenital atonic sclerotic muscular dystrophy. A case report. Journal of Neurology 236: 108

Dubowitz V 1971 Recent advances in neuromuscular disorders. Rheumatology and Physical Medicine 11: 126

Dubowitz V 1973 Rigid spine syndrome: a muscle syndrome in search of a name. Proceedings of the Royal Society of Medicine 66: 219

Dubowitz V 1978 Muscle disorders in childhood. Saunders, London

Dubowitz V, Brooke M H 1973 Muscle biopsy. A modern approach. Saunders, London

Eaton W L, Conkling W S, Daeschner C W 1957 Early myositis ossificans progressiva occurring in homozygotic tiwns. A clinical and pathologic study. Journal of Pediatrics 50: 591

Ebrahim G J, Grech P, Slavin G 1966 Myositis ossificans progressiva in an African child. British Journal of Radiology 39: 952

Engel W K 1977 Integrative histochemical approach to the defect of Duchenne muscular dystrophy. In: Rowland L P (ed) Pathogenesis of human muscular dystrophies. Excerpta Medica, Amsterdam, p 277

Engel W K, Gold G N, Karpati G 1968 Type 1 fibre hypotrophy and central nuclei. A rare congenital muscular abnormality with a possible experimental model. Archives of Neurology (Chicago) 18: 435

Fairbank H A T 1950 Myositis ossificans progressiva. Journal of Bone and Joint Surgery 32B: 108

Frame B, Azad N, Reynolds W A, Saeed S M 1972 Polyostotic fibrous dysplasia and myositis ossificans progressiva. A report of coexistence. American Journal of Diseases of Children 124: 120

Furukawa T, Toyokura Y 1977 Congenital, hypotonic-sclerotic muscular dystrophy. Journal of Medical Genetics 14: 426

Geschickter C F, Masteritz I H 1938 Myositis ossificans. Journal of Bone and Joint Surgery 20: 661

Goebel H H, Lenard H G, Görke W, Kunze K 1977 Fibre type disproportion in the rigid spine syndrome. Neuropaediatrie 8: 467

Goto I, Nagasaka S, Nagara H, Kuroiwa Y 1979 Rigid spine syndrome. Journal of Neurology, Neurosurgery and Psychiatry 42: 276

Goto I, Muraoka S, Fujii N, Ohta M, Kuroiwa Y 1981 Rigid spine syndrome: clinical and histological problems. Journal of Neurology 226: 143

Goto I, Ishimoto S, Yamada T, Hara H, Kuroiwa Y 1986 The rigid spine syndrome and Emery–Dreifuss muscular dystrophy. Clinical Neurology and Neurosurgery 88: 293

Gött H, Josten E A 1954 Beitrag zur kongenitalen atonisch-sklerotischen Muskeldystrophie (Typ Ullrich). Zeitschrift für Kinderheilkunde 75: 105

Grewal K S, Dass N 1953 Myositis ossificans progressiva. Journal of Bone and Joint Surgery 35B: 244

Hentzer B, Kobayasi T, Asboe-Hansen G 1977 Ultrastructure of dermal connective tissue in fibrodysplasia ossificans progressiva. Acta dermato-venereologica 57: 477

Joh M, Kogasaka R, Shinoda M 1976 A case of Ullrich syndrome. Clinical Neurology 16: 728

Kinoshita M, Satoyoshi E 1974 Type 1 fibre atrophy and nemaline bodies. Archives of Neurology (Chicago) 31: 423

Knoots A R 1927 Myositis ossificans progressiva. American Journal of the Medical Sciences 174: 406

Löwenthal A 1954 Une groupe hérédodégénératif nouveau; les myoscléroses hérédofamiliales. Acta neurologica belgica 54: 155

Ludman H, Hamilton E B D, Eade A W T 1968 Deafness in myositis ossificans progressiva. Journal of Laryngology and Otology 82: 57

Lutwak L 1964 Myositis ossificans progressiva. Mineral, metabolic and radio-active calcium studies of the effects of hormones. American Journal of Medicine 37: 269

McKusick, V A 1974 Fibrodysplasia ossificans progressiva. In: Heritable disorders of connective tissue. Mosby, St. Louis, p 687

Magruder L F 1926 Myositis ossificans progressiva. Case report and review of the literature. American Journal of Roentgenology 15: 328

Mahmud H R, Rumpf P, Sailer R, Ullrich B 1978 Zur Myositis ossificans nach Shädel-Hirntrauma. Langenbecks Archiv für Chirurgie 346: 265

Mastaglia F L, Gardner-Medwin D, Hudgson P 1971 Muscle fibrosis and contractures in a pethidine addict. British Medical Journal 4: 532

Maxwell W A, Spicer S S, Miller R L, Halushka, P V, Westphal M C, Setser M E 1977 Histochemical and ultrastructural studies in fibrodysplasia ossificans progressiva (myositis ossificans progressiva). American Journal of Pathology 87: 483

Miller R L, Maxwell W A, Spicer S S, Halushlea P V, Varner H H, Westphal M C 1977 Studies on alkaline phosphatase activity in cultured cells from a patient with fibrodysplasia ossificans progressiva. Laboratory Investigation 37: 254

Mishima K, Miyoshino S, Mine K, Nonaka I, Miike T 1973 Ullrich type of congenital muscular dystrophy: a case report with autopsy findings. Brain and Development (Tokyo) (Domestic Edition) 5: 530

Mitra M, Sen A K, Deb H K 1976 Myositis ossificans traumatica; a complication of tetanus. Journal of Bone and Joint Surgery 58A: 885

Muller S A, Winkelmann R K, Brunsting L A 1959 Calcinosis in dermatomyositis. Archives of Dermatology 79: 669

Mussini J-M, Mathe J F, Prost A, Gray F, Labat J-J, Feve J-R 1982 Le syndrome de la colonne raide. Un cas feminin. Revue Neurologique 138: 25

Naito M, Okada R, Segawa M, Tanabe H 1974 A case of Ullrich's disease. Clinical Neurology 14: 813

Nakano Y, Tochigi S, Kawaguchi S, Watanabe S 1976 A case of probable Ullrich congenital muscular dystrophy. Clinical Neurology 16: 597

Nihei K, Kamoshita S, Atsumi T 1979 A case of Ullrich's disease (Kongenitale, atonisch-sklerotische Muskeldystrophie). Brain and Development 1: 61

Nonaka I, Chou S M 1979 Congenital muscular dystrophy. In: Vinken P J, Bruyn G W (eds) Handbook of clinical neurology, vol 41. North-Holland, Amsterdam, p 27

Nonaka I, Ueno T, Miyoshino S, Miike T, Mishima K 1974 Clinical and pathological study of Ullrich-type of congenital muscular dystrophy. Brain and Development (Tokyo) (Domestic Edition) 6: 48

Nonaka I, Une Y, Ishihara T, Miyoshino S, Nakashima T, Sugita H 1981 A clinical and histological study of Ullrich's disease (congenital atonic-sclerotic muscular dystrophy). Neuropediatrics 12: 197

Paul J R 1925 A study of an unusual case of myositis ossificans. Archives of Surgery 10: 185

Plezia R A, Mintz S M, Calligaro P 1977 Myositis ossificans traumatica of the masseter muscle; report of a case. Oral Surgery 44: 351

Poewe W, Willeit H, Sluga E, Mayr U 1985 The rigid spine syndrome — a myopathy of uncertain nosological position. Journal of Neurology, Neurosurgery and Psychiatry 48: 887

Ricci E, Bertini E, Boldrini R et al 1988 Late onset scleroatonic familial myopathy (Ullrich disease): a study of two sibs. American Journal of Medical Genetics 31: 933

Rogers J G, Chase G A 1979 Paternal age effect in fibrodysplasia ossificans progressiva. Journal of Medical Genetics 16: 147

Rogers J G, Geho W B 1979 Fibrodysplasia ossificans progressiva; a survey of 42 cases. Journal of Bone and Joint Surgery 61A: 909

Rosenstirn J 1918 A contribution to the study of myositis ossificans progressiva. Annals of Surgery 68: 485, 591

Rotthauwe H W, Kowalewski S, Mumenthaler M 1969 Kongenitale Muskeldystrophie. Zeitschrift für Kinderheilkundes 106: 131

Rotthauwe H W, Mortier W, Beyer H 1972 Neuer Typ einer recessiv X-chromosomal verebten Muskeldystrophie: scapulo-humero-distale Muskeldystrophie mit fruhzeitigen Kontrakturen und Herzenrhythmussttörungen. Humangenetik 16: 181

Rowland L P, Fetell M, Olarte M, Hays A, Singh N, Wanat F E 1979 Emery–Dreifuss muscular dystrophy. Annals of Neurology 5: 111

Ryan K J 1945 Myositis ossificans progressiva. A review of the literature with report of a case. Journal of Pediatrics 27: 348

Santoro L, Marmo C, Gasparo-Rippa P, Toscano A, Sadile F, Barbieri F 1989 A new case of Ullrich's disease. Clinical Neuropathology 8: 69

Sasaki K, Shimoda M, Nakamura N 1985 An autopsy case of Ullrich's disease. Japanese Journal of Pediatrics 38: 411

Sastri V R K, Yadav S S 1977 Myositis ossificans progressiva. International Surgery 62: 45

Sato A, Sannomiya A 1970 A case of Ullrich's syndrome. Japanese Journal of Paediatrics 23: 1261

Schneider H 1957 Die atonisch-sklerotische Muskeldystrophie (Ullrich) im Rahmen mesodermaler Dysplasien. Zeitschrift für Orthopaedie und Ihre Grenzgebiete 88: 397

Seay A R, Ziter F A, Petajan J H 1977 Rigid spine syndrome. A type 1 fibre myopathy. Archives of Neurology (Chicago) 34: 119

Segawa M, Mizuno Y, Itoh K, Uono M 1973 Neuropathic and myopathic arthrogryposis multiplex congenita. In: Kakulas B A (ed) Clinical studies in myology. Excerpta Medica, Amsterdam, p 283

Serratrice G, Pellissier J F 1983 Une dystrophie musculaire oubliée: la maladie d'Ullrich Revue Neurologique (Paris) 139: 523

Smith D M, Zeman W, Johnston C C, Deiss W P 1966 Myositis ossificans progressiva. Case report with metabolic and histochemical studies. Metabolism 15: 521

Smith R 1975 Myositis ossificans progressiva: a review of current problems. Seminars in Arthritis and Rheumatism 4: 369

Smith R, Russel R G G, Woods C G 1976 Myositis ossificans progressiva. Clinical features of eight patients and their response to treatment. Journal of Bone and Joint Surgery 58B: 48

Stoeber E 1939 Über atonisch-sklerotische Muskeldystrophie (Typ Ullrich). Zeitschrift für Kinderheilkunde 60: 279

Stonham C 1892 Myositis ossificans. Lancet 2: 1485

Sympson T 1886 Case of myositis ossificans. British Medical Journal 2: 1026

Thery C I, Krivosic I, Dewailly Ph, Pirot J, Lablanche J M, Jaillard J 1981 Cardiomyopathie congestive associée a un syndrome de la colonne raide 'rigid spine syndrome'. Archives des Maladies du Coeur et des Vaisseaux 8: 985

Thomas N S T, Williams H, Elsas L J, Hopkins L C, Sarfarazi M, Harper P S 1986 Localisation of the gene for Emery–Dreifuss muscular dystrophy to the distal long arm of the X chromosome. Journal of Medical Ganetics 23: 596

Toyokura Y, Takasu T, Yanagisawa N, Tsukagoshi H 1966 Kongenitale atonischsklerotische Muskeldystrophie (Typ Ullrich): a case report. Clinical Neurology 6: 742

Tünte W, Becker P E, Knorre G V 1967 Zur genetik der myositis ossificans progressiva. Humangenetik 4: 320

Uehara M, Hara T, Uehara S, Senoo H, Nonaka I 1982 A histological and histochemical study on the biopsied muscles from a case with rigid spine syndrome. Neurological Medicine 16: 50

Ullrich O 1930a Kongenitale, atonisch-sklerotische Muskeldystrophie, ein weiterer Typus der heredodegenerativen Erkrankungen des neuromuskulären Systems. Zeitschrift für die Gesamte Neurologie und Psychiatrie 126: 171

Ullrich O 1930b Kongenitale, atonisch-sklerotische Muskeldystrophie. Monatsschrift für Kinderheilkunde 47: 502

van Munster E T L, Joosten E M G, van Munster-Uijtdehaage, H A M, Kruls H J A, ter Laak H J 1986 The rigid spine syndrome. Journal of Neurology, Neurosurgery, and Psychiatry 49: 1292

Vogel P, Goebel H H, Seitz D 1982 Rigid spine syndrome in a girl. Journal of Neurology 228: 259

Walter K, Eyrich K, Schimrigk K, Ricker K, Zwirner R 1974 Myositis ossificans nach Tetanus. Langenbecks Archiv für Chirurgie 335: 273

Wheeler C E, Curtis A C, Cawley E P, Grekin R H, Zheutlin B 1952 Soft tissue calcification, with special reference to its occurrence in the 'collagen diseases'. Annals of Internal Medicine 36: 1050

Wilkins W E, Regen E M, Carpenter G K 1935 Phosphatase studies on biopsy tissue in progressive myositis ossificans. American Journal of Diseasses of Children 49: 1219

Yates J R W, Affara N A, Jamieson D M et al 1986 Emery–Dreifuss muscular dystrophy: localisation to Xq 27.3 → qter confirmed by linkage to the factor VIII gene. Journal of Medical Genetics 23: 587

Index